tenth edition

Maingot's

ABDOMINAL OPERATIONS

Volume II

tenth edition

Maingot's

ABDOMINAL OPERATIONS

Volume II

Editors

Michael J. Zinner, MD, FACS
Moseley Professor of Surgery
Harvard Medical School
Surgeon-in-Chief
Brigham and Women's Hospital
Boston, Massachusetts

Seymour I. Schwartz, MD
Distinguished Alumni Professor and Chair
Department of Surgery
University of Rochester School
  of Medicine and Dentistry
Rochester, New York

Harold Ellis, CBE, DM, MCh, FRCS
Clinical Anatomist
Department of Anatomy
United Medical and Dental School
University of London
Emeritus Professor of Surgery
University of London
London, United Kingdom

Assistant Editors

Stanley W. Ashley, MD
Senior Surgeon
Brigham and Women's Hospital
Associate Professor of Surgery
Harvard Medical School
Boston, Massachusetts

David W. McFadden, MD
Professor of Surgery
Chief, Division of General Surgery
University of California Los Angeles
  School of Medicine
Los Angeles, California

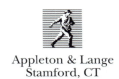

Appleton & Lange
Stamford, CT

Copyright © 1997 by Appleton & Lange
A Simon & Schuster Company

97 98 99 00 / 10 9 8 7 6 5 4 3 2 1

Prentice Hall International (UK) Limited, London
Prentice Hall of Australia Pty. Limited, Syndey
Prentice Hall of Canada, Inc., Toronto
Prentice Hall of Hispanoamericana, S.A., Mexico
Prentice Hall of India Private Limited, New Delhi
Prentice Hall of Japan, Inc., Tokyo
Simon & Schuster Asia Pte. Ltd., Singapore
Editora Prentice Hall do Brasil Ltda., Rio de Janeiro
Prentice Hall, Upper Saddle River, New Jersey

Library of Congress Cataloging-in-Publication Data
Maingot, Rodney, 1893–
    Maingot's abdominal operations.—10th ed. / [edited by] Michael
J. Zinner
      v.   cm.
    Includes bibliographical references.
    ISBN 0-8385-6106-3 (v. 1 & 2 : case : alk. paper).—ISBN
0-8385-6104-7 (v. 1 : case : alk. paper).—ISBN 0-8385-6105-5 (v.
2 : case alk. paper)
    1. Abdomen—Surgery.   I. Zinner, Michael.   II. Title.
    [DNLM: 1. Abdomen—surgery.   WI 900 M225 1997]
RD540.M24   1997
617.595—dc20
DNLM/DLC
for Library of Congress   96-28893
                                                              CIP

Managing Editor, Development: Kathleen McCullough
Production Service: York Production Services
Designer: Libby Schmitz

ISBN 0-8385-6106-3

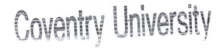

CONTRIBUTORS

Robin Abel, BSc, MB, BS, FRCS
Research Fellow
Department of Pediatric Surgery
Institute of Child Health
University of London
London, United Kingdom

Jack Abrahamson, MB, ChB, FRCS, FACS
Chairman of Surgery
Carmel Hospital
Haifa, Israel

Steven A. Ahrendt, MD
Assistant Professor of Surgery
The Johns Hopkins University School of Medicine
Baltimore, Maryland

John Alexander Williams, MD, FRCS
Consultant Surgeon
Birmingham, Nuffield, and Priory Hospitals
Professor of Gastrointestinal Surgery
University of Birmingham
Birmingham, United Kingdom

Stanley W. Ashley, MD
Senior Surgeon
Brigham and Women's Hospital
Associate Professor of Surgery
Harvard Medical School
Boston, Massachusetts

Stephen A. Barnes, MD
Chief Resident, Department of Surgery
The Johns Hopkins Hospital
Fellow, Department of Surgery
The Johns Hopkins University School of Medicine
Baltimore, Maryland

Robert W. Beart, Jr., MD
Professor of Surgery
Chairman, Colorectal Surgery
University of Southern California
Los Angeles, California

R. Daniel Beauchamp, MD
Associate Director of Clinical Programs
Vanderbilt Cancer Center
Associate Professor of Surgery and Cell Biology
Vanderbilt University School of Medicine
Nashville, Tennessee

Robert S. Bennion, MD
Associate Professor of Surgery
University of California Los Angeles School of Medicine
Los Angeles, California

Jonathan S. Berek, MD
Vice Chair, Department of Obstetrics and Gynecology
Chief, Gynecology and Gynecologic Oncology
Professor
Jonsson Comprehensive Cancer Center
University of California Los Angeles School of Medicine
Los Angeles, California

Scott M. Berry, MD
Surgery Chief Resident
University of Cincinnati School of Medicine
Cincinnati, Ohio

Elisa H. Birnbaum, MD
Assistant Professor of Surgery
Washington University School of Medicine
St. Louis, Missouri

Kirby I. Bland, MD
Executive Surgeon-In-Chief
Brown University Affiliated Hospitals
J. Murray Beardsley Professor and Chairman
Department of Surgery
Brown University School of Medicine
Providence, Rhode Island

Leslie H. Blumgart, MD, FACS, FRCS
Chief, Hepatobiliary Surgical Section
Director, Hepatobiliary Disease Program
Enid A. Haupt Chair
Memorial Sloan Kettering Cancer Center
Professor of Surgery
Cornell University Medical College
New York, New York

Scott J. Boley, MD, FACS
Chief of Pediatric Surgical Service
Montefiore Medical Center
Professor of Surgery and Pediatrics
Albert Einstein College of Medicine
Bronx, New York

David C. Brooks, MD, FACS
Surgeon
Brigham and Women's Hospital
Assistant Professor of Surgery
Harvard Medical School
Boston, Massachusetts

L. Michael Brunt, MD
Staff Surgeon
Barnes-Jewish Hospital
Assistant Professor of Surgery
Washington University School of Medicine
St. Louis, Missouri

John M. Burch, MD
Chief, General Surgery
Denver General Hospital
Professor of Surgery
University of Colorado Health Sciences Center
Denver, Colorado

Agustin A. Burgos, MD
Resident in Surgery
Tulane University School of Medicine
New Orleans, Louisiana

Ronald W. Bussutil, MD, PhD
Director, Dumont–UCLA Transplant Center
Professor of Surgery
Dumont Chair in Transplantation Surgery
University of California Los Angeles School of Medicine
Los Angeles, California

John L. Cameron, MD
Surgeon-in-Chief
The Johns Hopkins Hospital
Professor of Surgery
Chairman, Department of Surgery
The Johns Hopkins University School of Medicine
Baltimore, Maryland

Helena R. Chang, MD, PhD
Staff Surgeon
Roger Williams Hospital
Associate Professor in Surgery and Pathobiology
Brown University
Providence, Rhode Island

Nicholas J. W. Cheshire, MD, FRCS
Lecturer in Surgery
St. Mary's Hospital
Imperial College of Medicine
London, United Kingdom

Alfred Cushierei, MD, ChM, FRCS(Ed), FRCS(Eng), FRCS(Glas[Hon]), FRCSI(Hon)
Consultant Surgeon
Dundee Teaching Hospital
NHS Trust
Ninewalls Hospital and Medical School
Professor and Head
Department of Surgery
University of Dundee
Dundee, United Kingdom

John M. Daly, MD
Surgeon-in-Chief
New York Hospital
Lewis Atterbury Stimson Professor and Chairman
Cornell University Medical College
New York, New York

Haile T. Debas, MD
Dean, School of Medicine
The Mauric Galante Distinguished Professor of Surgery
University of California San Francisco
San Francisco, California

Malcolm M. DeCamp, Jr., MD
Associate Surgeon
Division of Thoracic Surgery
Brigham and Women's Hospital
Assistant Professor of Surgery
Harvard Medical School
Boston, Massachusetts

Tom R. DeMeester, MD
Professor and Chairman, Department of Surgery
University of Southern California School of Medicine
Los Angeles, California

Harold Ellis, CBE, DM, MCh, FRCS
Clinical Anatomist
Department of Anatomy
United Medical and Dental School
University of London
Emeritus Professor of Surgery
University of London
London, United Kingdom

S. T. Fan, MBBS, MS, FRCS(Glasg), FACS
Professor of Surgery
Division of Hepatobiliary Surgery
Department of Surgery
The University of Hong Kong
Queen Mary Hospital
Hong Kong

Douglas G. Farmer, MD
Fellow, Transplantation Surgery
Division of Pancreas and Liver Transplantation
Dumont–University of California Los Angeles
    Transplant Center
Los Angeles, California

Victor W. Fazio, MD
Rupert Turnbull Chairman
Department of Colorectal Surgery
Cleveland Clinic Foundation
Professor of Surgery
Ohio State University School of Medicine
Cleveland, Ohio

Carlos Fernandez-del Castillo, MD
Assistant Surgeon
Massachusetts General Hospital
Assistant Professor of Surgery
Harvard Medical School
Boston, Massachusetts

Aaron S. Fink, MD
Chief, Surgical Service
Atlanta Veterans Administration Medical Center
Decatur, Georgia
Associate Professor of Surgery
Emory University School of Medicine
Atlanta, Georgia

Josef E. Fischer, MD
Surgeon-in-Chief
University of Cincinnati Hospital Group
Christian R. Holmes Professor
Chairman, Department of Surgery
University of Cincinnati
Cincinnati, Ohio

James W. Fleshman, MD
Associate Professor of Surgery
Washington University School of Medicine
St. Louis, Missouri

Manson Fok, MBBS, FRCS(Edin)
Senior Lecturer
Department of Surgery
The University of Hong Kong
Queen Mary Hospital
Hong Kong

Eric W. Fonkalsrud, MD
Chief of Pediatric Surgery
University of California Los Angeles Medical Center
Professor of Pediatric Surgery
University of California Los Angeles School of
    Medicine
Los Angeles, California

Robert D. Fry, MD
Chief, Division of Colon and Rectal Surgery
Professor of Surgery
Thomas Jefferson University
Philadelphia, Pennsylvania

Geoffrey Glazer, MS, FRCS, FACS
Consultant Surgeon
St. Mary's Hospital
Honorary Senior Lecturer in Surgery
Imperial College of Medicine
London, United Kingdom

Steven L. Glorsky, MD
Attending Surgeon
Lower Florida Keys Health System

Key West, Florida
Former Clinical Instructor of Surgery
University of Southern California School of Medicine
Los Angeles, California

Jay L. Grosfeld, MD
Surgeon-in-Chief
J. W. Riley Hospital for Children
Lafayette Page Professor and Chairman
Department of Surgery
Indiana University School of Medicine
Indianapolis, Indiana

J. Michael Henderson, MD
Staff Surgeon
Chairman, General Surgery
The Cleveland Clinic Foundation
Cleveland, Ohio

Oscar J. Hines, MD
Resident in Surgery
University of California Los Angeles School of
    Medicine
Los Angeles, California

Darryl T. Hiyama, MD
Assistant Professor of Surgery
Division of General Surgery
University of California Los Angeles School of
    Medicine
Los Angeles, California

Edward R. Howard, MS, FRCS
Department of Surgery
King's College Hospital
Denmark Hill
London, England

Bernard M. Jaffe, MD
Professor and Vice-Chairman
Department of Surgery
Tulane University School of Medicine
New Orleans, Louisiana

David Johnston, MBChB, MD, ChM, FRCS
Consultant Surgeon
Leeds General Infirmary
Professor of Surgery
University of Leeds
Leeds, United Kingdom

Barbara M. Kadell, MD
Clinical Professor and Chief, Gastrointestinal
    Radiology
University of California Los Angeles Medical Center
Vice Chair, Department of Radiological Sciences
University of California Los Angeles School of
    Medicine
Los Angeles, California

Kim U. Kahng, MD
Associate Professor of Surgery
Vice Chairman, Administrative Affairs
Medical College of Pennsylvania
Hahnemann University
Philadelphia, Pennsylvania

Ronald N. Kaleya, MD
Associate Professor of Surgery
Montefiore Medical Center
Albert Einstein College of Medicine
Bronx, New York

Joseph A. Karam, MD
Research Fellow
Instructor in Surgery
The Medical College of Pennsylvania
Hahnemann University
Philadelphia, Pennsylvania

Seiji Kawasaki, MD
Professor and Chairman
First Department of Surgery
Shinshu University School of Medicine
Matsumoto, Japan

Keith A. Kelly, MD, FACS
Chair, Department of Surgery
Mayo Clinic Scottsdale
Scottsdale, Arizona
Professor of Surgery
Mayo Medical School
Rochester, Minnesota

Ira J. Kodner, MD
Chief, Section of Colon and Rectal Surgery
Jewish Hospital and Barnes Hospital
Professor of Surgery
Washington University School of Medicine
St. Louis, Missouri

Han C. Kuijpers, MD, PhD
Associate Professor of Gastroenterologic Surgery
University Hospital Nymegen
Nymegen, Netherlands

Keith D. Lillemoe, MD, FACS
Active Staff
The Johns Hopkins Hospital
Associate Professor of Surgery
The Johns Hopkins University School of Medicine
Baltimore, Maryland

Pamela A. Lipsett, MD
Co-Director, Surgical Intensive Care Unit
Attending Surgeon
Johns Hopkins Hospital
Associate Professor of Surgery, Anesthesia, Critical Care
    Medicine
Johns Hopkins University School of Medicine
Baltimore, Maryland

Michael Liptay, MD
Fellow in Thoracic Surgery
Brigham and Women's Hospital
Harvard Medical School
Boston, Massachusetts

Carson D. Liu, MD
Surgical Resident
University of California Los Angeles School of
    Medicine
Los Angeles, California

Edward H. Livingston, MD
Attending Surgeon
University of California Los Angeles School of
    Medicine
Assistant Chief, Surgical Service
Veterans Medical Center, West Los Angeles
Assistant Professor of Surgery
Assistant Dean
University of California Los Angeles School of
    Medicine
Los Angeles, California

David S. K. Lu, MD, CM
Attending Radiologist
University of California Los Angeles Medical Center
Assistant Professor of Radiology
University of California Los Angeles School of
    Medicine
Los Angeles, California

Masatoshi Makuuchi, MD, PhD
Chairman, Second Department of Surgery
Tokyo University Hospital
Professor of Hepatobiliary Pancreatic Surgery
    Divisionand of Artificial Organs and
    Transplantation Division
University of Tokyo, Faculty of Medicine
Tokyo, Japan

Iain Martin, MBChB, MD, FRCS
Consultant Surgeon
Leeds General Infirmary
Senior Lecturer
Leeds University
Leeds, United Kingdom

Miguel E. Martinez Noack, MD
Postdoctoral Fellow in Surgery
Tulane University School of Medicine
New Orleans, Louisiana

Jeffrey B. Matthews, MD
Associate Chief of General Surgery
Beth Israel Hospital
Associate Professor of Surgery
Harvard Medical School
Boston, Massachusetts

Emeran A. Mayer, MD
Director, Center for Functional Bowel and Motility
  Disorders
University of California Los Angeles Center for Health
  Sciences
Professor of Medicine and Physiology
University of California School of Medicine
Los Angeles, California

David W. McFadden, MD
Professor of Surgery
Chief, Division of General Surgery
University of California Los Angeles School of Medicine
Los Angeles, California

Howard R. Mertz, MD
Assistant Professor of Medicine
Division of Gastroenterology
Vanderbilt University School of Medicine
Nashville, Tennessee

J. Michael Millis, MD
Co-Director, Liver Transplant Program
University of Chicago Hospitals
Assistant Professor of Surgery
University of Chicago
Chicago, Illinois

Fredrick J. Montz, MD
Attending Surgeon
Gynecologic Oncology Service
University of California Los Angeles Center for Health
  Sciences
Associate Professor
Department of Obstetrics and Gynecology
University of California Los Angeles School of Medicine
Los Angeles, California

Ernest E. Moore, MD
Chief, Department of Surgery
Denver General Hospital
Professor and Vice Chairman of Surgery
University of Colorado Health Sciences Center
Denver, Colorado

Frederick A. Moore, MD
Director, General Surgery and Trauma and Critical
  Care
Hermann Hospital
Professor and Vice Chairman of Surgery
University of Texas–Houston Medical School
Houston, Texas

Sean J. Mulvihill, MD
Chief, Division of General Surgery
Associate Professor of Surgery
University of California San Francisco
San Francisco, California

Robert J. Myerson, MD
Associate Professor of Radiology
Radiation Oncology Center

Washington University School of Medicine
St. Louis, Missouri

David L. Nahrwold, MD
Surgeon-in-Chief
Northwestern Memorial Hospital
Loyal and Edith Davis Professor and Chairman
Department of Surgery
Northwestern University Medical School
Chicago, Illinois

L. K. Nathanson, FRACS
Consultant Surgeon
Royal Brisbane Hospital
Associate Professor of Surgery
University of Queensland
Brisbane, Queensland, Australia

Santhat Nivatvongs, MD, FACS
Consultant in Colon and Rectal Surgery
Mayo Clinic
Professor of Surgery
Mayo Medical School
Rochester, Minnesota

Jeffrey A. Norton, MD
Attending Surgeon
Barnes Hospital
Professor of Surgery
Chief of Endocrine and Oncologic Surgery
Washington University School of Medicine
St. Louis, Missouri

Marshall J. Orloff, MD
Professor of Surgery
University of California San Diego Medical Center
University of California San Diego School of Medicine
San Diego, California

Mark S. Orloff, MD
Associate Professor of Surgery
Section of Solid Organ Transplantation
Strong Memorial Hospital
University of Rochester
Rochester, New York

Thomas George Parks
Consultant surgeon
Belfast City Hospital
Professor of Surgical Science
Queen's University of Belfast
Belfast, Ireland

Edward Passaro, Jr., MD
Chief, Surgical Service
Veterans Administration Medical Center West Los
  Angeles
Professor of Surgery
University of California Los Angeles School of Medicine
Los Angeles, California

Carlos A. Pellegrini, MD
Professor of Surgery
Chairman, Department of Surgery
University of Washington School of Medicine
Seattle, Washington

Gary R. Peplinski, MD
Resident in Surgery
Barnes Hospital
Washington University School of Medicine
St. Louis, Missouri

Jeffrey H. Peters, MD
Chief, Section of General Surgery
University of Southern California University Hospital
Associate Professor of Surgery
University of Southern California School of Medicine
Los Angeles, California

Jack Pickleman, MD
Chief, Division of General Surgery
Loyola University Medical Center
Dr. and Mrs. John Igini Professor of Surgery
Loyola University Stritch School of Medicine
Maywood, Illinois

Henry A. Pitt, MD
Professor and Vice Chairman
Department of Surgery
Johns Hopkins University School of Medicine
Baltimore, Maryland

John H. C. Ranson, MD*
S. Arthur Localio Professor of Surgery
New York University
New York, New York

David W. Rattner, MD
Associate Visiting Surgeon
Massachusetts General Hospital
Associate Professor of Surgery
Harvard Medical School
Boston, Massachusetts

Robert A. Read, MD
Surgical Consultants
Denver, Colorado

Howard A. Reber, MD
Chief of Surgery
Sepulveda Veterans Administration Medical Center
Sepulveda, California
Professor and Vice Chairman
Department of Surgery
University of California Los Angeles School of Medicine
Los Angeles, California

John J. Ricotta, MD
Chairman, Department of Surgery
Millard Fillmore Hospital

Professor of Surgery
State University of New York at Buffalo
Buffalo, New York

Rolando H. Rolandelli, MD
Associate Professor of Surgery
Medical College of Pennsylvania
Hahnemann University
Philadelphia, Pennsylvania

Steven Rose, MD
Associate Professor of Radiology
University of California San Diego School of Medicine
Los Angeles, California

R. David Rosin, MS, FRCS, FRCS (Edin)
Chief Gastro-Intestinal and Soft Tissue Tumor Service
St. Mary's Hospital
Imperial College of Medicine
University of London
London, United Kingdom

Joel J. Roslyn, MD
Professor and Chairman
Department of Surgery
The Medical College of Pennsylvania
Hahnemann University
Philadelphia, Pennsylvania

Seymour I. Schwartz, MD
Distinguished Alumni Professor and Chair
Department of Surgery
University of Rochester School of Medicine and
    Dentistry
Rochester, New York

Mika N. Sinanan, MD, PhD
Attending Surgeon
University of Washington Medical Center
Assistant Professor of Surgery
University of Washington School of Medicine
Seattle, Washington

Peter W. Soballe, MD, FACS
Assistant Professor of Surgery
Head, Surgical Oncology
National Naval Medical Center
Bethesda, Maryland
Uniformed Services University of Health Sciences
Washington, DC

Nathaniel J. Soper, MD
Staff Surgeon
Barnes Hospital
Associate Professor of Surgery
Washington University School of Medicine
St. Louis, Missouri

*Deceased

David I. Soybel, MD
Associate in Surgery
Brigham and Women's Hospital
Associate Professor of Surgery
Harvard Medical School
Boston, Massachusetts

Lewis Spitz, MB, ChB, PhD, FRCS
Nuffield Professor of Pediatric Surgery
Consultant Surgeon
Great Ormond Street Hospital for Children
Professor
Institute of Child Health
University of London
London, United Kingdom

Bruce E. Stabile, MD
Chairman, Department of Surgery
Harbor–University of California Los Angeles Medical
    Center
Torrance, California
Professor of Surgery
University of California Los Angeles School of
    Medicine
Los Angeles, California

Michael J. Stamos, MD
Chief, Section of Colon and Rectal Surgery
Harbor–University of California Los Angeles Medical
    Center
Torrance, California
Assistant Professor of Surgery
University of California Los Angeles School of Medicine
Los Angeles, California

David J. Sugerbaker, MD
Chief, Surgical Services
Dana Farber Cancer Institute
Chief, Division of Thoracic Surgery
Brigham and Women's Hospital
Associate Professor of Surgery
Harvard Medical School
Boston, Massachusetts

Harvey J. Sugerman, MD
Vice Chairman, Department of Surgery
Virginia Commonwealth University
David M. Hume Professor of Surgery
Medical College of Virginia
Richmond, Virginia

James C. Thompson, MD
Surgeon, The University of Texas Medical Branch
    Hospitals
Ashbel Smith Professor of Surgery
The University of Texas Medical Branch
Galveston, Texas

Ronald K. Tompkins, MD, MSc
Chief, Section of Gastrointestinal Surgery
University of California Los Angeles Medical Center
Professor of Surgery
University of California School of Medicine
Los Angeles, California

Andrew L. Warshaw, MD
Chief, General Surgery
Massachusetts General Hospital
Harold and Ellen Danser Professor of Surgery
Harvard Medical School
Boston, Massachusetts

Karen W. West, MD
Associate Professor
Section of Pediatric Surgery
Indiana University School of Medicine
Indianapolis, Indiana

Edward E. Whang, MD
Assistant Resident, General Surgery
Department of Surgery
University of California Los Angeles
Los Angeles, California

**John Wong, MBBS, PhD, MD(Hon), FRACS,
    FRCS(Edin), FACS (Hon)**
Professor and Head
Department of Surgery
The University of Hong Kong
Queen Mary Hospital
Hong Kong

Charles J. Yeo, MD
Attending Surgeon
The Johns Hopkins Hospital
Professor of Surgery
Associate Professor of Oncology
The Johns Hopkins University School of Medicine
Baltimore, Maryland

Peter T. Zimmerman, MD
Assistant Clinical Professor of Radiology
University of California Los Angeles School of
    Medicine
Los Angeles, California

Michael J. Zinner, MD, FACS
Moseley Professor of Surgery
Harvard University Medical School
Surgeon-in-Chief
Brigham and Women's Hospital
Boston, Massachusetts

CONTENTS

PREFACE

It is an honor and a privilege to be given the opportunity to edit *Maingot's Abdominal Operations*. In the past five decades and through nine editions, this text has become the standard for all general surgeons and surgeons-in-training. The new edition of this textbook is a complete revision—a completely new book. We have expanded the focus of the book to include more operative procedures as well as new concepts in diagnosis and new management of diseases. As in past editions, we have drawn on internationally recognized groups of contributors who share their contemporary experience with the readers. This book is an up-to-date text on current diagnostic procedures and surgical techniques related to the management and care of patients with all types of abdominal disease and injury.

An extensive artwork program was undertaken for this 10th edition. More than 700 line drawings have been redone. They depict the chapter authors' preferred method for performing certain surgical procedures. Approximately 80% of all the illustrations in this edition are new, giving the book a more modern and consistent look.

Section I, Diagnostic and Interventional Procedures, deals with the symptoms and conditions that bring the patient to the surgeon. These include gastrointestinal bleeding, functional gastrointestinal syndromes, nausea and vomiting, constipation and diarrhea, and abdominal pain. The contributors bring newer concepts and treatment to these areas.

Many sections have been added, including contemporary endoscopic and laparoscopic techniques, since these are becoming an increasingly important operative tool for the practicing surgeon. In many sections of the book there are deliberate duplications to bring more than one perspective to an important disease entity. For example, in the section on peptic disease of the stomach and duodenum, two perspectives are given—one by David Johnston and Iain Martin, one by Bruce Stabile and Edward Passaro. This book is the work of distinguished international authors, and is intended to represent a complete and explicit account of the diseases and techniques for their treatment as are currently practiced in the world's finest teaching hospitals, large general hospitals, and surgical clinics.

In addition to adding new chapters, we have expanded old chapters. For example, we have extended the topic of operations on the esophagus into Benign Disorders of the Esophagus (Chapter 24) and Surgical Procedures to Resect or Replace the Esophagus (Chapter 26). We have added chapters on the Surgical Management of Ascites (Chapter 56), as well as on Gynecological Pelvic Procedures (Chapter 82) as they relate to the surgeon dealing with gastrointestinal disease. In each chapter, where appropriate, laparoscopic procedures have been added as they become more established in the practice of abdominal surgery.

In the preface to his sixth edition, Rodney Maingot noted: "As all literature is personal, the contributors have been given a free hand with their individual sections. A certain latitude in style and expression is stimulating to the thoughtful reader." Similarly, in this edition, we have tried to maintain consistency for the reader; however, the contributors have been given a free hand in their contributions.

I give my appreciation and grateful thanks to my co-editors, Seymour Schwartz and Harold Ellis for their assistance in the preparation of this edition. Without their support and cooperation, we would not have been able to publish this edition. I am also intensely grateful for the contributions of Stanley Ashley and David McFadden. They played an essential role in organizing early components of the text. They have generously given their time and made important contributions, not only as chapter contributors, but also as section editors.

At Appleton & Lange, I would like to thank Edward H. Wickland, Jr. for his unwavering support during the lengthy time of this project development. His support and the support of the publisher was critical to the success of this textbook. Also at Appleton & Lange, the support and help of Kathleen McCullough, Managing Editor of Development, and Cynthia Shepard, developmental editor, were invaluable in finally putting all this work into a single comprehensive textbook. Their suggestions and attention to detail made it possible to overcome the innumerable problems that occur in publishing such a large textbook.

I have had the good fortune to deal with outstanding illustrators during the development of this book. These include Gwynne Gloege, who was our in-house illustrator at the University of California, Los Angeles, as well as Philip Ashley, medical illustrator extraordinaire, who, in addition to creating quality illustrations, maintained a consistent stylistic theme throughout the entire book by coordinating a group of outstanding medical illustrators, including Tracie Aretz, Jessica Buchman, Juan Garcia, Nicole Mock, and Lynn Reynolds. A special thanks goes to Jessica Buchman for her commitment, professionalism, and tireless efforts throughout the entire project.

Finally, I owe a great debt of gratitude to my three assistants who have survived the trials of this book, Carole Dool, Karen Tyler, and Patrina Tucker. They have helped me with every step of the work, from helping type manuscripts, to reading and editing proof, and for their encouragement during the prolonged dry periods and preparation of this textbook.

To all of those who contributed, thank you very much.

Michael J. Zinner, MD, FACS

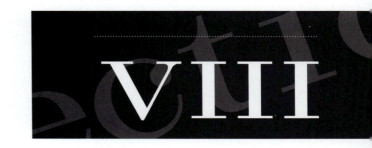

SMALL INTESTINE

35

Meckel's Diverticulum, Diverticulosis of the Small Intestine, Umbilical Fistula and Tumors

Harold Ellis

■ MECKEL'S DIVERTICULUM

HISTORICAL BACKGROUND

Soderlund gives an interesting account of the early history of this most common congenital abnormality of the gastrointestinal (GI) canal.[1] From the end of the 17th century, diverticula were observed as contents of hernial sacs, by Lavater in 1672, Littre in 1770, and Mery in 1701. To this day, a hernial sac containing a Meckel's diverticulum is termed Littre's hernia, although there is some debate as to whether the three cases he described where a portion of the intestinal circumference as strangulated in a hernial sac were, rather, examples of Richter's hernia, implicating a portion of the circumference of the small intestine, as described by Richter in 1777. Ruysch published a drawing of a diverticulum of the small intestine that he observed at autopsy and added two additional cases in 1701.

In 1808, Johann Friedrich Meckel, Professor of Anatomy at Halle, stated that the diverticulum comprised a remnant of the duct between the intestinal tract and the yolk sac.[2] As evidence he put forward the observation that more than one diverticulum with the same structure as the small intestine, is never found in the same embryo that the diverticulum is always situated on the distal part of the small intestine and on its outer circumference, and that coincidental malformations are often present. Meckel gave a more detailed account of his observations the following year.[3] He pointed out that although the duct generally disappears in the tenth week of fetal life, he had seen it persist past this period in two cases, and he described a case in which the duct persisted in its entirety as far as the umbilicus. His account of the origin of the diverticulum was so clear that his name has become eponymously and permanently attached to this abnormality.

In 1898, Kuttner described intussusception of a Meckel's diverticulum.[4] In 1904, Salzer described ectopic gastric mucosa in the diverticulum[5] and, in 1907, Deet noted the association of this aberrant gastric mucosa with ulceration of the adjacent ileum.[6]

INCIDENCE

Meckel's diverticulum has been reported, in various autopsy series, to have an incidence varying from 0.3% to 2.5%. This quite wide difference in the incidence figures is probably owing to the fact that pathologists vary in the enthusiasm with which they study the distal ileum. Soderlund reports the very careful study carried out in a series of 1954 children undergoing appendectomy in which at least the terminal 100 cm of the ileum was explored.[1] Meckel's diverticulum then was found in 63 of the children (3.2%).[1] In most reported series there is a male-to-female preponderance of approximately 3 to 2.

ANATOMY

Developmentally, the vitelline duct connects the yolk sac and the midgut of the embryo at an early stage in fetal life. Thus, in the 3 week old embryo, the yolk sac forms the ventral aspect of the gut and communicates through a wide, short vitelline duct, which gradually elongates and narrows. During the fifth week (at the 7-mm stage) the midgut normally closes off completely by atrophy of the vitelline duct to form a fibrous cord, which subsequently becomes absorbed. The blood supply to the vitelline duct comes from paired ventral branches of the abdominal aorta, the vitelline arteries. Normally, the left artery involutes while the right persists to form the superior mesenteric artery. Meckel's diverticulum receives its blood supply from a remnant of the right vitelline artery, usually as an end branch of the superior mesenteric. Occasionally, as stressed by Rutherford and Akers, the Meckel's diverticulum may be associated with a mesodiverticular band, which may represent an accentuation of the normal end artery that supplies the diverticulum and that comes to run in the separate mesentery, or may represent the persistence of the left vitelline artery.[7] The importance of this band, as will be discussed later, is that it creates a triangular hiatus under which a loop of intestine can become strangulated.[8]

Failure of all or a portion of the vitelline duct to become obliterated accounts for the various forms of this anomaly (Figs 35–1, 35–2, and 35–3):

1. There may be a completely obliterated duct persisting as a band between the umbilicus and the small intestine, or the cord may extend from the diverticulum to the umbilicus.
2. The vitelline duct remains patent throughout (persistent omphaloenteric fistula).
3. The duct may persist in part of its course as a sinus opening at the umbilicus, without attachment to the small intestine, or with the band passing to the ileum, or as an enterocystoma, an intermediate cyst attached by a fibrous cord to both the umbilicus and the small intestine.
4. Most commonly, a persistence of the proximal portion of the duct results in the formation of a Meckel's diverticulum (approximately 90% of cases).

The size and shape of the diverticulum varies greatly, between 1 and 26 cm in length, although it is usually between 3 and 5 cm long. Soderlund found that the diverticulum was situated from 10 to 150 cm from the ileocecal valve.[1] In children, it usually lays about 40 cm from the valve, and in adults, about 50 cm from the valve. The diameter is somewhat less than that of the ileum, but it may occasionally be a narrow appendix-like protrusion.

It possesses a mesentery, and it has an independent arterial supply from an arcade of the ileal vessels, except in those cases in which the diverticulum is unusually small. It may fold over on itself and lie by the side of the gut, and it may be covered by a filmy membrane when it lies flat on the mesentery of the intestine. Out pouchings or diverticula may be present on the diverticulum itself (Fig 35–4).

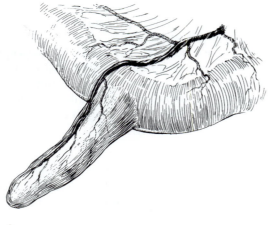

A

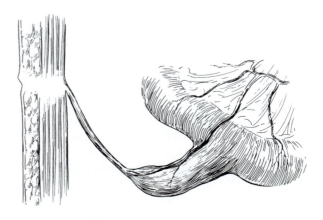

B

Figure 35–1. Meckel's diverticulum and its associated anomalies. **A.** The usual type; persistence of the proximal portion of the duct results in the formation of a Meckel's diverticulum (about 90% of cases). **B.** A fibrous cord extends from the diverticulum to the umbilicus. *Continued*

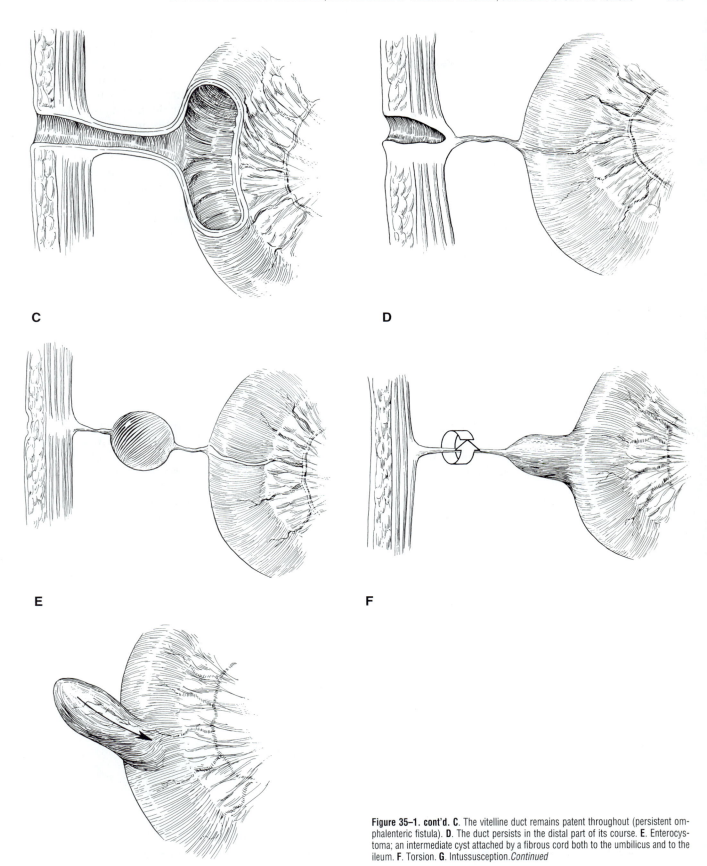

C

D

E

F

G

Figure 35–1. cont'd. C. The vitelline duct remains patent throughout (persistent omphalenteric fistula). **D**. The duct persists in the distal part of its course. **E**. Enterocystoma; an intermediate cyst attached by a fibrous cord both to the umbilicus and to the ileum. **F**. Torsion. **G**. Intussusception.*Continued*

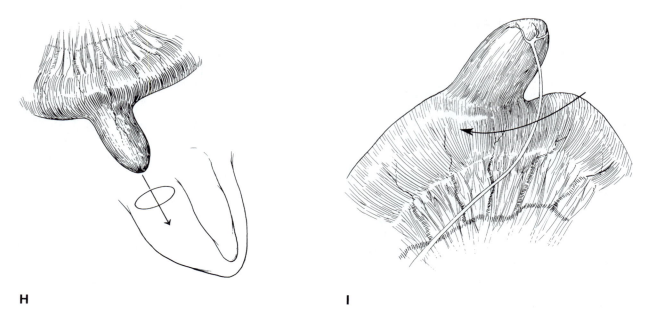

H

I

Figure 35–1. cont'd. H. Littre's hernia. **I.** Obstruction owing to mesodiverticular band.

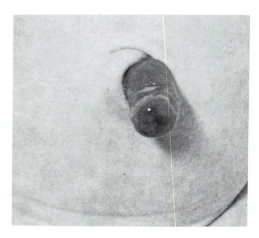

Figure 35–2. Enteric umbilical fistula. (Redrawn from Gracey LRH, Williams JA. Meckel's diverticulum in children. *Br J Clin Pract* 1963;17:315)

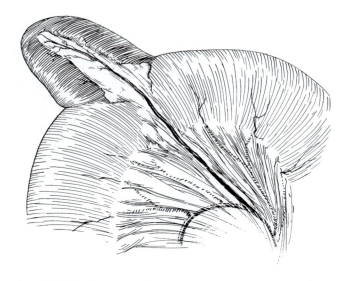

Figure 35–3. Meckel's diverticulum. Note blood supply to the diverticulum. (After RN Lane)

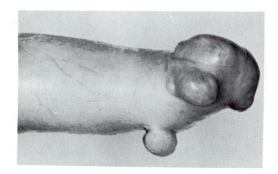

Figure 35–4. Outpouchings or diverticula of a Meckel's diverticulum. (Courtesy of Mr. L. Gracey)

ASSOCIATED CONGENITAL MALFORMATIONS

Simms and Corkery point out that Meckel's diverticulum occurs more commonly in individuals born with other congenital malformations, especially exomphalos, esophageal atresia, anorectal atresia, and gross malformations of the central nervous system or the cardiovascular system.[9] In Soderlund's study of 413 clinical cases, there were 22 congenital malformations in 19 of them.[1] Hemingway and Allison reported an interesting association between angiodysplasia of the cecum and ascending colon and Meckel's diverticulum in five patients aged 13 to 21.[10] Angiodysplasia had previously been reported only in patients over the age of 35.

Although isolated cases of Meckel's diverticulum among relatives have been described, there is no evidence that Meckel's diverticulum is an inherited trait.

HETEROTOPIC MUCOSA

The lining of the diverticulum is the same as that of the ileum in the majority of cases. However, heterotopic gastric, duodenal, colonic, or pancreatic tissue may occur, either singly or in combination. Mackey and Dineen carried out microscopic examinations of 140 symptomless Meckel's diverticula removed incidentally at operation.[11] In 23 (16.4%), heterotopic mucosa was identified: gastric mucosa was present in 15, pancreatic tissue was found in 3, another 3 had colonic mucosa, 1 contained jejunal mucosa, and 1 had both gastric and duodenal tissue. In a further 62 instances in which the Meckel's diverticulum was removed because of symptoms, the incidence of heterotopic mucosa was higher, identified in 21 patients (34%). Of these, 19 had gastric mucosa; 1 had pancreatic tissue; and 1 had colonic mucosa.

COMPLICATIONS

The complications of Meckel's diverticulum may be classified as follows:

1. *The peptic group,* in which the heterotopic gastric mucosa results in the development of a chronic peptic ulcer in the diverticulum itself or adjacent to its stoma. This may present with hemorrhage or, less frequently, acute perforation.
2. *The inflammatory group,* in which acute inflammatory changes take place that may result in gangrene and perforation. Perforation may also result from penetration by foreign bodies. In this group, the signs and symptoms closely mimic those of acute appendicitis.
3. *The obstructive group,* in which intestinal obstruction results from intussusception, volvulus, adhesions, bands, fibrous cord, foreign bodies, or concretions.

4. The umbilical group, which includes fistula, cyst, and granuloma.
5. *The tumor group,* which includes both benign (myoma, lipoma, neuroma, and adenoma) and malignant (adenocarcinoma, leiomyosarcoma, and carcinoid tumor), as well as cysts.

Rutherford and Akers found the following incidence of complications in a series of 80 children with symptomatic Meckel's diverticula: 43 had rectal bleeding, 26 presented with obstruction, 8 with inflammation, and 3 with perforation (2 from peptic ulceration and 1 from a pin).[7] Mackey and Dineen list the complications of 68 patients with symptomatic Meckel's diverticulum as follows: obstruction in 23, inflammation in 21, hemorrhage in 17, Littre's hernia in 8, umbilical fistula in 3, and 1 example each of multiple calculi torsion, and an abdominal wall abscess.[11] Soderlund, in a series of 142 patients with symptomatic Meckel's diverticulum, found the following distribution: peptic ulceration in 40, intussusception in 19, acute inflammation in 24, umbilical fistula in 15, and Littre's hernia in 4.[1]

Williams, in a review of 1806 collected cases, found the following incidence of complications:[12]

hemorrhage	31%
inflammation	25%
bowel obstruction owing to band, etc.	16%
intussusception	11%
hernial involvement	11%
umbilical sinus or fistula	4%
tumor	2%

There has been much discussion about the risk of a Meckel's diverticulum undergoing one or another of these complications. Soltero and Bill have carried out an estimation of this possibility by studying a stable population of over one million people during a 15 year period.[13] During this time 202 examples of complications of Meckel's diverticulum were encountered. The authors assume a 2%–3% incidence of diverticulum in the population, and, from life table calculations, they estimate that, in infancy, a child with a Meckel's diverticulum runs a 4.2% risk of developing symptoms, dropping to 3% in adults and almost zero in old age.

The presentation of Meckel's diverticulum in hospital practice is well reviewed by Mackey and Dineen.[11] During a 50 year period at the Cornell Medical Center in New York, a total of 402 examples of Meckel's diverticulum were recorded. Of these, 45% were incidental findings at postmortem, 35% were incidental findings at laparotomy, and 1.5% were incidental findings at radiologic examination. Definite symptoms attributable to the diverticulum accounted for 17% of the patients; another 1.5% had possible symptoms. In this study, patients most likely to develop symptoms from the diverticulum are those under 40 years of age, with a diverticulum 2 cm or more in length and probably, also male patients. The presence of heterotopic mucosa makes the diverticulum more likely to undergo complications, but in many cases it cannot be detected by gross findings. Indirect evidence is the presence of submucosal or mucosal nodularity, scarring, or inflammatory adhesions.

CLINICAL MANIFESTATIONS

In most cases a Meckel's diverticulum is an incidental finding at postmortem or laparotomy. When symptoms occur, the clinical manifestations vary with the type of complication present, and in most cases the diagnosis can be made with certainty only at operation.

Hemorrhage

The passage of blood per rectum, in a child, should always raise the possibility of hemorrhage from peptic ulceration of a Meckel's diverticulum. Bleeding can also occur in young adults; in Soderlund's series there were 24 such cases, with an age range from 6 months to 22 years (3 were adults).[1] Rutherford and Akers reviewed the nature of the rectal bleeding in 43 children.[7] Bright-red bleeding was recorded by history or direct observation in 47%. Dark-red or maroon stools were observed in 58%, and there was some overlap between the two. Tarry stools as the only evidence of bleeding were reported in only three patients (7%) and none presented with anemia or occult blood in the stools. A history of previous bleeding was elicited in 40% of the patients. Occult bleeding is, in fact, extremely rare. Farthing and associates report an example of this in a 14 year–old girl and state that an extensive search of previous publications failed to produce any other examples.[14]

Inflammation

Inflammation of the diverticulum closely simulates the clinical features of acute appendicitis and its complications. Therefore, the diverticulum should always be sought in a patient undergoing operation for appendicitis, but who is found to have a normal appendix, especially in children. The acutely inflamed diverticulum may proceed to perforation with localized abscess or general peritonitis (Fig 35–5). Peritonitis may also follow perforation of a peptic ulcer of the diverticulum or foreign body perforation. Rosswick reviewed 50 case reports of foreign body perforation of Meckel's diverticulum and no less than 28 of these were due to fish bones.[15] Other foreign bodies included a cherry stone, a knitting needle, a gramophone needle, a wooden splinter, and a chicken bone. Six of these patients were younger than 10 years of age, and three were older than 70 years of age. This author has records of three patients with this complication, the foreign body being a fish bone in two cases and a rolled-up piece of apple peel in the third (Fig 35–6); in this case, a boy 13 years of age had eaten an apple 33 hours previously. Three examples of gangrene of a Meckel's diverticulum owing to impaction of slow-release iron tablets also have been recorded. Layer and his colleagues report perfo-

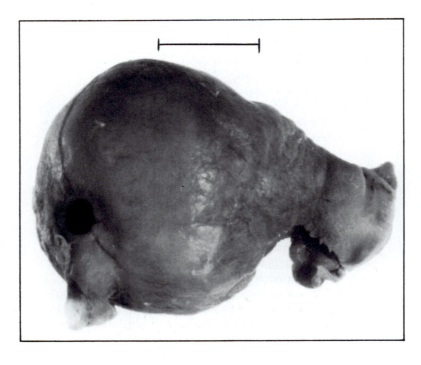

Figure 35–5. Perforated Meckel's diverticulum (Bar equals 1 cm.)

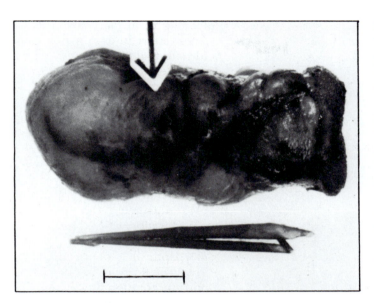

Figure 35–6. Meckel's diverticulum perforated by a rolled piece of apple peel (Bar equals 1 cm).

ration in a woman 65 years of age owing to impaction of a slow-release potassium tablet in the diverticulum.[16] A rare case of Meckel's diverticulitis fistulating into the bladder is reported by Hudson and colleagues.[17]

Intestinal Obstruction

This may result from intussusception (Fig 35–7), torsion, a band, or obstruction within a hernia. Rutherford and Akers reviewed 26 instances of this complication in children and found that volvulus around a vitelloumbilical cord occurred in 7 instances (with infarction in 5 instances), intussusception in 7, obstruction in an inguinal hernia in 2, and obstruction following inflammation with adhesions in 4.[7] In 6 patients, a segment of intestine had become trapped under a cord or band coursing between the diverticulum and the base of the mesentery, and half of these had progressed to infarction at the time of laparotomy. They observed such a band as an incidental finding in 6 other patients (Fig 35–8). They suggest that this mesodiverticular band represents a persistence of the vitelline arterial system; this author has observed this in one nonobstructed case.

Vellacott reports what appears to be a unique case of hemoperitoneum resulting from hemorrhage from the midpoint of such a mesodiverticular band, the Meckel's having the appearances of having undergone torsion.[18] Lawrence has recorded three case reports of obstruction owing to impacted food material in the ileum above the Meckel's diverticulum, caused by coconut, orange pulp, and sauerkraut.[19]

Umbilical Fistula

The presence of a fistula at the umbilicus suggests the presence of a patent vitelline duct. The diagnosis of fistula is certain when ileal contents ooze through the umbilicus.

Littre's Hernia

The presence of a Meckel's diverticulum in a hernia sac is rare and has, perhaps, received more attention in surgical publications than it deserves. This author has personally never seen a case. It may occur as an incidental finding in a nonstrangulated hernia or, an exceedingly rare phenomenon, as the content of a strangulated hernia. Castleden gives the incidence of the various hernias containing a Meckel's diverticulum as inguinal, 50%; femoral, 20%; umbilical, 20%; and incisional and other hernias, 10%.[20] A Meckel's diverticulum within an umbilical hernia is a particularly rare finding. The possibility of a coincidental Meckel's diverticulum should be borne in mind, however, in newborn infants with omphalocele. Soderlund notes that a diverticulum was present in 4 of 24 such cases in his study.[1] Apart from this rarity, it is, of course, impossible to diagnose the presence of a Meckel's diverticulum preoperatively, in either a simple or a strangulated hernia.

Further information can be found in a monograph by Watson, who presents a series of 259 examples of Lit-

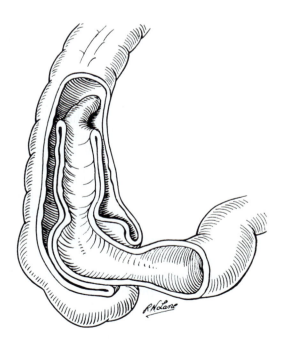

Figure 35–7. Intussusception of a Meckel's diverticulum.

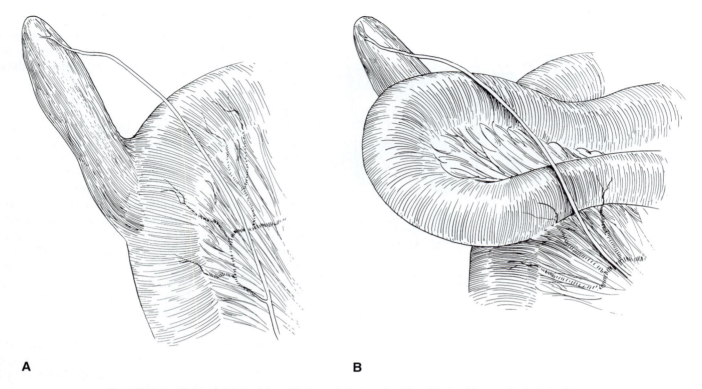

A

B

Figure 35–8. A and **B**. Intestinal obstruction resulting from volvulus around a vitelloumbilical cord (or mesodiverticular band).

tre's hernia,[21] and in an interesting account by Leslie and colleagues of a unique case of a small bowel fistula complicating a strangulated Meckel's diverticulum within a femoral hernia.[22] Perlman and colleagues review the 43 published cases in the English language of femoral hernia containing a strangulated Meckel's diverticulum.[23]

Neoplasm

Weinstein et al review this rarity.[24] In a collected series of 106 cases, 26 were benign; the most common was leiomyoma, followed by fibroma, hemangioendothelioma, neuroma, and lipoma. Of the 80 malignant cases, 35 were sarcomas, 29 were carcinoids, and 16 were adenocarcinomas. Nies and his colleagues have collected 104 published cases of carcinoid in Meckel's diverticulum and point out that they resemble ileal carcinoids in their biological behavior more than they do appendiceal carcinoids.[25] No less than three quarters of these tumors had metastasized at the time of presentation. Kusumoto and colleague review 30 cases of adenocarcinoma in this situation; their own case was the first to be diagnosed preoperatively, this by a combination of technetium scintigraphy and angiography.[26] Tumor formation appears to be the least common pathologic condition to which Meckel's diverticulum is prone. For example, there was not a single example in the extensive series that was reported by Soderlund of 413 clinical cases in adults and children.[1]

DIAGNOSTIC STUDIES

Rather surprisingly, a Meckel's diverticulum rarely is demonstrated on a routine barium meal follow-through; the reason for this is not obvious since jejunal diverticula show readily. However, a small bowel enema, carried out by an infusion of dilute barium through a nasogastric tube guided into the duodenum, will demonstrate the diverticulum in about 0.7% of all examinations. The injection of contrast material into an umbilical fistula differentiates a patent vitelline duct communicating with the ileum from a patent urachus communicating with the urinary bladder.

In 1970, Jewett and associates demonstrated that the ectopic gastric mucosa in a Meckel's diverticulum could be visualized by a technetium scan of the abdomen, using Tc 99m pertechnetate (^{99m}Tc). They reported two examples in children, both of whom presented with rectal bleeding. By 1982, this same group at the Children's Hospital in Buffalo were able to report a series of 270 such scans carried out in children with a calculated accuracy of 90%.[28] This is certainly a technique that is valuable in the investigation of obscure lower GI bleeding in children and young adults.[29] Fig 35–9 (author's

1 Hr.

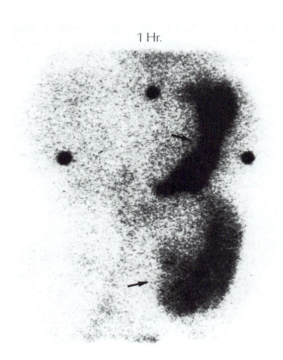

Figure 35–9. 1-hour technetium scan demonstrating a Meckel's diverticulum. The *upper arrow* points to the stomach image, the *lower arrow* to the visualized diverticulum.

case) demonstrates such a scan; this was a young man 30 years of age who had experienced central abdominal pains since he was a schoolboy. In the few months before admission to Westminster, he had had two episodes of melena, each requiring transfusion with four units of blood. A barium meal and follow-through, gastroscopy, barium enema, and colonscopy were all negative. The ^{99m}Tc scan showed a take-up in the lower left abdomen, and a diagnosis of a Meckel's diverticulum was made. At operation, there was indeed a large Meckel's diverticulum that contained no less than three ulcers. Following its resection in 1979, he has remained free from further symptoms.

TREATMENT

Resection of a Meckel's diverticulum is, of course, performed when it is the site of any of the complications already described. Most surgeons would advise the removal of an asymptomatic pouch when found incidentally at laparotomy, in infants, children, or young adults, if there is attachment either by bands to the umbilicus or by a mesodiverticular vascular strand, or if there is any palpable thickening or adhesions suggestive of ectopic tissue. A wide-mouthed, thin-walled unattached diverticulum in an adult patient can probably quite safely be left alone, a view supported by studies by Leijonmarck and his colleagues from Stockholm and by Demartines and his colleagues from Switzerland.[30,31] In

exploring the right iliac fossa for suspected acute appendicitis, a normal appendix is, or course, an indication for searching for an inflamed Meckel's diverticulum. However, most surgeons would agree that if an acutely inflamed appendix is found there is no need to search for a Meckel's diverticulum. Indeed, the association of acute appendicitis with an acute Meckel's diverticulitis, although recorded, is extremely rare.

There are two techniques for excision of the diverticulum, simple excision or resection with the segment of ileum containing the diverticulum.

Simple excision is satisfactory, in most cases. The diverticulum is clamped in the transverse axis of the ileum in order to avoid narrowing of the lumen when the defect is closed by means of two layers of 2/0 continuous catgut (Fig 35–10). Similarly, the diverticulum can be

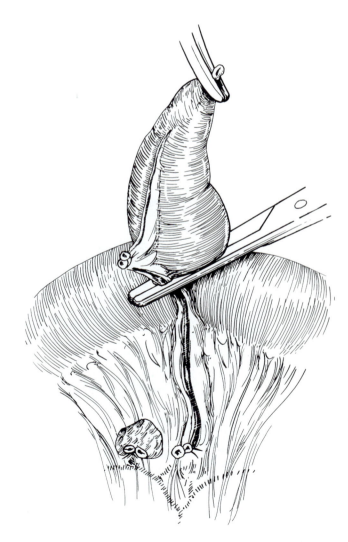

Figure 35–10. Excision of a Meckel's diverticulum. (Adapted from Gross RE. Meckel's diverticulum: diverticulectomy. In: Gross RE (ed), *An Atlas of Children's Surgery*. Philadelphia, PA: WB Saunders; 1970. After RN Lane.)

removed by a single firing of a stapling device. This can be oversewn to reinforce the staple line. It is important to divide the supplying artery on the ileal mesentery and to excise the distal segment that crosses the ileum. This will avoid the possibility of later band obstruction from fibrosis of the distal arterial segment.

Resection of a segment of the ileum containing the diverticulum, followed by end-to-end anastomosis, is reserved for patients with peptic ulceration (which may involve the adjacent ileum), a gangrenous diverticulitis affecting the base of the diverticulum, or in those rare cases of malignant disease. When the diverticulum has a mesentery, this should be isolated, clamped, divided, and ligated first. Following resection of the bowel containing the diverticulum, intestinal continuity is restored by a two layer anastomosis.

■ DIVERTICULOSIS OF THE SMALL INTESTINE

INCIDENCE

Solitary or multiple diverticula may occasionally be found in the jejunum or, much less commonly, in the ileum (Fig 35–11). The reported prevalance in autopsy studies is about 1%.[32] However, 12 (2.3%) of 519 patients were found to have small bowel diverticula when studied by a double-contrast examination following infusion of barium through a tube placed at the duodeno-jejunal junction.[33] Simultaneous involvement of both jejunum and ileum is rare. Shackelford and Marcus found only 1 example of 750 upper GI barium studies.[34] Males are affected more often than females and, although the condition can be seen in young adults, it is encountered clinically most often in elderly patients. Williams and associates, in a review of 34 patients with diverticula of the small intestine, found that 18 were male and 16 female.[35] The ages ranged from 26 to 87 years, with a mean age of 67. The distribution was as follows: 4 had a solitary diverticulum of the jejunum; 19 had multiple jejunal diverticula; 5 had a solitary ileal diverticulum; 5 had multiple ileal diverticula; and 1 had diverticula that affected the entire small intestine. Interestingly, 8 of the patients also had diverticula of the duodenum.

ANATOMY

The diverticula are usually situated on the mesenteric border of the intestine but diverticula of the antimesenteric border (apart from Meckel's diverticulum) have also been described. The condition usually is regarded as one of multiple pulsion mucosal herniations, but this

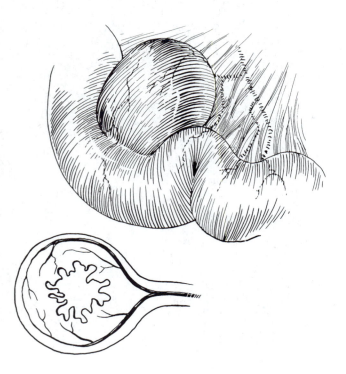

A

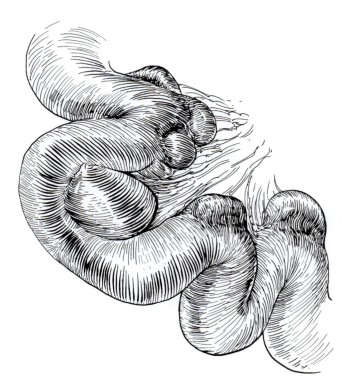

B

Figure 35–11. Solitary (**A**) and multiple (**B**) diverticula of the jejunum. Inset demonstrates the normal blood supply of the jejunum in transverse section.

is only true in a proportion of cases. A careful pathological study of 11 resected specimens of jejunal diverticulosis by Meagher and his colleagues suggests three patterns of diverticulum: pulsion, muscle coat defect, and congenital.[32] Four cases showed evidence of pulsion; they developed at the point of penetration of blood vessels that passed through the main muscle coat and had a narrow mouth with a thin or absent muscle layer over the diverticulum. In four cases, the diverticula were associated with an abnormality of the muscle coat. These diverticula were wide mouthed and the submucosal layer was preserved. The abnormal main muscle coat over each diverticulum, while thinned and partly fibrosed, was identifiable. The fibrosis, in some cases, was mainly at the mouth but, in others, was over the main part of the diverticulum. Two cases had diverticula with features of both pulsion and muscle coat defect. Ganglia cells were seen in the submucosal and main muscle coats of all cases. One congenital diverticulum was identified. It was wide mouthed and the main muscle coat was of normal thickness, although architecturally abnormal. The wall contained both ductal and glandular pancreatic tissue.

COMPLICATIONS

Diverticula of the small intestine are symptomless in the majority of cases. Eckhauser and associates estimate that complications occur only in 6% to 10% of cases.[36] These may be classified as in the following paragraphs.

Diverticulitis and Perforation

Inflammation in a diverticulum usually is the result of foreign body inspissation or the presence of an enterolith. When perforation occurs, it may result in a generalized peritonitis, a localized abscess, or intestinal fistula formation between adjacent loops of bowel. The perforated diverticulum may be partly hidden by the mesenteric fat and may be difficult to detect.

Hemorrhage

Hemorrhage from small bowel diverticula is a rare cause of melena, which may be massive and repeated. A diverticulum always should be sought in a severely bleeding patient who, at laparotomy, has no other obvious source. Its presence may be indicated by arteriography.

Obstruction

An intestinal diverticulum may produce obstruction by postinflammatory adhesions or by volvulus of the diverticulum-bearing loop of intestine.

Metabolic

Jejunal diverticulosis may result in the so-called blind-loop syndrome, which is better termed "the small intestine stasis syndrome." This is fully reviewed by Ellis and Smith and

comprises some or all of the following features: diarrhea, steatorrhea, abdominal pain, and anemia owing to vitamin B_{12} deficiency.[37] In 1930, Taylor noted an example of "pernicious anemia" in this condition.[38] Montuschi, in 1949, first reported the association of steatorrhea with jejunal diverticulosis.[39] A classic account of the jejunal diverticulosis syndrome, including the development of frank subacute combined degeneration of the cord, was given by Badenock and associates in 1955,[40] and Watkinson and associates gave the first report, in 1959,[41] of improvement both in stools and vitamin B_{12} level after resection of the affected segment of jejunal diverticulosis. Cooke and associates give an extensive review of this interesting metabolic association with jejunal diverticula.[42]

Miscellaneous

Various other complications have been described. Infestation with round worms or thread worms, neoplastic change, and association with pneumatosis cystoides have

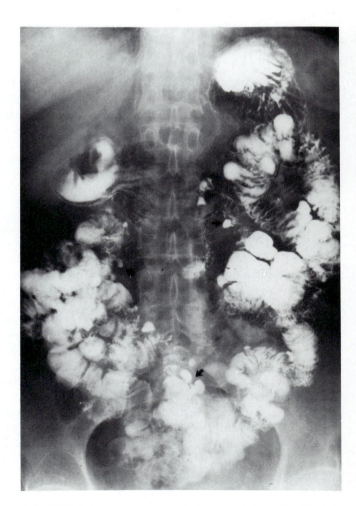

Figure 35–12. Barium follow-through examination demonstrating multiple jejunal diverticula (*arrows*).

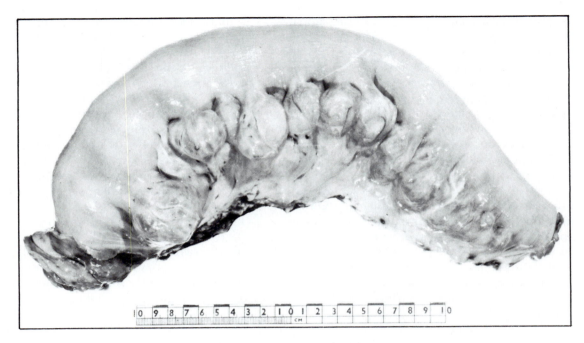

Figure 35–13. Resected specimen of localized segment of jejunal diverticulosis.

been reported. Craft and this author have recorded what is believed to be the first example of the latter, that is, a man of 63 years of age who presented with pneumoperitoneum and who, at laparotomy, was found to have multiple diverticula of the jejunum with superimposed areas of pneumatosis.[43] He recovered following resection of the affected segment.

DIAGNOSIS

Jejunal diverticula are symptomless in the great majority of cases. Vague abdominal discomfort may occur or there may be recurrent attacks of colicky abdominal pain, indicating a subacute obstruction. The symptoms are rather nonspecific and it may only be the onset of an unmistakable event such as hemorrhage or perforation that leads to the establishment of the correct diagnosis. Jejunal diverticula should also be suspected in patients presenting with megaloblastic anemia, steatorrhea, and the other features of the blind-loop syndrome.

Sometimes the diagnosis is suggested by a plain film of the abdomen that shows scattered pockets of air, but a careful barium-meal and follow-through examination of the small intestine will confirm the diagnosis in the majority of cases (Fig 35–12).

TREATMENT

As in the duodenum, the mere presence of a small intestinal diverticulum is not sufficient reason for its removal. A thorough search should be made for all other possible causes of symptoms, and treatment should be deferred until they have been excluded.

In patients presenting with steatorrhea or megaloblastic anemia, a sustained course of an intestinal antibiotic such as neomycin, together with vitamin B_{12} replacement, may keep the condition in check. When medical treatment fails, however, or in the presence of serious complications, operation must be considered the treatment of choice.

Severe hemorrhage, perforation, and obstruction are, of course, indications for urgent laparotomy.

In the case of a solitary diverticulum, simple diverticulectomy will suffice. Inversion of the diverticulum should not be carried out because of the possibility of subsequent intussusception. When the diverticula are confined to a small segment of the bowel, resection and end-to-end anastomosis should be undertaken (Fig 35–13). When the diverticula are scattered throughout the whole length of the small intestine, resection should be limited to the segments containing the largest diverticula. In an emergency situation, resections should be confined to the segment bearing the affected diverticulum.

OPERATIVE TECHNIQUE

Jejunoileal diverticula are often paper-thin and may lie concealed within the fat of the mesentery. It is not always easy to determine their presence in an empty bowel, despite the evidence of a barium-meal follow-through examination. In this situation, milking gas and fluid content from the ileum or stomach to distend the suspected segment helps to inflate the diverticula and make them evident.

For excision of a solitary diverticulum on the mesenteric border of the intestine, the affected segment should be emptied of its content and noncrushing clamps applied proximally and distally. An incision is made in the leaf of the mesentery over the diverticulum, care being taken to avoid cutting the adjacent vasa recta, although these may be divided and tied if they lie directly over the diverticulum. The diverticulum then is grasped gently with a tissue forceps and dissected out to its base, at which point it is excised with scissors. The resulting defect is closed transversely in two layers of 2/0 chromic catgut and further sutures repair the leaf of the mesentery.

For diverticula of the antimesenteric border, the technique of excision is exactly similar to that described for Meckel's diverticulum.

■ UMBILICAL FISTULAS AND TUMORS

Umbilical abnormalities (apart from hernia) may be classified as follows:

1. Anomalies of the vitellointestinal duct
   a. Patent duct (umbilical fistula)
   b. Umbilical granuloma
2. Anomalies of the urachus
   a. urachal cyst
   b. Patent urachus
3. Tumors of the umbilicus
4. Miscellaneous, including "umbolith," pilonidal sinus of the umbilicus, endometrioma, etc.

ANOMALIES OF THE VITELLOINTESTINAL DUCT

As already stated, the vitellointestinal duct may persist in whole or in part. Complete persistence is extremely rare and results in an external umbilical fistula. Such a fistula may discharge feces, but more commonly it discharges only a small amount of mucus. The absence of fecal discharge is due to peristalsis in the patent duct passing from the umbilicus toward the subjacent ileum and preventing any ileal reflux. The fistulous connection with the bowel may easily be demonstrated by sinography. The treatment of complete umbilical fistula is total excision of the patent duct via a paraumbilical incision.

Umbilical granuloma, sometimes known as raspberry tumor, represents the umbilical extremity of the duct. It appears as a bright red granulomatous swelling, and the persistent mucoid discharge from it may produce a considerable degree of umbilical dermatitis. Most commonly there is no connection between the umbilical granuloma and the underlying ileum, but in about one-third of cases a fibrous cord or narrow fistula connects the ileum to the umbilicus (Fig 35–14). Because of the danger of such a band causing acute intestinal obstruction, laparotomy is advised in all cases of umbilical granuloma.

ANOMALIES OF THE URACHUS

The allantois may very rarely persist between the fundus of the bladder and the umbilicus, forming a completely patent urachus. This produces a congenital urinary fistula and may occasionally be associated with membranous obstruction of the urethra. Equally rarely, the umbilical end may persist as an umbilical abscess. Another rarity is coexistence of a urachal and a vitellointestinal fistula.[44] Effective treatment involves drainage of the abscess in the acute stage, followed by complete excision of all urachal remnants when the infection has subsided.

TUMORS OF THE UMBILICUS

Such tumors are rare. Endometrioma may occur and occasionally a squamous cell carcinoma is found. Lymphatic spread from such a tumor may involve inguinal nodes in both groins. The primary tumor is best treated by wide local excision and the secondary nodes by block dissection. Secondary carcinoma of the umbilicus, the so-called Sister Mary Joseph's nodule, may occur by transcelomic spread. The primary tumor is almost always in some abdominal organ, for example, the stomach or ovary.

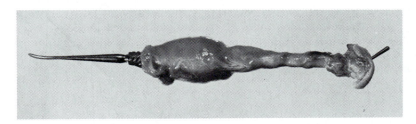

Figure 35–14. Umbilical granuloma with narrow fistulous connection to the underlying ileum. (Courtesy of Mr. L. Gracey).

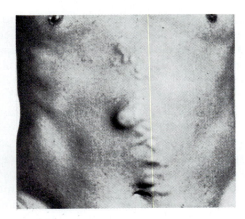

Figure 35–15. Distended umbilical veins in hepatic cirrhosis.

MISCELLANEOUS

Sebaceous material may collect in the umbilicus and then inspissate and form a sebaceous horn or "umbolith." These accretions may be easily lifted out intact, and this should be done preoperatively while the abdomen is being shaved and prepared for operation.

Very rarely, in patients with cirrhosis of the liver and severe portal hypertension, a mass of veins may form at the umbilicus, resembling a tumor, the so-called Cruveilhier-Baumgarten syndrome (Fig 35–15).

REFERENCES

1. Soderlund S. Meckel's diverticulum; a clinical and histologic study. *Acta Chir Scand* 1959;248(suppl):1
2. Meckel JF. *Beytrage zur Vergleichenden Anatomie.* Leipzig: Carl Heinrich Reclam; 1808:91
3. Meckel JF. Ueber die divertikel am darmkanal. *Arch Physiol* 1809;9:421
4. Kuttner H. Ileus durch intussusception eines Meckelschen divertikel. *Beitr Klin Chir* 1898;21:298
5. Salzer H. Ueber das offene Meckelsche divertikel. *Wien Klin Wochenschr* 1904;17:614
6. Deet E. Perforationsperitonitis von einem darmdivertikel mit Magenschleimhautbau ausgehend. *Dtsch Z Chir* 1907; 88:482
7. Rutherford RB, Akers DR. Meckel's diverticulum: a review of 148 pediatric patients, with reference to the pattern of bleeding and to mesodiverticular vascular bands. *Surgery* 1966;59:618
8. Pfalzgraf RR, Zumwalk RE. Mesodiverticular band and sudden death in children. *Arch Pathol Lab Med* 1988; 112:182
9. Simms MH, Corkery JJ. Meckel's diverticulum; a clinical and histologic study. *Acta Chir Scand* 1959;248(suppl 10):1
10. Hemingway AP, Allison AJ. Angiodysplasia and Meckel's diverticulum: a congenital association? *Br J Surg* 1982; 69:493
11. Mackey WC, Dineen P. A fifty year experience with Meckel's diverticulum. *Surg Gynecol Obstet* 1983;156:56
12. Williams RS. Management of Meckel's diverticulum. *Br J Surg* 1981;68:477
13. Soltero MJ, Bill AH. The natural history of Meckel's diverticulum and its relation to incidental removal. *Am J Surg* 1976;132:168
14. Farthing MG, Griffiths NJ, et al. Occult bleeding from Meckel's diverticulum. *Br J Surg* 1981;68:176
15. Rosswick RP. Perforation of Meckel's diverticulum by foreign bodies. *Postgrad Med J* 1965;41:105
16. Layer GT, Jupp RH, et al. Slow release potassium and perforation of Meckel's diverticulum. *Postgrad Med J* 1987; 63:211
17. Hudson HM, Millham FH, Dennis R. Vesicodiverticula fistula: a rare complication of Meckel's diverticulum. *Am Surg* 1992;58:784
18. Vellacott KD. Haemoperitoneum due to Meckel's diverticulum. *J R Coll Surg Edinb* 1981;26:89
19. Lawrence RE. A case of coconut bezoar and Meckel's diverticulum. *Postgrad Med J* 1982;58:119
20. Castleden WM. Meckel's diverticulum in an umbilical hernia. *Br J Surg* 1970;57:932
21. Watson LF. *Hernia*, 3rd ed. St. Louis, MO: CV Mosby; 1948: 547
22. Leslie MD, Slater ND, et al. Small bowel fistula from a Littre's hernia. *Br J Surg* 1983;70:244
23. Perlman JA, Hoover HC, et al. Femoral hernia with strangulated Meckel's diverticulum (Littre's hernia). *Am J Surg* 1980;139:286
24. Weinstein EC, Dockerty MB, et al. Neoplasms of Meckel's diverticulum. *Surg Gynecol Obstet* 1963;116:103
25. Nies C, Zielke A et al. Carcinoid tumours of Meckel's diverticula: report of two cases and review of the literature. *Dis Colon Rectum* 1992;35:589
26. Kusumoto H, Yoshida M et al. Complications and diagnosis of Meckel's diverticulum in 776 patients. *Am J Surg* 1993;164:382
27. Jewett TC, Duszynski DO, Allen JE. The visualization of Meckel's diverticulum with ⁹⁹ᵐTc-pertechnetate. *Surgery* 1970;68:567
28. Cooney DR, Duszynski DO, et al. The abdominal technetium scan (a decade of experience). *J Pediatr Surg* 1982; 17:611
29. Kusumoto H, Yoskitake H et al. Adenocarcinoma in Meckel's diverticulum: report of a case and review of cases in the English and Japanese literature. *Am J Gastroenterol* 1992;87:910
30. Leijonmarck CE, Bonman-Sandelin K, et al. Meckel's diverticulum in the adult. *Br J Surg* 1986;73:146
31. Demartines N, Herzog U, et al. Meckel's diverticulum: surgical complications. *Helv Chir Acta* 1992;59:325
32. Meagher AP, Porter AJ, et al. Jejunal diverticulosis. *Aust NZ J Surg* 1993;63:360
33. Maglinte DD, Chernish SM, et al. Acquired jejunoileal diverticular disease: subject review. *Radiology* 1986;158:577

34. Shackleford RT, Marcus WY. Jejunal diverticula-a cause of gastrointestinal hemorrhage. *Am Surg* 1960;151:930

35. Williams RA, Davidson DD, et al. Surgical problems of diverticula of the small intestine. *Surg Gynecol Obstet* 1981; 152:621

36. Eckhauser FE, Zelenock GB, et al. Acute complications of jejunal ileal pseudodiverticulosis: surgical implications and management. *Am J Surg* 1979;138:320

37. Ellis H, Smith ADM. The blind-loop syndrome. *Monogr Surg Sci* 1967;4:193

38. Taylor GW. Intestinal diverticulosis, pernicious anemia, bilateral suprarenal apoplexy: report of a case. *N Engl J Med* 1930;202:269

39. Montuschi E. Jejunal insufficiency with hypoproteinemic edema. *Proc R Soc Med* 1949;42:868

41. Watkinson G, Feather DB, et al: Jejunal diverticulosis with steatorrhea and megaloblastic anemia improved by excision of diverticula. *Br Med J* 1959;2:58

42. Cooke WT, Cox EV, et al. The clinical and metabolic significance of jejunal diverticula. *Gut* 1963;4:115

43. Craft I, Ellis H. Pneumatosis cystoides intestinalis associated with jejunal diverticula, presenting as pneumoperitoneum. *Proc R Soc Med* 1967;60:141

44. Alessandrini P, Derlon S. Congenital umbilical fistulas. a report of 12 cases. *Pediatrie* 1992;47:67

36

Crohn's Disease of the Small Intestine

John Alexander Williams

It is impossible to cure Crohn's disease by medical therapy or surgical excision. It is a panintestinal disease of unknown etiology that has a tendency to recrudescence throughout the life of the patient. Nevertheless, the majority of patients can be maintained in a good state of health by a combination of appropriate medical and surgical treatment.

■ PHILOSOPHY OF MANAGEMENT

We believe that almost all of the serious ill health and mortality associated with Crohn's disease is caused by mismanagement of complications rather than by the disease itself. Therefore, in recent years, we have adopted a conservative approach to the surgical treatment of all patients with Crohn's disease who do not respond rapidly to appropriate medical therapy or who require perpetual medication with potentially dangerous drugs.

■ MEDICAL THERAPY

This author recognizes that this brief, and possibly biased, account of drug therapy is written from the simplistic point of view of a surgical specialist used to being presented with end-stage disease for surgical management. Although I believe that many patients presented to us for surgical intervention have been treated medically for far too long, I am convinced of the value of appropriate medical management.

RATIONALE

We do not know the cause of Crohn's disease or even the primary precipitating factor. However, we know something about the pathophysiology. There may be an initial microbiological insult that results in an inflammatory response that damages tissue. Mucosal cellular damage leads to ulceration, allowing secondary tissue invasion of pathogenic microorganisms from the gut lumen. Chronic ulceration also provides a source of blood and protein loss. The healing response of granulation tissue produces fibrosis, which causes obstruction and predisposes to the penetration of deep fissured ulcers through the wall of the gut, with subsequent abscess and fistula. The stenosis also impairs gut motility, leading to alteration in gut microflora which, in turn, affect digestion and absorption.

The therapeutic armamentarium can be arranged into four groups: supportive, antimicrobial, antiinflammatory, and immunosuppressive. Some overlap may occur between that last two groups.

SUPPORTIVE

Monitoring of hematological and biochemical indices during patient surveillance will indicate the need for replacement or supplementation of hematinics such as iron, vitamin B_{12}, and folic acid. Trace element deficiency is less obvious clinically and more difficult to detect. Zinc, manganese, magnesium, calcium, selenium and other trace elements may need supplementation. The patient also may require other essential nutrients, such as amino acids and calories (see diet below).

ANTIMICROBIAL DRUGS

Although some claim that there is good evidence of infection with mycobacterium paratuberculosis in the pathogenesis of Crohn's disease, there is, as yet, no generally accepted evidence to support specific antimicrobacterial chemotherapy.

Nonspecific antibiotic or chemotherapeutic treatment is often effective, sometimes dramatically so. However, the benefit is almost invariably transient. The rationale for the temporary success of such therapy is probably that it combats secondary invasion of deeper layers by normal gut saporophytic organisms once the protective mucosal layer has been damaged.

A broad spectrum antibiotic seems to have a temporary beneficial effect during inflammatory exacerbations of the disease that is characterized by tenderness, fever, and leukocytosis. Antianaerobic therapy, particularly with metronidazole, seems particularly effective. However, it has many side effects that preclude its long-term use.

ANTI-INFLAMMATORY AND IMMUNOSUPPRESSIVE THERAPY

Steroids act in both capacities and are the most used therapy with undoubted efficacy in acute exacerbations of the disease. They reduce the inflammatory swelling and often relieve obstruction. However, long-term steroid therapy has inherent dangers and side effects. We routinely use steroids to treat acute exacerbations, but use as small a dose as is compatible with symptom relief. We review all patients on steroids for 12 weeks or more to consider whether surgical intervention could not more efficiently or safely relieve symptoms. For example, a patient with small bowel stenoses that can only be made tolerable by 20 mg of prednisolone daily often can be managed by a low morbidity surgical intervention such as stricturoplasty, enabling cessation of steroid therapy.

The beneficial effect of 5-aminosalicylic acid (ASA) compounds is probably related to their anti-inflammatory properties. However, they seem to have little place in the treatment of exacerbations. Evidence exists that they may have prophylactic value if used in asymptomatic patients after surgical relief.[1]

The beneficial effects of blood transfusion on patients with Crohn's disease exacerbations are probably the result of immunosuppression. More powerful immunosuppressive agents have been used to manage symptomatic disease, including 6-mecaptopurine, aza-

thioprine, and cyclosporine. All have undoubted efficacy that may take weeks to manifest. They are used mainly for their steroid-sparing effect and may be safer than steroids for long-term treatment. However, they, too, have their own inherent dangers. Our philosophy has been to seek safe surgical relief of symptoms.

DIET

Under supportive management, this author has listed provision of adequate calories and nutrients. There seems no doubt that a well-nourished patient is better able than a malnourished one to combat Crohn's disease and to recover more quickly from exacerbations. It is common to see a patient with repeated subacute obstruction from small bowel Crohn's disease who is undernourished to the point of having a compromised defense system. In such patients, a highly nutritious diet will exacerbate symptoms. To overcome this problem, some have advocated parenteral nutrition, others have advocated fine-bore nasogastric tube feeding of an elemental or a blended diet.

Central venous parenteral nutrition is prone to complications, whereas elemental diets are more expensive than simply finely blending a normal diet. If the patient has "the stomach" for a normal diet in blended form, this is preferable aesthetically and economically. If the patient is anorexic, then blended feeding slowly via a fine-bore tube may be advantageous. The rule we follow is to use the simplest, least complicated, least expensive means of providing balanced nutrition without solid particles of food that may obstruct the narrow lumen.

■ HISTORY OF SURGERY

Early attempts at surgical management of Crohn's disease in the 1930s and 1940s involved bypass procedures that were marred by serious complications, including sepsis, development of cancer, and an increased rate of recurrence. By the 1950s, resection became the preferred operation; however, there soon arose a controversy about the amount of bowel that should be removed. Some advocated radical excision, removing all diseased bowel with a large margin of apparently normal tissue on each side of the resection. Others found less radical resection safer, since it preserved gut and also had no apparent effect on the rate of recurrence of the disease. Although this argument continues, the balance has gradually shifted toward conservative surgery.

MINIMAL SURGERY

Many reports have shown Crohn's disease to be panintestinal with multifocal potential. Histological abnormalities have been demonstrated on routine rectal biopsies of apparently normal rectum from patients with small bowel disease.[2] We have found both histological and cellular changes in biopsies of the mucosa of the intestine well away from overt disease (Fig 36–1).[2,3] The incidence of anastomosis leakage and recurrence rates have been shown to be independent of the presence or absence of even microscopic disease at the suture line.[4–7] When we performed ileocecal resections and anastomosed ileum to abnormal, but not stenosed, large bowel, we found no higher incidence of anastomotic leakage than when performing anastomosis with macroscopically normal bowel ends.[8]

Most patients with small bowel Crohn's disease eventually require surgical intervention, with some requiring multiple bowel resections.[9,10] Data from our unit show that, in a mean follow-up of more than 10 years, 30% of patients with distal ileal disease needed more than one resection, and almost 5% required more than 3 resections.[11] Repeated wide resection in this last group of patients could lead to the development of the short gut syndrome and its consequences. Hellers reported a 1.5% incidence of this syndrome in his series in Stockholm County.[12] Hulten and associates in Goteborg consider it very rare to have to perform multiple wide resections. Some would consider an incidence of 1.5% rare.

In India in the 1970s, Kataria and associates reported that tuberculous enteric strictures were treated more safely and effectively by strictureplasty than by excision.[13]

In 1982, Lee and Papaioannou reported their experience from Oxford with "minimal surgery" for Crohn's disease.[14] Most patients had strictureplasty constructed through inactive disease. The procedure was reported to be safe and effective in relieving symptoms and improving health.

In 1981, we adopted strictureplasty as a treatment option for obstructing Crohn's disease. We believe that surgical intervention for Crohn's disease should be for complications only; it should be safe and it should preserve as much gut as possible. Furthermore, if most of the initial complications of small bowel Crohn's disease are stenotic, then only the stenosis needs to be treated.

INITIAL SURGICAL INTERVENTION

When Crohn's disease first presents, usually in the terminal ileum, it is our policy to perform a simple ileocecal resection of the abnormal segment of bowel with end-to-end anastomosis of macroscopically normal gut.[11] We include in the resection any segments containing multiple adjacent strictures, provided that it is not necessary to remove more than 50 cm of gut. We rarely perform strictureplasty for the initial operation. We prefer to have an adequate histological examination.

We perform strictureplasty in the following situations:

1. Recurrence after initial resection when there are single or multiple short fibrous strictures of the small bowel.
2. Duodenal strictures. Since it is not feasible to resect the duodenum, the recommended treatment used to be bypass by gastrojejunostomy plus vagotomy to reduce the risk of stomal ulceration. Whenever possible, we now prefer duodenal strictureplasty without vagotomy.
3. Skip lesions that are proximal to the resection

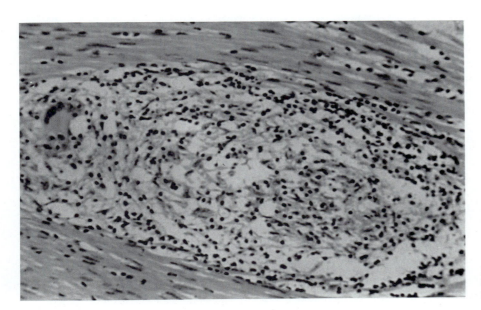

Figure 36–1. Typical histological picture of Crohn's disease in esophageal biopsy from a patient with symptomatic disease only in terminal ileum.

margin, in patients undergoing local ileal resection, and

4. Long continuous stricture (up to 30 cm) in patients with a short gut as a result of previous resections.

OPERATIVE PREPARATION AND TECHNIQUE

To reduce the risk of infection, all patients receive antibiotics, usually a 5 day course of cephalosporin and metronidazole.

Our routine antiembolic measures consist of elastic stockings on admission to hospital plus pneumatic compression leggings during the operation. We do not use routine prophylactic heparinization. We usually use a low transverse incision for a primary operation. However, in patients who have had previous surgery, we use a midline incision through the old scar. We recommend never to use a paramedian incision, since most patients with Crohn's disease have the potential for temporary or permanent ileostomy. Thus, stoma sites should be left free from scars.

We free all adhesions so that all the viscera and the whole gut can be inspected. This allows unexpected strictures to be identified and associated conditions, such as gallstones, to be treated. Freeing of the entire small bowel may involve a tedious and difficult dissection, but can be facilitated by CO_2 insufflation through a nasogastric tube.[15] If the entire bowel is not displayed, distal strictures may be missed with potentially disastrous consequences for a proximal anastomosis (Fig 36–2).

OPERATIVE TECHNIQUE

The gut is incised longitudinally on the antimesenteric border from normal gut proximally, through the stricture, to normal gut beyond. The incision is made with diathermy, since the gut is hyperemic and bleeds readily (Fig 36–3). The center of each side of the incision is distracted laterally with a stay suture or tissue forceps. This usually reveals luminal ulceration on the mesenteric border of the gut (Fig 36–4) and allows assessment of the length of the stricture. A horizontal mattress-stay suture secures the center of the wound and the gut then is closed transversely with one continuous layer of absorbable suture, such as Vicryl (Fig 36–5).

Before we suture the strictureplasty, we usually assess the luminal diameter of the rest of the small bowel by inserting a standard 18-Fr urinary balloon catheter through the initial enterotomy. We pass it along the whole length of the small bowel proximal and then distally, with the help of a catheter introducer (Fig 36–6). The balloon of the fully inserted catheter then is inflated with 8 mL of water to give a diameter of 25 mm, and the bladder is pulled back through the bowel until it becomes occluded by any stricture (Fig 36–7). The balloon then is deflated serially to allow accurate sizing of the diameter of the stricture, which is marked with a stay suture (Fig 36–8).

Once the stricture is passed, the balloon is reinflated and the whole small bowel is examined, giving a map of the stricture pattern throughout the gut. Based on trial and error observations, a luminal diameter of ≥ 20 mm

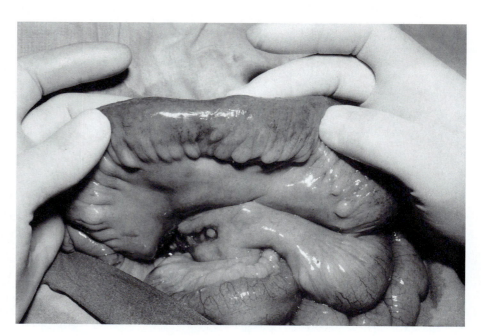

Figure 36–2. A. Most strictures can be detected by inspection or palpation. *Continued*

A

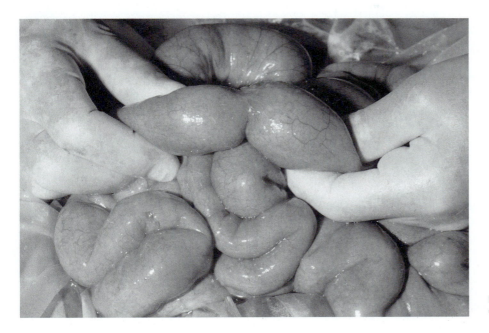

Figure 36–2. B. Inflating the gut with CO_2 simplifies the detection of quiescent strictures.

B

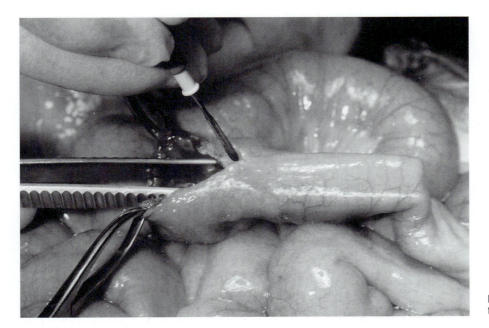

Figure 36–3. The gut is incised longitudinally with cutting diathermy.

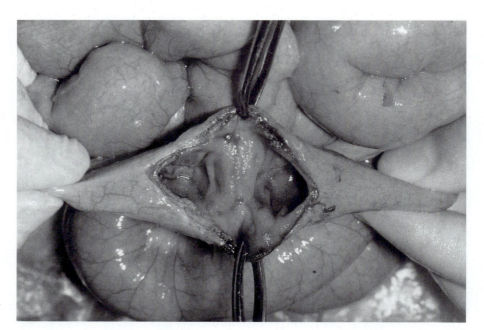

Figure 36–4. Transverse ulceration on mesenteric border of a stricture.

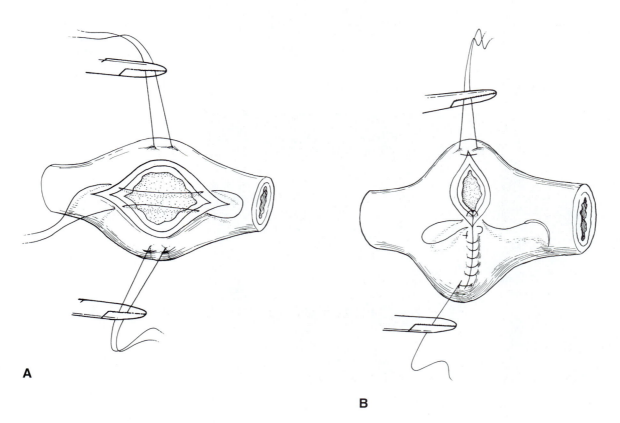

A

B

Figure 36–5. A. A central stay suture approximates the wound edges. **B**. The wound is then closed transversely. *Continued*

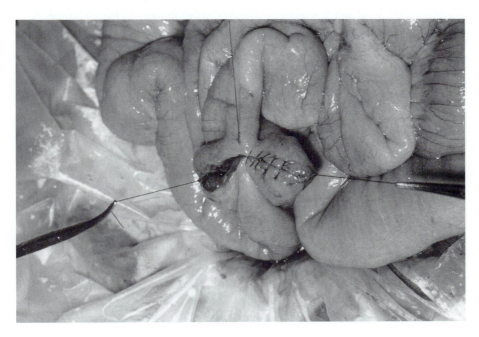

C

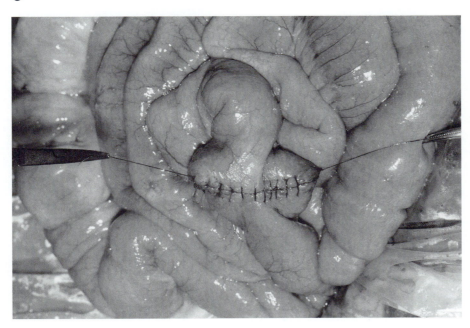

D

Figure 36–5. cont'd. C. A partially completed suture. **D**. A completed strictureplasty.

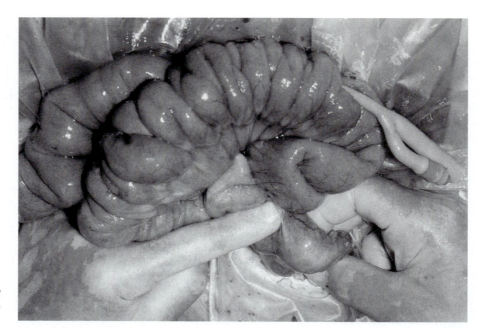

Figure 36–6. A balloon catheter is passed proximally through the small bowel and inflated with 8 mL of water. The balloon is held between finger tips.

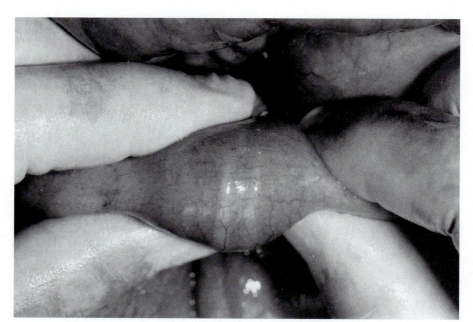

Figure 36–7. A 25-mm diameter balloon held up at a quiescent stricture.

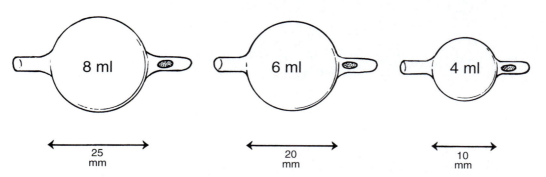

Figure 36–8. Diagram of balloon size when inflated with different volumes of water.

appears to be unlikely to produce any symptoms or sequelae. Our policy is that all strictures of a diameter <20 mm are treated. The maximal number of strictureplasties we have performed at any one operation was 16.

On completion of strictureplasties, all suture lines are checked with further CO_2 inflation to ensure that they are gas tight (Fig 36–9).[14] Finally, since the peritoneum inevitably is contaminated during the procedure, it is washed out with 3 to 4 L of saline.

Strictures of ≤10 cm in length have been treated with a Heineke-Mickulicz–type closure and those >10 cm in length are treated with a Finney closure. It could be argued that a long strictureplasty has no advantage over a side-to-side enteroenterostomy. However, cutting open the whole length of a long stricture enables it to be assessed and if necessary, biopsied. Complications have been no greater with a long strictureplasty than with a short strictureplasty (Fig 36–10).

COMPLICATIONS

Initially, we feared that a strictureplasty, constructed through grossly diseased bowel, would lead to a high rate of anastomotic leakage and enterocutaneous fistula. However, experience with strictureplasty has shown that bowel affected by Crohn's disease has a good blood supply and strong fibrous scar tissue to take sutures; it appears to heal well. There seems to be little evidence that the presence of active Crohn's disease hinders healing of anastomoses or suture lines.

Of the 90 operations in our series 9 (7.7%) were followed by an enterocutaneous fistula. This incidence rate is no greater than the rate we have found after re-

section for complicated Crohn's disease in ill patients. Fazio and associates reported enterocutaneous fistulas in 3 out of their 50 patients who underwent 225 strictureplasties.[16] Dehn and associates from Oxford performed 86 strictureplasties in 24 patients and reported no anastomotic leakage or fistula.[17] One explanation for the high incidence of postoperative enterocutaneous fistulas in our series is that we performed strictureplasty in all patients, even in the presence of severe intra-abdominal sepsis. On 13 occasions, when we found gross intra-abdominal sepsis (peri-intestinal abscess, enteroenteric and enterocutaneous fistula–related sepsis and psoas abscess), there were six (46%) resultant enterocutaneous fistula. The remaining seven patients healed without complications. Nutritional factors did not seem to influence postoperative recovery. Eight patients in the series had serum albumin levels between 16 and 23 g/dL; only one developed an anastomotic leak and enterocutaneous fistula.

RISK OF RECURRENCE AFTER STRICTUREPLASTY

Strictureplasty tends to be used for patients with multifocal Crohn's disease and often is used after multiple previous resections. A higher incidence of recurrence therefore might be expected than after resection, in which a single site of Crohn's disease is resected with an end-to-end anastomosis.

An appropriate, randomized prospective comparative trial of strictureplasty and resection does not seem to be feasible, but we have calculated the risk of recurrence at individual sites of stenosis that have been treated either by resection or by strictureplasty.[18] We an-

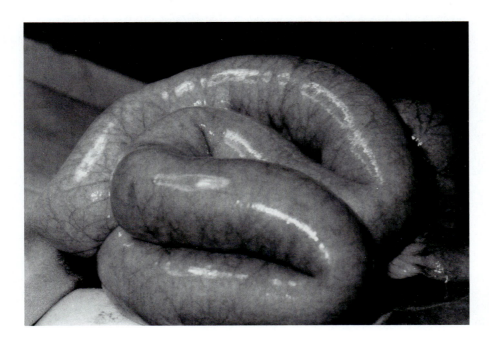

Figure 36–9. At completion of strictureplasties, the lumen of the gut is distended with CO_2 to ensure that no leaks have been missed.

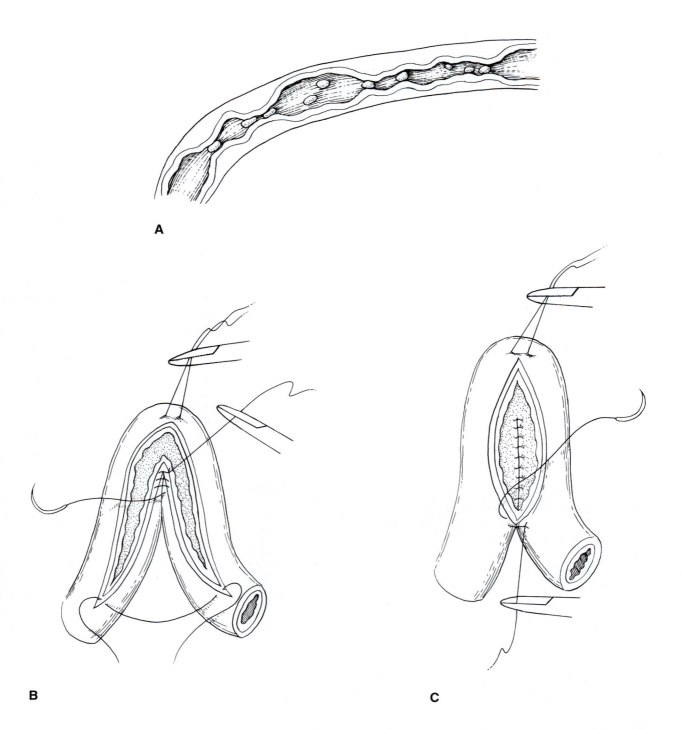

Figure 36–10. A 30 cm–long stricture or a series of strictures up to this length can be incised longitudinally, bent over as a pouch and sutured as in a Finney pyloroplasty. *Continued*

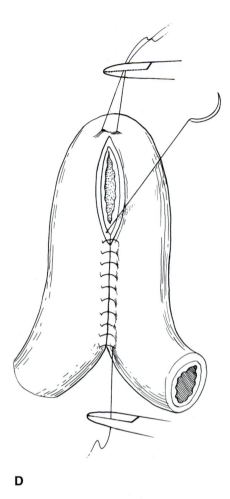

D

Figure 36–10, cont'd.

alyzed the follow-up data on 41 patients treated by resection only, in whom 93 separate resections had been performed, and compared them with those of 41 other patients whose treatment had included strictureplasty and in whom the outcome of 129 separate strictureplasty sites could be analyzed. The number of sites treated by either strictureplasty or resection that required further operation in the months and years following the first definitive operation were analyzed statistically. There appeared to be no significantly greater risks of recrudescence at any individual site where lesions had been treated by resection or by strictureplasty. It was concluded that strictureplasty was a reasonable alternative to multiple resections for multifocal stenotic small bowel disease.

Evidence from some of the patients who required subsequent operation months or years later for further stenotic complications suggests that the active disease process may become quiescent at the site of stricture-

plasty. It is not known whether there is a significant long-term risk of the development of small bowel carcinoma at the strictureplasty site, but the risk of carcinoma developing in such an area appears to be no greater than that found in residual areas of Crohn's disease in which there was no specific indication for surgical operation.

■ RESULTS

THE EXPERIENCE OF THE AUTHOR

Over a period of 9 years, 61 patients underwent 265 strictureplasties at 90 operations. The indications for surgery were recurrent intestinal obstruction in 81, enterocutaneous fistula in 8, and recurrent ileostomy bleeding in one. Bowel resection was undertaken in addition to strictureplasty, in 25 operations. We performed strictureplasty in the following sites: duodenum, 9 jejunum, 124 ileum, 108 and ileocolic anastomosis, 24. There was no postoperative mortality. Three patients have since died of carcinoma of the lung, uterus, and small bowel. Twenty-six patients (42.6%) have required reoperation during follow-up. All but two previous strictureplasties were unstrictured.

Twelve major complications developed in 9 patients; 7 enterocutaneous fistulas, 2 pulmonary emboli, 2 abdominal sepsis and 1 drug-induced hemoperitoneum.

At the 6 month review, there was a mean weight gain of 3.4 kg that was maintained on subsequent follow-up. Over a mean follow-up of 61 months, 53 of 58 survivors (91%) have complete symptomatic relief and satisfactory nutritional state. The remaining 5 patients have recurrent symptoms because of underlying diffuse small bowel disease.

Other centers have reported good quality of life after strictureplasty and have attested to the safety of the procedure.[19,20] We believe that strictureplasty is a useful and usually safe procedure. In the presence of established intra-abdominal sepsis, drainage and preliminary fecal diversion should be considered to reduce the risk of postoperative enterocutaneous fistula formation.

REFERENCES

1. Capnilli R, Andreoli A, Capurso L, et al. Oral mesalazine (5-aminosalicylic acid:Asacol) for prevention of postoperative recurrence of Crohn's disease. *Aliment Pharmacol Ther* 1994;8:35–43
2. Korelitz BI, Sommers SC. Rectal biopsy in patients with Crohn's disease: normal mucosa on sigmoidoscopy examination. *JAMA* 1977;237:2742–2744
3. Dunn WT, Cooke WT, Allen RN. Enzymatic and morpho-

metric evidence of Crohn's disease as a diffuse lesion of the gastrointestinal tract. *Gut* 1977;18:290–293

4. Lee ECG, Papaioannou N. Recurrences following surgery for Crohn's disease. *Clin Gastroenterol* 1980;9: 419–438

5. Pennington I, Hamilton SR, Bayless TM, et al. Surgical management of Crohn's disease: influence of disease at margin of resection. *Ann Surg* 1980;192:311–317

6. Heuman R, Boeryd B, Bolin T, et al. The influence of disease at the margin of resection on the outcome of Crohn's disease. *Br J Surg* 1983;70:519–521

7. Williams JG, Wong WD, Rothenberger DA, et al. Recurrence of Crohn's disease after resection. *Br J Surg* 1991; 78:10–19

8. Alexander-Williams J, Haynes IG. Conservative operations for Crohn's disease of the small bowel. *World J Surg* 1985; 9:945–951

9. Greenstein AJ, Sachar DB, Pasternack BS, et al. Reoperation and recurrence in Crohn's colitis and ileocolitis. *N Engl J Med* 1975;293:685–690

10. Mekhijian HS, Switz DM, Watts HD, et al. National cooperative Crohn's disease study: factors determining recurrence of Crohn's disease after surgery. *Gastroenterology* 1979;77:907–913

11. Andrews HA, Keighley MRB, Alexander-Williams J, et al. Strategy for management of distal ileal Crohn's disease. *Br J Surg* 1991;78:679–682

12. Heller G. Crohn's disease in Stockholm County 1955–1974: a study of epidemiology, results of surgical treatment and long term prognosis. *Acta Chir Scand* 1979; 490(suppl):31–69

13. Katariya RN, Sood S, Rao PG, et al. Strictureplasty for tubercular strictures of the gastrointestinal tract. *Br J Surg* 1977;64:496–498

14. Lee ECG, Papaioannou N. Minimal surgery for chronic obstruction in patients with extensive or universal Crohn's disease. *Ann R Coll Surg* 1982;64:299–333

15. Cabrol H, Griffiths C, Alexander-Williams J. Carbon dioxide insufflation in gastrointestinal surgery (Bity-pudema technique). *Br J Surg* 1991;78:499–500

16. Fazio VW, Galandiuk S, Jagelman DG, et al. Strictureplasty in Crohn's disease. *Ann Surg* 1989;210:621–625

17. Dehn TCB, Kettlewell MGW, Mortensen NJMcC, et al. Ten year experience of strictureplasty for obstructive Crohn's disease. *Br J Surg* 1989;76:339–341

18. Sayfan J, Wilson DAL, Allan A, et al. Recurrence after strictureplasty or resection for Crohn's disease. *Br J Surg* 1989;76:335–338

19. Silverman RE, McLeod RS, Cohen Z. Strictureplasty in Crohn's disease. *Can Assoc Clin Surgeons* 1989;32: 19–22

20. Kendall GP, Hawley PRF, Nicholls RJ, et al. Strictureplasty. A good operation for small bowel Crohn's disease? *Dis Colon Rectum* 1986;5:312–316

37

Small Bowel Obstruction

Jack Pickleman

Small bowel obstruction is defined as a partial or complete interference with the passage of stool distally in the small intestine. It is one of the more common acute abdominal emergencies and is associated with significant morbidity and mortality, especially if it progresses to bowel ischemia. Obstruction is to be differentiated from paralytic ileus, which is associated with a wide variety of intraperitoneal and extraperitoneal processes that interfere with the normal motility of the intestine. The latter will resolve spontaneously once the inciting cause has been eliminated.

In the United States, the cause of small bowel obstruction, in up to 70% of patients, is adhesions, usually secondary to prior abdominal operations.[1,2] Other less common causes of adhesions are those that are congenital, those associated with prior blunt trauma to the abdomen, inflammatory processes within the abdomen, or an indirect inguinal hernia with adhesion formation at the internal ring. Adhesion formation appears to be especially frequent following gynecologic surgery, total abdominal colectomy, or abdominoperineal resection.

The second most common cause of bowel obstruction is incarceration of the intestine in either an inguinal, femoral, or ventral hernia. While these are generally obvious on physical examination (Figs 37–1, 37–2, 37–3, and 37–4), the diagnosis of femoral hernia may be obscure, particularly in obese individuals. Malignant tumors of the colon frequently present with large bowel obstruction. However, obstructing tumors in the right colon may lead to a clinical and radiologic picture that is indistinguishable from that of small bowel obstruc-

tion (Figs 37–5 and 37–6). Metastases from any primary tumor likewise can cause small bowel obstruction (Fig 37–7), as can primary small intestinal lesions such as carcinoma, carcinoid, lymphoma, and benign and malignant soft-tissue tumors. These often present with obstruction secondary to intussusception (Fig 37–8).

Most patients with small bowel obstruction will manifest abdominal pain, nausea and vomiting, obstipation, and abdominal distention. Initially, the pain tends to be diffuse and poorly localized. It is generally intermittent or crampy in nature. With the onset of bowel ischemia, however, pain becomes constant. Vomiting may occur early in the course of the illness, and secondary to stimulation of intestinal stretch reflexes. Vomiting tends to occur earlier in proximal small bowel obstruction and later in more distal obstructions. Likewise, the character of the vomitus differs in high versus low obstructions, being more bilious in the former and more feculent in the latter. Although obstipation characteristically is seen, some patients may evacuate residual gas and stool initially, thus confusing the clinical picture. Distention may be mild or massive, but is often absent in proximal bowel obstructions. Bowel sounds will be high pitched and active, coming on in rushes, coincident with crampy pain. Thin people may manifest visible peristalsis. In simple small bowel obstruction, abdominal tenderness tends to be diffuse and mild, while in strangulation obstruction, it tends to be localized. Unless bowel ischemia has supervened, the stool will generally be negative for occult blood. Evidence of dehydration is frequent, with tachycardia, postural hypotension, and decreased uri-

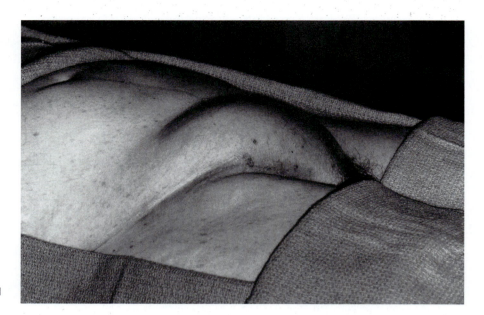

Figure 37–1. Female patient presenting with incarcerated right inguinal hernia.

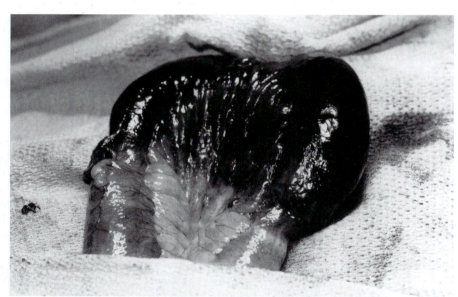

Figure 37–2. Operative findings demonstrating gangrenous bowel and ischemic constriction from the internal inguinal ring.

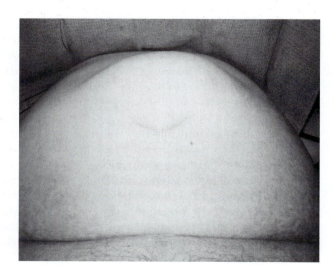

Figure 37–3. Incarcerated umbilical hernia in an obese female patient.

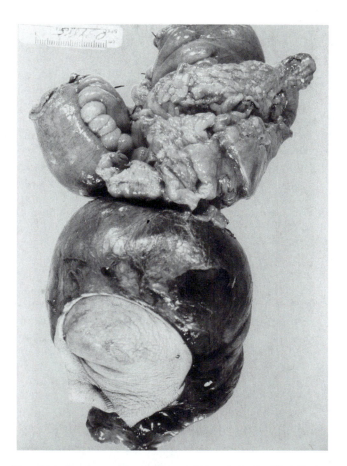

Figure 37–4. Operative specimen showing completely excised periumbilical skin, hernia sac containing gangrenous bowel, and entering and exiting intestinal loop.

ings have been stated to be more indicative of a strangulation obstruction, but elevations in the white blood cell count, creatine phosphokinase (CPK), phosphate, and amylase may occur in either form of obstruction. Similarly, conventional abdominal x-rays may be nondiagnostic owing to fluid-filled loops. The most immediately life-threatening aspect of small bowel obstruction results from the significant dehydration and electrolyte losses that accompany the condition. Normally, approximately 9L of upper gastrointestinal secretions are delivered into the proximal small bowel lumen every 24 hours. Of this, only 400 to 500 cc/day cross the ileocecal valve, with the small intestine normally absorbing the rest. The colon absorbs 200 to 300 cc/day, and therefore, the net stool water loss is 150 to 200 cc daily. The presence of small bowel obstruction disturbs this equilibrium and leads to increased extracellular fluid within the small bowel lumen, gut wall, and peritoneal cavity. The increased pressure within the bowel leads to an increased secretion from the intestine along with a decreased absorption of fluid. This fluid loss is further aggravated by reflex vomiting. In proximal small bowel obstruction, these fluid losses are accompanied by significant losses of hydrogen ion, potassium, and chloride, leading to a metabolic alkalosis. In more distal ob-

nary output. This is often confirmed by the findings of an elevated hematocrit, blood urea nitrogen (BUN), and serum sodium.

One of the major issues in managing a patient with suspected small bowel obstruction is determining which patients harbor ischemic or gangrenous bowel. Although this complication may be suggested by the presence of constant pain preceded by abdominal cramps, the symptoms and signs in a strangulation obstruction may be indistinguishable from those in simple obstruction.[2–5] Clinical findings that include increased abdominal pain and tenderness, decreased bowel sounds, and the presence of peritoneal signs, although suggestive of strangulation obstruction, also may be present in simple obstruction. Studies have indicated that few patients with strangulation obstruction will manifest *all* of these signs. One study indicated that no patient harbored ischemic small bowel if tachycardia, fever, localized pain, and leukocytosis were absent. The presence of any of these findings, however, increased the probability of ischemic bowel being present.[2] Various laboratory find-

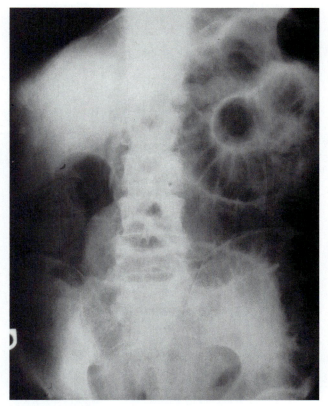

Figure 37–5. Supine abdominal x-ray of a small bowel obstruction in a man with no hernia or prior laparotomy.

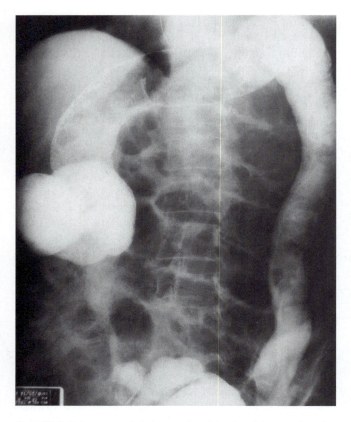

Figure 37–6. Barium enema disclosing complete obstruction of the ascending colon caused by carcinoma.

structions, fluid losses are similar, but are usually not accompanied by significant electrolyte losses.

The increased gas within the gut lumen mainly results from swallowed air, although CO_2 production from neutralization of bicarbonate, and organic gases from bacterial fermentation, are also present. Of these, however, swallowed air is most important because of its high nitrogen content. Nitrogen is not absorbed significantly by small intestine mucosa. Thus, about 70% of intestine gas remains as nitrogen. Although large quantities of carbon dioxide are produced, CO_2 contributes little to gaseous distention, since it is quickly absorbed. Studies have indicated that gastric suction will keep the stomach empty with no increase in small bowel distention, whereas patients without nasogastric tubes will have progressively increasing small intestinal gas.

In the presence of obstruction, stasis of bowel contents occurs, favoring aerobic and anaerobic bacterial overgrowth and the characteristic foul odor of obstructed small intestinal contents. Although the normal gut mucosa is relatively impermeable to bacteria, ischemic mucosa readily permits the transudation of bacteria and toxins prior to bowel perforation. Whether markedly distended, but nonischemic, bowel favors translocation of bacteria is controversial, but several studies have indicated that bacterial translocation occurs even in simple intestinal obstruction.[6,7]

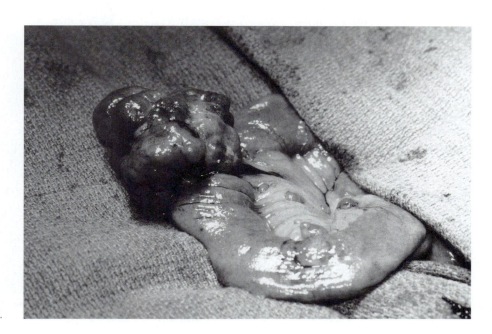

Figure 37–7. Renal cell carcinoma metastatic to bowel.

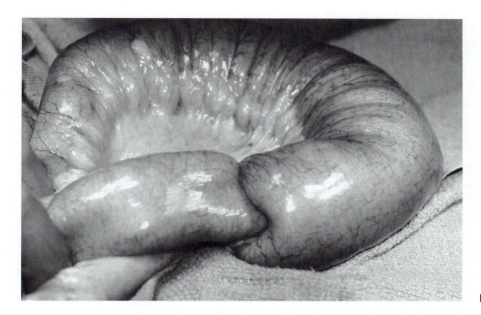

Figure 37–8. Intussusception causing bowel obstruction.

■ DIAGNOSIS

The presence of small bowel obstruction should be suspected in any patient presenting with abdominal pain, vomiting, distention, and obstipation. Most individuals will have either a visible hernia or a laparotomy scar, and the diagnosis becomes far more difficult if neither of these are present. The essential diagnostic test in all such patients is four x-ray views of the abdomen, including an upright chest, upright abdomen, supine abdomen, and a left lateral decubitus view. Often the supine views will disclose dilated small bowel, which is identified by the presence of valvulae conniventes, and is differentiated from colonic distention by the presence of haustral markings in the latter. Upright abdominal views often will show multiple air-fluid levels, although these also can be present in some patients with paralytic ileus (Fig 37–9). In ileus, however, the presence of gas throughout the gastrointestinal (GI) tract, including stomach, small intestine, and colon is more common. The presence of significant amounts of colonic gas should raise the suspicion of a large bowel rather than a small bowel obstruction.

There are no diagnostic laboratory tests to verify the presence of a small bowel obstruction; rather, most of these tests will give some evidence of the severity of the physiologic derangement or indicate the presence of ischemic bowel. The white blood cell count may be normal or mildly elevated in simple small bowel obstruction; higher white blood cell counts always should arouse the suspicion of ischemic bowel. The hematocrit and BUN often will be elevated, reflecting the degree of third space fluid losses and dehydration. Serum elec-

trolytes are generally normal in distal small bowel obstruction. However, in a proximal bowel obstruction, a pattern of metabolic alkalosis with hypokalemia and hypochloremia may be noted, which is similar to that found in patients with gastric outlet obstruction. Serum amylase may be abnormal in both simple and strangulated small bowel obstruction, and very high levels should suggest an alternate diagnosis, namely acute pancreatitis with resultant ileus. Other blood tests have been suggested as potentially useful in the differentiation of simple versus strangulated small bowel obstruction. These include phosphate levels, CPK, and serum glutanate oxalotransferase (SGOT), but in general, these are not helpful.

The role of radiologic contrast studies is controversial. A barium enema is indicated if the patient is thought to harbor a large rather than a small bowel obstruction. The presence of a large bowel obstruction may be suggested by a long history rather than an abrupt onset of symptoms, the presence of occult blood in the stool, or the presence of significant colonic gas on supine abdominal x-ray (Figs 37–10 and 37–11). In all such patients, an unprepped barium enema should be accomplished. Likewise, the patient who presents with signs and symptoms of obstruction and who has the radiologic picture of small bowel obstruction on conventional abdominal x-rays, but who has no scar on his abdomen nor external hernia present, should have a barium enema, since no apparent etiology is present (Figs 37–5 and 37–6). The usefulness of upper GI contrast studies is far more controversial. Several studies in the radiology literature have indicated that these x-rays are highly accurate in diagnosing small bowel obstruc-

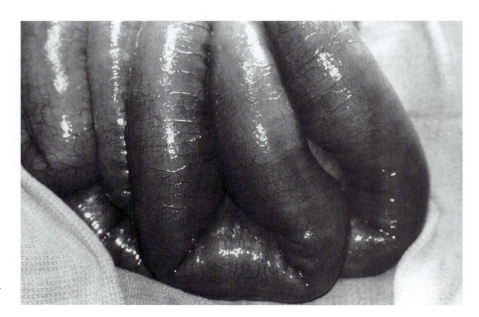

Figure 37–9. Operative photograph of obstructed intestine showing multiple air-fluid levels.

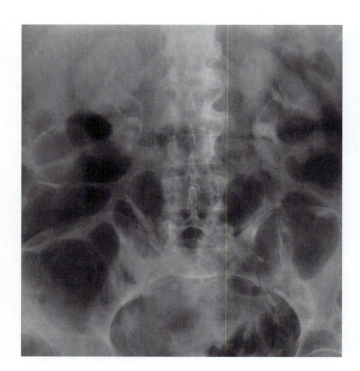

Figure 37–10. Supine abdominal x-ray in a patient presenting with distal large bowel obstruction.

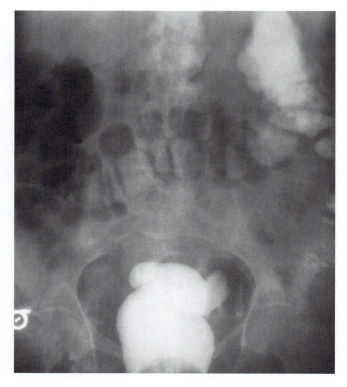

Figure 37–11. Barium enema disclosing near total obstruction of the rectosigmoid colon by carcinoma.

tion, and even in differentiating complete from incomplete obstruction. Most authorities recommend the use of barium, instead of water soluble Gastrografin, since the latter material rapidly dilutes within the luminal fluid and thereby yields a poor-quality study. Others have noted that upper GI contrast studies may provide misleading information, indicating an incomplete small bowel obstruction (barium passing throughout the length of the small intestine) in patients who ultimately required operation and indicating the presence of complete bowel obstruction in patients who subsequently recovered nonoperatively.[8] As a result, these studies are not routinely advised.

Strangulation obstruction of the small intestine may be one of the most difficult acute abdominal conditions to recognize, but is one of the most important, since it is life-threatening if diagnosis is delayed. These patients may have little vomiting or distention, but steady abdominal pain that appears out of proportion to the physical findings on abdominal examination. In addition, watery stools are frequent. Since the strangulated loop of intestine rapidly fills up with fluid, the usual radiographic signs of dilated bowel with air-fluid levels often are absent. Any patient with a scar on his abdomen who has such a clinical picture should be promptly operated upon after resuscitation.

■ TREATMENT

Once small bowel obstruction has been diagnosed, the most important initial step is to rehydrate the patient. Volume losses can be profound, and large quantities of lactated Ringers solution may be required. An indwelling Foley catheter is mandatory, since the production of an adequate volume of urine is the most useful sign of successful volume resuscitation. Resuscitation utilizing colloid solutions are not indicated because of the short-term nature of their intravascular effectiveness and their expense. Depending upon the clinical circumstances, a central venous pressure line or Swan-Ganz pulmonary artery catheter may be required. The use of antibiotics is controversial. Surely, any patient who is being prepared for operation should receive perioperative antibiotics, and any drug regimen effective against the more common gram-positive and gram-negative aerobic and anaerobic bacteria is sufficient. More controversial is the recommendation to utilize antibiotics in simple small bowel obstruction during the brief period of nonoperative management, while the decision to operate is still pending. Since the nonischemic but distended small intestine may allow the passage of bacteria and toxins into the portal circulation and peritoneal cavity, this author favors prophylactic antibiotics during the brief observation period prior to the decision to operate.

All patients should be operated on promptly following volume resuscitation, if there is any evidence or suspicion of ischemic bowel being present. Most, but not all, of these patients will have some of the following signs: tachycardia, localized tenderness, an abdominal mass, fever, or leukocytosis. However, some patients may harbor ischemic bowel despite the absence of these signs. Accordingly, the clinician must differentiate between the presence of complete versus incomplete small bowel obstruction. In complete small bowel obstruction, there has been no passage of significant flatus or stool in the previous 12 hours, and there is no significant colonic gas on abdominal x-rays (Fig 37–12). The percentage of patients with ischemic bowel is higher in this circumstance than in incomplete obstruction, and up to 80% of such patients will not resolve with intestinal suction alone.[1,3,4,9–11] Therefore, this author favors immediate operation on all patients with a complete small bowel obstruction. On the other hand, patients with an incomplete small bowel obstruction, and no evidence of ischemic bowel, may be safely treated for a period of time, since resolution in this group of patients may be expected in up to 80% of cases.[1,4,10] Most of

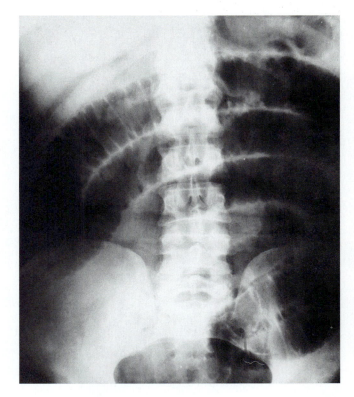

Figure 37–12. Supine abdominal x-ray in a patient with a complete small bowel obstruction.

these patients successfully treated nonoperatively will show definite signs of clinical improvement within 24 hours, and nearly all will show improvement by 48 hours (Figs 37–13 and 37–14).[1,10] Accordingly, this is the maximum period of observation. After this period, laparotomy is indicated.

Most authorities advocate a standard Levin tube as their choice for intestinal decompression, while others favor a long intestinal tube with a weighted balloon to promote passage through the loops of small intestine. The theory behind a long intestinal tube is that providing suction closer to the point of obstruction will decrease the luminal pressure and therefore, increase venous and arterial circulation adjacent to the obstructed loop, thereby hastening resolution. Although this is an appealing concept, the difficulties involved in placing and passing these tubes seem to far outweigh their theoretic advantages. Frequent positioning of the patient and advancement of the tube into the nares is required, with serial x-rays to gauge the progression of the tube (Figs 37–15 and 37–16). Also, some patients will simultaneously require a nasogastric tube, since the intestinal tube will not decompress a distended stomach. There are several published series of patients who have been treated with long intestinal tubes and in which usage of

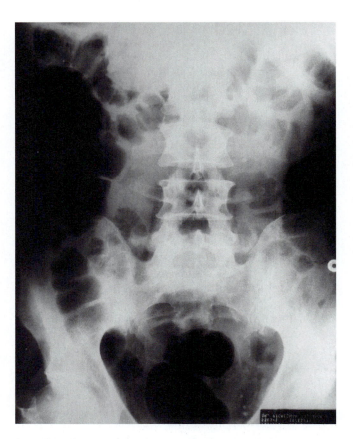

Figure 37–14. Supine abdominal x-ray taken eight hours later showing significant resolution of small bowel obstruction with large quantities of gas in the colon and rectum.

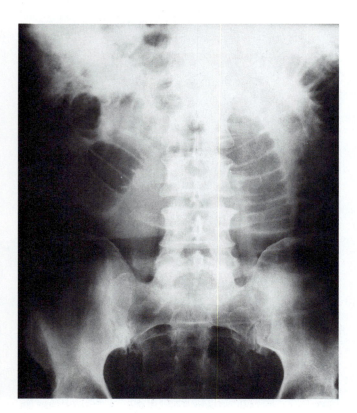

Figure 37–13. Supine abdominal x-ray in a patient with an incomplete adhesive obstruction.

the long tube led to a longer period of preoperative treatment, a higher incidence of ischemic bowel, and a longer period of postoperative hospitalization than in those patients in whom short tubes were utilized.[1,5,10,11] Thus, this author sees no advantage in the use of such tubes over the standard nasogastric tube.

The anesthesiologist plays a critical role in the operative management of these patients. Many will choose to perform endotracheal intubation with the patient awake, but lightly sedated, in an attempt to minimize the possibility of aspiration during anesthetic induction. Following this, excellent muscle relaxation is required not only to aid in the conduct of the exploration, but also to facilitate closure of the abdomen in the presence of markedly distended bowel.

The choice of the operative incision is critical. Remembering that adhesions are likely to form on the undersurface of previous incisions, in many instances it is wise to make a new incision. If the prior laparotomy incision is midline, a transverse incision just above or below the umbilicus will satisfy all the requirements for exposure within the abdomen and pelvis and provide a structurally sound incision. The other advantage of

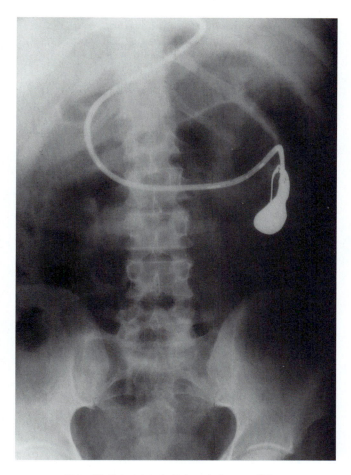

Figure 37–15. Long intestinal tube at the ligament of Trietz.

placing a new incision away from a scar is that the abdomen can be entered in a virgin area, hopefully minimizing the potential for bowel injury during the initial dissection. The character of the peritoneal fluid should be observed and noted as to whether it is serous, turbid, or bloody. The latter two characteristics tend to indicate the presence of ischemic bowel. Aerobic and anaerobic cultures of this fluid should be taken. If possible, the exploration should begin at the ileocecal valve and should continue proximally. In certain instances, a single obstructing band will be noted, with dilated bowel proximally and decompressed bowel distally (Fig 37–17). Following lysis of such a band, the cause of the obstruction has been eliminated. However, in other instances, it is far more difficult to ascertain the exact point of obstruction, since multiple segments of dilated and partially decompressed bowel will be present. In such a circumstance, it is essential to lyse all adhesions from the ileocecal valve to the ligament of Treitz. Often, it may be advantageous for the more experienced surgeon to act as the first assistant, since it is probably more difficult to

expose difficult tissue planes than it is to dissect them once exposed. There will be instances where it will be far safer to utilize sharp, even scalpel, dissection rather than blunt dissection, since the latter may tend to deserosalize bowel. When bowel is damaged by dissection, it should be repaired only if mucosa is visible. If only a serosal tear is involved, there is no need to repair this defect. Indeed, repair of such a defect may predispose to increased adhesion formation.

The determination of bowel viability may be extremely difficult in certain circumstances. Although color, the presence of motility, and arterial pulsations are reassuring, these are not definite indicators of viable bowel. Several intraoperative aids have been advocated to determine bowel viability, including intestinal Doppler studies, fluorescein staining, and bowel wall O_2 tensions. Although these will probably indicate the state of bowel viability in the majority of patients, there will be some patients in whom this determination cannot be accurately made. In such situations, placing the suspect loop of intestine in warm packs for about 15 minutes

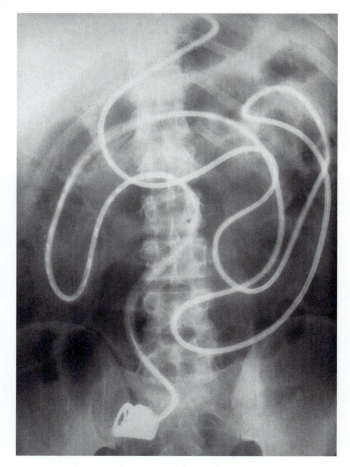

Figure 37–16. Long intestinal tube following passage distally.

and later observation may provide the answer. If the loop is still questionable, it should be resected and a primary anastomosis carried out. However, if the suspect loop is lengthy, and there is concern about creating a short gut syndrome, the bowel can be replaced in the peritoneal cavity, the abdomen closed, and a second-look operation carried out the following day.

At the end of the lysis of adhesions, if it is technically possible, the distended bowel should be emptied of its luminal contents. This will not only improve the blood supply of the bowel, but also facilitate abdominal closure. The two most practical ways to accomplish this are to milk the intestinal contents in a proximal direction, with aspiration by either a nasogastric tube or an intestinal tube that has been placed in the jejunum. Alternatively, milking of the intestinal contents distally into the right colon also may be accomplished. An enterotomy or colotomy to evacuate bowel contents is not suggested, since this may unnecessarily contaminate the peritoneal cavity.[2] Whether a viable segment of intestine that is densely adherent in the pelvis should be resected or bypassed remains a matter of judgment. Surely, in some circumstances, it will be obvious that attempts to dissect free such a loop will result in damage to the loop and surrounding structures, thereby resulting in the need for resection and anastomosis. In such a circumstance, it may be preferable to perform an enteroenterostomy or enterocolostomy to bypass a segment, providing the area bypassed is a short length of intestine. In case of irradiated bowel in the pelvis, bypass is often preferable to dangerous resection. Bypass of long segments of small intestine tend to yield poor long-term re-sults, with problems of stasis and bacterial overgrowth in the long segment and chronic intestinal symptoms.

Fascial closure of the abdomen should be accomplished in nearly every situation. Whether the skin should be closed will depend upon the presence of gangrenous bowel. In such a case, the skin and subcutaneous tissues should be left open and a delayed primary closure accomplished. In rare circumstances, edema and swelling will be so massive, that the intra-abdominal contents cannot be replaced into the peritoneal cavity. In such circumstances, a prosthetic silo can be constructed. This silo can be gradually shortened at the bedside over the next three or four days, until the intestines are within the peritoneal cavity (Fig 37–18). At that time, either the mesh can be sutured together, or the patient can be returned to the operating room for primary fascial closure.

■ SPECIAL CONSIDERATIONS

POSTOPERATIVE SMALL BOWEL OBSTRUCTION

Patients who develop signs and symptoms of a small bowel obstruction shortly following a laparotomy may be considered different from patients who develop an obstruction at a time remote from prior operation. Bowel ischemia is extremely uncommon in immediate postoperative obstruction, which characteristically is caused by filmy soft adhesions or inflammatory tissue. These may disappear in a short time, leading to resolution of the obstruction. Eighty to ninety percent of such

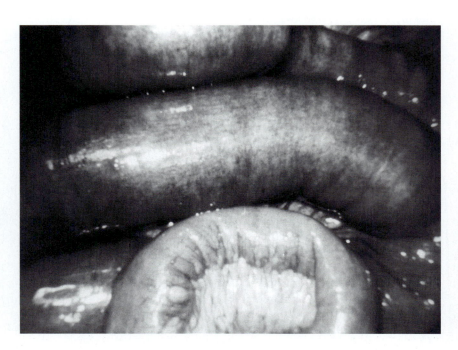

Figure 37–17. Operative photograph in a patient with a complete small bowel obstruction showing dilated proximal and decompressed distal intestine.

patients will resolve with nasogastric suction, with two-thirds of these resolving within 7 days, and the remainder by 14 days.[12] Spontaneous resolution is unlikely after this time period, and reoperation should be performed. Clearly, during this prolonged treatment time, total parenteral nutrition should be initiated.

RECURRENT SMALL BOWEL OBSTRUCTION

The patient presenting with a recurrent small bowel obstruction presents a challenge to the general surgeon. Many of these patients will undergo spontaneous resolution of the problem, only to sustain a future recurrence.[5,13,14] Others will remain relentlessly obstructed and require laparotomy that may be time consuming and technically demanding. The risk of serosal injury to the intestine and resultant intra-abdominal abscess and fistula formation will be present in the latter case. The patient with recurrent small bowel obstruction may have had many obstructions in the past, either treated operatively or nonoperatively. These patients with recurring obstructions differ from patients presenting with their second small bowel obstruction at a remote time from their initial obstruction. These latter patients are treated as a standard adhesive small bowel obstruction, with early operation reserved for those presenting evidence of ischemia or a complete obstruction. A trial of nasogastric suction is reserved for those who appear to have a clinically and radiologically incomplete obstruction.

Patients with multiple recurrences of small bowel obstruction are less likely to harbor ischemic bowel. This fact, coupled with the increased technical demands in such a circumstance, make nonoperative therapy preferable. No reliable figures exist as to the incidence of recurrent small bowel obstruction. It is felt that approximately 15% to 30% of patients who sustain an adhesive small bowel obstruction will develop another episode of obstruction in the future.[5,13,14] It is still unclear how many of these patients go on to develop multiple obstructions. However, these individuals represent a very small subset of patients with small bowel obstruction.

An understanding of the etiology of adhesion formation is necessary in order to formulate a strategy for dealing with these patients. Immediately postoperatively, there is an outpouring of fibrin in the peritoneal cavity. This may resolve completely or become organized by capillary and fibroblast ingrowth. Several factors are known to increase the amount of adhesion formation. Areas of ischemic or devitalized tissue within the peritoneal cavity, and foreign bodies, such as suture material, increase adhesion formation. As fibrin is removed by tissue macrophages, the adhesions become organized as collagen. The disappearance of fibrinous adhesions may be affected by the presence of local plasminogen activators found in the serosa of the intestine. Mature adhesions, however, are permanent.

Many eclectic treatments have been proposed for the prevention of adhesions. Most, however, have shown little consistent effect. Some investigators have attempted to decrease fibrin deposition by the use of heparin or dextran. Others have attempted to accelerate the removal of fibrin exudate with such adjuncts as peritoneal lavage, enzyme therapy, and fibrinolytic agents such as streptokinase or urokinase. Still others have approached the problem mechanically and have attempted to separate the surfaces of the serosa with either instillation of lubricants or oxygen into the peritoneal cavity, or by stimulation of peristalsis. Some have attempted to decrease fibroblast proliferation by administering either corticosteroids or cytotoxic drugs.

The patient with a recurrent small bowel obstruction should be treated with a nasogastric tube and intravenous fluids, with the decision for administration of total parenteral nutrition made early in the illness, if it appears that quick resolution is not likely. Some information in this regard may be gleaned from the behavior of prior obstructions in a given patient, since subsequent obstructions tend to mimic previous ones, in terms of symptoms and duration. Depending upon the clinical circumstances, 1 to 2 weeks of treatment may be indicated prior to considering operation. This is especially true if the patient appears to have a "boggy" abdomen on physical examination. This physical sign is indicative of dense adhesion formation, and experienced surgeons rely upon this finding to guide them away from operative intervention in such a circumstance.

In an attempt to prevent future obstruction, surgeons, in the past, advocated plication of either the intestine or the mesentery to form the intestine into gently curving loops. It was quickly found, however, that fistulas and recurrent obstruction ensued. For the most part, these procedures are no longer utilized. Currently, the best adjunct is internal plication utilizing a fairly rigid (C.R. Bard Co., New Jersey) tube that may be inserted distally into the intestine.[15,16] This may be inserted percutaneously into the stomach and passed around the duodenum or, alternatively, it may be inserted percutaneously into the jejunum. This author favors the former method. This internal stent may be sufficient to allow adhesion formation in gently formed curves so that the possibility of recurrent obstruction is minimized.

One specialized problem occurring in patients with recurrent obstruction, or in some patients with postoperative obstruction, is the entity described as obliterative peritonitis. Physical examination reveals a doughy-feeling abdomen and, if operation is performed on such a patient, a totally cemented mass of inflamed edematous intestines is encountered that defies separation without risking intestinal damage or devitalization. In such a cir-

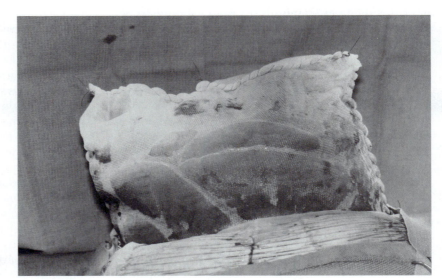

Figure 37–18. Marlex silo in a patient with massively distended and edematous small bowel, rendering fascial closure impossible.

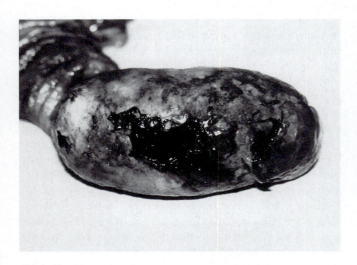

Figure 37–19. Primary small bowel leiomyosarcoma presenting as a small bowel intussusception.

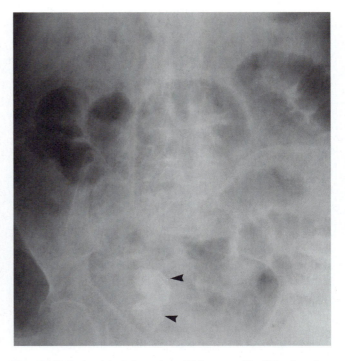

Figure 37–20. Supine abdominal x-ray in an elderly woman with gallstone ileus. Note two distally impacted gallstones and dilated small intestine. Air in the biliary tree is not clearly seen.

cumstance, the surgeon should immediately desist and place these patients on long-term parenteral nutrition, with either nasogastric suction or gastrostomy tube decompression, if anatomically possible. Ill-advised attempts to forge ahead in such a circumstance may well lead to fistula formation, abscess, or even the need for massive small bowel resection with resultant short bowel syndrome. Generally, after 2 to 10 weeks, the obstruction will disappear and alimentation can resume.[17]

CARCINOMATOSIS ASSOCIATED WITH SMALL BOWEL OBSTRUCTION

The patient harboring metastatic intraperitoneal carcinoma who presents with a bowel obstruction provides a unique challenge. In many, this event will merely herald the terminal phase of their illness. In others, however, successful surgical treatment can provide long-term survival. In most published series, it has been noted that nearly one-third of these patients harbor an adhesive rather than a malignant obstruction, and so it would appear prudent to operate on most of these patients, if their symptoms do not promptly resolve.[18–21] Certain cancers, such as breast, renal cell carcinoma, and melanoma often will give rise to solitary metastatic deposits within the peritoneal cavity, leading to a bowel obstruction. Such obstructions are easily dealt with by resection of the metastatic mass, along with a segment of intestine (Fig 37–7).

The patient who truly has carcinomatosis presents a much greater problem, since often there are multiple sites of potential obstruction that are not amenable to either resection or bypass. In such a circumstance, the provision of a tube gastrostomy may be worthwhile, since it may enable the patient to live without a nasogastric tube or vomiting, and thus provide the potential to leave the hospital and receive home or hospice care. In a patient presenting with such an obstruction, treatment with either chemotherapy or radiation therapy will rarely be of benefit, and so the mainstay of management must be surgical.

Radiation Enteritis

When a patient who has received prior abdominal radiation therapy presents with a bowel obstruction, it is often unclear whether this is an adhesive obstruction, one owing to radiation damage, or a malignant obstruction. When there is doubt, an upper GI series with a small bowel follow-through will generally clarify the matter. If a fixed obstruction is noted, operation is indicated and, if possible, the segment is resected and primary anastomosis carried out. The anastomosed ends should be relatively free of visible radiation changes, although sometimes this is not possible and anastomosis is still feasible. In other circumstances, it may be wiser to perform a by-

pass of the obstructed segment if it cannot be removed, but only if such a bypass does not involve a long segment of intestine.

Intussusception in the Adult

Adults who present with a bowel obstruction and no prior history of abdominal operation sometimes will be found to harbor a spontaneous intussusception. In nearly all cases in adults, these are the result of preexisting small bowel pathology serving as a lead point for the intussusception. Conditions such as Crohn's disease, benign and malignant small bowel tumors, and metastatic tumors to the small intestine are not infrequent. Treatment in such a case is resection of the intussuscepted mass without prior attempt to reduce it, since, unlike children with intussusception, nearly all adults have pathology causing the condition (Figs 37–8 and 37–19).

Obturation Obstruction

Any ingested object can lodge in the small intestine and cause an obstruction. Usually, these are ingested foreign bodies or bezoars that form in the stomach. Such foreign objects will lodge at the narrowest point in the small intestine, usually the ileum. Perhaps the most common obturation obstruction is gallstone ileus, whereby a large

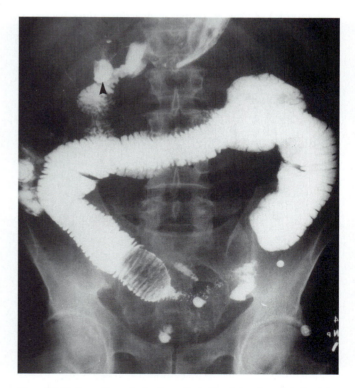

Figure 37–21. Upper GI examination in a patient with gallstone ileus. Note the cholecystoduodenal fistula and the proximally impacted gallstone.

gallstone erodes from the gallbladder into the duodenum and passes distally. Such patients will present with distal bowel obstruction and, if looked for carefully, will have radiologic evidence of air within the biliary tree (Figs 37–20 and 37–21). Treatment consists of laparotomy, enterotomy, and stone removal followed by cholecystectomy, only if there is no dense inflammation in the right upper quadrant. If inflammation is present, cholecystectomy should be omitted. If gallbladder symptoms persist, or if the patient does well postoperatively, an interval cholecystectomy can be performed.

REFERENCES

1. Brolin RE. The role of gastrointestinal tube decompression in the treatment of mechanical intestinal obstruction. *Am Surg* 1983;49:131

2. Stewardson RH, Bombeck CT, Nyhus LM. Critical operative management of small bowel obstruction. *Ann Surg* 1978;187:189

3. Cheadle WG, Garr EE, Richardson JD. The importance of early diagnosis of small bowel obstruction. *Am Surg* 1988; 54:565

4. Peetz DJ, Gamelli RL, Pilcher DB. Intestinal intubation in acute mechanical small bowel obstruction. *Arch Surg* 1982; 117:334

5. Turner DM, Croom RD. Acute adhesive obstruction of the small intestine. *Am Surg* 1983;49:126

6. Deitsch EA, Bridges SM, Ma JW. Obstructed intestine as a reservoir for systemic infection. *Am J Surg* 1990;159:394

7. Deitsch EA. Simple intestinal obstruction causes bacterial translocation in man. *Arch Surg* 1989;124:699

8. Dunn JT, Halls JM, Berne TV. Roentgenographic contrast studies in acute small bowel obstruction. *Arch Surg* 1984; 119:1305

9. Sarr MG, Bulkley GB, Zuidema GD. Preoperative recognition of intestinal stangulation obstruction. *Am J Surg* 1983;145:176

10. Brolin RE, Krasna MJ, Mast BA. Use of tubes and radiographs in the management of small bowel obstruction. *Ann Surg* 1987;206:126

11. Hofstetter SR. Acute adhesive obstruction of the small intestine. *Surg Gynecol Obstet* 1981;152:141

12. Pickleman J, Lee RM. The management of patients with suspected early postoperative small bowel obstruction. *Ann Surg* 1989;210:216

13. Landercasper J, Cogbill T, Merry W, et al. Long-term outcome after hospitalization for small bowel obstruction. *Arch Surg* 1993;128:765

14. Montefusco RP, Ward RJ, Geiss AC. Recurrent adhesive small bowel obstruction. *Contemp Surg* 1985;27:98

15. Brightwell NL, McFee AS, Aust JB. Bowel obstruction and the long tube stent. *Arch Surg* 1977;112:505

16. Weigelt JA, Snyder WH, Norman JL. Complications and results of one hundred sixty Baker tube plications. *Am J Surg* 1980;140:810

17. Selby RR, Mertz GH, Gilsdorf RB. Spontaneous resolution of intestinal obstruction while receiving home parenteral nutrition. *Am J Surg* 1983;146:742

18. Spears H, Petrelli NJ, Herrera L, et al. Treatment of bowel obstruction after operation for colorectal carcinoma. *Am J Surg* 1988;155:383

19. Osteen RT, Guyton S, Steele G, et al. Malignant intestinal obstruction. *Surgery* 1980;87:611

20. Greenlee HB, Aranha GV, De Orio A. Obstruction of the small and large intestine due to malignancy. In: Hickey, RC, Clark, RL (eds) *Current Problems in Cancer.* Chicago, IL: Yearbook Medical; 1979:IV(2)

21. Aranha GV, Folk FA, Greenlee HB. Surgical palliation of small bowel obstruction due to metastatic carcinoma. *Am Surg* 1981;47(3):99

38

Tumors of the Small Intestine

Agustin A. Burgos ▪ *Miguel E. Martinez* ▪ *Bernard M. Jaffe*

Tumors of the small intestine are remarkably rare. Even though the small intestine accounts for 80% of the length and 90% of the mucosal surface of the gastrointestinal tract, only 3% to 6% of the gastrointestinal tumors and 1% of the gastrointestinal malignancies arise from the small bowel.[1] Most small bowel tumors are incidental findings at operation or autopsy. In fact, the rarity of small bowel tumors, paucity of specific symptoms, and diversity of tumor types all contribute to the frequent delay in diagnosis and poor prognosis when the tumors are malignant.

The first reported case of a small bowel tumor was a duodenal carcinoma described by Hamburger in 1746. In 1876, Liechtenstein published the first collected series of malignancies, and the first review of benign lesions was published by Hearteaux in 1899. Since then, there has been considerable progress in understanding the nature and diversity of small bowel tumors. However, further study is essential to achieve earlier detection and improved survival.

■ INCIDENCE AND EPIDEMIOLOGY

The average age at the time of diagnosis of small bowel tumors is 59.5 years, with a range of 14 to 84 years. The average age at presentation with benign tumors is 62.2 years and for malignant tumors, 56.8 years. Adenocarcinoma is usually diagnosed in the 7th decade, whereas carcinoids and leiomyosarcomata, in the 6th.[1] Lymphoma is the most common malignant tumor of the small intestine, in children.

Overall, there is no significant gender preference, although some investigators report a slight male predominance for intestinal malignancies.[2–4]

Small bowel adenocarcinoma appears to have an increased incidence in developed Western countries and a positive correlation with prevalence rates of colon carcinoma.[5] Mediterranean lymphoma (α-chain disease or immunoproliferative small intestinal disease) is very common in the Middle East and North Africa; this tumor occurs in lower socioeconomic classes and younger patients.[6] In the United States, 70% of carcinoids occur in blacks, while lymphomas are twice as common in whites.[5]

■ ETIOLOGY

When compared with the esophagus, stomach, and colorectum, the remarkably low incidence of small bowel tumors has focused attention on possible antineoplastic characteristics of this segment of the alimentary tract. These include the relatively rapid transit time, when compared with the stomach or colon,[7] an alkaline environment that appears protective,[8] liquid content rather than solid stool,[9] a high level of benzopyrene hydroxylase, an enzyme that may detoxify potential carcinogens,[10] and a lower bacterial population and different bacterial metabolism in the colon, producing fewer carcinogens.[11] The high concentration of IgA in the lumen neutralizes potential carcinogenic viruses, which is consistent with the increased incidence of small bowel malignancy in immunosuppressed or IgA-deficient patients, such as those with Crohn's disease, Wiskott-Aldrich syndrome, and acquired immunodeficiency syndrome (AIDS).[5,11] Finally, the high incidence of Mediterranean lymphoma in this specific geographic area is caused by defective gastrointestinal immune surveillance.

On the other hand, the mucosa of the small intestine appears susceptible to carcinogens. Adenocarcinoma occurs mostly in the proximal intestine, as is adenocarcinoma induced by azoxymethane in rats.[12] This correlates with increased exposure of the bowel to biliary and pancreatic secretions, possibly implicating them in the carcinogenic process.[13,14]

Specific premalignant conditions and risk factors play a role in the pathogenesis of small bowel tumors. The adenoma-carcinoma sequence appears as important in the small intestine as in the large intestine.[15] This has special importance for patients with familial adenomatous polyposis, in which some patients have adenomatous polyps in the small intestine. Another condition suggested as premalignant is diffuse nodular lymphatic hyperplasia of the small intestine. It was observed to be associated with the development of jejunal malignant lymphoma in a patient with common variable hypogammaglobulinemia.[16]

In patients with preexisting Crohn's disease, mucosal dysplasia has been considered premalignant. This also applies to the small bowel, if it has been affected by the inflammatory bowel disease.[17]

In addition to the premalignant conditions, risk factors for small intestinal malignancies include longstanding celiac disease, despite compliance with a gluten-free diet. Affected patients are at increased risk of developing T cell lymphoma of the small intestine,[18] and have a poor prognosis because of the delay in diagnosis.[19] Patients with Peutz-Jeghers syndrome who have multiple benign hamartomas have an increased incidence of malignancy because of the concurrent presence of adenomatous components.[20] The hamartoma-carcinoma sequence has been verified by several investigators.[21] These patients must be followed for life, including regular (biannual) polypectomies.[21]

Patients with von Recklinghausen's neurofibromatosis often (12% to 25%) have small bowel tumors, predominantly neurofibromas, ganglioneuromas, and schwannomas.[22,23] A number of malignancies have been described associated with von Recklinghausen's disease, including neurofibrosarcoma,[24] leiomyosarcoma,[25] adenocarcinoma,[23] and carcinoid.[26]

Other risk factors are related to immunosuppression. Transplant recipients receiving immunosuppressive drugs and patients with AIDS, autoimmune diseases (rheumatoid arthritis, Wegener's granulomatosis, systemic lupus erythematosus), and congenital immunodeficiencies (X-linked agammaglobulinemia and Wiskott-Aldrich syndrome) all are at increased risk of developing malignancy, especially lymphomas and sarcomas. Oncogenic viruses have been implicated in the pathogenesis of malignancies in these patients, including cytomegalovirus with Kaposi's sarcoma and Epstein Barr Virus with Burkitt's lymphoma.[27–29]

Finally, in patients with defective immune surveillance and small bowel malignancies, there is a high incidence of other primary neoplasms elsewhere. Alexander and Altemeier reported that 83 out of 112 patients with small bowel tumors had a second primary elsewhere at time of their death.[30]

■ PRESENTATION

Except for those that present as emergencies, the symptoms of small bowel tumors are nonspecific, of insidious onset, and slow in progression until the diagnosis is established. The surgeon needs to be "small-bowel conscious," in other words, think of these rare tumors when the diagnosis is not obvious.

The benign tumors are usually asymptomatic, whereas malignant ones usually cause some symptoms. Benign tumors may present with pain secondary to intermittent incomplete obstruction, usually the result of intussusception. Ten percent of patients present with evidence of gastrointestinal bleeding, ranging in severity from anemia as the result of occult bleeding to frank hemorrhage, although the latter is very rare.

The most frequent presenting symptoms of malignant tumors are weight loss, anorexia, and abdominal pain. The severity and nature of the pain depends on the site and size of the lesion, whether partial or complete obstruction is present, or if perforation has occurred.

Pain described as dull may be caused by pressure from a large mass, as occurs with lymphomas and sarcomas. Cramps are associated with partial obstruction caused by a luminal mass, such as a partially occluding annular adenocarcinoma, or by intussusception. If total obstruction occurs, the likeliest diagnoses are adenocarcinoma and carcinoid. An acute abdomen may be caused by perforation, especially of lymphomas, which are characterized by the absence of desmoplastic reaction surrounding the tumor. Should the surgeon attempt a primary closure, this will surely result in failure. Some carcinoids are characteristically located at the base of the mesentery, causing fixation and shortening, and leading to obstructive symptoms. Volvulus also has been described as a result of a malignancy of the small bowel.

Bleeding is not as common in the face of malignant tumors as with benign lesions. Leiomyosarcoma has been reported to cause massive bleeding, but this manifestation is rare. At the Massachusetts General Hospital, only 0.2% of cases with massive upper gastrointestinal bleeding were due to small bowel tumors.[31] In both benign and malignant tumors, the bleeding is usually occult.

An abdominal mass is most frequently associated with lymphomas and leiomyosarcomas. Jaundice may be the result of a duodenal or periampullary mass, made more likely if there is evidence of associated gastrointestinal bleeding. Pancreatic carcinomas are not as commonly associated with occult bleeding. Malabsorption and steatorrhea may be secondary to extensive intestinal lymphoma.

The carcinoid syndrome causes a specific set of symptoms, although by the time it appears, the patients usually have liver metastases. The symptoms include diarrhea, flushing, evidence of right-sided heart failure, and bronchoconstriction.

Because of the lack of specificity of the symptoms, there is a delay in diagnosis of small intestinal tumors. In patients with malignancy, almost 80% of which cause late symptoms,[11] one-third of the patients developed complaints within 6 months prior to diagnosis, another third within 6 to 12 months, and another third in 5 years.[32] In carcinoids, the average time from onset of symptoms to diagnosis, usually when the syndrome ensues, is about 9 years.[33]

■ DIAGNOSIS

The diagnosis of small bowel tumors requires a high index of suspicion. The history and physical examination, although essential, are usually nonspecific and unrevealing. Laboratory data may reveal anemia owing to intestinal bleeding, but most lesions do not bleed. In patients with the carcinoid syndrome, urinary excretion of 5-hydroxyindole-acetic acid (5-HIAA) often is increased and circulating levels of serotonin are elevated.

Plain films may confirm the presence of partial or complete bowel obstruction, or suggest a volvulus, but they are generally nonspecific. Contrast radiography is one of the most frequently used modalities. Although hypotonic duodenography using glucagon has been replaced by endoscopy, enteroclysis or selective-intubation contrast studies of the small bowel are invaluable for evaluation of more distal intestine. Small bowel series may reveal mucosal abnormalities or ulcerating lesions, suggesting adenocarcinoma or lymphoma; intramural masses, suggesting sarcomas or lymphomas; or intraluminal lesions, such as polyps or leiomyomas. A 50% preoperative diagnostic rate has been reported based on contrast studies.[34] Reflux from a barium enema could reveal a distal ileal tumor.

Endoscopy is essential for evaluation of the duodenum. Colonoscopy may allow visualization of distal ileal lesions in some patients. Surgical ostomies can provide easier access for evaluation of intestinal segments, using a colonoscope. The ability to perform biopsies and therapeutic maneuvers is a definite advantage of endoscopy.

Enteroscopy, endoscopic evaluation of the small bowel, is now being developed. It has already proven useful in cases of occult bleeding. Two techniques have been reported, "push" and sonde-type enteroscopy. Sonde-type enteroscopy uses a balloon-tipped endoscope to help the passage into the intestine; however, this technique takes several hours to perform, requires fluoroscopy, and biopsies cannot be performed. Push enteroscopy uses a special enterscope that is passed orally down to almost 60 to 100 cm distal to the ligament of Treitz.[35] Biopsies can be performed, but fluoroscopy may be needed for passage. In the report by Lewis and colleagues, the technique identified 13 tumors as causes of occult gastrointestinal (GI) bleeding, whereas routine x-ray, endoscopic, and nuclear medicine studies were negative.[35]

Enteroscopy is useful in cases of occult bleeding, but it may be complemented by a "bleeding scan" or arteriography. As the technique of enteroscopy is improved, its role in the diagnosis of small bowel tumors will be better defined.[36]

Angiography is useful in cases of vascular tumors, where the presence of "parasitic" vascular supply suggests malignancy. These are feeder branches that usually are absent, if there is no malignancy. Angiography may identify the site of a bleeding tumor. However, if the bleeding is slow (<0.1 mL/min), a bleeding scan may be more helpful in localizing the area of oozing. After the scan, angiography then may be performed to further define the site. It is essential to localize the lesion preoperatively because of the frequent difficulty in finding it intraoperatively.

Computer tomography (CT) scanning is a useful modality for identifying extraluminal lesions, such as sarcomas and lymphomas, for which preoperative staging is essential. This technique is also helpful for evaluating the presence or absence of mesenteric and liver metastases.

If preoperative evaluation does not provide adequate information, it is appropriate to explore the abdomen, using either laparoscopy or celiotomy. As Thompson and associates suggested, early exploratory laparotomy may have a high yield in cases of occult bleeding in young patients.[37] In these patients, the most probable causes are small bowel tumors or Meckel's diverticula, whereas in older populations, the most likely lesions are arteriovenous malformations.

In the future, newer diagnostic techniques like endoscopic ultrasound[38] and somatostatin receptor scintigraphy[39] will undoubtedly play a role in achieving an earlier diagnosis, better management, and improved survival.

■ BENIGN TUMORS

About one-half of benign tumors remain asymptomatic and are discovered at autopsy.[1] In most series, two-thirds of small bowel tumors are found to be malignant, mainly because benign lesions are usually silent.[40] However, at autopsy, benign tumors account for more than three-fourths of all tumors.

The most common presentation of benign small bowel tumors is pain owing to partial obstruction, often caused by intussusception. Occult bleeding is the second most common symptom.

The most common small bowel benign tumor is the leiomyoma (30% to 35%), followed in sequence by adenoma (20% to 22%), lipoma (14% to 16%), hemangioma (12%), fibroma (6%), and others (14%).[40,41]

The frequency of benign small bowel tumors generally increases from duodenum to ileum. However, per unit area, the proximal 15 to 20 cm of intestine have the greatest number. In the review of Ashley and Wells,[40] leiomyomas were mostly jejunoileal, adenomas were equally distributed among the 3 intestinal segments, and lipomas were mostly ileal. The duodenum, comprising 8% of the length of the small bowel, contributes 10% to 20% of all tumors.

LEIOMYOMA

Leiomyoma is the most common symptomatic benign lesion. It usually is diagnosed in the fifth decade of life, although it may occur at any age. There is no sex predilection. Mostly jejunoileal, there is a disproportionately high incidence of smooth muscle neoplasms in Meckel's diverticula, followed by the duodenum, if the unit area is considered.[5]

Leiomyoma has 4 types of growth patterns: extraluminal (65%), intramural (16%), dumbbell shaped (into and out of the lumen) (11%), and intraluminal (8%).[42] Grossly, leiomyomas are white-gray lesions. Microscopically, they contain well-differentiated smooth muscle cells and no mitoses, which differentiates them from their malignant counterpart. On x-ray studies, they appear as ovoid filling defects. A fluid-filled cavity may appear when they grow large. This central necrosis is the result of the tumor outgrowing its vascular supply.

The major concern is bleeding, either into the lumen or the peritoneal cavity. Two-thirds of patients present with evidence of bleeding, whereas only one-fourth present with obstructive symptoms.[42]

The treatment of leiomyoma is segmental resection with clear margins, since differentiation from leiomyosarcoma is difficult, even on pathological examination. Lymph node resection is not routinely performed because leiomyosarcoma does not commonly spread via the lymphatics.

ADENOMA

Adenomas are usually asymptomatic, pedunculated, and amenable to endoscopic or operative polypectomy. When sessile, these tumors require segmental resection.

The distribution of adenomas in the small intestine is equal in each of the three segments.[40] Three types are usually described: adenomatous polyps, villous adenomas, and Brunner's gland adenomas. It now is believed that adenomas in the small bowel behave like those in the colorectum, regarding their potential for malignant degeneration. Moreover, when symptomatic adenomas are excised, they are very likely to exhibit malignant changes.[15] Adenomas are the most common benign lesions of the duodenum and in this location, they are mostly periampullary.

Adenomatous Polyp

Adenomatous polyps usually occur in the duodenum and generally remain asymptomatic. Commonly pedunculated, polyps are usually amenable to endoscopic polypectomy; if not, segmental resection or polypectomy via an enterotomy are indicated. They have low malignant potential, but they can bleed or cause obstruction, especially intussusception, which is the most common presenting symptom. Intussusception with a polyp as the lead point requires resection.

Villous Adenomas

Villous tumors have a distinct malignant potential. They are generally sessile and solitary. Villous adenomas are rare, comprising 1% of duodenal tumors.[43] When in the duodenum, the lesions are generally periampullary. Malignancy arises in about 30% of duodenal villous adenomas and resection is indicated, especially if they are >3 cm in diameter. The presence or absence of associated symptoms does not alter the decision to resect these lesions.

Villous adenomas may present with bleeding, obstruction, or jaundice. If an endoscopic polypectomy specimen contains adenocarcinoma, the tumor requires wider resection. Therapeutic recommendations from Bjork and associates are: for tumors with invasive carcinoma in the 1st and 2nd portions of the duodenum, pancreatoduodenectomy should be performed and provides a reported 5 year survival rate of 45%; for malignant tumors in the third and fourth portions and tumors on the antimesenteric wall with no pancreatic involvement, segmental resection is advocated; transduodenal submucosal local excision is preferred over endoscopic polypectomy for tumors without invasive carcinoma regardless of their location; for benign periampullary lesions, ampullary reconstruction, including bile duct sphincteroplasty and pancreatic duct septectomy should be performed as the initial treatment.[43] They also reported no mortality and very low rates of morbidity and tumor recurrence. In their series, two patients with large obstructing benign lesions required Whipple procedures.

Brunner's Gland Adenoma

These tumors represent hyperplasia of the exocrine glands in the mucosa of the proximal duodenum, and present as polyps. Usually asymptomatic, they too can bleed and obstruct, if large. Brunner's gland adenomas have only a tiny malignant potential. Limited resection is the procedure of choice. Even if the mass is large, bypass should be considered, rather than a Whipple procedure, to avoid the associated morbidity and mortality.[1,40] Carcinoma arising from Brunner's gland adenomas has been described, and any change in the gross appearance or size is suspicious of malignancy and requires excision.[44] Regular follow-up is implicated.

LIPOMA

Lipomas are the third most common benign tumors of the small intestine, following leiomyomas and adenomas. In a review by Ashley and Wells, most lipomas were ileal, then duodenal, and the lowest percent were in the jejunum.[40] More than 80% of lipomas are intraluminal and asymptomatic. They may rarely obstruct or bleed. Excision is required if the tumors are symptomatic. If found incidentally, and if the appearance is benign and the tumor is so small as not to cause symptoms, they may be left alone. When larger than 4 cm, 86% cause symptoms,[45] such as intussusception, pain, and bleeding. Fat necrosis is not uncommon and can make the differentiation from liposarcoma difficult. Malignant degeneration has not been reported. Their radiolucency establishes the diagnosis on barium studies; so, too, does its gross globular yellowish appearance on endoscopy. CT scan can detect their nature by measuring density.

HEMANGIOMA

Hemangiomas can involve the mucosa, submucosa, or muscle. Together with lymphangiomas, they comprise 7% of the benign lesions.[1] A hereditary form involving large segments of the intestine is known as Olser-Weber-Rendu disease. These lesions arise from the submucosal vascular plexus, and when symptoms appear, bleeding (70%) and pain (30%) predominate. They are mostly sessile, but polypoid forms also exist.

Angiography can localize the tumor, sometimes even in the absence of bleeding. Segmental resection is the procedure of choice. Association with hemangiomas elsewhere in the body is not uncommon.

LYMPHANGIOMA

Much less frequent than hemangiomas, these tumors also are associated with other lymphangiomas elsewhere in the body. Like hemangiomas, lymphangiomas are probably developmental anomalies rather than neoplasms.[1] Most are incidental findings at surgery or autopsy.

NEUROGENIC TUMORS

Benign neurogenic tumors of the small bowel are very rare. They originate from the nerve sheath (neurilemmoma and neurofibroma) or from components of the sympathetic nervous system (ganglioneuroma). Neurofibromas, probably hamartomatous malformations rather than neoplasms, are usually isolated when they occur in the gastrointestinal tract, and are not associated with von Recklinghausen's disease. Segmental resection is indicated for isolated tumors because of the risk of obstruction, bleeding, or intussusception.[1]

■ POLYPOSIS SYNDROMES IN THE SMALL INTESTINE

There are several polyposis syndromes with involvement of the small intestine. Those that involve adenomatous polyps have a definite risk for cancer, while those with hamartomas have low malignant potential.

These include:

- *Bessauds-Hillmand-Augier Syndrome* Intestinal polyposis and sexual infantilism.[46]
- *Carter-Horsley-Hughes Syndrome* Diffuse polyposis described in one family.[47]
- *Cronkhite-Canada Syndrome* Nonhereditary diffuse polyposis with ectodermal defects (alopecia, hyperpigmentation, nail atrophy) and protein loss through the intestine.[48]
- *Cowden's Syndrome* Hamartomas in the stomach, colon and small intestine.[49] This autosomal dominant condition is associated with tumors of thyroid and breast.[50]
- *Devon Family Syndrome* Multiple recurrent inflammatory polyps in the stomach and ileum. These polyps have significant malignant potential.[51]
- *Familial Adenomatous Polyposis* Previously thought to involve only the colon, diffuse polyposis is now described. This autosomal dominant disease is

associated with malignancies elsewhere (thyroid, liver, gallbladder, adrenal). It has a nearly 100% rate of malignant degeneration.[52]

- *Familial Juvenile Polyposis* Hamartomas transmitted by autosomal dominant genetic transmission.

- *Gardner's Syndrome* Usually colorectal, but polyps also are described in the small bowel. This autosomal dominant condition is associated with malignancies elsewhere, like familial adenomatous polyposis. Affected patients also develop epidermoid cysts, fibromas, desmoids, retroperitoneal fibrosis, and osteomas. It has a very high malignant potential.[53]

- *Gordon's Disease* Protein-losing gastroenteropathy with which a diffuse polyposis has been described.[54]

- *Juvenile Polyposis* Nonfamilial hamartomas, usually colonic, but diffuse cases involving the small intestine have been observed. Extremely low malignant potential,[55] this syndrome is associated with protein-losing enteropathy.

- *Peutz-Jeghers Syndrome* Hamartomatous polyposis associated with abnormal mucocutaneous pigmentation. First described by Peutz[56] and then by Jegher,[57] it has a high familial penetrance. The average age at diagnosis is in the third decade.

The hamartomatous polyps are found mainly in the jejunum, but are present throughout the gut. While the hamartomas are benign, there is significant malignant potential for this syndrome.[21,58] There is also an apparent risk of other malignancies. Twenty-two percent of Spigelman and associates[1] patients developed a neoplasm other than the polyps, 56% of these of gastrointestinal origin. In this series, the risk of dying of a malignancy by age 57 was 48%.[21]

Most commonly, affected patients are identified by screening of relatives. Symptomatic presentations include attacks of intermittent obstruction owing to intussusception or gastrointestinal bleeding. The recommended management is as limited a resection as possible to include the symptomatic polyps. In view of the high incidence of ovarian tumors, these glands should be examined at surgery.

- *Pseudoxanthoma Elasticum (Gronblad-Strandberg Syndrome)* A generalized connective tissue disorder associated with arterial degeneration causing blindness. Benign vascular lesions have been observed in the intestine.[59]

- *Rendu-Osler-Weber Disease* This is familial; telangiectasia of the gastrointestinal tract has been described, as well as its presence in the nasopharynx, and its association with vascular lesions on the face, lips and fingers.[59]

- *Torres Syndrome* This syndrome includes sebaceous adenomas, fibromas, lipomas, fibrosarcomas, leiomyomas with visceral cancers.[60]

- *Turcet's Syndrome* These are multiple adenomas, usually colorectal, but also observed in the small bowel, and are associated with brain tumors. It has a similar malignant potential as familial adenomatous polyposis.[51]

- *Turner's Syndrome* Seven percent of patients with the syndrome have intestinal telangiectasia.[61]

- *von Recklinghausen's Disease* Gastrointestinal involvement described includes leiomyosarcoma[20] and other tumors already mentioned above.

■ MALIGNANT TUMORS

Small intestinal malignancies are very rare, accounting for 0.3% of all malignancies and 1% to 3% of gastrointestinal malignancies.[1] Rather than one major type of malignancy, like that affecting the stomach and colon, several types of tumors dominate the spectrum in the small bowel. More than 35 different neoplasms have been described, with all cells of origin well represented. The premalignant conditions and risk factors for malignancies have already been described. To further complicate the picture, 29% of patients with small bowel malignancies develop a second primary malignancy,[43] implying the need for lifelong follow-up.

Most malignancies of the small bowel are diagnosed in the seventh decade. In order of reported frequency, the most common types are adenocarcinoma (40% to 50%), carcinoid (30%), lymphoma (14%), and sarcoma (11%).

Most malignancies arise in the ileum (almost 50%), with the remaining being equally divided between duodenum (25%) and jejunum (25%). Adenocarcinomas are more common in the duodenum, while the remaining tumors occur more common distally, especially carcinoids, 80% of which arise in the distal ileum.

Adenocarcinomas carry the worst prognosis, while carcinoids offer the best rates of survival; the 5 year survival rates are 20% to 30% and 60% to 70%, respectively.[41,62,63]

Malignant tumors usually become symptomatic, but generally late in the course of the disease. Two-thirds of all small bowel tumors are considered to be malignant because of the frequency of symptoms allow their diagnosis. The average time from the onset of symptoms to diagnosis is 6 to 8 months, and even longer (years) in carcinoid. At the time of diagnosis, two-thirds of tumors have metastatic disease.[2,3,63]

The most common symptoms are pain and weight loss. Obstruction is usually partial, since the bowel wall is distensible and its content is fluid. Intussusception is not as common as with benign tumors. Obstruction is secondary to tumor growth or kinking of the mesentery by carcinoids.

A palpable mass usually represents a dilated proximal intestinal segment obstructed by malignancy. Lymphoma may present as aneurismal dilatation of the bowel owing to infiltration of the wall; this can readily be felt as a mass. Perforation is the presenting manifestation of 10% of tumors, usually lymphoma or sarcoma. The resultant peritonitis may be localized or diffuse.[40]

A preoperative diagnosis is reached in only 17% to 50% of cases.[64,65] Contrast radiography and endoscopy are the most helpful modalities. CT scanning may help identify metastases, a thickened wall in the case of lymphoma, or other abdominal masses.

ADENOCARCINOMA

Adenocarcinomas are the most common malignant tumors in the small bowel, constituting 30% to 50% of all small bowel cancers. They tend to occur in the sixth and seventh decades of life and correlate, in distribution, with colonic carcinomas, with which they share several risk factors,[66] such as Crohn's disease. For patients with Crohn's disease, a number of risk factors for small bowel cancer have been described, including chronic disease (>20 years), surgically excluded loops, proximal disease, the use of 6-mercaptopurine, exposure to carcinogens (hazardous occupations),[67] and male sex. Because of the risk of malignancy in chronic fistulas and strictures, Ribeira and associates recommend frozen sections at the time of stricteroplasty and fistula resection.[68] Senay and associates described the typical Crohn's patient with small bowel cancer: a late recrudescence after a long quiescent period, a delay in diagnosis owing to confusion with inflammatory symptoms, and rapid deterioration.[69]

In fact, small bowel cancer behaves differently in patients with Crohn's disease. The Chron's patients are younger (average age 48 vs 64 years), and carry a male:female ratio of 3:1 (rather than is 1:1), have an ileal location, and carry worse prognosis because of the delay in diagnosis. Usually Crohn's patients present with obstruction, perforation, or bleeding. The 2 year disease-free survival rate in patients with Crohn's disease and small bowel cancer is 9%, whereas the mean 5 year survival rate in patients with no inflammatory bowel disease is 15% to 25%.[70]

Adenocarcinomas occur primarily in the proximal gut. Almost one-half arise in the duodenum, and in that site, two-thirds are periampullary. They usually cause pain in the upper abdomen owing to partial obstruction. Anemia and guaiac-positive stools are frequent manifestations of periampullary lesions, and jaundice is common. The diagnosis of a duodenal lesion is suspected from an upper gastrointestinal series and con-

firmed with endoscopy and biopsy. Treatment of duodenal adenocarcinomas depends on the size, location, and presence or absence of metastases. Periampullary lesions usually require a radical pancreatoduodenectomy (Whipple procedure), whereas small lesions in the first and fourth portions may be amenable to segmental resection, including the draining nodal system.

Zollinger and associates reported that only palliative procedures were possible in one-third of the patients.[2] Moreover, up to 70% of patients have microscopic metastases, even though the resection was believed to be curative. As a result, the surgeon must weigh the survival rate as well as the morbidity and mortality of a radical operation versus the results of a wide segmental resection with a corresponding regional lymphadenectomy, especially in tumors in the third and fourth portions of the duodenum. There is no clear evidence that pancreatoduodenectomy results in better survival than segmental resection, if the latter is technically possible.[70]

Palliative procedures include gastrojejunostomy to bypass the duodenal obstruction, and biliary bypasses or stenting to overcome ampullary biliary obstruction.

The prognosis is improved by early diagnosis. Duke's modified B1 lesions (Table 38–1) showed a 5 year survival rate of up to 80%.[4] However, overall, the survival rate is poor (Table 38–2), averaging 20% to 30% at 5 years.[41]

Adenocarcinomas of the jejunoileum present later than those in the duodenum. Complete obstruction and intussusception are rare; partial obstruction is the most common presentation, occurring in 50% to 74% of patients. Blood loss occurs in 30% to 60%.[12,65] The diagnosis can be suspected on small bowel barium follow-through studies or CT scans, but the majority of cases are diagnosed intraoperatively.

For jejunoileal adenocarcinomas, wide segmental resection, encompassing the regional mesentery and lymphatics, is the treatment of choice. However, the extent of resection may be limited by the superior mesenteric artery. A tumor in the distal ileum requires a right hemicolectomy.

The rates of survival are also poor for jejunoileal tu-

TABLE 38–1. ASTLER COLLER MODIFIED DUKE'S STAGING SYSTEM

Stage	
A	limited to submucosa negative nodes
B1	invading muscularis propria negative nodes
B2	through muscularis propria negative nodes
C1	B1 with positive nodes
C2	B2 with positive nodes
D	distant metastases

(From Ouriel KK, Adams JT: Adenocarcinoma of the small bowel. Am J Surg 1984;147:56–71)

TABLE 38–2. 5 YEAR SURVIVAL RATES IN PATIENTS WITH ADENOCARCINOMA

	Period (yr)	Patients	Survival (%)
Awrich et al, 1980[71]	25	26	25
Mittal and Bodzin, 1980[66]	21	10	62
Norberg and Emas, 1981[72]	34	11	0
Waterhouse et al, 1981[73]	28	24	18
Adler et al, 1982[74]	43	338	17
Lanzafame et al, 1982[75]	40	29	35
Barclay and Schapira, 1983[76]	30	74	22
Williamson et al, 1983[12]	64	68	14
Ouriel et al, 1984[4]	31	65	30
Cooper and Read, 1985[77]	15	25	0
Johnson et al, 1985[78]	28	16	6
Zollinger et al, 1986[2]	20	18	17
Martin, 1986[79]	38	87	21
Cicarelli et al, 1987[64]	14	17	12
Brophy and Cahoe, 1989[80]	14	18	36
Lioe and Biggart, 1990[81]	34	25	16
Desa et al, 1991[82]	15	7	20
Kusumoto et al, 1992[62]	15	19	10
Baillie and Williams, 1994[83]	20	11	15
DiSario et al, 1994[84]	25	80	25
Bhutani et al, 1989[63]	6	35	0

(Updated from Coit DG. Cancer of the small intestine. In: DeVita VT Jr, et al (eds), Cancer: Principles and Practice of Oncology. 4th ed Vol 1. Philadelphia, PA: Lippincott; 1993:915–928)

mors, averaging 20% at 30 months.[82] Positive prognostic factors include jejunal location, absence of nodal metastases, and well-differentiated type. The roles of radiotherapy and chemotherapy in small bowel adenocarcinoma still are undefined.

CARCINOID

Carcinoid tumors are the most common intestinal endocrine tumors. They account for 13% to 34% of all tumors of the small bowel and 17% to 46% of the malignancies.[33] This malignant tumor was first described by Lubarsch in 1888,[85] and the term "carcinoid" was coined by Oberndorfer in 1907.[86] In 1930, Kramer described a similar tumor in the Kultchitzky cells in the bronchial mucosa.[87] Rappaport and colleagues isolated serotonin in 1948[88]; Thorson and associates described the carcinoid syndrome[89]; and in 1952, Erspamer and Asero reported the production of serotonin by the carcinoid tumors.[90]

Carcinoids grow slowly, and usually remain silent for years before presenting with the carcinoid syndrome (average, 9 years).[33] The likelihood of metastases is related directly to the tumor size, under 2% if the lesion is <1 cm in diameter, but 100% if it is >2 cm.

The most common site of carcinoid is the appendix. The small bowel is second, especially in the ileum. Eighty percent of intestinal carcinoids arise in the distal

2 feet of ileum. Several carcinoid tumors have been described in Meckel diverticula.[91] Carcinoids have been divided into foregut, midgut, and hindgut derivatives, each with different clinical features.

Foregut carcinoids arise in the stomach, duodenum, pancreas, and bronchial tree. They produce a small amount of serotonin, secreting 5-hydroxytryptophan instead. Their functional manifestations include atypical carcinoid syndrome, Zollinger-Ellison syndrome, acromegaly, Cushing's syndrome, and other endocrine disorders including those of somatostatinoma. Midgut carcinoids develop from the jejunum to the ascending colon, including Meckel's diverticula. They also arise in the ovary and remnants of neural crest tissue. These carcinoids produce serotonin, bradykinin and tachykinins, prostaglandins and substance P, among others. The classic carcinoid syndrome is their functional manifestation.

Hindgut carcinoids, from the transverse colon to rectum, rarely secrete any hormones and therefore, are not usually associated with the carcinoid syndrome.[33]

Midgut carcinoids are usually asymptomatic, or may present with vague pain, especially if associated with mesenteric kinking and shortening owing to infiltration into the mesentery.

A syndrome of pain as a result of chronic ischemia, called elastic vascular sclerosis, has been described.[92] On arteriogram, occlusion of the nutrient arcades are observed.

Ten percent of patients develop the carcinoid syndrome, although two-thirds of all patients experience some of the symptoms at some point during their course.[33] The syndrome includes flushing of the head and neck, secretory diarrhea, right-sided valvular heart disease, and bronchial asthma. By the time patients develop the syndrome, hepatic metastases are generally present, and the diagnosis may be confirmed by increased rates of urinary 5-H1AA excretion and elevated levels of circulating serotonin. The symptoms can be prompted by stress, alcohol, and certain foods.[33]

Diagnosis of carcinoid tumors in patients without the syndrome is more difficult. Rates of urinary excretion of 5-H1AA are not elevated. Radiographic studies are not specific and CT scan may only reveal mesenteric infiltration. The absence of liver metastases does not preclude the carcinoid syndrome, since the manifestations can still occur without them.

Treatment of carcinoid tumors is wide resection of the primary tumor, mesenteric metastases, and compromised bowel segments. Debulking as much tumor as technically possible is useful in controlling symptoms of carcinoid syndrome, which also responds to treatment with somatostatin analog. Hepatic dearterialization has been also recommended, although only as short-term treatment.[93] Response rates to chemotherapy are in the range of 20% to 40%, but no effect on the course of the disease has been documented.

The prognosis of carcinoids is better than that of adenocarcinomas (Table 38–3). Survival rates depend on tumor size, degree of invasion, and the presence or absence of metastatic disease. Without metastatic disease, complete resection offers up to 95% 5 year survival, whereas the survival rate is 19% to 54% in patients with liver metastases.[93]

Carcinoids in the ampulla of Vater have a better prognosis. These tumors do not present with the previously described syndrome and may be treated by Whipple procedure or wide local resection. The 5 year survival rate is close to 90%.[106]

LYMPHOMA

Primary lymphomas of the small bowel are rare, accounting for <2% of all gastrointestinal malignancies and 10% to 20% of the small bowel malignancies.[41] They arise from lymphoid tissue in the small bowel, and are more common in the ileum, consistent with the higher number of lymphocytes in the distal gut. For small bowel lymphomas to be categorized as primary, the criteria described by Dawson[107] include no mediastinal or peripheral lymphadenopathy, a normal white blood cell count and differential, predominant intestinal involvement, and no splenic or hepatic involvement. The risk factors for development of small bowel lymphoma have been described above.

Gastrointestinal lymphomas are staged using a modified Ann Arbor classification:

IE   **tumor confined to small intestine**
IIE   **spread to regional lymph nodes**
IIIE **spread to nonresectable nodes beyond regional nodes**
IVE   **spread to other organs.**

According to Amer and El-Akhad, rates of 5 year survival average 63% to 95%, 38% to 75%, 15% to 53%, and 8% to 31% respectively.[6]

Four main types of lymphomas have been described, the Western type, the Mediterranean type, childhood lymphoma, and Hodgkin's lymphoma.

In general, the presentation of lymphoma is nonspecific. Fever and night sweats are uncommon, as is diffuse lymphadenopathy. A mass is palpable only rarely. Patients are usually in the seventh decade of life with the Western type, while the Mediterranean type affects younger patients. One-fourth of the patients present as an emergency, due either to perforation, obstruction, or bleeding.[19]

The typical patient with Western-type lymphoma is male, presents with abdominal pain, and has an abdominal mass. Anemia is present in 20% of patients and perforations present in 10% of patients.[108] The diagnosis may be suspected by identification of thickening of the intestinal wall on CT scan, although inflammatory bowel disease must be ruled out. Most of the time, the diagnosis is made intraoperatively. Perforation can occur with no surrounding desmoplastic reaction and therefore, primary closure is not therapeutic; resection of the affected segment with its mesentery is the only acceptable procedure.

The grade of most small bowel lymphomas is intermediate or high. They usually have a diffuse rather than a nodular growth pattern, and are of B-lymphocyte origin.[19] B-cell tumors are annular, exophytic, or polypoid masses, generally in the distal ileum. In contrast, lymphomas associated with celiac disease are of T-lymphocyte origin and involve the proximal small intestine with strictures or ulcerated plaques.[18]

Pancreatoduodenectomy may be required for patients with primary duodenal lymphoma. In any operation for suspected lymphoma, the procedure should also provide staging, including biopsy of the liver and resection of paraaortic, mesenteric, and regional nodes en bloc.

In patients with evidence of residual lymphoma after resection, chemotherapy is recommended.[108] It also is recommended for all high-grade tumors, even at stage IE.[109]

TABLE 38–3. 5 YEAR SURVIVAL RATES IN PATIENTS WITH CARCINOID

	Period (yr)	Patients	Survival (%)
Awrich et al, 1980[71]	25	28	47
Mittal and Bodzin, 1980[65]	10	9	87
Norberg and Emas, 1981[72]	34	8	63
Waterhouse et al, 1981[73]	28	26	69
Lanzafame et al, 1982[75]	40	18	44
Collin et al, 1982[94]	15	16	33
Zeitels et al, 1982[95]	37	28	62
Barclay and Schapira, 1983[76]	30	94	64
Peck et al, 1983[96]	10	30	31
Strodel et al, 1983[97]	20	82	59
Dawes et al, 1984[98]	18	32	80
Thompson et al, 1985[99]	10	66	62
Giuliani et al, 1985[100]	34	4	67
Olney et al, 1985[101]	44	75	33
Johnson et al, 1985[78]	28	22	50
Zollinger et al, 1986[2]	20	10	60
Martin, 1986[79]	38	89	51
O'Rourke et al, 1986[102]	10	43	52
Sjoblom, 1988[103]	19	48	77
Cicarelli et al, 1987[64]	14	20	35
Brophy and Cahoe, 1986[80]	14	8	83
Nwiloh et al, 1990[104]	22	11	44
McDermott et al, 1991[105]	18	42	66
Desa et al, 1991[82]	15	7	64
Baillie and Williams, 1994[83]	20	12	50
DiSario et al, 1994[84]	25	136	83
Bhutani et al, 1994[63]	6	26	75

In the review by Amer and El-Akkad, multimodality treatment was superior to surgery or chemotherapy alone.[6] Debulking is recommended, if technically feasible, because it might lead to improved survival.

The best prognosis for intestinal lymphoma is for B-cell lymphomas of low grade (75% 5 year survival), while the worst is for T cell lymphomas (25% 5 year survival).[19]

Most series report 5 year survival rates of about 50% with multimodality therapy (Table 38–4). Prognostic factors include the stage at presentation, the presence or absence of perforation, tumor resectability, the histologic subtype, and the use of multimodality therapy.[108,109]

Mediterranean lymphoma, now known as immunoproliferative small intestinal disease, is the most common type of intestinal lymphoma in the Middle East and North Africa, especially in low socioeconomic classes. Patients are usually younger and present with symptoms of malabsorption (weight loss, diarrhea, steatorrhea, and abdominal cramps). Some patients have an abdominal mass. There is a high concentration of free alpha heavy-chain protein in the serum and jejunum; as a result, this disease also is known as alpha chain disease. However, identification of this protein is not essential for the diagnosis.

The involvement of the bowel with Mediterranean lymphoma is diffuse, with widespread lymphoplasmacytoid infiltration associated with mucosal atrophy. The diagnosis usually is confirmed by peroral jejunal biopsy. Eighty-five percent of patients have lymph node involvement.[6] Treatment is with systemic chemotherapy and/or radiation, but the prognosis is poor.

The third form of lymphoma is the type that occurs in children. These tumors usually present with abdominal pain, but perforation and intussusception are not uncommon. Most of these lymphomas are of the Burkitt's type. The initial therapy includes surgical correction of the acute problem followed by chemotherapy and radiotherapy.

Hodgkin's lymphoma of the small bowel is very rare. It, too, presents as an abdominal illness requiring surgery for diagnosis and initial treatment. The mainstay of treatment is systemic chemotherapy.

SARCOMA

Sarcomas of the small intestine comprise about 9% of all the tumors and 11% of the malignancies in the small bowel.[41] There is a slight male predominance, and the diagnosis is generally made in the sixth decade of life.

Most sarcomas arise from intestinal smooth muscle, although they can arise from any mesodermal component of the bowel wall (nerve, connective tissue, vessels, fat). Leiomyosarcomas are by far the most common of the sarcomas. Other types include fibrosarcoma, hemangiopericytoma, neurofibrosarcoma, and rhabdomyosarcoma.

Infectious, genetic, and toxic mechanisms have been postulated as causative agents, and sarcomas have been observed after abdominal radiotherapy.[119] A genetic basis has been suggested by the description of a syndrome consisting of gastrointestinal leiomyosarcoma, pulmonary chondroma, and paragangliomas.[120]

The distribution of leiomyosarcomas is uniform throughout the small bowel, although there is a disproportionately high incidence in Meckel diverticula. As with other small bowel tumors, sarcomas have been described in patients with other primary tumors elsewhere.

Sarcomas can grow as intraluminal, serosal, or circumferential lesions. They are highly vascular and tend to bleed into the lumen, even though they are not mucosal. Obstruction is not as common as with adenocarcinoma. Leiomyosarcomas may grow extrinsically and eventually outgrow their vascular supply, causing central necrosis and leading to intraluminal or intraperitoneal bleeding. However, as most other intestinal malignancies, the symptoms are vague and nonspecific, resulting in a low likelihood of preoperative diagnosis.

Recurrent melena is the most common symptom. Ten percent present as an acute abdomen.[41] Unusual

TABLE 38–4. 5 YEAR SURVIVAL RATES OF PATIENTS WITH LYMPHOMA

	Period (yr)	Patients	Survival (%)
Awrich et al, 1980[71]	25	18	33
Mittal and Bodzin 1980[65]	10	5	80
Contreary et al, 1980[108]	32	24	27
Rosenfelt and Rosenberg 1980[109]	9	12	40
Waterhouse et al, 1981[73]	28	8	12
Lanzafame et al, 1982[75]	40	4	50
Weingrad et al, 1982[110]	30	15	44
Collin et al, 1982[94]	15	3	33
Williamson et al, 1983[12]	64	41	15
Al-Bahrani et al, 1983[111]	14	132	23
Rao et al, 1984[112]	12	15	42
Skudder and Schwartz, 1985[113]	15	12	33
Giuliani et al, 1985[100]	34	14	40
Dragosics et al, 1985[114]	8	13	32
Martin, 1986[79]	38	8	62
O'Rourke et al, 1986[102]	10	36	56
Shepherd et al, 1988[115]	13	7	57
Sweentenhaus et al, 1989[116]	12	19	58
Brophy and Cahoe, 1989[80]	14	7	20
Bhutani et al, 1989[63]	6	16	50
Fleming et al, 1990[117]	25	54	76
Auger and Allan, 1990[118]	8	22	50
Desa et al, 1991[82]	15	13	10
Kusumoto et al, 1992[62]	15	11	32
Baillie and Williams, 1994[83]	20	12	27
DiSario et al, 1994[84]	25	72	62

presentations have been described, including hyperemesis secondary to a BHCG-producing leiomyosarcoma,[121] ichthyosis that resolved after tumor resection,[122] and torsion of the small bowel around a sarcoma in a Meckel's diverticulum.[123]

The mean duration of symptoms before the diagnosis is established is 1 year.[119] Pain and weight loss, plus a palpable abdominal mass, suggest the possibility of sarcoma. The diagnosis is suggested by a mass effect on a barium gastrointestinal series. A fluid-filled cavity seen on CT scan may indicate the presence of central necrosis. Angiography may help localize the tumor, if bleeding is present.

Treatment involves wide resection. Extended lymphadenectomy is not routinely done because of the rarity of lymphatic spread of leiomyosarcoma. In fact, regional lymph node involvement occurs in <11% of patients.[119] A duodenal lesion may require a Whipple procedure because of the size or location of the tumor. If possible, segmental resection of leiomyosarcomas is preferred. Palliative surgery may also be indicated in selected patients. Removal of solitary lung or liver metastases should be considered, although it is not certain that these procedures improve survival.[42] Twenty to forty percent of patients have distant metastases at the time of operation.[124]

The prognosis of sarcomas depends on the tumor grade determined by the mitotic index.[125,126] Five year survival rates for low-grade tumors is 55% to 58% and 5% to 20% for high-grade tumors (Table 38–5). Adjuvant chemotherapy and radiotherapy have not proven to be of benefit.

Kaposi's sarcoma is one of the major manifestations of acquired immunodeficiency syndrome (AIDS).[130–132] Approximately one-half of homosexual men with AIDS develop Kaposi's sarcoma of the gastrointestinal tract. The involvement is multifocal, with submucosal violaceous nodules. Although these lesions are usually asymptomatic, if numerous or large, they may cause obstruction or bleeding. However, when an AIDS patient presents with abdominal pain, one also must consider a concurrent infection as the causative agent. The diagnosis of Kaposi's sarcoma of the intestine should be suspected from barium contrast studies, endoscopy, or CT scanning. The treatment is conservative, unless there is certainty that the lesions are the sole cause of significant abdominal symptoms.

MISCELLANEOUS MALIGNANCIES

The tumors already mentioned comprise more than 95% of the small bowel malignancies. Other tumors sporadically reported include fibrosarcoma, angiosarcoma, rhabdomyosarcoma, liposarcoma, and neurogenic tumors. The principles of diagnosis and treatment are similar to those already mentioned, including wide segmental resection with the mesentery.

Neuroendocrine tumors of the duodenum (gastrinomas, insulinomas, and somatostatinomas) also warrant comment. Gastrinomas have been shown to be quite common in the duodenum in patients with Zollinger-Ellison syndrome. Thompson and associates have recommended duodenotomy as one component of the exploration for sporadic gastrinoma, if no pancreatic tumor is found, and in patients with the MEN-I syndrome, regardless of pancreatic findings.[133] If a duodenal tumor is found, local enucleation plus regional lymph node excision is recommended. Although a discussion of the management of these tumors is far beyond the scope of this chapter, new diagnostic techniques involving radiolabeled somatostatin scintigraphy and endoscopic ultrasound will undoubtedly increase the number of these tumors identified in the proximal small intestine.

■ METASTATIC DISEASE

Melanoma is the most common tumor that metastasizes to the small bowel. Other tumors with the potential to spread to the bowel include carcinomas of the lung, breast, cervix, and kidney. Tumors that often metastasize to the small bowel transperitoneally include colorectal, ovarian, gastric, pancreatic, and bladder cancers.

Treatment of these metastatic diseases is purely for palliative purposes, and the prognosis is very poor.

TABLE 38–5. 5 YEAR SURVIVAL RATES OF PATIENTS WITH SARCOMA

	Period (yr)	Patients	Survival (%)
Awrich et al, 1980[71]	25	10	38
Mittal and Bodzin, 1980[65]	10	3	33
Norberg and Emas, 1981[72]	34	9	11
Waterhouse et al, 1982[73]	28	12	50
Lanzafame et al, 1982[75]	40	15	33
Chiotasso et al, 1982[125]	30	28	42
Shiu et al, 1983[127]	25	18	32
Johnson et al, 1985[78]	28	12	25
Zollinger et al, 1986[2]	20	10	10
Martin, 1986[79]	38	33	18
Cicarelli et al, 1987[64]	14	8	12
McGrath et al, 1987[128]	34	14	40
Brophy and Cahoe, 1989[80]	14	11	40
Bhutani et al, 1989[63]	6	8	50
Kimura et al, 1991[129]	24	16	50
Dougherty et al, 1991[126]	24	14	18
Kusumoto et al, 1992[62]	15	8	57
DiSario et al, 1994[84]	25	36	45

■ CONDITIONS MIMICKING SMALL BOWEL NEOPLASMS

Several conditions may have the appearance, and mimic the symptoms of small bowel neoplasms. One of the most important of these is endometriosis, which can cause obstruction, adhesions, and serosal thickening. Endometriosis usually is identified at laparoscopy or laparotomy, and the diagnosis is established by biopsy. The treatment of endometriosis is nonoperative, unless mechanical obstruction mandates surgical intervention.

Other such conditions include Crohn's disease, which can present as an inflammatory mass in the small bowel. Malacoplakia is a granulomatous process usually described in the bladder, but which is seen rarely in the intestines. Grossly, there are ulcers with yellow-brown plaques. Malacoplakia may cause abdominal pain and diarrhea, and in rare advanced cases, may obstruct, perforate, or cause fistulas.[51]

Whipple's disease, a storage disorder of accumulation of fat in the lymphatic channels, causes nodularity or cysts in the proximal gut. It may cause malabsorption symptoms and simulate a picture of small intestinal neoplasia.[51]

Another such condition is radiation enteritis, manifest by scarring and stenosis of the intestine. This process may be accompanied with symptoms of obstruction, malabsorption, and/or blood loss.

Finally, other conditions simulating intestinal tumors are splenosis, congenital pancreatic rests, and enteric duplications.

REFERENCES

1. Herbsman H, Wetstein L, Rosen Y, et al. Tumors of the small intestine. In: Ravitch MM (ed), *Current Problems in Surgery,* vol 17. Chicago, IL: Yearbook Medical; 1980
2. Zollinger RM, Sternfeld W, Schreiber H. Primary neoplasms of the small intestine. *Am J Surg* 1986;151:654–658
3. Cabano F, Cebrelli C, Barbiggia C, et al. 1 tumori maligni primitivi del piccolo intestine. *Minerva Chirurgica* 1990; 45(11):821–826
4. Ouriel KK, Adams JT. Adenocarcinoma of the small bowel. *Am J Surg* 1984;147:56–71
5. Sarr MG. Small intestinal neoplasms. In: Greenfield LJ, et al. (eds), *Surgery: Scientific Principles and Practice,* 1993: 753–763
6. Amer MH, El-Akkad D. Gastrointestinal lymphoma in adults: clinical features and management of 300 cases. *Gastroenterology* 1994;106:846–858
7. Wattenberg LW. Carcinogen-detoxifying mechanisms in the GI tract. *Gastroenterology* 1966;51:932
8. Feldman M. Multiple primary carcinomas of the small intestine. *Am J Digest Dis* 1953;20:1
9. Lowenfils AB. Why are small bowel tumors so rare? *Lancet* 1973;1:24
10. Wattenberg LW. Studies of polycyclichydrocarbon hydroxylases of the intestine possibly related to cancer. *Cancer* 1971;28:99
11. Wilson JM, Melvin DB, Gray GF, et al. Primary malignancies of the small bowel: a report of 96 cases and review of the literature. *Ann Surg* 1974;180:175–179
12. Williamson RC, Welch CE, Malt RA. Adenocarcinoma and lymphoma of the small intestine. *Ann Surg* 1983; 197:172–178
13. Ross RK, Hartnett NM, Bernstein L, et al. Epidemiology of adenocarcinomas of the small intestine: is bile a small bowel carcinogen? *Br J Cancer* 1991;63:143–145
14. Scudamore CH, Freeman HJ. Effects of small bowel transection, resection, or bypass in 1,2-dimethylhydrazine-induced rat intestinal neoplasia. *Gastroenterology* 1983; 84:725–731
15. Sellner F. Investigations on the signficance of the adenoma-carcinoma sequence in the small bowel. *Cancer* 1990;66:702–715
16. Castellano G, Moreno D, Galvao O, et al. Malignant lymphoma of jejunum with common variable hypogammaglobulinemia and diffuse nodular hyperplasia of the small intestine: a case study and literature review. *J Clin Gastroenterol* 1992;15(2):128–135
17. Simpson S, Traube J, Riddell RH. The histologic appearance of dysplasia (precarcinomatous change) in Crohn's disease of the small and large intestine. *Gastroenterology* 1981;81:492–501
18. Trier JS. Celiac sprue. *N Engl J Med* 1991;325(24):1709–19
19. Domizio P, Owen RA, Shepherd NA, et al. Primary lymphoma of the small intestine: a clinicopathological study of 119 cases. *Am J Surg Pathol* 1993;17(5):429–442
20. Altemeier WA. In: Discussion of Dozois RR, Judd ES, Dahlia OC, et al. The Peutz-Jeghers syndrome: is there a predisposition to the development of intestinal malignancies? *Arch Surg* 1969;98:509–517
21. Spigelman AD, Murday V, Phillips RKS. Cancer and the Peutz-Jeghers syndrome. *Gut* 1989;30:1588–90
22. Schaldenbrand JD, Appelman HD. Solitary solid stromal gastrointestinal tumors in von Recklinghausen's disease with minimal smooth muscle differentiation. *Hum Pathol* 1984;15:229–232
23. Jones TJ, Marshall TL. Neurofibromatosis and small bowel adenocarcinoma: an unrecognized association. *Gut* 1987;28:1173–1176
24. Hochberg FH, DaSilva AB, Galdabini J, et al. Gastrointestinal involvement in von Recklinghausen's neurofibromatosis. *Neurology* 1974;24:1144–1151
25. Ishizaki Y, Tada Y, Ishida T, et al. Leiomyosarcoma of the small intestine associated with von Recklinghausen's disease: report of a case. *Surgery* 1991;111:706–710
26. Fernandez MT, Puig L, Capella G, et al. von Recklinghausen neurofibromatosis with carcinoid tumor and submucosal leiomyomas of the duodenum. *Neurofibromatosis* 1988;1:294–298
27. Drew WL, Miner RC, Ziegler JL, et al. Cytometalovirus and Kaposi's sarcoma in young homosexual men. *Lancet* 1982;1:125
28. Hanto WH, Frizzera G, Purtillo DT, et al. Clinical spectrum of lymphoproliferative disorders in renal transplant

recipients and evidence for the role of Epstein Barr virus. *Cancer Res* 1981;41:4253–4261

29. Ioachim HL, Cooper MC, Hellman GC. Lymphomas in men at high risk for acquired immunodeficiency syndrome (AIDS). *Cancer* 1985;55:2831–2842

30. Alexander JW, Altemeir WA. Association of primary neoplasms of the small intestine with other neoplastic growths. *Ann Surg* 1968;167:958–964

31. Darling RC, Welch CE. Tumors of the small intestine. *N Engl J Med* 1959;260:397

32. Pagtalunan RJG, Mayo CW, Dockerty MB. Primary malignant tumors of the small intestine. *Am J Surg* 1964;108:13–18

33. Vinik AI, McLeod MK, Fig LM, et al. Clinical features, diagnosis and localization of carcinoid tumors and their management. *Gastroenterol Clin North Am* 1989;18(4): 865–897

34. Silberman H, Crichlow RW, Caplan HS. Neoplasms of the small bowel. *Ann Surg* 1974;180:157–161

35. Lewis BS, Kornbluth A, Waye JD. Small bowel tumors: yield of enteroscopy. *Gut* 1991;32:763–765

36. Nakamura S, Iida M, Nakao Y, et al. Diagnostic value of push-type jejunal endoscopy in primary jejunal carcinoma. *Surg Endosc* 1993;7(3):188–190

37. Thompson JN, Hemingway AP, McPherson GAD, et al. Obscure gastrointestinal hemorrhage of small bowel origin. *BMJ* 1984;288:1663–1665

38. Trible W, Hoffman BJ, Cunningham JT. Use of endoscopic ultrasonography for evaluation of painless jaundice (Review). *Southern Medical J.* 1993;86(3):358–360 (Abstract)

39. Dorr U, Rath U, Schurmann G, et al. Somatostatin receptor scintigraphy: a new imaging procedure for the specific demonstration of carcinoids of the small intestine. *Rofo. Fortschritte auf dem Gebiete der Rontgenstrahlen und der Neven Bildgebenden Verfahren.* 1993;158(1):67–73 (Abstract)

40. Ashley SW, Wells SA Jr. Tumors of the small intestine. *Semin Oncol* 1988;15(2):116–128

41. Coit DG. Cancer on the small intestine. In: DeVita VT Jr, et al (eds), Cancer: Principles and Practice of Oncology, 1993 (4th ed) Vol 1, p. 915–928

42. Starr GF, Dockerty MB. Leiomyomas and leiomyosarcomas of the small intestine. *Cancer* 1955;8:101–111

43. Bjork KJ, Davis CJ, Nagorney DM, et al. Duodenal villous tumors. *Arch Surg* 1990;125:961–965

44. Itsuno M, Makiyama K, Omagari K, et al. Carcinoma of duodenal bulb arising from the Brunner's gland. *Gastroenterol Jpn* 1993;28(1):118–125 (Abstract)

45. Mayo CW, Pagtalunan RJG, Brown DJ. Lipoma of the alimentary tract. *Surgery* 1963;53:598

46. Ravitch MM. Discussion of: Carter BN, Horsley GW, Horsley JS, et al. A new form of diffuse familial polyposis. *Ann Surg* 1968;167:942–948

47. Carter BN, Horsley GW, Horsley JS, et al. A new form of diffuse familial polyposis: a probable genetic explanation. *Ann Surg* 1968;167:942–946

48. Cronkhite LW, Canada WJ. Generalized gastrointestinal polyposis, pigmentation, alopecia and onychotrophia. *N Engl J Med* 1955;252:1011

49. Gold BM, Bagla S, Zarrabi MH. Radiologic manifestations of Cowden's disease. *AJR Am J Roentgen* 1980;135:385–387

50. Burnett JW, Goldner R, Calton GJ. Cowden disease. Report of two additional cases. *Br J Dermatol* 1975;93: 329–336

51. Fenoglio-Preiser CM, Pascal RR, Perzin KH. Tumors of the intestines. In: *Atlas of Tumor Pathology*, 2nd Series, Fascicle 27. Washington, DC: Armed Forces Institute of Pathology; 1990

52. Ross JRE, Mara JE. Small bowel polyps and carcinoma in multiple intestinal polyposis. *Arch Surg* 1974;108:736

53. Gardner EJ. Genetic and clinical study of intestinal polyposis: predisposing factor for carcinoma of colon and rectum. *Am J Hum Genet* 1951;3:167

54. Gill WJ, Wilken BJ. Diffuse gastrointestinal polyposis associated with hypoproteinemia. *JR Coll Surg Endinb* 1967; 12:149

55. Sachatello CR, Pickren JW, Grace JT. Generalized juvenile gastrointestinal polyposis: a hereditary syndrome. *Gastroenterology* 1970;58:699–708

56. Peutz JLA. Very remarkable case of familial polyposis of mucous membranes of the intestinal tract and nasal pharynx accompanied by peculiar pigmentation of skin and membrane. *Ned M Aandschr Geneeskd* 1921;10:134

57. Jegher H, McKusick VA, Katz KH. Generalized intestinal polyposis and melanin spots of oral mucosa, lips and digits. *N Engl J Med* 1949;241:993

58. Flageole H, Raptis S, Trudel JL, et al. Progression toward malignancy of hamartomas in a patient with Peutz-Jeghers Syndrome: case report and literature review. *Can J Surg* 1994;37:231–236

59. Manley KA, Skyring AP. Some heritable causes of gastrointestinal disease. *Arch Intern Med* 1961;107:182

60. Torres D. Multiple sebaceous tumors. *Arch Dermatol* 1968; 98:549

61. Haddad HM, Wilkins L. Congential anomalies associated with gonadol aplasia: review of 55 cases. *Pediatrics* 1958; 23:885

62. Kusumoto H, Takahashi I, Yoshida M, et al. Primary malignant tumors of the small intestine: analysis of 40 Japanese patients. *J Surg Onc* 1992;50:139–143

63. Bhutani, Manoop S, Gopalswamy N. Letter to the Editor. *Am J Gastroenterol* 1994;89:460

64. Ciccarelli O, Welch JP, Kent G. Primary malignant tumors of the small bowel: the Hartford Hospital Experience, 1969–1983. *Am J Surg* 1987;153:350–354

65. Mittal VK, Bodzin JH. Primary malignant tumors of the small bowel. *Am J Surg* 1980;140:396

66. Neugut AI, Santos J. The association between cancers of the small and large bowel. *Cancer Epidemiol Biomarkers Prevent* 1993;2(6):551–553

67. Lashner BA. Risk factors for small bowel cancer in Crohn's disease. *Dig Dis Sci* 1992;37(8):1179–1184

68. Ribeiro MD, Greenstein AJ, Heiman TM, et al. Adenocarcinoma of the small intestine in Crohn's disease. *Surg Gynecol Obstet* 1991;173:343–349

69. Senay E, Sachar DB, Keohane M, et al. Small bowel carcinoma in Crohn's disease: distinguishing features and risk factors. *Cancer* 1989;63(2):360–363

70. O'Rourke MGE, Lancashire RP, Vattoune JR. Lymphoma of the small intestine. *Aust NZJ Surg* 1986;56:351–355

71. Awrich AE, Irish CE, Vetto RM, et al. A twenty-five year ex-

perience with primary malignant tumors of the small intestine. *Surg Gynecol Obstet* 1980;151:9–14

72. Norberg K, Emas S. Primary tumors of the small intestine. *Am J Surg* 1981;142:569–573

73. Waterhouse G, Skudlarick J, Adkins RB. A clinical review of small bowel neoplasms. *South Med J* 1981;74:1202–1203

74. Adler SN, Lyon DT, Sullivan PD. Adenocarcinoma of the small bowel clinical features, similarity to regional enteritis, and analysis of 338 documented cases. *Am J Gastroenterol* 1982;77:326–330

75. Lanzafame RJ, Long JE, Hinshaw JR. Primary cancer of the small bowel. *NY State J Med* 1982;8:1325–1329

76. Barclay THC, and Schapira DV. Malignant tumors of the small intestine. *Cancer* 1983;51:878–81

77. Cooper BT, Read AE. Small intestinal lymphoma. *World J Surg* 1985;9:930–937

78. Johnson AM, Harman PK, Hanks JB. Primary small bowel malignancies. *Am Surg* 1985;51:31–36

79. Martin RG. Malignant tumors of the small intestine. *Surg Clin North Am* 1986;66:779–785

80. Brophy C, Cahow CE. Primary small bowel malignant tumors. *Am Surg* 1989;55:408–412

81. Lioe TF, Biggart JD. Primary adenocarcinoma of the jejunum and ileum: clinicopathological review of 25 cases. *J Clin Pathol* 1990;43:533–536

82. Desa L, Bridger J, Grace PA, et al. Primary jejunoileal tumors: a review of 45 cases. *World J Surg* 1991;15:81–87

83. Baillie CT, Williams A. Small bowel tumors: a diagnostic challenge. *J R Coll Surg Edinb* 1994;39(1):8–12

84. DiSario JA, Burt RW, Vargas H, et al. Small bowel cancer: epidemiological and clinical characteristics from a population-based registry. *Am J Gastroenterol* 1994;89(5):699–701

85. Lubarsch O. Uber den primaren Krebs des ileum nebst bemerkungen uber das gleichzeitige vorkommen von Krebs und tuberculos. *Virchows Arch Pathol* 1888;111:281

86. Obendorfer S. Karzinoide tumoren des dunndarms. *Z Pathol* 1907;1:426

87. Kramer R. Adenoma of bronchus. *Ann Otol Rhinol Laryngol* 1930;39:689

88. Rappaport MM, Green AA, Page H. Partial purification of the vasoconstrictor in beef serum. *J Biol Chem* 1948;174:735–741

89. Thorson AH, Biorck G, Bjorkman G, et al. Malignant carconoid of the small intestine with metastases to the liver, valvular disease of the right side of the heart, peripheral vasomotor symptoms, bronchoconstriction, and an unusual type of cyanosis: a clinical and pathologic syndrome. *Am Heart J* 1948;47:795–817

90. Erspamer V, Asero B. Identification of enteramine, the specific hormone of the enterochromaffin cell system, as 5-hyeroxytryptamine. *Nature* 1952;169:800

91. Kusumoto H, Yoshitake H, Mochida K, et al. Adenocarcinoma in Meckel's diverticulum: report of a case and review of 30 cases in the English and Japanese literature. *Am J Gastroenterol* 1992;87:910–913

92. Makridis C, Oberg K, Juhlin C, et al. Surgical treatment of midgut carcinoid tumors. *World J Surg* 1990;14:377–385

93. Moertel CG. Treatment of the carcinoid tumor and the malignant carcinoid syndrome. *J Clin Oncol* 1983;1(11)727

94. Collin CF, Amerson JR, et al. Primary malignant small bowel tumors: clinical imitators of benign disease. *Surg Gastroenterol* 1982;1:203–211

95. Zeitels J, Naunteim K, Kaplan EL, et al. Carcinoid tumors—a 37 year experience. *Arch Surg* 1982;117:732–737

96. Peck JJ, Shields AB, Boyden AM, et al. Carcinoid tumors of the ileum. *Am J Surg* 1983;146:124–132

97. Strodel WE, Talpos G, Eckhauser F, et al. Surgical therapy for small bowel carcinoid tumors. *Arch Surg* 1983;118:391–397

98. Dawes L, Schulte WJ, Condon RE. Carcinoid tumors. *Arch Surg* 1984;119:375–378

99. Thompson GB, vanHeerden JA, Martin JK, et al. Carcinoid tumors of the gastrointestinal tract: presentation, management and prognosis. *Surgery* 1985;98:1054–1063

100. Giuliani A, Caporale A, Teneriello F, et al. Primary tumors of the small intestine. *Int Surg* 1985;331–334

101. Olney JR, Urdaneta LF, Al-Jurf AS, et al. Carcinoid tumors of the gastrointestinal tract. *Am Surg* 1985;51:37–41

102. O'Rourke MGE, Lancashire RP, Valtoune JR. Carcinoid of the small intestine. *Aust NZJ Surg* 1986;56:405–408

103. Sjoblom SM. Clinical presentation and prognosis of gastrointestinal carcinoid tumors. *Scand J Gastroenterol* 1988;23:779–787

104. Nwiloh JO, Phillarisetty S, Moscovic EA, et al. Carcinoid tumors. *J Surg Oncol* 1990;45:261–264

105. McDermott E, Guduric B, Brennan MF. Prognostic variables in gastrointestinal carcinoid tumors. *Brit J Surg* 1991;81(7):1007–1009

106. Hatzitheoklitos E, Buchler MW, Friess H, et al. Carcinoid of ampulla of Vater: clinical characteristics and morphological features (Review). *Cancer* 1994;73(6):1580–1588

107. Dawson IMP, Cornes JS, Morson BC. Primary malignant lymphoid tumors of the intestinal tract: report of 37 cases with a study of factors influencing prognosis. *Br J Surg* 1961;49:80–89

108. Contreary K, Nance FC, Becker WF. Primary lymphoma of the gastrointestinal tract. *Ann Surg* 1980;191:593–598

109. Rosenfelt F, Rosenberg SA. Diffuse histiocytic lymphoma presenting with gastrointestinal tract lesions—the Stanford experience. *Cancer* 1980;45:2188–2193

110. Weingrad DN, Decosse JJ, Sherlock P, et al. Primary gastrointestinal lymphoma: a 30 year review. *Cancer* 1982;49:1258–1265

111. Al-Bahrani ZR, Al-Mondhiry H, Bakir F, et al. Clinical and pathologic subtypes of primary intestinal lymphoma. *Cancer* 1983;52:1666–1672

112. Rao AR, Kagan AR, Potyk D, et al. Management of gastrointestinal lymphoma. *Am J Clin Oncol* 1984;7:213–219

113. Skudder PA Jr, Schwartz SI. Primary lymphoma of the gastrointestinal tract. *Surg Gynecol Obstet* 1985;160:5–8

114. Dragosics B, Bauer P, Radaszkierwicz T. Primary gastrointestinal non-Hodgkin's lymphoma—a retrospective clinicopathologic study of 150 cases. *Cancer* 1985;55:1060–1073

115. Shepherd FA, Evans WK, Kutas G, et al. Chemotherapy following surgery for stages IE and IIE non-Hodgkins

lymphoma of the gastrointestinal tract. *J Clin Oncol* 1988; 6:253–260

116. Sweentenhaus JW, Mead GM, Wright DH, et al. Involvement of the ileocecal region by non-Hodgkin's lymphoma in adults: clinical factors and results of treatment. *Br J Cancer* 1989;60:366–369

117. Fleming ID, Turk PS, Murphy SB, et al. Surgical implications of primary gastrointestinal lymphoma of childhood. *Arch Surg* 1990;125:252–256

118. Auger MJ, Allan NC. Primary ileocecal lymphoma. *Cancer* 1990;65:358–361

119. Licht JD, Weissman LB, and Antman K. Gastrointestinal sarcomas. *Semin Oncol* 1988;15(2):181–188

120. Carney JA. The triad of gastric epitheloid leiomyosarcoma, pulmonary chondroma, and functional extradrenal paraganglioma: a five year review. *Medicine* 1983; 62:159–169

121. Meredith RF, Wagman LD, Piper JA, et al. Beta-chain human chorionic gonadotropin producing leiomyosarcoma of the small intestine. *Cancer* 1986;58: 131–135

122. Majekodunmi AE, Femi-Pearse D. Ichthyosis: early manifestation of intestinal leiomyosarcoma. *Br J Med* 1974; 3:724

123. Niv Y, Abu-Avid S, Kopelman C, et al. Torsion of leiomyosarcoma of Meckel diverticulum. *Am J Gastroenterol* 1986;81:288–291

124. Akwari OE, Dozois RR, Weiland LH, et al. Leiomyosarcoma of the small and large bowel. *Cancer* 1978;42: 1375–1384

125. Chiotasso PJP, Fazio VW. Prognostic factors of 28 leio-

myosarcomas of the small intestine. *Surg Gynecol Obstet* 1982;155:197–202

126. Dougherty MJ, Compton C, Talbert M, et al. Sarcomas of the gastrointestinal tract: separation into favorable and unfavorable prognostic groups by mitotic count. *Ann Surg* 1991;214:569–574

127. Shiu MH, Farr GH, Egeli RA, et al. Myosarcomas of the small and large intestine: a clinicopathological study. *J Surg Oncol* 1983;24:67–72

128. McGrath PC, Neifeld JP, Lawrence W, et al. Gastrointestinal sarcomas: analysis of prognostic factors. *Ann Surg* 1987;206:706–710

129. Kimura H, Yonemura Y, Kadoya N, et al. Prognostic factors in primary gastrointestinal leiomyosarcoma: a retrospective study. *World J Surg* 1991;15:771–777

130. Saltz RK, Kurtz RC, Lightdale CJ, et al. Kaposi's sarcoma: gastrointestinal involvement correlation with skin findings and immunologic function. *Dig Dis Sci* 1984;29: 817–823

131. Giraldo G, Beth E, Huang ES. Kaposi's sarcoma and its relationship to cytomegalovirus: III. CMV DNA and CMV-early antigens in Kaposi's sarcoma. *Int J Can* 1980; 26:23–29

132. Friedman SL, Wright TL, Altman DF. Gastrointestinal Kaposi's sarcoma in patients with acquired immunodeficiency syndrome: endoscopic and autopsy findings. *Gastroenterology* 1985;89:102–108

133. Thompson NW, Pasieka J, Fukuuchi A. Duodenal gastrinomas, duodenotomy and duodenal exploration in the surgical management of Zollinger-Ellison syndrome. *World J Surg* 1993;17:455–462

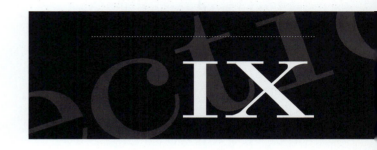

APPENDIX AND COLON

39

Appendix and Appendectomy

Harold Ellis ▪ *L. Keith Nathanson*

■ HISTORY

The first appendicectomy was performed by Claudius Amyand, surgeon to Westminster and St. George's Hospitals and Sergeant Surgeon to George II. In 1736, he operated on a boy 11 years of age who had a right scrotal hernia accompanied by a fistula. Within the scrotum was found the appendix, perforated by a pin. The appendix was ligated and all or, more likely, part of it was removed, with recovery of the patient.

In 1755, Heister recognized that the appendix might be the site of acute primary inflammation. He described an autopsy on the body of a criminal who had been executed and wrote:

> When about to demonstrate the large bowel, I found the vermiform appendix of the cecum preternaturally black. As I was about to separate it, its membranes parted and discharged two to three spoonfuls of matter. It is probable that this person might have had some pain in the part.

In 1824, Loyer-Villermany gave a presentation to the Royal Academy of Medicine in Paris, entitled "Observations of Use in the Inflammatory Conditions of the Cecal Appendix," in which he described two examples of acute appendicitis leading to death. In both cases, the appendix was found at autopsy to be black and gangrenous, whereas the cecum was scarcely involved. Three years later, these observations were confirmed by Melier. Unfortunately, at this stage the pathologic picture became obscured. The writings of Husson and

Dance in 1827, Goldbeck in 1830 and, most powerfully of all, Dupuytren, in 1835, developed the concept of inflammation arising in the cellular tissue surrounding the cecum; it was Goldbeck who invented the term *perityphlitis*, which did much to delay the progress of the understanding of this disease.

The first textbook to give a description of the symptoms that accompanied inflammation and perforation of the appendix was published by Bright and Addison in 1839. The terms "typhlitis" and "perityphlitis" remained in use until the end of the nineteenth century. It was Fitz, professor of medicine at Harvard, who in 1886 gave a lucid and logical description of the clinical features and described in detail the pathologic changes of the disease; he was also the first to use the term *appendicitis*. He wrote:

> In most fatal cases of typhlitis, the caecum is intact whilst the appendix is ulcerated and perforated. The question should be entertained of immediate opening. If any good result is to arise from such treatment it must be applied early.

The evolution of the operative treatment of appendicitis proceeded significantly when Hancock, in London, successfully drained an appendix abscess in a female patient, 30 years of age, who was in her eighth month of pregnancy. In 1848, he wrote:

> It may be premature to argue from the result of one case, but I trust that the time will come when this plan will be successfully employed in other cases of peritonitis terminating in effusion, which usually end fatally.

Parker of New York advocated earlier incision of appendix abscesses in 1867; after the publication of his paper, many similar accounts were published.

From the priority point of view, Shepherd showed, in 1880, that Tait of Birmingham, England operated on a patient with gangrenous appendicitis and removed the appendix, with recovery of the patient. Tait, however, did not record this case until 1890. Credit for the first published account of appendectomy must go to Kronlein in 1886, although the patient, 17 years of age, died 2 days later. In 1887, Morton of Philadelphia successfully diagnosed and excised an acutely inflamed appendix lying within an abscess cavity. Two years later, McBurney, in New York, pioneered early diagnosis and early operative intervention, and also devised the muscle-splitting incision named after him.[2] Early intervention was still further popularized by the teachings of Murphy, of Chicago. Both these surgeons pioneered the removal of the appendix before perforation had taken place.

It soon became evident that, although the results of appendectomy for the acutely inflamed unperforated appendix were satisfactory, the operative death rate for the later cases of perforated appendix with peritonitis was distressingly high. Ochsner, in Chicago, and Sherren, at The London Hospital, were both advocates of conservative treatment in late cases, in the early years of the 20th century. The discovery of antibiotics, fortunately, resolved the controversy between the schools of conservative and active surgery in these cases.

For detailed accounts of the history of appendicitis, the reader is referred to the fascinating books by Sir Zachary Cope and Dr. Ralph Major.[1a,1b]

■ ANATOMY

The appendix arises from the posteromedial aspect of the cecum, about 2.5 cm below the ileocecal valve. It is the only organ in the body that has no constant anatomic position; in fact, its only constant feature is its mode of origin from the cecum, where it arises from the site at which the three teniae coli coalesce. It varies considerably in length, from 1 to 25 cm, but it averages 5 to 10 cm. The various positions of the appendix are as follows: paracolic (the appendix lies in the sulcus on the outer side of the cecum), retrocecal (the organ lies behind the cecum and may even be totally or partially extraperitoneal), preileal, postileal, promontoric (the tip of the organ points toward the promontory of the sacrum), pelvic (the appendix dips into the pelvic cavity), and midinguinal (subcecal). The retrocecal position is the most common at autopsy. Wakeley, in an analysis of 10 000 cases at postmortem examination, gave the location of the appendix as follows: retrocecal,

65.28%; pelvic, 31.01%; subcecal, 2.26%; preileal, 1%; and right paracolic and postileal 0.4%[3] (Fig 39–1). However, we have demonstrated at computerized tomography that the retroileal appendix appears to occur much more frequently in living subjects.[4]

Williamson and associates found that of 105 retrocecal appendixes removed at operation, 12 (11.4%) extended retroperitoneally.[5] In this position the appendix may extend upward as far as the kidney and indeed, in 2 of these 12 cases, the patient experienced pain in the right flank.

The appendix may be situated in the left lower quadrant of the abdomen, in cases of transposition of the viscera. Here the clue may be the observation that the patient has dextrocardia; this author has correctly diagnosed and operated on such a case. A particularly long appendix also may extend over into the left side of the abdomen and, if inflamed, produce left iliac fossa pain. In cases of malrotation of the bowel, where the cecum fails to descend to its normal position, the appendix may be found in the epigastrium, abutting against the stomach or beneath the right lobe of the liver.

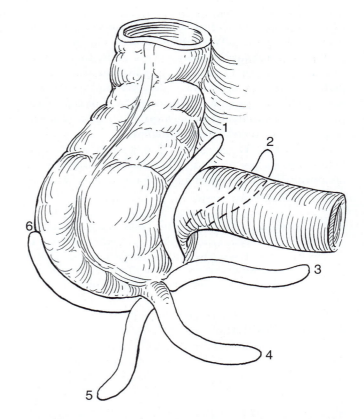

Figure 39–1. Top: Various positions that the appendix can occupy: (1) preileal; (2) postileal; (3) promontoric; (4) pelvic; (5) subcaecal; (6) paracolic or precaecal. (Redrawn from Wakeley CP. The position of the vermiform appendix as ascertained by analysis of 10 000 cases. *J Anat* 1933;67:277). After Waldron.

Robinson, in reporting a case of congenital absence of the appendix, was able to collect only 68 other examples, a figure sufficiently indicative of the great rarity of this condition.[6]

Duplication of the appendix, a subject well reviewed by Khanna,[7] is an anomaly of extreme rarity: fewer than 100 cases have been reported. Wallbridge classified duplication of the appendix into three types: type A comprises partial duplication of the appendix on a single cecum[8]; type B has a single cecum with two completely separate appendixes (this is further subdivided into type B1, which is also called "birdlike appendix" because of its resemblance to the normal arrangement in birds, where there are two appendixes symmetrically placed on either side of the ileocaecal valve, and type B2, in which one appendix arises from the usual site on the cecum, with another rudimentary appendix arising from the cecum along the line of one of the teniae coli); and type C, where there are two ceca, each of which bears an appendix. Tinckler described a unique case of a triple appendix, associated with a double penis and ectopia vesicae.[9]

Embryologically, the appendix is part of the cecum, of which it forms the distal end and which, histologically, it closely resembles, with the exception that it contains an excess of lymphoid tissue in the submucous layer. The mesentery of the appendix is contiguous with the lower leaf of the mesentery of the small intestine, and it passes behind the terminal ileum. The appendicular artery runs in the free border of the mesentery of the appendix and is a branch of the ileocolic artery (Fig 39–2). This artery represents the entire arterial supply of the organ and therefore, thrombosis of this artery, in acute appendicitis, inevitably results in gangrene and subsequent perforation. This situation is in contrast to acute cholecystitis, in which the rich collateral blood supply of the gallbladder, from its bed in the liver, accounts for the comparative rarity of gangrene.

The veins from the appendix drain into the ileocolic vein, which in turn empties into the superior mesenteric vein. A variable number of slender lymphatic channels traverse the mesoappendix to empty into the ileocecal nodes.

■ ACUTE APPENDICITIS

INCIDENCE

Acute appendicitis is the most common cause of "acute surgical abdomen" in the United Kingdom, but because notification of the disease is not required, the exact incidence is unknown.

The Hospital Inpatient Inquiry, which estimates the total hospital inpatient discharges in England and Wales,

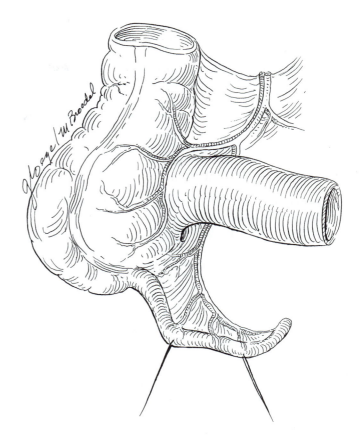

Figure 39–2. The appendix and its blood supply.

gave the annual estimated total of acute appendicitis, based on a one-tenth sample, as 50 115.[10]

Pieper and Kager, in a careful study from Sweden, estimated a yearly incidence of 1.33 cases of appendicitis per thousand of the male population and 0.99 per thousand of the female population (this difference is statistically significant, $P=.002$).[11] In this study of 971 cases, the ages of the patients ranged from 1 to 89 years, with a median of 22 years. Twenty-five percent of the patients were younger than 14 years, and 75% younger than 33. Although these authors found no evidence of a fall in the incidence of acute appendicitis, other studies have indicated a steady decline in appendicitis and appendectomy. Noer reported a decrease in the incidence of acute appendicitis from 1.3 per thousand to 0.5 per thousand over a 30 year period, from 1943 to 1972, in a study of a well-defined population in Norway.[12]

Burgess and Done studied the total number of appendectomies performed over a 15 year period from 1972 to 1986 at one large general hospital in the North of England.[13] During this period there was >50% reduction in the number of these operations, from approximately 1000 cases annually to between 400 to 500.

Such figures need cautious interpretation. Many

studies do not differentiate between all cases of appendectomy and those in which the diagnosis of acute appendicitis was confirmed. Others do not confirm the diagnosis by pathological examination. A decline in the rate may reflect a change in operative policy or may reflect an improvement in diagnostic ability of the surgical team. All these factors must be taken into consideration before a true decline in the incidence of acute appendicitis is established.

GEOGRAPHIC DISTRIBUTION

Appendicitis is most frequently observed in North America, the British Isles, Australia, New Zealand, and among white South Africans. It is rare in most of Asia, Central Africa, and among the Eskimos. When people from these areas migrate to the Western world or change to a Western diet, appendicitis becomes prevalent, suggesting that the distribution of this disease is determined environmentally rather than genetically. It is undoubtedly much more common among meat-eating white races and relatively rare in those races that habitually live on a bulk cellulose diet.

Many surgeons believe that there is a familial tendency in this disease that could be explained by an inherited malformation of the organ. However, the incidence of a large number of cases in the same family can equally be explained by the common nature of this disease. Andersson and associates compared 29 children between 5 and 15 years of age who had acute appendicitis with 29 control subjects. Twenty in the study group and four of the control subjects gave a history of appendicitis in parents or siblings.

PATHOLOGY

Cases of appendicitis are best classified as (1) acute appendicitis without perforation, and (2) acute appendicitis with perforation. The latter includes acute appendicitis with peritonitis, and acute appendicitis with local abscess (appendix mass).

Acute appendicitis is not associated with any specific bacterial, viral, or protozoal invader. The bacteria in the inflamed organ are those of the normal bowel flora, suggesting secondary invasion of damaged tissue from the lumen of the bowel. A detailed study of the bacterial population of 50 inflamed appendixes gave both aerobic and anaerobic isolates from all cases.[15] Anaerobic bacteria were found more frequently than aerobic (1412 versus 96 isolates). *Escherichia coli* was the most common aerobic bacterium (47 out of 50 patients). Ten patients also harbored other aerobic gram-negative rods, including *Klebsiella, Proteus,* and *Pseudomonas.* Enterococci (*Streptococcus faecalis* and *S faecium*) were found in 15 patients, and other streptococci (*S mitior, S milleri,* and *S salivarius*) were found in 21 patients. Of the anaerobic strains, *Bacteroides fragilis* predominated. Anaerobic gram-positive cocci were next in frequency, and *Clostridium perfringes* was cultivated from nine patients.

Examination of a series of fresh specimens of acutely inflamed appendixes will show that types of inflammation fall into two groups. The first is a "catarrhal" inflammation of the whole organ, and the second is characterized by an obstruction of the appendix beyond which there is acute inflammation, distention with pus, and, in later cases, progression to gangrene and eventually, perforation.

Catarrhal appendicitis is initially a mucosal and submucosal inflammation. In early cases, the appendix may appear normal externally or may merely show hyperemia. When the appendix is slit open, however, the mucosa will be seen to be thickened, edematous, and reddened; later it becomes studded with dark brown hemorrhagic infarcts, patches of grey-green gangrene, or small ulcers. Eventually the whole appendix becomes swollen and turgic, and the serosa becomes roughened, loses its healthy sheen, and becomes coated with a fibrinous exudate. The probable cause of this condition is bacterial invasion of the lymphoid tissue in the appendix wall. Some cases are probably localized manifestations of a generalized enteritis. Because the lumen of the appendix is not obstructed, these cases rarely progress to gangrene. In many instances, the acute inflammatory attack will resolve spontaneously. In other cases, however, swelling of the lymphoid tissue in the appendix wall may lead to obstruction of the lumen and the condition then may proceed to obstructive appendicitis and gangrene. Even when the acute inflammatory process subsides, the appendix probably never regains its pristine state; adhesion formation and kinking of the appendix may lead to a final episode of acute obstructive appendicitis. An episode of gangrenous appendicitis may well be preceded by several milder and resolving attacks (Fig 39–3).

Obstructive appendicitis is the dangerous type, since the appendix becomes a closed loop of bowel containing decomposing fecal matter. The changes after the sudden blocking of the lumen of the appendix depend on the amount and character of the content distal to the obstruction. If the lumen is empty, the appendix distends with mucus to form a mucocele (Fig 39–4). When the appendix becomes obstructed, the process of events begins with accumulation of normal mucus secretion, proceeds to proliferation of the contained bacteria and pressure atrophy of the mucosa, which allows bacterial access to the deeper tissue planes, and continues with inflammation of the walls of the appendix with vessel thrombosis that, because the blood supply is an end-artery system, leads inevitably to gangrene and then to perforation of the necrotic appendix wall. On other occasions, bacterial invasion occurs through pressure ero-

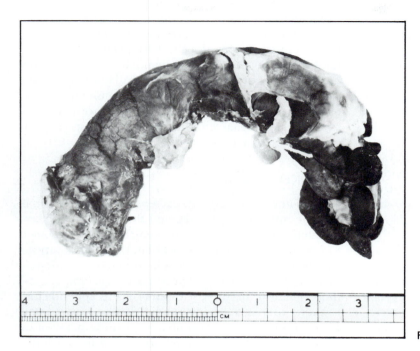

Figure 39–3. An acutely inflamed appendix; the distal half is gangrenous.

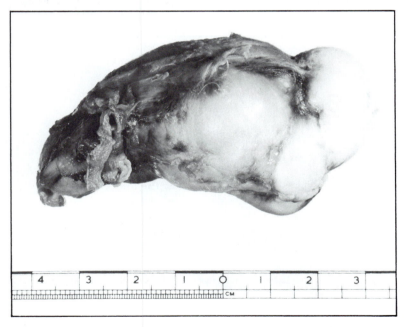

Figure 39–4. Mucocele of the appendix.

sion of a contained fecalith, which may discharge into the peritoneal cavity through the perforation.

The relationship between obstruction of the appendix and gangrenous appendicitis was demonstrated in 1914 by Wilkie, who showed that acute appendicitis followed ligation of the appendix in the rabbit.[16] In 1937, Wangensteen and associates documented that combined obstruction and bacterial infection resulted in acute appendicitis, whereas, if the appendix was first washed free of faecal material and then ligated, a mucocele developed as mucus continued to be secreted within the bacteria-free lumen of the appendix.[17] These classic studies were elegantly extended by Pieper and associates, who showed that obstruction of the appendix in the rabbit, with the use of a balloon catheter introduced via a cecostomy, resulted, within 12 hours, in the inflammatory changes that histologically were similar in all respects to appendicitis in man.

Obstruction may be owing to a large number of possible causes. Inflammatory swelling of the lymphoid tissue in the appendix wall may, as we have noted, occlude the lumen. Kinks and adhesions may result from congenital bands or from previous episodes of inflammation. One or more fecaliths are commonly found within the appendix lumen in the normal organ; in about two-thirds of all gangrenous appendixes, a fecalith is found firmly impacted at the junction between the uninflamed proximal and the gangrenous distal part of the appendix. Other foreign bodies, such as food debris, worms, or even a gallstone, have been found to obstruct the appendix lumen.

Perhaps the rarest cause of obstructive appendicitis is strangulation of the appendix within a hernial sac. Thomas and associates reported seven such cases.[19] The most common hernia to be involved is the right femoral, followed by the right inguinal. However, cases also have been reported of an acutely inflamed appendix within a left inguinal, an umbilical, an incisional, and an obturator hernia. The usual diagnosis is, of course, a strangulated hernia, and the correct diagnosis virtually has never been made before operation.

APPENDICEAL FECALITH

Fecal material is commonly present in both the normal and the inflamed appendix, and this should be differentiated from the true fecalith, which is ovoid, about 1 to 2 cm in length, and fecal colored. Unlike ordinary feces, the true fecalith shows a well-ordered lamination in section. The great majority of these fecaliths are radiopaque and, in 10% of cases of acute appendicitis, contain sufficient calcium to be demonstrated on a plain x-ray film of the abdomen.[20] In a study of 240 cases of acute appendicitis, in which the appendix specimen was x-rayed, fecaliths were demonstrated in 33% of cases. When a fecalith was present, 77% of the specimens were gangrenous, compared with 42% when there was no evidence of a stone (Fig 39–5).

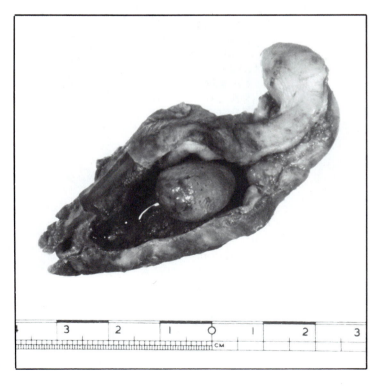

Figure 39–5. Gangrenous appendix containing a large fecalith.

EFFECTS OF PERFORATION

The appendix may rupture at any spot, but most frequently the site of perforation is along the antimesenteric border. After perforation, a localized abscess may form in the right iliac fossa or the pelvis, or diffuse peritonitis may ensue. Whether the peritonitis remains localized or becomes generalized depends on many factors, including the age of the patient, the virulence of the invading bacteria, the rate at which the inflammatory condition has progressed within the appendix, and the position of the appendix.

It is usually stated that poorer localization of the infection occurs in infants because the omentum of the child is filmy and less able to form a protective sheath around the inflamed appendix. A more likely explanation is that delays in diagnosis are more proven to occur in infants. Similar delays occur in the management of elderly persons. In the nonobstructed type of acute appendicitis, the disease is comparatively limited in its course, and there is ample time for inflammatory peritoneal adhesions to form. In contrast, in the acute obstructive form, the rapidity of the process gives little time for defensive adhesions to develop before the sudden flood of infected contents. An appendix situated in the retrocecal or pelvic location is probably more likely to form a local abscess than one in the preileal or subcecal position.

CLINICAL MANIFESTATIONS

The diagnosis and management of acute abdominal pain remains one of the last bastions of clinical medicine. There is no other common situation where clinical features, accurate diagnosis, and immediate decision are of such importance.[21] In most other fields, an initially tentative, or even incorrect, clinical diagnosis is not necessarily harmful; we can wait until it is confirmed or refuted by laboratory investigations or by the clinical progress of the case. In an acute abdominal emergency, however, a treatment delay of even a few hours may result in a stormy course. Additionally, an early case of acute appendicitis undiagnosed overnight, with the patient well sedated with morphine, may mean a missed opportunity of an almost certain smooth recovery. In dealing with the patient with acute abdominal pain, the surgeon must realize that reliance is almost entirely on clinical features, rather than on laboratory and radiologic investigation. Surgeons have become so accustomed, in recent years, to being able to skimp on history and examination in other situations that it comes as something of a shock to realize, in dealing with an acute abdominal emergency, that dependence is on the five senses for diagnosis. It is a very good aphorism that, in the diagnosis of an acute condition of the abdomen, special investigations can be used only to reinforce a clinical diagnosis; seldom, if ever, can they establish or refute it. This aphorism is particularly apt in the case of acute appendicitis.

It is important to remember that abdominal pain may result from disease of almost any organ of the body. Apart from the abdominal and retroperitoneal viscera themselves, including, of course, the pelvic organs, one also must consider diseases of the chest, of the central nervous system, and even of the ears and throat. Metabolic disorders, particularly diabetes, may result in acute abdominal symptoms and finally, the psychologic disturbance of the Munchausen syndrome provides us with an occasional diagnostic difficulty. The novice may well smile at the long list of differential diagnoses for acute appendicitis given in textbooks until, as personal experience grows, the chagrin of slowly ticking off mistakes one by one from the list comes to pass. It has been said that nothing can be so simple, nor yet so difficult, as the diagnosis of acute appendicitis.

The classic story of acute appendicitis is the onset of central colicky abdominal pain followed by nausea or one or more episodes of vomiting, with the pain, after several hours, shifting to the lower right abdomen. The pain becomes continuous and severe, so that the patient finds movement uncomfortable and wishes to lie still, often with the legs flexed. Sleep is impossible. With progression of the disease process, the pain spreads diffusely over the abdomen.

The explanation of the pain distribution is that the central colicky pain is the result of stretching of the inflamed appendix wall. When the inflammatory process extends to the serosa, the parietal peritoneum is involved and the pain shifts to the site of the appendix. Later, diffuse spread of the pain corresponds with the development of generalized peritonitis.

Occasionally, there is no history of this classic shift of pain. The onset of central pain might have occurred during sleep or, because of its relatively mild nature, may be forgotten by the patient preoccupied by the much more intense parietal pain. The severity and time relationships of the pain are also extremely variable; rapid progression to gangrene and peritonitis may take place within 12 hours, whereas in other instances, an acutely inflamed, but nonperforated, appendix may be removed after 3 or 4 days. The patient may give a history of several previous mild attacks of what undoubtedly must have been appendicitis but which were overlooked as a mild stomach ache.

The bowels usually are constipated, but there may be accompanying diarrhea, which is a confusing symptom because the condition may be diagnosed as enteritis and treatment may, in consequence, be delayed. This situation is said to occur particularly when the appendix lies in the retroileal position. The appendix at this site is likely to be deceptive. It produces less overlying peritoneal irritation and less marked shift of pain than does acute inflammation of an appendix lying in one or another of its more usual positions.

Examination commences with a careful inspection of the patient; the patient usually is flushed and in obvious pain, which is aggravated by movement. Pain becomes progressively worse as the disease progresses. Movement is avoided and the knees are often flexed. The tongue is at first lightly furred; it then becomes progressively coated, and the breath becomes foul. Nevertheless, there is no absolute finding in acute appendicitis, so one should not be surprised to find a patient with a perfectly clean, moist tongue who has an acutely inflammed appendix. Temperature and pulse both usually are raised, and the rise progresses during the course of the disease. In adults, the usual finding is a temperature elevated about 1°C above normal; higher temperatures can be expected in children, but a very high pyrexia, although occasionally seen in acute appendicitis, suggests some other diagnosis, such as a pyelitis or respiratory infection.

An interesting study by Smith of 100 consecutive patients with acute appendicitis showed that only 60 had a temperature of 37.2°C or more and only 75 had a coated tongue.[22]

The abdomen is now systematically and gently palpated with the warmed hand of the examiner. In early cases, this examination reveals localized tenderness, slight guarding, and release tenderness over the region of the appendix. Classically, this area coincides with the McBurney point, but if the appendix is lying in one of its less common positions, this localized tenderness may be in the right flank, low in the abdomen, towards the umbilicus, or even in the left iliac fossa. When the unperforated appendix is hanging over the brim of the pelvis or is lying wholly within the pelvis, abdominal rigidity and tenderness may be absent. However, rectal examination will reveal definite tenderness anteriorly on the right side. In late cases with generalized peritonitis, the abdomen is diffusely tender, rigid, and silent on auscultation, and the patient is obviously extremely ill. Later still, the abdomen is distended, and the patient shows all the features of advanced peritonitis.

If the perforated appendix has become walled off by surrounding structures into an appendix abscess, palpation will reveal tender swelling in the right iliac fossa; there also may be a boggy mass on rectal examination. There may be mucous diarrhea owing to irritation of the rectum and frequency of micturition caused by congestion of the wall of the bladder by the pelvic abscess. However, the remainder of the abdomen will be soft, with no evidence of generalized peritonitis. Bowel sounds also will be present.

It should be stressed, of course, that the physical signs of acute appendicitis are not specific but are merely those produced by local peritoneal irritation in the right iliac fossa, the most common cause of which is acute inflammation of the appendix. Exactly the same clinical features are seen in other causes of lower right-sided inflammatory disease, for example, an acute Meckel's diverticulitis or an acute terminal ileitis. The most constant and reliable signs of local peritoneal irritation are local tenderness and guarding; a completely soft abdomen is most unlikely to harbor any serious intra-abdominal catastrophe.

DIFFICULTIES IN DIAGNOSIS

Difficulties in diagnosis are likely to be encountered in the patient with diarrhea whose condition mimics enteritis, or in the patient whose appendix is in the pelvic position. In such cases, abdominal signs are minimal in the early hours, and the diagnosis may be missed if a rectal examination is not performed. Patients who are obese disguise the physical signs of localized tenderness and guarding under their body fat, and poor historians are their own worst enemies. However, any experienced surgeon would say that the greatest difficulties lie with young children, elderly persons, and pregnant women.

Appendicitis in Children
Because the appendix has a relatively wide lumen in infants, appendicitis is rare before the age of 2 years. However, it has been recorded in babies only a few days old and even in premature babies.[23,24] Ayalon and associates reported a case in a 31 week old premature infant and collected 23 previously published cases.[25] From the age of 2 years, the incidence of appendicitis rises to a peak at about 11 years of age and then declines gradually at 15 years before dropping rapidly thereafter.[26]

Both the mortality and morbidity rates for appendicitis are higher in preschool children than in children >5 years of age. The most likely explanation is that, because delays in diagnosis are more likely in infants, a higher proportion are admitted to the hospital with established peritonitis. Jackson studied 313 children up to 12 years of age with acute appendicitis in Newcastle.[27] Almost 50% had a perforated appendix at the time of admission. Perforation could be correlated closely with parental delay in seeking a physician. Details were available in 285 of these cases. In 73 cases, the delay was up to 12 hours, and 24% had perforation. In 80 cases, the delay was up to 24 hours, and 42% had perforation. In 80 cases, children did not reach the hospital until the second day, and 60% had perforation. A further 52 children had delays of more than 48 hours, and of these no fewer than 83% had perforation. One-third of the children had been given purgatives by the parents, and 62% of these had a perforated appendix, compared with 42% of the nonpurged group. Fortunately, there was only one death in this series (0.3%). A study of 7000 patients with acute appendicitis at all ages in Los Angeles, found that 22% had perforation by the time of admission; the overall mortality was 2.4%.[28] In this series, 30 cases occurred in infants 3 years of age or less. Eighteen of these had perforation and, in four more, the appendix was gangrenous but had not yet ruptured. There were two deaths among these 30 children.

It is important to recognize that the clinical picture of acute appendicitis in young children is often atypical. Rather than a story of a shift of pain, there is frequently only the complaint of generalized abdominal pain. It is a good rule that if there is localized tenderness and muscle guarding in the right iliac fossa, in a previously healthy child, then the chances are very strong indeed that the diagnosis is one of acute appendicitis. Thus, in a group of 153 children who were subjected to surgery for acute abdominal pain, no fewer than 114 had confirmed acute appendicitis.[29] A further 21 operated on after this diagnosis were found to have a normal appendix, and most of these had acute mesenteric adenitis. Of the remaining 18 children, 11 had intestinal obstruction (mostly intussusception) and 7 had visceral injuries.

Appendicitis in Elderly Persons

Appendicitis is undoubtedly a more serious situation in elderly patients than in younger ones. Peltokallio and Jauhianen showed that the clinical features of patients more than 60 years of age with acute appendicitis are similar to those of younger age groups in the pattern and duration of symptoms, the temperature changes, and the leukocyte responses.[30] However, at operation both gangrenous changes and perforation had occurred five times as often in the older age group. These findings suggest that poorer localization of the infection and diminished blood supply of the appendix are important factors in allowing rapid progression of the disease. Similar findings have been reported by other investigators. For example, Andersson and Bergdahl found that half of their 68 patients older than 60 years of age with acute appendicitis had perforations, and postoperative complications occurred in one-third of these patients.[31] Owens and Hamit reviewed 68 appendectomies in patients between 65 and 99 years of age. The appendix was normal in four of these patients but in three-quarters, the appendix had ruptured at the time of surgery. Six of the patients died, all with perforated appendixes. In 21 of the cases, delays of 48 hours or more took place before surgical consultation.

There are other problems that face the surgeon dealing with an elderly patient with suspected acute appendicitis. First, there is, inevitably, a higher incidence of associated diseases that affect the general condition of the patient. Second, because the number of alternative causes of intra-abdominal emergencies is greater, the differential diagnosis is more difficult. Finally, there is little doubt that most elderly patients are less likely to complain of pain than are younger people, and their stoic attitude is probably a powerful component in delay in seeking surgical treatment.

Appendicitis in Pregnancy

This is not an infrequent occurrence, because the pregnant woman is neither more nor less prone to appendicitis than a nonpregnant young adult. Black analyzed 373 such cases and noted that the incidence was equally distributed through the three trimesters.[33] Diagnosis is undoubtedly more difficult in the pregnant woman. In the first trimester, the history of amenorrhea and the local physical signs may lead to a diagnosis of ruptured ectopic pregnancy. The nausea and vomiting may be thought to be physiologic "morning sickness," consequently delaying accurate diagnosis. As the pregnancy progresses, the uterus enlarges and the appendix is pushed upward and more laterally. Thus, the pain, tenderness, and guarding are situated in the mid or upper abdomen, which may lead to confusion with pyelitis or cholecystitis. Moreover, the stretched abdominal muscles in the later stages of pregnancy make the detection of guarding or rigidity difficult.

Doberneck reported a series of 29 appendectomies carried out during pregnancy without maternal or fetal death.[34] However, the risk of death of mother or fetus increases considerably in cases of perforation of the appendix. It is the peritonitis, and not the appendectomy, that poses the risk to mother and fetus alike, and therefore, early operation is advised in the pregnant woman with suspected appendicitis.

Appendicitis in the Appendiceal Stump

Francis pointed out that not even a clear history of a previous appendectomy invariably rules out the diagnosis of acute appendicitis.[35] He described a woman, 44 years of age, who had undergone a previous appendectomy for acute appendicitis and who subsequently had perforation of an appendix stump 1 cm in length. It is possible to carry out a subtotal appendectomy and to overlook the stump if the appendix is kinked, bound to the cecum by adhesions, or obscured by edema of the adjacent cecum.

DIAGNOSTIC STUDIES

It must be stressed that acute appendicitis is essentially a clinical diagnosis; there is no laboratory or radiologic test yet devised that is 100% diagnostic of this condition.

White Blood Cell Count

A polymorphic leukocytosis is stressed by some authors as an important feature for diagnosing acute appendicitis. The leukocyte count is raised above 12 000 in about three-fourths of patients with acute appendicitis. However, it is only slightly raised or is entirely normal in the remainder, and one must not discount the diagnosis under these circumstances. In a detailed study of 493 patients with acute appendicitis, Pieper and associates, in 1982, noted that only 66.7% had a leukocyte count of 11 000 or more, and only 5.5% had a raised count of more than 20 000.[15] Doraiswamy pointed out that the combination of a raised leukocyte count and neutrophilia is useful in the diagnosis of appendicitis in children, particularly when these figures are age adjusted.[36] He found that in 225 children with acute appendicitis, 96% had neutrophilia and 42% had a raised leukocyte count. As a comparison, these figures were 30% and 4%, respectively, in 50 children who were found at operation to have a normal appendix, and 32% and 3%, respectively, in 100 children whose acute abdominal pain resolved without surgery. Bower and associates found that only 15 of 382 children with histologically inflamed appendixes had both a normal leukocyte count and a normal differential cell count.[37]

Urine Examination

This, of course, should be routine in every patient with acute abdominal pain. The presence of hematuria or pus cells in the urine points to a urinary tract infection but by no means excludes acute appendicitis. In an important study, Graham quantitatively analyzed midstream urine specimens in 71 patients with a diagnosis of acute appendicitis who underwent surgery. Of these, 62 had an acutely inflamed appendix removed; in the remaining 9 patients, the organ was normal (3 of these had mesenteric adenitis and the other 6 had no abnormality at operation). In the whole group of patients, microscopic pyuria was found in nine, all of whom were female and one of whom also had hematuria. One male patient with acute appendicitis had microscopic hematuria. Graham noted that the distribution of microscopic pyuria was approximately as expected in the normal population. If pus cells or erythrocytes are found in the urine, the clinical features should be reviewed carefully. If the surgeon is satisfied that appendicitis cannot be ruled out, operation under such circumstances is entirely justified; often the inflamed appendix will be found to be adherent to the right ureter or to the bladder.

Radiography

Plain x-ray films of the abdomen with the patient in the erect and supine positions are of value in the differential diagnosis of acute abdominal pain, but the radio-logic features are often nonspecific and must be interpreted with caution (Fig 39–6 and 39–7). Thus, free intraperitoneal gas may be demonstrated, suggesting a perforated peptic ulcer, but, as is mentioned later, this radiologic sign occasionally is seen in cases of perforated appendix.

A number of radiologic signs have been described in plain x-ray films of the abdomen in patients with acute appendicitis. Brooks and Killen list the signs as follows: (1) fluid levels localized to the cecum and to the terminal ileum, indicating local inflammation in the right lower quadrant of the abdomen, (2) localized ileus, with gas in the cecum, ascending colon, or terminal ileum, (3) increased soft-tissue density in the right lower quadrant, (4) blurring of the right flank stripe, the radiolucent line produced by fat between the peritoneum and transversus abdominis, (5) a fecalith in the right iliac fossa that may be confused with a ureteric stone, a gallstone, or a calcified mesenteric lymph node, (6) blurring of the psoas shadow on the right side, (7) a gas-filled appendix, (8) free intraperitoneal gas, and (9) deformity of the cecal gas shadow owing to an adjacent inflammatory mass. This is difficult to interpret because there may be disturbance of cecal gas from intraluminal fluid or feces.

Without knowing the diagnosis, Brooks and Killen reviewed the x-ray films of 200 patients who had under-

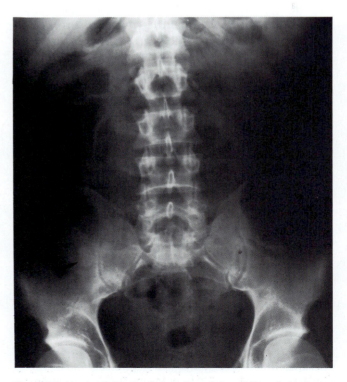

Figure 39–6. An unusually large fecalith in the appendix (*arrow*). The patient had a gangrenous appendix.

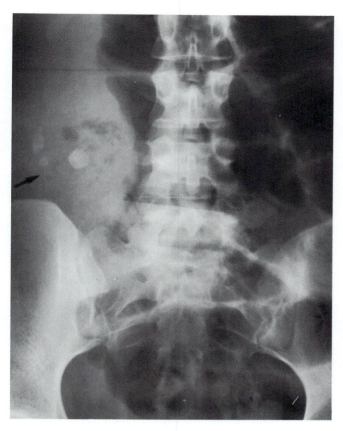

Figure 39–7. Plain x-ray film of the abdomen—an appendiceal abscess. There is a large soft-tissue mass (*arrow*) that displaces the large bowel medially and contains fecaliths and free gas.

gone laparotomy for acute appendicitis.[39] Fifty-four percent of the cases of acute appendicitis without perforation had one or more of these signs, and the figure rose to 80% in advanced cases. However, 14 of 41 cases in which the appendix was not acutely inflamed (37%) had similar x-ray findings, 12 of these had another acute lesion, including ruptured ovarian follicle or intestinal obstruction, but 3 had no abnormal findings at surgery.

Saebo reported three examples of pneumoperitoneum associated with a perforated appendix and found about 40 published reports of this condition.[40] He points out that because appendectomy often is performed without prior radiography of the abdomen, more such cases may occur than appear in published reports. I recently encountered such a case for the first time.

It is rare for gas to be seen in a normal appendix or in the appendix distended because of large bowel obstruction. Killen and Brooks added five examples of a gas-filled gangrenous appendix to the four cases previously reported.[41]

The use of an emergency barium enema examination is almost confined in practice to the United States and is rarely, if ever, ordered in the United Kingdom. Smith and associates enumerated the radiologic signs of appendicitis after barium enema as (1) persistent nonvisualization of the appendix (although this occurs in 5% to 10% of barium enema examinations of normal appendices), (2) partial visualization of the appendix, (3) pressure defect on the cecum, and (4) irritability of the cecum and terminal ileum on screening.

In rare cases, even the acutely inflamed appendix has been filled, on radiologic examination. The authors who reported these cases have pointed out that perforation of the inflamed appendix owing to the x-ray examination is unlikely and also have stressed that they would advise a barium enema only in equivocal cases.

Ultrasonography

Ultrasonography may be useful in the differentiation of gynecological causes of acute abdominal pain, for example, in the detection of an ovarian mass. With improving techniques, the acutely inflamed appendix itself can be visualized.

Pearson reviewed recent interesting studies of the use of high-resolution ultrasonography with graded compression; this technique achieves deep penetration of the transducer.[43] The ultrasonographic appearances of acute appendicitis are of a noncompressible, aperistaltic tubular structure with a central dilated lumen, surrounded by an inner echogenic mucosal layer and an outer, edematous wall that shows few echoes. Although some investigators report a high degree of accuracy, others report false-negative results of up to 25%.

Ooms and associates report a considerable experience in this field.[44] In a study of no less than 525 patients with clinical signs of acute appendicitis, the inflamed appendix was visualized sonographically in 91% of cases of nonperforated appendicitis and 55% of cases of perforated appendicitis. Of 155 patients with a subsequently confirmed alternative diagnosis, ultrasonography made the correct diagnosis in 140. These cases included ileocecitis, mesenteric lymphadenitis, gynecological and urological conditions, perforated peptic ulcers and cecal diverticulitis. Of 139 patients in whom no definite diagnosis was made, ultrasonography showed no abnormality in 138. In only four patients was a false-positive diagnosis of appendicitis made and in two patients with appendicitis, an alternative condition was incorrectly diagnosed. During the last three years of the study, the negative appendectomy rate was only 7% and delay beyond 6 hours after admission occurred in only 2% of patients with surgically proven appendicitis. These authors conclude that, when used to complement clinical diagnosis, ultrasonography improves the diagnostic accuracy and patient management in those suspected of having acute appendicitis.

There seems little doubt that this method of investigation will be used increasingly in the future, especially in equivocal cases and where skilled ultrasonographers are available. Because both false-positive and false-negative findings are obtained even by the most skilled examiners, the ultimate decision remains, as ever, with the clinician.

Laparoscopy

As more and more general surgeons become skilled in laparoscopy, this investigation now has a useful role in the equivocal case of appendicitis. This is especially so if the surgeon is skilled in this procedure and, of course, suitably equipped.

An interesting study by Paterson-Brown and his associates showed that after laparoscopy, only 3 out of 40 patients (7.5%) had an unnecessary appendectomy compared with 11 of 60 patients (22%) operated on without this investigation. This was particularly useful in female patients. Excellent results, of course, can only be obtained under ideal conditions. If the widespread use of laparoscopy is to be advocated as an essential investigation in the management of the acute abdomen, general surgeons require training to become expert laparoscopists.[46]

DIFFERENTIAL DIAGNOSIS

The clinical features and special investigations are all nonspecific, and the list of differential diagnoses is long indeed. In many instances, a diagnosis of acute appendicitis is made but at laparotomy some other acute abdominal condition, which itself requires urgent surgery, is discovered (ie, an acute Meckel's diverticulitis or a perforated peptic ulcer). A small proportion of patients will be found to have a normal appendix, and the exact cause of the pain may never be found. Provided that the proportion of such cases remains small, the surgeon must accept a number of such noninformative laparotomies, placing their risk against the risk of leaving a possibly early, acutely inflamed appendix within the abdomen. Some children will have acute mesenteric adenitis, and the differential diagnosis between the two conditions is, in my opinion, impossible to make with any accuracy. The tragedy comes when an appendectomy is performed in a patient who has some medical condition, such as diabetes or pleurisy, that is responsible for the pain and in whom operation can only aggravate the condition.

The differential diagnosis can be considered under the following headings: (1) other intra-abdominal causes of acute pain, (2) acute pain of gynecologic origin, (3) urinary tract conditions, (4) thoracic conditions, (5) diseases of the central nervous system, and (6) other medical conditions.

Other intra-abdominal diseases that commonly mimic acute appendicitis are perforated peptic ulcer, acute cholecystitis, acute intestinal obstruction, gastroenteritis, acute sigmoid diverticulitis, acute regional ileitis, and, in children, intussusception, acute Meckel's diverticulitis, and mesenteric adenitis. In women, acute salphingitis, a ruptured ecoptic pregnancy, ruptured cyst of the corpus luteum, and a twisted ovarian cyst need to be considered.

Colic from a right-sided ureteral calculus or acute pyelonephritis usually includes radiation of the pain from the loin to the groin. A calculus may be seen on a plain x-ray film of the abdomen and confirmed on an emergency pyelogram. The urine must be tested for blood and pus cells in every case of acute abdominal pain, but as already noted, the presence of either of these abnormalities does not exclude acute appendicitis.

A basal pneumonia and pleurisy may result in referred abdominal pain that may be surprisingly difficult to differentiate from an acute condition of the abdomen, especially in children. Jona noted in 1976 that 12 of 250 children with acute abdominal pain had basal pneumonia as the only cause, and only two of these had abnormal physical findings when the chest was examined.[47] However, the abdominal pain was severe and was associated with abdominal tenderness and even, on occasion, with absent bowel sounds. This author stresses that a chest x-ray film is invaluable and should include a lateral film because the basal consolidation may be hidden by the diaphragm in the posteroanterior film.

A coronary thrombosis may be accompanied by marked epigastric pain, but generalized abdominal pain and rigidity are rare and the condition is only occasionally confused with appendicitis.

Diseases of the central nervous system should be kept in mind in the differential diagnosis. The lightning pains of tabes dorsalis have all but disappeared from clinical practice, but abdominal pain and local tenderness may occur in the 2 or 3 days before the rash of herpes zoster appears. In this group, simulated abdominal pain, the so-called Munchausen syndrome, may be suggested by the presence of multiple abdominal scars, a bizarre history, no fixed address, and occasionally, the telltale scars over the veins of the antecubital fossae of the drug addict.

Medical conditions that may be confused with acute appendicitis include infective hepatitis in the preicteric phase, gastroenteritis, sickle cell crisis (which should always be considered in black children) and, very rarely, acute porphyria. In young children, tonsillitis, acute respiratory tract infection, otitis media, and meningitis can all be associated with acute abdominal pain. Undiagnosed diabetes can undoubtedly mimic an acute abdominal emergency, especially in children. Valerio stressed three important clinical clues: a history of polyuria, polydipsia, and anorexia that precede the abdominal pain; deep sighing and rapid respirations; and severe dehydration.[48] The abdominal pain is usually generalized, in contrast to the localized tenderness and pain of acute appendicitis. It may be difficult to get a urine specimen to test for sugar because of the dehydration, and an immediate blood sugar estimation should be performed. The abdomen will become pain free and soft within a few hours of appropriate treatment for diabetes, but obviously, very close observation is required during this critical period.

The accuracy of diagnosis of acute appendicitis was carefully studied by Pieper and associates.[49] They reviewed 1018 appendectomies carried out in Stockholm in patients whose ages ranged from 1 to 89 years. The diagnosis was correct in 67.6% of the cases (77.7% of the male patients and 58% of the female patients). The diagnostic accuracy was low in the female group, 10 to 39 years of age, in whom it fell to 52.7%. In this group, gynecologic disorders were found in 15.5% of cases. In patients <10 years of age, appendicitis was confirmed in 72.9% of cases, and in those older than 60 years of age, in 66.7%. Surgical diseases that mimic acute appendicitis accounted for 4.1% of cases in this study. Of the patients on review, 28.3% did not require surgery. Of these 288 patients, 149 had no disease at all at operation. The remaining 139 had a variety of conditions, including mesenteric adenitis (63 patients), gynecologic disorders (26 patients), gastroenteritis (24 patients), and urinary tract infection or stones (12 patients).

TREATMENT

The correct treatment of appendicitis in all its aspects is one of the most important subjects in abdominal surgery because it is the most common major abdominal condition necessitating emergency operation.

The treatment of acute appendicitis is appendectomy. The sooner it is done, the better. There are four exceptions to this excellent rule: (1) the patient is moribund with advanced peritonitis; here the only hope is to improve the condition by intravenous fluids, nasogastric suction, antibiotics, and blood transfusion in an attempt to get the patient fit for operation, (2) the attack has already resolved; in such a case, appendectomy can be advised as an elective procedure to prevent recurrence, but there is no immediate emergency, (3) circumstances make operation difficult or impossible (ie, in a small boat at sea). Here reliance must be placed on a conservative regimen in the hope that resolution will occur, or a local appendix mass may form. If available, morphine, antibiotic therapy, and intravenous fluids are given; this is preferable to attempting surgery in less than optimal conditions, and (4) an appendix mass has formed without evidence of general peritonitis.

Preoperative Preparation

If the diagnosis is one of a straightforward acute appendicitis, no special steps need be taken apart from those of any routine abdominal operation. Broad spectrum antibiotic therapy is commenced to cover both aerobic and anaerobic organisms. My current practice is to use cefuroxime and metronidazole.

If the diagnosis of a generalized peritonitis is made, intravenous fluid therapy and nasogastric aspiration are commenced.

CHOICE OF INCISION

Experience should enable the surgeon to determine with a fair degree of accuracy the position of the appendix and its pathologic changes before operation. When the patient is fully anaesthetized, the surgeon should once again systematically palpate the abdomen in an endeavor to locate the position of the appendix. A circumscribed lump may be felt, a diffuse thickening made out, or a movable tumor identified. The incision then can be carefully planned to give adequate, but not excessive, exposure.

A right iliac fossa, skin-crease, muscle-split incision is used (Fig 39–8), commencing just above and medial to the anterior superior iliac spine. It is a mistake to place the incision too far medially; this brings the surgeon down onto the anterior rectus sheath and not over the oblique muscles in the lines of their fibers (Fig 39–9). The muscles are retracted and the peritoneum is exposed. Moist packs are placed around the wound and the peritoneum is opened cautiously. In a true case of

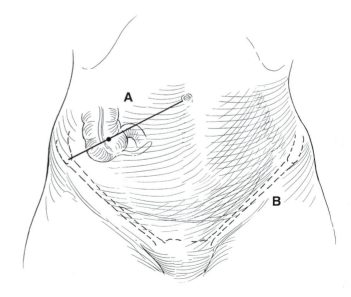

Figure 39–8. The appendectomy incision. The classic oblique McBurney incision **(A)** is usually replaced by the cosmetically better skin crease incision **(B)**.

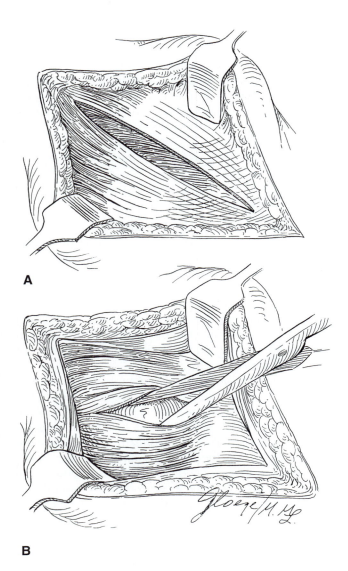

A

B

Figure 39–9. A. A gridiron incision. The aponeurosis of the external oblique has been divided in line with its fibers. **B.** McBurney incision. Internal oblique and transversus muscles are split. The skin incision should be placed transversely or obliquely to lie in one of the Langer lines.

appendicitis, there is usually at least a serous exudate in the peritoneal cavity, or frank pus may be present. A swab is taken for bacteriologic study and the fluid is sucked away.

A well-placed incision should bring the surgeon immediately onto the cecum. It is picked up with the fingers and slowly and carefully drawn through the incision. The index finger may be used to lift the appendix and coax it onto the surface, but whenever this maneuver is necessary, it must be performed with the greatest care. There is nothing more dangerous than the so-called hooking out, or blind dissection, with the fingers of a friable gangrenous appendix, especially when it

happens to be fixed to the lateral wall of the pelvis or embedded in coils of small intestine. In such cases, the appendix is not uncommonly ruptured or torn in half by clumsy manipulations. If any difficulty is encountered in localizing the appendix, it can be found by tracing the teniae coli along the cecum to their junction at the appendix base.

If careful palpation indicates that the delivery of the appendix is going to be difficult, the surgeon ascertains whether further access is needed medially or laterally. In the former case, the incision may be extended inward through the sheath of the rectus muscle; in the latter case, the oblique muscles are divided transversely or obliquely in line with the incision. The transverse division affords an excellent approach to an appendix lying far out in the loin above the level of the anterosuperior iliac spine, even in the most hidden, adherent retrocecal situation in an obese patient.

In discussing the extension of an incision, it is worth noting that some surgeons advise a lower right paramedian incision for appendectomy, particularly if the diagnosis is in some doubt or, in female patients, if there is a question of a gynecologic cause for the acute abdominal pain. However, there is no doubt that the right iliac fossa incision gives the most direct access to the appendix even in the most difficult cases. Even if the diagnosis proves to be incorrect, most other local abnormalities can be dealt with through this incision, especially if it is extended as described above. On numerous occasions, I have dealt with a ruptured ectopic pregnancy, acute Meckel's diverticulitis, acute cecal diverticulitis, and even, in one case, a mucocele of the gallbladder through this approach. If, however, it is found that the cause of the acute abdominal condition is out of reach of this incision (eg, perforated duodenal ulcer), then the incision is left open, the appropriate vertical incision is performed, and the emergency is dealt with appropriately. Both incisions then are closed at the end of the laparotomy.

After delivery of the appendix, it is removed under direct vision, with all intra-abdominal manipulations reduced to a minimum. The appendix is held up by tissue forceps applied around the appendix in such a manner as to encircle the organ and yet not inflict any damage. In some instances, it may be preferable to grasp the mesoappendix with the forceps.

The appendix may be long, in which case appendectomy is a simple procedure, or the appendix may be found closely bound to the cecum by congenital adhesions or inflammatory bands that require preliminary mobilization before one can deal with vessels in the mesoappendix. If the mesoappendix is long, thin, and rather redundant, it may be simply transfixed and ligated with thread, after which it is divided close to the appendix at the base of the organ (Fig 39–10). It is more usual

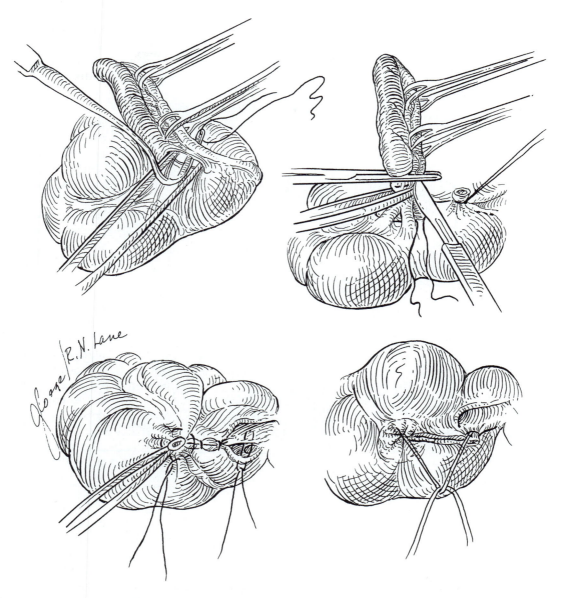

Figure 39–10. Appendectomy by the purse-string method. Note how the Babcock forceps are applied to the mesoappendix to avoid any damage to the acutely inflamed appendix.

to have to divide the mesoappendix by clipping and dividing it seriatim, section by section, until the base of the appendix is reached. When the mesentery of the appendix is fatty, edematous, or frankly gangrenous, the ligatures have to be applied with special care, because they are likely to cut through this friable, buttery structure. If there is any difficulty, the vessels should be cautiously oversewn with interrupted atraumatic thread sutures.

The mobilized appendix is held upward and its base crushed with two artery forceps. After removal of the first (close to the cecal wall), the crushed appendix area is ligated with thread, the ends of which are cut short. A purse-string suture of 2/0 chromic catgut is next inserted about 1 cm from the appendix. This suture passes through the seromuscular coat, especially at the longitudinal bands, and great care is taken to avoid puncturing the gut or pricking a blood vessel.

The appendix is divided close to the artery forceps (Fig 39–11) and the stump invaginated by the purse-string suture. This procedure is reinforced by a second purse-string or Z stitch to secure inversion of the stump even further.

When the cecal wall is sodden with edema, it may be impossible to invaginate the stump. In such cases, two

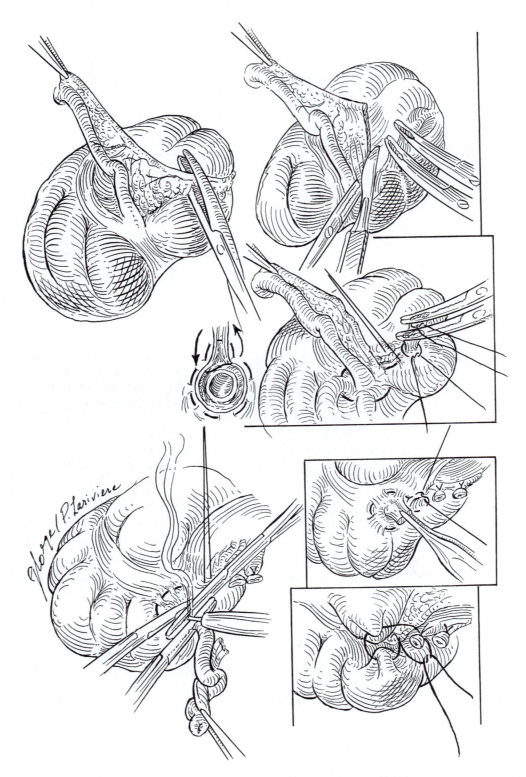

Figure 39–11. Appendectomy. Intraluminal invagination of the stump. (Redrawn from Ochsner A, Lilly G. The technique of appendectomy. *Surgery* 1937;2:532.)

thread ligatures are applied to the base of the appendix; the ligatures may then, with advantage, be left long to anchor a portion of the mesoappendix over the vulnerable spot (Fig 39–12).

The safety of foregoing invagination of the stump is demonstrated by an interesting study reported by Engstrom and Fenyo; in a randomized trial, they compared 374 appendectomies with ligation and double invagination of the stump with 361 appendectomies in which simple ligation alone was performed. There were no differences in wound infection, postoperative pyrexia, or hospital stay between the two groups. Indeed, there were six postoperative obstructions in the invaginated group within 2 months of surgery (1.6%), compared with only one in the noninvaginated group (0.3%). This difference was significant at the $P=.05$ level. Many surgeons now routinely leave the stump uninvaginated.

It is tempting to draw the handy, bloodless fold of Treves and to stitch it over the appendix stump; however, doing so may lead to angulation and subsequent obstruction of the last inch or so of the ileum. Care also must be taken not to hitch up the terminal ileum with one of the purse-string sutures.

Retrograde Appendectomy

Occasionally, the inflamed appendix in the retrocolic position is firmly bound down along the length of the ascending colon and cannot be delivered into the wound.

It is of the utmost importance to have the whole length of the appendix in view during the operation; otherwise, the tip of the appendix may be overlooked. Under such circumstances, retrograde appendectomy is performed. The base of the appendix is freed until the whole circumference of the organ near its cecal junction can be visualized. Tissue forceps are applied around the appendix base, and the first inch or so of the appendix is freed. It is then a simple matter to ligate the base of the appendix, insert a purse-string suture, clamp and divide the appendix, and invaginate its stump. The surgeon then proceeds to define the remainder of the mesoappendix and to clip, cut, and tie small portions of it at a time until the entire mesoappendix is divided and the organ is removed in toto (Fig 39–13).

Occasionally, the appendix will be found firmly wrapped in adherent omentum. In such a case, the appendix should be removed together with its protective omental sheath. Attempts to free the omentum may result in spillage of a collection of pus into the peritoneal cavity.

Closure of the muscle split incision is simplicity itself. The peritoneum is closed with chromic catgut, the transversus and internal oblique muscles are left unsutured, and one or two catgut sutures are used to appose the external oblique aponeurosis. The skin then is sutured with interrupted nylon stitches (Fig 39–14).

Drainage is not generally advised after appendec-

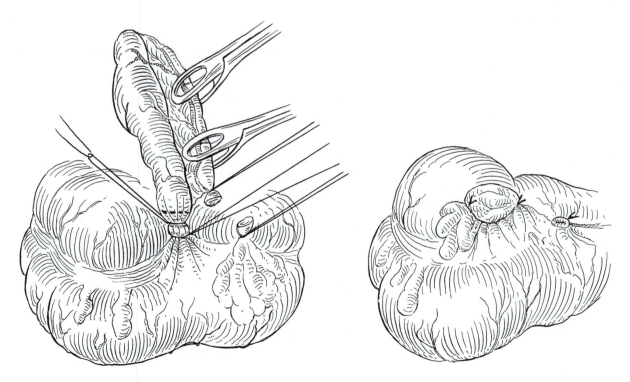

Figure 39–12. Appendectomy. Simple double ligation of the crushed area of the stump without inversion of the stump. After RN Lane.

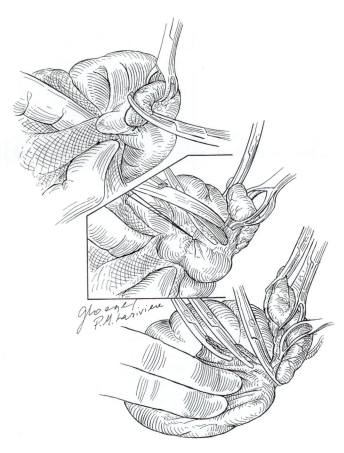

Figure 39–13. Retrograde appendectomy. (Redrawn from Maingot R. *The Management of Abdominal Operations,* 2nd ed. HK Lewis (ed), 1957)

tomy. Where there has been a local abscess, leaving behind a shaggy, granulating cavity, or where difficulty has been encountered in dealing with the appendix stump, closed-suction drainage may be advised.

The Appendiceal Mass

Occasionally, a walled-off perforated appendix will form an inflammatory mass. Usually there is a history of 4 or 5 days of pain. The condition probably is being seen less commonly now as a result of improved health education. In various series, the incidence ranges from 2% to 6% of cases.[51]

The clinical features are a shifting temperature with an increased pulse rate. There is a tender mass in the right iliac fossa that can often also be palpated on rectal examination. However, there is no evidence of a generalized peritonitis, in that the rest of the abdomen is soft and bowel sounds are present. The white blood cell count usually is raised considerably.

Pathologically, the mass may represent a spectrum that ranges from phlegmon to an abscess. The former is

an inflammatory mass made up of the inflamed appendix, the adjacent viscera, and the greater omentum. The latter is a pus-containing mass. Differentiation between the two can be difficult.[52] On ultrasonography, an abscess is diagnosed as a rounded or irregularly outlined sonolucent structure containing small echogenic particles close to the cecum. If only thick-walled liquid-containing intestine or nothing abnormal is noted, the mass can be regarded as a phlegmon. However, the sonographic appearance may be variable with an echogenic abscess or sonolucent phlegmon. Other authorities advise contrast-enhanced computed tomography, where the phlegmon appears as a soft tissue high-density mass while an abscess is significantly lower in density.

Treatment. The initial treatment should be conservative. The patient is placed on a regimen of bed rest and maintained on fluids only. A careful watch is kept on the general condition of the patient, temperature, and pulse, and, above all, on the size of the mass, which is marked out on the abdominal wall with a skin pencil. Metronidazole is given intravenously, but a prolonged course of antibiotics should be avoided because of the risk of development of a honeycomb of chronic abscess cavities.

On this regimen, the majority of appendix masses resolve, but if the swelling is obviously enlarging over the next day or two or if the pyrexia becomes more elevated, the appendix should be drained through a small incision over the apex of the mass; the surrounding adhesions allow for this to be performed extraperitoneally (Fig 39–15).

After the patient has been anesthetized, the surgeon should carefully palpate the swelling and make an incision over the most projecting and superficial part of the abscess. The oblique muscles are split, as in an appendectomy approach. If possible, the surgeon exposes the lateral edge of the peritoneum and, by stripping it medially with the finger, reaches the mass retroperitoneally. If this is impossible, the peritoneum is opened gently and the peritoneal cavity is cautiously packed with gauze before the index finger is inserted down to the most prominent and cystic portion of the abscess wall. This procedure frees the abscess contents for rapid aspiration. If the appendix readily comes to hand, it should be excised by one of the techniques previously described. More often, appendectomy is impossible and the abscess cavity should be drained by means of a perforated tube brought out through the lateral extremity of the wound. With increasing expertise in imaging techniques, CT or ultrasound-guided percutaneous drainage of the abscess is now frequently performed.[52] This procedure is particularly likely to be successful where there is a large unilocular abscess.[53]

Occasionally, the appendix abscess occurs in the pelvis. The characteristic feature is diarrhea, with the

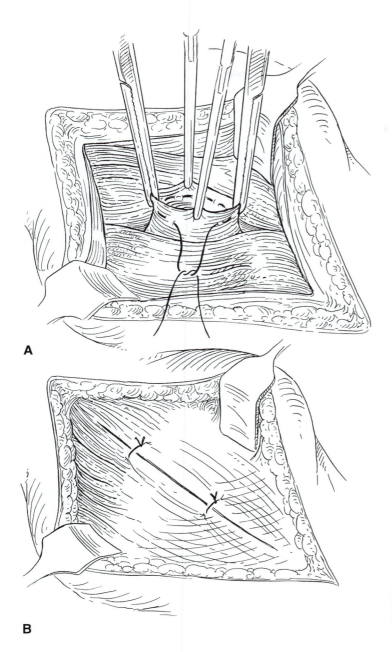

A

B

Figure 39–14. Closure of the muscle split incision. **A**. The peritoneum is closed with a purse-string suture. **B**. One or two catgut sutures close the external oblique aponeurosis.

passage of mucus in the stools. The abscess may be felt to bulge into the rectum or into the posterior vaginal fornix in the female. If the abscess actually points into the vagina, it should be drained through an incision in the posterior fornix, but in most cases, rectal drainage is preferred. The bladder is emptied with a catheter and the patient is placed in the lithotomy position. The surgeon's index finger then locates the site of maximum point softening in the anterior rectal wall, and through this area, the points of a closed artery forcep are gently and evenly forced in an upward direction. This procedure also can be performed under direct vision with the use of a lighted proctoscope (Fig 39–16 and 39–17).

Some surgeons attempt to keep a drainage tube within the pelvic abscess cavity, but this author finds that it dislodges almost immediately. Its use has been abandoned.

Whether resolution occurs or whether drainage is required, elective appendectomy should be recommended after an interval of about 8 weeks, a time sufficient to allow the inflammatory condition to settle down. This procedure is recommended because of the significant risk of further episodes of acute appendicitis, if the damaged appendix is not removed. Useful accounts of series of cases were published in 43 adult patients and in 59 children.[54,55] Skoubo-Kristensen and Hvid reviewed 193 patients treated conservatively for an

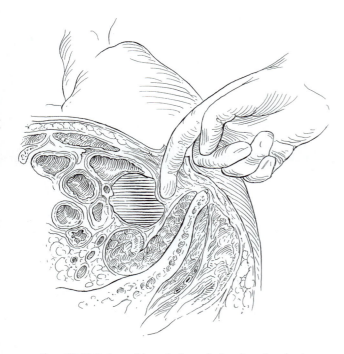

Figure 39–15. Drainage of appendix abscess by the extraperitoneal route.

appendix mass over a 10 year period in Aarhus, Denmark.[56] One hundred and seventy (88%) became quiescent. Of the 23 patients who required early operation, 6 had small bowel obstruction, 14 had unresolved abscesses, and 3 had a suspected perforated abscess; 1 of these abscesses was confirmed at operation. The one death was of a female patient 86 years of age. Of the 170 patients discharged after conservative treatment, 12 were readmitted within 3 months, with either a further abscess or an attack of appendicitis. An elective appendectomy was carried out at 3 months on the remaining patients. These authors noted that there are wide variations in the recurrence rate after conservative treatment of appendix abscess, varying from 7% to 46% in different series, but the majority of recurrences are likely to occur in the early months, after resolution of the mass.

Rarely, the appendix abscess may rupture into the bladder, producing an appendicovesical fistula, or into the intestine, or onto the skin to produce an appendic-ocutaneous fistula (Fig 39–18). In a 1978 review of such fistulae, a case associated with a fecal fistula in the right buttock was reported.[57]

Laparoscopic Appendectomy

Visualization of the peritoneal cavity using videolaparoscopy allows excellent exposure of the appendiceal region. Much has been written regarding the merits of the standard open incision versus the benefits of videolaparoscopic access. As will be discussed, there are situations where the laparoscopic approach has definite advantages. It allows a wide view of the peritoneum with-

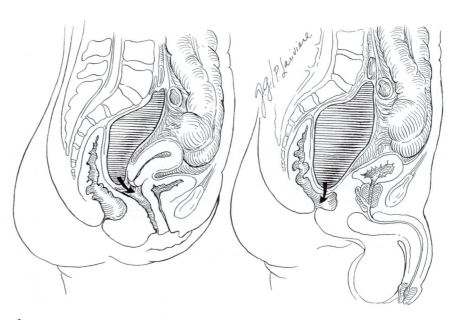

Figure 39–16. Pelvic abscess. **A**. The abscess is bulging into the posterior vaginal fornix. **B**. The abscess is pointing into the rectum.

A

B

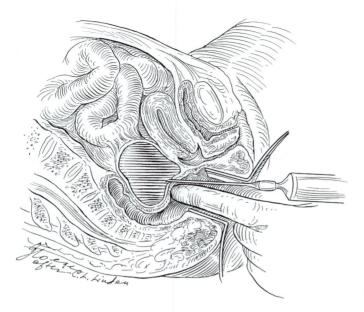

Figure 39–17. Drainage of a pelvic abscess.

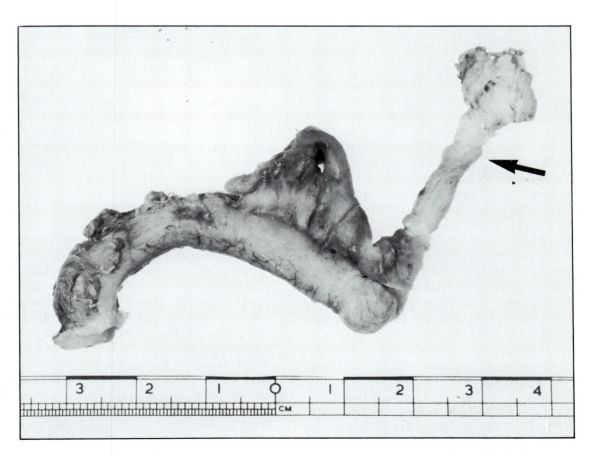

Figure 39–18. Appendicocutaneous fistula cured by appendectomy. The *arrow* indicates the fistulous tract, which led to the skin surface.

out excessive handling of tissues. With care and patience, the small bowel can be followed to detect other pathology. The ovaries, fallopian tubes, and uterus can be seen easily and manipulated. Other causes of lower abdominal pain are often better dealt with by laparoscopy.

At open appendectomy, the appendix is removed even if not inflamed. This is desirable because early appendicitis has, on occasion, only been apparent on histologic examination, to avoid a second laparotomy at some stage in the future, and to prevent subsequent diagnostic confusion resulting from a scar in the right iliac fosa with the appendix in situ. These considerations are not as clearly relevant with the laparoscopic approach. The risks associated with removal of a normal appendix are low, but are essentially the same as those encountered when removing the inflamed appendix. Probably of most concern is the incidence of long-term adhesive bowel obstruction. For all these reasons, this author believes that only when the other organs within the peritoneum do not account for the symptoms and the question of mucosal appendicitis is raised does it seem in order to perform laparoscopic appendectomy to remove an ostensibly normal appendix.

Indications

Appendectomy should be undertaken when the diagnosis of acute appendicitis is suspected. The clinical probability of being correct in this clinical judgment is highest in young adult males and lowest in females of child-bearing age and in children. In many of the latter group, the pathology is diagnosed easily laparoscopically, and either needs no further operative intervention or is easily dealt with laparoscopically.

Contraindications to a laparoscopic approach are few. In pregnancy, both because the uterus may hinder exposure and because reservations remain about the possible deleterious effects of intraperitoneal insufflation on uterine blood flow, the open approach may be preferable. However, as experience with mechanical elevation of the abdominal wall (gasless laparoscopy) increases, laparoscopy during pregnancy may well prove safe and useful. A localized appendiceal abscess in the right iliac fossa, if treated operatively, is approached best by an incision over that area and drainage, with or without concurrent appendectomy. If the appearance of the appendix suggests malignancy, or the lumen of the appendix is obstructed by a cecal polyp, a standard en bloc right hemicolectomy is the correct approach. It must be emphasized that laparoscopic appendectomy should not be performed without the correct instrumentation, or without experience in laparoscopic surgical techniques.

Instrumentation

By its nature, viewing the peritoneum using a laparoscope with a camera conveying an image to a distant screen takes the performance of the operation to a level where detailed knowledge of the endoscopic equipment by the surgeon is essential. The basics of this has been covered elsewhere, but the surgeon must be familiar with the many techniques of ligature application, endoscopic knot tying and tissue extraction.

Instruments recommended, if not actually required, in all cases include a 30° forward oblique viewing laparoscope, bipolar forceps, atraumatic bowel graspers, atraumatic tubal graspers to manipulate appendix, scissors, suction/irrigation device, endoloop ligatures, clip applier, appendix extractor (reducing sleeve), lap sac (or equivalent waterproof strong tissue extraction bag), linear stapler/cutter, and an S-shaped skin retractor.

The principles of the surgical procedure remain similar to those of open surgery: (1) handle inflamed friable tissue gently, (2) reduce manipulation of the bowel to a minimum, (3) minimize wound contamination during appendix removal, and (4) avoid extension of peritoneal contamination.

Patient Preparation

Antibiotic prophylaxis, using intravenous aminoglycoside and metroindazole, for instance, is given during induction of anesthesia. High tissue levels are maintained for the duration of the operation.

The supine position is used, with the lower body restrained by well-padded straps connected to the table rails below the level of the pelvis. This positioning allows the patient to be tilted laterally, without fear of slippage or pressure on unprotected sites. In females, the legs may be abducted in Allen stirrups to allow access to the perineum. By avoiding flexion of the hips, instrument manipulation via the inferior ports remains unhindered.

The bladder should be emptied just prior to induction of anesthesia, thus avoiding the potential morbidity of bladder catheterization. Open laparoscopy with visual dissection to the peritoneal cavity is advocated. The initial skin incision is vertically within the umbilicus. The linea alba is exposed with the aid of the S-shaped retractors, incised, and the edges elevated with hemostats. An anchoring fascial suture holds the seal of the Hasson cannula and provides closure of the defect on completion of the appendectomy. After previous surgery, choosing a site away from scars may require initial port placement at a site higher up or in the left upper quadrant, away from the umbilicus. Open dissection to the peritoneum through a small incision in these sites is more time consuming, but becomes easy with experience and the aid of the S-shaped retractors. This approach to initial access, insufflation, and initial trocal placement will avoid injuries to major blood vessels, decrease the likelihood of gas embolism, and avoid un-recognized bowel injury.

Exposure of the Appendix

The principle of safe laparoscopic access is a multi-puncture approach. Reports using a single port at the umbilicus are interesting and may be useful for very thin mobile appendixes, but are limited for practical purposes.[58] Alternatively, the laparoscopically visualized appendix can be used to direct a subsequent incision to allow exteriorization of the entire appendix through the abdominal wall and the performance of appendectomy outside the peritoneum.[59] Both these techniques have limitations with single-instrument mobilization in the presence of a two dimensional image. Additionally, both techniques are susceptible to undesirable wound contamination in the presence of acute inflammation. Mobilization of adherent or retrocecal appendixes using these techniques may well be more hazardous than the multipuncture approach.

With the umbilical Hasson cannula in place, the pneumoperitoneum is created. The laparoscopic view within the peritoneum guides insertion of all accessory cannulae. Special care is taken to avoid the inferior epigastric vessels running up from the internal ring in the extraperitoneal fat and visible through parietal peritoneum (Fig 39–19). All 11-mm right inguinal cannula is used to allow controlled extraction of the appendix. Care must also be exercised to avoid injury to the inguinal canal by initial upward insertion through subcutaneous fat before penetrating the muscles. An additional 5-mm cannula in the right upper quadrant may be required for cases where more extensive dissection is necessary.

Videolaparoscopy

The advances in tissue dissection using the laparoscope have been much facilitated by the exposure obtained when a videocamera is attached to the endoscope. The high-quality image conveyed to the screen allows all the operating room staff to view and assist. The image can be controlled by an assistant who can magnify structures by moving the laparoscope closer or achieve panoramic views by withdrawing it. Both the surgeons' hands remain free to operate instruments so that tissue manipulation closely simulates that achieved in open surgery, with the exception of tactile sensation.

After an initial survey of the peritoneum, the appendix is exposed by displacing ileum and cecum using atraumatic grasping forceps. Placing the patient in an adequate Trendelenburg (head down) position, supplemented by left-lateral tilt, encourages gravitation of the small bowel towards the upper abdomen. When the fallopian tubes, ovaries and uterus need to be viewed,

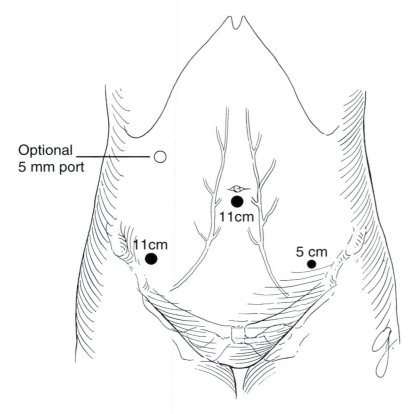

Optional 5 mm port

11cm

11cm

5 cm

Figure 39–19. Three cannula technique for laparoscopic appendectomy. Note the course of the inferior epigastric artery which must be visualized by the telescope from the peritoneal aspect to guide the insertion of the inferior ports. These are conveniently placed low in the hair line, but carefully tunneled upwards subcutaneously to avoid damage to the inguinal canal or ilioinguinal nerve.

the assistant's fingers placed in the fornices of the vagina allow upward displacement of the uterus and so provide excellent exposure. Greater control of the uterus is achieved with a cervical tenaculum, but this requires cannulation of the cervical os and is best used in conjunction with a gynecologic colleague.

Mobilization of the inflammed appendix follows the same principles as open surgery. The appendix is handled gently with an atraumatic grasping forceps and the mesoappendix displayed by dissecting the peritoneal leaves with scissors. When the appendix is very friable, manipulation is aided by a ligature around the tip of the appendix or by grasping the mesoappendix alone.

When the appendix lies behind the cecum, the cecum may, in some cases, need to be freed from its lateral peritoneal reflection. Even if the appendix initially appears normal for some of its length, it is essential that the entire length of the organ be viewed before accepting that it is not inflamed. The mesoappendix is controlled by either ligature, clips, or bipolar coagulation (Fig 39–20, and 39–21). The latter technique allows safe coaptation and coagulation of vessels within fat, with documented safety.[60] A minimum of mesoappendix should be included with the appendix to facilitate its subsequent extraction.

The base of the appendix is ligated by two catgut lig-

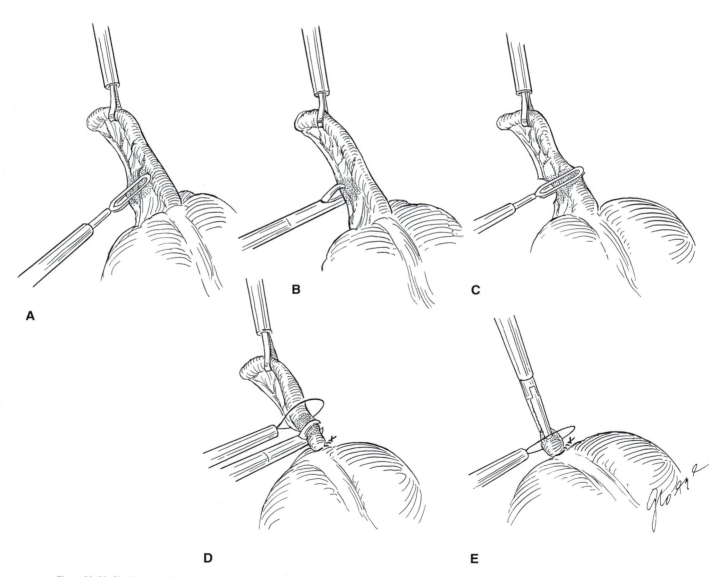

Figure 39–20. Bipolar coagulation technique appendectomy. **A**. The mesoappendix is exposed and coagulated using bipolar electrosurgery. **B**. The mesoappendix is then divided with scissors; if fat laden this may require a number of coagulations to completely transect. **C**. The base of the appendix is sealed using bipolar coagulation. **D**. Endoloop ligatures are placed proximally and distally, and the appendix is transected and extracted. **E**. A second endoloop is placed over the first to ensure secure ligation. A purse-string to bury the stump is not advocated.

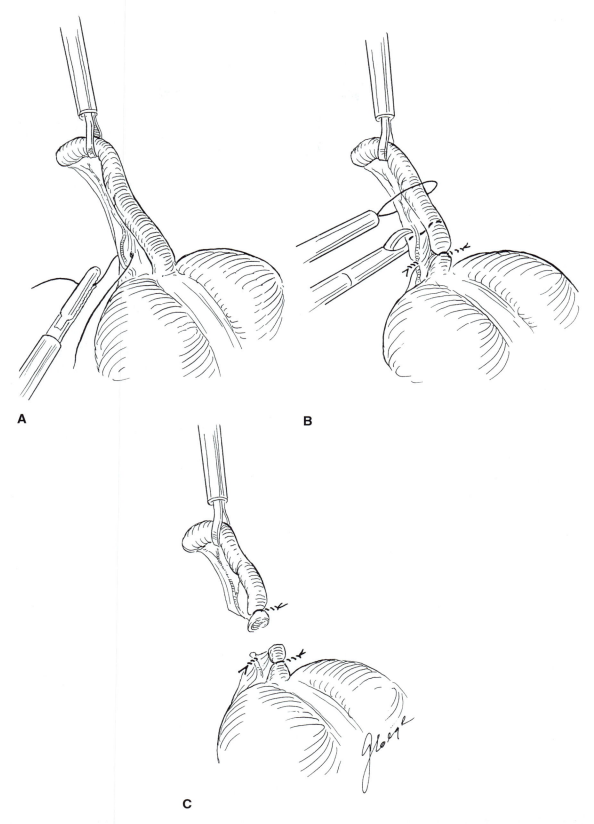

A

B

C

Figure 39–21. Ligation technique appendectomy. **A**. After creation of a window through the mesoappendix, a ligature passed through the left inguinal port is knotted externally (Roeder knot) and tightened down with a pushrod. **B**. The mesoappendix is then divided. **C**. Pretied endoloops are placed proximally and distally, and the appendix is transected and extracted.

atures tied with the Roeder knot or by external ligatures snugged down with a knot pusher. It is ligated or sealed using bipolar coagulation 12 mm distally and then transected. The appendix stump is not buried.[61]

Alternative Techniques

These may well be most useful for a heavily fat laden mesoappendix or in situations of difficult access, such as the retrocecal position.

The appendix is grasped at the tip, its base displayed and then coagulated with bipolar forceps about 1 cm from the cecum (Fig 39–22). The appendix then is tran-

sected with application of two endoloops to the base and one distally. The mesoappendix then is secured with an endoloop or clip and the appendix excised. For a retrocecal appendix, this initial approach to the base allows division of the appendix, and then retrograde dissection of the inflamed organ with improved visualization.

In the occasional patient where inflammation has extended beyond the base of the appendix to involve the wall of the cecum, the transection across the cecum is most safely and cleanly achieved using the linear stapler/cutter (Fig 39–23). If this instrumentation is not available, conversion to an open approach is required.

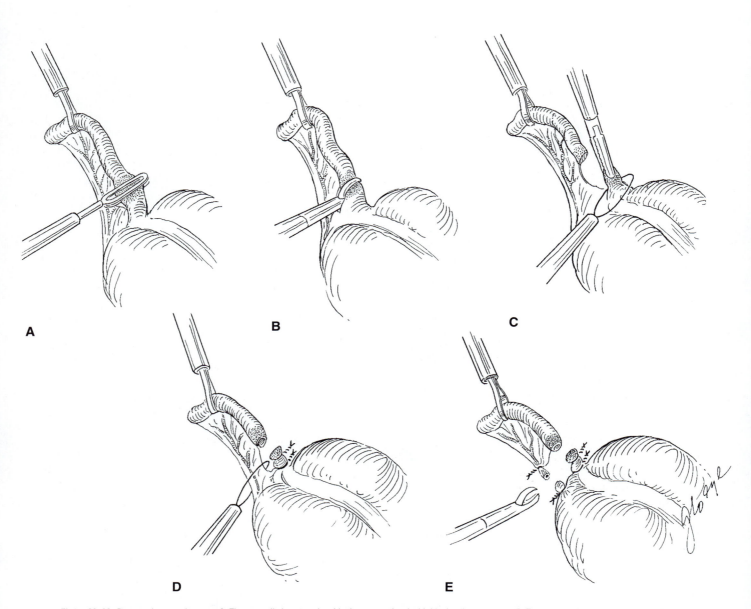

Figure 39–22. Retrograde appendectomy. **A**. The appendix is grasped and its base coagulated with bipolar electrosurgery. **B**. Transection of the sealed appendix. **C**. Placement of endoloops to securely ligate the stump. **D**. The mesoappendix is displayed, often only after scissor mobilization of the cecum, and **E**. Secured with an endoloop (or bipolar coagulation).

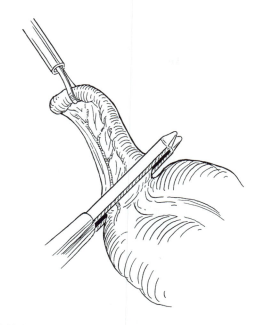

Figure 39–23. Linear cutter/stapler transection across the cecum for inflammation extending beyond the base of the appendix. An initial application of the stapler to transect the mesoappendix may often be required.

The appendix is extracted prior to final washout and peritoneal toilet. This must be achieved without contact with the wound and not by dragging it through a small puncture hole with infected exudate being expressed into surrounding tissue. A thin appendix may be withdrawn into the appendix extractor (so called 5/11 metal reducer) and removed through the 11-mm cannula. If the mesoappendix is fat laden or edematous, this tissue can be excised and extracted separately to expedite appendix removal. A bulky friable appendix will not be removed easily this way and is better inserted into a strong impermeable sac introduced for this purpose (Fig 39–24). The layers of the wound are protected as the entire bag is withdrawn out of the peritoneum through the 11-mm cannula site.

Hemostasis is checked and the remaining serum and blood aspirated using the combination suction/lavage instrument. In patients with perforated appendicitis, special care must be taken to find and remove a fecalith extruded at the time of perforation. To leave it behind will surely result in a peritoneal abscess. The peritoneum finally is lavaged with warm Ringer's solution and then sucked dry.

Drainage is not generally required or useful. On occasion, where a pelvic abscess is encountered, drainage may be desirable. Insertion of a soft-tube drain down a port allows its placement under vision, prior to desufflation.

For small pediatric patients, consideration should be given to using smaller ports. A 5-mm telescope often will give adequate views. In planning the use of smaller ports, the surgeon must remember the port size required for use of staples and wound dimensions needed to extract the appendix. In many circumstances, an intermediate sized 7-mm port may be useful.

After complete removal of carbon dioxide and withdrawal of the cannulae, the wounds are closed. Care is taken to close the fascia of the larger 11-mm port sites with polyglactin. Failure to do so will result in early small bowel entrapment or an incisional hernia, in significant numbers of patients. Closure of the peritoneum is not necessary. Difficulty exposing the fascia can most simply be overcome with the S-shaped retractors. Skin approximation is satisfactorily accomplished using steristrips. Wound infiltration, using 0.5% bupivicaine, allows a more comfortable early return to mobility and minimizes the immediate requirements for narcotic analgesia.

Postoperative Care

Fluids are encouraged as soon as desired and diet started once normal appetite has returned. Immediate ambulation after the operation is encouraged. Analgesia can be supplemented by using indomethacin, either orally or in suppository form. This will minimize the requirement for narcotics that have been implicated in postoperative nausea and ileus.

Reported Results of Laparoscopic Appendectomy

Since publication of the technique of endoscopic appendectomy in 1983,[62] one of the largest experiences reported has been that of Pier, Got and Backer (625 cases).[60] They used bipolar coagulation to control the mesoappendix and appendicular vessels. Eighty-six percent of the appendixes showed evidence of inflammation on histologic examination. Three patients developed postoperative intra-abdominal collections of pus requiring subsequent laparotomy. Wound infection occurred in 2.2%. Routine perioperative antibiotic prophylaxis was not used, but was reserved for those cases with perforation.

Fourteen cases required conversion to open procedures. Eight of these were because the appendix could not be mobilized, and three had uncontrolled bleeding. Most of these conversions were among the first 50 cases of the series. Operative time averaged 20 minutes. Patients were discharged on average 1 week postoperatively. These results suggested that the procedure was safe, but experience in other centers was needed to confirm this.

Several aspects of the current management of patients with acute, severe, lower abdominal pain are highlighted by laparoscopic exposure. In the group with progressing signs, exposure with accurate diagnosis will allow their appropriate management, without

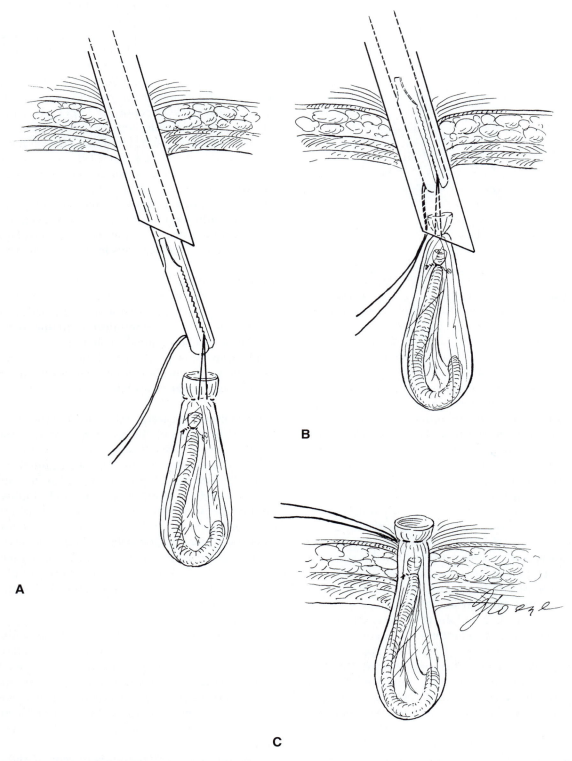

Figure 39–24. Extraction of a large appendix using a strong impermeable bag. **A**. The bag is introduced through an 11-mm port and the appendix placed within it. The drawstring is held by a strong grasper. **B**. The neck of the bag then is drawn into the cannula, which then is withdrawn, delivering the top of the bag out of the wound. **C**. Firm external traction on the bag allows delivery of the appendix with complete protection of the wound from contamination.

mandatory removal of the normal appendix. In those patients, most of whom are young adult females, where clinical signs during observation do not subside quickly or completely, early laparoscopy allows a definitive diagnosis to be established and, in most cases, early discharge from hospital. This approach may well be of most benefit to patients in whom evidence of low-grade tubal inflammation is more easily detected laparoscopically. Bacteriologic swabs can be taken and appropriate antibiotics prescribed. It is my suspicion that, in the past, a normal appendix was removed in these circumstances, and tubal sepsis was left undiagnosed and untreated with subsequent tubal scarring blamed on the appendectomy.

The benefits or otherwise of removal of the normal appendix are unclear. Can we be certain which appendixes are normal? The accuracy of visual assessment of the appendix both at open and laparoscopic surgery has been the subject of some recent scrutiny. These data are illustrated in Table 39–1.[63–65] It would appear from these data that the magnified laparoscopic view allows as good an assessment of the diagnosis of acute inflammation as open surgery. Grunewald and Keating make the telling observation that, in the subgroup of patients where no other cause for their symptoms is found at the time of the operation and the appendix appears normal, 9 out of 31 cases (29%) had histologic evidence of inflammation.[63] It must be emphasized that the entire length of the appendix, especially the tip, should be visible for proper evaluation. This may entail extensive mobilization of the cecum and terminal ileum, on occasion. Because of the extensive dissection required, which results in significant local scarring, my own view is that the routine removal of the appendix has not been demonstrated to be of benefit to the patient.

Concern remains regarding the adequacy of laparoscopic exposure to treat severe sepsis. The documented prospective data on the incidence of postoperative intraperitoneal sepsis, comparing open with laparoscopic appendectomy, is listed in Table 39–2.[66–69] The trends

TABLE 39–2. INCIDENCE OF POSTOPERATIVE SEPSIS IN OPEN COMPARED WITH LAPAROSCOPIC APPENDECTOMY

Number of Patients	Open	Laparoscopic
64[66]	2%	7%
109[67a]	0%	0%
155[68]	0%	6%
200[69]	1%	0%

[a]Denotes a prospective randomized series.

in these series are not clear and numbers of patients are small. It is imperative that, after removal of the appendix, the paracolic gutters and pelvis are adequately lavaged and aspirated dry. In those cases with extensive peritoneal pus, great care must be taken to clean out all the pockets collected between loops of bowel and the subphrenic areas. In all perforated cases, a diligent search for a fecalith should be made.

Wound complications have been documented in a number of recent comparative series and are listed in Table 39–3.[65–70] The number of patients in each study was not large and the trend toward lower wound infection rates is of interest. Long-term follow-up by Nowzaradan showed no incisional hernia in the laparoscopic series after 1.5 years, but 3 incisional hernias required repair in the open group.[69]

Postoperative recovery has been carefully evaluated in two prospective studies listed in Table 39–4.[67,70] These two small randomized series give some evidence of benefit in hospital stay but more significant differences in return to work and social activities.

Another area of possible benefit is the possible decrease in adhesive bowel obstruction. Adhesions between the omentum, cecum, small bowel, and abdominal wall occur in approximately 80% of patients after appendectomy for appendicitis.[71] In a randomized study of 40 patients having either open or laparoscopic appendectomy, a planned second-look laparoscopy at 3 months documented adhesions in 16 out of the 20 open

TABLE 39–1. ACCURACY OF OPEN VERSUS LAPAROSCOPIC DIAGNOSIS OF ACUTE APPENDICITIS

	Positive Predictive Value (%)	False Positive (%)	Negative Predictive Value (%)	False Negative (%)
Open Exposure (n=175)[63]	91	1	74	26
Laparoscopic Exposure (n=53)[64]	100	0	100	0
(n=122)[65]	93	0	90	10

TABLE 39–3. INCIDENCE OF WOUND COMPLICATIONS IN OPEN VERSUS LAPAROSCOPIC APPENDECTOMY

Number of Patients	Open	Laparoscopic
62[70]	1%	0%
64[66]	2%	0%
109[67a]	8.8%	0%
116[65]	9.4%	4.3%
155[68]	12%	2%
200[69]	1.1%	15.6%

[a]Denotes a prospective randomized series.

TABLE 39–4. ANALYSIS OF POSTOPERATIVE RECOVERY IN PROSPECTIVE RANDOMIZED TRIALS

	Laparoscopic (n=26)[a]	Open Appendectomy (n=28)[a]	p Value Wilcoxon
Hospital Stay	2 (1–7)	3 (1–7)	.01
To Work	10 (1–25)	16 (2–84)	.001
Full Fitness	21 (5–120)	38 (5–150)	.02
	Laparoscopic (n=52)[b]	**Open Appendectomy (n=57)[b]**	**t-test**
Hospital Stay	3.2 (0.6)	4.2 (1)	
Full Home Activity	16.7 (5)	30.1 (10)	p < 0.01
Full Social Activity	19.1 (6)	32.2 (12)	p < 0.05

[a]Numbers are in days (median/range):
[b]Numbers are days (mean ± SD). Adapted from references 67, and 70, with permission.

versus 2 out of the 20 laparoscopic appendectomies (P<.01).[72] This strongly supports the concept of a reduction in late bowel obstruction in those cases treated laparoscopically; however, data to prove the point may take years to accumulate.

There are substantial drawbacks to the introduction of laparoscopic appendectomy for routine clinical use. These include the inexperience of both senior and junior surgeons with the technique and equipment in what may be, for them, a very routine open procedure. Sufficient equipment is expensive and its introduction needs careful organization. However, this is made easier if the staff have previous experience with diagnostic laparoscopy and laparoscopic cholecystectomy. Experienced nursing personnel are essential to clean and maintain the equipment and keep it readily available for emergency surgery. While surgeons are learning the technique, a laparoscopic appendectomy takes about one-and-a-half times as long as a conventional operation.

However, the potential for decreased wound complications, more rapid recovery and earlier return to work following laparoscopic appendectomy has been validated by early randomized trials. The translation of these potential advantages to the broader community of surgeons awaits further evaluation.

ANTIBIOTIC THERAPY

Before the antibiotic era, sepsis was a common complication after appendectomy. Wound infection rates would vary from about 5% in cases of early inflammation to 75% if the appendix was gangrenous or perforated. Other septic complications (pelvic abscess, sub-

phrenic abscess, portal pyemia, and septicemia) were not uncommon in advanced cases and accounted for most of the deaths from this disease. Controlled studies have demonstrated the value of antibiotics in greatly reducing the mortality rate.

Infection in acute appendicitis is produced by a mixed inoculum of aerobic and anaerobic organisms, and there is good evidence that synergy exists between these two groups. Dealing with the anaerobic organisms alone is highly effective in preventing the development of postoperative sepsis. Metronidazole alone, given either as a suppository or intravenously, is probably sufficient prophylaxis in cases of early appendicitis, but when the appendix is gangrenous or perforated, best results are obtained by using a broad spectrum antibiotic against the aerobic organisms, in combination with metronidazole. In a controlled study, Saario and associates could demonstrate no difference between cefuroxime and gentamicin in combination with metronidazole; of 42 patients with peritonitis owing to perforation of the appendix who were randomly assigned to one of the two regimens, there were four wound infections in each group.[73] My choice of antibiotic therapy is metronidazole in combination with cefuroxime, an antibiotic that avoids the nephrotoxic and ototoxic risks of gentamicin.

POSTOPERATIVE COMPLICATIONS

The enormous difference between the usually smooth postoperative course after appendectomy in a case of early acute appendicitis and the stormy recovery that so often accompanies removal of a gangrenous, perforated appendix in a patient with generalized peritonitis emphasizes the importance of early diagnosis and treatment.

Paralytic Ileus

Paralytic ileus invariably accompanies general peritonitis. It is treated by means of regular doses of morphine, gastric aspiration, careful fluid and electrolyte replacement by intravenous drip, and antibiotic therapy using metronidazole and cefuroxime, while guided by bacteriologic study of the peritoneal exudate. Careful watch must be maintained to differentiate mechanical obstruction as a result of early postoperative adhesions because continued ileus requires conservative therapy, whereas mechanical obstruction calls for urgent laparotomy.

Septic Complications

These complications include *local wound abscess,* which is dealt with by removal of a suture and gentle probing of the wound to release the pus. A *pelvic abscess* is particularly likely to occur after removal of a perforated pelvic appendix. In addition to fever, there is often diarrhea with mucus discharge through the rectum. Rectal examination reveals a tender pelvic mass, which, in most cases, drains spontaneously into either the vagina or the rectum. Occasionally, drainage needs to be performed through the rectum or the posterior fornix of the vagina, with the patient under general anesthesia (Figs 39–16 and 39–17). *Subphrenic abscess* is now much less commonly associated with a perforated, gangrenous appendix than it was in the preantibiotic era. Wang and Wilson, for example, reviewing 93 cases occurring between 1955 and 1975, found that only 8% occurred after appendicitis.[74]

Rupture of the Stump or Cecal Wall

This tragedy is rare, but it occurs when a portion of the cecal wall or the appendix stump gives way in the first few days after appendectomy. Probably the most common cause is administration of an enema, which unduly distends the gut and causes it to rupture at some weakened spot. Enemas should never be prescribed postoperatively in bowel surgery since the general peritoneal cavity at once becomes flooded with fecal contents and enema fluid. The only hope of saving the patient's life is immediate laparotomy and the performance of a cecostomy. Metronidazole and cefuroxime are administered by the intravenous route.

Hemorrhage

Sudden abdominal pain and shock at any time during the first 72 hours after appendectomy may mean either leakage from the stump or a slipped arterial ligature, both of which now are rare. More often, bleeding is gradual and arises from a blood vessel in the mesoappendix or in a divided adhesion not noticed at the time of operation. On reexploration of the wound, after removal of a mass of clotted blood from the hollow of the pelvis and right paracolic gutter, it is exceptional to locate the site of the hemorrhage. At best, the mesoappendix is ligated once more and the wound closed with a generous tube drain.

Late Complications

Late complications after appendectomy are unusual. It is rare to see a hernia through a right iliac fossa muscle-splitting incision. When this does occur, there is almost invariably a history of prolonged sepsis and of the use of a large drain at what is now the site of the hernia. Probably the most common late complication is intestinal obstruction due to a local adhesive band.

There have been few accurate studies of the risk of infertility as a complication of a perforated appendicitis in young women. Recently, Puri and associates reviewed case reports of 134 girls who, at less than 13 years of age, had undergone appendectomy for a perforated appen-

dix; 103 of these subjects, now adults, were traced.[75] Of these, 59 were married and had had one or more children (as had two of the unmarried women). Of the nine women with no children, one had miscarried and five had been married for less than a year. Two further patients consented to be investigated; one had a sterile husband, and the other had patent tubes. The remaining patient refused to be studied. These authors concluded (1) that pelvic peritonitis and abscess in childhood resolve in the majority of cases after appendectomy and appropriate antibiotic therapy without permanent tubal damage, and (2) that these complications during childhood do not result in salpingitis or endometriosis in the adult.

MORTALITY RATE

The dramatic effect of antibiotics on the mortality rate from sepsis is well illustrated by the statistics related to appendicitis. Until 1938, more than 3000 deaths from acute appendicitis took place in England and Wales each year; the number had fallen to 1774 by 1945, to 498 by 1964, and to 375 by 1969. By 1985, the annual deaths amounted to only 147, of which 10 were recorded in children between 1 and 14 years of age (four male and three female deaths per million of the population). The statistics quoted by one of the most expert surgeons of his day, when antibiotics were not available, are of great interest: Turner, reviewing over 2500 personal appendectomies, found a mortality of 0.68% in cases of early acute appendicitis.[76] However, this rose to nearly 10% in cases with local peritonitis, and to 29% in cases with diffuse peritonitis. The overall mortality in the whole series was 3.5%. In contrast, Peltokallio and Tykka reviewed nearly 10 000 cases of appendectomy from Helsinki, with only 29 deaths (0.27%).[77] In the nonperforated group, this amounted to 0.12%, and in the perforated group to 1.18%. Pieper and associates found only 2 deaths in their review of 1018 appendectomies (0.2%).[78] One of these deaths was of a woman, 73 years of age, who died of a pulmonary embolism and the other, of a woman 84 years of age, who died of a myocardial infarction.

The deaths that do occur as a result of appendicitis are usually of infants or elderly persons, and are associated with delays in diagnosis and the presence of advanced peritonitis. These deaths also are associated with other serious medical conditions, particularly myocardial or pulmonary disease.

■ CHRONIC APPENDICITIS

No one will deny that patients can experience *recurrent* attacks of appendicitis. Indeed, it is not unusual for one or more such episodes to precede a full-blown acute appendicitis. Chronic, or grumbling, appendicitis as an entity is still a subject of controversy. Today, there are many more skeptics than believers, and this author is convinced that there is no such organic entity. It has been well said that "the appendix does not grumble—it either screams or remains silent."

It was once fashionable to attribute many of the psychosomatic conditions that beset the abdomen, of which the irritable bowel syndrome is the most common, to chronic appendicitis and to remove the offending organ. The results, however, are not at all good. An interesting study by Ingram and Evans reviewed 118 young women who had undergone appendectomy a year previously.[78] Of those treated for acute appendicitis, 90% were perfectly well and satisfied at review, but 55% of those whose appendix was normal at operation were still experiencing symptoms at the time of follow-up.

■ UNUSUAL CONDITIONS OF THE APPENDIX

DIVERTICULUM

A diverticulum, or diverticulosis, of the appendix is occasionally found (Fig 39–25). It was documented in detail by Wilson.[79]

INTUSSUSCEPTION

Intussusception of the appendix is rare, with only about 160 cases reported since McKidd described the first example in 1858.[80] Fraser reported 7 new cases and reviewed 75 previously published examples.[81] The disease may occur at any age, although the majority are seen in the first two decades of life. Occasionally, a mucocele of the appendix, an adenomatous polyp, a carcinoid tumor, or a foreign body may precipitate the condition.

The intussusception may start either at the tip or at the base of the appendix, with complete inversion into the cecum being the final result in either case. In most of the collected cases, the intussusception was of the simple form (ie, inversion into the cecum), but in some instances, the appendicular inversion was associated with cecocolic or ileocolic intussusception. Rarely, the intussuscepted appendix first has been detected on rectal examination.

Cleland noted six reported case in which the stump of the recently amputated appendix formed the apex of a colic intussusception.[82] The main symptom is colic and the outstanding physical sign is a palpable mass in the right iliac fossa that is slightly tender by freely movable. The intussusception can be visualized on barium enema examination, but the exact nature of the intussusception is rarely guessed at.

It is usually possible to reduce the intussusception by operative manipulation. When reduction is complete,

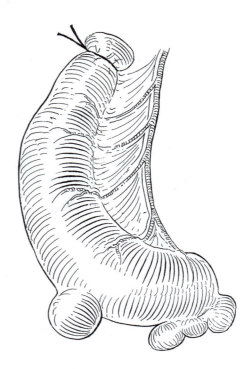

Figure 39–25. Diverticulosis of the appendix.

the appendix is excised in the usual way. If it is not possible to effect reduction, a local resection with ileocolic anastomosis is performed.

TORSION

Torsion of the appendix was first described by Payne in 1918.[83] Since then, only a few cases have been described.[84] In the majority of cases, the appendix was in the pelvic position and had undergone torsion in a counterclockwise direction. The etiologic factors are unknown, but a lax, fan-shaped mesoappendix, and the presence of foreign bodies in the appendix, have both received attention. The signs and symptoms are those of acute appendicitis, and the treatment is expeditious appendectomy.

Endometriosis

The appendix is affected in <1% of cases of pelvic endometriosis. Rarely, the appendix alone is affected.[85]

■ TUMORS

Tumors of the appendix are unusual, probably because of the small surface area of mucosa that is available for malignant change. Therefore, the appendix is probably just as likely to develop cancer as any other part of the large bowel, of which it represents an adnexa. It is true, however, that the distribution of tumor type is in rather sharp contrast to the rest of the large bowel. By far the most common neoplasm of the appendix is the carcinoid tumor, which accounts for some 85% of all tumors of this organ and which is found in about 0.1% of all appendixes subjected to careful histologic examination. As with the rest of the large bowel, villous tumors and carcinomas also may occur.

Benign tumors of the appendix are rare, but include adenomatous polyps, mucous cystadenoma, leiomyoma, fibroma, and neuroma. The mucous cystadenoma, while uncommon, may obstruct the lumen of the appendix and distend the organ with mucus to form a mucocele. The other benign lesions, because they develop in the wall of the appendix, do not obstruct its lumen, are rarely of clinical significance, and usually are detected only as an incidental observation in an appendectomy specimen or at postmortem.

The malignant tumors comprise malignant carcinoid, villous adenocarcinoma, and what has been termed the colonic type of adenocarcinoma.

CARCINOID TUMOR

Carcinoid tumor is the most common of all tumors of the appendix and the only one likely to be encountered by a general surgeon in routine practice. It is usually a solitary finding, although occasionally it may be associated with carcinoids of the ileum. In the detailed study by Moertel and colleagues in 1968, at the Mayo Clinic, 71% of these tumors, from a total of 144 specimens, occurred in the tip, 22% in the body, and 7% at the base of the appendix.[86] The tumor may occur at any age, including childhood, although it tends to affect patients in their thirties and forties. When the tumor occurs in the tip of the appendix, it is usually identified easily by the surgeon at laparotomy, but those in the body or at the base may mimic a fecalith.

Pathology

Carcinoid tumors arise from the argentaffin cells, which are situated in the bases of the crypts of the intestinal mucosa. These cells are often termed Kulchitsky cells, in honor of the histologist who gave the original description. Characteristically, the cells contain silver-staining granules in their cytoplasm; hence the alternative name of argentaffinoma.

To the naked eye, the tumor in the appendix forms a hard, greyish-yellow nodule arising in the deep aspect of the mucosa, with a diameter varying between 0.5 and 3.5 cm. On microscopic examination, the muscle wall is invaded and, in many cases, the overlying peritoneum is involved. Metastatic spread, however, is rare. In the study by Moertel and associates, metastases were present in 1.4% of cases and were practically confined to lesions

that were >2 cm in diameter.[86] Such tumors account for only 1% of carcinoids of the appendix. In the study by Svendsen and Bülow of 64 patients with carcinoid tumors of the appendix who were <40 years of age, only one patient had local metastases, and in this case the tumor was 2 cm in diameter.[87] Anderson and Wilson studied 147 patients with carcinoid tumors of the appendix.[88] Two of these patients had metastatic spread at the time of presentation, and both had tumors >2 cm in diameter. Parkes and associates reviewed 40 children with this condition who were under the age of 15.[89] All the tumors were incidental findings. There were no recurrences, metastases or deaths. They estimate an incidence of 0.08% of appendectomies in children, or a rate of 1.14 per million children per year.

The majority of carcinoids are found incidentally on routine histologic study of appendixes removed during the course of laparotomy for other procedures. Because of the usual location of the tumor at the tip of the organ, acute appendicitis does not usually develop. However, the lumen may be occluded by a tumor at the base or in the body of the appendix, and the carcinoid then may present as a case of acute appendicitis or even as an appendiceal abscess (Fig 39–26).

The carcinoid syndrome, resulting from the secretion of 5-hydroxytryptamine into the portal circulation, is seen only in cases of extensive malignant carcinoid, nearly always associated with hepatic metastases. In these instances, the appendix is rarely the primary site, and the tumor is usually situated in the terminal ileum (see Chapter 38).

VILLOUS TUMORS

Villous tumors of the appendix may be papillary or adenomatous. The majority are noninvasive but have a propensity to fill the appendix with mucus and to make a differentiation from a benign mucocele of the appendix difficult. If unruptured, the tumor will rarely metastasize, but perforation of a malignant mucocele may result in the development of *pseudomyxoma peritonei*.

ADENOCARCINOMA

The first case of carcinoma of the appendix was described by Berger in 1882.[90] Menon,[91] in a 1980 report of two cases presenting as appendicular masses, was able to collect fewer than 200 examples in English-language publications and presents a valuable clinical review of the subject. Gilhome and associates found only 10 confirmed examples amount 9380 appendixes submitted to pathologic examination, while Burgess and Done noted 11 carcinomas found at 10 526 appendectomies; of these, eight were removed as emergencies and three at elective operations.[13]

The histologic appearance of adenocarcinoma of the

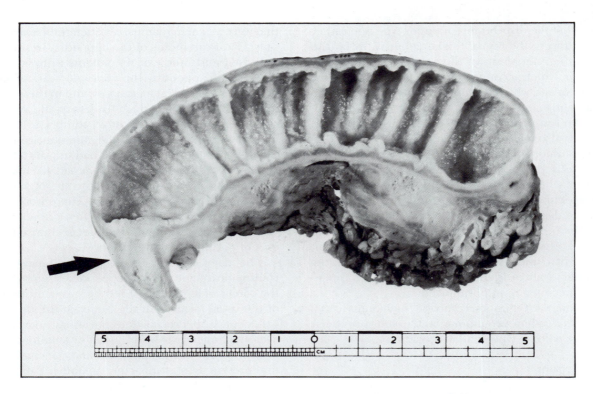

Figure 39–26. Carcinoid tumor (*arrow*) at the base of the appendix, producing acute appendicitis.

appendix is similar to that of tumors elsewhere in the large bowel, except that mucus secretion is rather more prominent. The lesion may be polypoid or ulcerative and may cause hemorrhage or obstruction of the appendix. Typically the tumor arises at the base of the appendix in patients over 50 years of age. It may be an incidental finding or may be thought to be acute appendicitis or an appendiceal abscess. If the tumor invades the cecum, it may be difficult to differentiate it from a primary carcinoma of cecal origin. Hesketh, in a study of a collected series of 95 cases, found that the majority were thought to be acute appendicitis, appendiceal abscess, or chronic right iliac fossa pain.[93] In 14% the tumor was detected as an incidental finding at laparotomy, and in another 11% widespread metastases were found at presentation.

MANAGEMENT

It would be rare indeed for a surgeon to make a diagnosis of tumor of the appendix before operation. If the tumor is discovered at laparotomy, either in dealing with an acutely inflamed appendix or as an incidental finding, then fine judgment is required in its management. If a confident diagnosis of carcinoid tumor is made, the rest of the small intestine should be carefully examined for other carcinoid tumors, which oc-

casionally may be multiple. The mesoappendix and right mesocolon are examined carefully for lymph node involvement, and the liver is accurately palpated. In the vast majority of cases, the findings will be completely negative, and under such circumstances, particularly if the carcinoid tumor is <2 cm in diameter, nothing more needs to be done but to carry out appendectomy. If, however, involved nodes are found, then a right hemicolectomy is the treatment of choice. Right hemicolectomy is indicated also in the rare instances when the carcinoid tumor is >2 cm in diameter. When the tumor of the appendix is obviously malignant, then a right hemicolectomy is performed (Fig 39–27).

Sometimes the diagnosis is not established until the postoperative examination of the specimen. If a carcinoid tumor is found and the resection has been adequate, no further procedure need be contemplated. If the carcinoid involved the bases of the appendix, and histologic examination showed that the resection had been incomplete, then there is certainly a case for reoperation, with excision of an adequate cuff of surrounding cecal wall. If the specimen shows the presence of an undoubted adenocarcinoma, then even if resection had been adequate, the patient should be advised to submit to a formal right hemicolectomy.

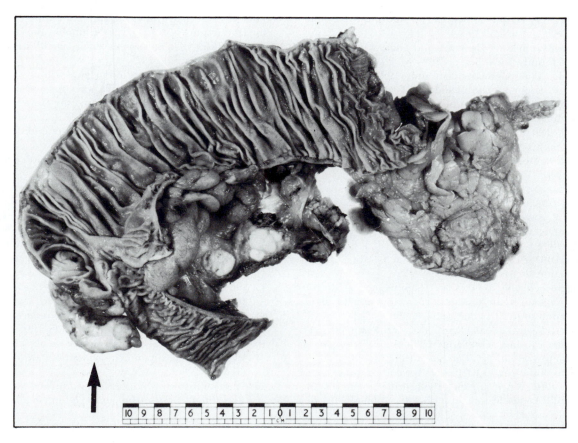

Figure 39–27. Adenocarcinoma of the appendix (*arrow*) removed by right hemicolectomy. Note enlarged and involved lymph nodes in the mesocolon.

PROGNOSIS

With rare exceptions, carcinoid tumor of the appendix is cured by appendectomy. The only exceptions are those unusual cases in which the tumor is >2 cm in diameter or there is evidence of lymphatic or hepatic spread at the time of operation.

With regard to the prognosis of carcinoma of the appendix, it is difficult to give accurate figures when the total number of cases reported is in the region of 200. Andersson and associates, in a well-documented paper, pointed out that the prognosis of malignant mucocele of the appendix is excellent after appendectomy, provided that the mucocele had not perforated, had not invaded the submucosa, and was confined to the tip.[31] Of six patients submitted to appendectomy, all six achieved 5 year survival. In a review of 51 cases of primary adenocarcinoma of the appendix of the colonic type, these authors noted that of 26 patients treated by appendectomy alone, 12 (46%) were still alive 5 years after the operation, compared with 15 (60%) of 25 patients subjected to right hemicolectomy.[94]

REFERENCES

1a. Cope Z. *A History of the Acute Abdomen.* London, England: Oxford University Press; 1965

1b. Major RH. *Classic Descriptions of Disease,* 3rd ed. Springfield, IL: Charles C Thomas; 1944

1. Fitz RH. Perforating inflammation of the veriform appendix with special reference to its early diagnosis and treatment. *Trans Assoc Am Physicians* 1886;1:107

2. McBurney C. Experience with early operative interference in cases of disease of the vermiform appendix. *NY Med J* 1889;50:676

3. Wakeley CP. The position of the vermiform appendix as ascertained by an analysis of 10 000 cases. *J Anat* 1933; 67:277

4. Pickens G, Ellis H, et al. The normal vermiform appendix at computed tomography: visualization and anatomical location. *Clin Anat* 1993;6:9

5. Williamson WA, Bush RD, et al. Retrocecal appendicitis. *Am J Surg* 1981;141:507

6. Robinson JO. Congenital absence of vermiform appendix. *Br J Surg* 1952;39:344

7. Khanna AK. Appendix vermiformis duplex. *Postgrad Med J* 1983;59:69

8. Wallbridge PH. Double appendix. *Br J Surg* 1962;50:346

9. Tinckler LF. Triple appendix vermiformis—a unique case. *Br J Surg* 1968;55:79

10. Office of Population Censuses and Surveys: Hospital In-patient Inquiry 1984, Series MB4 No. 25. London, England: Her Majesty's Stationery Office; 1984

11. Pieper R, Kager L. The incidence of acute appendicitis and appendectomy: an epidemiological study of 971 cases. *Acta Chir Scand* 1982;148:45

12. Noer T. Decreasing incidence of acute peritonitis. *Acta Chir Scand* 1975;141:431

13. Burgess P, Done HJ. Adenocarcinoma of the appendix. *J R Soc Med* 1989;82:28

14. Andersson N, Griffiths H, et al. Is appendicitis familial? *Br Med J* 1979;2:697

15. Pieper R, Kager L, et al. The role of *Bacteroides fragilis* in the pathogenesis of acute appendicitis. *Acta Chir Scand* 1982;148:39

16. Wilkie DPD. Acute appendicitis and acute appendicular obstruction. *Br Med J* 1914;2:959

17. Wangensteen OH, Bowers WF. Significance of the obstructive factor in the genesis of acute appendicitis: an experimental study. *Arch Surg* 1937;34:496

18. Pieper R, Kager L, et al. Obstruction of the appendix vermiformis causing acute appendicitis: an experimental study in the rabbit. *Acta Chir Scand* 1982;148:63

19. Thomas WEG, Vowles KDJ, et al. Appendicitis in external herniae. *Ann R Coll Surg Engl* 1982;64:121

20. Shaw RE. Appendix calculi and acute appendicitis. *Br J Surg* 1965;52:451

21. Ellis H. Diagnosis of the acute abdomen. *Br Med J* 1968;1:491

22. Smith PH. The diagnosis of appendicitis. *Postgrad Med J* 1965;41:2

23. Coetzee T. Acute appendicitis in an infant. *S Afr Med J* 1958;32:890

24. Fields IA, Naiditch MJ, et al. Acute appendicitis in infants: ten-year survey at the Los Angeles County Hospital. *Am J Dis Child* 1957;93:287

25. Ayalon A, Mogilner M, et al. Acute appendicitis in a premature baby. *Acta Chir Scand* 1979;145:285

26. Leffall LD, Cooperman A, et al. Appendicitis: a continuing surgical challenge. *Am J Surg* 1967;113:654

27. Jackson RH. Parents, family doctors and acute appendicitis in childhood. *Br Med J* 1963;2:277

28. Fields IA, Cole NM. Acute appendicitis in infants thirty-six months of age or younger: ten-year survey at the Los Angeles County hospital. *Am J Surg* 1967;113:269

29. Winsey HS, Jones PF. Acute abdominal pain in childhood: analysis of a year's admissions. *Br Med J* 1967;1:653

30. Peltokallio P, Jauhianen K. Acute appendicitis in the aged patient: study of 300 cases after the age of 60. *Arch Surg* 1970;100:140

31. Andersson A, Bergdahl L, et al. Primary carcinoma of the appendix. *Ann Surg* 1976;183:53

32. Owens BJ, Hamit HF. Appendicitis in the elderly. *Ann Surg* 1978;187:392

33. Black WP. Acute appendicitis in pregnancy. *Br Med J* 1960;1:1938

34. Doberneck RC. Appendectomy during pregnancy. *Am Surg* 1985;51:265

35. Francis D. The grumbling appendix. *Br Med J* 1979;2:936

36. Doraiswamy NV. Leucocyte counts in the diagnosis and prognosis of acute appendicitis in children. *Br J Surg* 1979;66:782

37. Bower RJ, Bell MJ, et al. Diagnostic value of the white blood count and neutrophil percentage in the evaluation of abdominal pain in children. *Surg Gynecol Obstet* 1981;152:424

38. Graham JA. Urinary cell counts in appendicitis. *Scot Med J* 1965;10:126

39. Brooks DW, Killen DA. Roentgenographic findings in acute appendicitis. *Surgery* 1965;57:377

40. Saebo A. Pneumoperitoneum associated with perforated appendicitis. *Acta Chir Scand* 1978;144:115

41. Killen DA, Brooks DW. Gas-filled appendix: a roentgenographic sign of acute appendicitis. *Ann Surg* 1965;161:474

42. Smith DE, Kirchmer NA, et al. Use of barium enema in the diagnosis of acute appendicitis and its complications. *Am J Surg* 1979;138:829

43. Pearson RH. Ultrasonography for diagnosing appendicitis. *Br Med J* 1988;297:309

44. Ooms HW, Koumans RK, et al. Ultrasonography in the diagnosis of acute appendicitis. *Br J Surg* 1991;78:315

45. Paterson-Brown S, Thompson JN, et al. Which patients with suspected appendicitis should undergo laparoscopy? *Br Med J* 1988;296:1363

46. Paterson-Brown S, Vipond MN. Modern aids to clinical decision-making in the acute abdomen. *Br J Surg* 1990;77:13

47. Jona JZ. Basilar pneumonia simulating acute appendicitis in children. *Arch Surg* 1976;111:552

48. Valerio D. Acute diabetic abdomen in childhood. *Lancet* 1976;1:66

49. Pieper R, Kager L, et al. Acute appendicitis: a clinical study of 1,018 cases of emergency appendectomy. *Acta Chir Scand* 1982;148:51

50. Engstrom L, Fenyo G. Appendectomy: assessment of stump invagination versus simple ligation—a prospective randomized study. *Br J Surg* 1985;72:971

51. Arnbjornsson E. Management of appendiceal abscess. *Curr Surg* 1984;41:4

52. Nitecki S, Assalia A, Schein M. Contemporary management of the appendiceal mass. *Br J Surg* 1993;80:18

53. Goletti O, Lippolis PV, et al. Percutaneous ultrasound-guided drainage of intra-abdominal abscesses. *Br J Surg* 1993;80:336

54. Foran B, Berne TV, et al. Management of the appendiceal mass. *Arch Surg* 1978;113:1144

55. Gästrin U, Josephson S. Appendiceal abscess—acute appendectomy or conservative treatment? *Acta Chir Scand* 1969;135:539

56. Skoubo-Kristensen E, Hvid I. The appendiceal mass: results of conservation management. *Ann Surg* 1982;196:584

57. Hedner J, Jansson R, et al. Appendico-cutaneous fistula: a case report. *Acta Chir Scand* 1978;144:123

58. Pelosi MA, Pelosi MA III. Laparoscopy using a single umbilical puncture (minilaparoscopy). *J Repro Med* 1992;37:588–594

59. de Kok HJ. A new technique for resecting the non-inflamed not adhesive appendix through a minilaparo-

tomy with the aid of the laparoscope. *Arch Chir Neerl* 1977; 29:195–198

60. Pier A, Got F, Backer C. Laparoscopic appendectomy in 625 cases: from innovation to routine. *Surg Laparosc Endosc* 1991;1:8–13

61. Engstom L, Fenyo G. Appendectomy: assessment of stump invagination versus simple ligation—a prospective randomized study. *Br J Surg* 1985;72:971

62. Semms K. Endoscopic appendectomy. *Endoscopy* 1983;15: 59–64

63. Grunewald B, Keating J. Should the "normal" appendix be removed at operation for appendicitis? *J R Coll Edinb* 1993;38:158–160

64. Cox MR, McCall JL, Wilson TG, et al. Laparoscopic appendectomy: a prospective analysis. *Aust NZ J Surg* 1993; 63:840–847

65. Schirmer BD, Schmieg RE Jr, Dix J, et al. Laparoscopic versus traditional appendectomy for suspected appendicitis. *Am J Surg* 1993;165:670–675

66. Gilchrist BF, Lobe TE, Schropp KP, et al. Is there a role for laparoscopic appendectomy in pediatric surgery. *J Pediatr Surg* 1992;27:209–214

67. Kum CK, Ngoi SS, Goh PMY, et al. Randomized controlled trial comparing laparoscopic and open appendicectomy. *Br J Surg* 1993 (in press).

68. Tate JJT, Chung SCS, Dawson J, et al. Conventional versus laparoscopic surgery for acute appendicitis. *Br J Surg* 1993;80:761–764

69. Nowzaradan Y, Barnes JP, Westmoreland J, et al. Laparoscopic appendectomy: treatment of choice for suspected appendicitis. *Surg Laprosc Endosc* 1993;5:411–416

70. Attwood SEA, Hill ADK, Murphy PG, et al. A prospective randomized trial of laparoscopic versus open appendectomy. *Surgery* 1992;112:497–501

71. Semms K, Freys I. Endoscopic appendectomy: technical operative steps. *Minim Invas Ther* 1991;1:41–50

72. De Wilde RL. Goodbye to late bowel obstruction after appendicectomy. *Lancet* 1991;338:1012

73. Saario I, Arvilommi H, et al. Comparison of cefuroxime and gentamicin in combination with metronidazole in the treatment of peritonitis due to perforation of the appendix. *Acta Chir Scand* 1983;149:423

74. Wang SMS, Wilson SE. Subphrenic abscess: the new epidemiology. *Arch Surg* 1977;112:934

75. Puri B, Guiney EJ, et al. Effects of perforated appendicitis in girls on subsequent fertility. *Br Med J* 1984;288:25

76. Turner GG, Rogers LC (eds). *Modern Operative Surgery*, vol 1, 4 ed. London, England: Cassell; 1956:1142

77. Peltokallio P, Tykka H. Evolution of the age distribution and mortality of acute appendicitis. *Arch Surg* 1981; 116:153

78. Ingram PW, Evans G. Right iliac fossa pain in young women. *Br Med J* 1965;2:149

79. Wilson RR. Diverticula of appendix and certain factors in their development. *Br J Surg* 1950;38:65

80. McKidd J. Case of invagination of caecum and appendix. *Edinb Med J* 1858;4:793

81. Fraser K. Intussusception of the appendix. *Br J Surg* 1943; 31:23

82. Cleland G. Caecocolic intussusception following appendicectomy. *Br J Surg* 1953;41:108

83. Payne JE. A case of torsion of the appendix. *Br J Surg* 1918;6:327

84. Peterson KR, Brooks L, et al. Torsio appendicis veriformis: report of an unusual case. *Acta Chir Scand* 1982; 148:383

85. Langman J, Rowland R, et al. Endometriosis of the appendix. *Br J Surg* 1981;68:121.

86. Moertel GC, Dockerty MB, et al. Carcinoid tumors of the vermiform appendix. *Cancer* 1968;21:270

87. Svendsen LB, Bülow S. Carcinoid tumours of the appendix in young patients. *Acta Chir Scand* 1980;146:137

88. Anderson JR, Wilson BG. Carcinoid tumours of the appendix. *Br J Surg* 1985;72:545

89. Parkes SE, Muir KR, et al. Carcinoid tumours of the appendix in children. *Br J Surg* 1993;80:502

90. Berger A. Ein Fall von Krebs des Wurmfortsatzes. *Berl Klin Wochenschr* 1882;19:616

91. Menon NK. Primary adenocarcinoma of the appendix. *Postgrad Med J* 1980;56:448

92. Gilhome RW, Johnston DW, et al. Primary adenocarcinoma of the vermiform appendix: report of a series of 10 cases and review of the literature. *Br J Surg* 1984; 71:553

93. Hesketh KT. The management of primary adenocarcinoma of the vermiform appendix. *Gut* 1963;4:158

94. Andersson A, Bergdahl L. Acute appendicitis in patients over sixty. *Am Surg* 1978;44:445

40

Diverticular Disease of the Colon

Thomas George Parks

■ HISTORICAL BACKGROUND

Credit for the earliest detailed description of diverticular disease of the colon is usually ascribed to Cruveilhier.[1] Virchow, in 1853, described a condition of "isolate circumscribed adhesive peritonitis" and, although he also described colonic diverticula, he did not associate the two lesions.[2] Habershon, a physician at Guy's Hospital, London, is credited with publishing the first account of colonic diverticula in the English language, in 1857.[3] Two years later, Jones reported a case of diverticulitis complicated by fistulization into the urinary bladder.[4]

Toward the end of the 19th century, in Germany, Graser emphasized the pathologic significance of the condition when he described the hyperplastic stenosing form of the disease known as peridiverticulitis and emphasized its stimulation to carcinoma of the sigmoid colon.[5] Moynihan reported a case of peridiverticulitis and underlined the difficulties in the differential diagnosis.[6] Wilson, in 1911, after careful pathologic study, suggested that chronic inflammation could be responsible for the segregation of colonic epithelium from which carcinoma might subsequently develop.[7] Although this view was held for a time by Mayo and others, little concrete evidence was put forward to support it.[8]

Spriggs and Marxer stressed the importance of radiology in establishing a diagnosis and assessing the extent and degree of involvement.[9] They described in detail what they called "the prediverticular state," although Marxer had earlier introduced the term in his writings.[10]

The place of surgery in the treatment of diverticular disease was emphasized by Mayo and associates who recommended the use of a temporary colostomy, followed by resection, for the treatment of obstruction associated with inflammation.[11] However, it was not until Smithwick showed that surgery could be carried out with an acceptable mortality that resection of the diseased segment was frequently undertaken as a planned procedure.[12]

The term "diverticulosis" was proposed independently in 1914 by Case and de Quervain to describe the condition characterized by the presence of uncomplicated and noninflamed colonic mucosal pouches[13,14] (Fig 40–1). The terms "diverticulitis" and "peridiverticulitis" indicate inflammation in and around diverticula. The distinction between diverticulosis and diverticulitis is not always clear; thus, it is helpful to adopt the nomenclature "diverticular disease" to encompass the complicated as well as the uncomplicated state.

■ INCIDENCE

It is difficult to assess accurately the frequency with which diverticular disease occurs in the community, since it often remains symptomless, and many patients with the disorder do not present for investigation at the hospital.

The prevalence of diverticular disease of the colon varies considerably in different parts of the world. In rural Africa and Latin America and certain areas of Asia,

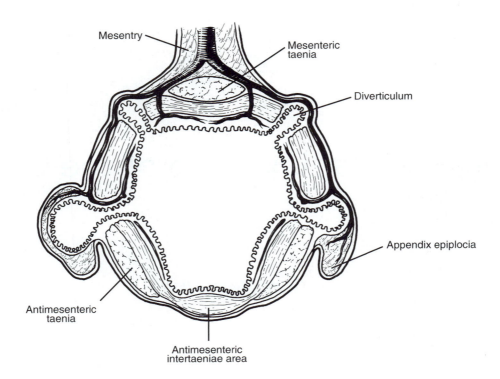

Figure 40–1. Diagrammatic representation of the relationship of diverticula and blood vessels to the teniae coli.

the incidence is very low compared with that in the Western countries. Coode and colleagues recorded only a 5% incidence of diverticula in an autopsy study in Hong Kong; half of these cases were solitary diverticula of the cecum.[15] In West Africa, the native who ingests a bulky diet rarely suffers from diverticular disease. On the other hand, volvulus of the excessively large colon is relatively common. Colonic diverticula are not uncommon among those of African extraction who live in North America.

There is a considerable amount of evidence relating dietary fiber intake to the prevalence of diverticular disease of the colon. When more refined techniques for milling of grain were introduced in Great Britain about 100 years ago, the fiber content of flour dropped to about one tenth of its former level. Subsequently, the incidence of diverticula began to rise in the community in which the intake of fiber was markedly reduced. It is now widely accepted that an adequate intake of dietary fiber in the form of wholemeal bread, fruit and vegetables, and a reduced intake of refined carbohydrates considerably reduces the tendency to develop colonic diverticula.[16]

Colonic diverticula are uncommon in patients under 40 years of age. In this country about 5% of patients in the fifth decade of life have colonic diverticula, and by the eight or ninth decade, up to 50% of individuals are affected.

DIVERTICULAR DISEASE IN THE ELDERLY

The incidence of diverticular disease increases with longevity. Furthermore, if complications develop in elderly patients, the associated mortality is higher than for those of a younger age group. Older patients also suffer from a higher incidence of concurrent disease and, if inflammatory complications ensue, the sufferers are less likely to withstand the adverse effects of this disease. Colonic hemorrhage in the elderly hypertensive subject is not infrequently associated with diverticulosis.

DIVERTICULAR DISEASE IN YOUNG SUBJECTS

Diverticular disease presenting in younger individuals tends to be a more aggressive form of disease and is associated with more troublesome recurrent episodes of inflammation. Hannan and associates reported that an operative procedure was required in more than 60% of younger patients with symptomatic diverticular disease, compared with only 20% to 30% of all patients with diverticular disease who came under their care.[17] High complication and readmission rates were reported by Ouriel and Schwartz, in patients under 40 years of age suffering from diverticular disease of the colon.[18] Fig 40–2 demonstrates marked muscle abnormality in a patient who had perforated diverticular disease when 25 years of age. Fig 40–3 shows consid-

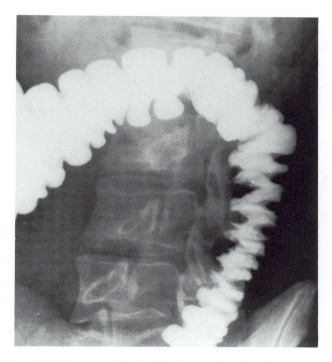

Figure 40–2. Barium enema of a male patient 25 years of age who had had a previous pelvic abscess secondary to acute peridiverticulitis confirmed at laparotomy and treated by drainage alone. A few diverticula were present and marked zig-zag deformity owing to muscle thickening and shortening was demonstrable in the sigmoid and descending colon.

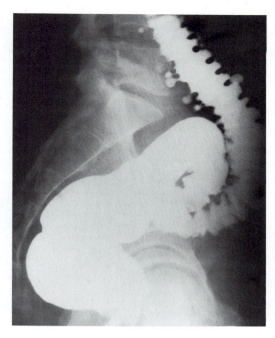

Figure 40–3. Radiograph of the same patient as illustrated in Fig 40–2, taken after an interval of 8 years, when the patient was 33 years of age. Considerable progress of the disease process with marked diverticular formation.

erable diverticular formation by 33 years of age, in the same patient.

■ PATHOLOGY

MORPHOLOGIC FEATURES

Although the circular muscle fibers of the colon form a complete layer, the outer longitudinal fibers are concentrated into three bands of teniae, leaving much of the colonic wall devoid of a distinct longitudinal coat. Thus, when diverticula develop, they occur in the areas between the teniae (Fig 40–1), in other words, in the lateral interteniae areas and, much less commonly, in the antimesenteric interteniae area. The herniations of the mucous membrane tend to occur along arteries that penetrate the muscle wall en route to the submucosa and mucosa. Vessels larger than those that reach the antimesenteric region penetrate the muscle wall in the lateral areas. Fig 40–4 shows a segment of sigmoid colon in which large diverticula are present in the lateral areas, whereas small pouches at an early stage of development are seen in the area between the two antimesenteric teniae.

For the most part, colonic diverticula are false diver-

ticula, the wall being made up of mucosa and muscularis mucosae covered by serosa. Initially, the diverticula are covered by muscle but as they enlarge, the investing muscle thins and atrophies and virtually disappears except perhaps for an area around the neck. Early lesions are small protrusions into which, and from which, fecal material can pass readily. As they enlarge, they become flask-like in shape with a relatively narrow neck. It is inevitable that fecal stasis will occur in these diverticula, particularly because there is a lack of muscle in the wall (Fig 40–5).

Morson demonstrated that one of the most consistent features of the diverticular colon is the thickening of the muscle coats[19] (Fig 40–6). Further light has been thrown on the pathogenesis of the condition in a fascinating study by Whiteway and Morson who demonstrated excessive amounts of elastin in the teniae, but not in the circular muscle of the colon in diverticular disease.[20] They considered the increase in formation of elastin, which they termed "elastosis," to be a progressive age-related phenomenon. As the elastin molecules are being laid down, they adopt a spiral contracted state that resists lengthening. The tissue is thought to be derived from the fibroblasts or even the muscle cells, possibly in response to inter-

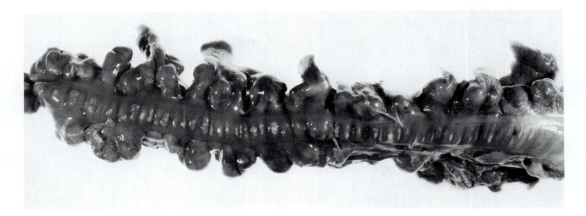

Figure 40–4. Specimen showing numerous large diverticula in the lateral interteniae areas. Early diverticular formation between the antimesenteric teniae.

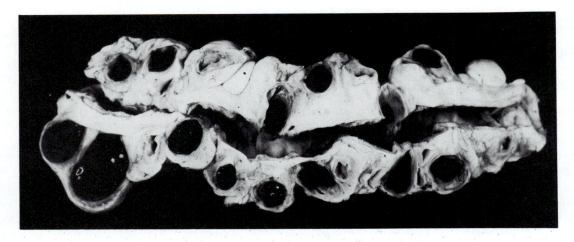

Figure 40–5. Specimen demonstrating numerous fecaliths in sigmoid diverticula.

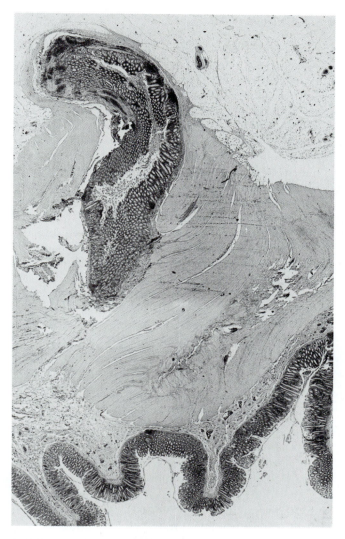

Figure 40–6. Photomicrograph demonstrating numerous fecaliths in sigmoid diverticula.

mittent increases in pressure. These electron microscopic findings in the longitudinal teniae help to explain the distinctive macroscopic features found in the musculature of the colonic wall, which are an integral part of the diverticular disease. As a result of thickening and shortening, the colonic wall looks like a concertina. This leads to the formation of thick circular muscle folds that project into the lumen of the bowel, causing considerable narrowing (Fig 40–2). The mucosa and submucosa also are heaped up, thus causing further encroachment on the lumen. The mesocolon of the diverticular colon also tends to be shortened. Although the majority of patients with diverticular disease have this muscle abnormality as a main feature, there are some patients who have diverticula widely scattered and densely concentrated

along the colon and who have no evidence of muscular thickening.

■ INFLAMMATORY ASPECTS

The earliest signs of inflammation often occur in lymphoid tissue at the apex of a diverticulum. This may result from abrasion of the mucosal lining of the pouch by inspissated feces that form a fecalith (Fig 40–5).

Low-grade inflammation extends readily to involve adjacent peritoneum, pericolic fat, and mesenteric fat, since the diverticula are thin walled and lie mainly outside the muscular wall of the colon.

The inflammation commonly spreads a considerable distance from a single diverticulum along the outer aspect of the colonic muscular tube. Thus, the bowel becomes encased and involved in an acute inflammatory reaction, culminating in the development of a large and often palpable tender mass.

Because the peritoneum usually is involved in the inflammatory process, adhesion of the involved segment to the parietes or to other organs is common. This may help to wall off infection and localize an abscess on the one hand, or allow the development of an internal fistula on the other. If prior adherence of colonic visceral peritoneum to parietal peritoneum or other viscera has not occurred, then an open breach in the diverticular wall will lead to free communication between the colonic lumen and the peritoneal cavity, and hence, generalized peritonitis.

In some instances, spread of inflammation occurs between the mesenteric leaves or into the retroperitoneal area. If an abscess develops and subsequently ruptures, then an indirect communication with the colonic lumen may establish itself.

Resolution of pericolic inflammation results in fibrosis, although residual walled-off chronic abscesses may occur. Recurrent episodes of acute inflammation are common. Narrowing of the lumen of the bowel owing to a combination of muscular hypertrophy and fibrosis is inevitable.

■ COLONIC MOTILITY

Arfwidsson reported significant increases in intraluminal pressure activity in patients with colonic diverticular disease, compared with control subjects under resting conditions, after food intake, and following cholinergic stimulation.[21] Painter and Truelove found no major difference in diverticular disease and normal colons during basal motility recordings, but they noted an enhanced response to morphine and prostigmine in diverticula-bearing segments.[22] An exaggerated response to food intake and prostigmine was demonstrated by Parks and Connell.[23] Additionally, these authors demonstrated fast wave activity similar to that recorded in some patients with irritable bowel syndrome. Although such pharmacologic stimuli are relatively uncommon in normal life, the frequently recurring physiologic stimulus of eating may be relevant in the pathogenesis of colonic diverticula.

Following simultaneous manometric and cineradiographic studies, Painter and Truelove postulated that contraction of interhaustral rings, which effectively can occlude the bowel lumen, leads to the formation of multiple isolated short segments along the colon.[22] The tendency to develop temporary occlusion of the lumen is accentuated by the prominence of the crescentic folds of circular muscle and the folds of redundant mucosa. It is evident that further contraction of the walls of the closed segments thus formed sets the scene for considerable rise in intraluminal pressure.

When motility was assessed in colons manifesting the prediverticular state, Arfwidsson claimed that the pressures generated were higher than normal and suggested that these findings supported the view that an abnormality in the muscle is the primary defect in diverticular disease.[21] Furthermore, the fact that the motility index is reduced after eating bran supports the hypothesis that narrowing of the colonic lumen associated with a low food residue may predispose to diverticular formation. Administration of methylcellulose or ispaghula leads to a reduction of rectal and colonic pressures in patients with diverticular disease.

Following resection of the sigmoid colon for diverticular disease, we have shown that the apparently normal segments that remain may exhibit abnormal motility response to stimuli, similar to, but less in degree, than regions of established disease. These findings suggest that there is a primary muscular abnormality that exists in segments of the colon that are free from diverticula.

COMPLIANCE STUDIES OF THE COLONIC WALL

Although increased intracolonic pressure may be important in the etiology of diverticular disease, it does not appear to be the only factor. Our studies of compliance of the sigmoid colon in patients with uncomplicated diverticular disease demonstrated that the colonic muscle, in spite of its thickness, is unable to resist pressure as well as normal colonic muscle in control subjects. We also demonstrated that a lower threshold for distension-type pain exists in diverticular disease, indicating an increased sensitivity of the colonic muscle to stretch. This weakness, or loss of compliance of the wall, could be relevant in the etiology of diverticular disease.

■ CLINICAL MANIFESTATIONS

It is estimated that only 10% to 20% of persons with colonic diverticula develop symptoms related to their presence. Diverticular disease of the colon may be associated with quite troublesome symptoms even in the absence of inflammation. Recurring episodes of lower abdominal cramps can result from a degree of functional obstruction secondary to the narrowing and excessive segmentation of the sigmoid. In clinical practice, the clinician may find it difficult to differentiate between painful noninflammatory and inflammatory diverticular disease. In some patients with a presumptive diagnosis of diverticulitis who have undergone operation, the resected specimens have shown multiple diverticula, thickening of the wall, and narrowing of the lumen, but without microscopic evidence of inflammation.

Abdominal pain, especially in the left lower quadrant, is a cardinal feature and is the most common symptom requiring hospital admission. Persistent pain is suggestive of an inflammatory origin. Central and lower abdominal cramps may signify a degree of obstruction.

Intermittent diarrhea or alternating constipation and diarrhea are common symptoms. Constipation may become troublesome in patients with a significant degree of narrowing in the sigmoid segment as the result of either the muscular abnormality or to fibrosis.

Nausea and vomiting of a reflex nature may be associated with an acute inflammatory reaction. Alternatively, these symptoms may be mechanical in nature owing to large or small bowel obstruction. Urinary symptoms owing to irritation of the ureter or bladder are not infrequent.

On physical examination, the abdomen may be tender in the left lower quadrant. Guarding and rebound tenderness may be present. A palpable mass is not uncommon in the left iliac fossa. Occasionally, rectal examination may reveal a tender mass or even a pelvic abscess. Abdominal distension also may be present.

Sigmoidoscopy will help to rule out other conditions, particularly neoplasm of the rectum. Hyperemic, edematous mucosa is sometimes visible in the rectosigmoid region. Straight and erect x-ray films of the abdomen may reveal a soft tissue mass in the left iliac fossa, air under the diaphragm, or dilatation of the colon, indicating obstruction.

EXTENT OF COLONIC INVOLVEMENT

In approximately 65% of cases, the sigmoid colon alone is affected. However, in about 95% of cases, other segments are also affected (Fig 40–7). Although there are some patients in whom only the sigmoid is affected initially, and in whom other regions subsequently become involved, this does not necessarily occur. It would seem

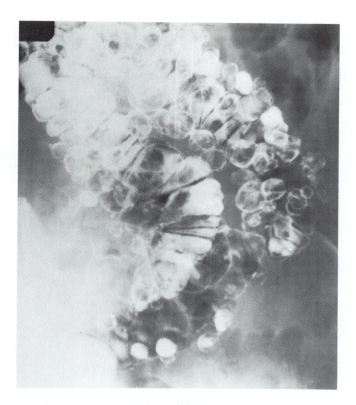

Figure 40–7. Barium enema showing the colon studded with numerous large diverticula.

that if a segment of colon is prone to be affected, this is often determined early in the course of the disease. Progression is more often within the segment or segments initially involved rather than occurring in a stepwise fashion, segment by segment, along the length of the colon. In the majority of patients with disease initially localized to the distal colon, disease does not generally progress to involve additional segments. Two-thirds of patients with colonic diverticula do not have relentless advance of the disease along the colon.

In the experience of this author, severe inflammatory complications occur as commonly in patients with distal disease as in patients with total colonic involvement.

Diverticular disease of the colon may simulate other abdominal conditions, including carcinoma of the colon, irritable bowel syndrome, acute appendicitis, Crohn's disease and ulcerative colitis, ischemic colitis, urinary tract disorders, and pelvic inflammatory disease. In addition to disorders that simulate diverticular disease, lesions may coexist simultaneously or even be masked by the condition. Small benign polyps anywhere along the colon, or small malignant tumours, particularly those in the diverticular segment, may not be evident on barium enema examination. The more frequent use of colonoscopy as a diagnostic aid has led to

an increased awareness of the frequency of coexistent pathologic conditions, which may in fact be responsible for the symptoms of the patient.[24] As discussed later, vascular ectasia, a not uncommon cause of hemorrhage in the elderly patient, may be diagnosed colonoscopically and treated by electrocoagulation or laser obliteration.

CARCINOMA OF THE COLON

Of all the conditions that may simulate diverticular disease, one of the most important and, on occasion, one of the most difficult to differentiate is carcinoma of the colon. Within the colon itself both conditions have a predilection for the sigmoid segment. Furthermore, both conditions can occur coincidentally in the same area. Clinical features associated with the two disorders are often remarkably similar. Symptoms such as alteration of bowel habit, lower abdominal pain, and rectal bleeding readily occur in either condition. However, the typical patient with inflammatory diverticular disease is more likely to have severe abdominal pain, tenderness, fever, and leucocytosis. With carcinoma, bleeding is often occult or mild, whereas in diverticular disease it may be mild, moderate, or severe. Hughes estimated that up to one-fifth of cases of so-called perforated diverticulitis were eventually diagnosed as carcinoma.[25]

The prognosis in patients with carcinoma is diminished by the coexistence of diverticular disease. Not infrequently, definitive surgery is delayed to allow the inflammatory process to subside, based on the premise that the clinician is dealing with benign disease alone. If the segment of colon harbors carcinoma, then the opportunity for cure of that patient may be considerably lessened by the delay (Fig 40–8). Furthermore, when carcinoma arises in a patient who has already been diagnosed as having symptomatic diverticular disease, malignancy may go unrecognized, since it is all too often assumed that the symptoms are the result of diverticular disease. Careful double-contrast barium enema and, if necessary, colonoscopy are of prime importance in reaching an accurate diagnosis.

The following points help in the radiologic differentiation of diverticular disease from colonic cancer.

1. Typically the stricture owing to diverticular disease is longer and more tapered at both ends than carcinoma (Fig 40–9).
2. The colonic mucosa remains intact in diverticular strictures and it is eroded in carcinoma.
3. Propantheline bromide administration during barium enema examination may help to relieve spasm associated with diverticular disease but has no effect in carcinomatous strictures.
4. A repeat radiologic examination after a short interval to allow resolution to occur may help clarify the situation in doubtful cases.

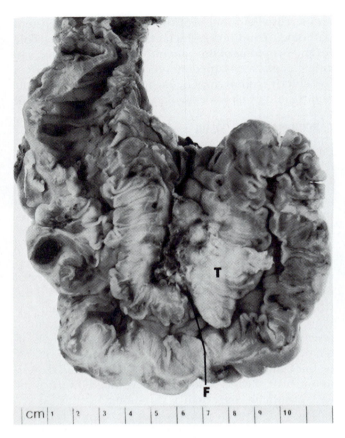

Figure 40–8. Resected specimen of sigmoid colon showing gross muscle thickening with narrowing of the lumen and concertina-like effect of advanced diverticular disease. A coexisting tumor (T) was confirmed as a moderately well-differentiated invasive adenocarcinoma, and a colovesical fistula was also present; the colonic component is shown by *arrow* F.

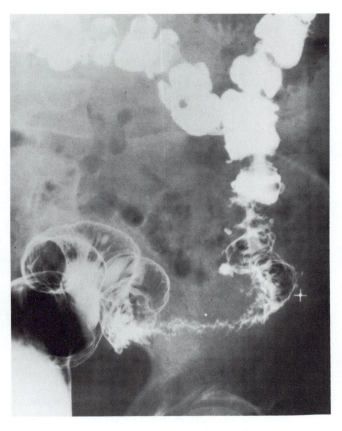

Figure 40–9. A long sigmoid stricture with tapered ends and intact mucosa associated with diverticular disease.

IRRITABLE BOWEL SYNDROME

The patient with irritable bowel syndrome is usually younger than the diverticular patient and typically presents with a longer history of abdominal pain and alteration in bowel habit. The pain tends to be more diffuse and is often referred to the upper or right side of the abdomen. Pellet-type stools and mucus may be passed. Passage of stool or flatus may relieve symptoms.

ACUTE APPENDICITIS

Diverticular disease may be confused with acute appendicitis in the following circumstances:

1. When acute inflammation occurs at the apex of a redundant sigmoid loop lying to the right of the midline.
2. When acute inflammation occurs in a cecal diverticulum.
3. When a patient presents with a pelvic abscess and it is feasible that the lesion could have

arisen from either a pelvic appendix or from an inflamed diverticulum in a sigmoid loop lying in the pelvis.

ULCERATIVE COLITIS

The persistence and the severity of the diarrhea typical of ulcerative colitis is noteworthy. Rectal bleeding is greater and abdominal pain much less in ulcerative colitis compared with diverticular disease. Sigmoidoscopy and biopsy readily establish the diagnosis of inflammatory bowel disease because the rectum is almost always involved.

Crohn's Disease

Crohn's disease of the colon may simulate the symptoms of diverticular disease, since left lower quadrant pain and tenderness associated with altered bowel habit may be present in either condition. In Crohn's disease, however, the diarrhea tends to be unremitting over a longer period of time. Moreover, patients with the disease tend to be younger, although older persons are sometimes affected. The coexistence of anorectal disease or perianal inflammation points toward the correct diagnosis.

Errors in diagnosis are more likely to occur when the two diseases coexist. Schmidt and associates reported 26 cases of coexistence of diverticular and Crohn's disease of the colon. The combined disease abnormalities usually were present in the rectal mucosa on sigmoidoscopy. The incidence of postoperative complications was much higher in patients with combined disease than in those with diverticular disease alone.

Ischemic Disease of the Colon

Ischemic colitis and diverticular disease affect similar age groups. However, the sudden onset of acute diarrhea and hemorrhage associated with left-sided pain and tenderness in elderly patients is suggestive of colonic ischemia. An early barium enema helps to clarify the diagnosis. The more severe forms of colonic ischemia presenting with acute peritoneal signs may progress to gangrene. Efforts should be made to differentiate these cases from perforated diverticular disease.

■ DIETARY AND MEDICAL MANAGEMENT OF UNCOMPLICATED DIVERTICULAR DISEASE

It is now generally accepted that increasing the amount of fiber in the diet is beneficial to patients suffering from uncomplicated diverticular disease. The additional fiber ingested leads to the passage of a softer and bulkier stool. The increased volume of feces is partly owing to the additional residue of indigestible fiber and partly to the entrapment of water in the stool. The changes in the volume and consistency of the stool help to maintain a greater diameter of colonic lumen and lead to a reduction in segmental activity, a lower intraluminal colonic pressure, and an increase in the transit rate through the intestine.

Fruit and vegetables vary considerably in the proportion of indigestible fiber that they contain and hence, in the amount of water retained by the fibrous material. Each gram of fiber from fruit and vegetables, such as apples, oranges, carrots and brussels sprouts retains 2 to 3 gm of water.

The addition of bran to the diet helps to ensure that the fecal residue is more voluminous and that the stools are softer and passed more easily without straining. The fiber derived from wheat bran has also a laxative effect, which is greater than fiber derived from fruit and vegetables. Each gram of unprocessed bran binds with approximately four times its own weight of water. Because of its bulking properties it is not unusual for patients who

commence taking bran to develop a bloated sensation in the abdomen. For a time they may complain of the passage of excess gas and also complain of flatulence. When adaptation to the new regimen takes place over the ensuing weeks, these symptoms gradually settle.

Initially, an intake of about 5 or 10 gm of bran daily is advised, the amount being increased to 20 gm over a 3 or 4 week period. Coarse bran has been shown to be more effective than fine bran in increasing the stool weight, regulating the transit time, and reducing the motility index. There seems little doubt that patients with diverticular disease are helped symptomatically by the ingestion of a high-fiber diet, although the efficacy of this moiety in the diet has been questioned by some authors. A high-fiber diet also seems to afford some protection against the development of further complications after acute inflammatory attacks. Findlay and associates have shown that although basal motility remains unchanged during bran therapy, the colonic response to food and prostigmine is reduced.[27]

One of the disadvantages of unprocessed bran is that it lacks palatability for some patients who prefer to take other vegetable fiber. It should be remembered that wholemeal bread and several palatable breakfast cereals can provide a good complement of dietary fiber. Several pharmaceutical bulk additive preparations have an important hydrophilic property, thereby maintaining an increased volume of fecal residue. For example, methylcellulose (Celevac) absorbs about 25 times its own weight in water. Ispaghula husk (Isogel, Fybogel, or Regulan) retains about 40 times its own weight in water. Sterculia (Normacol or Movicol) and psyllium seed powders (Metamucil) act in a similar fashion.

Patients who suffer from the pain of colonic spasm may be relieved by mebeverine hydrochloride (Colofac). This drug acts directly on the smooth muscle of the colonic wall and is preferable to anticholinergic drugs, such as probantheline bromide (Probanthine), which act through the autonomic nervous system. Anticholinergic drugs have the drawback that they cause dryness of the mouth and mucous membranes, blurring of vision, and even urinary retention.

■ COMPLICATIONS

The complications of diverticular disease fall broadly under two headings, inflammatory complications and hemorrhage. Inflammation around diverticula may lead to peridiverticulitis and pericolitis, which may progress to the formation of an inflammatory mass, particularly in the sigmoid region. The inflammation may gradually subside but, in some cases, it progresses to form a localized paracolic abscess. Alternatively, sepsis may spread to cause generalized peritonitis of a purulent or fecal nature, depending on whether there is a direct breach in the colonic wall. Inflammation may culminate in the formation of an internal or external fistula. It can also lead to obstruction of the large intestine or even of the small intestine, if the latter becomes involved in the inflammatory mass.

Hemorrhage related to colonic diverticula may be mild, moderate, or severe. In the majority of cases bleeding ceases spontaneously but occasionally, persistent bleeding may require intensive investigation and emergency surgery.

■ MANAGEMENT

ACUTE DIVERTICULITIS, LOCALIZED PERITONITIS, AND PERICOLIC ABSCESS

Persistent and severe pain in the lower abdomen, especially in the left lower quadrant, but sometimes also in the hypogastrium extending to the right of the midline, is accompanied by acute tenderness. Localized guarding and rigidity are present and, not uncommonly, a mass is palpable in the left iliac fossa. Tachycardia, pyrexia, and leucocytosis are to be expected.

Initial Management

Bedrest is advised and, depending on the severity of the inflammatory process, intravenous fluids may be required. In addition, in more acute cases, nasogastric suction may need to be instituted. Antibiotic therapy, such as metronidazole, together with a cephalosporin is recommended. An analgesic (eg, pethidine), is given for the relief of pain. Morphine is best avoided, in view of its tendency to increase intracolonic pressures. Purgatives, wash-outs, and barium enema examinations are avoided early in the course of management of patients with these complications.

With a conservative regimen as outlined, symptoms and signs may be expected to subside, in a high percentage of cases. After such time, the colon may be examined by barium enema to confirm the diagnosis of diverticular disease and to exclude other large bowel pathology (Fig 40–10). Careful sigmoidoscopy also should be undertaken when the acute phase has passed.

During the period of observation, careful watch is kept for evidence of spreading peritonitis or adverse changes in the vital signs that would indicate the need for surgical intervention.

A patient with a phlegmonous mass or a small paracolic abscess may improve symptomatically, with concomitant subsidence of inflammation while on a conservative regimen. Likewise, a small abscess situated between the leaves of the mesentery may remain confined and gradually resolve. However, the majority of

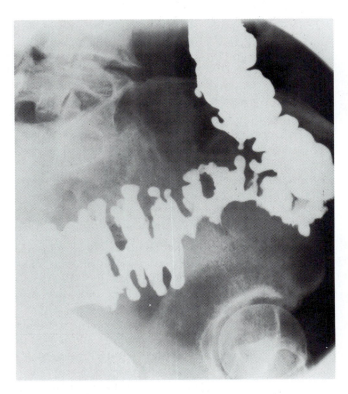

Figure 40–10. A large paracolic abscess associated with severe diverticular disease of the sigmoid colon.

patients with paracolic abscesses will require surgical drainage.

A localized collection of pus may be demonstrable on ultrasonography or on CT scanning. If the abscess is walled off, it is often feasible to drain it by an ultrasound-guided percutaneous approach. However, operative intervention sometimes is required to achieve adequate drainage.

In recent years, many surgeons believe that a more aggressive approach is indicated, and there has been an increasing number of encouraging reports in which excision of the perforated segment has been undertaken at initial operation.

PERFORATION WITH GENERALIZED PERITONITIS

When a colonic diverticulum ruptures directly into the peritoneal cavity, widespread contamination ensues with resultant fecal peritonitis. Rupture of a paracolic abscess may lead to widespread purulent peritonitis.

Initial Management

If the patient is seriously ill and in a state of shock, the initial aim is to institute resuscitative measures and seek to reestablish and maintain an adequate circulation. Patients suffering from fecal peritonitis are often in profound shock and it may be difficult or impossible to obtain optimal circulatory stability prior to surgery. Intravenous fluids and intravenous antibiotics against aerobic and anaerobic bacteria are started. My preference is to give a combined initial dose of metronidazole (500 mg) and cefuroxime (1.5 gm), preoperatively so that a high serum level is achieved to help combat the initial infection and any further contamination occurring during the operative phase. Antibiotic therapy (metronidazole, 500 mg; cefuroxime, 750 mg, 8 hourly) is continued for 5 to 7 days.

Operative Approaches

A wide range of surgical procedures have been tried in an effort to cope with this highly lethal complication. The prognosis is related to the age and state of the patient. Elderly patients and those with concomitant disorders have a worse prognosis.

In the last two decades there have been gradual changes in the operative policy at many centers. The emphasis is now on more radical procedures for treatment of perforation associated with localized or generalized peritonitis. The initial surgical procedures fall broadly into two groups: those in which the diseased segment is left in situ at the time of the first operation, and those in which the diseased segment is removed from the peritoneal cavity at the time of the original surgery (Fig 40–11).

Operations in Which the Diseased Segment is Left in Situ at the Initial Operation. In the past, a number of more conservative approaches were in vogue whereby the diseased segment was left in situ at the time of initial operation. Interventional procedures included suture of perforation, drainage of region of perforation, peritoneal toilet and the formation of a transverse colostomy. These procedures are associated with a high mortality, particularly if the peritonitis is of the fecal variety. A distinct disadvantage is that the septic focus still remains within the peritoneal cavity, with this seat of inflammation continuing to cause toxicity. Furthermore, it may lead to further contamination of the peritoneal cavity.

Attempts to suture an edematous, inflamed, friable, and perforated colon is an unsatisfactory procedure. The wall surrounding the perforation is unyielding and lacks pliability. The risk of subsequent breakdown is high. The formation of a proximal colostomy, although beneficial, is no guarantee against further leakage at the site of the original perforation because it is apparent that there is often considerable fecal loading between

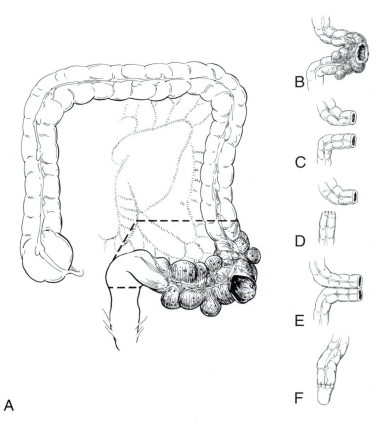

Figure 40–11. A. A diagrammatic representation of operations in which the perforated segment is removed from the peritoneal cavity. **B.** Exteriorization. **C.** Surgical excision, end colostomy, mucous fistula. **D.** Hartmann operation. **E.** Paul Mickulicz procedure. **F.** Primary resection anastomosis.

the site of the closed perforation and the site of the transverse colostomy.

The above operations are only the first phase of the classical three-stage procedure, the second stage being resection of the involved segment, and the third stage, the closure of the colostomy. There are considerable drawbacks to the three-stage approach, which for many years held a foremost place in the management of acute complications of diverticular disease.

Some valid criticisms of the three-stage approach are worthy of consideration. Of prime concern is the high mortality and morbidity. In a collective survey, reported by Painter, of 15 groups of reputable surgeons who treated patients suffering from perforated diverticulitis by laparotomy and drainage, with or without proximal colostomy, the overall mortality was 37.7%.[28] These reports relate to the period between 1957 and 1971. Although the prognosis has improved considerably today because of better resuscitative measures and much more effective antibiotic regimens, particularly relating to gram-negative infection, the results of this policy are still not as good as patients and their surgeons would desire. A retrospective review of 1353 cases with acute perforated diverticulitis, treated surgically, was made by Greif and associates.[29] They reported a mortality of 29% in patients treated by colostomy without resection, compared with 12% for those treated by primary resection or exteriorization of the diseased segment.

The fistula rate following proximal colostomy with drainage varies from 5% to 20% in different series and is equally high in patients who have closure of the perforation along with concomitant transverse colostomy. A chronic colocutaneous fistula is likely to prolong the hospital stay considerably.

In some patients the inflammatory process is slow to subside after the first phase. There is also the added risk of leaving the perforated sigmoid carcinoma in situ for an unduly long period before the second stage. A further disadvantage of the three-stage procedure is the length of time for which transverse colostomy may be present and for the patient to cope with a malodorous fluid effluent from the proximal stoma. In fact, a significant number of patients do not proceed to the second and third stages. It is clear that the three-stage approach necessitates considerable hospitalization, and each operation carries with it a potential morbidity and mortality.

Operations Designed to Remove the Perforated Segment. Surgical procedures to remove the diseased or perforated segment of bowel from the peritoneal cavity have a major role and play an increasingly important part in the management of perforated diverticulitis. First, they minimize continuing toxemia that would otherwise result from the continuing inflammation. Second, they remove the potential hazard of further leakage and contamination of the peritoneal cavity by colonic content. There can be little argument that excisional surgery is the procedure of choice in coping with a direct open perforation associated with fecal peritonitis. Even in patients with generalized purulent peritonitis associated with an inflamed sigmoid loop, the patient is likely to make a more rapid recovery if the septic focus is removed.

Exteriorization. Although this operation, in which the sigmoid loop is exteriorized and a colostomy formed in the left iliac fossa, removes the septic focus from the peritoneal cavity, thereby avoiding further contamination of the peritoneum, it does not exclude the toxins from the inflamed portion of bowel entering the circulation and thus, adversely affects the general condition of the patient. Furthermore, the lesion tends to be malodorous and not easily cared for by the nursing staff.

Surgical Excision, End Colostomy, Mucous Fistula. When the inflamed or perforated segment has been mobilized, it takes little extra time to excise it compared with the exteriorization method and, in my view, this should be done. The question of what should be done with the proximal and distal ends of the colon is a separate issue. Various alternatives exist. If there is a reasonable length of sigmoid colon, it may be possible to bring the distal end out as a mucous fistula while the proximal end of the colon is used in the formation of an end colostomy.

This procedure has gained a distinct place in the management of complicated diverticular disease, although it requires more expertise than is required for the first stage of a classical three-stage approach. It involves mobilization and resection of an inflamed colon in a potentially hemorrhagic field.

Concern has often been expressed about the technical problems associated with the procedure. The inflamed colon may be adherent to other pelvic organs, although, with care, it usually can be safely separated. Edema may facilitate dissection of the tissue planes and mobilization of the colon.

Segmental Excision, End Colostomy, Closure of Distal Stump (Hartmann Operation). Because the mesentery of patients with diverticular disease tends to be short, it is often not possible to bring out the distal end to the surface of the abdomen as described above. This is especially true if the patient is obese or if the perforation is low down in the sigmoid colon. In such circumstances, the distal end can be oversewn, as in the Hartmann operation, and the proximal colon brought out as an end colostomy. In all of these procedures, it is best to avoid opening up the retrorectal space in an attempt to achieve extra length because this mobilization predisposes to the potential hazard of sepsis spreading to the retrorectal area.

Einenstat and associates reported their experience of the use of the Hartmann procedure in the surgical management of complicated diverticular disease (perforation, abscess formation, obstruction, and fistula formation).[30] The mortality rate in 44 patients treated by this method was 4.5%. Tudor and associates recorded four deaths in 33 cases.[31]

The primary aim of the above mentioned procedures is to save the life of an ill and often elderly patient in the midst of an emergency situation. A further aim is to achieve a satisfactory state of health to allow restoration of the bowel continuity at a subsequent date. A bonus associated with these methods is that the number of stages is reduced to two.

Primary Resection and Anastomosis. Numerous surgeons have advocated this approach on the premise that it not only eradicates the septic focus but achieves bowel continuity at the time of the initial operation. It is true that in some series good results have been achieved by experienced surgeons who have been operating on well-selected cases. This procedure has a distinct role in the surgical management of a patient with an acute phlegmonous mass, and even has a limited place in the management of perforated diverticular disease, such as cases in which there is a small localized abscess between the leaves of the mesentery.

It cannot, however, be too strongly emphasized that the risk of anastomotic breakdown and leakage is considerable if primary anastomosis, unprotected by a proximal colostomy, is undertaken in the presence of frank sepsis in a shocked and hypotensive patient. Mortality rates in patients who developed an anastomotic leak after a single-stage resection and anastomosis have been high.

In view of the clinical and experimental evidence confirming that an anastomosis undertaken in a septic field has a greatly increased risk of dehiscence, most surgeons avoid single-stage resection and anastomosis in these circumstances. Furthermore, lack of preoperative mechanical bowel preparation adversely affects the anastomosis in the postoperative phase.

It is true that concomitant transverse colostomy gives a measure of protection to the anastomosis, but it does not eliminate the risk of anastomotic leak because considerable fecal material may be present between the site of anastomosis and the colostomy. The operation of primary resection and anastomosis also takes longer than the surgical options mentioned above.

To acquire adequate lengths of residual bowel to achieve a join-up without tension, it may be necessary to mobilize the splenic flexure, thus increasing the

risk of further subphrenic contamination. Opening up the presacral space during mobilization of the rectum is liable to increase the incidence of sepsis in that region. In addition, if a protective colostomy is included, the procedure can no longer be classified as one-stage and thus has limited advantage over a policy of immediate resection but delayed anastomosis until the time of the second operation. However, in a series reported by Gregg, the ultimate mortality was lower following resection and primary anastomosis with a proximal stoma than with a Hartmann operation.[32] Furthermore, the likelihood of achieving complete restoration of colonic continuity was higher in the former group.

Suggested Policy. My recommendation, applicable in most cases, is to excise the perforated segment as expeditiously as possible, bringing out the proximal colon as an end colostomy. The distal transection is made just below the rectosigmoid junction and is stapled or oversewn, the closed end of the rectum being hitched to the sacral promontory. If fecal material is present, it should be removed from the peritoneal cavity using moist sponges. Any friable necrotic tissue is excised, and the peritoneal cavity is thoroughly irrigated with copious amounts of warm saline. The toilet process is completed by irrigation of a solution of tetracycline is saline at a concentration of 1 gm/L. Administration of systematic antibiotics that normally has been initiated preoperatively should be continued in the postoperative phase. My practice is to give a combination of metronidazole (500 mg) and cefuroxime (750 mg) every 8 hours for 5 to 7 days.

The wisdom of this policy of resection of the perforated segment is underlined by the recent review by Krukowski and Matheson of 57 publications dealing with a total of 1282 patients undergoing emergency surgery for perforative diverticulitis.[33] Of these, 61% had some form of conservative operation (drainage, perforation closure, proximal colostomy), with a 25% mortality. In contrast, those patients undergoing resection of the perforated segment had an 11% mortality.

When the time comes to reestablish bowel continuity, this is achieved most readily using a circular stapling device from which the anvil has been removed to allow the passage of the shaft through the top of the rectal stump, eliminating the need for a purse-string suture at the rectal end. When the central shaft of the instrument has penetrated the upper end of the rectal stump, the anvil is reattached for its insertion into the mobilized descending colon in which a purse-string suture has been inserted. This approach simplifies the restoration of bowel continuity after the Hartmann procedure, which admittedly is not always the most straightforward of operations.

■ FISTULA

Fistulas associated with diverticular disease of the colon may communicate with internal organs or the external body surface. They may arise spontaneously as a result of the inflammatory complications of the disease itself or they may result from operative intervention in the disease process.

COLOCUTANEOUS FISTULA

An external fistula may arise spontaneously on those extremely rare occasions when a paracolic abscess points and ruptures in the left iliac fossa. More often, the fistula occurs after incision and drainage of a left lower quadrant abscess that is, itself, in communication with the colonic lumen via a ruptured diverticulum. A rare variety of colocutaneous fistula may arise when a paracolic abscess spreads downward and ruptures through the levator ani into the ischiorectal fossa, necessitating drainage. In patients who have had resection of the colon for diverticular disease, a colocutaneous fistula may result from the breakdown of the anastomotic line.

The management of a colocutaneous fistula depends on the nature of the circumstances under which it has arisen. If the leakage is slight and there is no evidence of spreading peritonitis, then a conservative approach is desirable. If, however, the leakage is considerable, then a transverse colostomy should be established without delay. Most fistulas will heal if there is no distal obstruction. When the inflammatory reaction has settled, examination by barium enema will clarify whether or not there is narrowing at the site of the defect. It is important to determine if an adequate colonic lumen has been maintained before considering colostomy closure.

COLOVESICAL FISTULA

The most common internal fistula associated with diverticular disease is the colovesical variety (Fig 40–12). The patient is usually a male in whom interconnection has occurred between the apex of an inflamed, fairly mobile sigmoid loop and the bladder. In women, interposition of the uterus between the sigmoid colon and the bladder has a protective role. The patient may present with symptoms suggestive of urinary tract infection or, in more advanced cases, may describe the actual passage of air or feces per urethra.

Cytoscopy usually reveals an inflamed area in the upper part of the bladder but a fistula is not always seen. Occasionally, a large intercommunication between the colon and the bladder may be visualized.

A barium enema will confirm the presence of diverticular disease and, in some cases, will demonstrate the passage of contrast medium into the bladder. If the fis-

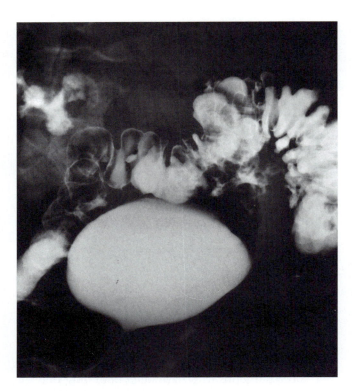

Figure 40–12. Colovesical fistula. Barium has passed from the sigmoid colon through a distinct tract (*arrow*) into the urinary bladder.

tula is small, contrast may not pass into the bladder. Likewise, contrast medium may fail to pass from the bladder into the colon during cystographic examination but, in some instances, contrast medium may outline the large intestine (Fig 40–13). Because these fistulas rarely heal spontaneously, surgical correction usually is advisable in all cases that are suitable for major surgical intervention. It is often possible to undertake a one-stage resection, particularly if the inflammatory reaction is limited and noninflamed, pliable bowel is available proximally and distally for the formation of a colonic anastomosis. After mobilization of the colon from the bladder, the latter is sutured with chromic catgut, and urethral catheter drainage is maintained for 10 days.

In rare instances, the inflammatory reaction in the pelvis is too advanced to proceed to one-stage resection and anastomosis. In such circumstances, a preliminary proximal colostomy is carried out and a period of 2 or 3 months allowed to elapse before resection. Although the preliminary operation does facilitate the resolution of associated pelvic inflammation, the fistula rarely heals until resection has been undertaken.

In the treatment of colovesical fistulas, it is vitally important to excise the affected segment of the colon with reanastomosis of healthy colonic tissue because lesser

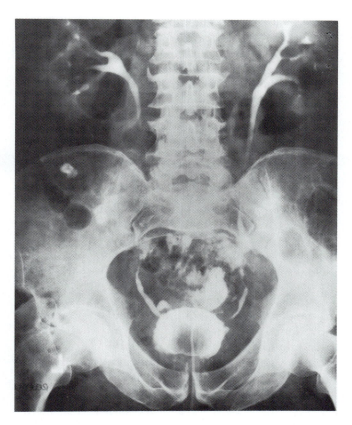

Figure 40–13. Intravenous urogram demonstrating a communication between the urinary bladder and the large intestine in a patient with diverticular disease of the colon.

procedures, such as division of the fistulous track combined with simple closure of the bladder and colon, are almost certain to fail.

COLOENTERIC FISTULA

When the colon becomes inflamed with diverticular disease, it is not uncommon for a loop of the small bowel to become adherent and to become part of an inflammatory mass, particularly if a paracolic abscess has developed. In these circumstances, an intercommunication may develop between the large and small intestines (Fig 40–14).

In the surgical management of such fistulas, an en bloc resection of the segments of affected colon and small bowel is undertaken, and anastomosis of both the enteric and colonic components is completed. It is only in cases of advanced sepsis and gross abscess formation that it may be prudent to delay the colonic anastomosis until a later date. However, even in these circumstances, it is evident that the small bowel continuity should be restored at initial operation.

COLOVAGINAL FISTULA

This rare variety of fistula may arise spontaneously following sepsis in the pelvis secondary to diverticular disease or alternatively, it may be the sequel to operative procedures. Depending on the circumstances, it may be possible to resect the diverticular segment and perform an end-to-end anastomosis as an initial procedure with or without a temporary transverse colostomy.

■ INTESTINAL OBSTRUCTION

Intestinal obstruction associated with diverticular disease of the colon may be partial or complete and may involve either the colon or the small bowel. It is not uncommon for an acute inflammatory stenosing type of lesion or a large paracolic abscess associated with mural inflammation to lead to marked narrowing or complete occlusion of the sigmoid colon. Alternatively, an enteric loop may become adherent to or incorporated in a diverticular inflammatory mass, resulting in small bowel obstruction.

Patients with complete intestinal obstruction will require surgery after electrolyte correction and fluid replacement have been achieved. The choice of surgical procedure depends on the operative findings. The most widely practiced initial procedure has been formation

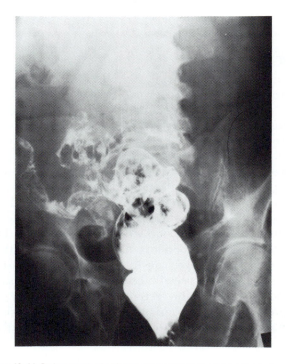

Figure 40–14. Barium enema of a 79 year–old man showing a fistula between the pelvic colon and the ileum, about 15 cm from the ileocecal junction. Multiple diverticula are present in the pelvic colon. There is considerable stenosis at the site of the fistula (*arrow*) and little barium passed into the colon proximal to it.

of a right transverse loop colostomy, with resection of the stenosed diverticular segment as a second stage and colostomy closure usually as a third stage. In recent years there has been a move by numerous surgeons to proceed at the time of the initial operation to the excision of an obstructing inflammatory sigmoid mass. This having been achieved, it has been common practice to delay an anastomosis until a subsequent date. Dudley and associates have described a method of on-table orthograde irrigation of the proximal colon following resection to clear if of feces and hence, proceed to primary anastomosis.[34]

When a mass is found in the sigmoid region at laparotomy, it may be difficult to determine whether the lesion is owing to diverticular disease alone or to carcinoma of the colon, or even to coexistent carcinoma in a diverticular segment. Sometimes it is not possible to make the distinction with confidence until the lesion has been resected and the excised segment of colon opened.

If a decision has been made to perform a transverse colostomy as the initial step in the management of an obstructing mass in the distal colon, and doubt remains as to the exact nature of the lesion, then an early barium enema, when the patient has recovered sufficiently, may help to clarify the problem. Further information may be obtained by colonoscopy in the postoperative period. If there is still lingering doubt about the differential diagnosis, then undue delay before the second stage should be avoided.

■ HEMORRHAGE

Acute massive hemorrhage may be alarming for the patient and family. A large amount of blood varying in color from a fairly bright red to dark maroon may be passed. In patients over 60 years of age, angiodysplasia now is thought to cause massive colonic hemorrhage more often than diverticular disease. These two conditions, together with malignancy, account for about 90% of cases of severe lower intestinal hemorrhage in this age group. Acute bleeding also may occur in ischemic colitis, although the blood loss is seldom massive. Less severe degrees of blood loss may be the result of infective or inflammatory causes, internal hemorrhoids, polyps, or solitary rectal ulceration. The possibility of blood collecting in the rectum above a competent anal sphincter should be kept in mind. The presence of diverticula in a patient presenting with rectal bleeding may be coincidental and not necessarily the actual cause of the hemorrhage. Hence, care must be taken to make a correct diagnosis and to include in the differential diagnosis the possibility of the upper gastrointestinal source. Patients with severe colonic bleeding require blood replacement by intravenous transfusion. The diagnostic approach depends on a number of factors: (1) the severity of the blood loss, (2) whether the bleeding ceases spontaneously or is persistent or recurrent, (3) the age and general state of the patient, and (4) the availability of sophisticated investigative procedures.

A suggested diagnostic scheme for the investigation of severe lower intestinal bleeding is outlined in Table 40–1. It must be emphasized, however, that it may be unclear, initially, whether the hemorrhage originates from the upper or lower intestinal tract.

Proctoscopy and sigmoidoscopy will aid in the elimination of other acutely bleeding lesions in the distal large bowel. A well-functioning suction device may be necessary if a reasonably adequate view is to be obtained. If these investigations do not reveal a source of hemorrhage, and if upper gastrointestinal bleeding has been excluded by nasogastric suction or esophagogastroduodenoscopy, or both, a series of more complex procedures may be required, the time and order of which vary with the circumstances.

In cases of continuous bleeding, radionuclide scanning using technetium 99m (^{99m}Tc)-labeled red blood cells is a safe, noninvasive test that may help to identify the site of bleeding in about half the cases. If technetium scanning results are negative, it is more efficacious to proceed directly to colonoscopy rather than to selective arteriography, since the latter also may have negative results unless blood loss is continuing at a rate of >0.5 mL/min. The above tests are best done prior to barium studies because the contrast medium obscures endoscopic or radiologic visualization of the bleeding site.

In those patients in whom bleeding has ceased, total colonoscopy is the procedure of choice initially. In addition to revealing diverticula, colonoscopy may reveal mucosal lesions such as polyps anywhere along the length of the large bowel or angiodysplastic lesions,

TABLE 40–1. DIAGNOSTIC SCHEME FOR INVESTIGATION OF SEVERE LOWER INTESTINAL BLEEDING

Bleeding Active	Bleeding Ceased
Coagulation studies	Coagulation studies
Blood urea nitrogen	Blood urea nitrogen
Nasogastric aspiration	Nasogastric aspiration
Radionuclide scanning	Total colonoscopy
Colonoscopy	Barium studies
Selective arteriography	Double-contrast enema
Barium studies	Upper gastrointestinal and small
Double-contrast enema	bowel series
Upper gastrointestinal	Selective arteriography
and small bowel series	

particularly in the right colon. Angiography aids in the differentiation from angiodysplasia in which vascular tufts may be seen, particularly in the cecal region or right colon during the capillary phase. Premature filling of veins may be demonstrable during the venous phase. A barium enema may be expected to demonstrate the colonic diverticula, when present. However, they may not be the source of bleeding. Diverticula are present in about 25% of patients who have angiodysplasia as a cause of the colonic bleeding. In patients with bleeding owing to diverticular disease, the hemorrhage is as likely to come from the right colon as from the left, and it frequently occurs in the absence of inflammation.

CONTROL OF HEMORRHAGE

The intra-arterial infusion of vasopressin into the appropriate mesenteric vessel via the angiographic catheter is often effective in controlling, at least temporarily, the bleeding associated with diverticular disease. Administration is continued for 24 to 48 hours. Alternatively, transcatheter embolization, using Gelfoam or Oxycel, has been advocated by Goldberger and Bookstein, but this procedure is not without risk because it may cause intestinal ischemia.[35]

Surgery is indicated in cases of continuing or recurrent severe hemorrhage. The procedure undertaken depends on the general condition of the patient and whether or not the site of bleeding has been accurately determined during preoperative investigations.

If the bleeding site has been clearly identified preoperatively, an operation to resect the appropriate segment is the procedure usually undertaken. If the exact site of origin within the colon has not been determined, then subtotal colectomy is recommended. However, a more radical approach in good-risk patients was advised in 1980.[36] These authors recommended subtotal colectomy in the following circumstances: (1) diverticular bleeding in which the diverticula are scattered throughout the colon, (2) angiodysplasia of the right colon and extensive diverticulosis of the left colon, and (3) massive bleeding from an undetermined site within the colon.

A mortality of 11% among 43 patients who underwent subtotal colectomy with massive rectal bleeding was reported,[37] and death rates of up to 50% have been recorded in some series. Although this extensive procedure is necessary for bleeding from an undetermined colonic site, it seems preferable to undertake a more limited procedure with a lower mortality and morbidity when localization has been possible. Patients who have had considerable blood loss and blood replacement and who undergo emergency resection of unprepared bowel loaded with fecal material are prone to a higher than usual complication rate, in any event.

■ ELECTIVE SURGERY

RESECTION

When acute complications occur, there may be no reasonable alternative to urgent surgical intervention. In nonacute circumstances, the indications for surgery also may be clear cut, but sometimes they are less well defined and, indeed, may be relative rather than absolute. Numerous factors such as the patient's general state of health, age, as well as the local clinical features and radiologic findings, may dictate the best policy.

Some surgeons advocate surgical resection of the diseased segment after one episode of acute diverticulitis. However, it must be stressed that many patients make an excellent recovery following an acute attack of diverticulitis and may have few symptoms or even remain completely asymptomatic for several years afterward.

Those patients who have two or more inflammatory attacks within a few years should normally be considered for surgery unless there are clear contraindications on other grounds.

Patients who develop a palpable phlegmonous mass in the left lower quadrant or in the left side of the pelvis often require surgery. Although this type of lesion may respond to a conservative regimen, it is not uncommon for such patients to require subsequent removal of the affected segment. Gross deformity of the sigmoid colon on radiologic examination, especially if associated with significant clinical features, weighs in favor of a surgical extirpation.

Most patients with internal fistulas are treated with surgery electively. A high proportion are suitable for one-stage resection, but as described earlier, a minority of cases require preliminary diversionary colostomy.

The development of urinary symptoms in a patient with diverticular disease may indicate irritation of the bladder or of the ureter by an inflamed sigmoid colon and may be a premonitory warning that a colovesical fistula is developing.

Resection should be considered in those cases with repeated episodes of mild to moderate hemorrhage, especially if coexisting with other symptoms such as left lower quadrant pain or altered bowel habit.

Specific consideration also should be given to the patient who presents earlier in life, that is, under the age of 55 years, with signs of acute inflammation. Many of these individuals will require operation.

A clear indication for surgery exists in those patients in whom it has not been possible to exclude, with certainty, the possibility of a carcinoma in the diverticular segment. With improved radiology and the aid of colonoscopy, such cases are less numerous now. However, when doubt exists, surgical intervention must be undertaken. Initially, a decision is made as to whether the lesion found at laparotomy is owing to diverticular disease alone or whether the segment also could be the seat of a carcinoma. When the case evidently is one of diverticular disease, then a less radical dissection of the mesentery and lymphatic drainage field is undertaken. If doubt exists as to the possibility of carcinoma, this can be clearly assessed when the specimen has been removed and opened up so that the mucosal aspect can be inspected. If there is any indication of malignancy, the operative field can be reexamined and, if necessary, a wider excision may be undertaken.

MORBIDITY FOLLOWING OPERATIONS FOR DIVERTICULAR DISEASE

The postoperative morbidity following resection for diverticular disease tends to be higher than that of a comparable group of patients with carcinoma. This may be accounted for by a number of factors. First, the diverticula may be associated with considerable inflammation, adherence, and chronic fibrosis, and there also may be an existing paracolic abscess. Second, shortening of the colon and mesocolon means that there is less remaining colon for anastomosis following resection, unless the splenic flexure is mobilized. It is important to avoid tension on the anastomosis. Third, the muscle abnormality associated with diverticular disease leads to narrowing of the lumen and friability of the wall. Hence, attempts to anastomose the abnormal thickened segment is fraught with danger. The importance of the proper choice of the proximal and distal lines of section cannot be overemphasized. Fourth, it is evident that in many instances diverticula are present in the proximal portion of the colon; the presence of one of these at the level of the line of anastomosis may compromise the safety of the junction. Finally, leakage after resection for diverticular disease is more hazardous than dehiscence after resection for carcinoma. This increased risk may be owing, in part, to the inherent muscle abnormality or, alternatively, to the prior existence of sepsis.

SIGMOID MYOTOMY

The operation of longitudinal colomyotomy introduced by Reilly[38] and the operation of transverse teniamyotomy described by Hodgson[39] never gained widespread acceptance and are not considered obsolete.

■ CECAL DIVERTICULA

Diverticula of the cecum may occur in association with widespread colonic diverticulosis, as part of it as well, and, therefore, as an acquired lesion. Alternatively, a distinct entity of congenital origin known as solitary diverticulum of the cecum may be encountered. The pouch, which has smooth muscle in its wall, is usually situated medially, near the ileocecal valve. It is usually symptomless unless diverticulitis occurs.

The differential diagnosis of cecal diverticulitis include appendicitis, right-sided colonic carcinoma, solitary cecal ulcer, Crohn's disease, actinomycosis, carcinoid, tuberculosis, and chronic cholecystitis.

Right-sided diverticulitis may closely mimic appendicitis. Patients with diverticulitis tend to have a longer symptomatic period with intermittent or chronic symptoms. The pain of cecal diverticulitis begins and remains in the right side of the abdomen or the right lower quadrant rather than commencing in the periumbilical region. Vomiting is uncommon in acute right-sided diverticulitis. Massive hemorrhage may occur. If a mass is present, the differential diagnosis includes carcinoma, appendix abscess, Crohn's disease, and actinomycosis.

Schapira and associates emphasized the features essential to making a diagnosis of cecal or right-sided diverticulitis on barium contrast examination:[40]

1. Discrete extramural or intramural filling defect
2. Limited distensibility of the bowel wall
3. Spasm, edema, and fixation of the bowel wall
4. Demonstration of a diverticulum or diverticula
5. An intact mucosal pattern without intraluminal filling defect
6. Absence of a constant intraluminal filling defect

The correct diagnosis of cecal diverticulitis is not often made preoperatively. If at laparotomy a mass is present, it may be difficult or impossible to exclude malignancy until resection has been undertaken. Right hemicolectomy is the treatment of choice for patients in whom doubt exists as to the possibility of malignancy. Even if malignancy can be confidently excluded, and removal of an inflammatory lesion is being undertaken, it is preferable to excise the cecum and reconstitute bowel continuity by ileocolic anastomosis rather than attempting diverticulectomy.

If an uncomplicated solitary diverticulum is discovered at the time of operation for some other condition, then it may be simply invaginated and buried using a purse-string suture inserted in the cecal wall.

REFERENCES

1. Cruveilhier J. *Traité d'Anatomie Pathologique Général,* vol 1. Paris, France: Bailliére; 1849: 593
2. Virchow R. Virchows Archiv für Pathologische Anatomie und Physiologie und für. *Klinische Medizin* 1853; 5:335
3. Habershon SO. *Observations on Diseases of the Alimentary Canal.* Philadelphia, PA: Blanchard and Lea; 1857.

4. Jones S. Transactions of the Pathological Society of London. 1859;10:131

5. Graser E. Uber multiple falschi Darmdivertikel in der Flexina Sigmoidea. *Munch Med Wschr* 1899;46:721

6. Moynihan BFA. The mimicry of malignant disease in the large intestine. *Edinb Med J* 1907;21:228

7. Wilson LB. Diverticula of the lower bowel: their development and relationship to carcinoma. *Ann Surg* 1911; 53:223

8. Mayo WJ. Diverticulitis of the large intestine. *JAMA* 1917; 69:781

9. Spriggs EI, Marxer OA. Multiple diverticula of the colon. *Lancet* 1927;1:1067

10. Marxer OA. *Duff House Papers,* vol 1. London, England: OUP; 1923:165

11. Mayo WJ, Wilson LB, et al. Acquired diverticulitis of the large intestine. *Surg Gynecol Obstet* 1907;5:8

12. Smithwick RH. Experience with surgical management of diverticulitis of the sigmoid. *Ann Surg* 1942;115:969

13. Case JT. The roentgen demonstration of multiple diverticula of the colon. *AJR Am J Roentgenol* 1914;2:654

14. de Quervain F. Zur Diagnose der erworbenen Dickdarmdivertikel und der sigmoiditis diverticularis. *Deutsche Ztschr f Chir* 1914;128:67

15. Coode PE, Chan KW, et al. Polyps and diverticula of the colon: a necropsy study in Hong Kong. *Gut* 1985;26:1045

16. Heaton KW. Diet and diverticulosis, new leads. *Gut* 1985; 26:541

17. Hannan CE, Knightly JJ, et al. Diverticular disease of the colon in younger age group. *Dis Colon Rectum* 1961;4:419

18. Ouriel K, Schwartz SI. Diverticular disease in the young patient. *Surg Gynecol Obstet* 1983;156:1

19. Morson BC. The muscular abnormality in diverticular disease of the sigmoid colon. *Br J Radiol* 1963;36:385

20. Whiteway J, Morson BC. Elastosis in diverticular disease of the sigmoid colon. *Gut* 1985;26:258

21. Arfwidsson S. Pathogenesis of multiple diverticula of the sigmoid colon in diverticular disease. *Acta Chir Scand* 1964;342(suppl)

22. Painter NS, Truelove SC, et al. Segmentation and localisation of intraluminal pressures in the human colon with special reference to the pathogenesis of colonic diverticula. *Gastroenterology* 1965;49:169

23. Parks TG, Connell AM. A comparison of the motility in the irritable colon syndrome and diverticular disease of the colon. *Rendic Di Gastroenteriol* 1972;4:12

24. Boulos PB, Karamanolis DG, et al. Is colonoscopy necessary in diverticular disease? *Lancet* 1984;1:95

25. Hughes LE. Complications of diverticular disease: inflammation, destruction and bleeding. *Clin Gastroenterol* 1975; 4:147

26. Schmidt GT, Lennard-Jones JE, et al. Crohn's disease of the colon and its distinction from diverticulitis. *Gut* 1968;9:7

27. Findlay JM, Smith AN, et al. Effects of unprocessed bran on colon function in normal subjects and in diverticular disease. *Lancet* 1974;1:146

28. Painter NS. *Diverticular Disease of the Colon.* London, England: Heinemann Medical; 1975

29. Greif JM, Fried G, et al. Surgical treatment of perforated diverticulitis of the sigmoid colon. *Dis Colon Rectum* 1980; 23:483

30. Einenstat TE, Rubin RJ, et al. Surgical management of diverticulitis: the role of the Hartmann procedure. *Dis Colon Rectum* 1983;26:429

31. Tudor RG, Oates GD, et al. Outcome after Hartmann procedure for complicated diverticular disease. *Gut* 1986; 27:626

32. Gregg RO. An ideal operation for diverticulitis. *Am J Surg* 1987;153:285

33. Krukowski ZH, Matheson NA. Emergency surgery for diverticular disease complicated by generalized and fecal peritonitis. *Br J Surg* 1984;7:921

34. Dudley HA, Radcliffe AG, et al. Intraoperative irrigation of the colon to permit primary anastomosis. *Br J Surg* 1980;67:80

35. Goldberger LE, Bookstein JJ. Transcatheter embolization for the treatment of diverticular hemorrhage. *Radiology* 1977;122:613

36. Welch CE, Ottinger LW, et al. Hemorrhage from the colon and rectum. In: Manual of Lower Gastrointestinal Surgery. New York, NY: Springer-Verlag; 1980:204

37. Drapanas T, Pennington DG, et al. Emergency subtotal colectomy: preferred approach to management of massively bleeding diverticular disease. *Am Surg* 1973; 177:519

38. Reilly M. Sigmoid myotomy. *Proc R Soc Med* 1964;57:556

39. Hodgson J. Transverse tenia myotomy: a new surgical approach for diverticular disease. *Ann R Coll Surg Engl* 1974;55:80

40. Schapira A. Leichtling JJ, et al. Diverticulitis of the cecum and right colon: clinical and radiographic features. *Am J Dig Dis* 1958;3:351

41

Inflammatory Bowel Disease of the Colon

Victor W. Fazio

The term inflammatory bowel disease (IBD) has, by common usage, become synonymous with ulcerative colitis and Crohn's disease. Inflammation and ulceration of the intestine may be the result of several known and definable causes. When these are excluded, there remains this group, with intestinal inflammation of unknown cause, ulcerative and Crohn's colitis. Yet in recent years, a third category has emerged, indeterminate colitis, which has assumed importance because of prognostic and therapeutic implications. This category is evidence of our inability to label neatly all forms of nonspecific IBD. Thus, this chapter will deal with granulomatous (Crohn's) colitis and ulcerative colitis, and where pertinent, reference will be made to indeterminate colitis. In the past, distinctions between the two major varieties of colitis (a better term would be proctocolitis rather than ulcerative colitis, since the rectum is invariably involved) were made with several practical surgical implications to be noted:

1. Ulcerative colitis is cured by proctocolectomy; however, recurrence of inflammation may occur in the ileostomy or proximal small bowel after the same operation is done for Crohn's disease.
2. The cancer risk in ulcerative colitis is far greater than in Crohn's colitis.

3. Restorative operations following subtotal colectomy, such as ileorectal anastomosis, have higher failure rates in Crohn's colitis than in ulcerative colitis.
4. Perianal disease, such as fistula, abscess, and fissure, is largely a feature of Crohn's disease.

In the past 15 years, a further and, indeed, more pertinent point has arisen with respect to distinguishing these two forms of colitis—choice of operation. The ileal pouch–anal anastomosis (IPAA) following proctocolectomy for ulcerative colitis has become the new "gold standard" operation for ulcerative colitis, based upon patient acceptance, acquisition of necessary skills by surgeons, a track record for good to reasonable function and an acceptably low complication and conversion-to-ileostomy rate. However, the failure rate of IPAA and early complication rates, when done inadvertently for Crohn's disease, may be quite high. Since "failures" may necessitate sacrifice of extra amounts of small intestine, there is some concern about the risk of short bowel syndromes.

In practice, there is no perfect method of distinguishing between the two forms of colitis. However, there are clinical and histological clues that may alert the clinician to a diagnostic dilemma being present and that may facilitate distinction between these two entities.

■ INFLAMMATORY BOWEL DISEASE

GRANULOMATOUS COLITIS (CROHN'S DISEASE OF THE LARGE BOWEL)

Perhaps the better term is Crohn's colitis, since some patients may have only the rectum or only the anus affected by the condition. Equally important, fewer than half of such patients have granulomas on microscopic examination of the affected large bowel. Crohn's disease is a chronic inflammatory disorder that may affect any part of the alimentary canal from the mouth to the anus. It is a focal disease with diseased segments separated by "healthy" segments or segments that are invariably inflamed in severity (Fig 41–1). All coats of the bowel wall may be involved (ie, transmural disease), and one of the characteristic features is the presence of granulomas. In the large bowel, part or all of the colon, may be affected.

ULCERATIVE COLITIS

Ulcerative colitis characteristically affects young individuals, although a variant exists that affects patients in their 40s, 50s, or later. The disease usually begins in the distal colon and rectum and, in many cases, extends proximally to affect the entire colon. Distal disease (ie, proctosigmoiditis), may be treated successfully with nonoperative means such as anti-inflammatory drugs. In the past, surgery was reserved for patients with universal or total colitis (disease extending to, or proximal to, the hepatic flexure). Yet left-sided colitis may produce disabling symptoms, requiring the same amounts and variety of medication. An appreciable incidence of

poor response to medical therapy is seen, with operation by no means an uncommon outcome.

The disease appears as a diffuse, nonpatchy inflammation extending proximally from the dentate line in a more or less evenly affected manner, and topical steroid enemas may give a picture of relative rectal sparing. The mucosa is granular, friable and lacks the longitudinal deep ulcers seen in Crohn's disease. Likewise, although diffuse superficial ulcers may be seen, the aphthoid ulcer typical of Crohn's disease, appearing as it commonly does in a background of relatively spared mucosa, is not present.

HISTORICAL ASPECTS

In 1806, Charles Combe and William Saunders described autopsy findings on a man with stricturing of the terminal ileum and three constricted inflamed segments of the colon, each about 5 to 8.5 cm long.[1] There were several centimeters of normal colon between the strictures. In their seminal paper, Crohn, Ginzburg and Oppenheimer reported 14 cases of regional ileitis.[2] The pathology findings were characterized by thickened intestinal wall, enlarged mesentery, linear ulceration of the bowel, stenosis and fistulae. Not all cases had granulomas. It was not until two decades later that Lockhart-Mummery and Morson reported on 25 cases seen between 1955 and 1959, in which the features of Crohn's disease were confined to the colon.[3] Earlier, in 1952, Wells pointed out that Crohn's disease could affect the colon as a "segmental colitis."[4]

■ PATHOLOGY OF INFLAMMATORY BOWEL DISEASE

CROHN'S DISEASE

The prevailing view for the past several decades is that Crohn's disease and ulcerative colitis are separate entities. As early as 1930, in a paper entitled "Regional Migratory Chronic Ulcerative Colitis," Bargen and Weber described 23 patients with such a condition, 17 of whom had a normal rectum and therefore, probably represented cases of Crohn's disease.[5] Slater and Ausfes gave an account on how Crohn and his colleagues believed that patients with both ileal and colonic inflammation had *both* granulomatous ileitis and ulcerative colitis.[6] Originally, Crohn's disease was regarded as a chronic granulomatous inflammatory disease of the terminal ileum. However, it is recognized that all parts of the intestine may be affected and that frequently the disease is *not* granulomatous. In its active phase, aphthoid ulceration is common, as is a chronic inflammatory process that is usually, but not always, transmural. This inflammation may be both acute and chronic and is associated with lymphoid aggregates and occasionally, with granu-

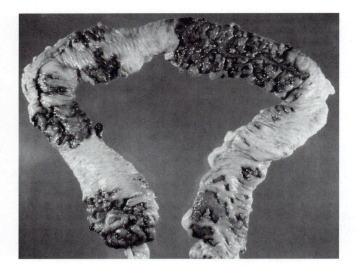

Figure 41–1. Colonic Crohn's disease, with patchy ulceration in the cecum, hepatic flexure, distal transverse colon, and sigmoid colon. The diseased areas are separated by apparently normal segments, a feature characteristic of Crohn's disease.

lomas. As linear ulceration develops, macroscopic serpiginous "rake" or "bear-claw" ulcers appear and penetrating fissures are seen (Figs 41–2, 41–3). As these fissures penetrate to and through the serosa to an adjacent viscus or wound, localized abscess formation and fistulas develop. With chronic disease, acute inflammation is replaced by fibrosis, scarring and stricture formation (Fig 41–4). Characteristically, the disease is focal or multifocal, as opposed to the diffuse and more or less even distribution of ulcerative colitis.

Strictures may be tight, short or long and multiple in the colon. Generally, however, they do not approach the frequency or severity of small bowel strictures. Serositis is common but, although penetrating fissures are common, free perforation of the colon is unusual, except in cases of toxic megacolon. The combination of linear ulcers with transverse narrow fissures produce a cobblestone appearance in late stage disease where edematous mucosal folds are thrown into relief (Fig 41–5). Pseudopolyps also may be seen, usually in a background of relatively quiescent colitis. Occasionally a sea of polyps, called "colitis polyposa", may be seen. Fat wrapping may occur but is less common than in small bowel.

Lymph node enlargement is typical in Crohn's disease, and suppuration may occur. Aphthoid ulcers are characteristic of active Crohn's disease. These are small (1 to 5 mm in diameter), superficial, pale with a pink or red halo, distinct from the background "normal" mucosa and occasionally migratory. These may be clearly visible on the outer surface of an ileostomy but disappear or migrate to another quadrant 1 or 2 weeks later. There is a propensity for such ulcers to form over an epithelium covering lymphoid aggregates. Areas of previous ulceration can be recognized by distortion of the architecture, pyloric metaplasia, and thickened or duplicated muscularis mucosa, with subjacent submucosal fibrosis.

Granulomas do not reflect disease activity and, while characteristic of Crohn's disease, may not be totally specific. Granulomas may arise secondary to suture material or to buried vegetable matter, especially if the granuloma is close to an area of ulceration. The granulomas are noncaseating and rarely necrotic. They consist of localized, well-formed aggregates of epithelial histiocytes, with or without giant cells, or a surrounding cuff of lymphocytes. Granulomas commonly appear in the submucosa, but also may occur in all coats of the bowel wall as well as in adjacent lymph nodes. The frequency of occurrence of granulomas depends upon the diligence of searching for such lesions, in other words, the number of sections taken and examined. A 30% to 50% incidence usually is reported.

Commonly, endoscopic biopsies of colonic mucosa are reported as acute and chronic nonspecific inflammation, even in patients in whom numerous clinical features suggest Crohn's disease as the diagnosis. Thus, clinical features are important in adding to the diagnostic accuracy of a particular problem case. Such clinical factors include (1) normal appearing rectum with proximal colonic disease, (2) perianal fistula(s), (3) velvety or indurated, "elephant-ear" skin tags, (4) aphthoid ulcers, (5) broad, indolent, large or lateral fissures or anal canal ulcers, (6) ileal disease or endoscopy, and (7) skip lesions. These features point to the diagnosis of Crohn's disease, notwithstanding the uncertainty of the pathologist in reviewing the slides. The corollary of this

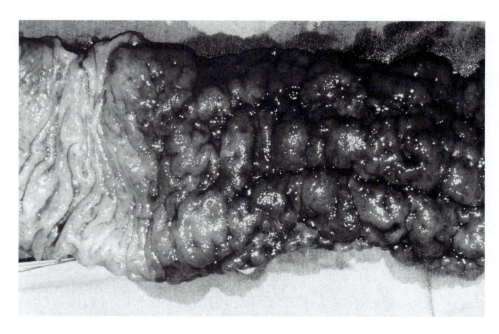

Figure 41–2. Rake or bear-claw linear ulceration is a common feature of Crohn's colitis. A sharp cut-off is seen between diseased and "normal" bowel.

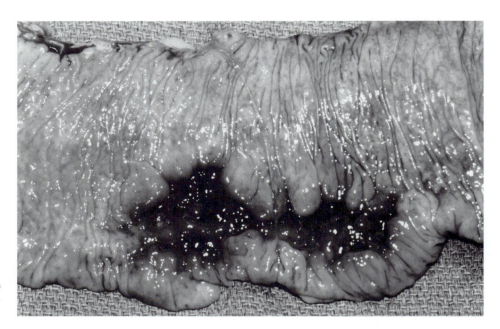

Figure 41–3. Serpiginous longitudinal ulcer of Crohn's disease, in a background of apparently normal colon.

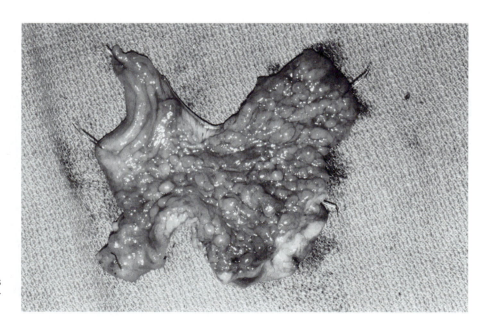

Figure 41–4. Section of colon stricture. Mural fibrosis and thickening of muscularis mucosa occurs. Cobblestoning is apparent.

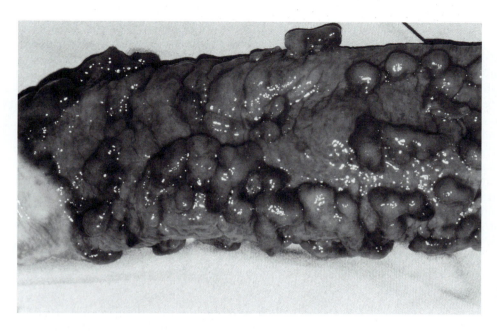

Figure 41–5. Cobblestone appearance in late-stage Crohn's colitis.

situation is that the presence of the above features will be strong deterrents to the performance of a pelvic or Kock pouch, since recurrences of Crohn's disease in such pouches may lead to early reoperative resectional surgery for complications, especially septic complications.

COLITIS INDETERMINATE

In a sizable number of cases, perhaps 7% to 10%, the clear differentiation between ulcerative colitis and Crohn's disease cannot be made. The clinical features, as well as the histologic findings, may be ambiguous. Relative rectal sparing may be seen in ulcerative colitis, when topical anti-inflammatory agents are used. Deep ulcers may be found in patients with fulminant ulcerative colitis. Both perianal fistula and rectovaginal fistula may be observed in ulcerative colitis, albeit rarely. Ileal disease or inflammation may represent the "backwash" ileitis of ulcerative colitis, as opposed to Crohn's disease of the ileum. In these and other ambiguous cases, careful discussion with the pathologist is needed. In turn, a candid and full discussion with the patient then is required, specifying the positive and negative aspects of performing procedures such as restorative proctocolectomy with pelvic ileal pouch, *and* the relative likelihood of such events happening. These cases have been called *colitis indeterminate*. Further discrimination may be engendered by the IBD pathologist, who may have three subcategories: (1) indeterminate colitis, without modifier, (2) indeterminate colitis, with the modifier favor Crohn's disease, and (3) favor ulcerative colitis. In

practice, these categories are useful for this author, since I can relate the dilemma and degrees of uncertainty of diagnosis to the intelligent patient with reasonable assurance of their comprehension that sphincter-saving operations may carry risks of later developing overt features of Crohn's disease.

In the past, indeterminate colitis was a term used for patients with fulminant disease where the colitis was unclassifiable. Essentially, this was a temporary diagnosis until more material or more information was obtained. Yet in recent times, there is increasing use of the term as a final diagnosis, when the exact nature of the disease is obscure even after full histologic examination of the resected colon. Indeterminate colitis is commonly diagnosed following urgent surgery for fulminant disease, usually after a short period of medical management.[7,8]

Fulminant colitis is a difficult entity to analyze pathologically since many of its features, such as deep penetrating ulcers, are, in the nonacute case, strongly suggestive of Crohn's disease. As Riddell has stated, it is essential that these changes be interpreted in context.[9] Indeed, other features of indeterminate colitis that do not necessarily equate with a diagnosis of Crohn's disease and that can be seen in fulminant disease of any cause include rectal sparing, patchy distribution, hemorrhagic ulceration with relatively little inflammation, cobblestoning of mucosa, and deep fissuring ulcers. However, gross skip lesions, granulomas unrelated to local ulcers and lymphoid aggregates in the subserosa or submucosa, especially if unrelated to overlying ulceration, are strongly suggestive of a diagnosis of Crohn's disease.

ULCERATIVE COLITIS

In active ulcerative colitis, mucosal superficial ulceration is seen with a diffuse acute and chronic inflammatory infiltrate in the mucosa and submucosa. Goblet cell depletion is the rule, although it may return when resolution occurs. Crypt abscesses are nonspecific but common findings in ulcerative colitis. If all crypts are involved, then this is an important diagnostic differentiation from Crohn's disease where crypt abscesses tend to be isolated or areas of crypts are seen without abscesses, but with neutrophil infiltration of the lamina propria. In ulcerative colitis, resolution of chronic inflammation may give a patchy infiltrate suggestive of microscopic skip lesions of Crohn's disease. While sarcoid-like granulomas are not seen in ulcerative colitis, granulomas may be seen in ulcerative colitis, resulting from a reaction to leaked mucin or foreign material.

■ CLINICAL FEATURES OF INFLAMMATORY BOWEL DISEASE

CROHN'S DISEASE OF THE COLON

The spectrum of the disease is wide. The most common pattern is that of right-sided colitis combined with ileal Crohn's disease (ileocolitis). Other patterns include pancolitis with sparing of the rectum, proctitis, anal canal and perianal manifestations, pan-proctocolitis, and that rare entity, Crohn's disease confined to the appendix. The clinicoanatomic pattern, in turn, produces a particular set of clinical features. Ileocolitis, for example, most commonly is manifested by septic phenomenon such as fever, right lower quadrant mass, leukocytosis, abdominal pain and tenderness. Additionally, obstructive symptoms are common owing to the associated narrowing of the terminal ileum. As in all forms of inflammatory bowel disease, diarrhea, weight loss, failure to thrive, bleeding, or features of anemia may be seen. In children, growth retardation or fever of unknown origin may be associated features. In the patient with extensive colitis or proctocolitis of either Crohn's disease or ulcerative colitis origin, the clinical features are frequently diarrhea with episodic bleeding, malnourishment, abdominal pain and extraintestinal manifestations of disease. Such manifestations include pyoderma gangrene, erythema nodosum, arthritis or arthralgia, and a variety of liver and ophthalmic complications. More threatening is the occurrence of emergencies such as toxic megacolon and massive colonic hemorrhage. There are other variations of presentation, such as anorectal and perianal Crohn's disease, which exhibit such features as bleeding, fistula/abscesses, fissure-ulcers, painful skin tags, stricture, and in-

continence. Digital rectal examination will help in the assessment of rectal stricturing as well as tone of the anal sphincter.

ULCERATIVE COLITIS

Typically, the presenting symptom is diarrhea, which is often watery and bloody. Subacute or chronic loss anemia may occur. Chronic active colitis or severe attacks are frequently associated with hypoproteinemia. Abdominal cramps, urgency, tenesmus and even incontinence may occur. Strictures may develop in the colon, although, if seen within the first ten years of symptom onset, these strictures are almost always benign. Carcinoma may occur and, in the absence of a surveillance program for identification of dysplasia, is insidious in onset. If advanced, obstruction and perforation of the colon, as well as distant metastases, may occur. Toxic megacolon may occur with either ulcerative colitis or Crohn's disease. The patient is acutely ill and, in addition to colonic distention, has two or more of the following features: tachycardia, fever, leukocytosis, anemia, or hypoalbuminemia. In addition, electrolyte abnormalities, shock, and hypotension may occur. If the bowel has perforated, features of peritonitis are present. Extraintestinal manifestations also may be seen in ulcerative colitis. Sclerosing cholangitis, portal triaditis and even bile duct cancer occur in association with ulcerative colitis.

■ DIAGNOSIS

ENDOSCOPY

Whenever endoscopy of the large bowel is done, local pain and tenderness, as occurs in association with perianal lesions of Crohn's disease, may thwart the performance of a good examination. Especially in this circumstance, a careful examination is required, frequently under anesthesia. Particular attention to the perianal area and anal canal is useful in picking up occult fistulas, anorectal thickening, stricture or anal canal ulceration. Typically, fissures that are wide, lateral (as opposed to posterior or anterior lesions), indolent, and relatively painless are characteristic of Crohn's disease. Vulval and vaginal fistulae may be present at colonoscopy. Particular attention is paid to the presence or absence of rectal inflammation, distensibility of the rectum on air insufflation, confluence or evenness of distribution of inflammation, which is diffuse in the case of ulcerative colitis and commonly patchy or associated with skip lesions in Crohn's disease. Deep ulceration is a common feature of Crohn's disease, although it also may be seen in toxic or fulminant ulcerative colitis (Fig 41–6). Earlier, aphthoid ulcers were described in associ-

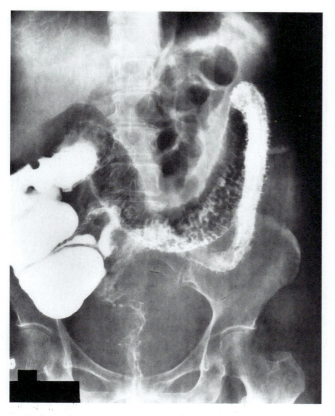

Figure 41–6. Extensive ulceration of the colon, particularly left-sided, in ulcerative colitis. Barium enema is contraindicated in toxic colitis as dilation frequently follows.

lated segments, such as transverse or sigmoid colon, may be affected by Crohn's disease. Reflux of colon contents into the small bowel may demonstrate ileal Crohn's disease or backwash ileitis. In ulcerative colitis, a diffuse ground-glass appearance is commonly seen (Fig 41–7). Shortening of the colon is seen in chronic disease, which leaves a lack of haustral pattern, or "lowering" of the flexures, the so-called lead-pipe appearance. Filling defects are produced by pseudopolyps. Strictures are usually symmetrical, although irregularity may suggest a malignant change (Fig 41–8). In Crohn's disease, a nodular appearance is produced by the cobblestoning referred to in the pathology section. Extracolonic barium may be seen in an abscess cavity or extending into an adjacent viscus, such as small bowel (ileosigmoid fistula) or urinary bladder (colovesical fistula).

Rose thorn ulceration or spiculation is a feature suggesting the presence of penetrating transmural ulcers of Crohn's disease. Occasionally, a long extramural tract that runs parallel with the bowel is seen. This tract is termed Marshak's sign (Fig 41–9). With good quality air-contrast studies, even small ulcers may be identified. Small bowel studies are recommended in patients with colitis to look for evidence of small bowel or duodenal involvement.

Other studies that may be used in the assessment of

ation with Crohn's disease. In these cases, the background mucosa may appear almost normal. Asymmetric involvement of the bowel wall also is seen in Crohn's disease. Colonscopy is particularly useful intraoperatively. In such cases, it may be difficult for the surgeon to identify the precise distal margin of large bowel involvement. This is best determined by intraluminal visualization.

In ulcerative colitis, the rectum typically is involved. Pseudopolyps may be present in both ulcerative colitis and Crohn's disease when advanced disease is present. Ulceration may be present in ulcerative colitis, but is not linear as a rule nor do the ulcers appear with a normal or near normal background mucosa. Biopsy information is important, especially if focal skip lesions or granulomas are identified, which favor a diagnosis of Crohn's disease. In ulcerative colitis, dysplasia may be identified and may be an important indication for surgery.

RADIOLOGICAL STUDIES

Lesions may be distributed throughout the entire colon and rectum or may involve specific segments that leave intervening normal-appearing mucosa. Iso-

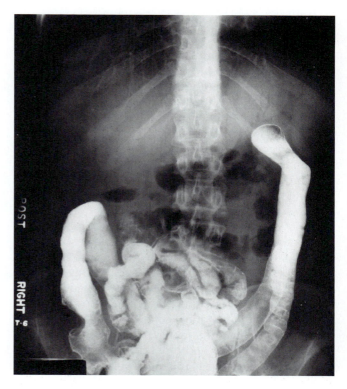

Figure 41–7. Lack of haustration in chronic ulcerative colitis.

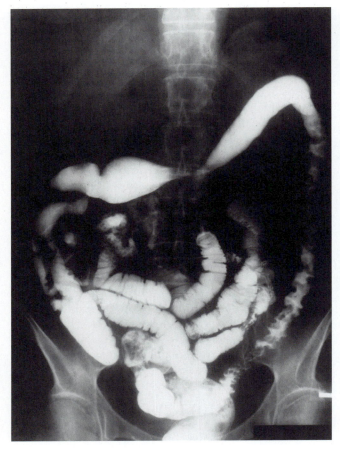

Figure 41–8. Smooth stricture of the transverse colon in Crohn's disease.

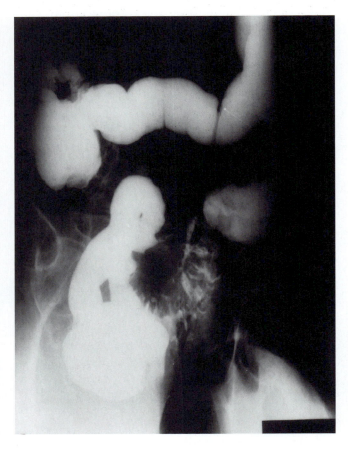

Figure 41–9. Extramural tracking of barium in Crohn's disease of the sigmoid colon (Marshak's sign).

patients with inflammatory bowel disease include CT, ultrasound, scintiscanning and physiological tests of anal function. CT is used when there is suggestive evidence of intra-abdominal abscess (eg, psoas abscess secondary to ileocecal perforation). CT is also useful in clarifying pelvic or anorectal septic/fistula phenomena and is valuable in the postoperative setting, when investigating a septic state. Endoluminal rectal ultrasound testing is useful in assessing rectal strictures, incontinence states and suspected extrarectal pelvic collections. The indium 3-labeled autologous leukocyte scan has been reported to be accurate in localizing the site of inflammatory involvement in the colon, both in ulcerative colitis and in Crohn's disease. Anal physiological studies are useful in the assessment of patients with questionable sphincter function, when anticipating a sphincter-saving operation such as the ileoanal pull-through operation. Additionally, in patients with Crohn's colitis and rectal sparing, compliance assessment, as determined by maximum tolerated volume of fluid instilled into the rectum, is of prognostic importance when advising patients on the performance of colec-

tomy with ileorectal anastomosis. The more distensible or compliant the wall of the rectum, the better the functional outcome of ileoproctostomy.

■ TREATMENT

MEDICAL TREATMENT OF INFLAMMATORY BOWEL DISEASE

Medical treatment, like all current therapy of inflammatory bowel disease, is empiric and targeted to a particular individual. Symptomatic management of abdominal pain, diarrhea, and anemia is used where feasible. Sulfasalazine, antibiotics, steroids and immunosuppressive agents are the commonly used medications.

SYMPTOMATIC TREATMENT

This type of treatment will lessen the need for use of steroids. Antispasmodic measures, antidiarrheal measures, and mild sedatives will lessen the irritable colon component that frequently accompanies inflammatory bowel disease. Anticholinergic drugs are best avoided, especially in toxic cases, since megacolon may be induced. Diphenoxylate or loperamide are frequently used antidiarrheal drugs. Bulking agents, especially psyllium compounds, are also useful as bowel normalizers. Cigarette smoking is vigorously condemned for patients with Crohn's disease.

DIETARY MANAGEMENT

Diarrhea commonly abates with reduced intake of seasoned foods, fruit juice concentrate, caffeine, fatty foods and raw vegetables. Patients with lactose intolerance are placed on a lactose-reduced diet. Nutritional deficiencies, particularly iron, protein, and trace elements, may occur and restoration is attempted.

SULFASALAZINE AND 5-AMINO-SALICYLATE (5-ASA)

Efficacy for sulfasalazine in the treatment of both Crohn's colitis and ulcerative colitis was shown in the National Cooperative Crohn's Disease Study (4 g/day).[10] For the patient experiencing side effects of the drug, mostly due to the sulfa component (sulfapyridine), 5-ASA is useful in inhibiting inflammatory reaction, although side effects occur in 20%. In patients who experience a good response to sulfasalazine treatment, prolonged use is recommended. Local therapy with 5-ASA enemas can be helpful for proctitis. Sulfasalazine is most effective for mild to moderately active colitis.

ANTIBIOTICS

Antibiotic therapy is used in specific situations in Crohn's disease patients. Metronidazole is particularly useful for perianal sepsis (eg, abscess and fistulas), especially in combination with ciprofloxacin. There is a lag period before a response is observed when metronidazole is used. The agent is also useful in managing patients with nonhealing of the perineal wound after proctocolectomy. Additionally, metronidazole may result in lessening the inflammatory features of Crohn's colitis. A major side effect of prolonged use in peripheral neuropathy. Alternative antibiotics include tetracycline, ampicillin, cephalexin, erythromycin and sulfamethoxazole-trimethoprim. These agents are useful for patients who are intolerant of sulfasalazine or metronidazole. Blichfeldt and colleagues compared metronidazole with placebo as an adjuvant to prednisone or sulfasalazine.[11] The group of patients with disease limited to the large intestine was the only subset who showed marked clinical improvement.

CORTICOSTEROIDS

In Crohn's disease, remission of acute flares commonly will occur, although there is little evidence that long-term therapy produces beneficial effects. In ulcerative colitis, steroids are valuable for acute flares of the disease, and in certain chronic intractable cases, benefit from a course of steroids may be realized. Many clinicians use steroids as a "bridge" to suppress colitis activity until the effect of immunosuppressives is obtained.

IMMUNOSUPPRESSIVES

In Crohn's disease, the role of azathioprine and 6-mercapto-purine is controversial. The NCCDS failed to show clinical improvement when azathioprine was compared with placebo.[10] Present and associates, however, found a significant (67% vs 8%) improvement with 6-mercapto-purine over placebo.[12] Thus, immunosuppressants are used in treating certain patients with Crohn's disease: those who have responded well to the drug, those who will have regular surveillance blood counts drawn, and those with no firm indication for surgery. In ulcerative colitis, the same drugs are used in patients who are not at high risk for developing colorectal carcinoma. Many surgeons would recommend operation for the ulcerative colitis patient rather than recommend immunosuppressives.

Cyclosporine has been reported to have possible beneficial effects in both Crohn's disease and in ulcerative colitis in the short term. However, the mechanism of action is unknown. Side effects can be very significant. At present, there is some enthusiasm among gastroenterologists to use cyclosporine in cases of toxic colitis to avoid urgent surgery.

■ SURGERY OF CROHN'S DISEASE OF THE LARGE BOWEL

Unlike the case in ulcerative colitis, colectomy or proctocolectomy may not prove to be curative. A majority of patients result with a permanent ileostomy. Many will undergo alternatives to ileostomy, temporizing as they may be. This is especially true for those patients with perianal disease. About two-thirds of patients with Crohn's colitis undergo surgery within ten years of diagnosis.

INDICATIONS FOR SURGERY

Indications for surgery are outlined in Table 41–1. Poor response to medical therapy or intractability is found to be the primary indication for surgery in about 25% of patients with Crohn's colitis, as compared with the 8% to 10% rate for patients with Crohn's ileitis or ileocolitis. Extraintestinal manifestations of Crohn's disease may be classified as (1) colitis related, (2) related to the pathophysiology of the small intestine (malabsorption, gallstones, kidney stones) and (3) nonspecific (osteoporosis, liver disease, peptic ulcer, amyloidosis). Joint, skin and eye complications are colitis related. In gen-

TABLE 41–1. INDICATIONS FOR SURGERY IN CROHN'S DISEASE OF THE LARGE BOWEL

Medical intractability
    failure to thrive
    steroid dependency
    complications of medication
    disabling diarrhea
    resistent anemia
    fecal incontinence
Extraintestinal manifestations
Malnutrition, growth retardation
Bowel obstruction
Stricture
Cancer
Obstructive uropathy
Hemorrhage
Intra-abdominal abscess
Fistula—internal and external
Fulminant colitis—toxic megacolon
Perianal disease
Recurrent Crohn's disease (with complications)

eral, those patients that respond well or fairly well to steroid therapy also respond well to surgery. Liver complications, such as sclerosing cholangitis, and ankylosing spondylitis respond poorly to both medical and surgical treatment. About one-third of patients with Crohn's disease have extraintestinal manifestations. Bowel obstruction is relatively uncommon in colonic Crohn's disease, occurring in 12% of patients at the Cleveland Clinic. When ileocolitis is considered, 37% of such patients undergo surgery for bowel obstruction. Typically, in colonic Crohn's disease, obstruction is rarely acute and relates to stricturing, especially in the anorectum.

Colonic Stricture

Colonic stricture (Fig 41–8) may or may not be associated with obstructive symptoms. Usually the stricture is benign and can be managed nonoperatively if relatively asymptomatic. Surgery is indicated where there is high-grade obstruction, inability to keep the proximal colon under surveillance, or if carcinoma cannot be excluded from the differential diagnosis. Yamazaki and colleagues reported on 132 patients with colonic strictures due to Crohn's disease; nine (6.8%) had cancer in a strictured segment.[13] Although the benign strictures tended to be of greater length than the malignant ones, the symptoms were similar. Strictureplasty for colonic strictures, even when short, cannot be recommended since there is little compulsion to preserve colonic length (compared with small bowel) and postoperative sepsis rates are likely to be high. Anastomotic stricture of the colon is another indicator.

In one series of 40 patients who underwent resection

for ileocolitis with follow-up over a 20 year interval, 69% had symptomatic stricturing.[14] For the most part, these are treated by re-resection, although strictureplasty has been very successful when the stricture is short. Endoscopic dilation has been used successfully with two-thirds of patients free of symptoms at 15 months, in one series.[15,16] However, bowel perforation and intestinal hemorrhage occurred in 1 and 2 patients, respectively, of the 27 treated cases. At present there are no definite rules about the appropriateness of dilation. Relative points for dilation include early development of anastomotic stricture (eg, within one year), short segment (<2.0 cm) stricture, and low-level (eg, ileorectal anastomosis) stricture.

Colonic Carcinoma

Colonic carcinoma in Crohn's disease occurs more frequently than small bowel cancer. Site distribution is similar to that of non-Crohn's disease colonic carcinoma.[17–21] In longstanding Crohn's disease with extensive colonic involvement, the Cancer Epidemiology Research Unit in Birmingham, U.K., found a four-fold increase in alimentary tract cancer compared with a nondiseased cohort.[22] Risk of cancer was directly related to the duration of Crohn's disease. We and others have noted that colonic cancers in patients with Crohn's disease are not necessarily located in visibly diseased segments.[23] Additional, excluded segments, such as the distal rectum after subtotal colectomy and ileostomy, may develop cancer.[24]

Ekbom and colleagues reported the relative risk of colorectal malignancy in 1655 Swedish patients with Crohn's disease.[17] With follow-up during 30 years, this group determined that disease distribution at diagnosis was an important determinant of the increased risk. With disease confined to the ileum, the relative risk for cancer was 1.0. For ileocolitis and colitis patterns at the time of diagnosis, the relative risk was 3.2 and 5.6, respectively.

The difficulties facing the clinician relate to the fact that cancer of the colon in Crohn's disease is not easy to diagnose. Colonic strictures may be malignant, but biopsy and even cytology of the stricture may not be diagnostic. Hence, the risk exists on the one hand of "excessive" surgery if all strictures are resected versus the risk of neglecting a malignant stricture if surgery is withheld. To minimize the risks, one could advocate a policy or provide the following guidelines.

1. Resect any excluded segment of bowel (eg, bypassed ileum or an excluded rectum), provided the patient is fit for surgery and future restoration involving that segment is unlikely.

2. If the patient declines resection of an excluded colon or rectum, then recommend annual co-

lonoscopy with multiple biopsies as for ulcerative colitis surveillance.

3. In patients whose duration of Crohn's disease is longer than 10 years, and in whom colonic strictures are present, recommend resection.

4. In patients in whom a colonic or rectal stricture precludes adequate surveillance of the proximal large bowel, recommend resection.

5. All patients with colonic strictures should undergo colonoscopy, multiple biopsies of the stricture, and/or cytology.

6. If dysplasia or adenoma is identified, recommend resection. Note however, that the dysplasia-cancer sequence is not as clear-cut as in ulcerative colitis.

7. For longstanding chronic fistula-in-ano patients, curettage of tracts and Tru-cut deep biopsy of any indurated skin or subcutaneous tissue is recommended.

Colonic Hemorrhage

Colonic hemorrhage due to Crohn's disease produces bleeding that is generally diffuse. Additionally, the colon is often affected by fulminant disease, even toxic megacolon. In such cases, urgent colectomy is required. The blow-hole colostomy/ileostomy procedure is contraindicated since hemorrhage will likely continue despite diversion. There are three options for colectomy. Subtotal colectomy and end ileostomy is usually successful, but there is a small chance of bleeding from the rectal stump. Since one can rarely be certain of the diagnosis (ulcerative colitis vs Crohn's disease) in fulminant hemorrhagic colitis, one should be especially circumspect about performing a total proctocolectomy. Even though this procedure will eliminate the risk of rectal bleeding, there is an increased risk of impotence in urgent cases. Thus, the possibility of a pelvic pouch operation in the future is negated. My preference over the years has been subtotal colectomy, with careful inspection of the rectum via proctoscope to ensure no active rectal bleeding is occurring. If later bleeding occurs, one can use intrarectal adrenalin for control. A solution of adrenalin is prepared (1:200 000) and 25 to 50 cc are instilled into the rectum via a Foley catheter. This regimen is repeated every hour while monitoring pulse and blood pressure and is usually successful. If this regimen is unsuccessful, completion proctectomy can be done, leaving the anal canal and sphincters in case the diagnosis is ulcerative colitis.

Internal Fistula

These are common in Crohn's disease, but most arise from small bowel and secondarily involve an adjacent, otherwise normal viscus (eg, ileosigmoid, ileotransverse, ileoileal fistula). Nonetheless, fistulas from diseased colon to normal small bowel, duodenum, stomach, urinary bladder, fallopian tubes, uterus and vagina may occur. The principles of surgery include resection of the diseased part and detachment of the "normal" anatomical structure from the diseased segment. The defect in the normal tube or viscus then is freshened and repaired.

Rectovaginal Fistula

When small and minimally symptomatic, rectovaginal fistula (RVF) requires no treatment. If rectal Crohn's disease is present, as well as symptoms of RVF, then no curative treatment is feasible short of ileostomy and proctectomy. However, patients may be managed successfully for long periods, even in such circumstances, with steroids, long-term low-dose metronidazole, vaginal hygiene and occasionally, immunosuppressives such as azathioprine. With rectal sparing, alternative curative approaches include advancement rectal flap, transsphincteric division and repair, transvaginal repair and, for the patient with associated anal canal ulceration, advancement sleeve operation similar to a limited Altemeir operation.

Colocutaneous fistulas are relatively uncommon, but may occur spontaneously after drainage of an abscess secondary to colonic disease and perforation. Alternatively, they may occur as a sequel to abdominal surgery. If the segment of colon is affected by Crohn's disease, the same principles of fistula surgery will apply.

Abdominal Abscess

Most abscesses usually arise secondary to penetrating ulceration through the bowel wall. Escape of enteric contents then may be localized by an adjacent viscus or peritoneal surface, producing containment. If not contained, a free perforation and peritonitis result. Abscesses may spontaneously drain into an adjacent viscus or along a drain tract or former incision, producing a fistula. Manifestations of abscess formation therefore may vary from the classic acute signs to an occult smoldering presentation as the result of partial spontaneous drainage internally, or the result of the masking effect of steroids.

The varieties of abscess include enteroparietal, interloop, intramesenteric and retroperitoneal. Most of these abscesses relate to the ileitis or ileocolitis pattern of Crohn's disease. However, psoas abscesses may result from posterior perforation of the cecum or sigmoid, and presacral abscesses may arise from rectal or sigmoid Crohn's disease, even presenting as ischiorectal abscesses via an extrasphincteric or intersphincteric fistulous communication. The principles of management include preoperatively draining of all pus by CT-guided needle, where feasible, and performing surgery electively to resect the diseased segment that acts as the source of the infection. With retroperitoneal sepsis or phlegmon of the cecum or sigmoid colon, ureteric compression may occur. Such obstructive uropathy is rapidly relieved with bowel resection. Ureterolysis rarely is required.

Toxic Colitis and Megacolon

Although usually associated with ulcerative colitis, this condition is increasingly seen in Crohn's disease. By its nature, toxic colitis, in which penetrating ulcers extend through the bowel wall and, in some cases, produce free perforation, is a transmural process. Hence, there is usually great difficulty for both the clinician and the pathologist to characterize this entity as ulcerative colitis or Crohn's colitis with high confidence levels. Toxic colitis is defined as being present when inflammatory colonic disease is associated with two or more of the following: tachycardia, fever, hypoalbuminemia, leukocytosis, and anemia. Shock, hypotension, electrolyte abnormalities, toxic psychosis, and peritonitis may be present but are not necessary for the diagnosis.

Megacolon is added to the entity of toxic colitis when the haustral pattern is absent and the colon is dilated beyond 5 cm (Fig 41–10).

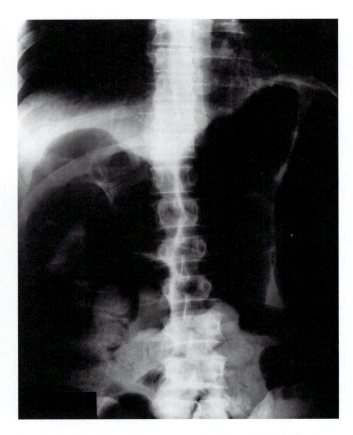

Figure 41–10. Toxic megacolon. Dilation is usually most prominent in the distal transverse colon.

Following resuscitation of the patient with toxic colitis or megacolon, the clinician will check for certain associated features that indicate a need for urgent surgery. These include pneumoperitoneum, endotoxemia, massive hemorrhage, general peritonitis, and severe, localized abdominal tenderness.

The mortality of toxic colitis, with or without colonic dilation, is related to sepsis. The most devastating type of sepsis is that of spontaneous or iatrogenic perforation of the colon. Thus, the strategy for approaching the entity of toxic colitis is that of early recognition of perforation, early recognition of impending perforation, early recognition of inadequate or failed response to medical therapy, recognition of factors that promote colonic dilation or perforation, preoperatively and intraoperatively, recognition of factors (other than perforation) that carry an adverse prognosis for the patient, and selection of the operative procedure that maximizes survival rate and minimizes morbidity rate.

Early recognition of colonic perforation may be difficult owing to the effects of steroids, or other immunosuppressives or narcotics that may mask features of peritonitis. Plain x-rays of the abdomen are taken daily if there are features of colonic dilation. Frequent abdominal examinations also are performed. In a few cases, the evidence for pneumoperitoneum may be subtle, such as a thin rim of gas under one or another diaphragm. Rarer still is the linear collection of free air in the mid-abdomen, where trapping has occurred between the inferior edge of the transverse colon and the transverse mesocolon.

Impending perforation may be suspected by the development of increasing abdominal pain. Severe pain usually is absent in toxic colitis. Additionally, signs of increasing toxicity may be evident: increased tachycardia, leukocytosis, fever, chills, hypotension, and oliguria. Localized abdominal tenderness is a sinister sign, indicating a probable contained perforation. Radiographically, the presence of small, 1-cm diameter opacities in the distal transverse colon, seen in relief against a background of a gas-filled, radiolucent colon, indicates very deep ulceration occurring around an edematous mound of mucosa and impending perforation.

Medical therapy is instituted in patients with toxic colitis or megacolon where there is no indication for urgent surgery. The rationale of treatment is that the colitis may go into remission and provide long-term freedom from surgery or that elective surgery may be later considered, with a lessened rate of complications compared with urgent operation. The components of medical therapy include intravenous fluid, steroids, correction of correctable deficiencies, and nasogastric suction, in certain cases. Somewhat controversial is the use of broad-spectrum antibiotics, although it is our practice to do so. The Mt Sinai Hospital group in New York described the use of cyclosporin-A as an adjunctive treatment in severe ulcerative colitis, refractory to conventional therapy.[25] Colectomy was avoided in 81% of 32 patients. However, this modality remains controversial. As well, Present and associates, from the same institution, have advocated conservative therapy for toxic megacolon; the basis of treatment invokes decompression of the dilated colon by colonic intubation and repositioning of the patient at intervals.[26] This method also remains controversial. The common dilemma facing the surgeon is the patient in whom conservative therapy has been started, but in whom there is no improvement after a period of observation. For how long should therapy be given before deciding that there has been an inadequate response to medical therapy? There is no clear answer to this question, however, Go-ligher and associates showed improved survival when operating for ulcerative colitis within 7 days of the onset of the acute attack.[27] It is likely that this experience applies also to Crohn's colitis.

Certain factors have been described as associations or promoters of dilation of the bowel in cases of toxic colitis. These include anticholinergic agents, antidiarrheal medication, hypokalemia and contrast roentgenographic studies, especially barium enema.[28] One would also add to this list colonic endoscopy during which distention of the colon with air insufflation may occur. Raised intracolonic pressure may be the final straw in converting a near transmural ulcer or contained perforation of the bowel into a free perforation.

At operation, mobilization of a fragile, distended, stool-laden colon, especially the flexures, may be accompanied by iatrogenic perforation with its accompanying increased mortality and complication rate. Thus, intraoperative needle decompression of the colon, quarantining of the flexures with packs, and cautious colonic mobilization may help minimize the risk of perforation.

The major factors associated with an adverse outcome in the surgery of toxic colitis include free perforation with peritonitis, hypoalbuminemia and accompanying massive hemorrhage. In emergencies, there is little that can be done to alter these states. However, for free perforation, one will, after peritoneal toilet, usually perform subtotal colectomy, making an end ileostomy and leaving a generous rectosigmoid segment that will easily reach the lower end of the incision for exteriorization, if the bowel is very fragile, or for stapling and extraperitonealization (see below). Completion proctectomy then may be deferred to an elective time. Although for permanent treatment hypoalbuminemia requires removal of the cause of the protein losing enteropathy (the diseased colon), colloid osmotic pressure may be improved transiently and intraoperatively by albumin transfusion, supplemented by postoperative total parenteral nutrition. Any coagulopathy may be addressed perioperatively.

The strategy of surgical choices for toxic colitis and megacolon is based on the premise that one performs the least complicated procedure promising a reasonable prospect of recovery. In most cases, this procedure will be subtotal colectomy and ileostomy. The rectal stump, often the distal sigmoid stump, is managed by one of three methods: (1) simple suture or staple oversew, (2) creation of a mucus fistula, or (3) exteriorization and gauze wrapping of the distal sigmoid segment through the lower end of the incision.

Each of these approaches are appropriate depending upon, and in increasing order of, the severity of the local disease and fragile nature of the bowel wall.

In certain cases a lesser procedure, such as blow-hole colostomy and ileostomy, is appropriate. This operation, pioneered by Rupert B Turnbull Jr, was commonly used by our group for toxic megacolon of both Crohn's disease and ulcerative colitis etiology. This preference was mostly in an era, the 1960s to mid 1970s, when patients presenting for treatment were very debilitated with gross malnutrition, and major delays in surgical referral were common. Thus, the operative mortality was high owing to preoperative debility. Intraoperative perforation with abdominal colectomy was identified as a problem contributing significantly to morbidity and mortality. Turnbull's response was to avoid manipulation of the colon and perform a staged procedure, namely, ileostomy (to divert the fecal stream) and cutaneous, skin-level transverse colostomy (to vent the dilated colon). In current times, a few patients are so debilitated, and the vast majority can withstand subtotal colectomy safely. The exceptions are patients in whom colectomy may be risky owing to the fragile nature of the colon (eg, the neglected patient with longstanding toxicity), patients with a high splenic flexure, or pregnant patients. In these patients, there is value in performing ileostomy/colostomy. At six months, definitive surgery, usually proctocolectomy, is done.

Perianal Disease

In longstanding, advanced cases of sepsis due to complex fistulae, especially where rectal Crohn's disease is present, proctectomy and fecal diversion is required. However, other treatments may provide satisfactory palliation for long periods (eg, periodic incision and drainage of abscesses, setons, antibiotics, and selective fistulotomy).

PREPARATION FOR SURGERY

Counseling

There is no substitute for a frank discussion by the physician about the natural history of Crohn's disease, the specific clinicoanatomical type in the individual patient, the alternatives (medical and surgical), and the risks, benefits, sequelae and possible complications of treatment. Volunteers from lay organizations such as the Crohn's and Colitis Foundation of America, carefully selected former patients, and the enterostomal therapy nurse are particularly useful.

Stoma Site Marking

Patients with proctocolitis, severe anorectal disease, or incontinent sphincters will frequently need a permanent ileostomy. In others, the stoma may be temporary (eg, certain cases of toxic colitis, malnutrition, or as an adjunct to distal bowel resection with anastomosis). Critical to rehabilitation of the patient is accurate preoperative siting of the stoma. The "rules" for this ideal care include:

1. Marking out the site with the patient in the sitting and supine position
2. Site is visible to the patient while sitting
3. Site is away from bony prominences, skin creases, scars or distended skin
4. Placement at the summit of the infraumbilical fat mound
5. Surface marking is within the boundaries of the rectus abdominis muscle

Restoration of Physiologic Defects

Many deficits can be remedied quickly, such as anemia, electrolyte imbalance, dehydration, and coagulation deficits, even in emergencies. Malnutrition is a complex issue, since contained colonic and protein losses may occur despite supplements. Hyperalimentation may improve certain nutritional parameters, but there is very little data indicating that outcome is improved or that complications of surgery are fewer.

Medication Withdrawal Including Steroids

Where feasible, immunosuppressive drugs are withdrawn for as long as possible before elective surgery. Aspirin compounds are stopped a week before surgery. Stress-dose steroids in the form of intravenous hydrocortisone are given preoperatively, intraoperatively, and postoperatively.

Mechanical Preparation

For elective cases, in the absence of obstruction, polyethylene glycol is used and is supplemented with rectal irrigation in the operating room until clear effluent is seen. For toxic cases, no preparation other than withholding of solid foods is used.

Antibiotics

Cephalosporin combined with metronidazole are given preoperatively and continued postoperatively for 24 hours. If intraoperative sepsis is found or contamination occurs, a 5-day course is given.

STRATEGIES AND TACTICS IN SURGERY OF CROHN'S DISEASE OF THE LARGE BOWEL

In general, the following principles or guidelines will be operative.

1. Make the operation as safe as possible with preoperative planning and preparation.
2. Mark out ostomy sites preoperatively.
3. Use midline incisions.
4. Do not make anastomoses in strictured or grossly ulcerated bowel.
5. Do not resect bowel *just* because Crohn's disease is identified.
6. Do not leave bowel segments out-of-circuit, unless adequate long-term surveillance is possible and likely to occur.
7. Drain/treat septic foci before resective surgery is done.
8. Favor resection of bowel to bypass.

The specific procedures for Crohn's disease at specific sites in the large bowel are summarized in Tables 41–2 and 41–3.

OPERATIVE PROCEDURES FOR SITE SPECIFIC DISEASE

Ileocecal Crohn's Disease

This disease is commonly associated with bowel obstruction, perforation and abscess or fistula formation (Fig 41–11). Resection of ileum and cecum, as opposed to right colon, with anastomosis is the preferred treatment. Quarantine of septic areas by omental interposition is advisable. Similar interposition of omentum is recommended if right colectomy and ileotransverse colon anastomosis is required for extensive right colonic disease (Fig 41–12). Thus, if recurrence of Crohn's disease occurs, there is less likelihood of penetration into the duodenum. With right and transverse colonic disease, subtotal colectomy and ileosigmoid anastomosis is performed (Fig 41–13).

Colonic Crohn's Disease

Operative selection depends upon the age of the patient, comorbidity, rectal sparing and compliance, extent of disease and severity, previous small bowel resection, adequacy of the anal sphincters presence, extent of concomitant small bowel disease, and presence and type of perineal disease. The procedures used are discussed below.

Subtotal Colectomy and Ileostomy

For acutely ill patients, where colitis may be complicated by associated features such as hemorrhage, contained or full perforation, or where comorbid conditions such as serious medical illness or malnutrition are present, the preferred treatment is subtotal colectomy and ileos-

TABLE 41–2. ELECTIVE SURGERY FOR CROHN'S DISEASE OF THE LARGE BOWEL

Site	Indication or comment	Procedure
Appendix	(a) Acute ileitis, no Crohn's disease (included in elective resection for convenience)	(a) Appendectomy, biopsy adjacent lymph node
	(b) Ileocecal resection, anastomosis, usually ileal or cecal disease as well	b) Appendiceal Crohn's disease, rare
Ileocecal	Common situation	Ileocecal resection, anastomosis
Right colon	After resection, anastomosis overlies duodenum; risk of complex fistula, if anastomotic recurrence	Right colectomy, ileo distal–transverse anastomosis, and wrap anastomosis with omentum
Right and transverse colon	Ileo-descending anastomosis makes for difficulty in closing mesenteric defect	Extended colectomy and ileo-sigmoid anastomosis
Segmental (transverse descending or sigmoid)	(a) High recurrence rates but allows maximal preservation of colonic absorptive surface. Older patients, previous significant (>30 cm) small bowel resection.	(a) Segmental resection, colo-colic anastomosis, and cecorectal anastomosis (if transverse *and* left colon disease)
	(b) Younger (<50 yrs) patients. Minimal or no previous SB resection	b) Resect disease segment *plus* proximal colon and ileosigmoid or ileorectal anastomosis
Rectum with colonic sparing	(a) Young patient, minimal or no ileal disease; no previous SB resection	(a) Proctocolectomy and ileostomy
	(b) Older patient, previous significant SB resection	(b) Proctosigmoidectomy and colostomy
Total colon disease	Rectum normal or minimal inflammation; good rectal compliance; adequate anal sphincters; absence of active perianal sepsis	Total colectomy, ileorectal anastomosis (IRA)
	PLUS disease in upper third of rectum; anastomosis possible, but function may be impaired without enhancing compliance. Higher risk (vs. colectomy/ ileostomy) of recurrence	Total colectomy, partial proctectomy, ileo low–rectal anastomosis, ±small (10-cm limbs) J-pouch
	Rectum spared; active perianal or rectovaginal fistula. (a) Fistula repair possible.	(a) Total colectomy, IRA, repair fistula, and temporary loop ileostomy.
	(b) Fistula repair *not* possible or desirable.	(b) Proctocolectomy and ileostomy (TPC).
	PLUS rectal disease plus or minus perianal sepsis/fistula. (a) Able to tolerate major operation.	(a) Proctocolectomy and ileostomy.
	(b) Ability to tolerate TPC is questionable.	(b) Subtotal colectomy and ileostomy.

From Fazio VW, Strong SA. Surgical management of Crohn's disease. In: Kirsner (ed), Inflammatory Bowel Disease, *4th ed. Baltimore, MD: Williams & Wilkins; 1995.*

TABLE 41–3. NON-ELECTIVE SURGERY FOR CROHN'S DISEASE OF THE LARGE BOWEL

Site	Indication or comment	Procedure
Ileocecal	With mesenteric or retroperitoneal abscess, drain preoperatively if possible; elective resection after 2 to 4 weeks	Ileocecal resection and anastomosis ± further drainage; quarantine anastomosis with omentum
	(a) If preoperative drainage *not* possible, consider temporary stoma after resection	(a) ± temporary stoma
	(b) If free perforation or peritonitis	(b) Resection, no anastomosis, and temporary ileostomy
Right or segmental colitis	Toxic, severely malnourished patient with colonic perforation and peritonitis	Resect disease, exclude distal segment, proximal diversion (usually ileostomy)
Rectal	Perforation or abscess with systemic signs of sepsis	Drain abscess, colostomy; latera proctectomy or TPC
Total colonic disease	(a) Malnourished, septic, toxic megacolon (perforation due to disease)	(a) Subtotal colectomy, ileostomy, and close rectosigmoid stump or mucus fistula
	(b) Toxic megacolon and contained perforation; colectomy very hazardous due to high splenic flexure, pregnancy, general condition of patient	(b) Staged operation; blow-hole colostomy and ileostomy; elective colectomy or TPC at 6 months
	(c) Colonic hemorrhage	(c) Same as (a); if rectum source of bleeding, TPC
	(d) Colonoscopic perforation in patient with quiescent colitis	(d) Exteriorize perforation of oversew/resect perforation and ileostomy

From Fazio VW, Strong SA. Surgical management of Crohn's disease. In: Kirsner JB (ed), Inflammatory Bowel Disease, *4th ed. Baltimore, MD: Williams & Wilkins; 1995*

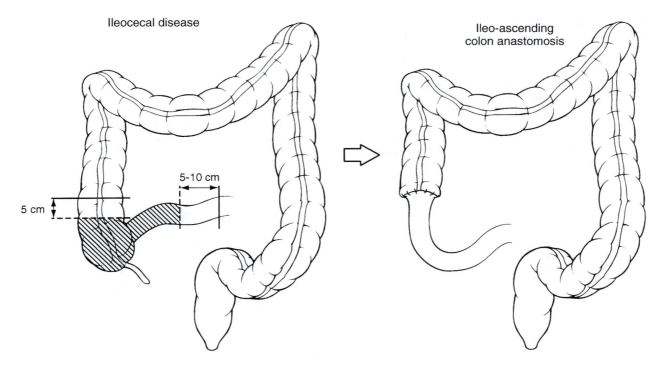

Figure 41–11. Ileocecal resection and ileoascending colon anastomosis for ileocecal Crohn's disease.

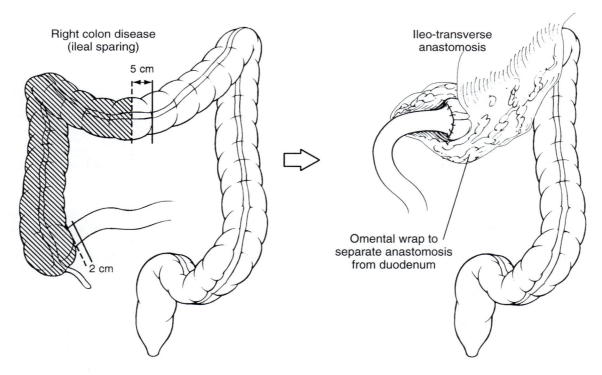

Figure 41–12. Right colectomy and ileotransverse anastomosis for right-sided Crohn's disease.

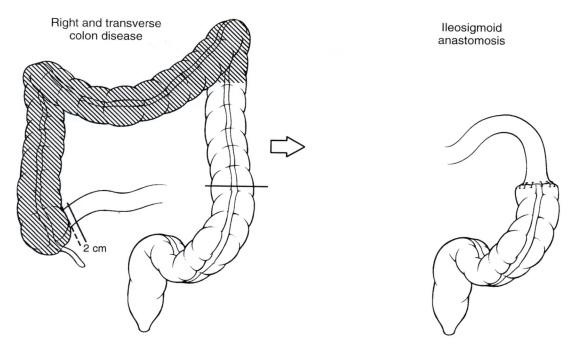

Right and transverse
colon disease

Ileosigmoid
anastomosis

2 cm

Figure 41–13. Extensive Crohn's colitis with sigmoid and rectal sparing. Extended right colectomy and ileosigmoid anastomosis.

tomy (STC) (Fig 41–14). If the rectal stump is spared of disease and is distensible, then later ileorectal anastomosis usually is performed after an interval of 6 months or longer. In performing the operation, there is no need for high-vascular ligations. The ileocolic vessels are usually preserved. Opinions vary whether to preserve omentum; it is our practice to do so. The ileostomy aperture is made through the rectus fascia using a muscle-splitting technique. A 3.5-cm aperture is used and the stoma primarily is matured to the skin with 3-0 chromic catgut sutures. It is important to make the stoma as perfectly as one can since this may very well prove to be the permanent stoma. Before eversion, the cut edge of ileum should exhibit active bleeding. The internal mesenteric defect is closed by suturing the mesentery to the anterior abdominal wall, about 2 cm lateral to the wound edge.

The alternative techniques for management of the rectal stump were discussed in the section dealing with toxic colitis (Fig 41–15).

Ileorectal Anastomosis

Ileorectal anastomosis (IRA) (Fig 41–16) may be done in several settings. In patients with partial or total involvement of the colon, *but* with rectal sparing *and* without comorbid conditions, one-stage total colectomy and ileorectal anastomosis is done. Second, the procedure may be done as a restorative operation following abdominal colectomy and ileostomy. In this situation, ile-

orectal anastomosis is done *after* the comorbid conditions associated with the earlier procedure have abated. Third, there is a small group of patients in whom there are *some* concerns about the suitability of a one-stage colectomy and IRA: those patients who have been on a prolonged course of high-dose steroids, patients with moderate hypoalbuminemia (eg, 2.0 to 2.5 g/dL), or patients with other significant medical conditions, such as diabetes. Here the surgeon may judge that a loop ileostomy added to the STC and IRA is an appropriate precaution. This may represent a fine point of distinction regarding the virtues and drawbacks of a later "simple" ileostomy closure versus a more complete laparotomy, takedown of ileostomy, and IRA.

All anastomoses to the rectum are leak tested by air or betadine insufflation intraoperatively. If a circular stapler is used, the tissue rings are checked. If a temporary loop ileostomy is placed upstream of an anastomosis, Gastrografin enema testing is done to check on anastomotic integrity immediately prior to stoma closure.

In cases where there is extensive proximal colitis with relative sparing of the sigmoid colon as well as the rectum, one will preserve as much distal bowel as one can. In fact, it is very useful to have intraoperative colonoscopy performed when checking distal lines of resection for colonic Crohn's disease; otherwise, there is often great difficulty in selecting this margin accurately. The presence of aphthoid ulcers in a noninflamed sigmoid colon would not justify sigmoid resection.

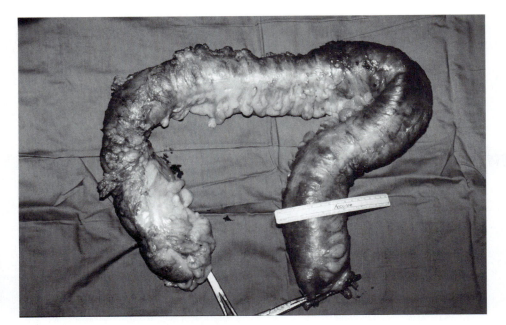

Figure 41–14. Subtotal colectomy specimen. Operation done for toxic megacolon. Final pathology report—ulcerative colitis. Completion proctectomy and ileal pouch-anal anastomosis was later performed successfully.

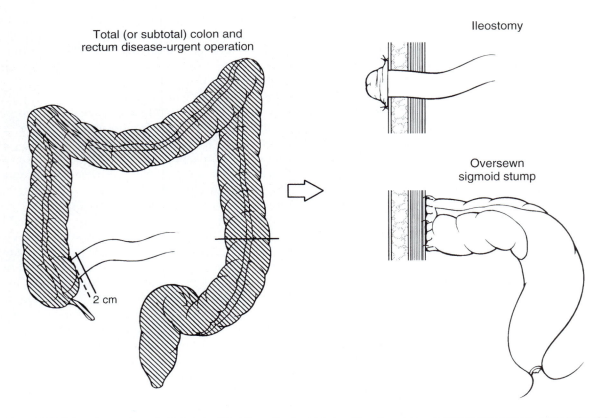

Figure 41–15. Schema for urgent operation in Crohn's colitis, with or without rectal disease. Where the rectal or rectosigmoid stump is fragile, exteriorization of the bowel end is done, otherwise, stapling or oversewing the stump is performed, with extraperitoneal positioning of the closed end.

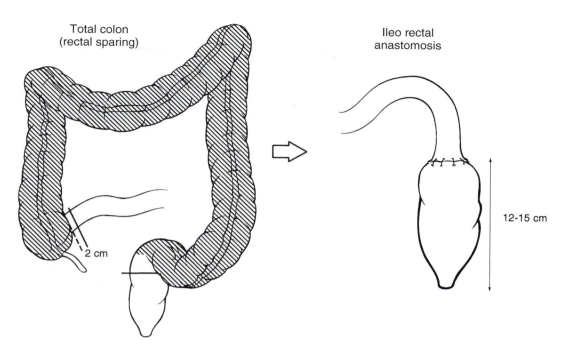

Figure 41–16. Total colectomy and ileorectal anastomosis.

The other side of this coin is in situations where the proximal half of the rectum is significantly involved with Crohn's disease. "Significant" means deep or linear ulcers or stricturing. Thus, the patient with just 7 to 8 cm of normal distal rectum (ie, ampulla) may be advised to have total proctocolectomy and ileostomy *or* to have an extended total colectomy with ileo low–rectal anastomosis. How does one choose? There is good data on this fine point, but a reasonable approach seems to be to offer restoration of continuity in the patient who is young, well-motivated (ie, strong, desires to avoid a stoma) and very well-informed about the recurrence risks.

Ileorectal anastomosis has a relatively poor reputation, associated with a high risk of recurrent disease and reoperation. We reviewed our experience with ileorectal anastomosis in 118 patients over a 26 year period.[29] At 10 years following surgery, 61% of patients had a functioning IRA. A successful outcome was independent of age or duration of symptoms. However, patients with synchronous small bowel disease fared worse than patients who were free of ileitis.

In selecting patients for IRA, there is evidence that the more pliable the rectum is, the better the outcome. Thus, a rigid, walled rectum that distends poorly on air insufflation probably acts like a conduit rather than a reservoir and augers poorly for future function. Experienced clinicians may judge this well enough on air insufflation. Objective testing, by infusing saline into the rectum and finding a maximum tolerated volume less than 150 mL, has been associated with a poor outcome.[30]

Segmental Resection of the Colon

Certain patterns of colitis, limited to a specific part of the colon, are encountered from time to time (Figs 41–17, 41–18). These patterns include right-sided colonic involvement, transverse and sigmoid colon involvement. A fourth variety is skip lesions affecting the cecum and transverse colon with normal intervening bowel. In patients exhibiting the first, second, and third varieties, a strong case for segmental resection and anastomosis can be made on the basis of preserving as much of the bowel as possible, thereby enhancing water and mineral resorption. The case against this practice is the very high rate of recurrence; reported to be as high as 100% in the earlier literature.[31,32] The trend of opinion has shifted from that of subtotal colectomy and IRA for sigmoid Crohn's disease (Fig 41–19) to that of sigmoid resection or left colectomy and anastomosis. While recurrence occurs in two-thirds of such patients at 5 to 15 years of follow-up, continuity is frequently preserved.

RECTAL CROHN'S DISEASE WITH AND WITHOUT COLONIC INVOLVEMENT

Total proctocolectomy and ileostomy

Total proctocolectomy and ileostomy (TPC) (Fig 41–20) is done as a primary procedure in several situations.

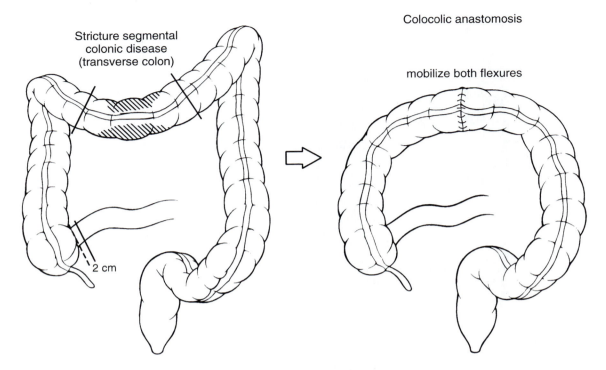

Figure 41–17. Resection of transverse colon and anastomosis for segmental Crohn's disease.

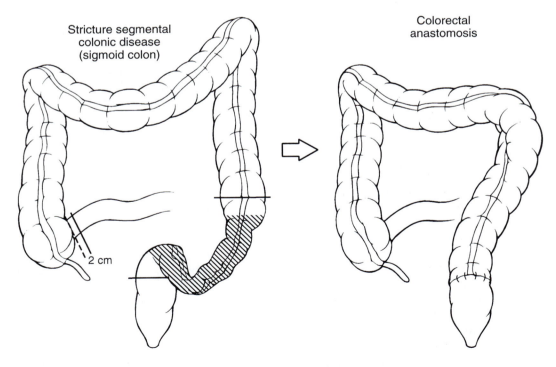

Figure 41–18. Segmental resection of the sigmoid colon for Crohn's disease.

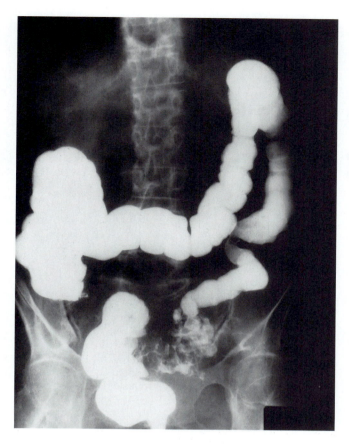

Figure 41–19. Crohn's disease of the sigmoid colon.

These situations include patients with significant disease affecting the rectum or distal bowel, including panproctocolitis. Additionally, TPC is used when restorative procedures are unwise, even with a normal-appearing rectum, because of significant fecal incontinence or complex perianal disease that is disabling despite treatment. The techniques of surgery are outlined in other chapters. The principles of TPC include

1. Presacral mobilization of the rectum in the plane between the investing layer of fascia of the rectum and Waldeyer's fascia.
2. Lateral mesorectal incisions are united anteriorly on the rectum, not the bladder or cul-de-sac.
3. Ligate superior rectal vessels below the sacral promontory to avoid sympathetic nerve injury (retrograde ejaculation).
4. For the lower one-third of the rectum, keep the dissection close to the rectal wall and avoid exposure of the seminal vesicles, to avoid induction of impotence.
5. Use an intersphincteric dissection with primary closure of the perineal wound.
6. Sump drainage of the presacral space.

7. Pack omentum into the pelvic cavity where possible.

In patients who have had a right colectomy or subtotal colectomy, completion proctocolectomy may be required because of recurrent disease in the distal bowel, development of stricture, dysplasia or cancer in the distal bowel, or inability to keep the distal bowel under surveillance.

Proctectomy or Proctosigmoidectomy

An unusual pattern of Crohn's disease occurs when the disease is confined to the distal rectum or rectum and sigmoid colon. No firm conclusions have been drawn regarding the procedure of choice in such circumstances, and opinion is divided between TPC and ileostomy versus proctosigmoidectomy and colostomy. The latter alternative would be favored strongly, however, should there be synchronous small bowel disease mandating resection or a history of previous small bowel resection.

ANAL AND PERIANAL CROHN'S DISEASE

Manifestations of Crohn's disease include skin tags, typified by an indurated pink mass of tissue called an "elephant-ear" tag; cyanotic discoloration of anal ulcers or fissures; perianal, rectovaginal, rectourethral fistula/abscesses; and anorectal stricture (Fig 41–21). These symptoms occur in 28% to 80% of cases depending on the inclusion criteria and length of follow-up.[33–35]

Intestinal symptoms and signs usually antedate the perianal lesions, but in 4% to 5% of cases, perianal lesions may be the sole manifestation of Crohn's disease. Usually, intestinal features of disease will appear within 5 years of onset of perianal disease. The colorectal pattern of Crohn's disease is the one most likely to be associated with perianal disease; the small bowel pattern is least likely to have that association. The diagnosis is established by inspection, endoscopy, and biopsy. Frequently, examinations under anesthesia are required for accurate assessment. Other imaging tests were discussed in the earlier part of the chapter. Similarly, medical therapy was discussed. The operative management of perianal Crohn's disease is discussed below.

Resection of Proximal Disease

Most patients with perianal disease have Crohn's disease in the proximal intestine. There is a certain logic to the hypothesis that control or removal of active proximal disease may encourage healing or improvement in the anorectal lesions. In a Scandinavian study of 43 pediatric patients, spontaneous healing of perianal fistulas occurred in 47% of patients who had undergone resection of diseased intestine.[36] Others have noted no significant similar improvement after resection.[37]

Our practice has been to treat medically active prox-

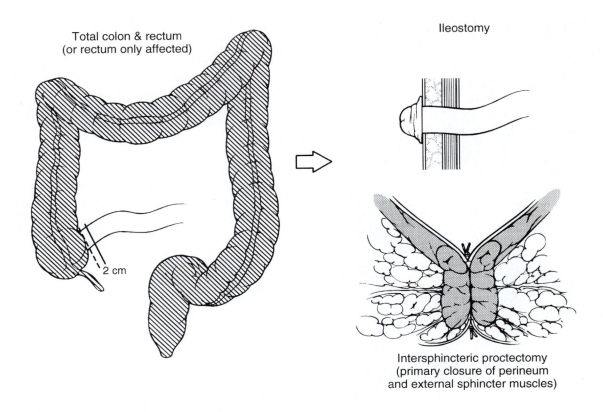

Total colon & rectum
(or rectum only affected)

Ileostomy

2 cm

Intersphincteric proctectomy
(primary closure of perineum
and external sphincter muscles)

Figure 41–20. Proctocolectomy and ileostomy for Crohn's disease of the large bowel involving the rectum.

imal Crohn's disease when treating anorectal disease. If sophisticated reconstruction procedures are used (eg, advancement flap repair), or the proximal disease merits surgery anyway, resection is carried out.

Skin Tag Excision; Hemorrhoidectomy

These procedures generally are avoided because of the risk of nonhealing of the wound. This is especially true when the lesions are painless. In a few very selected cases, a conservative excision of a painful tag is appropriate. In a St. Mark's Hospital report of 20 patients who had undergone hemorrhoidectomy and had Crohn's disease, six required late proctectomy.[38]

By contrast, it is not uncommon for patients with ulcerative colitis to have surgery for symptomatic hemorrhoids. In such cases, hemorrhoidectomy is appropriate, although this is done, in the case of restorative protocolectomy, *after* pelvic pouch surgery and at, or before, the time of ileostomy closure.

Operations for Fissure

Most fissures are painless and should be left alone. Painful fissures may respond to sitz baths, topical anti-inflammatory agents, bulking medication, or anal dilation. In selected patients, dilation under anesthesia, or

internal sphincterotomy may be required. For painful anal ulceration, intralesional steroids and immunosuppressives may be helpful (Fig 41–22).

Operations for Abscess/Fistula

Abscesses are treated by periodic incision and drainage, similar to the principles of management of abscesses secondary to cryptic glandular infection. Drainage catheters are removed after 2 to 3 weeks. If the fistula/abscess is chronically recurrent and a definitive operation is not feasible, then chronic drainage with mushroom-shaped catheters or noncutting setons is used.

Anal fistulas is Crohn's disease are one of the major therapeutic challenges in this disorder (Fig 41–23). For many patients, conservative management is appropriate, since the fistulas remain relatively quiescent or, if active and suppurate, do so at infrequent intervals. These fistulas earned a reputation, some would say a well-deserved reputation, for disastrous sequelae when subjected to the operations traditionally done for non-Crohn's disease patients, namely, fistulotomy and extensive unroofing of tracts. Thus, therapeutic nihilism held sway for several decades, treatment being confined to symptomatic measures or to long-term or intermittent drainage measures. Thus, patients would have a

continence is that of excising the external component of the fistula up to the external sphincter and excising the internal os and that portion of the internal sphincter underlying it. A seton is left around the remaining external sphincter component superficial to the fistula. Alternatives then include using a cutting action seton, or simply removing the seton after 6 months. Frequently, the fistula will heal without the need for external sphincter division.

Advancement Rectal Flap Repair of Fistula

The appeal of this procedure is that no sphincter division is required. Anorectal stenosis or fistula associated with a large adjacent cavity are contraindications. This approach may be used for transsphincteric, suprasphincteric, and even selected extrasphincteric fistulas. Success rates range from 50% to 75%. However, even if a failure occurs, there is no significant risk of worsening of the condition of the patient. Redo operation is feasible and, generally, this will be done with a covering diverting stoma. This same procedure is used for recto-

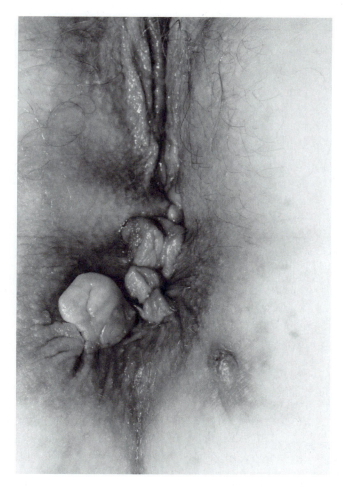

Figure 41–21. Indurated, large skin tags, typical of Crohn's disease of the perineum. A posterolateral fistulous tract is also present.

chronic fistula that was rendered less painful by the tract being maintained in an open state with a loosely placed seton, preventing redevelopment of an abscess. In practical terms, these conservative measures still hold, especially for the patient whose rectum is overtly involved with Crohn's disease. But for the apparently (endoscopically) normal rectum, fistulas may be approached in a definitive way, depending upon the complexity or height of the fistula.

Fistulotomy

Fistulotomy is appropriate for low or intersphincteric fistulas and for certain low transsphincteric fistulas, especially where there are no other risk factors for incontinence (eg, multiparity or anterior location of fistula).

Staged Fistulotomy

Staged fistulotomy can be done in several ways. A common method used for transsphincteric fistulas where one-stage fistulotomy will likely produce significant in-

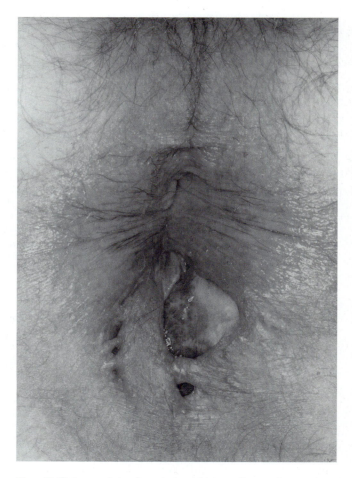

Figure 41–22. Large anal ulcer. Several external fistulous orifices are also present.

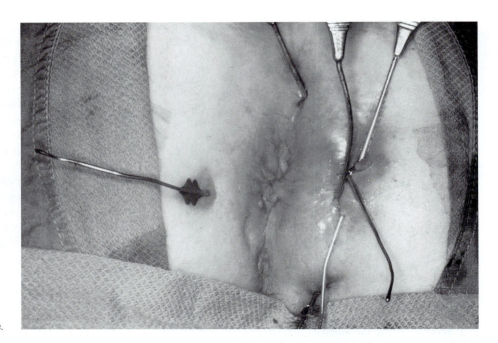

Figure 41–23. Multiple fistulas in Crohn's disease.

vaginal and rectourethral fistulae in Crohn's disease, provided the rectum is endoscopically normal.

■ SURGERY OF ULCERATIVE COLITIS

The evolution of surgery of ulcerative colitis has been one characterized by the quest for restoring fecal continence after removal of the diseased colon and rectum. Unlike Crohn's disease, ulcerative colitis is cured by proctocolectomy. In the 1950s and 1960s, the challenges for patients and physicians, when considering surgery for ulcerative colitis, were those of providing a form of severity for themselves or their patients with the incontinent ostomy. Panproctocolectomy was then the only realistic alternative. Ileostomy problems were commonplace as the result of many reasons. The principles of accurate preoperative siting of the ostomy were largely unknown except in specialized centers. The "rules" of fashioning of the ileostomy were in a similar state. Pouching materials, especially skin barriers, were in the infancy stages of development.

It was not until 1951 that Brooke in the United Kingdom, and Crile and Turnbull in the United States, independently solved the problem of ileostomy dysfunction when, for the first time, an ileostomy was matured to the skin with primary mucocutaneous suturing. The advent of Karaya washers and Stomahesive skin barriers coincided with the development of enterostomal therapy, a term coined by Rupert B Turnbull Jr, in the United States. These seminal events firmly established proctocolectomy as the "gold standard" or operations for ulcerative colitis, since now there was a curative operation for which reasonable and reliable rehabilitation was possible. Notwithstanding this, there were some patients and surgeons alike who, by disposition or bad experience, regarded an ileostomy as an affront that was difficult to bear. Aylett in the United Kingdom pioneered the first real alternative to an incontinent stoma by means of his operation, the abdominal colectomy and ileorectal anastomosis. This procedure and its main protagonist, Stanley Aylett, were roundly disparaged by traditionalists since leaving behind a diseased rectal segment seemed to fly in the face of basic good sense, with predictable problems of continued rectal inflammation and persistent symptoms. It was a further decade or two before collective reports from Europe, the United States and Australia gave support to Aylett's thesis. This thesis, simply put, was that although a diseased rectum was left behind and, indeed, produced significant and sometimes disabling symptoms in many, these symptoms went into abeyance after 6 months. The concerns about anastomotic leaks, continued proctitis and cancer development in the rectum were valid, although much debated as to incidence.

No sooner had "respectability" of sorts been given to ileorectal anastomosis, however, when the next restorative procedure emerged in the late 1970s, the ileal pelvic pouch operation. This operation has, in essence, rendered obsolete Aylett's procedure.

Before the development of the pelvic pouch, however, another unique contribution was made to the surgeons armamentarium in the late 1960s and early 1970s: Nils Kock's continent ileostomy. This procedure achieved for patients much of the desiderata of the perfect operation for ulcerative colitis, namely, total cure of ulcerative colitis, freedom from use of medication, one-stage procedure, minimal follow-up requirements, freedom of cancer risk, and no need for ileostomy pouching equipment. The drawbacks included a very complex operation, high reoperation rate, need for tubes for pouch drainage, and vulnerability of the pouch to become inflamed. As discussed in succeeding pages, the role of the Kock pouch has been much reduced since restorative proctocolectomy (RP) was introduced, but there is still a place for continent ileostomy.

The modern "gold standard" operation, for most clinicians, is that of the pelvic ileal pouch procedure, commonly referred to as the "pull-through", ileoanal "pull-through", or restorative proctocolectomy (RP).

INDICATIONS FOR SURGERY OF ULCERATIVE COLITIS

These indications (Table 41–4) follow closely the indications for surgery of Crohn's disease of the colon and, in broad terms, can be defined as urgent or elective. The specifics of these indications and preparation for surgery are almost identical for both conditions. However, colonic cancer and dysplasia occur far more commonly in ulcerative colitis than in Crohn's disease and merit further discussion.

Colorectal Cancer and Dysplasia in Ulcerative Colitis

There is no consensus regarding the relative risk of cancer development in ulcerative colitis. Community-based studies have reported values as low as 0.07% annual risk and a cumulative risk of 1.4% after 18 years of disease.[39] Others, in reviewing hospital-based populations, noted that 10% had developed cancer of the colon with a cumulative incidence of 60% after 40 years of disease.[40] It is probable that studies on hospital-based patients overestimate relative risk of colonic carcinoma in ulcerative colitis. One study that seems to give a more accurate assessment of risk is that of a community-based study from three defined geographic areas (West Midlands, Oxford

and Stockholm County).[41] This study showed an eight-fold increased risk overall and nineteen-fold risk if pancolitis was present. The cumulative risk of cancer in patients with extensive colitis was 7.2% and 16.5% after 20 and 30 years of disease, respectively. Ekbom and colleagues, in a population-based cohort study, found a 30% absolute risk of colorectal cancer in patients after 35 years of total colitis that increased to 40% for those diagnosed at under 15 years of age.[42] Particular risk factors for development of colorectal cancer include extensive nature of the colitis; early age of onset (in teens); and duration of colitis. Activity of the colitis is not a risk factor. Colorectal cancer is frequently multifocal (26% in our own series). Prior to colonic endoscopic and histologic surveillance in ulcerative colitis, decisions for prophylactic proctocolectomy were based upon the presence of risk factors mentioned above. In addition, the occurrence of colonic strictures in a patient with ulcerative colitis, while usually benign, constituted an indication for surgery, even if biopsy of the stricture proved benign.

Dysplasia

There is considerable controversy about several aspects of colonic dysplasia. First, there is a certain amount of subjective interpretation of specific cases of dysplasia. Recognizing all these problems, however, the clinician will generally place credence on a report of a particular specimen showing high-grade dysplasia. If that sample is reviewed and the diagnosis confirmed, the clinician will strongly recommend panproctocolectomy. This is especially true if the dysplasia is associated with a mass or ulcerated lesion. With low-grade dysplasia, the recommendation for surgery is probably not as strongly made but, nonetheless, *is* made. Some authorities recommend a *repeat* confirmation biopsy if the dysplasia is low grade before surgery is recommended. In current times, the major disadvantage of proctocolectomy, namely a permanent ileostomy, rarely is applicable with the emergence of RP. Second, one should keep in mind that the absence of dysplasia does not equate with the absence of coexisting cancer. In one study of 80 colorectal specimens with colitis-related adenocarcinoma, nearly 20% had no associated dysplasia.[43]

STRATEGIES AND TACTICS IN THE SURGERY OF ULCERATIVE COLITIS

The general principles are the same as for Crohn's disease: make the operation as safe as possible for the patient with preoperative preparation; use midline incisions and mark out ostomy sites preoperatively.

The specific strategies or principles of surgery of ulcerative colitis include

1. Remove all colorectal epithelium. An exception to this is made in certain cases, such as ileorec-

---

TABLE 41–4. INDICATIONS FOR SURGERY IN ULCERATIVE COLITIS

Inadequate response to medical therapy
Extraintestinal manifestations
Malnutrition, growth retardation
Stricture
Dysplasia
Colorectal cancer
Hemorrhage
Toxic colitis and megacolon (±perforation of colon).

tal anastomosis and RP done with double stapling technique (discussed below).

2. If large bowel epithelium is left after a curative operation (ie, no metastatic cancer), then the residual large bowel is kept under routine endoscopic/histologic surveillance.

3. If dysplasia or colonic cancer is present, wide mesenteric excision with high lymphovascular pedicle ligation is done.

4. Prevent genitourinary complications by dissecting close to the rectum in its distal one-third.

5. With proctocolectomy and end ileostomy, use primary closure of the perineal wound.

OPERATIVE PROCEDURES FOR ULCERATIVE COLITIS

Tables 41–5 and 41–6 summarize the indications, contraindications, advantages, and disadvantages of spe-cific operations done for emergency or elective situations in ulcerative colitis. Several of these are discussed in detail in later chapters.

Proctocolectomy and Ileostomy

This procedure still is regarded by some as the standard operation for ulcerative colitis. If the patient is indifferent to having an ostomy or has a prohibitive concern about the outcome of more complex procedures, such as the Kock pouch or pelvic reservoir, then total proctocolectomy and Brooke ileostomy is the procedure of choice. Most patients adapt well to an ileostomy. In large series of pelvic pouch procedures where a temporary ileostomy is used, a number of patients choose *not* to have ileostomy reversal despite eligibility to do so. They have become so impressed by their improved quality of life with the proctocolectomy operation, and so tolerant of an ileostomy, that they would prefer not to

TABLE 41–5. ELECTIVE OPERATIVE PROCEDURES FOR ULCERATIVE COLITIS

Procedures	Indications	Contraindications	Advantages	Disadvantages
TPC with *mucosectomy* and hand-sewn IPAA and temporary loop ileostomy.[a]	Most cases? Dysplasia Colonic cancer Excellent sphincters	Low rectal CA Obesity Poor sphincters	Restorative Eliminates cancer risk and need for surveillance	Difficult operation Two-stages Anastomotic tension Septic complications may be high. Nocturnal incontinence Pouchitis 20% to 30% Use of perineal pads
TPC with stapled IPAA and temporary loop of ileostomy.*	Most cases? Can be used in obese pts Can be used if low/normal sphincter pressure	Low rectal CA Synchronous colon CA High-grade dysplasia	Compared with mucosectomy Faster Less anastomotic tension Fewer septic problems Better anal function	Two-stages Leaves 0.5 to 2.0 cm Distal mucosa with dysplasia/cancer risk and risk of inflammation. Pouchitis 20% to 30%
TPC and ileostomy.	Older pt Poor sphincter Rectal CA Pt. preference	Toxic megacolon Toxic colitis Major comorbid disease (then do STC + ileostomy)	One-stage Cures disease No further drugs OK if Crohn's disease is possibility Least complex	10% reop. rate on ileostomy 10% pt with perineal sinus 10% SBO Permanent ileostomy Strictureplasty 1% to 5%
STC + IRA	Indeterminate colitis with relative rectal sparing Colonic cancer with metastasis	Poor rectal compliance ie, rigid, poor insufflation Poor sphincter Synchronous cancer or *dysplasia* of colon Perianal disease Severe rectal inflammation	May be one-stage Stoma avoidance No risk of sex dysfunction	Anastomotic leak 2% to 3% 25% conversion to ileostomy 5% risk of CA of rectal stump Need for surveillance
TPC + Kock pouch	Pt anxious to avoid external bag Poor sphincters	Obesity Multiple abdominal operations Short bowel or high output stoma	Avoid ileostomy equipment Sense of body image improved	Complex operation Valve complication 5% to 25% Pouchitis risk

[a]TPC + IPAA with ileostomy avoidance may be done when patient is nontoxic; no serious comorbid conditions; steroid dose less than 15 mg/day; no anastomotic tension; no blood loss or transfusion. Operation is particularly smooth and effortless. SBO = small bowel obstruction; Pt = patient

TABLE 41–6. URGENT PROCEDURES FOR ULCERATIVE COLITIS

Procedure	Indications	Contraindications	Advantages	Disadvantages
Subtotal colectomy and ileostomy	Toxic colitis Toxic megacolon Colonic hemorrhage Colonic perforation	Confined ie, sealed *colonic* perforation Very high splenic flexure; fragile colon Rectal hemorrhage ? Pregnancy	Relatively safe Preserves options regarding rectum Allows for better definitive histological diag (than nonresective surgery) Pt can get off steroids and lose weight	Two-stages May develop rectal bleeding Mucous fistula may be needed (ie, two ostomy bags)
Blow-hole colostomy and ileostomy	High-risk pt with toxic megacolon eg, pregnancy, high flexure, contained perforation	Colonic perforation Colonic hemorrhage	Quick Safe Rapid detoxification Reserves later surgery options	Two-stages Colonic hemorrhage
Proctocolectomy and ileostomy.	Colorectal hemorrhage (or completion proctectomy after STC and rectal bleeding points)	Most cases unless "indications" are present Some experienced surgeons will do for moderate toxicity in good risk patients Rectal perforation	One-stage	Eliminates later restorative operation Some risk of impotence Unhealed perineal wound, enterocutaneous fistula and pelvic sepsis

risk possible adverse sequelae of reversal. The operation may be done in one or two stages, after subtotal colectomy. In the latter event, the surgeon is well-advised to leave a long rectosigmoid stump that easily reaches the lower end of the wound. This then eliminates the risk of a complicated pelvic operation, as is likely when the stump has been amputated and oversewn at the level of peritoneal reflection. This leads often to great difficulty in finding the stump, risking ureteric injury and avoiding injury to the nervi erigentes. Bleeding is often excessive. The principles of pelvic dissection were outlined earlier. The operation is particularly appropriate for patients who have poor sphincter function, synchronous colorectal cancer, significant comorbid illness, >60 years of age, and obesity. The major complications of surgery are ileostomy problems, requiring reoperation in 10% to 15% of cases; perineal wound sinus, requiring reoperation in 10% to 15% of cases; sexual dysfunction, requiring reoperation in 1% to 4% of cases; dyspareunia; and small bowel obstruction, requiring reoperation in 5% to 20% of cases.

Colectomy and Ileorectal Anastomosis

Aylett popularized this procedure as the first realistic alternative to a permanent ileostomy for ulcerative colitis.[44] The operation has largely been replaced by restorative proctocolectomy using the ileal pelvic pouch. This has helped offset several of the concerns about ileorectal anastomosis in that the retained rectal mucosa is eliminated, thus negating the risk of inflammation (with its attendant urgency), severe diarrhea, and 25% rate of return to an ostomy. Additionally, the risk of cancer/dysplasia in the rectal segment, with the requisite need for regular surveillance endoscopy and biopsy is avoided. Nevertheless, there is still a role for IRA, in certain circumstances. The patient in whom a diagnostic dilemma exists (ulcerative colitis versus Crohn's disease) perhaps may be treated best by colectomy and IRA, when there is relative rectal sparing. Additionally, in the uncommon situation in which colonic cancer has metastasized in a patient with ulcerative colitis, colectomy and IRA, as a one-stage procedure, is indicated. Thus, the patient can be spared an ostomy and have a palliative one-stage procedure. Contraindications to elective curative surgery include synchronous colorectal cancer, poor sphincter tone, and a poorly distensible rectum, as measured by maximum-tolerated volume or as assessed on endoscopy. Should a patient with an established IRA for ulcerative colitis require proctectomy, a pelvic pouch procedure usually can be done.

For the established ileorectal anastomosis, function can be quite satisfactory. The authors reported our experience at the Cleveland Clinic with 92 patients who had an average of 4.3 bowel movements (range 1 to 10) per day.[45] Only five patients had nocturnal bowel movements. Antidiarrheal medications were used in 23%, sulfasalazine in 33% and steroids in 8% of patients. Rectal cancer occurred in 3.5% of the group.

The Continent Ileostomy

Kock pioneered this operation in 1969 as a method of fashioning a continence mechanism for patients who required an ileostomy. Two or three 12 to 15 cm loops of terminal ileum were united to construct a reservoir, and

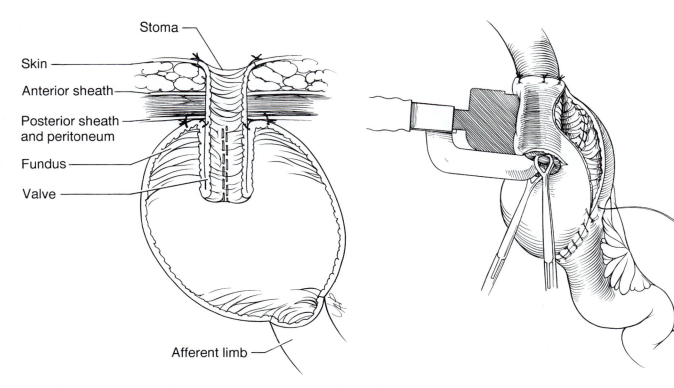

Figure 41–24. The continent ileostomy, or modified Kock pouch.

Figure 41–25. Technique designed to prevent nipple valve slippage—the most common serious complication of the continent ileostomy. The linear stapler is advanced through a pouchotomy, and the valve is *stapled* to the pouch wall. This procedure reduced our valve slippage rate to 3% (one of 34 patients).

the continence mechanism was supplied by adding a valve. This valve was fashioned by intussuscepting a 12-cm segment of the efferent loop of ileum into the pouch, thus creating a 5- to 6-cm valve (Fig 41–24).

The operation is complex, and the learning curve is long. Valve-related complications occur in 5% to 25% of patients, and it is surprising to see the enthusiasm patients have for reoperative surgery when complications occur. Few choose to revert to a conventional ileostomy. The main reason patients desire this operation is the enhanced sense of worth and body image that occurs when an external fecal collecting appliance is replaced by a small gauze pad and tape. Patients need to have a constant draining catheter attached to a leg bag for 3 to 4 weeks postoperatively before a regular catheterizing schedule is instituted. This is done 3 to 4 times a day. A major advance in avoidance of valve slippage has been the technique of stapling the valve to the pouch itself (Figs 41–25 and 41–26). Indications and contraindications to the procedure are listed in Table 41–5.

Proctocolectomy with Ileal Pouch–Anal Anastomosis

This procedure is reported in detail in a later chapter. Table 41–5 outlines, in summary form, the indications, contraindications, advantages and disadvantages of this procedure. The restorative proctocolectomy has

emerged as the new "gold standard" operation for ulcerative colitis, achieving as it does most of the desiderata for an excellent operation. Mortality rate is low, most series citing frequencies of <0.5%. In our experience (1983 to 1993), there were three deaths in 1005 pelvic pouch cases. Only one was attributed to a pouch-related complication. Pouch excision rates average 5%, most commonly the result of a late emergence of Crohn's disease features. In the Mayo Clinic series, the status of patients in the early, postileostomy closure period was evaluated.[46] Seventy-nine percent of patients were completely continent, 19% were mostly continent, with occasional daytime and nocturnal soilage, and 2% were incontinent. In later follow-up significant fecal incontinence, more than twice a week, occurred in 5% of patients during the day and in 12% during sleep.

The lessons learned with restorative proctocolectomy, over the past decade include the following:

1. Rectal muscle preservation is unnecessary to continence; thus, a lengthy mucosectomy is avoided by distal amputation of the rectum at the anorectal ring.
2. Thus, bleeding from the muscle sleeve is eliminated, as is the entity of cuff abscess.

3. Presacral space dissection can be done in the upper two-thirds of the pelvis, within the bloodless plane anterior to Waldeyer's fascia. Close dissection to the rectum is necessary only from the lower one-third of rectum.

4. An ileal-pouch reservoir is mandatory if early bowel function is to be optimal.

5. Selected patients may undergo safe IPAA without a protecting loop ileostomy. The criteria includes lack of anastomotic tension, lack of toxicity, an effortless operation without blood loss, and no or low-dose ($\leq$ 10 mg) prednisone. The vast majority of patients having RP will still have temporary ostomies.

6. Wait at least 3 months before closing temporary ileostomies. This reduces the risk of postoperative adhesive obstruction.

7. Shape of pouch (**J**, **S**, **W**) probably has little significance in terms of outcome or function.

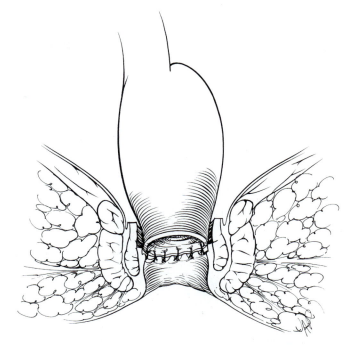

Figure 41–27. Ileal pouch–anal anastomosis; mucosectomy with hand-sewn anastomosis.

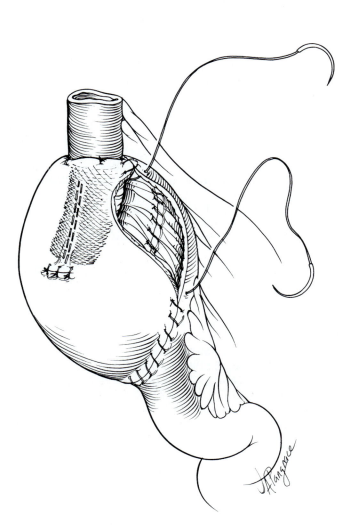

Figure 41–26. The pouch opening is closed.

The major technical controversy at present relates to the debate over mucosectomy and hand-sewn anastomosis (Fig 41–27) vs. the double- or tripled-stapled anastomosis of the pouch to the upper anal canal (Fig 41–28). Protagonists of mucosectomy point to the certainty of eliminating cancer or dysplasia prone epithelium. Surgeons favoring the stapling technique respond that, provided patients with synchronous cancer or dysplasia of the colon are excluded (ie, undergo mucosectomy), the incidence of dysplasia is low in the short-term and, unlike the "traditional" mucosectomy procedure, as yet no case of cancer in the anal canal has been reported. We have found three cases of dysplasia in about 300 patients undergoing stapled IPAA. All had transanal excision of the residual large bowel epithelium with pouch preservation.

On the other hand, the advocates of stapled IPAA point to their operation being speedier, safer and associated with better functional outcome (ie, less nocturnal seepage and less wearing of perineal pads). These points are all contested by those practicing mucosectomy and hand-sewn anastomosis. Table 41–5 lists some of the points favoring one operation over another. No resolution of the debate seems imminent.

The operation is appropriate therapy for carcinoma-associated ulcerative colitis, provided the lower one-third of the rectum is not involved by the malignancy. At the Cleveland Clinic, of 631 patients undergoing

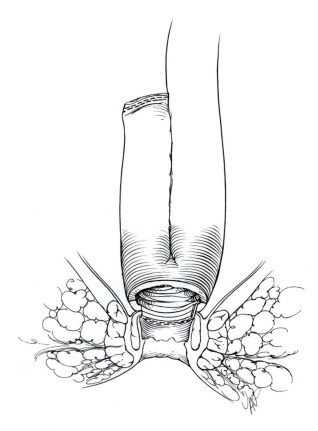

Figure 41–28. Ileal pouch–anal anastomosis double-stapled technique.

proctocolectomy and pelvic pouch surgery for ulcerative colitis from 1983 to 1992, 27 had invasive colorectal cancer. At a mean follow-up of 4.3 ± 2.6 years, cancer recurred in two patients. Pouch function was good to excellent in surviving patients.[47]

Pouchitis is the main late complication of pelvic pouch surgery for ulcerative colitis. The cause remains obscure and treatment is largely empiric using antibiotics effective against anaerobic bacteria. Refractory pouchitis may be treated by long-term antibiotics such as metronidazole but treatment failures will often require pouch excision.

REFERENCES

1. Myren J. Inflammatory bowel disease: a historical perspective. In: deDombal FT, Myren J, Boucier AD, et al (eds), *Inflammatory Bowel Disease,* 2nd ed. Oxford, England: Oxford Medical, University Press; 1993;17–41
2. Crohn BB, Ginzburg L, Oppenheimer GD. Regional ileitis: a pathological and clinical entity. *JAMA* 1932;99:1323–1329
3. Lockhart-Mummery HE, Morson BC. Crohn's disease (regional entities) of the large intestine and its distinction from ulcerative colitis. *Gut* 1960;1:87
4. Wells C. Ulcerative colitis and Crohn's disease. *Ann R Coll Surg Engl* 1952;11:105
5. Bargen JA, Weber HM. Regional migratory chronic ulcerative colitis. *Surg Gynec Obstet* 1930;50:964–972
6. Slater G, Ausfes AH. Granulomatous colitis and ulcerative colitis. In: Schwartz SI, Ellis H (eds), *Maingot's Abdominal Operations,* 9th ed. Stamford, CT: Appleton & Lange; 1989:1023–1032
7. Price AB. Overlap in the spectrum of nonspecific inflammatory bowel disease "colitis indeterminate." *J Clinic Pathol* 1978;38:567–577
8. Lee KS, Medline A, Shockey S. Indeterminate colitis in the spectrum of inflammatory bowel disease. *Arch Pathol Lab Med* 1979;103:173–176
9. Tanaka M, Riddell RH. The pathological diagnosis and differential diagnosis of Crohn's disease. *Hepatogastroenterology* 1990;37:18–31
10. Summers RW, Switz DM, Sessions J, et al. National Cooperative Crohn's Disease Study results of drug treatment. *Gastroenterology* 1979;77:847–869
11. Blichfeldt P, Blomhoff JP, Myhre E, et al. Metronidazole in Crohn's disease. *Scand J Gastroenterol* 1978;13:123–127
12. Present DH, Korelitz BI, Wisch N, et al. Mercaptopurine: a long-term randomized double blind study. *N Engl J Med* 1982;302:981–987
13. Yamazaki Y, Ribeiro MB, Sachar DB, et al. Malignant strictures in Crohn's disease. *Am J Gastroenterol* 1991;86:881–885
14. Trnka YM, Glotzer DJ, Kasdon EJ, et al. The long-term outcome of restorative operation in Crohn's disease. Influence of location, prognostic factors, and surgical guidelines. *Ann Surg* 1982;196:345–355
15. Blomberg B, Roiny P, Jarnerot G. Endoscopic treatment of anastomotic strictures in Crohn's disease. *Endoscopy* 1991;23:195–198
16. Breysen Y, Janssens JF, Coremans G, et al. Endoscopic balloon dilation of colonic and ileocolonic Crohn's strictures: long-term results. *Gastrointest Endosc* 1992;38:142–147
17. Ekbom A, Helmick C, Zack M, et al. Increased risk of large bowel cancer in Crohn's disease with colonic involvement. *Lancet* 1990;336:357–359
18. Greenstein AJ, Sachar DB, Smith H, et al. Patterns of neoplasia of Crohn's disease and ulcerative colitis. *Cancer* 1980;46:403–407
19. Gyde SN, Prior P, McCartney JC, et al. Malignancy in Crohn's disease. *Gut* 1980;21:1024–1029
20. Weedon DD, Shorter RG, Ilstrup DM, et al. Crohn's disease and cancer. *N Engl J Med* 1975;289:1099–1103
21. Savoca PE, Ballantyne GH, Cahor CE. Gastrointestinal malignancies in Crohn's disease: a 20-year experience. *Dis Colon Rectum* 1990;33:7–11
22. Faintuch J, Levin B, Kirsner JB. Inflammatory bowel disease and their relationship to malignancy. *Crit Rev Oncol Hematol* 1985;2:323–353
23. Hawker PC, Gyde SN, Thompson H, et al. Adenocarcinoma of the small intestine complicating Crohn's disease. *Gut* 1982;23:188–193
24. Lavery IC, Jagelman DG. Cancer in the excluded rectum

following surgery for inflammatory bowel disease. *Dis Colon Rectum* 1982;25:522–524

25. Lichtiger S, Present DH. Cyclosporin A in the treatment of severe ulcerative colitis. *Gastroenterology* 1992;102:A653

26. Present D, Wolfson D, Gelernt I, et al. The medical management of toxic megacolon: technique of decompression with favorable long-term follow-up. *Gastroenterology* 1981;80:A1255

27. Goligher JC, Hoffman DC, de Dombal FT. Surgical treatment of seven attacks of ulcerative colitis with special reference to the advantage of early operation. *Br Med J* 1970;4:703–706

28. Fazio VW. Toxic megacolon in ulcerative colitis and Crohn's colitis. *Clin Gastroenterol* 1980;9:389–407

29. Longo E, Oakley JR, Lavery IC, et al. Outcome of ileorectal anastomosis for Crohn's colitis. *Dis Colon Rectum* 1992; 35:1066–1071

30. Keighley MRB, Buchmann P, Lee JR. Assessment of anorectal function in selection of patients for ileorectal anastomosis in Crohn's colitis. *Gut* 1982;23:102–107

31. Longo WE, Ballantyne GH, Cahon E. Treatment of Crohn's colitis: segmental or total colectomy. *Arch Surg* 1988;123:588–590

32. Allan A, Andrews MR, Hilton CJ, et al. Segmental colonic resection is an appropriate operation for short skip lesions due to Crohn's disease in the colon. *World J Surg* 1989;13:611–616

33. Fielding JF. Perianal lesions in Crohn's disease. *J R Coll Surg Edinb* 1972;17:32–33

34. Rankin GB, Watts HP, Melnyk CS, et al. National Cooperative Crohn's Disease Study: extraintestinal manifestations and perianal complications. *Gastroenterology* 1979;77: 914–920

35. Keighley MRB, Allan RN. Current status and influence of operation on perianal Crohn's disease. *Int J Colorectal Dis* 1986;1:104–107

36. Hellers G, Bergstrand O, Ewerth S, et al. Occurrence and outcome after primary treatment of anal fistula in Crohn's disease. *Gut* 1980;21:525–527

37. Buckman P, Keighley MRB, Allan RN, et al. Natural history of perianal Crohn's disease: ten-year follow-up: a plea for conservatism. *Am J Surg* 1980;140:642–644

38. Jeffery PJ, Ritchie JK, Parks AG. Treatment of hemorrhoids in patients with inflammatory bowel disease. *Lancet* 1977;i:1084–1085

39. Hendrickson C, Kreiner S, Binder V. Long-term prognosis in ulcerative colitis—based on results from a regional patient group from the County of Copenhagen. *Gut* 1985; 26:158–163

40. Sachar DB, Smith H, et al. Cancer in universal and left-sided ulcerative colitis: factors determining risk. *Gastroenterology* 1979;77:290–294

41. Gyde SN, Prior P, Allan RN, et al. Colorectal cancer in ulcerative colitis: a cohort study of primary referral from three areas. *Gut* 1988;29:206–217

42. Ekbom R, Helmick A, Zack C, et al. Ulcerative colitis and colorectal cancer. a population-based study. *N Engl J Med* 1990;323:1228–1233

43. Riddell RH. The precarcinomatous phase of ulcerative colitis. *Current Top Pathol* 1976;63:179–219

44. Aylett SO. Diffuse chronic ulcerative colitis and its treatment by ileorectal anastomosis. *Ann R Coll Surg Engl* 1960;27:260

45. Oakley JR, Jagelman DG, Fazio VW, et al. Complications and quality of life after ileorectal anastomosis for ulcerative colitis. *Am J Surg* 1985;149:23–30

46. Grotz R, Pemberton JH. The ileal pouch operation for ulcerative colitis. *Surg Clin North Am* 1993;5:909–932

47. Ziv Y, Fazio VW, Strong SA, et al. Ulcerative colitis and co-existing colorectal cancer: recurrence rate after restorative proctocolectomy, *Ann Surg Oncol* 1994;1: 512–515

42

Tumors of the Colon

Helena R. Chang ▪ *Kirby I. Bland*

The physiologic functions, water absorption, and stool storage of the colon are simplistic. However, this organ can be involved in a variety of disease processes. Tumors of the colon are important because they are frequent and associated with significant mortality. The most common benign tumors of the colon are polyps. Approximately 14 million Americans have colonic polyps. Some have no malignant potential and others are premalignant. The former group consists of non-neoplastic polyps, such as hamartomas and inflammatory and hyperplastic polyps. The latter group consists of neoplastic polyps, such as tubular, tubulovillous, villous adenomas, and hereditary adenomatous polyposis. Malignant tumors are the most serious of colon pathologies. Adenocarcinoma is the most common malignancy, while lymphoma, sarcoma, and carcinoid are all rare.

▪ BENIGN COLONIC POLYPS

Polyp is a morphologic description of tissue growth protruding beyond the luminal surface of the gastrointestinal tract. There are two general types of benign polyps: non-neoplastic and neoplastic polyps. The former group consists of hamartomas, hyperplastic and inflammatory polyps. The latter group includes various adenomatous polyps and hereditary polyposis coli.

BENIGN NON-NEOPLASTIC POLYPS

Hamartomas

Hamartomas are characterized by the overgrowth of normal components of colon, such as epithelium and connective tissue. Hamartomas do not have malignant potential and lack atypia or invasion. Juvenile polyps, and the Cronkhite-Canada and Peutz-Jeghers syndromes all are characterized as hamartomas.

Juvenile Polyps. Isolated juvenile polyps occur during childhood and only occasionally in adults. Clinical symptoms include bleeding, prolapse, and abdominal pain secondary to autoamputation of the polyps or intussusception. The polyps have a bright-red color with a smooth and round contour, or a stalk-like shape following autoamputation. Multiple polyps should be removed for pathologic examination to establish the diagnosis. Microscopically, the polyp has a smooth contour with cystic dilation of the glands and edematous lamina propria.

Generalized juvenile polyposis, on the other hand, may occur at any age. This condition is transmitted as an autosomal dominant trait. These polyps have both juvenile and adenomatous components. The symptoms may be more serious, including anemia, finger clubbing, and failure to thrive. Other family members may have cancer of the stomach, duodenum, or pancreas. The treatment should be aggressive colonoscopic polypectomy or abdominal colectomy.[1] Familial screening should be considered.

Cronkhite-Canada Syndrome. Cronkhite-Canada syndrome is characterized by generalized gastrointestinal polyposis, cutaneous hyperpigmentation, alopecia, and nail dystrophy.[2,3] This disorder is not linked genetically. The mean age of onset is 60 years. Frequent sites for polyps are the stomach and colon. The small intestine and esophagus rarely are involved. Microscopically, the widespread mucosal changes are characterized by an intact epithelial surface containing tortuous glands with cystic dilation, in some cases, and a chronically inflamed lamina propria. Remission may occur spontaneously, or after either medical treatment or partial gastrectomy. Major symptoms include abdominal pain, diarrhea, bleeding, and anorexia with consequential weight loss, malabsorption, and anemia. Management includes polypectomy for diagnosis and supportive treatment.

Peutz-Jeghers Syndrome. The Peutz-Jeghers syndrome consists of generalized gastrointestinal polyposis and mucocutaneous melanin spots. Peutz-Jeghers appears to be transmitted via a dominant gene with a high degree of penetration.[4,5] The entire gastrointestinal tract may be involved, but the small intestine is the most frequently involved. Macroscopically, these polyps resemble the lobulared surface of adenomas. Microscopically, an arborized muscularis mucosa is covered by mucosa containing mature glands, with intervening lamina propria. Onset is at an early age, ranging from 10 to 30 years.

Symptoms include vomiting, bleeding, and abdominal pain. Surgery is conservative and directed to relieving the symptoms secondary to the ulcerated polyps, obstruction, or intussusception. Many of these patients may eventually develop extracolonic malignancies.[6,7] Surveillance for gastrointestinal, pancreatic, breast, and ovarian cancers is appropriate.

Inflammatory Polyps

This type of polyp may be single or multiple. When multiple, inflammatory bowel disease usually is present. Microscopically, inflammatory polyps are characterized by the submucosal lymphoid infiltration and regenerative changes. Polyps should be removed for pathologic examination. Active ulcerative colitis should be treated, if present.

Hyperplastic Polyps

Hyperplastic polyps also are known as metaplastic polyps. This type may be the most common colonic polyp. Hyperplastic polyps themselves are non-neoplastic, but they appear frequently in patients with colon cancer.[8,9] The etiology is not clear, although a viral nature has been suggested. Endoscopically, these polyps appear to be slightly raised nodules with the color of normal mucosa. Although some gross features may suggest this diagnosis,[10] one cannot reliably distinguish hyperplastic from adenomatous lesions.[11] Therefore, polypectomy and pathologic confirmation are recommended. Routine colorectal cancer screening is adequate for following hyperplastic polyps.[12]

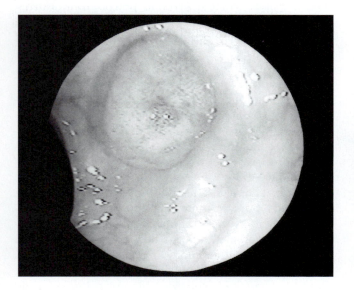

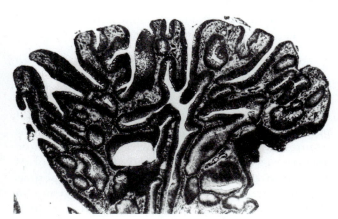

A

Figure 42–1. A. Tubular adenoma: Left: macroscopic, Right, microscopic (x44); *Continued*

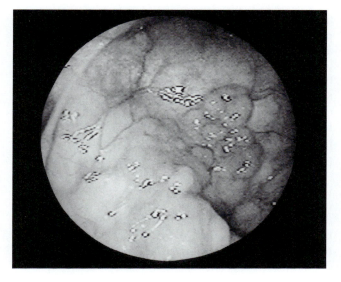

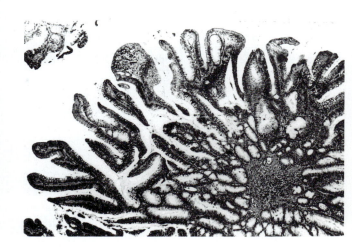

B

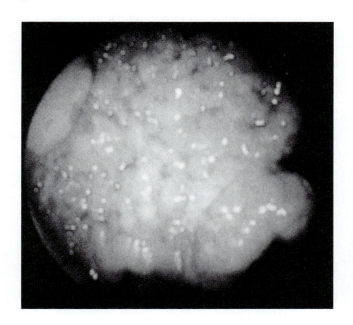

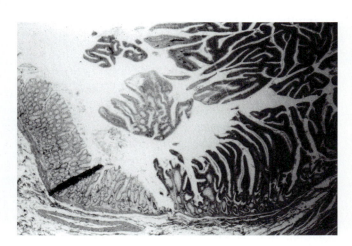

C

Figure 42–1, cont'd. B. Tubulovillous adenoma: Left: macroscopic; Right: microscopic (x44); **C**. Villous adenoma: Left: macroscopic, Right: microscopic (x44). (**A, B,** and **C**, left: courtesy of Drs. A Epstein and S Degli-Esposti, Brown University. A and B, right: from Robert Lev, *Adenomatous Polyps of the Colon: Pathobiological and Clinical Features*, New York, NY: Springer-Verlag; 1990. C, right: courtesy of Dr. Robert Lev.)

BENIGN NEOPLASTIC POLYPS

Adenomatous Polyps

Colonic adenomas are neoplastic polyps. Approximately one-third to two-thirds of Americans over age 65 have adenomatous polyps. Adenomas of the colon can be classified into three types according to their histopathologic appearances: tubular, tubulovillous, and villous adenomas (Fig 42–1). The most common type is tubu-lar adenoma, which accounts for 75% of all colonic adenomas. Most of these polyps are small, with 75% <1 cm, and only 4% >2 cm.[13] They can be either pedunculated or sessile. Small polyps tend to have smooth, round contours, while large tumors are frequently lobulated. Microscopically, tubular adenomas are characterized by branching and enfolding of the glandular epithelium.[14] Villous adenomas are less frequent and account for 10% of the colonic adenomas. These polyps are generally

TABLE 42–1. HISTOLOGY, SIZE, DISTRIBUTION AND INCIDENCE OF CANCER AMONG ADENOMAS.

	Histology			Size (cm) %			Incidence of Cancer
Adenomas	Tubular (%)	Villous (%)	Incidence	<1	1–2	>2	(%)
Tubular	75–100	0–25	75	76	20	4	5
Tubulovillous	26–74	26–75	15	25	47	28	23
Villous	0–24	76–100	10	14	26	60	41

larger, with only 14% of the tumors <1 cm and 60% >2 cm.[13] Villous adenomas are frequently sessile and velvety soft. Microscopically, villous adenomas are characterized by finger-like projections containing epithelial cell-covered core lamina propria.[14] Atypia frequently is observed in villous adenomas. Tubulovillous adenomas characteristically have properties intermediate between tubular and villous adenomas. The large size, villous type, and presence of atypia are associated with an increased risk of malignancy[13,15] (Table 42–1). The pathophysiology of the adenoma is characterized by an excessive proliferation coupled with retarded cell maturation. Normally, the surface epithelial cells of the colonic mucosa are replaced every 4 to 8 days,[14] with a balanced cell loss and cell division and migration from the basal two-thirds of the colonic crypts. In adenomas, proliferation also occurs in the upper crypt region with cells accumulated at the luminal surface.

Management of Adenomatous Polyps. Many patients with adenomatous polyps are asymptomatic; however, they may present with hematochezia, obstruction, pain, mucus discharge, or diarrhea. Most of these polyps are incidental findings. The fecal occult test (FOT) for blood is not sensitive for adenomas of small size or proximal location.[16] When a polyp is found at sigmoidoscopy, a complete polypectomy should be performed for pathologic evaluation, unless the polyp is too large or sessile. In these cases, multiple endoscopic biopsies correlate better with the eventual histologic diagnosis obtained from a subsequent surgical specimen. Colonoscopy still is required because of the possibility of synchronous colon cancer or adenomas at proximal sites. The major morbidity of colonoscopic polypectomy is the failure of retrieval. In this case, stool should be strained to recover specimens for pathologic examination. The more serious complications of colonoscopy are bleeding and perforation, although the incidence needing surgical intervention is extremely low, ranging from 0.1% to 0.3%.

In general, total polypectomy is both diagnostic and therapeutic. However, an invasive carcinoma may be present in a colorectal polyp. By definition, invasive carcinoma in a pedunculated polyp is one with invasion through the muscularis mucosa. Because of the lymphatics present at the submucosal level,[17] the question arises as to whether a surgical resection of colon and lymph nodes is necessary. The incidence of such spread beyond the muscularic mucosa is low, ranging from 2% to 9% of polyps, with a mean of 5%.[18–22] The incidence of lymph node metastases associated with this condition has been reported to be between 8% and 16%.[23] The pathologic features that predict nodal metastasis are positive or close margins, poorly differentiated tumor, or the presence of vascular and lymphatic invasion[23–28] (Fig 42–2). Invasive carcinoma in sessile polyps of the colon almost invariably requires colonic resection. In the absence of such adverse factors, complete polypectomy is considered to be the definitive procedure. Multiple studies have shown no patient mortality from colon cancer or recurrent cancer with a follow-up time of 5 years.[20,27,28] Conversely, colectomy with nodal removal is indicated if any of the high-risk features are present. A difficult condition may be encountered such as a polyp located at the rectosigmoid junction or a lower level. The appropriate level of resection may be difficult to identify after a polypectomy. One approach is to repeat the sigmoidoscopy as soon as possible to visualize the polypectomy scar and inject the site with 1 to 2 cc of India ink. This procedure would identify the concerned area for the surgeon and the pathologist. The pitfalls of India ink injection are occasional perforation and the possible nonvisible marks at the time of surgery. The alternative approach is to perform the resection within 1 to 2 weeks, so that the polypectomy site can be clearly seen during the surgery, and thoroughly examined by the pathologist.

Following complete colonoscopy and therapeutic polypectomy, the follow-up may vary based on the pathologic assessment of the polyp. If the adenoma contains invasive carcinoma, colonoscopy should be repeated at 3 months, 1 year and subsequently, ever 3 years. If the adenoma contains in situ carcinoma or is completely benign, endoscopy is repeated 1 year later to ensure the absence of polyps, and every 3 years thereafter. A recent study suggested that the first follow-up at 3 years are equally effective and less costly.[29]

The rationale behind such a surveillance program is the suspected adenoma-carcinoma sequence. The currently accepted hypothesis is that most colon cancers originate from previously benign adenomas. The indirect supporting evidence is strong. Distal bowel and cecum are frequent sites[30] for both adenomas and cancer, suggesting a similar distribution of the two conditions. Cancer may arise from untreated adenomas.[13] The cumulative risk of developing subsequent cancer among patients having adenomas for more than 15 years is significant.[31,32] Frequent coexistence of the adenomatous remnants in large bowel cancer also has been re-

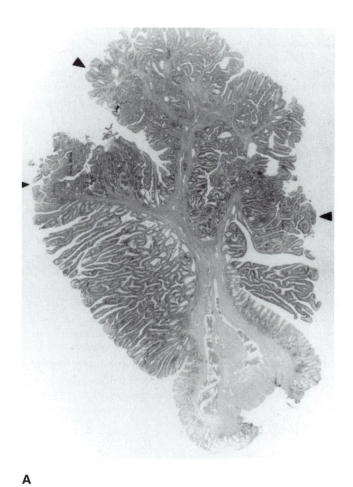

A

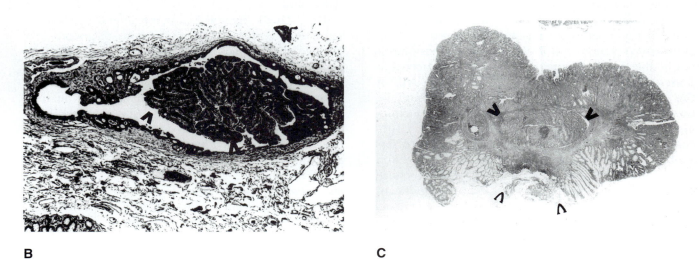

B

C

Figure 42–2. Malignant polyps. **A**. Tubulovillous adenoma (x11) with an invasive carcinoma (*arrows*). Margins are clear. (From Dr. Robert Lev, *Adenomatous Polyps of the Colon: Pathobiological and Clinical Features,* New York, NY: Springer-Verlag; 1990). **B**. Malignant polyp (x22) with tumor in vein (*arrows*). **C**. Malignant polyp with invasive carcinoma (*heavy arrows*) close to margin (*light arrows*). B and C: courtesy of Dr. Robert Lev).

ported.[13,33–35] Molecularly, the protein kinase C is reduced in the particulate fraction of both adenomas and colon cancer. The decrease progresses as the adenoma advances in size and progresses in colonic carcinomas.[36] Based on the similarities of anatomic distribution, temporal sequence of the neoplastic progression, coexistence of adenomas in carcinomas, and qualitatively similar disturbance in cellular proliferation, developments of colonic adenoma and carcinoma are regarded as sequential events. Although this stepwise progression does not exclude a de novo pathway of carcinoma development, the early detection and removal of adenomatous polyps is expected to reduce the incidence of large bowel cancer.[37]

Neoplastic Hereditary Polyposis

Familial Adenomatous Polyposis. Familial polyposis is an inherited disorder in which the main feature is diffuse adenomatous polyps of the entire lower gastrointestinal tract. The clinical presentation was first described by Corvisart[38] and the familial pattern first suggested by Cripps.[39] The autosomal dominant feature was established by Dukes and Lockhart-Mummery.[40,41] The genetic localization demonstrated that the defect resides on the long arm of chromosome 5.[42] Familial polyposis commonly occurs in the second decade of life, but occasionally may occur earlier. The malignant potential of this condition was first reported by Handford.[43] The incidence of malignant transformation approaches 100%, if left untreated. The mean age of cancer diagnosis is approximately 40[44]; however, it may be diagnosed as early as the first decade of life. The nature of this disease dictates early and aggressive prophylaxis by removing the involved bowel before the onset of malignancy.[45–47] Total proctocolectomy with ileal pouch–anal anastomosis fulfills the goals of preventing colorectal cancer and preserving transanal and defecation.[48] The pitfalls of this procedure are the frequent pouchitis, multiple bowel movements with possible nighttime incontinence,[49] and temporary ileostomy with a 5% to 10% chance of permanence.[50,51] The alternative approach is a subtotal colectomy with ileoproctostomy, if the rectum can be rendered polyp-free. Although this procedure does not require temporary ileostomy, a significant number of patients must have the residual rectum removed, either owing to numerous polyps or the development of cancer at follow-up.[49]

Many of these patients may not have the option of ileoanal anastomosis because of fibrosis and shortening of the small bowel mesentery or because of previous colectomy, abdominoperineal resection, and permanent ileostomy. Subsequent cancer develops in 3% to 30% of patients treated by subtotal colectomy and ileoproctostomy.[44,47,51]

The other significant issue in familial polyposis is the treatment of the family. The optimal surveillance includes annual proctoscopy of family members starting at age ten, since early diagnosis and appropriate surgical prophylaxis may completely prevent subsequent cancer of the colon and rectum. Diagnosis by the symptoms is associated with a high incidence of cancer.

Gardner's Syndrome. Extracolonic manifestations of familial polyposis were first described by Gardner.[52] The syndrome is a variant of familial adenomatous polyposis, consisting of diffuse polyposis of the lower intestine, osteomas, epidermoid cysts, congenital hypertrophy of the retinal pigment epithelium, polyps of the stomach, small intestine, pancreas, thyroid, adrenal, and parathyroid, as well as retroperitoneal fibrosis and desmoid tumor following abdominal surgery.[44,53–56] Treatment of Gardner's polyposis is identical to that of familial polyposis coli.

Turcot's Syndrome. Turcot's syndrome is characterized by the association of familial polyposis and tumors of the central nervous system.[57] The most common brain tumors are medulloblastoma and glioblastoma.[58] Turcot's syndrome is a phenotypic variant of familial polyposis and Gardner's syndrome; however, it is transmitted by an autosomal recessive gene.

■ MALIGNANT DISEASES OF THE COLON

CARCINOMA OF THE COLON

Epidemiology

In 1993, it was estimated that, in the United States, there were 109 000 new colon cancer cases diagnosed and 50 000 patients died of their disease. This disorder affects both genders equally.[59] Internationally, the incidence of colon cancer is higher in industrialized and Western European countries. The variations in incidence suggest the possible influence of environmental and genetic factors in its development.[60,61] In the United States, the incidence of colon cancer in blacks and whites is similar within a given geographic area.[62,63] Native Americans, on the other hand, have significantly less disease.[64] The 5 year relative survival rate for American blacks and whites is 48% and 59%, respectively. Although the trend of survival has shown a steady improvement since 1960, disease-related death has been consistently higher in the black population.[59]

Etiology

Diet. Among the environmental factors, diet has been implicated most frequently in colon cancer carcinogenesis.[65,66] High dietary fiber content was reported to be the key factor responsible for the low incidence of colorectal cancer in native Africans.[67] The hypothesis is that a high-fiber diet is associated with a shorter fecal transit time and rapid evacuation, thus allowing only a brief contact of dietary carcinogens with the mucosa. Experiments have shown that increasing dietary fiber decreases the incidence of colon cancer induced by dimethyl-hydrazine (DMH) in rats.[68] Other biochemical mechanisms that may be induced by fiber require better characterization. Fecal bile acid concentration has been studied in colon cancer patients and controls. It was found that a higher concentration of fecal bile acid is common in patients with colorectal cancer and uncommon in normal individuals.[69] Fecal bile acid is increased by dietary fat and lowered by fiber.[70] It also is postulated that fecal bacteria are altered in high-risk populations[71,72] as a result of diet and bile acid, as well as other neutral steroles that may be converted by the selected fecal flora into cancer promoters or carcinogens. Alcohol also has been linked to the development of colon cancer.[73–74] The mechanism responsible for the alcohol association is unclear at the present time.

Genetics

With increasing biomarker research, genetic influences have been shown to be closely linked to the development of colon cancer.[75] The hereditary nature of this disease first was observed in patients with familial adenomatous polyposis (FAP). While this condition accounts for <1% of all colorectal cancers, it provides a model for genetic analysis.[76,77] The APC gene responsible for FAP has been located on the long arm of chromosome 5. Hereditary nonpolyposis colorectal cancer (HNPCC) is another form of familial aggregation of colorectal cancer. HNPCC has been even more useful in genetic mapping of the genes predisposing to colon cancer. HNPCC kindreds commonly are defined as those in which three or more family members have colorectal cancer, with one member having been diagnosed at <50 years of age.[78] This condition also is known as Lynch's syndrome I and is characterized by an autosomal dominant transmission, the early onset of colon cancer (particularly in the right colon), the lack of polyposis, and frequent synchronous and metachronous colonic cancers. In addition to the colon, other organs such as kidney, ureter, bladder, small bowel, bile duct, stomach, breast, ovary, and endometrium are at high risk for cancer development. HNPCC, with both colonic and extracolonic manifestation of cancer, has been described as Lynch's syndrome II.[79–80] The gene that is responsible for familial colon cancer (FCC) has recently been mapped to chromosome 2 p15–16 by in situ hybridization, linkage, and somatic cell hybrid analysis.[81–84] The defect has been described as an inaccuracy of DNA replication, secondary to the presence of microsatellite DNA markers.[23–26] The FCC gene also may play a role in some sporadic colon cancers.

Genes other than FCC and their associated chromosomes that have been implicated in colon cancer development are APC on chromosome 5q myc on chromosome 8, K-ras on chromosome 12, p53 and neu/HER2 are chromosome 17, and DCC on chromosome 18q. K-ras, neu/HER 2 and myc are known as oncogenes. APC, DCC and p53 are tumor suppressor genes. The interplay of various genes and sequential events is not fully understood at the present time, although there seems to be a progression of alterations in the adenoma-carcinoma sequence.

Prevention and Early Detection

While an effective method of preventing colorectal cancer is not available at the present time for asymptomatic individuals at risk, periodic screening may lead to removal of precancerous polyps and to the detection of colon cancer at an early stage. The guidelines proposed by the American Cancer Society for screening asymptomatic Americans with average risk are as follows: (1) yearly FOT for Americans 50 years of age and more, and (2) sigmoidoscopy, preferably flexible sigmoidoscopy (FS), to be started in the same population and repeated every 3 to 5 years thereafter.[85]

Regarding the proposed screening tests, the FOT has been widely used and appears to be effective. The false-positive rate is low (0.5%), when performed properly. The incidence of positive results in large screening series is reported to be between 1% and 4%. Approximately 10% to 20% of the positive findings are due to adenomatous polyps, and 5% to 10% result from colorectal cancer.[86–88] Approximately 75% of patients with colorectal cancer detected by FOT have localized disease. The 5 year survival rates for cancers detected in this way are anticipated to be better than those of the national statistics of colon cancer mortality.[86,89–92] The cost of screening was reported to be $3800 per cancer case identified.[87]

The benefits of sigmoidoscopy in detection of polyps and early cancer also have been demonstrated. A prospective, nonrandomized study of the patients in the Kaiser Permanente Multiphasic Health Checkup Program showed 10 year survival rates of scoped and control groups as 80% and 48%, respectively.[93,94] Similar benefits were shown by the studies from Minnesota's Cancer Detection Center,[95] Memorial Sloan–Kettering Cancer Center and Strang Clinic.[96,97] Muller and Lopez,[98] as well as Atkin and associates.[99]

Rectal examination should be part of a general physical examination. This examination would provide for detection of low, and probably some middle, rectal growths. Serologic tumor markers are of no value in screening for colon cancer at the present time. When

TABLE 42–2. MODIFIED SURVEILLANCE PROGRAM FOR INDIVIDUALS WITH INCREASED RISK OF DEVELOPING COLORECTAL CANCER

Groups	Surveillance
FAP and associated syndromes	FS every 6 to 12 months from teens. Colonoscopy every 3 years. Colectomy if polyposis found.
Pancolitis, longstanding	Annual colonoscopy after 7 years. Colectomy if progressive or severe dysplasia found.
Left-sided colitis, longstanding	Annual colonoscopy after 15 years.
Previous adenomatous polyps	Colonoscopy in 1 year if adenomas are villous type or greater than 1 cm. If negative, repeat every 3 to 5 years. Yearly FOT.
Lynch Syndrome	Yearly FOT and colonoscopy every 3 years from the 3rd decade.
Pelvic irradiation	Yearly FOT. FS every 3 years.
History of breast, endometrial or ovarian cancer	Yearly FOT, rectal exam. FS every 3 years. Periodic UGI study

any of these screening procedures is positive, a full colonoscopy is indicated to complete the examination and to establish the tissue diagnosis of an abnormality. When colonoscopy is not readily available, a double-contrast barium enema is the alternative choice. Those individuals with increased risk are followed on different schedules.[86] Surveillance should be started earlier than 50 years of age and follow-up should be more frequent in certain individuals. In the cases of polyposis coli and long-standing active ulcerative colitis, colonoscopy instead of sigmoidoscopy should be used for screening. The FOT is ineffective in these individuals. The modified surveillance program for individuals with increased risk of developing colorectal cancer is summarized in Table 42–2.

Anatomy

The colon is defined topographically as the large bowel, starting at the cecum and ending at the inferior margin of the sigmoid colon. Embryonically, the colon can be divided into proximal and distal portions, with the former segment derived from the midgut and the latter segment from the hindgut. Blood supplies to the proximal and distal colon are obtained from the superior mesenteric artery (SMA) and the inferior mesenteric artery (IMA), respectively (Fig 42–3A). The venous and lymphatic drainages are parallel to the SMA. The inferior mesenteric vein, however, passes vertically in the retroperitoneum and joins with the splenic vein en route to the portal venous system (Fig 42–3A). The lymphatics parallel the IMA distribution. The nodes are subdivided into four groups: epicolic, paracolic, intermediate, and principal nodes, with the epicolic right on the colonic wall and the principal nodes on the superior

mesenteric or inferior mesenteric vessels (Fig 42–3B). The subsequent lymphatic drainages extend to the paraaortic chains and cisterna chyli.

Cecum and Ascending colon. The right colon extends from the cecum to the right colic flexure (hepatic flexure). It overlies the iliacus and quadratus lumborum muscle and right kidney, and crosses over and indents the inferior surface of the right lobe of the liver. It receives blood supply from the iliocolic and right colic arteries, branches of the superior mesenteric artery.

Transverse Colon. The transverse colon starts at the right hepatic flexure and extends obliquely toward the left upper abdomen to form the splenic flexure. The transverse colon is an intra-abdominal viscus with the exception of the first 8 cm of retroperitoneal location. Anatomically, it lies anterior and inferior to the duodenum, pancreas and inferior pole of the spleen. The major blood supply comes from the middle colic artery, which branches into right and left divisions. A watershed occurs at the distal two-thirds of the transverse colon, the junction of the SMA and IMA. Collateral circulation occurs via the marginal artery of Drummond which receives blood from the middle colic and left colic arteries.

Descending Colon. The descending colon extends from the splenic flexure to the true pelvis. It overlies the left kidney and quadratus, psoas, and iliac muscles. It is bound to the retroperitoneum by the peritoneal investment and turns medially to begin the sigmoid colon. The descending colon is supplied by the left colic artery.

Sigmoid Colon. The sigmoid colon extends from the lower margin of the descending colon, passes medially into the midline of the pelvis, and terminates in the upper rectum at the S3 vertebra. The sigmoid colon also is invested with peritoneum and forms a fan-shaped mesentery. The length of the sigmoid is highly variable because of the redundancy. In the female, the uterus, and, in the male, the bladder, lies immediately in front of the sigmoid colon. This anatomical relationship predisposes the sigmoid colon to the formation of colovaginal or colovesical fistula when the sigmoid colon is diseased with diverticulitis, cancer, inflammatory bowel disease, or severe radiation damage. The sigmoid colon is also in close contact with the abdominal and pelvic ureter. The ureter courses retroperitoneally along the medial aspect of psoas muscle, and crosses over the bifurcation of left iliac artery to become the pelvic ureter. Below this level, it passes posteriolaterally. The left ureter may adhere to the diseased sigmoid colon at the level of iliac bifurcation, and an injury to the ureter may occur as a result of dissection.

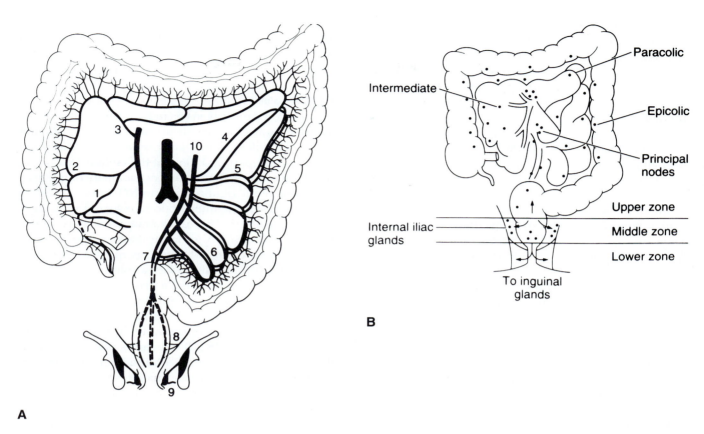

Figure 42–3. A. Arterial and venous supply of the colon. Branches of superior mesenteric artery: (1) ileocolic, (2) right colic, (3) middle colic. Branches of inferior mesenteric artery: (4) ascending left colic, (5) left colic, (6) sigmoid, (7) superior rectal, (8) middle rectal, (9) inferior rectal, and (10) inferior mesenteric vein. **B**. Lymphatic drainage of colon. Principal, intermediate, paracolic and epicolic nodal sites of colon and rectum. (From Bland KI. Malignant diseases of the colon. In: Levine B et al (eds), *Current Practice of Surgery,* vol 3. New York, NY: Churchill-Livingston, 1993:1–45)

Microscopic Anatomy

The large bowel wall is composed of six layers: mucosa, muscularis mucosa, submucosa, muscularis propria, subserosal fat and serosa. The rectum has similar histological features but lacks a serosa. The appendices epiploicae represent peritoneal pouches filled with fat. The *mucosa* is the innermost layer of the large intestine and rectum; it is smooth, pale and contains crypts (glands) arranged in an orderly fashion. To be differentiated from the small bowel mucosa, colorectal mucosa has no villi, but instead contains colonic crypts of Lieberkühn that are deeper than their enteric histologic counterpart. The large bowel is lined by a single layer of columnar epithelial cells that rest on a delicate basement membrane containing variable quantities of mucin.

The *muscularis mucosae* represents an external longitudinal layer that is continuous and thin, with an intercircular configuration. In the abdominal colon, its outer layer is thickened to form three longitudinal bands of approximately 5 to 10 mm width that are termed the *teniae coli.* At the level of each tenia is an in-

terchange of muscle bundles between circular and longitudinal layers. Of note, at the level of the distal rectal wall, the circular muscle thickens to form the valves of Houston; the teniae are replaced by anterior and posterior longitudinal musculature.

Between the circular muscle and the muscularis mucosae is the submucosa. The *submucosa* is considered the strongest microscopic layer and is thus the anatomic subunit that surgeons target for suture placement in colonic and rectal anastomoses. This layer contains a vast network of blood vessels and the autonomic nervous *plexus of Meissner.* Submucosa is incompletely developed in the appendix.

The *muscularis propria* is comprised of an inner circular layer and an outer longitudinal layer of smooth musculature. It has clinical importance in that lymphatic channels traverse it in a circumferential pattern, between the two muscle layers and the subserosal fat. This subanatomical relationship, in part, explains the morphological pattern of annular submucosal spread of colonic and rectal cancer.

The most external layer of the large intestine is the

serosa which conveniently continues, in part, to the upper one-third of the rectum. This coat invests a variable portion of the circumference of the intestine and represents the visceral peritoneum. All microscopic layers of the colon and rectum are significant in defining clinical and pathological tumor staging which guides the therapeutic approaches.

Symptoms and Signs of Colon Cancer

The clinical manifestations of colon cancer are influenced by the location and size of the lesion. Lesions on the right side tend to be bulky and ulcerating. The frequently associated symptoms are anemia and dull aching pain in the right lower quadrant. Nausea, anorexia and a palpable abdominal mass in the right lower quadrant may be other manifestations of cancer of the cecum and ascending colon. Obstruction is an infrequent presentation. Transverse colon cancer is frequently manifested by signs of obstruction or pain at the tumor location. A mass effect of gastrocolic fistula may be other presenting symptoms. The left side of the colon, consisting of descending and sigmoid colon, frequently harbors annular and scirrhous lesions. The most frequent symptoms are an alteration in bowel habits and a decrease in stool caliber as a result of the narrower colonic lumen and the solid stool in the left colon. Mucus and blood mixed with bowel movements are other frequent complaints. Signs and symptoms of obstruction or involvement of the urinary tract may occur. A painless mass may be felt in the left lower quadrant or suprapubic area. Low back pain, with or without sciatica, signifies locally advanced disease. The anatomic distribution of colon cancer and associated symptoms are summarized in Table 42–3. Other complaints, such as cachexia, excessive weight loss, jaundice, or ascites, are suggestive of metastatic disease.

Findings of colon cancer on physical examination may include hemoccult-positive stool, an abdominal

mass, an umbilical nodule, hepatomegaly, ascites, a Bloomer's shelf or a Virchow's node. With the exception of a positive FOT, the remaining findings are all suggestive of an advanced stage of colon cancer.

Diagnostic Studies

When colon cancer is suspected, colonoscopy is the diagnostic study of choice. It provides access to examine the entire colon, allows polypectomy for therapeutic purposes and permits biopsy of the colonic lesion. The pitfalls of colonoscopy are an occasional incomplete examination of the right colon (5 to 10% of cases) and the necessity of surgical intervention for significant complications of 0.1% to 0.3% of examinations. Rarely, mortality may occur.[100] Alternative diagnostic procedures are the double-contrast barium enema (BE) and proctosigmoidoscopy. In BE studies, a colon cancer may appear as an apple-core lesion, a stricture with mucosal irregularity, a polypoid lesion, or a large filling defect. The endoscopic and radiographic appearances of various types of colon cancer are shown in Figure 42–4. The perforation rate of BE is low, ranging between 0.04 and 0.008%.[101] The disadvantages of radiographic imaging are that it is nontherapeutic, provides no tissue diagnosis, and may miss small, flat mucosal lesions that can represent a synchronous cancer.

If a diagnosis of colon cancer is made, the patient is evaluated for operability and resectability. The operability is determined by the cardiopulmonary condition and performance status. A detailed history and thorough physical examination, EKG, CXR, and laboratory studies such as a complete blood count, renal function studies, and a blood sugar will provide a reasonable assessment of the general medical condition of the patient. The resectability is governed by the extent of disease. A CT scan of the abdomen and pelvis will provide information regarding any liver involvement and local extension of a sigmoid colon cancer. A CXR is sufficient evaluation for pulmonary metastasis in an asymptomatic patient who does not have evidence of other metastases. Liver function tests, serum alkaline phosphatase, serum gamma-gutamyl transferase (SGGT), serum glutamic-oxaloacetic transaminase (SGOT), serum glutamic pyruvic transaminase (SGPT),[60,102] and lactic dehydrogenase (LDH),[60] have been shown to have predictive value for possible hepatic metastasis.

Tumor markers such as CEA, CA 19-9 and CA-50 have been used in the care of patients with colorectal cancer.[103] The carcinoembryonic antigen (CEA), first described by Gold and Freedman,[104] has been widely used. The markers CA 19-9 and CA-50 are not routinely used, although anti-CA 19-9 antibody was originally produced against human colon cancer.[105,106] CEA has been shown to be valuable as part of the preoperative evaluations. It correlates well with tumor staging[107,108] and with pre-

TABLE 42–3. ANATOMIC LOCATIONS AND CLINICAL MANIFESTATIONS OF COLON CANCER

Distribution (%)	Ascending/ Cecum[24]	Transverse[13]	Descending/ Sigmoid[34]
	Anatomic Location		
Manifestations	Bleeding: anemia, melana, abdominal pain, mass obstruction, diarrhea	Abdominal pain obstruction mass	Changing bowel habit/stool caliber mucus and blood in stool Abdominal pain mass obstruction/ perforation low back pain

dictions of subsequent survival and recurrence.[109–111] The CEA of normal individuals ranges from 0 to 2.5 ng/mL, although many benign conditions are associated with an elevated CEA. Benign elevations of CEA are in general <10 ng and reversible. Known benign conditions associated with CEA elevation are biliary obstruction, hepatocellular dysfunction, cigarette smoking, bronchitis, gastric ulcer, gastritis, inflammatory bowel disease, diverticulitis, adenomatous polyps, renal disease, and benign prostatic hyperplasia.[112–115] The CEA is also elevated in patients with carcinoma other than colon cancer.

CT scans are not routinely performed preoperatively. However, in patients with an elevated CEA, abnormal liver function tests, weight loss, a palpable mass, or large sigmoid cancers, a preoperative CT scan of the abdomen and/or the pelvis is advised.

A recent development in diagnostic tools utilizes the radiolabeled antibody to target tumors for imaging or detection. The development of immunoscintigraphy is aimed at a more specific and sensitive tumor imaging. A glycoprotein, TAG 72, has been found to be a useful target antigen in colorectal cancer. The expression of TAG 72 was reported to be as high as 94% in colon adenocarcinoma. A study using indium 111 (^{111}In)-labeled anti-TAG 72 for imaging colon cancer showed a sensitivity of 70%, specificity of 90% and accuracy of 72%.[116] Twelve percent of patients with occult disease were detected by preoperative immunoscintigraphy only. Subsequent study showed that the antibody scan was more sensitive than the CT scan for pelvic tumors and other extrahepatic sites. The CT scan was superior to the antibody scan for liver metastasis, regardless of the type of antibody used (ie, anti-TAG 72 vs anti-CEA).[117,118] The side effects from radiolabeled mouse antibody are infrequent and reversible. Two major limitations are that a large percentage of patients who received mouse antibody developed human antimouse antibody and 10% of patients showed false positivity.[119] Radioimmunoguided surgery (RIGS) also utilizes the radiolabeled antibody to localize the tumors. The detection is achieved by a hand-held gamma-detecting probe during the surgery. Studies suggested that more thorough surgery is done with the probe-assisted exploration. The upstaging may qualify patients for postoperative adjuvant therapy.[120] Areas that require more studies are the exclusion of false positivity and its association with unnecessary extra procedures, and the prolongation of operative time. Some investigators believe that the inability to detect tumors in some RIGS-positive tissues is a result of the limitations of conventional microscopic examination. However, this belief should be regarded as a preliminary suggestion. The supportive evidence is weak and indirect, at present.[121,122] Demonstration

of tumor cell binding by ^{111}In-CC49 in tissues that are RIGS-positive and hematoxylin-eosin-negative is a minimal requirement to prove the true positivity of the RIGS. With continuous development and additional experience, RIGS may become a complementary tool to our standard diagnostic studies.

Treatment of Colon Cancer

After a thorough evaluation of the patient's health and the extent of the tumor, the next step is treatment. The principal treatment for colon cancer is anatomical resection. The details concerning colon resection, including preoperative preparation, extent of colon resection, and postoperative follow-up, will be discussed.

Preoperative Preparation. Operations performed on the unprepared colon have a wound infection rate of 40%. A combined approach of mechanical washout and oral antibiotics was reported to decrease the wound infection rate to 9%.[123] With additional parenteral antibiotic prophylaxis, the infection rate can be further reduced to 5% or less.[124]

In elective colon resections, most patients are candidates for bowel preparation as outpatients, with the exception of those patients with confusion, significant cardiac or renal disease, or the elderly (80 years of age or older). Bowel preparation consists of a special diet, whole-bowel lavage and oral antibiotics. Two days before surgery, the patient begins a diet of clear liquids. The day before surgery, the patient is instructed to take one gallon of Golytely for washing the entire colon.[125] The formula consists of Na^+, 125 mEq/L; SO_4, 80 mEq/L; Cl, 35 mEq/L; HCO_3, 20 mEq/L; K^+, 10 mEq/L; and 80 mM polyethylene glycol-3350 which does not cause water or electrolyte absorption or secretion. The mechanical cleansing takes approximately 3 hours to complete. Lavage alone, however, does not lower the incidence of wound infection.[123,126–128] Addition of a poorly absorbed oral antibiotic with both aerobic and anaerobic coverage significantly reduces the incidence of infection. Erythromycin base (1 g) and neomycin sulfate (1 g), at 1, 2, and 11 PM the day before surgery are employed frequently. On the day of surgery, parenteral prophylaxis is given within an hour of the surgery and extended for a full 24 hour coverage. Cefotetan (1 g) every 12 hours, and cefoxitin (2 g) every 6 hours, are both effective regimens.

To prevent deep vein thrombophlebitis and subsequent pulmonary embolism, the intermittent pulsatile compression device is used intraoperatively and postoperatively until the patient is fully ambulatory. A Foley catheter should be inserted in all cases of formal colon resections, particularly those involving the sigmoid colon and rectum. Selective placement of a ureteric catheter should be considered when hydronephrosis

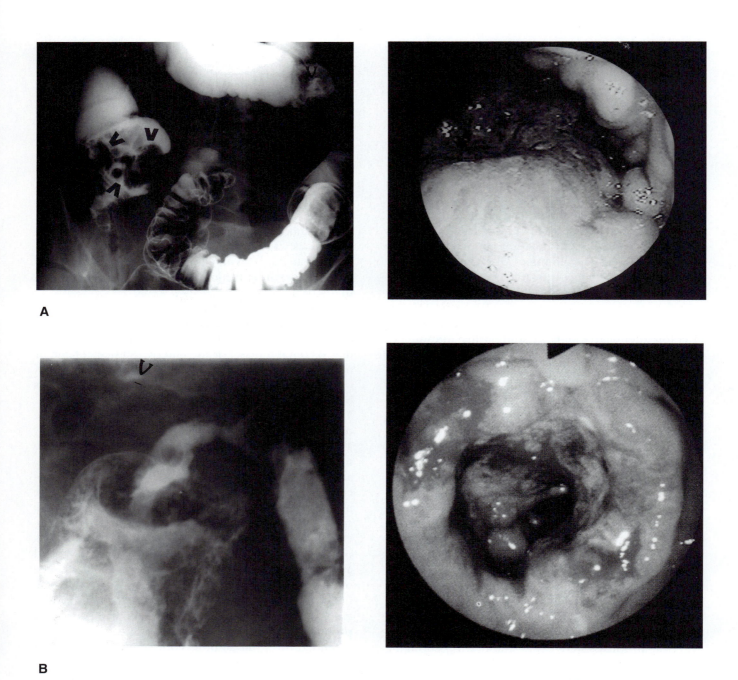

Figure 42–4. Colon cancer. **A**. Large lobulared cecal cancer (*arrows*) seen on barium enema (left) and colonscopy (right). Left: A synchronous cancer is shown by barium enema in the transverse colon. A small *arrow* points to the central ulceration of the transverse colon carcinoma. (A, right: courtesy of Dr. Amer Malik, Department of Medicine, Gastrointestinal Division, Brown University, Providence, Rhode Island; A, left: courtesy of Dr. William Colaiace, Department of Radiology, Brown University, Providence, Rhode Island). **B**. Annular lesions. Left: radiographic view, by barium enema. The annular carcinoma seen on barium enema also reveals a colo-gastric fistula (*arrows*). Right: Annular carcinoma, endoscopic view. (B, left: courtesy of Dr. William Colaiace, Department of Radiology, Brown University, Providence, Rhode Island). B, right: In: Silverstein FE, Tytgat G. (ed), *Atlas of Gastrointestinal Endoscopy*, New York, NY: Gower Medical, 1992.) *Continued*

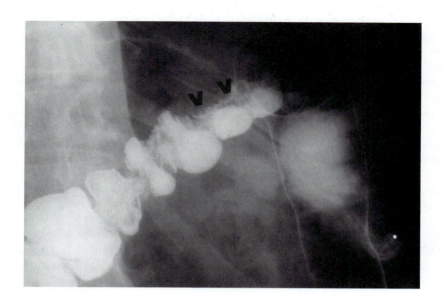

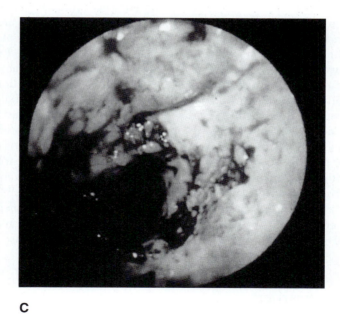

C

Figure 42–4,cont'd. C. Infiltrative carcinoma. Left: by barium enema; right: by colonoscopy. (C, left: courtesy of Dr. William Colaiace, Department of Radiology, Brown University, Providence, Rhode Island; C, right: In: Silverstein FE, Tytgat G (eds), *Atlas of Gastrointestinal Endoscopy*. New York, NY: Gower Medical; 1992.)

and hydroureter are present, or the tumor mass is contiguous to the ureter.

Operative Treatment. A midline abdominal incision allows full exploration and further extension for additional needs. The extent of the resection is determined by the location of the primary colon cancer, as well as the absence or presence of invasion into adjacent structures and distant metastasis. When there is no incidence of colon invasion into surrounding organs or metastasis, a segmental colon resection is the main treatment. The principles of segmental colonic resection for cancer include ligation of the major vascular pedicles, with dissection of mesenteric lymph nodes and the achievement of tumor-free margins. Anatomical resections of colon cancer at different sites are summarized in Table 42–4.

Tumor-free margins are easily achievable for colon cancer because mucosal spread of the disease rarely exceeds 4 cm.[129] In the case of low anterior resection, a minimal distal margin of 2 cm for well-differentiated tumor is acceptable.[130] When synchronous colon cancers are found at different sites in the colon, a subtotal colectomy is the preferred procedure.[131]

Resection of contiguous organs for locally invasive colorectal cancer is necessary in approximately 10% of cases.[132–135] The most frequently involved organs are the bladder, ovary, ureter, and abdominal wall.[136–138]; less frequently involved are the small intestine, spleen, pancreas, stomach, and uterus.[136,137] It is neither important nor possible to accurately differentiate malignant and benign adhesions intraoperatively.[137] En bloc resection with negative soft tissue margins is the choice of surgery. Patients with B3 lesions were shown to have a 67% 5 year survival rate, although C3 lesions were reported to have a much worse prognosis, with a 5 year survival rate of 22%.[136] In patients with known locally advanced disease, preoperative irradiation with 4500 cGy may be beneficial in terms of increasing the resectability and improving the chance of margin-free resection.[139,140] This is especially true for those patients who will have pelvic exenteration. Pelvic exenteration should be considered only with a curative intent, with clear margins critical for the outcome.

Ovarian involvement with colon cancer may not be a direct extension, but instead may represent microscopic metastasis. The true incidence is difficult to evaluate and has been reported to be between 2% to 10%.[141–145] The frequency of ovarian metastases increases with the stage of disease[141,142,146] and a premenopausal status.[142,146] Thus, in patients with either of these conditions, an oophorectomy should be considered.

Patients presenting with malignant obstruction of the colon deserve special attention to surgical planning. The incidence has been estimated to be 16%.[147] The surgical mortality and morbidity are high[148,149] and 5 year survival rates are low.[149–152] Emergency surgery is recommended for patients with complete obstruction and pending rupture. Minimal surgery, such as proximal colostomy, is recommended only for patients with extreme age and high APACHE II (Acute Physiology and Chronic Health Evaluation) scores.[153] Primary resection is preferred for patients in stable condition.[154,155] Both segmental and subtotal colectomy have been performed.[147,156] The latter approach is preferred because of (1) the increased incidence of synchronous colon cancer in these patients,[157,158] and the inability of intraoperative palpation and preoperative examination to detect synchronous colon lesions; (2) anastomosis between the size-matched proximal ileum and nonobstructed distal colon is facilitated; and (3) the reduced possibility of spillage of liquid stool during the anastomosis. However, segmental resection is more appropriate in elderly patients and those who may not tolerate lengthy resection. A protective ileostomy or colostomy is made when primary anastomosis is performed in the obstructed and nonprepared bowel.

Colonic perforation may develop in 3% to 8% of patients with colon cancer.[154,159–163] Perforation is often a result of obstructing cancer of the colon. The combination of these two conditions occurs in approximately 2% of colorectal cancer cases.[159,160] When a competent

---

TABLE 42–4. ANATOMICAL RESECTION OF COLON CANCER

Tumor Location	Vascular Ligation	Colon Resection	Anastomosis
Cecum, ascending colon	Ileocolic, right colic	Right hemicolectomy	Ileotransverse colostomy
Hepatic flexure, proximal transverse colon	Ileocolic, right, middle, colic	Extended right hemicolectomy with omentectomy	Ileodescending colostomy
Distal transverse colon, splenic flexure	Ileocolic, right, middle or left branch of middle colic, left colic	Extended right hemicolectomy with omentectomy or left hemicolectomy	Ileosigmoid colostomy or transverse-sigmoid colostomy Transverse sigmoid colostomy
Descending colon	Inferior mesenteric or left colic	Left hemicolectomy	Transverse colorectal anastomosis
Sigmoid colon	Inferior mesenteric or sigmoid	Left hemicolectomy or sigmoid resection	or descending colorectal anastomosis

ileocecal valve is present, a free perforation associated with obstruction frequently occurs in the dilated, thin-walled cecum, with a clinical presentation of fecal peritonitis. Perforation also may develop at the site or proximal to the tumor.[160] Perforation also may be manifested as a local sepsis, such as abscess or fistula.[164,165] Identification of enteric organisms in an abscess should raise the suspicion of a colonic origin.

Free perforation is a life-threatening condition requiring emergency surgery. Thorough exploration is essential. Resection of perforated tumor-bearing colon is preferred. Primary anastomosis is to be avoided when generalized peritonitis and hemodynamic instability are present.[166] Abscess and fistula, on the other hand, may be managed initially by antibiotics, fluid replacement, drainage, and decompression. The definitive resection may be performed when the condition of the patient improves and stabilizes. The operative mortality of perforated colon cancer is high, ranging from 10% to 50%.[167] Long-term survival is poor, with a reported 5 year survival rate of 0% to 15%.[154,160]

Laparoscopic surgical intervention in colon cancer is a recent development in treatment. With improved instruments, it is possible to perform laparoscopic colon resection.[168–170] Sigmoid resection and right colectomy are the most frequently performed procedures. Tumors of the transverse colon, two flexures and rectum are technically more difficult using laparoscopic resection. The advantage of this form of surgery appears to be a shorter hospital stay. However, there are many problems yet to be worked out. Longer operating time and capital investments for equipment have increased the cost. Complications of laparoscopic colectomy have not been fully documented because of limited experience and follow-up. The multiple port sites and significant incisions required for the removal of the specimen and assisted anastomosis make it less attractive. Finally, the most critical issue is the uncertainty of the adequacy of oncologic treatment with laparoscopic colectomies. At this point, this approach remains experimental and unproven for standard care of colon cancer patients.

Other conditions that might be encountered during the colectomy for colon cancer are liver metastases, cholelithiasis and abdominal aortic aneurysm. When an isolated liver metastasis is found at the periphery of the liver, it may be removed by a wedge resection, with a margin. If the number, location or size of the liver mass(es) dictates a formal hepatectomy, it is usually performed through a separate procedure with a delay of 6 to 12 weeks from the colon surgery. An incidental cholecystectomy for cholelithiasis during an elective colectomy procedure does not change the operative risk.[171] Finding a small abdominal aortic aneurysm during the elective colon resection need not change the operative plan. Only the planned bowel resection should be performed. A large or symptomatic abdominal aortic aneurysm almost always is found preoperatively. This situation can be addressed preoperatively with the assistance of a vascular surgeon; resection of the aneurysm may take priority. Simultaneous colon resection and aneurysmal surgery is discouraged.

The operative mortality for colon cancer surgery in elective cases is 5% or less.[172–174] The colon resection with curative intent carries lower surgical mortality than palliative resections.

Staging of Colon Cancer—The Prognosticator in Colon Cancer

Staging of colon cancer is used to assess the prognosis and to tailor the treatment according to the risk of recurrent disease. The most commonly used staging system is the Dukes' classification which was originally described in 1932.[175] Dukes' A cancer is tumor with invasion of the bowel wall but not beyond the muscularis propria, Dukes' B cancer is transmural invasion of the bowel wall, and Dukes' C cancer is any degree of bowel wall invasion with nodal metastasis. The C stage was subsequently divided into C1 and C2, with C1 representing epicolic and paracolic lymph node metastases and C2 representing intermediate and proximal nodal involvement. Despite the simplicity of the classification, the Dukes' stage predicts survival across time and geographic differences.[172,176] Five year survival rates are reported to be 80%, 60% and 30% for Dukes' A, B, and C, respectively.

Astler and Coller's modified Dukes' classification also is employed often in clinical practice.[177] The differences between the original Dukes' and Astler-Coller's modification are: the latter system defines the stage A cancers as those confined to the submucosal invasion; B1 cancers as those invading the muscularis propria; B2 cancers as cancers invading all layers of bowel wall; and C1 cancers as limited to the bowel wall with nodal involvement, whereas C2 cancers have full thickness invasion through the serosa and nodal involvement. Fisher and associates reported that survival was comparable among patients with Astler and Coller A and B1 and TNM T1 or T2 N0M0. Astler-Coller C1 and C2, however, provide a striking prognostic prediction that is independent of the number of lymph node metastases, the distance between involved nodes and the primary tumor and the degree of tumor differentiation. They concluded that Dukes' staging is the simplest and most consistent algorithm for prognosis.[178]

To avoid the confusion between the Dukes' and modified Dukes' systems, a newer classification of TNM clearly defines the precise anatomic extent of the tumor (Table 42–5).[179] The National Institutes of Health Consensus Committee on Adjuvant Therapy for Patients with Colon and Rectal Cancer recommended the use of the TNM staging system for evaluating these patients

TABLE 42–5. TUMOR/NODE/METASTASIS (TNM) STAGING

T

Tx:	Primary tumor cannot be assessed
T0:	No evidence of primary tumor
Tis:	Carcinoma in situ[a]
T1:	Tumor invades the submucosa
T2:	Tumor invades the muscularis propria
T3:	Tumor invades the subserosa, serosa or into pericolic/perirectal fat
T4:	Tumor invades the visceral peritoneum and adjacent organs/structures

N

Nx:	Lymph nodes cannot be assessed
N0:	No evidence of lymph node metastasis
N1:	Metastasis in 1 to 3 adjacent mesenteric lymph nodes
N2:	Metastasis in ≥4 mesenteric lymph nodes
N3:	Metastasis into the lymph nodes along the course of a named vascular trunk

M

Mx:	Presence of distant metastasis cannot be assessed
M0:	No evidence of metastasis
M1:	Distant metastasis

[a]Tis includes cancer cells confined within the glandular basement membrane (intraepithelial) or lamina propria (intramucosal) with no extension through the muscularis mucosa into the submucosa.
Modified from Beahrs OH, Henson DE, Hutler RVP, et al (eds). Colon and Rectum. In: Handbook of Staging of Cancer, 4th ed. Phildelphia, PA: JB Lippincott, 1992:95

and the translation of all other systems into a standard format (Table 42–6).

The significance of TNM staging in predicting survival for cancer of the colon was shown clearly by its correlation with survival.[179,180]

Other Prognosticators In Colon Cancer

Degree of Tumor Differentiation. The trend toward better survival is observed in patients with well-differentiated colon cancer. The 5 year survival rate of well-differentiated colon and colorectal cancers is reported to be 71% and 55%, respectively.[181] The difference, however, was statistically insignificant. In another study analyzing 306 patients with nodal positive colon cancer, the degree of tumor differentiation was shown to be a significant prognosticator in a univariate analysis, but not in a multivariate analysis.[182] Similar observations were made in a group of 745 patients with rectal cancer.[178]

Tumor Cell DNA Content. Determination of DNA ploidy was shown to be a better prognosticator of recurrence and survival rates than the degree of tumor differentiation.[183–187] Subgroup analysis showed ploidy exerted an effect in patients with stage B tumors, mobile tumors, better-differentiated tumors, and in patients over 65

years of age.[187] The definitive role of ploidy determination in prognosis, however, has not been established.

Lymphatic/Blood Vessel Invasion. In a population-based study including 134 patients with colorectal cancer, the lymphatic infiltration was found to be insignificant in affecting survival.[181] Cohen and associates observed similar findings.[182] In contrast, blood vessel invasion was found by Corman and associates to adversely affect the survival of patients with colorectal cancer. The effect is particularly prominent in patients with Dukes' B lesions.[172] Michelassi and associates found vascular and lymphatic microinvasion to be one of the independent prognosticators of survival in 603 patients with colon cancer.[188]

Obstructing and Perforating Colon Cancer

These conditions are associated with high perioperative morbidity, mortality and poor long-term survival.[148,149,154,160]

Age

Young individuals with colorectal cancer are thought to have poor prognosis. Recalde and associates reported a 5 year survival rate of 13% in a group of colon cancer patients 35 years of age or younger.[189] Sanfelippo and Beahrs reported a slightly better 5 year survival rate of 39% among 118 patients 40 years of age or younger.[190] Very few young patients are diagnosed at an early stage. A majority of young colorectal cancer patients were found to have Dukes' C and D disease. Thus, delayed diagnosis may play an important role in the poor survivorship among young patients. Another mechanism that has been suggested is the intrinsic aggressiveness of the disease in young individuals.[191–193] Many young patients were found to have poorly differentiated tumor of the mucinous type. DNA content does not seem to play a role in young patients with colorectal cancer.[183]

TABLE 42–6. COMPARISON OF VARIOUS STAGE CLASSIFICATIONS WITH TNM SYSTEM

TNM Stage[180]	T	N	M	Dukes'[175]	Astler-Coller[177]
0	Tis	N0	M0		
I	T1	N0	M0	A	A
	T2	N0	M0		B1
II	T3	N0	M0	B	B2
	T4	N0	M0		
III	Any T	N1	M0	C	C1, C2
	Any T	N2, N3	M0		
IV	Any T	Any N	M1	D	D

Blood Transfusion

Studies suggest that the recurrence rate and survivals are adversely affected by the number of units of blood transfused.[194,195] Opinions as to whether the adverse effect of blood transfusion is independent of other covariants are divided. Stephenson and associates, and others, reported that the risk from blood transfusion was significant even when other variables such as type of resection, extent of disease, age, gender, Dukes' stage and tumor differentiation were controlled.[194,196,197] Others found no direct link between significant transfusions and prognosis.[198–200]

Although there is no consensus regarding the impact of blood transfusion on survival, hemostasis during surgery should be secured maximally to avoid blood transfusion. While all other prognosticators are determined by the disease or the patient, blood transfusion may be partially controlled by surgeons.

Adjuvant Treatment for Colon Cancer

From the survival statistics of colon cancer, it is clear that curative surgery alone is not sufficient in individuals at increased risk of recurrence. The National Institutes of Health Consensus Conference on Colorectal Cancer Treatment suggested that the pathologic staging is the most important determinant of the risk of recurrence and survival. Stage II colon cancer with an elevated CEA preoperatively and stage III colon cancer are indications for adjuvant chemotherapy. The other prognosticators, such as ploidy and S-phase fraction are not used as indicators for adjuvant therapy. Colon cancer and rectal cancer are considered differently in adjuvant therapy, because patterns of failure are different. Colon cancer tends to recur in the peritoneal cavity, liver, or in distant sites. The most common adjuvant therapy for colon cancer is chemotherapy. Immunotherapy also has been employed, but is more experimental.

Adjuvant treatment with 5-FU and levamisole was shown to be effective for colon cancer, particularly Dukes' C disease. A prospectively randomized trial was conducted by the North Central Cancer Treatment Group and the Mayo Clinic (Protocol #784852). The study included three arms: surgery alone, surgery with levamisole, and surgery with 5-FU and levamisole. Among 408 patients with Dukes' B2, 3 and C1–3, 387 patients had colon cancer. Levamisole was given at 150 mg orally 3 days a week every other week for 1 year. 5-FU was given at 450 mg/m^2 daily for 5 days as a loading dose, followed by a weekly injection of 5-FU starting on day 28. The study showed improved overall and disease-free survival (DFS) in patients treated with either levamisole or 5-FU and levamisole (Table 42–7, Figs 42–5A, B).[201,202] The results of this study were subsequently confirmed by a national intergroup study with participation of the

NCCTG, the Eastern Cooperative Oncology Group, and the Southwest Cooperative Oncology Group. Rectal cancers were excluded. After enrollment of 1300 patients and a median follow-up of 3 years., Moertel and associates reported that the combination of levamisole plus 5-FU resulted in a statistically significant reduction in tumor recurrence. The DFS was 63% vs 47% for surgery alone. The survival was improved as well (71% vs 55% for surgery alone). The estimated reduction in cancer recurrence was 41% and the reduction of the overall death rate was 33%.[203] Subsequent studies including the National Surgical Adjuvant Breast and Bowel Project (NSABP): C03, C04 and C05 were designed to determine the benefit of adding leucovorin to 5-FU and levamisole and of adding interferon to 5-FU-leucovorin in patients with Stages B2 and C colon cancer.

Other innovative treatments, such as the adjuvant immunotherapy in the form of tumor targeting monoclonal antibodies and autologous tumor vaccines, have been studied in patients with colorectal cancer. In such carcinomas, many tumor-associated antigens (TAA) have been described. These include CO 17-1A, TAG72, CA 19-9, CEA, L6, and 28A32. The monoclonal antibodies against these TAAs all have been studied clinically.[204–208] All of the antibodies employed were of mouse origin, with the exception of 28A32, which is a monoclonal human IgM. Although the toxicities of antibody treatment were shown to be minimal, the therapeutic effect was also marginal, with a reported response rate of 20% to 30%.[209,210] The proposed mechanisms of antibody-mediated tumor cell cytotoxicities are antibody-dependent cellular cytotoxicity, complement-dependent cytotoxicity and anti-idiotypic responses. Antibodies conjugated with toxins, drugs, and radioisotopes may prove to be more effective than the antibody alone.

Another form of adoptive immunotherapy is the administration of in vitro expanded cytotoxic T cells with

TABLE 42–7. DISEASE-FREE SURVIVAL (DFS) AND SURVIVAL RATES IN NCCTG-784852

	3 Year			5 Year		
		Levamisole			*Levamisole*	
	Control	*(L)*	*L/5-FU*	*Control*	*(L)*	*L/5-FU*
DFS						
Total	54	61	67	45	58	59
Dukes' B	73	78	84	58	78	78
Dukes' C	44	54	57	37	48	48
SURVIVAL						
Total	66	74	79	55	59	62
Dukes' B	89	86	96	78	78	80
Dukes' C	66	68	70	42	59	61

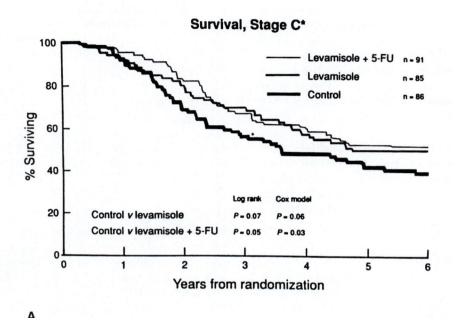

A

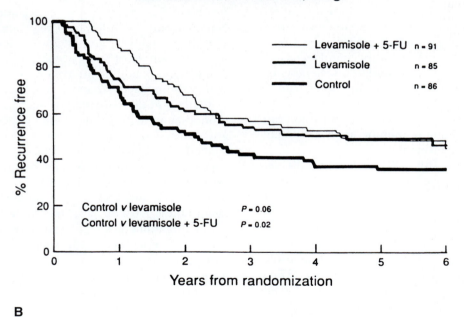

B

Figure 42–5. Survival of patients with Dukes' C colon cancer by postoperative adjuvant therapy consisting of 5-FU and levamisole. **A**. Improved overall survival. **B**. Disease-free survival. (From Laurie JA, Moertel CG, Fleming T, et al. Surgical adjuvant therapy for large bowel carcinoma: an evaluation of levamisole and the combination of levamisole and 5-fluorouracil. A study of the North Central Cancer Treatment Group and Mayo Clinic. *J Clin Oncol* 1989;7:1447)

cytokine.[211] A recent study used a combination of in vivo and in vitro stimulation of LAK cells by IL-2.[212] The overall response rate in patients with advanced colorectal carcinoma was 16%. The mortality was reported to be 1%; treatment-associated toxicities were significant.[213] The proposed mechanisms of the antitumor effects of IL-2 and LAK therapy are MCH class II-associated tumor cell kill and macrophage activation.[214,215]

Active specific immunizations also were studied in patients with colorectal cancer. One study reported a vaccine combination of neuraminidase-modified autologous tumor cells and BCG[216] and another study used the autologous tumor cells modified by Newcastle disease virus.[217] Both studies failed to show any effect on the disease-free survival or overall survival. Hoover and Hana used cryopreserved autologous tumor cells admixed with BCG as the vaccine in patients with stages II and III disease after curative surgery.[218] They were able to demonstrate a significant improvement in disease-free survival in patients with colonic cancer. The beneficial effect may be associated with the induction of cell-mediated antitumor immunity. The major drawback of using autologous tumor cells is the source of vaccines that restricts the clinical applicability. Cell-free vaccines or genetically engineered vaccines are being developed to substitute for the vaccines using tumor cells.

Adjuvant radiation has a more limited role in treating colonic cancer than in rectal cancer. Recent studies suggest that local failure after resection of colon cancer increases with fixation of the colon cancer, B3, C2, or C3 disease.[219,220] The experience of the Massachusetts General Hospital showed that among 533 patients with curative colon resection, the local failure was closely correlated to the stage of disease.[221–223] Postoperative tumor-bed irradiation may have a role in decreasing the intra-abdominal recurrence.[224–226] Obstructing and perforating colon cancer may be another indication for postoperative irradiation.[227]

Treatment of Metastatic Disease

Treatment for Liver Metastases. The use of CEA measurement and CT scanning, and recently MRI, in the follow-up of patients with colon cancer has identified an increasing number of liver metastases. If the disease is anatomically resectable with good margins and allows the preservation of enough liver function after hepatectomy, liver resection is the treatment of choice. In well-selected patients, the 5 year survival rate after a curative hepatectomy is approximately 25%, and the surgical mortality is reported to be 5% or less.[228–234] On the other hand, when multiple, bilobar tumors or extrahepatic metastases are present, liver resection is not indicated.

The long-term survival of patients with liver metastases is affected by the extent of liver involvement, the number of metastases, and the pathologic stage of the primary colon cancer.[228–235] Diffuse liver metastases are commonly treated by systemic chemotherapy.[236,237] Portal vein infusion has been shown to be ineffective. Hepatic arterial infusion of 5-FU or FUDR, on the other hand, has been shown to achieve a greater response than systemic treatment or portal vein infusion.[238–249] Occasionally, cryosurgery may play a role in treating patients with unresectable liver metastases.[250–253]

Treatment for Extrahepatic Metastases. The nonhepatic intra-abdominal recurrence of carcinoma of the colon accounts for 15% to 20% of first recurrences.[254,255] Isolated local-regional recurrence accounts for 5% to 19% of colon recurrences.[256–258] Complete resection may result in a 5 year survival rate of 30%.[259] Isolated pulmonary metastases occur in 2% of 4% of patients with recurrences. Approximately half of these patients may have pulmonary metastases resected. Long-term survival is influenced by the disease-free interval, stage of primary tumor, number, and size of the lung metastases. The 5 year survival rates were reported at 20 to 40%.[260–265]

Follow-up of Colon Cancer

The objective of follow-up is for early detection of a recurrence or a metachronous carcinoma that can be treated surgically for cure. The follow-up program in general consists of a periodic history and physical examination, FOB, CBC, liver function tests, tumor markers, colonoscopy, and CXR. CT scans of the abdomen and pelvis are not part of the routine follow-up. They may be included if the primary tumor appears to be locoregionally advanced or when the tumor markers or liver function is abnormally elevated.

The clinical check-up, including history, physical examination,[266] FOB[267] and blood studies, is usually scheduled every 3 months, in the first 3 years, and every 6 months for an additional 2 years. The serum or plasma tumor markers are studied every 8 weeks by some investigators[268] and monthly by others[269] for 3 years and then every 3 months for 2 more years. Beart and O'Connell suggest that the CEA level is the most sensitive indicator of recurrence.[267] Sugarbaker and associates demonstrated that CEA elevation was the first sign of recurrence in 67% of the cases.[270] The optimum frequency of CEA measurement has not been determined. Other tumor markers, such as CA 19-9 and TAG72,[271] also were studied. The role of these tumor markers in the follow-up program has not been clearly established. Colonoscopy is an important component of the program. Colonoscopy is a safeguard for detecting anastomosis recurrence, missed synchronous lesion, and metachronous tumors at an early stage. Again, different schedules have been employed. The first postoperative colonsocopy should be performed within 6 to 12 months of the surgery, with subsequent yearly examinations for two additional years. The examination may become less frequent, every 2 to 3 years thereafter. The most important time for follow-up is the first 2 to 3 years after colon resection, which includes 80% to 90% of all recurrences.[269,272] For distant sites, yearly CXR is required.[272] Others advocate more frequent studies.[267,273,274] There has been no definitive study to show that a more frequent CXR is associated with an improved survival.

NONADENOCARCINOMA MALIGNANCIES OF THE COLON

Carcinoid

Carcinoid tumor has been found throughout the gastrointestinal tract. The most common sites are the appendix, jejunum, and ileum, which account for 65% of all carcinoids. The rectum is the next most frequent site, accounting for 18% of cases. Other gastrointestinal tract sites, including the duodenum, stomach, colon, and Meckel's diverticulum, account for approximately 10% of carcinoid tumors. The extragastrointestinal sites of the bronchus, thyroid, pancreas, ovary and testes account for the rest. Malignant carcinoid syndrome of colonic origin does not occur unless there are liver metastases.[275] This is due to the draining of serotonin from the gastrointestinal tract to the liver, where it becomes inactivated. Vasoactive substances released from the liver metastases pass directly into the hepatic vein and cause systemic manifestation of the malignant carcinoid syndrome. The local symptoms are intestinal obstruction and bleeding. When carcinoid tumor is suspected, the chemical markers, such as serum serotonin and urinary 5-hydroxyindole acetic acid, should be measured. A small bowel series and colonoscopy also should be part of the workup. Most carcinoids are completely submucosal. Biopsy, therefore, may not be diagnostic. A CT scan of the abdomen is helpful for evaluating liver metastases. Colon resection is indicated for carcinoids of the colon. When liver metastases are present, curative resection is preferred. Palliative debulking is beneficial when the tumor is nonresectable. The 5 year survival rate was reported to be 57% for patients with localized carcinoid tumors of the gastrointestinal tract,[276] and from 21% to 38% for patients with metastatic carcinoid. Other treatment modalities include hepatic arterial embolization and chemotherapy with streptozotocin and 5-fluorouracil.

Sarcoma

Sarcomas of the colon are rare and account for less than 0.1% of all colorectal malignancies. The most common type of colonic sarcoma is leiomyosarcoma.[277–281] Other types, such as fibrosarcoma and angiosarcoma are rare.[282,283] A low-grade desmoid tumor may involve the large bowel.[284] Kaposi's sarcoma of the large bowel, associated with the AIDS virus, also have been reported recently.[285]

Wide resection of colon sarcoma is the treatment of choice. The incidence of mesenteric nodal metastases has been reported to be between 5% and 8%. Omental resection also has been advocated because of the evidence of metastasis.[286] The dominant sites of metastases are the liver and peritoneum. Lung metastases are relatively rare. Patients with sarcomas of the colon are likely to have metastatic disease and high-grade tumor[277,287]; hence, the prognosis is poor. Berkeley reported a 1 year survival rate of 33%.[287] Rao and associates demonstrated a 5 year survival rate of 10%.[288] A similarly low 5 year survival rate of 25% was recently reported by Meijer and associates.[277] The role of adjuvant chemotherapy in patients with curative resection of colonic sarcoma is uncertain because of the rarity of the disease.

Lymphoma

Primary lymphoma of the colon accounts for 0.5% of colonic malignancies. Seventy percent of lymphomas of the colon are found in the cecum. The next most common sites are the rectum and ascending colon.[289–291] The gross appearance of the tumor may be annular or just thickened bowel wall. The majority of the colon lymphomas are single (86%), but can be multiple or diffuse in nature.[289]

The symptoms are similar to those of colon cancer: abdominal pain, change in bowel habits, bleeding and obstruction. Colonoscopy with submucosal biopsy may be diagnostic. Once the diagnosis is suspected or made, staging should include a CBC, liver function tests, CXR, bone marrow biopsy, CT scan of the abdomen and lymphangiogram, in addition to a thorough history and physical examination. All primary lymphomas of the colon should have the involved colon and mesentery resected. In addition, liver biopsy, splenectomy, and biopsy of nonmesenteric lymph nodes are recommended. Radiation is beneficial for incomplete resection or nonresectable disease. Chemotherapy is recommended for patients with nodal spread or systemic disease. Histologically, lymphomas of the colon are similar to lymphomas of other parts of the gastrointestinal tract. Most of them are non-Hodgkin's lymphoma. The frequencies of histocytic type, lymphocytic type, mixed type and Hodgkin's disease are reported to be 43%, 29%, 14%, and 3.5%, respectively. The survival of patients after curative resection in patients with Hodgkin's lymphoma was reported to be 100%. This rate is in contrast to a ten year survival rate of 21.9% in patients with mixed-cell type. The patients with either histocytic or lymphocytic lymphomas were reported to have a 10 year survival rate of 40%.[292] The other poor prognosticators are nonresectability, tumor diameter >5 cm, extraluminal involvement, and nodal metastases.

REFERENCES

1. Grosfeld JI, West KW. Generalized juvenile polyps coli. *Arch Surg* 1986;121:530

2. Cronkhite LW Jr, Canada WJ. Generalized gastrointestinal polyposis. *N Engl J Med* 1955;252:1011

3. Johnson GK, Soergel KH, Hensley GT, et al. Cronkhite-Canada syndrome: gastrointestinal pathophysiology and morphology. *Gastroenterology* 1972;63:140

4. Jeghers H, McKusick VA, Katz KH. Generalized intestinal polyposis and melanin spots of the oral mucosa lips and digit. *N Engl J Med* 1949;41:933

5. Dormandy TL. Gastrointestinal polyposis with mucocutaneous pigmentation (Peutz-Jegher's syndrome). *N Engl J Med* 1957;256:1093

6. Spigelman AD, Murdey V, Phillips RKS. Cancer and the Peutz-Jegher's syndrome. *Gut* 1989;30:1588

7. Giardiello FM, Welsh SB, Hamilton SR, et al. Increased risk of cancer in Peutz-Jegher's Syndrome. *N Engl J Med* 1987;316:1511

8. Cappell MS, Forde KA. Special clustering of mutliple hyperplastic adenomatous and malignant colonic polyps in individual patients. *Dis Colon Rectum* 1989;32:641

9. Kusunoki M, Fujita S, Sakanoue Y, et al. Disappearance of hyperplastic polyposis after resection of rectal cancer. *Dis Colon Rectum* 1991;34:829

10. Waye JD, Bilotta JJ. Rectal hyperplastic polyps: now you see them, now you don't—a differential point. *Am J Gastroenterol* 1990;86:1557

11. Church JM, Fazio VW, Jones IT. Small colorectal polyps: are they worth treating. *Dis Colon Rectum* 1988;31:50

12. Corman ML. Polypoid disease. In: Corman ML (ed), *Colon and Rectal Surgery,* 3rd ed. Philadelphia, PA: JP Lippincott; 1993:436

13. Muto T, Bussey HJ, Morson BC. The evolution of cancer of the colon and rectum. *Cancer* 1975;36:2251

14. Day DW, Morson BC. The polyp problem, In: Morson BC (ed), *The Pathogenesis of Colorectal Cancer.* Philadelphia, PA: WB Saunders; 1978:43

15. Shinya H, Wolff WI. Morphology, anatomic distribution and cancer potential of colonic polyps: an analysis of 7,000 polyps endoscopically removed. *Ann Surg* 1979; 190:679

16. Herzog P, Holtermuller KH, Preiss J, et al. Fecal blood loss in patients with colonic polyps: a comparison of measurement with 51-chromium labeled erythrocytes and with hemoccult test. *Gastroenterology* 1982;83:957

17. Fenoglio CM, Kay GI, Lane I. Distribution of human colonic lymphatics in normal, hyperplastic and adenomatous tissue. *Gastroenterology* 1973;64:51

18. Gordon MS, Cohen AM. Management of invasive carcinoma in pedunculated colorectal polyps. *Oncology* 1989; 3:99

19. Colacchio TA, Forde KA, Scantlebury VP. Endoscopic polypectomy: Inadequate treatment for invasive colorectal carcinoma. *Ann Surg* 1981;194:704

20. Cranley JP, Petras RE, Carey WD, et al. When is endoscopic polypectomy adequate therapy for colonic polyps containing invasive carcinoma? *Gastroenterology* 1986;91: 419

21. Kaneko M. On pedunculated adenomatous polyps of the colon and rectum with particular reference to their malignant potential. *Mt Sinai J Med* 1972;39:103

22. Coutsoftides T, Sivak MV, Benjamin SP. Colonoscopy and management of polyps containing invasive carcinoma. *Ann Surg* 1978;188:638

23. Coverlizza MD, Risio M, Ferrari A, et al. Colorectal adenomas containing invasive carcinoma. *Cancer* 1989;64: 1937

24. Ellis LM, Bland KI, Copeland EM. Benign and premalignant lesions of the colon and rectum. In: Moody FG, Carey LC, Jones RS, et al (eds), *Surgical Treatment of Digestive Disease.* 2nd ed. Chicago, IL: Yearbook Medical; 1990

25. Fenoglio CM, Pascal RR. Colorectal adenomas and cancer: pathologic relationships. *Cancer* 1982;50:2600

26. Hermanek P. Polypectomy in the colorectum: histologic and oncological aspects. *Endoscopy* 1983;15:158

27. Morson BC, Whiteway JE, Jones EE, et al. Histopathology and prognosis of malignant colorectal polyps treated by endoscopic polypectomy. *Gut* 1984;35:437

28. Haggitt RC, Glotzbach RE, Soffer EE, et al. Prognostic factors in colorectal carcinomas arising adenomas: implication for lesions removed by endoscopic polypectomy. *Gastroenterology* 1985;89:328

29. Winawer S, Zauber AG, O'Brien MJ, et al. Randomized comparison of surveillance intervals after colonoscopic removal of newly diagnosed adenomatous polyps. *N Engl J Med* 1993;328:901

30. Ekelund GR. On cancer and polyps of colon and rectum. *Acta Pathol Microbiol Immunol Scand* 1963;59:165

31. Morson BC, Bussey HJR. Magnitude of risk for cancer in patients with colorectal adenomas. *Br J Surg* 1985; Sept 72 Suppl: 523

32. Stryker SJ, Wolff BG, Culp CE, et al. Natural history of untreated colonic polyps. *Gastroenterology* 1987;93:1009

33. Shimada T, Ikegami M, et al. Early colorectal carcinoma with special reference to the development de novo. *Cancer* 1989;64:1138

34. Kune GA, Kune S, Watson LF. History of colorectal polypectomy and risk of subsequent colorectal cancer. *Br J Surg* 1987;74:1064

35. Eide TJ. Remnants of adenomas in colorectal carcinomas. *Cancer* 1983;51:1866

36. Kusunoki M, Sakanoue Y, Hatada T, et al. Protein kinase C activity in human colonic adenoma and colorectal carcinoma. *Cancer* 1992;69:24

37. Gilbertsen VA. Proctosigmoidoscopy and polypectomy in reducing the incidence of rectal cancer. *Cancer* 1974;34: 936

38. Corvisart L. Hypertrophic partielle de la muquese intestine. *Bull Soc Anat Paris* 1874;22:400

39. Cripps. Two cases of disseminated polyposis of the colon. *Trans Pathol. Soc. Lond* 1882;33:165

40. Dukes CE. The hereditary factor in polyposis intestine or multiple adenomata. *Cancer Rev Br* 1930;5:241

41. Lockhart-Mummery JP. Cancer and heredity. *Lancet* 1925; i:427

42. Bodmer WF, Bailey CJ, Bodmer J, et al. Localization of the gene for familial adenomatous polyposis on chromosome 5. *Nature* 1987;328:614

43. Handford H. Disseminated polyps of the large intestine. *Tas Pathol Soc Land* 1890;41:133

44. Bussey HJR. Familial Polyposis Coli. Baltimore, MD: The Johns Hopkins University Press; 1975:47

45. Gingold BS, Jagelman DG. Sparing the rectum in familial polyposis: causes for failure. *Surgery* 1981;89:314

46. Bussey HJR, Eyers AA, Ritchie SM, et al. The rectum in adenomatous polyposis: the St. Mark's policy. *Br J Surg* 1985;72:529

47. Skinner MA, Tyler D, Branum GD, et al: Subtotal colectomy for familial polyposis: A clinical series and review of the literature. *Arch Surg* 1990;125:621

48. Ambroze WL, Dozois RR, Pemberton JH, et al. Familial adenomatous polyposis: results following ileal pouch-anal anastomosis and ileorectostomy. *Dis Colon Rectum* 1992; 35:12

49. Morgan RA, Manning PB, Coran AG. Experience with the straight endorectal pull through for the management of ulcerative colitis and familial polyposis in children and adults. *Ann Surg* 1987;206:595

50. Shoetz DJ, Coller JA, Veidenheimer MC. Ileo-anal reservoir for ulcerative colitis and familial polyposis. *Arch Surg* 1986;121:404

51. Bess MA, Adson MA, Elvebach LR, et al. Rectal cancer following colectomy for polyposis. *Arch Surg* 1980;115:460

52. Gardner EJ: A genetic and clinical study of intestinal polyposis: a predisposing factor for carcinoma of the colon and rectum. *Am J Hum Genet* 1951;3:167

53. Wennstrom J, Pierce ER, McKusick VA. Hereditary benign and malignant lesions of the large bowel. *Cancer* 1974; 34:850

54. Welch CE, Hedberg SE. *Polypoid Lesions of the Gastrointestinal Tract.* vol II, 2nd ed. Philadelphia, PA: Saunders; 1975:186

55. Painter TA, Jagelman DG. Adrenal adenomas and adrenal carcinoma in association with hereditary adenomatosis of the colon and rectum. *Cancer* 1985;55:2001

56. Jagelman DG. Extracolonic manifestations of familial adenomatous polyposis. *Oncology* 1991;5(2):23

57. Turcot J, Despres JP, St. Pierre F. Malignant tumors of the central nervous system associated with familial polyposis of the colon and rectum. *Dis Colon Rectum* 1959;2:465

58. Kropilak M, Jagelman DG, Fazio VW, et al. Brain tumors in familial adenomatous polyposis. *Dis Colon Rectum* 1989; 9:778

59. Boring CC, Squires TS, Tong T. Cancer statistics, 1993. *CA Cancer J Clin* 1993;43:7

60. Bland KI. Malignant diseases of the colon, In: Levine B. et al. (ed) *Current Practice of Surgery,* vol 3. New York, NY: Churchill, Livingstone: 1993:1–45

61. Corman ML. Carcinoma of the colon, In: Corman ML (ed) *Colon and Rectal Surgery,* 3rd ed. Philadelphia, PA: Lippincott; 1993:487

62. Cutler SJ, Young JL Jr. The third national cancer survey: incidence data. cancer morbidity. Natl Cancer Inst Monograph 1975;41:1

63. Young JL Jr. Devesa SS, Cutler SJ. Incidence of cancer in the United States blacks. *Cancer Res* 1975;35:3523

64. Creagan ET, Fraumini JF Jr. Cancer mortality among American Indians. *J Natl Cancer Inst* 1972;49:959

65. Willet WC, MacMahon B. Diet and cancer—an overview. *N Engl J Med* 1984;310:697

66. Willet WC. The search for the cause of breast and colon cancer. *Nature* 1989;338:389

67. Painter NS, Burkitt DP. Diverticular disease of the colon: a deficiency disease of Western civilization. *Br Med J* 1971;2:450

68. Fleiszer D, MacFarlane J, Murray D, et al. Protective effect of dietary fiber against chemically induced bowel tumors in rats. *Lancet* 1978;ii:552

69. Hill MJ, Drasar BS, Aries V, et al. Fecal bile-acids and clostridia in patients with cancer of the large bowel. *Lancet* 1975;i:535

70. Nigro ND. A strategy for prevention of cancer of the large bowel. *Dis Colon Rectum* 1982;25:755

71. Hill MJ, Draser BS, Aries V, et al. Bacteria and etiology of cancer of large bowel. *Lancet* 1971;i:95

72. Burkitt DP. Epidemiology of cancer of the colon and rectum. *Cancer* 1971;28:3

73. Pollack ES, Nomura AMU, et al. Prospective study of alcohol consumption and cancer. *N Engl J Med* 1984; 310:617

74. Phillips RL. Role of lifestyle and dietary habits in risk of cancer among Seventh-Day Adventists. *Cancer Res* 1975; 35(suppl H, part 2):3513

75. Lynch HT. The surgeon and colorectal cancer genetics. *Arch Surg* 1990;125:698

76. Mulvihill JJ. The frequency of hereditary large bowel cancer. In: Ingall JR, Mastromarino AJ (eds), *Prevention of Hereditary Large Bowel Cancer.* New York, NY: Liss; 1983:61

77. Jdrvinen HJ. Epidemiology of familial adenomatous polyposis in Finland: impact of family screening on the colorectal cancer rate and survival. *Gut* 1992;33:357

78. Vasen HFA, Mecklin J-P, Kahn PM, et al. The international collaborative group on hereditary nonpolyposis colorectal cancer. *Dis Colon Rectum* 1991;34:424

79. Lynch HT, Lanspa S, Smyrk T, et al. Hereditary nonpolyposis colorectal cancer (Lynch syndrome I & II). Genetics, pathology, natural history, and cancer control. Part 1. *Cancer Genet Cytogenet* 1991;53:143

80. Mecklin JP, Jdrvinen HJ. Tumor spectrum in cancer family syndrome (hereditary nonpolyposis colorectal cancer). *Cancer* 1991;68:1109

81. Marx J. New colon cancer gene discovered. *Science* 1993; 260:751

82. Peltomiiki P, Aaltonen LA, Sistonen P, et al. Genetic mapping of a locus predisposing to human colorectal cancer. *Science* 1993;26:810

83. Aaltonen LA, Peltomdki P, Leach FS, et al. Clues to pathogenesis of familial colorectal cancer. *Science* 1993;260:812

84. Thibodeau SN, Bren G, Schaid D. Microsatellite instability in cancer of the proximal colon. *Science* 1993;260:816

85. Levin B, Murphy GP. Revision in American Cancer Society recommendations for the early detection of colorectal cancer. *CA* 1992;42:296

86. Chang HR. Cancer Screening, In: Moosa AR, Schimpff SC, Robson MC (eds), *Comprehensive Textbook of Oncology,* 2nd ed, Baltimore, MD: Williams and Wilkins;1992:188

87. Petrelli N, Palmer M, Michalek A, et al. Massive screening for colorectal cancer. *Arch Surg* 1990;125:1049

88. Wanebo HJ, Fang WL, Mills AS, et al. Colorectal cancer—a blueprint for disease control through screening by primary care physicians. *Arch Surg* 1986;121:1347

89. Winawer SJ, Andrews M, Flehinger B, et al. Progress report on controlled trial of fecal occult testing for the detection of colorectal cancer neoplasia. *Cancer* 1980;45:2959

90. Gilbertsen VA, McHugh R, Schuman L, et al. The early detection of colorectal cancers: a preliminary report of the results of the occult blood study. *Cancer* 1980;45:2899

91. Hardcastle JD, Armitage NC, Chamberlin D, et al. Fecal occult blood screening for colorectal cancer in the general population: results of a controlled trial. *Cancer* 1986;58:397

92. Johnson MG, Jolly PC. Analysis of mass rectal cancer screening program for cost effectiveness. *Am J Surg* 1987;154:261

93. Iales LG, Friedman GD, Collen MF. Evaluating periodic multiphasic health checkup: a controlled trial. *J Chron Dis* 1979;32:385

94. Friedman GD, Collen MF, Friedman BH. Multiphasic health checkup evaluation: a 16 year follow-up. *J Chron Dis* 1986;38:453

95. Gilbertsen VA. Proctosigmoidoscopy and polypectomy in reducing the incidence of rectal cancer. *Cancer* 1974;34:936

96. Hertz RE, Deddish MR, Day E. Value of periodic examinations in detecting cancer of the rectum and colon. *Postgrad Med* 1960;29:290

97. Hertz RE. International symposium on colorectal cancer, New York, March 1979. *Int J Cancer* 1978;21:418

98. Muller CA, Lopez JL. Routine and periodic sigmoidoscopy in the detection and prevention of malignancies of the large bowel. In: Nieburgs HE (ed), *Prevention and Detection of Cancer. Part II Detection*, vol 2. *Cancer Detection in Specific Sites*, 1980:2115

99. Atkin WS, Cuzick J, Nonhover JMA, et al. Prevention of colorectal cancer by once-only sigmoidoscopy. *Lancet* 1993;341:736

100. Gilbert DA, Shaneyfeld SL, Mahler AK. The National ASGE colonoscopy survey: preliminary analysis of complications of colonscopy. *Gastrointest Endosc* 1983;29:191

101. Gelfand DW. Complications of gastrointestinal radiologic procedures: II. complications of routine fluoroscopic studies. *Gastrointest Radiol* 1980;15:293

102. Beart RW, O'Connel MJ. Postoperative follow-up of patients with cancer of the colon. *Mayo Clin Proc* 1983;58:361

103. Durand-Zaleski I, Rymer JC, Roudot-Thoraval F, et al. Reducing unnecessary laboratory use with new test form: example of tumor markers. *Lancet* 1993;342:150

104. Gold P, Freedman SO. Demonstration of tumor-specific antigens in human colonic carcinoma by immunologic tolerance and absorption techniques. *J Exp Med* 1965;121:439

105. Itzkowitz SH, Kim YS. New carbohydrate-tumor markers. *Gastroenterology* 1986;92:491

106. Ravikumar TS, Steele G Jr. Conventional and new tumor markers in the diagnosis and therapy of colorectal cancer. *Surg Rounds* 1987;10:30

107. Beatty JD, Romero C, Brown PW, et al. Clinical value of CEA: diagnosis prognosis and follow-up of patients with cancer. *Arch Surg* 1979;114:563

108. Midire G, Amanti C, Consorti F, et al. Usefulness of preoperative CEA levels in the assessment of colorectal cancer patient stage. *J Surg Oncol* 1983;22:257

109. Staab HJ, Anderer FA, Brummendorf T, et al. Prognostic value of preoperative serum CEA level compared to clinical staging—I. colorectal carcinoma. *Br J Cancer* 1981;44:652

110. Wanebo HJ, Rao B, Pinsky CM, et al. Preoperative carcinoembryonic antigen level as a prognostic indicator in colorectal cancer. *N Engl J Med* 1983;299:257

111. Goslin R, Steel G, MacIntyre J, et al. The use of preoperative plasma CEA levels for the stratification of patients after curative resection of colorectal cancer. *Ann Surg* 1980;192:747

112. Moore TL, Dhar P, Zamcheck N, et al. Carcinoembryonic antigen(s) in liver disease—I. clinical and morphologic studies. *Gastroenterology* 1972;63:88

113. Lurie BB, Loewenstein MS, Zamcheck N. Elevated carcinoembryonic antigen levels and biliary tract obstruction. *JAMA* 1975;233:326

114. Zamcheck N. Carcinoembryonic antigen. Quantitative variations in increasing levels in benign and malignant digestive tract diseases. *Adv Intern Med* 1974;19:413

115. Stevens DP, Mackay IR. Increased carcinoembryonic antigen in heavy cigarette smokers. *Lancet* 1973;i:1238

116. Doerr RJ, Abdel-Nabi H, Krag D, et al. Radiolabeled antibody imaging in the management of colorectal cancer. Results of a multicenter clinical study. *Ann Surg* 1991;214:118

117. Collier BD, Abdel-Nabi H, Doerr RJ, et al. Immunoscintigraphy performed with In-111-labeled CYT-103 in the management of colorectal cancer: comparison with CT. *Radiology* 1992;185:179

118. Beatty JD, Hyams DM, Morton BA, et al. Impact of radiolabelled antibody imaging on management of colon cancer. *Am J Surg* 1989;157:13

119. Tempero M. Pitfalls in antibody imaging. *Cancer* 1993;71:4248

120. Amold MW, Schneebaum S, Berens A, et al. Radioimmunoguided surgery challenges traditional decision making in patients with primary colorectal cancer. *Surgery* 1992;112:624

121. Houchens D, Cote R, Saad A, et al. Presence of occult tumor detected by injected iodine125 labelled monoclonal antibody CC49. Proceedings of the Eighty-Third Annual Meeting of the American Association of Cancer Research 1992:317

122. Houchens D, Cote R, Nines R, et al. Radioimmunoguided surgery in colorectal cancer; histologic and immunohistochemical analysis of lymph nodes from patients injected with iodine-125 labelled monoclonal antibody CC49. Presented at the International Conference on Monoclonal and Immunoconjugated Antibodies. San Diego, CA March 5–7, 1992.

123. Clarke JS, Condon RE, Bartlett JG, et al. Preoperative oral antibiotics reduce septic complications of colon operation. *Ann Surg* 1977;186:251

124. Condon RE, Bartlett JG, Greenlee H, et al: Efficacy of

oral and systemic antibiotic prophylaxis in colorectal operations. *Arch Surg* 1983;118:496

125. Davis GR, Santa Ana CA, Morawski SG, et al. Development of a lavage solution associated with minimal water and electrolyte absorption on secretion. *Gastroenterology* 1980;78:991

126. Washington JA, Dearing WH, Judd ES, et al. Effect of preoperative antibiotic regimen on development of infection after intestinal surgery. *Ann Surg* 1974;180:567

127. Goldring J, McNaught W, Scott A, et al. Prophylactic oral antimicrobial agents in elective colon surgery. *Lancet* 1975;ii:997

128. Hojer H, Wetterfors J. Systemic prophylaxis with doxycycline in surgery of the colon and rectum. *Ann Surg* 1978;187:362

129. Grinnell RS, Distal intramucosal spread of carcinoma of the rectum and rectosigmoid. *Surg Gynecol Obstet* 1954;99:421

130. Williams NS. The rationale of preservation of the anal sphincter in patients with low rectal cancer. *Br J Surg* 1984;71:575

131. Brief DK, Brener BJ, Goldenkranz R, et al. An argument for the increased use of subtotal colectomy in the management of carcinoma of the colon. *Ann Surg* 1983;49:66

132. VonProhaska J, Govostis MC, Wasick M. Multiple organ resection for advanced carcinoma of the colon and rectum. *Surg Gynecol Obstet* 1953;97:177

133. Polk HC. Extended resection for selected adenocarcinoma of the large bowel. *Ann Surg* 1972;175:892

134. McGlone TP, Bernie WA, Elliot DW. Survival following extended resection for extracolonic invasion by colon cancer. *Arch Surg* 1982;117:595

135. Bonfanti G, Bozzetti F, Doci R, et al. Results of extended surgery for cancer of the rectum and sigmoid. *Br J Surg* 1982;69:305

136. Heslov SF, Frost DB. Extended resection for primary colorectal carcinoma involving adjacent organs or structures. *Cancer* 1988;62:1637

137. Curley SA, Carlson GW, Shumate CR, et al. Extended resection for locally advanced colorectal carcinoma. *Am J Surg* 1992;163:553

138. Landercasper J, Stolee RT, Steenlage E, et al. Treatment and outcome of right colon cancers adherent to adjacent organs of the abdominal wall. *Arch Surg* 1992;127:841

139. Lopez MJ, Manofo WW. Role of extended resection in the initial treatment of locally advanced colorectal carcinoma. *Surgery* 1993;113:365

140. Mendenhall WM, Bland KI, Pfaff WW, et al. Initially unresectable rectal adenocarcinoma treated with preoperative irradiation and surgery. *Ann Surg* 1987;205:41

141. Birnkrant A, Sampson J, Sugarbaker P. Ovarian metastasis from colorectal cancer. *Dis Colon Rectum* 1986;29:767

142. Mackeigan JM, Ferguson JA. Prophylactic oophorectomy and colorectal cancer in premenopausal patients. *Dis Colon Rectum* 1979;22:401

143. Cutait R, Lesser M, Enker W. Prophylactic oophorectomy in surgery for large bowel cancer. *Dis Colon Rectum* 1983;26:6

144. Stearns MW, Deddish M. Five year results of abdomino-

145. O'Brien PH, Newton BB, Metcalf JS, et al. Oophorectomy in women with carcinoma of the colon and rectum. *Surg Gynecol Obstet* 1981;153:827

146. Quan SHQ, Sehdev MK. Pelvic surgery concomitant with bowel resection for carcinoma. *Surg Clin North Am* 1974;54:882

147. MacKenzie S, Thompson SR, Baker LW. Management options in malignant obstruction of the left colon. *Surg Gynecol Obset* 1992;174:338

148. Greenlee HB, Pienkos EJ, Vanderbilt PC, et al. Acute large bowel obstruction. *Arch Surg* 1974;108:470

149. Vieder L, Tzur N, Huber M, et al. Management of obstructive carcinoma of the left colon. *Arch Surg* 1985;120:825

150. Buechter KJ, Boustany C, Caillouette R, et al. Surgical management of the acutely obstructed colon. *Am J Surg* 1988;156:163

151. Ohman U. Prognosis in patients with obstructing colorectal carcinoma. *Am J Surg* 1982;143:742

152. Dutton JW, Hreno A, Hampson LG, et al. Mortality and prognosis of obstructing carcinoma of the large bowel. *Am J Surg* 1976;131:36

153. Knaus WA, Draper EA, Wagner DP, et al. APACHE II: a severity of disease classification system. *Crit Care Med* 1985;13:818

154. Phillips RKS, Hittinger R, Fry JS, et al. Malignant large bowel obstruction. *Br J Surg* 1985;72:296

155. Fielding LP, Wells BW. Survival after primary and after staged resection for large bowel obstruction caused by cancer. *Br J Surg* 1974;61:16

156. Halevy A, Levi J, Orda R. Emergency subtotal colectomy: a new trend for obstructing carcinoma of the left colon. *Ann Surg* 1989;210:220

157. Cunliffe WJ, Hasleton PS, Tweedle DEF, et al. Incidence of synchronous and metachronous colorectal carcinoma. *Br J Surg* 1984;71:941

158. Bat L, Neumann G, Shemesh E. The association of synchronous neoplasm with occluding colorectal cancer. *Dis Colon Rectum* 1985;28:149

159. Crowder VH Jr, Cohn I Jr. Perforation in cancer of the colon and rectum. *Dis Colon Rectum* 1967;10:415–420

160. Glenn F, McSherry CK. Obstruction and perforation in colorectal cancer. *Ann Surg* 1971;92:173(6):938–992

161. Goligher JC, Smiddy FG. The treatment of acute obstruction or perforation with carcinoma of the colon and rectum. *Br J Surg* 1957;45:270

162. Kelly WE Jr, Brown PW, Lawrence W Jr, et al. Penetrating, obstructing and perforating carcinomas of the colon and rectum. *Arch Surg* 1981;116:381

163. Umpleby HC, Bristol JB, Rainey JB. Survival of 727 patients with single carcinomas of the large bowel. *Dis Colon Rectum* 1984;27:803

164. Feldman MA, Cotton RE, Gray WM. Carcinoma of the colon presenting as a left perinephric abscess. *Br J Surg* 1968;55:21

165. Finlay DB, Jones RY, James DC. Carcinomas of the colon presenting as a remote abscess. *Br J Surg* 1982;69:479

166. Krukowski ZH, Matheson NA. Emergency surgery for di-

verticular disease complicated by generalized fecal peritonitis: review. *Br J Surg* 1984;71:921

167. Umpleby HC, Williamson RCN. Survival in acute obstructing colorectal carcinoma. *Dis Colon Rectum* 1984;27: 299

168. Fowler DL, White SA. Laparoscopy-assisted sigmoid resection. *Surg Laparosc Endosc* 1991;1:183

169. Jacobs M, Verdja JC, Goldstein HS. Minimally invasive colon resection (laparoscopic colectomy). *Surg Laparosc Endosc* 1991;1:144

170. Greene FL, Olsen D, Petelin JB. Laparoscopic colectomy. *Laparosc Focus* 1992;1(3):1

171. Biggers OR, Ready RL, Beart RW. Risk of additional intraabdominal procedures at the time of colectomy. *Dis Colon Rectum* 1982;15:185

172. Corman ML, Veidenheimer MC, Coller JA. Colorectal carcinoma: a decade of experience at the Lahey Clinic. *Dis Colon Rectum* 1979;22:477

173. Turunen MJ, Peltokillio P. Surgical results in 657 patients. *Dis Colon Recum* 1983;26:606

174. Botsford TW, Aliapoulios MA, Curtis LE. Results of treatment of colorectal carcinoma at the Peter Bent Brigham Hospital. *Am J Surg* 1965;109:566

175. Dukes CE. The classification of cancer of the rectum. *J Pathol* 1932;35:323

176. Dukes CE, Bussey HJ. The spread of rectal cancer and its effect on prognosis. *Br J Cancer* 1958;12:309

177. Astler VA, Coller FA. The prognostic significance of direct extension of carcinoma of the colon and rectum. *Ann Surg* 1954;139:846

178. Fisher ER, Sass R, Palekar A, et al. Dukes' classification revisited: findings from the National Surgical Adjuvant Breast and Bowel Projects (NSABP Protocol R-01). *Cancer* 1989;64:2354

179. Beahrs OH, Henson DE, Hutler RVP, et al (eds): Colon and rectum. In: *Handbook for Staging of Cancer* 4th ed. Philadelphia, PA: JB Lippincott; 1992:95

180. Hutler RV, Sobin L. A universal staging system for cancer of the colon and rectum: let there be light. *Arch Pathol Lab Med* 1986;110:567

181. Ponz de Leon M, Sant M, Micheli A, et al. Clinical and pathologic prognostic indicators in colorectal cancer. *Cancer* 1992;69:626

182. Cohen AM, Tremiterra S, Candela F, et al. Prognosis of node positive colon cancer. *Cancer* 1991;67:1859

183. Heimann TM, Martinelli G, Szporn A, et al. Prognostic significance of DNA content abnormalities in young patients with colorectal cancer. *Ann Surg* 1989;210:792

184. Emdin SO, Stenling R, Roos G. Prognostic value of DNA content in colorectal carcinoma: a flow cytometric study with some methodologic aspects. *Cancer* 1987; 60:1282

185. Armitage NC, Robins RA, Evans DF, et al. The influence of tumor cell DNA abnormalities on survival in colorectal cancer. *Br J Surg* 1985;72:828

186. Armitage NC, Ballantyne KC, Sheffield JP, et al. A prospective evaluation of the effect of tumor cell DNA content on recurrence in colorectal cancer. *Cancer* 1991;67:2599

187. Galandiuk S, Wieand HS, Moetrel CG. Patterns of recurrence after curative resection of carcinoma of the colon and rectum. *Surg Gynecol Obstet* 1992;174:27

188. Michelassi F, Ayala JJ, Balestracci T, et al. Verification of a new clinicopathologic staging system for colorectal carcinoma. *Ann Surg* 1991;214:11

189. Recalde M, Holyoke ED, Elias EG. Carcinoma of the colon, rectum and anal canal in young patients. *Surg Gynecol Obstet* 1974;139:909

190. Sanfelippo PM, Beahrs OH. Carcinoma of the colon in patients under forty years of age. *Surg Gynecol Obstet* 1974;138:169

191. Palmer M, Petrelli NJ, Herrera L. Colorectal carcinoma in patients less than 40 years of age. *Dis Colon Rectum* 1991;34:343

192. Pitluk H, Poticha SM. Carcinoma of the colon and rectum in patients less than 40 years of age. *Surg Gynecol Obstet* 1983;157:335

193. Adloff M, Arnaud J-P, Schloegel M, et al. Colorectal cancer in patients under 40 years of age. *Dis Colon Rectum* 1986;29:322

194. Stephenson KR, Steinberg SM, Hughes KS, et al. Perioperative blood transfusions associated with decreased time to recurrence and diseases survival after resection of colorectal liver metastases. *Ann Surg* 1988;208:679

195. Wobbes T, Joosen KHG, Kuypers HHC, et al. The effect of packet cells and whole blood transfusions on survival after curative resection of colorectal carcinoma. *Dis Colon Rectum* 1989;32:743

196. Beynon J, Davies PW, Billings PJ, et al. Perioperative blood transfusion increases the risk of recurrence in colorectal cancer. *Dis Colon Rectum* 1989;32:975

197. Parrott NR, Lennard TWJ, Taylor RMR, et al. Effect of perioperative blood transfusion on recurrence of colorectal cancer. *Br J Surg* 1986;73:970

198. Tang R, Wang JY, Chien CRC, et al. The association between perioperative blood transfusion and survival of patients with colorectal cancer. *Cancer* 1993;72:341

199. Mecklin JP, Jdrvinen HJ, Ovaska JT. Blood transfusion and prognosis in colorectal carcinoma. *Scand J Gastroenterol* 1989;24:33

200. Weiden PL, Bean MA, Schultz P. Perioperative blood transfusion does not increase the risk of colorectal cancer recurrence. *Cancer* 1987;60:870

201. Laurie J, Moertel C, Fleming T, et al. Surgical adjuvant chemotherapy of poor prognosis colorectal cancer with levamisole alone or the combination of levamisole and 5-fluorouracil. *Proc ASCO* 1986;5:81

202. Laurie JA, Moertel CG, Fleming T, et al. Surgical adjuvant therapy for large bowel carcinoma: an evaluation of levamisole and the combination of levamisole and 5-fluorouracil: a study of the North Central Cancer Treatment Group and Mayo Clinic. *J Clin Onol* 1989; 7:1447

203. Moertel CG, Fleming TR, MacDonald JS, et al. Levamisole and fluorouracil for adjuvant therapy of resected colon carcinoma. *N Engl J Med* 1990;322:352

204. Koprowski H, Steplewski J, Mitchall K, et al. Colorectal carcinoma antigens detected by hybridoma antibodies. *Somat Cell Genet* 1979;5:957

205. Dillman RO. Antibody therapy. In: Oldham RK (ed),

Principles of Cancer Biotherapy, New York, NY: Raven Press; 1987:291

206. Hellstrom J, Hom D, Linsley P, et al. Monoclonal mouse antibodies raised against human lung carcinoma. *Cancer Res* 1986;46:3917

207. Steis R, Smith J, Bookman M, et al. *Evaluation of a human anticolorectal carcinoma monoclonal antibody in patients with metastatic colorectal cancer, P42.* Second Int Conf MoAB Immunoconj for Cancer, San Diego, March 12–14, 1987.

208. Steis RG, Carrasquillo JA, McCabe R, et al. Toxicity, immunogenicity and tumor radioimmunodetecting ability of two human monoclonal antibodies in patients with metastatic colorectal carcinoma. *J Clin Oncol* 1990;8:476

209. Mellstedt H, Frodin JE, Masucci G, et al. Clinical status of monoclonal antibodies in the treatment of colorectal carcinoma. *Oncology* 1989;Dec. 3(12):25

210. Mellstedt H, Frodin JE, Masucci G, et al. Monoclonal antibodies (MAB 17-1A) for the treatment of patients with metastatic colorectal carcinomas. *Acta Chir Scand Supp* 1989;549:63

211. Beatty JD. Immunotherapy of colorectal cancer. *Cancer* 1992;70:1425

212. Hawkins MJ. IL-2/LAK: current status and possible future directions. *PPO Updates* 1989;3:2

213. Vetto JT, Papa MZ, Lotze MT, et al. Reduction of toxicity of interleukin-2 and lymphokine-activated killer cells in humans by the administration of corticosteroids. *J Clin Oncol* 1987;5:496

214. Rubin JT, Elwood LJ, Rosenberg SA, et al. Immunohistochemical correlates of response to recombinant interleukin-2-based immunotherapy in humans. *Cancer Res* 1989;49:7086

215. Boccoli G, Masciulli R, Ruggeri EM, et al. Adoptive immunotherapy of human cancer: the cytokine cascade and monocyte activation following high dose interleukin-2 bolus treatment. *Cancer Res* 1990;50:5795

216. Gray BN, Walker C, Andrewartha L, et al. Controlled clinical trial of adjuvant immunotherapy with BCG and neuraminidase-treated autologous tumor cells in large bowel cancer. *J Surg Oncol* 1989;40:34

217. Lehner B, Schlag P, et al. Postoperative active specific immunization in curatively resected colorectal cancer patients with a virus modified autologous tumor cell vaccine. *Cancer Immunol Immunother* 1990;32:173

218. Hoover HC Jr, Hana HC Jr. Active immunotherapy in colorectal cancer. *Semin Surg Oncol* 1987;5:436

219. Gunderson LL, Sosin H. Areas of failures found at reoperation (second or symptomatic) following "curative surgery" for adenocarcinoma of the rectum. *Cancer* 1974; 34:1278

220. Rich T, Gunderson LL, Lew R, et al. Clinical and pathological factors influencing local failure after curative resection of carcinoma of the rectum and rectosigmoid. *Cancer* 1983;52:1317

221. Willett CG, Tepper JE, Cohen AM, et al. Local failure following curative resection of colonic adenocarcinoma. *Int J Radiat Oncol Biol Phys* 1984;10:645

222. Willett CG, Tepper JE, Cohen AM, et al. Failure patterns following curative resection of colonic carcinoma. *Ann Surg* 1984;200:685

223. Willett CG, Tepper JE, Cohen AM, et al. Obstruction and perforative colonic carcinoma: patterns of failure. *J Clin Oncol* 1985;3:379

224. Duttenhaver JR, Hoskins RB, Gunderson LL, et al. Adjuvant postoperative radiation therapy in the management of adenocarcinoma of the colon. *Cancer* 1986;57:955

225. Willett CG, Tepper JE, Skates SJ, et al. Adjuvant postoperative radiation therapy for colonic carcinoma. *Ann Surg* 1987;206:694

226. Willett CG, Tepper JE, Skellito PC, et al. Indications for adjuvant radiotherapy in extrapelvic colonic carcinoma. *Oncology* 1989;(July) 3(7):25

227. Loeffler RK. Postoperative radiation therapy for Dukes' C adenocarcinoma of the cecum using two fractions per day. *Int J Radiat Oncol Biol Phys* 1984;10:1881

228. Fortner J, Silver J, Golbry R, et al. Multivariate analysis of a personal series of 247 consecutive patients with liver metastases from colorectal cancer. *Ann Surg* 1984; 306:316

229. Logan S, Meier S, Ramming P. Hepatic resection of metastatic colorectal carcinoma: A ten-year experience. *Arch Surg* 1982;117:25

230. Adson MA. Resection of liver metastases: when is it worthwhile? *World J Surg* 1987;11:511

231. Gennari L, Doci R, Bozzetti F, et al. Surgical treatment of hepatic metastases from colorectal cancer. *Ann Surg* 1986;205:49

232. Wagner J, Adson M, van Heerdan J, et al. The natural history of hepatic metastases from colorectal cancer. *Ann Surg* 1984;199:502

233. Hughes KS, Simon R, Songhorabodi S, et al. Resection of the liver for colorectal carcinoma metastases: A multi-institutional study of patterns of recurrence. *Surgery* 1986;100:278

234. Steele G Jr, Ravikumar TS. Resection of hepatic metastases from colorectal cancer. *Ann Surg* 1989;210:127

235. Ballantyne GH, Quin J. Surgical treatment of liver metastases in patients with colorectal cancer. *Cancer* 1993; 71:4252

236. Wasserman TH, Comis R, Goldsmith M, et al. Tabular analysis of clinical chemotherapy in the treatment of solid tumors. *Cancer Chemother Rep* 1975;6:399

237. Baker LH, Talley RW, Matter R, et al. Phase III comparison of the treatment of advanced gastrointestinal cancer with bolus weekly 5-FU versus methyl-CCNU plus weekly 5-FU: a Southwest Oncology Group Study. *Cancer* 1976;38:1

238. Lokich JJ, Skarin AT, Mayer RJ, et al. Lack of effectiveness of combined 5-FU and methyl-CCNU therapy in advanced colorectal carcinoma. *Cancer* 1977;40:2792

239. Ensminger WD, Rosowsky A, Raso V, et al. A clinical-pharmacological evaluation of hepatic arterial infusions of 5-fluoro-2-deoxyuridine and 5-fluorouracil. *Cancer Res* 1978;38:3784

240. Ensminger WD, Frei E. High-dose intravenous and hepatic artery infusions of thymidine. *Clin Pharmacol Therap* 1978;24:610

241. Garnick NM, Ensminger WD, Israel M. A clinical-pharmacological evaluation of hepatic arterial infusion of adriamycin. *Cancer Res* 1979;39:4105

242. Balch CM, Urist MM, Soong SJ, et al. A prospective phase

II clinical trial of continuous FUDR regional chemotherapy for colorectal metastases to the liver using a totally implantable drug infusion pump. *Ann Surg* 1983;198:567

243. Niederhuber JE, Ensminger W, Gyves J, et al. Regional chemotherapy of colorectal cancer metastases to the liver. *Cancer* 1984;53:1336

244. Kemeny N, Daly J, Oderman P, et al. Hepatic artery pump infusion: toxicity and results in patients with metastatic colorectal carcinoma. *J Clin Oncol* 1984;2:595

245. Kemeny NM, Goldberg D, Beatty JD, et al. Results of a prospective randomized trial of continuous regional chemotherapy and hepatic resection as treatment of hepatic metastases from colorectal primaries. *Cancer* 1986; 57:492

246. Cohen AM, Schaeffer N, Higgins J. Treatment of metastatic colorectal cancer with hepatic artery combination chemotherapy. *Cancer* 1986;57:1115

247. Kemeny N, Cohen A, Bertino JR, et al. Continuous intrahepatic infusion of floxuridine and leucovorin through an implantable pump for the treatment of hepatic metastases from colorectal carcinoma. *Cancer* 1990; 65:2446

248. Kemeny N, Daly J, Reichman B, et al. Intrahepatic or systemic infusion of fluorodeoxyuridine in patients with liver metastases from colorectal carcinoma. *Ann Intern Med* 1987;107:459

249. Daly JM, Kemeny N, Sigurson E, et al. Regional infusion for colorectal hepatic metastases. *Arch Surg* 1987;122: 1273

250. Ravikumar TS, Kane R, Cady B, et al. A 5 year study of cryosurgery in the treatment of liver tumors. *Arch Surg* 1991;126:1521

251. Onik G, Rubinsky B, Zemel R, et al. Ultrasound-guided hepatic cryosurgery in the treatment of metastatic colon carcinoma. *Cancer* 1991;67:901

252. Zhou X-D, Tang Z-Y, Yu Y-Q, et al. Clinical evaluation of cryosurgery in the treatment of primary liver cancer: report of 60 cases. *Cancer* 1988;61:1889

253. Kuramoto S. *Hepatic cryosurgery for unresectable tumors.* Presented at the American College of Cryosurgery, Caracas, Venezuela; June 6–9, 1989.

254. Galandiuk S, Wieand HS, Moertel CG, et al. Patterns of recurrence after curative resection of carcinoma of the colon and rectum. *Surg Gynecol Obstet* 1992;174:27

255. Winchester DP, McBride CM. Cancer of the colon: a comparison of survival factors. *South Med J* 1974;67:1025

256. Vassilopoulos PP, Yoon JM, Ledesma EJ, et al. Treatment of recurrence of adenocarcinoma of colon and rectum at the anastomotic site. *Surg Gynecol Obstet* 1981;152:777

257. Phil E, Hughes ES, McDermott FR, et al. Recurrence of carcinoma of the colon and rectum at the anastomotic suture line. *Surg Gynecol Obstet* 1981;153:495

258. Welch JP, Donaldson GA. Detection and treatment of recurrent cancer of the colon and rectum. *Am J Surg* 1978;135:505

259. Turk PS, Wanebo HJ. Results of surgical treatment of non-hepatic recurrence of colorectal carcinoma. *Cancer* 1993;71(12 suppl):4267

260. Goya T, Miyasawa N, Kondo H, et al. Surgical resection of pulmonary metastases from colorectal cancer. *Cancer* 1989;64:1418

261. Pihl E, Hughes ES, McDermott FR, et al. Lung recurrence after curative surgery for colorectal cancer. *Dis Colon Rectum* 1987;30:417

262. Brister SJ, Varennes B, Gordon PH, et al. Contemporary operative management of pulmonary metastases of colorectal origin. *Dis Colon Rectum* 1988;31:786

263. Mansel JK, Zinmeister AP, Pairolero PC, et al. Pulmonary resection of metastatic colorectal adenocarcinoma: a 10 year experience. *Chest* 1986;89:109

264. McCormack PM, Attiyeh FF. Resected pulmonary metastases from colorectal cancer. *Dis Colon Rectum* 1979; 22:553

265. Mori M, Tomoda H, Ishida T, et al. Surgical resection of pulmonary metastases from colorectal adenocarcinoma: special reference to repeated pulmonary resections. *Arch Surg* 1991;126:1297

266. Beart RW, Metzger PP, O'Connell MJ, et al. Postoperative screening of patients with carcinoma of the colon. *Dis Colon Rectum* 1981;24:585

267. Beart RW, O'Connell MJ. Postoperative follow-up of patients with carcinoma of the colon. *Mayo Clin Proc* 1983; 58:361

268. Minton JP, Martin EW Jr. The use of serial CEA determinations to predict recurrence of colon cancer and when to do a second-look operation. *Cancer* 1978;42: 1422

269. Kelly CJ, Daly JM. Colorectal cancer: Principles of postoperative follow-up. *Cancer* 1992;70:1397

270. Sugarbaker PH, Granola FJ, Dwyer A, et al. A simplified plan for the follow-up of patients with colon and rectal cancer supported by prospective studies of laboratory and radiological test results. *Surgery* 1987;102:79

271. Ohuchi N, Taira Y, Sakai N, et al. Comparison of serum assays for TAG-72, CA 19-9 and CEA in gastrointestinal carcinoma patients. *Jpn J Clin Oncol* 1989;3:242

272. Safi F, Link KH, Beger HG. Is follow-up of colorectal cancer patients worthwhile? *Dis Colon Rectum* 1993;36:636

273. Elkmann CA, Gustavson J, Henning A. Value of a follow-up study of recurrent carcinoma of the colon and rectum. *Surg Gynecol Obstet* 1977;145:895

274. Törnquist A, Ekelund G, Leandoer L. The value of intensive follow-up after curative resection for colorectal carcinoma. *Br J Surg* 1982;69:725

275. Wilson H, Cheek RC, Sherman RT, et al. Carcinoid tumors. *Curr Prob Surg I* 1970;1:17

276. Morgan J, Marks C, Hearn D. Carcinoid tumors of the gastrointestinal tract. *Ann Surg* 1974;189:720

277. Meijer S, Peretz T, Gaynor JJ, et al. Primary colorectal sarcoma: a retrospective review and prognostic factor study of 50 consecutive patients. *Arch Surg* 1990; 125:1163

278. Coit D, Raaf JH. Gastrointestinal leiomyosarcoma. In: Raaf JH (ed), *Soft Tissue Sarcomas—Diagnosis and Treatment.* Chicago, IL: Mosby; 1991:139

279. Chaok C, Smith TR. Multiple leiomyosarcoma of the transverse colon: report of a case and discussion. *Dis Colon Rectum* 1980;23:118

280. Feldtman RW, Oram-Smith JC, Teears RJ, et al. Leiomyo-

sarcoma of the rectum: the military experince. *Dis Colon Rectum* 1981;24:402

281. Khalifa AA, WL Bong, Rao VK, et al. Leiomyosarcoma of the rectum: report of a case and review of the literature. *Dis Colon Rectum* 1986;29:427

282. Bonser RS, McMaster P, Acland PC, et al. Fibrosarcoma of the transverse colon. *J Surg Oncol* 1986;31:34

283. Taxy JB, Battifora H. Angiosarcoma of the gastrointestinal tract: a report of three cases. *Cancer* 1988;62:210

284. Posner MC, Shiu MH, Newsome JL, et al. The desmoid tumor: not a benign disease. *Arch Surg* 1989;124:191

285. Lustblader I, Sherman A. Primary gastrointestinal Kaposi sarcoma in a patient with acquired immune deficiency syndrome. *Am J Gastroenterol* 1987;82:894

286. Scandalakis JE, Gray SE, Sheperd D, et al. *Smooth Muscle Tumors of the Alimentary Tract.* Springfield, IL. Thomas CC, 1962.

287. Berkeley KM. Leiomyosarcoma of the large intestine, excluding the rectum. *Int Surg* 1981;66:177

288. Rao BK, Kapur MM, Roy S. Leiomyosarcoma of the colon: a case report and review of literature. *Dis Colon Rectum* 1980;23:184

289. Walker MJ. Rare tumors of the colon and rectum. In: Nelson RL (ed), *Problems in Current Surgery. Controversies in Colon Cancer.* Philadelphia, PA: JB Lippincott; 1987:141

290. Henry CA, Berry RE. Primary lymphoma of the large intestine. *Am J Surg* 1988;54:262

291. Jinnai D, Iwasa J, Watanuki T. Malignant lymphoma of the large intestine—operative results in Japan. *Jpn J Surg* 1983;13:331

292. Gordon PH. Malignant neoplasms of the colon. In: Gordon PH, Nivatvongs S (eds), *Principles and Practice of Surgery for the Colon, Rectum and Anus.* St Louis, MO: Quality Medical, 1992:501

43

Surgery of the Small and Large Bowel

David C. Brooks ■ *Michael J. Zinner*

■ GENERAL PRINCIPLES

The philosophy and tenets of safe abdominal surgery awaited the waning years of the 19th century to be set forth. The introduction of anesthesia 30 or 40 years earlier had finally made intra-abdominal surgery possible, but until William Stewart Halsted at Johns Hopkins Hospital elucidated his principles of asepsis, gentleness, and hemostasis, surgery remained a tour de force relying on speed and technical virtuosity. Halsted demonstrated that a long operation need not be a danger to the patient. Instead, speed and its attendant disregard for the sanctity of tissue caused significantly more trauma. The century of surgery that has followed Halsted's principles has witnessed an unprecedented evolution in the management of disease, particularly of the intra-abdominal contents. Although Halsted did not have the benefit of antibiotics, his precepts allowed relatively reliable surgical approaches to the large and small bowel. Indeed, the principles he introduced had far more to do with safe surgery than the pharmacology that followed.

Today, the idea that tissues should be respected, handled gently and precisely and that blood supply is central to effective healing is a viable as it was 100 years ago. The surgeon operating in any part of the abdomen who follows Halsted's precepts will go a long way towards performing safe and effective surgery.

Bowel handling should at all times be gentle and respectful. In most cases of exploratory laparotomy or general abdominal procedures, the small bowel should be run from the ligament of Treitz. This can be done by identifying the ligament of Treitz at the base of the transverse mesocolon, gently lifting the bowel and placing the index and middle finger on either side of the bowel, with the V of the web space of the fingers on the antimesenteric border in a continuous manner. The bowel then can be run sequentially from ligament of Treitz to ileocecal valve. This will allow identification of both palpable and visual abnormalities. At no time should the bowel be grasped with sharp metallic instruments, unless a specific dissection is intended in that area. All bowel instruments have the potential for injury to the bowel, including laceration of the serosa and even penetration of the entire seromuscular wall.

Likewise, manual palpation of the colon should begin at the cecum and progress in an orderly fashion through the right, transverse, splenic flexure, descending and sigmoid colon. The bowel should be gently palpated between fingers to identify intraluminal lesions. This also will allow identification of woody, thickened areas of the bowel such as are seen in diverticulosis. In patients with particularly bulky or thickened mesentery, the overlying fat may obscure intraluminal lesions, making this less effective. Nonetheless, it should be part of the routine examination of the colon at all times. The virginal abdomen presents little problems for the attentive surgeon but in situations in which adhesions have formed as a result of previous operations, the surgeon may be presented with difficult dissections and dense adhesions that require lysing prior to fully examining the bowel. Adhesions should be lysed sharply with Metzenbaum scissors, utilizing a blunt tip. The sur-

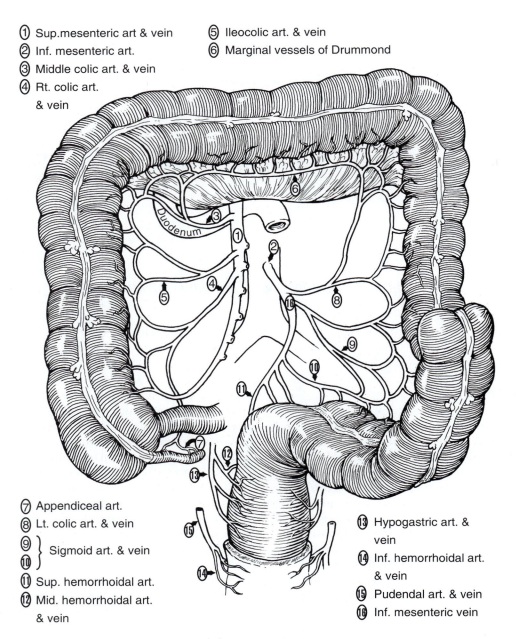

① Sup.mesenteric art & vein
② Inf. mesenteric art.
③ Middle colic art. & vein
④ Rt. colic art. & vein

⑤ Ileocolic art. & vein
⑥ Marginal vessels of Drummond

⑦ Appendiceal art.
⑧ Lt. colic art. & vein
⑨ ⑩ } Sigmoid art. & vein
⑪ Sup. hemorrhoidal art.
⑫ Mid. hemorrhoidal art. & vein

⑬ Hypogastric art. & vein
⑭ Inf. hemorrhoidal art. & vein
⑮ Pudendal art. & vein
⑯ Inf. mesenteric vein

Figure 43–1. Anatomy of the large intestine.

geon should incise along avascular planes wherever possible. The key principles of tension and retraction permit safe dissection when adhesions are present. Retraction is maintained by the operator's nondominant hand held behind tissue through filmy veils of adhesions or by gentle traction using a moistened sponge on the available surface of the bowel. Atraumatic forceps, if necessary, should be used judiciously with care being taken not to exert inordinate force on the tissues. The operator may opt to use electrocautery with a cutting current to lyse certain adhesions. This technique is similar to cold cutting and requires precise placement of the cautery wand so as not to injure underlying bowel or tissue.

■ ANATOMY OF THE SMALL AND LARGE BOWEL (Fig 43–1)

The small and large bowel are derived from the midgut and hindgut respectively, with the midgut portion extending throughout the small bowel, into the right and transverse colon. The small bowel originates at the ligament of Treitz, traveling approximately 20 to 30 ft until it terminates in the cecum. It is divided into two parts, the jejunum proximally and the ileum distally. Although there is no distinct transition, the jejunum has somewhat simpler arterial arcades, as opposed to the more complex arcades of the ileum. The vascular attachments of the entire small bowel derive from a 5 to 6 inch origin in the retroperitoneum, which runs obliquely from upper left to lower right, across the aorta and vena cava. The wall of the jejunum is somewhat thicker than the ileum and the lumen is slightly larger, although these differences are not immediately obvious when examining the isolated gut.

The large bowel originates in the right lower quadrant at the termination of the ileum in the ileocecal valve. The total length of the colon is approximately 5 to 6 ft and it runs from the cecum and appendix, in the right lower quadrant, to the right upper quadrant, across the upper abdomen, as the transverse colon; it then curves downwards at the splenic flexure in the left upper quadrant to become the left colon, then the sigmoid colon, diving into the pelvis and finally becoming the rectosigmoid and rectum below the pelvic floor.

Of considerable importance, when discussing the surgical anatomy of the large bowel, is the ureter. The ureter lies in harm's way whenever a colonic resection involving the pelvis from the brim to the peritoneal reflection is anticipated. The abdominal ureter exits the pelvis at the kidney and runs along the medial border of the psoas major muscle. The right ureter lies lateral to the inferior vena cava. The testicular or ovarian vessels cross over it, as do the right and ileocolic vessels. The left ureter also is crossed by the testicular or ovarian and left colic vessels. Both ureters enter the pelvis at the bifurcation of the common iliac artery into the internal and external branches. This is the ureter's most reliable landmark and initial efforts to identify it (which should be done in every case involving surgery in this area) should be directed to this location. The pelvic ureter edges laterally to the pelvic sidewalls before coming anterior and entering the bladder. The ureter of the male is above the seminal vesicle and in the female it lies above the lateral fornix of the vagina, 2 to 3 cm lateral to the cervix, as it exits the vagina.

■ VASCULAR SUPPLY (Fig 43–2)

The blood supply to the small and large bowel comes directly from the aorta via the superior and inferior mesenteric arteries. The blood supply to the small bowel is relatively straight forward. The superior mesenteric artery emanates from the aorta high in the upper abdomen, just caudal to the celiac axis. A few collateralizing branches are given off to the pancreas, followed by the middle colic artery which originates just inferior (caudal) to the inferior surface of the pancreas. The remaining superior mesenteric artery supplies the entire small bowel, the right colon and, via the middle colic, the transverse colon.

The entire blood supply of the small bowel enters at the mesenteric attachment. The mesentery is mobile and relatively free to move throughout the peritoneal cavity. The large bowel, on the other hand, is tethered on the right and left sides with avascular attachments to the lateral walls of the abdomen. These avascular attachments can be divided and the right and left colon can be brought to the midline. The exceptions to this are the vascular attachments at the hepatic flexure and splenic flexure that must be mobilized with care to avoid bleeding and injury to adjacent structures such as the duodenum on the right, which is in close proximity to the hepatic flexure, and the spleen on the left.

The colon develops from both the midgut and the hindgut and because of this its blood supply derives from both the superior and inferior mesenteric arteries. The majority of the blood supply to the right colon and transverse colon comes from the superior mesenteric, either via the previously mentioned middle colic artery or via the right colic and ileocolic arteries which are, respectively, the next major branches from the superior mesenteric. The middle colic artery itself branches into two vessels, one supplying the right transverse colon and the other communicates with the distal vessels of the inferior mesenteric artery in the watershed area known as the marginal artery of Drummond.

The inferior mesenteric artery originates from the aorta distal to the ligament of Treitz, midway between the area where the fourth portion of the duodenum crosses the aorta and the bifurcation of the aorta. The inferior mesenteric then branches, in order, into the left colic, several sigmoidal branches, and the superior hemorrhoidal artery. These vessels supply the left colon, sigmoid colon, and proximal rectosigmoid. Caudal to this, the inferior hemorrhoidal vessels, emanating from the hypogastric or internal iliac arteries, supply the remainder of the colon/rectum complex.

The inferior mesenteric artery is typically smaller than the superior mesenteric artery and more likely to be involved in atherosclerotic processes, in the older patient. Thus, the communications between the middle colic and the left colic arteries are important in maintaining the viability of anastomoses involving the left and sigmoid colon.

When performing a resection of the rectum or the rectosigmoid, the inferior mesenteric artery can be divided and ligated at the aorta or just distal to the margin of the left colic artery. The former is referred to as a "high tie" and the later a "low tie" technique. For years the "high tie" has been advocated because of the belief that it would

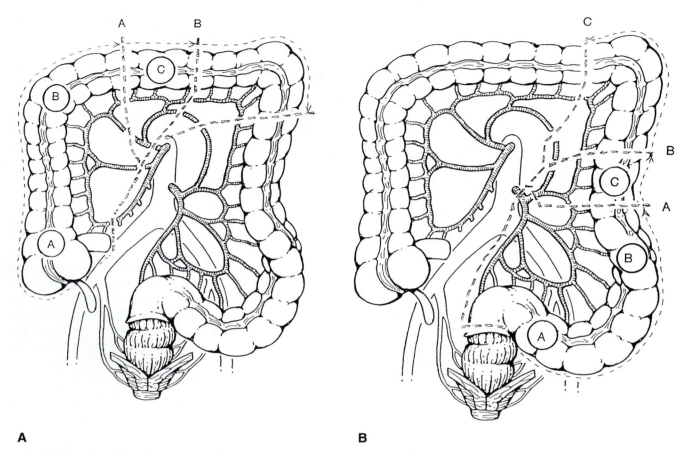

A

B

Figure 43–2. A. Surgical management of proximal colon cancer; extent of distal resection relative to tumor location. *O:* location of cancer; *dotted line:* extent of distal resection. **B.** Surgical management of distal colon cancer; extent of proximal resection relative to tumor location. *O:* location of cancer; *dotted line:* proximal extent of distal resection. (Courtesy of John Craig, MD)

provide a greater lymphatic harvesting and would diminish the likelihood of local or distant recurrence; this was first proposed by Moynihan in the early part of this century. A recent study reviewed over 1250 patients to compare the advantages or disadvantages of these two approaches to the inferior mesenteric artery.[1] As part of a multivariant analysis of this cohort, the level of ligation did not alter survival as predicted on the basis of the tumor's Dukes' classification. Thus, high ligation does not appear to improve long-term survival in patients.

More important than the named regional blood vessels mentioned above are the specific vessels supplying or draining the individual segments of the small or large bowel to be resected. Meticulous dissection of these vessels, clamping and ligating small arteries and veins with fine suture material, is necessary to maintain the viability of the cut ends of small or large bowel used in any anastomosis. Mass ligature always should be avoided, for it not only compromises the blood supply of the anastomosis but also foreshortens the mesentery sufficiently

to compromise bowel length when bringing two segments together. This tension is an important additional consideration when any anastomosis is created. This is rarely, if ever, a problem in the small bowel, but it consistently is noted as a problem in colonic anastomoses. Wide mobilization of the lateral attachments to the right and left colon can permit significant mobilization towards the midline. The cecum can even be moved to its embryological position in the left abdomen with adequate mobilization of the avascular peritoneal attachments known as the white line of Toldt. Sigmoid resections, particularly sleeve resections are rarely done under any tension because of the significant mobility and redundancy in the sigmoid colon. The same is not true, however, for left colectomies. When left colectomies are performed, the splenic flexure must be fully mobilized. These vascular attachments must be taken precisely and meticulously by serially clamping and ligating vessels, avoiding injury to adjacent structures and fully freeing all attachments that prevent mobilization.

The venous and lymphatic drainage of the small bowel and colon parallels the arterial supply. The distal colon/rectum drains into the iliac veins, the sigmoid and left colon into the inferior mesenteric vein, and the transverse, right, and small bowel into the superior mesenteric vein. The two major mesenteric veins tend to run in a cranial-caudal axis, overlying the midline until they reach the upper abdomen, where the inferior mesenteric vein deviates to the left to join the splenic vein beneath the pancreas. The splenic vein then courses to the right and, at its confluence with the superior mesenteric vein beneath the pancreas, becomes the portal vein, emptying into the liver.

■ ANTIBIOTICS

Postoperative infection accounts for the greatest morbidity following colon surgery. The lessons of infection in colon surgery were learned long before the 20th century. Infection has accompanied colonic surgery since it was first attempted in the 18th century. Techniques such as Mikulicz's double-barrel colostomy and exteriorization evolved to obviate many of these problems, but infections still occurred in many colon procedures. Today, however, surgeons can reliably operate with a low incidence of infection by preoperatively clearing the colon of as much bacteria as possible.[2] The use of antimicrobial agents to sterilize the gut became popular in the late 1960s and early 1970s. Although used as early as the late 1940s, available antibiotics at that time had an insufficient spectrum to cover the vast majority of colonic flora.

There are two methods for minimizing the possibility of infection in colon surgery. These are (1) mechanical cleansing of the bowel and (2) antibiotic sterilization of the bowel. Most surgeons currently use a combination of both techniques. An important study from the Veteran's Administration in the 1970s demonstrated that the use of magnesium sulfate cathartic and a cleansing enema schedule significantly decreased postoperative infections.[3] A later study by the same group examined the role of a mechanical bowel preparation in conjunction with oral antibiotics.[4] Patients treated with oral antibiotics (neomycin and erythromycin base) in conjunction with a mechanical bowel preparation had significantly fewer septic complications than those receiving a placebo. Quantitative colon cultures taken at the time of surgery demonstrated that patients receiving the antibiotic preparation had decreased concentrations of both aerobes and anaerobes. These findings were confirmed further by wound irrigation specimens, which were significantly lower in patients receiving antibiotics. The most common postop-

erative infections involved mixed aerobic and anaerobic flora; *Bacteroides fragilis* was responsible for approximately 75% of the bacteremic episodes. The colon contains 10^9 aerobes/gm of feces and 10^9 anaerobes/gm of feces. *E coli* is the most common aerobe and *Bacteroides fragilis* is the most common anaerobe. By mechanically preparing the bowel and by administering oral antibiotics, both sepsis and wound infections can be significantly reduced.[5] Importantly, the Veteran's Administration Cooperative Study demonstrated that microbial resistance did not increase in any of the regimens espoused by the Veteran's Administration Cooperative Study.

The mechanical preparation used in these studies consisted of a two-day regimen utilizing clear liquids, magnesium sulfate, and enemas. This preparation can lead to dehydration of the patients and can be unpleasant for patients to maintain for several days. An alternative to this longer regimen is the use of an unabsorbed electrolyte solution (Golytely) which is given in large doses, approximately 1 gal on the night before surgery, and effectively cleanses the entire intestine without the need for cathartics and enemas. Unfortunately, this preparation is often unpalatable and patients may become noncompliant because of the large volume that must be drunk on the evening before surgery. With proper compliance, however, this technique decreases the potential for fluid and electrolyte depletion that can be seen in a more typical mechanical bowel preparation using osmotic agents or cathartics.

Currently, the most common bowel preparations are either the three-day liquid diet/cathartic regimen or the one-day regimen using an electrolyte solution such as Golytely administered the night before surgery. Both are given in conjunction with oral erythromycin base and neomycin. The oral antibiotics are each given in three 1 gm doses, although some surgeons prefer to halve the dose and administer them in a longer period of time. Erythromycin can cause significant gastric distress and it has been the impression of some surgeons that a lower dose leads to less patient discomfort.

Although the above mentioned regimen may represent overkill, most surgeons are creatures of habit, with vivid memories of their most recent complication. For that reason, and knowing the cost and morbidity associated with postoperative wound and deep abdominal infections, most surgeons favor a course of over- rather than under-treatment.

In addition to the oral regimens discussed, parenteral antibiotics are administered at the time of anesthesia induction. The choice of antibiotics, the timing of their administration, and the duration of their administration have been the subject of a number of studies in the last 25 years. In 1969 Polk demonstrated that a parenteral antibiotic administered prior to the onset of the incision decreased wound infections.[6] This could be achieved without the administration of oral antibiotic solutions. It was further demonstrated by Stone that antibiotics begun after the operation had commenced failed to achieve the same salutary results, suggesting the need for an adequate therapeutic level at the time the incision was made.[7] Most surgeons now favor a broad spectrum of cephalosporin with sufficient coverage of colinic bacteria at the time of induction of anesthesia. To date, no studies have demonstrated the efficacy of additional doses of parenteral antibiotics after the single dose given at the induction of anesthesia. Nonetheless, many surgeons favor one or two doses postoperatively as an insurance policy.

■ OUTPATIENT BOWEL PREPARATION

As more and more procedures are performed as same-day admit cases rather than following a preoperative hospital night, a reliable outpatient bowel preparation has become important in the preparation of patients for surgery. A typical protocol was developed at Johns Hopkins Hospital in the early 1990s.[8] This preparation involves a 40 hour liquid diet prior to surgery, coordinated with administration of a buffered oral saline laxative containing sodium phosphate and sodium biphosphate. Additionally, bisacodyl preparation with oral erythromycin and neomycin is administered. No clearing enemas are used. This protocol has been remarkably successful with limited complications and an acceptable degree of bowel clearance.

■ EMERGENCY BOWEL PREPARATION

In certain situations, particularly those in which operations are emergent, there is insufficient time to adequately prepare the bowel through the means mentioned above. Intraoperative bowel irrigation has been shown to be successful and can markedly diminish postoperative wound infections[9] (Fig 43–3). A Foley catheter is placed via an enterotomy in the terminal ileum. The catheter should be of sufficient size to allow a relatively high flow of fluids. A colotomy is made at the point of distal resection and large corrugated tubing is inserted and held in place with umbilical tapes. Approximately 3 L of sterile fluid is washed into the bowel, using hydrostatic pressure, until the irrigate becomes clear. In the above mentioned paper, this technique was used in more than 60 patients, with an infection rate under 10%, significantly lower than would be expected in these potentially catastrophic patients.

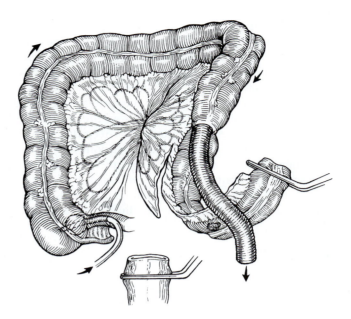

Figure 43–3. Technique for on-table cleansing of unprepared bowel.

■ TECHNICAL CONSIDERATIONS

INCISIONS

There are essentially four types of incisions available for performance of small bowel or colon resection. These include (1) midline incisions, (2) paramedian incisions, (3) subcostal incisions and (4) oblique lower quadrant incisions (Fig 43–4). The most popular incision for entering the abdomen at the present time is a generous midline incision placed through the avascular linea alba. It was not always so. Paramedian incisions were, at one time, the most common approach to the abdomen because of their strength, mobility and the low incidence of herniation. Additionally, oblique incisions based in the subcostal region, and transverse incisions for the midabdomen and lower abdomen also have enjoyed popularity from time to time.

The advantages of a midline incision are the speed with which it can be opened and closed and its ability to provide access to the entire abdomen. However, it is clear that approaches to the hepatic flexure and splenic flexure are somewhat compromised when a midline incision is used, regardless of the length of that incision. Despite this, the midline incision is currently the favored incision because of its ease, speed, and versatility. It may be limited to the upper abdomen (between the xyphoid and the umbilicus), the lower abdomen (umbilicus to pubic pubis), or it may be a combination of both. It allows access to all quadrants of the abdomen and also provides excellent and rapid access to the peritoneum in the event of emergencies.

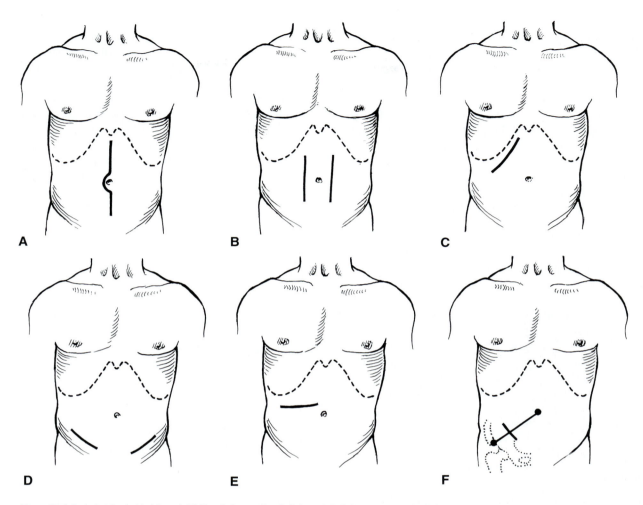

Figure 43–4. Typical abdominal incisions. **A.** Midline. **B.** Paramedian. **C.** Subcostal. **D.** Oblique lower quadrant incisions (right and left). **E.** Right lateral transverse incision. **F.** McBurney.

The single biggest disadvantage of midline incisions is incisional hernias that may develop in as many as 5% to 7% at one year.[10,11] The potential for hernia is increased if the sutures are placed close to the midline as opposed to at the lateral margin of the confluence of the rectus sheaths, if sutures are placed under excessive tension and if sutures are placed too closely. The linea alba itself has less strength than that point of the abdominal wall slightly lateral where the posterior and anterior rectus sheaths become conjoined in the upper portion of the abdomen. The incidence of wound herniation increases with time and may be as high as 10% at 5 years.

Nonetheless, the advantages of the well-performed midline incision include no muscle weakness and no interference with cutaneous innervation. The speed with which this incision can be opened and the access to all portions of the abdomen make it the preferred choice.

Subcostal incisions have been used for many years to gain access to the gallbladder on the right and the spleen on the left. It has long been thought that this incision provided excellent exposure and it had fewer respiratory complications than midline incisions. It also was thought to have a lower incidence of incisional hernias. These presumed advantages, however, have never been documented and, in fact, the incidence of respiratory complications does not appear to be significantly different when a subcostal rather than a midline incision is used to access the upper abdomen.[12] Although excellent visualization is available with both subcostal incisions, significant muscle denervation can occur to the abdominal wall that will lead to permanent weakness and numbness if the incision is taken too far laterally. This can be particularly problematic when a bilateral incision is made, such as a chevron incision. For limited resections around the hepatic and splenic flexures, however, these incisions may be useful.

Oblique lower quadrant incisions have recently gained significant enthusiasm, largely through the experience of renal transplantation. By using an approach comparable to an extended Rocky Davis incision on the right-hand side, a generous incision can be made, staying towards the lateral portion of the rectus muscle and allowing excellent access to limited portions of the proximal right colon and the pelvis or, on the left-hand side, allowing access to the sigmoid colon and the rectosigmoid. These incisions are cosmetically attractive, give an excellent repair, and, if the epigastric vessels are spared or only marginally effected, muscular function and sensory innervation is maintained.

The greatest drawback to oblique incisions is their lack of versatility and the inability to reach other portions of the abdomen that may be necessary after exploration, at the time of opening the peritoneum. Nonetheless, for limited procedures, these incisions should be kept in mind.

Finally, paramedian incisions, which have enjoyed great popularity in the past, must be mentioned as an excellent, albeit longer, approach to the abdomen. Indeed, close evaluation of paramedian incisions suggest that if constructed properly, they may lead to a lower rate of incisional hernia and wound dehiscence.[13] When a lateral paramedian incision is made through the anterior fascia on the lateral half of the rectus, significant devascularization of the muscle is eliminated, cutaneous innervation is maintained, and the rectus shutter mechanism between the anterior and posterior fascial sheets is preserved while providing secure closure of the abdomen. Unfortunately, when paramedian incisions are placed closer to the midline, the incidence of herniation increases as a direct relationship to that proximity. The paramedian incision has certain drawbacks. These include a somewhat longer time to create and slightly increased blood loss as the rectus muscle is split. Furthermore, closure requires more layers and this may increase operative time. This trade-off may be worth the diminished incidence of postoperative hernias or wound dehiscence.

WOUND CLOSURE

Closure of all the above mentioned incisions can be performed safely and effectively using standard techniques that emphasize gentleness of tissue handling, asepsis, and hemostasis. The closure may be running or interrupted. At our institution, the most common closure for midline incisions is a single-layer running suture using nonabsorbable material such as either 0 or 2 polypropylene. Subcostal incisions generally are closed in layers using a stout absorbable suture on the peritoneum and posterior fascia followed by a running closure of the anterior rectus fascia. 0 polyglycolic (PGA) sutures are preferred on the peritoneum and 0 PGA or 0 polydioxanone sutures on the fascia. Alternatively, the anterior

fascia may be closed with nonabsorbable 0 polypropylene sutures. The same technique is used for oblique lower quadrant incisions. Paramedian incisions should be closed with absorbable sutures on the posterior fascia and peritoneum and running closure of the anterior fascia using somewhat smaller sutures, such as 0 polypropylene. The importance of peritoneal closure continues to be debated with both sides of the argument having strong proponents. In general, this decision is ultimately based on the preference of the surgeon.

ANASTOMOTIC TECHNIQUE

There are two different anastomotic techniques for reconstructing the small or large bowel: sutured or stapled. Sutured anastomoses can be separated into two basic types: single layered or double layered. Stapled anastomoses can be subdivided into end-to-end or side-to-side techniques.

Sutured Anastomoses

Suture Material. Virtually all types of suture material have been used in the construction of small and large bowel anastomoses. Ultimately, the type of material used in an anastomosis is of little importance. Of far more importance are gentleness in the handling of tissue, adequate blood supply, and lack of tension on the anastomosis. For two-layer inverting anastomoses, the most common inner layer is an absorbable material such as PGA or chromic catgut. This typically is performed with a 4-0 or 3-0 suture. The catgut has been tanned to give it greater stability and a longer life span prior to reabsorption. Because most anastomoses have achieved their greatest durability within the first 6 weeks after anastomosis, the continued presence of foreign material within the lumen of the gut makes little sense and is of limited utility in maintaining viability of the anastomosis. For that reason, there has been little enthusiasm for synthetic nonabsorbable sutures such as polyglycolic and polyglycolitic acid (Vicryl and Dexon). There have a longer half-life than chromic catgut and do not appear to offer any improvement in the strength of the anastomosis. Newer synthetic absorbable sutures such as polydioxinone have not undergone adequate trials and because of their long half-life, there does not appear to be any useful advantage to using these materials except in single-layer hand-sewn anastomoses.

Braided silk continues to be used with great frequency for both single-layer anastomoses and as a seromuscular layer to further invert an inverted anastomosis. Typically, these sutures are either 4-0 or 3-0, depending on the surgeon's preference. They also are used for single-layer anastomoses and, in particular, for single-layer low colonic anastomoses in the setting of low anterior resection.

Other surgeons prefer 3-0 or 4-0 polypropylene sutures because of the ease with which they pass through tissue. This also can have a significant drawback because the suture material may cut through tissues once it has been placed. Furthermore, the very low coefficient of friction associated with polypropylene means that individual knots may not have uniform tension throughout the anastomosis. The higher coefficient of friction seen with silk obviates that problem and may be an easier material for the surgeon to work with.

In all cases of hand-sewn anastomosis there are certain principles that must be followed. The suture should always be fine. Manipulation of the bowel wall should be kept to a minimum and any forceps used should have fine teeth.

Two-layer Anastomoses. Historically, the inverted anastomosis, constructed in two layers has been the standard of practice. The technique is shown in Fig 43–5 and 43–6 and is created with an inner layer of 3-0 catgut or

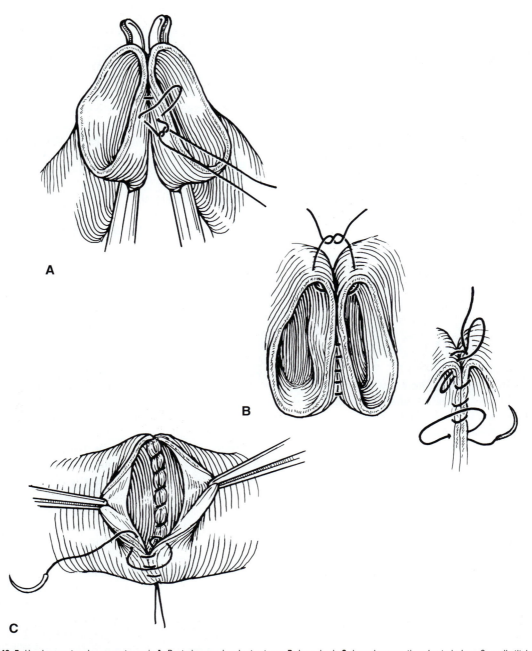

Figure 43–5. Hand-sewn, two-layer anastomosis **A.** Posterior row, Lembert sutures. **B.** Inner back. **C.** Inner layer continued anteriorly as Connell stitch.

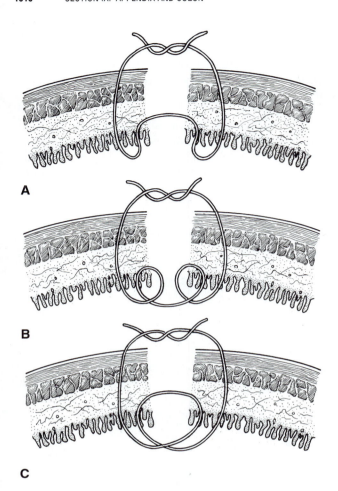

Figure 43–6. A. One-layer inverting anastomosis. **B.** Gambee single-layer stitch. **C.** Modified Gambee single-layer stitch.

other absorbable suture applied as a looping or a locking stitch posteriorly and as a Connell suture anteriorly. This inner layer is reinforced further with an outer seromuscular layer of interrupted 3-0 silk Lembert sutures. The posterior outer row of sutures is placed first, followed by the posterior inner row, the anterior inner row and finally, an anterior outer row. The inner layer is full thickness while the outer layer is seromuscular only. It is thought to have a particular advantage in diminishing anastomotic dehiscence. The hallmark of an inverting anastomosis is the creation of a precise serosa to serosa apposition. This is achieved by the outer, seromuscular layer, while the inner layer, created by using an absorbable, running full-thickness suture, brings opposing mucosal edges together. Inversion of the mucosa reestablishes integrity of the lumen so as to prevent both leakage during the early healing process and stricture during the later phases.

Single-layer Anastomoses. Single-layer anastomosis have been discouraged because of the apparent higher dehiscence rate. However, many surgeons have employed single-layer anastomoses without adverse effect and there is experimental evidence demonstrating that a single-layer technique causes the least reduction in mucosal blood flow, a consideration that may improve anastomotic healing.[14] A single-layer anastomosis is constructed by aligning the two segments of bowel and placing full-thickness sutures through the posterior walls that are subsequently tied on the inside; the anterior row is closed by a series of Gambee sutures which create mucosal apposition and inversion (Fig 43–7). In the Gambee technique, a single stitch is taken through full-thickness of the bowel wall, then back through the mucosa and submucosa of the same limb. It then reverses that pattern on the opposite limb. A modification of this includes full thickness of one limb, mucosa and submucosa of the opposite limb, back to the original limb with submucosa and mucosa, and then full thickness in the opposite side. This creates an inverting anastomosis with the advantages of both single- and double-layer technique. The sutures used are 3-0 absorbable or nonabsorbable material (Fig 43–8).

Stapled Anastomosis

The Use of Staplers in Gastrointestinal Surgery. Modern stapling devices and techniques were first developed in the Soviet Union in the 1950s through the work of the Scientific Research Institute for Experimental Surgical Apparatus and Instruments in Moscow.[15] Their development was based on a long history of investigations into mechanical surgical instruments dating back to the early years of the century when staples were first used and the principle of the B closure of staples was developed. Modern stapling techniques were first introduced to the United States in the late 1960s by the United States Surgical Corporation. Although these instruments have gone through a variety of evolutionary changes, the basic instruments remain the same. Furthermore, the theory and mechanical techniques involved also have remained essentially the same. The surgical stapling instruments now are made by several manufacturers and each has some slight differences.

The following instruments are available for use in surgical stapling and will be described using the nomenclature of the United States Surgical Corporation.

Thoracic Anastomosis Instruments. The thoracic anastomosis (TA) instruments (Fig 43–9) are available in a variety of sizes from approximately 30 mm to 90 mm. They place a double line of staggered staples in a linear, everting fashion. Staple sizes are variable depending on the thickness of the tissues to be used. They can be used

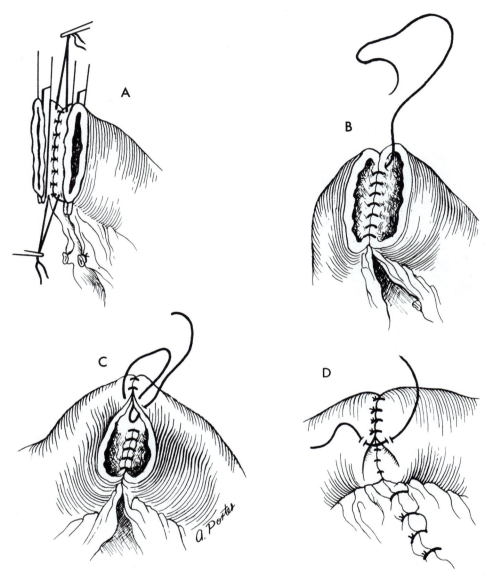

Figure 43–7. Open end-to-end anastomosis. **A.** Closure of outer posterior seromuscular layer. **B.** Placement of continuous inner posterior layer. **C.** Continuation of posterior layer anteriorly with Connell suture. **D.** Closure of seromuscular layer with interrupted silk sutures. (From Schirmer B, Jones RS. Small intestine. In: Nora PF (ed), *Operative Surgery: Principles and Techniques,* 3rd ed. Philadelphia, PA: WB Saunders; 1990)

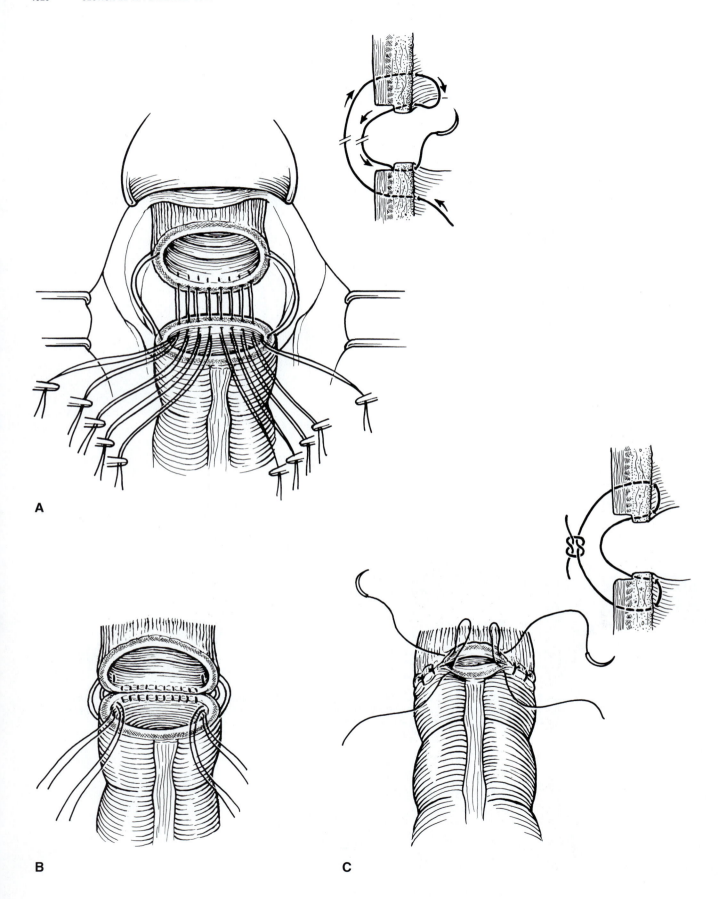

A

B

C

Figure 43–8. Single-layer hand-sewn anastomosis (low anterior). **A.** Interrupted posterior row vertical mattress sutures. **B.** Detail of vertical mattress sutures (Gambee modification). **C.** Knots tied on the colonic mucosa. *Inset.* Lateral knots turn-in corners. **D.** Anterior layer closed by interrupted Gambee sutures.

efficaciously to swiftly close various portions of the gastrointestinal tract, including stapled anastomoses, but also are used extensively in thoracic surgery because of their ability to provide a hemostatic, hydrostatic, and air-tight closure.

Gastrointestinal Anastomosis Instruments. The gastrointestinal anastomosis (GIA) instruments (Fig 43–10), also available in several sizes, place two double staggered rows of staples and simultaneously divide the tissue in the jaws of the stapler, with a knife mounted within the instrument. Typically, it is used to divide bowel on the proximal and distal ends of a resection site. It was designed, however, to create side-to-side anastomoses between two segments of bowel. By placing each limb of the instrument into the organs to be anastomosed, a side-to-side minimally inverting serosa-to-serosa anastomosis is formed. The two openings through which the instrument is applied subsequently become a single orifice that is closed with TA staplers. Both the GIA and the TA instruments have also been adapted to laparoscopic usage.

End-to-End Instruments. The end-to-end anastomosis (EEA) instrument (Fig 43–11) is a tubular device that is employed for creating either an end-to-end or an end-to-

side inverting anastomosis. It is attractive, particularly for low pelvic and rectal anastomoses, and is much favored by surgeons because it provides an inverting, serosa-to-serosa anastomosis that is performed in an end-to-end manner. This is exactly similar to hand-sutured anastomoses. The tubular instrument has a detachable anvil that is inserted into one limb of the bowel while the shaft and head of the instrument are inserted into the other. The head and the anvil of the instrument are brought together, screwed down until the head and the anvil are in close apposition and a double layer of staples are fired, creating an inverting anastomosis.

Types of Stapled Anastomoses

End-to-End Anastomosis. Stapled anastomoses can be constructed in either the direct, end-to-end fashion (Fig 43–12) or in the side-to-side, functional end-to-end fashion. The former is created using the circular, intraluminal stapler. This is ideal for low anterior resection of the rectum but can also be used from above when creating a colocolostomy, providing there is an appropriate proximal site through which the stapler may be inserted into the bowel. The circular stapler typically comes in three sizes ranging from approximately 25 to 33 mm in diameter. Each manufacturer uses different sizes. The

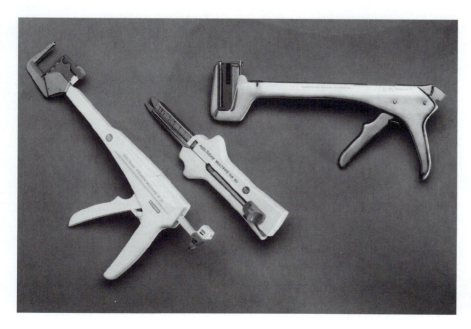

Figure 43–9. TA instrument. (United States Surgical Corp, Norwalk, CT)

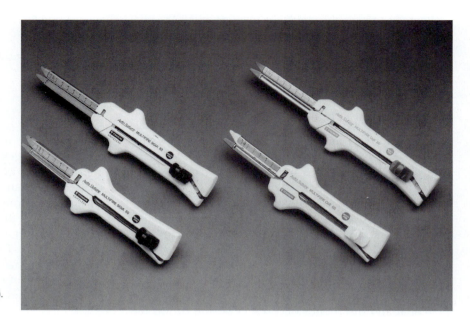

Figure 43–10. GIA instrument (60 and 80 mm lengths). (United States Surgical Corp, Norwalk, CT)

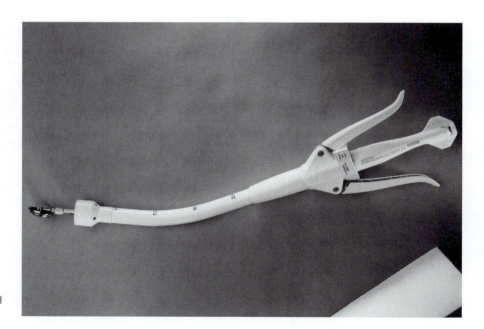

Figure 43–11. EEA instrument. (United States Surgical Corp, Norwalk, CT)

Figure 43–12. Technique of EEA anastomosis in low anterior resection. **A.** Transection of the rectum. **B.** Purse-string apparatus used to secure proximal limb. Bowel is opened longitudinally in preparation for insertion of stapler. **C.** Instrument introduced through proximal colon, anvil attached in preparation for insertion into the rectal stump. **D.** Anvil of EEA introduced into the rectal stump. **E.** Cross-section of stapler in place prior tightening the instrument. **F.** Picture of finished anastomosis. (Redrawn from Stapling Techniques: General Surgery, 2nd ed. Norwalk, CT: United States Surgical Corp; 1980. After W Baker.)

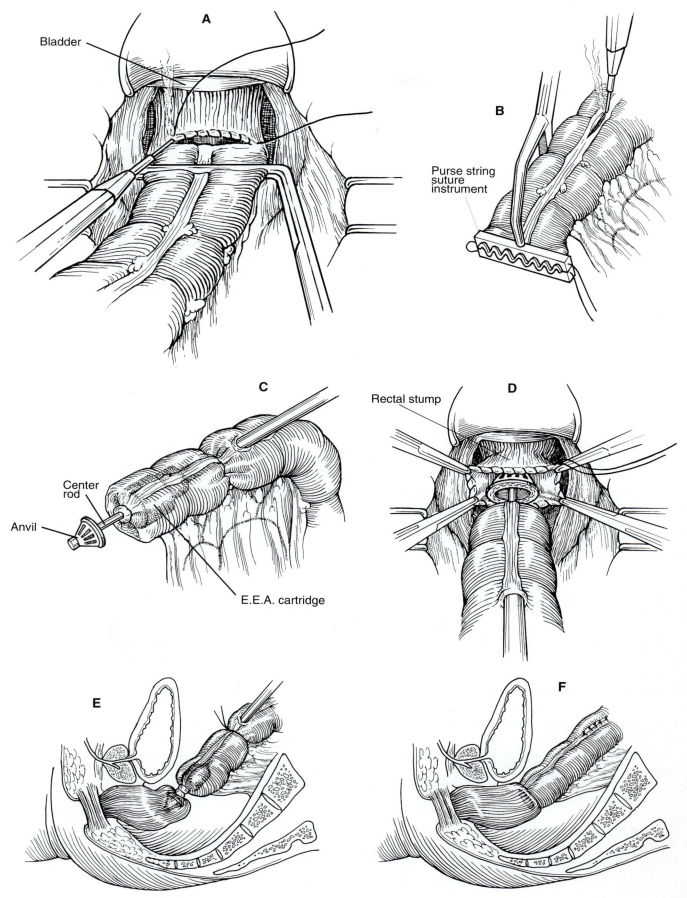

A

Bladder

B

Purse string suture instrument

C

Center rod

Anvil

E.E.A. cartridge

D

Rectal stump

E

F

1323

manufacturer supplies sizing instruments with which the surgeon may determine the appropriate anvil head.

The bowel is cleared approximately 1 cm from the cut margin. Proximal and distal margins each require a purse-string to secure the bowel around the anvil and shaft. The purse-string suture should be of sufficiently strong nonabsorbable material to allow a secure closure, generally 2-0 or 0 polypropylene suture is used. The suture can be placed in an over-and-over, baseball-type stitch around the circumference, or a true purse-string stitch mattressed serosa to mucosa to serosa without turning in the cut edge. Alternatively, nondisposable and disposable appliances are available that will place a purse-string suture on the cut edge of the bowel.

The anvil is inserted into one limb of the bowel and secured to the head of the shaft. The purse-string sutures are snugged down over the instrument ends and the anvil and head are brought together. A color-coded gauge on the instrument assists in adjusting the height of the staples and can be adjusted depending on the thickness of the bowel wall. After firing the circular stapler, the screw mechanism is undone for one-half or one-quarter turn by gently twisting the instrument, it can be removed from the bowel. It is important to check the "doughnuts" of bowel to ensure that two complete mucosal rings are present.

The EEA-type stapled anastomosis creates a completely inverting anastomosis in several different sizes. The stricture or leak rate reported with these does not differ significantly from those in everting two-layer anastomoses.

Side-to-Side Anastomosis. Side-to-side, functional end-to-end anastomoses are fashioned using a GIA instrument, which creates a serosa to serosa, inverting anastomosis of two layers (Fig 43–13 and Fig 43–14). The two limbs of bowel to be anastomosed are brought together at their antimesenteric margin. Stay sutures are placed and the GIA instrument is inserted into each limb via small enterotomies. The stapler arms are brought tightly together and the bowel is checked on each side to ensure that no mesentery will be included in the staple line. The instrument is fired, laying down 6 rows of staples and cutting between them. The arms of the instrument are opened and removed. The confluent staple entry sites on either segment of the bowel are closed with one or two firings of a TA stapler. The TA stapler creates an everting margin; thus, the stapled anastomosis is a combination of inverting and everting.

Sutured Versus Stapled Anastomoses

Stapled anastomoses, both the circular and linear, have been thoroughly compared with sutured anastomoses in both experimental and clinical series. When com-

pared directly, Brolin demonstrated that a two-layer inverted manual anastomosis compared favorably with a stapled anastomosis from the standpoint of anastomotic dehiscence and stricture.[16] In a variety of anastomoses, including enteroenterostomy, ileocolostomy and colocolostomy leaks occurred in only one of sixty animals with both the stapled and two-layer anastomoses. Single-layer simple and mattress-stitch everting anastomoses also were studied and both had prohibitively high leakage rates (>20%). In all animals, leaks were higher in the colocolostomy anastomoses as opposed to enteroenterostomies or ileocolostomies. This experimental study is confirmed by a clinical study by Goligher.[17] This prospective series was abandoned because of an unexpectedly high anastomotic leak rate in the single-layer everted technique. The mattress technique may cause increased ischemia at the suture site and may account for the high associated leak rate. McAdams found similar anastomotic disruption in another clinical series.[18] A 25% leak rate was seen in colocolostomies using the single-layer technique as compared to an 8% incidence with a standard two-layer anastomosis. Despite the higher dehiscence rate, the theoretical potential for stricture with everting anastomoses does not appear to be increased in either of the above mentioned studies compared to an inverting technique. Strictures were no more prevalent in everted than in inverted anastomoses.

The ultimate viability of any small bowel or large bowel anastomosis depends on a number of critical functions, including the nutritional status of the patient, the vascular integrity of the anastomosis, and the tension under which the anastomosis is created.[19] Doppler velocimetry was used to study experimental anastomoses that were created using either one- or two-layered sutured anastomoses, stapled anastomoses in three different heights, and stapled anastomoses reinforced with sutures. The blood flow to various areas of mucosa was measured before and after anastomosis, allowing each segment to act as its own control to determine the reduction of mucosal blood flow in each group. Single-layer sutured anastomoses had the least reduction in mucosal blood flow, at approximately 27%. Stapled anastomoses diminished blood flow by approximately 43%, and a traditional two-layer anastomosis, using chromic and silk, produced a nearly 60% reduction in blood flow. The greatest degree of ischemia was seen when staples were set at a closure height half the combined wall thickness of the two segments of bowel. A reduction of blood flow of approximately 70% was seen in this setting. Thus, it is important for surgeons to adjust the staple closure height to the appropriate thickness of the bowel being stapled to minimize the likelihood of ischemia at the sight of anastomosis. Clinical confirmation of this seems to be available in other areas of the

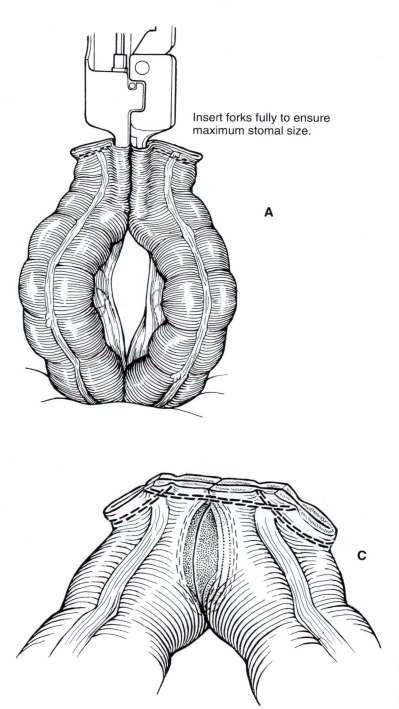

Insert forks fully to ensure maximum stomal size.

A

Care must be taken to overlap the ends of the previous staple lines.

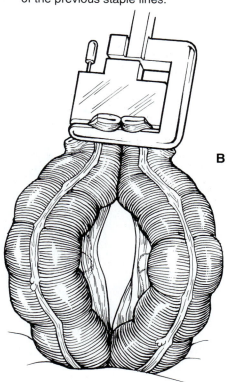

B

C

Figure 43–13. A. Instrument placed, handles locked and fired. **B.** Three sutures are placed to assist in closure of the confluent enterotomies, TA instrument in place to close defect. **C.** Completed anastomosis. (Redrawn from *Stapling Techniques: General Surgery,* 2nd ed. Norwalk, CT: United States Surgical Corp; 1980. After W Baker.)

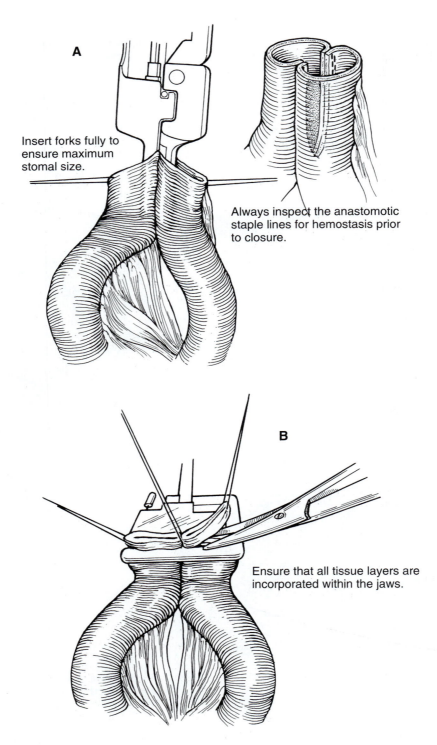

A

Insert forks fully to
ensure maximum
stomal size.

Always inspect the anastomotic
staple lines for hemostasis prior
to closure.

B

Ensure that all tissue layers are
incorporated within the jaws.

Figure 43–14. Small bowel resection using the GIA instrument (functional end-to-end). (Redrawn from *Stapling Techniques: General Surgery,* 2nd ed. Norwalk, CT: United States Surgical Corp; 1980. After W Baker.)

bowel. Specifically, in a comparison of hand-sutured and stapled subtotal gastrectomies, a nearly 5% leak rate was seen using hand-suture technique compared to a 2.5% leak rate for those with staples closure of the duodenum stump. In anastomoses of the stomach to the small bowel, a similar disparity was noted between hand-sutured and stapled anastomoses.[20]

A further variable revolves around the question of whether or not sutured or stapled anastomoses lead the higher recurrence rates of malignant lesions of the colon. In one study, nearly 300 patients who underwent presumably curative colorectal cancer resections were randomly allocated, after resection, to have either a sutured or stapled anastomosis.[21] Tumor recurrence in the sutured group, 2 years after surgery, was approximately 30%, as compared to 19% of the stapled group. It is difficult to understand these differences based entirely on anastomotic technique, but they may be a function of the adherence of micrometastases to suture or staple material. Certainly, in a micrometastases are more likely to adhere to a braided material as opposed to steel or titanium used in the staples.

POSTOPERATIVE DRAINS

Colonic and small bowel resections done for elective indications do not typically require postoperative drainage. Surgical teaching has long held that there is no role for drainage of the free peritoneal space in the absence of a drainable collection. The one exception to this rule, however, is closed-suction drainage following low anterior resection of the colon. Postoperatively, blood may accumulate adjacent to anastomoses low in the pelvis and provide a media for culture of bacteria. In one study,[22] anastomotic leakage was identified in 69% of the patients who underwent low anterior resection when studied with a barium enema two weeks after surgery. Not all were clinically significant. Many surgeons believe that the major cause of anastomotic dehiscence is infected hematomas that have developed in the perirectal spaces. The desirability of emptying the pelvis of blood and foreign media has encouraged the use of suction irrigation drains of the pelvis when performing low anterior resections.

One or two closed-suction drains such as a Jackson-Pratt drain are placed on either side of the low anterior resection anastomosis and brought out through separate stab wounds on either side of the abdomen. They are placed in the most dependent portion of the pelvis in order to absorb any hematoma that may develop. The drains are left in place until the irrigant becomes serosanguinous or the volume is diminished and then removed. It is unnecessary to wait for complete restoration of gastrointestinal (GI) function. Most studies to date have demonstrated the efficacy of this in retrospective studies.[23]

USE OF NASOGASTRIC TUBE FOLLOWING SMALL AND LARGE BOWEL RESECTION

Classic surgical teaching has encouraged the use of routine nasogastric drainage for any resection and reanastomosis of the small and large bowel. The rationale has been that the use of such a tube decompressed the stomach and prevents both vomiting and the accumulation of gas and fluid in the small bowel. In turn, this minimizes abdominal distention and minimizes wound dehiscence. Several recent studies suggest that the necessity of placing a nasogastric tube has been incompletely evaluated.[24] When patients have been allocated randomly to either nasogastric tube or no nasogastric tube, it was found that there were no significant differences in hospitalization, onset of oral intake, vomiting, nausea, or anastomotic leak and wound dehiscence. Decompression of the stomach does not appear to be important in resolving postoperative ileus. This suggests that there is no rationale for continued routine use of the tube. Moreover, other studies suggest that oral intake of solid foods may be begun immediately after surgery, at the discretion of the patient and depending on their appetite.[25,26]

■ SPECIFIC OPERATIVE PROCEDURES

SMALL BOWEL RESECTION

Small bowel resection (Fig 43–15) is employed in a variety of situations including ischemic segments, strictured segments, as part of a right colectomy, or to create a Roux-en-Y anastomosis for reconstruction following an upper GI procedure such as gastrectomy or biliary diversion.

A generic resection of the small bowel requires the following basic principles: isolation of the segment to be divided or resected, clearance of the bowel wall, isolation of the vascular arcade supplying the bowel, division of the bowel, and division of the mesentery.

The bowel is isolated and brought into the wound. Uninvolved segments of the small bowel are packed out of the field. The surgeon determines the afferent and efferent limbs so that anatomic reconstitution is reliable. Frequently, this consideration may be difficult to determine and may require a wide-ranging search for the proximal and distal segments. Proximal and distal resection sites are selected and marked with a suture or the brief application of electrocautery to the serosal surface. The bowel is lifted and held against the light in order to transilluminate the mesentery and determine where the arterial arcades will be divided. Electrocautery or scissors are used to make a small window through the mesentery in an avascular area adjacent to the bowel wall. This window is enlarged by sharply dividing the mesentery prox-

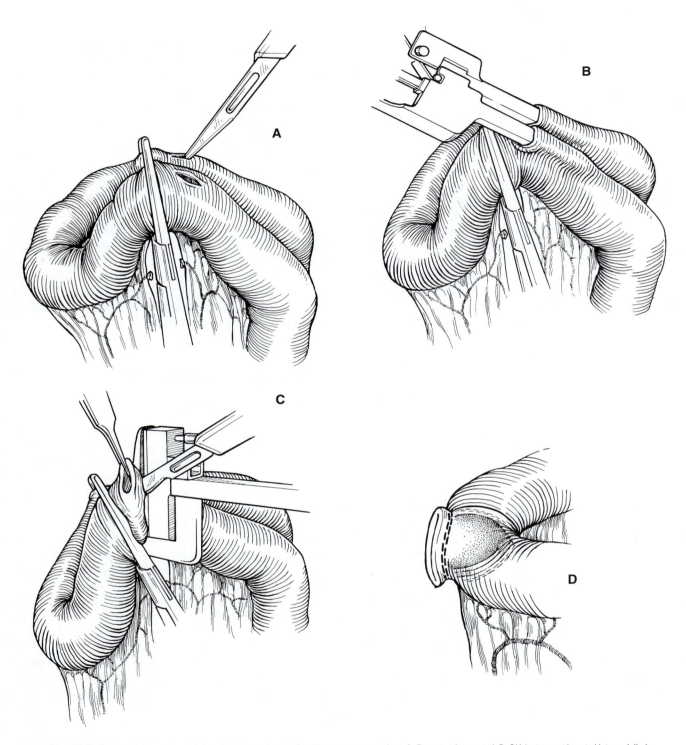

Figure 43–15. Alternative one-stage small bowel anastomosis, used for short segment resections. **A.** Enterotomies created. **B.** GIA instrument inserted into each limb. **C.** Placement of the TA instrument across the anastomosis. **D.** Completed anastomosis. (Redrawn from *Stapling Techniques: General Surgery*, 2nd ed. Norwalk, CT: United States Surgical Corp; 1980. After W Baker.)

imally towards the base of the mesentery until the first prominent vessels are encountered. The peritoneal surface of the mesentery should be incised first to facilitate placement of hemostats and to map out the proposed mesenteric resection line. Two hemostats are placed across this vessel and it is divided and tied with fine sutures. These sutures can be either absorbable or nonabsorbable, although the latter generally are preferred. The same process is performed on the other side of the small bowel segment to be excised. The mesenteric segment will be shaped like a wedge, with the narrowest portion closest to the base of the mesentery.

When the mesentery has been fully divided, attention is turned to the small bowel segment itself in preparation for division. The bowel should be cleared of small feeding vessels to a point approximately 1 cm from the proposed resection site. This allows precise application of sutures during the anastomosis and minimizes bleeding from the cut surface of the bowel. Clearance of these small vascular structures can be performed with electrocautery or fine sutures. The former is preferred because of its ease and precision. The method by which the bowel is divided is largely dependent on the proposed type of anastomosis to be performed. If a side-to-side anastomosis using staplers is planned, the bowel should be divided with the stapler applied at a right angle to the long axis of the bowel. If a sutured anastomosis is anticipated, noncrushing clamps are applied slightly oblique to the axis of the bowel, pointed away from the area to be resected. This accomplishes two purposes: it ensures a better blood supply to the antimesenteric border and it creates a slightly larger lumen in the completed anastomosis. Throughout this process the color of the cut ends of the bowel must be inspected and observed to ensure that it is viable.

The reanastomosis can be performed using either sutures or staples, and the sutured anastomosis may be either single or double layer. Stapled anastomoses generally are performed side-to-side. This results in a functional end-to-end anastomosis.

Once the anastomosis has been created, regardless of which form, it is tested by pinching between the thumb and index finger to ensure an adequate lumen. There will be a resulting mesenteric defect that must be attended to. Although some surgeons prefer not to close this for fear of compromising the fine vasculature along the cut edges, most feel that a defect in the mesentery may allow postoperative herniation of small bowel loops. In general, most surgeons close the defect with precisely placed sutures.

ENTEROSTOMY

When prolonged inability to feed via the upper gastrointestinal tract is anticipated, a tube enterostomy may be performed. This may be used for continuous nutrient delivery which is preferable to prolonged intravenous feedings whenever possible.

An enterostomy can be performed via laparotomy or via laparoscopy, if the sole intent is to place a feeding jejunostomy. The latter is appealing because of its diminished trauma to the patient, but in reality, most patients who will require feeding jejunostomy have had sufficient upper abdominal surgery that this approach may be impossible. Nonetheless, the technique is straightforward (Fig 43–16). Access to the peritoneum is gained in the usual fashion at the umbilicus. A second port (5 mm) is placed in the left lower quadrant and a third port can be placed at the proposed feeding catheter site (left hypogastrium) or in the right upper quadrant. The patient is rolled to the right and placed in steep reverse Trendelenberg to allow the distal small bowel to fall out of the field. The ligament of Treitz is identified at the base of the transverse mesocolon. A point 20 cm distal to this is grasped on the antimesenteric border with atraumatic grasping forceps introduced through the upper left port. The bowel segment is brought to the abdominal wall and percutaneously placed T fasteners are introduced into the lumen of the bowel and deployed. These hold the bowel against the abdominal wall. A Seldinger technique is employed to introduce the feeding catheter into the bowel and thread it distally for a distance of 5 to 6 cm. The catheter is secured to the abdominal wall with 2-0 or 0 silk sutures.

There are two methods for introducing the catheter into the bowel when a feeding jejunostomy is performed via laparotomy. The first, a Stamm enterostomy, is similar to the laparoscopic technique. A segment of proximal jejunum is brought into the wound and two concentric purse-string sutures are placed into the seromuscular layer of the bowel using 3-0 silk. An enterotomy is made using electrocautery through the center of the concentric sutures. A 14- or 16-French (Fr) whistle-tip latex catheter is inserted through the enterotomy and threaded distally for a distance of 5 to 6 cm. The purse-string sutures are secured around the catheter. The catheterized segment is brought to the abdominal wall some distance from the laparotomy incision. A 1 cm stab wound is made and a Kelly or tonsil clamp is inserted through the abdominal wall, the catheter tip is brought through the abdominal wall and 3 or 4 additional 2-0 silk sutures are placed to affix the segment to the underside of the abdominal wall. The catheter is secured at the skin with stout silk sutures.

A Witzel enterostomy is an alternative to the Stamm and may be preferred because it not only provides a slight valve-like effect but also more reliably prevents feeding solution or bowel contents from leaking around the catheter (Fig 43–17). The site of the catheterization is selected and a single concentric purse-string suture is

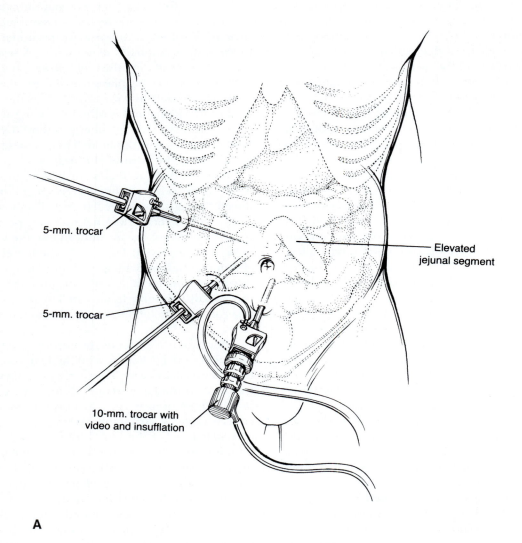

5-mm. trocar

5-mm. trocar

10-mm. trocar with
video and insufflation

Elevated
jejunal segment

A

Figure 43–16. A. Under either general anesthesia or generous intravenous sedation, carbon dioxide is insufflated into the abdomen to 15 mm Hg via an insufflator needle inserted just below the umbilicus by means of standard techniques. A 10-mm trocar is passed into the abdomen, and the camera is inserted. Two 5-mm trocars
are inserted under direct vision, one through the right midabdomen and one through the right lower quadrant. *Continued*

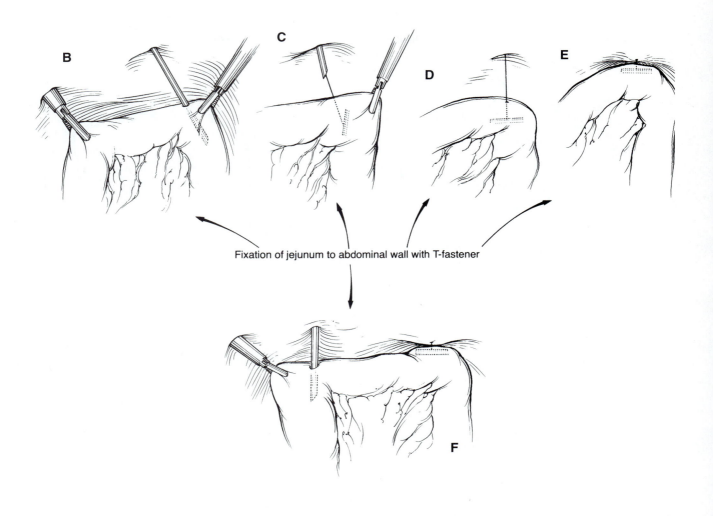

Fixation of jejunum to abdominal wall with T-fastener

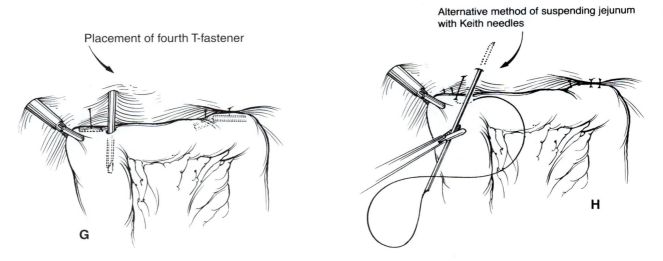

Placement of fourth T-fastener

Alternative method of suspending jejunum with Keith needles

Figure 43–16, cont'd. B through H. Four retraction sutures are placed with either T fasteners or 3-0 nylon sutures on Keith needles. *Continued*

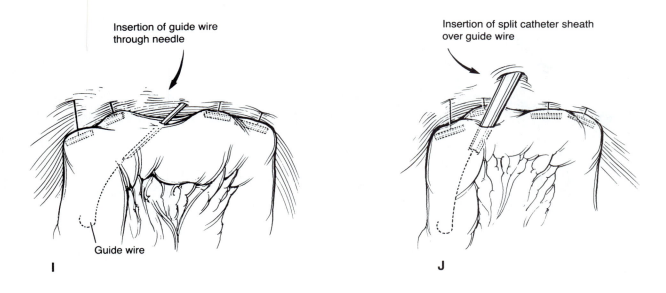

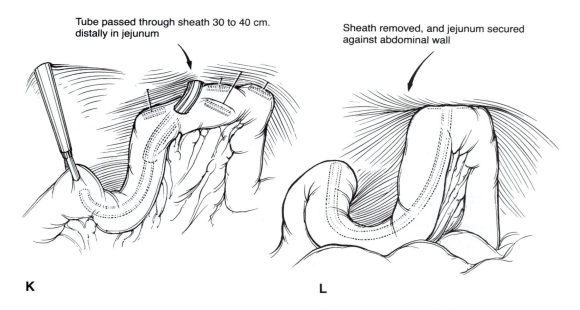

Figure 43–16, cont'd. I. A 14-gauge needle is passed through the abdominal wall and into the jejunum in the center of the four retention sutures. A guidewire is passed through the needle and directed distally into the bowel. The needle is removed. **J.** A 16-Fr split catheter sheath and dilator are passed over the guidewire and advanced into the small bowel. **K.** The guidewire and introducer are removed, and a 14-Fr jejunostomy tube is passed through the sheath into the small bowel. **L.** The sheath is removed. Gas is allowed to escape, reducing the intra-abdominal pressure to 8 to 10 mm Hg and the small bowel is drawn up and secured against the abdominal wall under minimal tension with the four retention sutures. The jejunostomy tube is anchored to the skin at the exit site with a 3-0 nylon suture. The tube is tested for patency by injection of a saline solution. All of the gas is then allowed to exit from the abdomen, the trocars are removed, the fascia at the 10-mm trocar site is approximated with an absorbable suture and sterile dressing are applied. The jejunostomy can be used immediately. The retention sutures are left in place for 3 to 4 weeks and then removed. (From Grant JP. Laparoscopic jejunostomy. In: Sabiston DC Jr (ed), *Atlas of General Surgery.* Philadelphia, PA: WB Saunders; 1994. Illustrations by Robert G Gordon.)

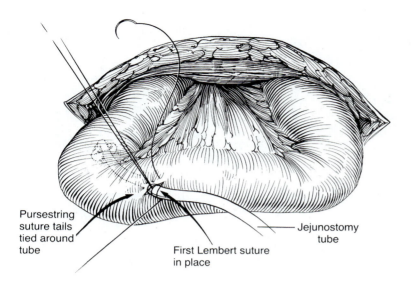

Pursestring
suture tails
tied around
tube

First Lembert suture
in place

Jejunostomy
tube

A

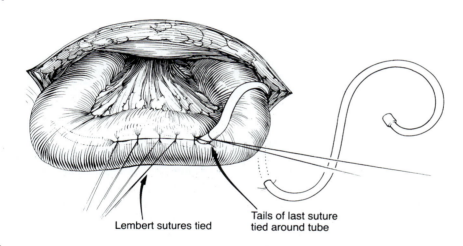

Lembert sutures tied

Tails of last suture
tied around tube

B

Jejunal loop sutured to
abdominal wall to prevent twisting

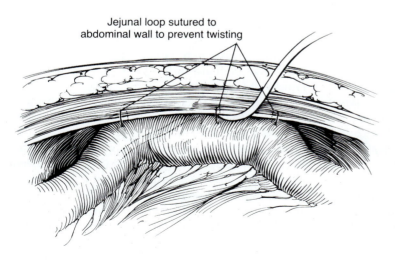

C

Figure 43–17. A. A stab wound is placed in the center of the purse-string, and a feeding jejunostomy tube (8 to 16 Fr) is passed distally into the bowel. The purse-string suture is secured around the tube. **B.** Four to six vertical mattress sutures of 4-0 silk are placed, beginning at the entrance site of the tube and extending proximally on the jejunum to create a serosal tunnel over the tube. The tails of the last suture are tied around the tube to secure it in place. A stab wound is made in the left upper quadrant of the abdomen, and the feeding tube is drawn through the stab wound with a Kelly clamp. **C.** The jejunum is sutured to the anterior abdominal wall with three 3-0 silk sutures. One suture is placed at the tube exit site, one just proximal to it, and another just distal to it. These sutures prevent torsion. The tube is secured to the abdominal wall and flushed with saline to ensure patency. The posterior rectus sheath and peritoneum are closed with 1-0 chromic catgut suture, and the anterior rectus sheath is closed with 1-0 or 2-0 permanent suture. Sterile dressings are applied. The jejunostomy may be used as soon as bowel sounds return. (From Grant JP. Witzel jejunostomy. In: Sabiston DC Jr (ed), *Atlas of General Surgery.* Philadelphia, PA: WB Saunders; 1994. Illustrations by Robert G Gordon.)

placed through the seromuscular segment of the bowel wall. The same catheter is inserted and the suture is secured. The tubing is run along the proximal antimesenteric portion of the jejunum for a distance of approximately 6 cm. Lembert-type sutures are placed on either side of the catheter tube and secured. This places the catheter in a serosal tube which acts as a valve and minimizes the possibility of leakage. The potential disadvantage of this technique involves narrowing the proximal lumen of the bowel with the inverting Lembert stitches. Care must be taken to use the right-sized catheter and to limit the inversion to avoid this complication. The tubing is anchored to the underside of the abdominal wall in a similar fashion to the Stamm technique.

Feedings can be begun immediately, using a hypotonic solution to limit the osmotic cathartic effect of full-strength solutions. Feedings are continuous. Volume and concentrations are increased gradually until adequate caloric intake is achieved. Catheters should not be removed until at least 4 weeks after placement. This ensures adequate healing of the jejunal loop to the abdominal wall. When catheters become dislodged or fall out, they should be replaced immediately. These enterostomies will heal over rapidly if they are not re-intubated within 12 to 18 hours.

ROUX-EN-Y ANASTOMOSIS

The Roux-en-Y anastomosis (Fig 43–18) is named after Caesar Roux, a Swiss surgeon who popularized, although he did not publicize, the operation in the 1880s. The operation was first performed because of the significant problems of bilious vomiting which occurred after simple gastrojejunostomy done for unresectable cancer of the stomach. Roux's original description of a gastrojejunostomy created as a Y subsequently fell into some disrepute because of the high likelihood of stomal ulceration. The Roux-en-Y anastomosis, however, was resurrected after World War II and has become a standard method for draining a variety of organs in which straight organ to small bowel anastomosis would be undesirable.

The current indications for Roux-en-Y anastomosis include the dumping syndrome, the afferent loop syndrome, reflux gastritis, and reflux esophagitis. It also is used to reconstruct the upper gastrointestinal tract after total gastrectomy or distal esophagectomy. It is equally important for surgical treatment of the biliary tract and that has become perhaps the common use of the Roux-en-Y anastomosis. It also is used for drainage of the pancreas in the form of Roux-en-Y pancreaticojejunostomy or for pancreatic cyst jejunostomy for pseudocyst. Finally, it has been used in the past for bariatic surgical treatment for gastric bypass of obesity. When a small gastric pouch is created, it generally is drained using the Roux-en-Y anastomosis.

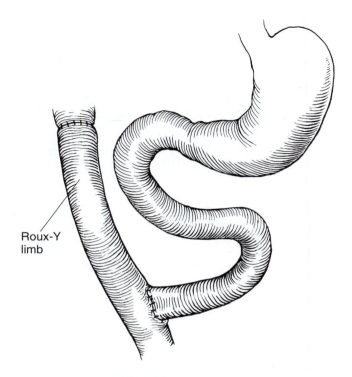

Figure 43–18. Basic anatomy of Roux-en-Y loop.

An important consideration in the creation of a Roux limb is the protection of adequate blood supply to the anastomosis. The Roux limb is created at a point approximately 15 to 20 cm distal to the ligament of Treitz. The jejunum is divided at this point. In current usage, simple division of the jejunum with the GIA stapler provides a quick and effective way of separating the bowel. Care must be taken to protect the vascular arcades that supply this area and after precisely identifying the vascular arcades, the mesentery is incised, the vessels doubly clamped, divided, and ligated until the base of the mesentery is reached. Great care must be taken at this point to re-evaluate both cut ends of the jejunum for adequacy of blood supply.

The length of the Roux limb has gradually increased with time. In the early years of the century, the limb was generally in the vicinity of 10 cm. As experience has been gained, most feel that the optimal length of a Roux limb should be approximately 30 to 40 cm. Depending on the organ to be reanastomosed, the cut distal end of the jejunum is brought through an antecolic or retrocolic position. For benign disease with long-term prognosis, a retrocolic limb placed on either side of the middle colic vessels will provide greater length and less chance of partial obstruction owing to the colon and the omentum. For malignant disease such as pancreatic cancer in which the Roux limb is for gastric bypass or biliary bypass, an antecolic position may be chosen in order to prevent tumor encroachment on the jejunal limb. Our current understanding of reflux suggests that the length of the Roux limb is relatively unimportant in preventing reflux. The reanastomosis, created as an end-to-side jejunojejunostomy is performed at a comfortable place in the distal segment. The exact method of reanastomosis is left to the preference of the surgeon. When adequate blood supply is present and there is no tension on the anastomosis, virtually all techniques used in reanastomosis are considered satisfactory.

Roux-en-Y anastomoses are not without complications. Stomal ulceration has been alluded to and is clearly the most obvious complication. Jejunal ulcer will occur in up to 15% of patients treated with a Roux-en-Y gastrojejunostomy. Because the jejunal mucosa is directly in contact with acid from the stomach without significant amounts of alkaline secretions from the biliary and pancreatic tree, ulcerations may occur.[27] Complete vagotomy can prevent this complication. The high incidence of ulceration is sufficiently reproducible so that this technique of gastrojejunostomy is used in a number of experimental conditions and is quite similar to the Mann-Williamson pouch.

A further complication is the Roux-en-Y syndrome. This results from inadequate emptying of the stomach into Roux-en-Y anastomosis and is characterized by nausea, vomiting, and pain with bloating. This may be particularly significant if a vagotomy has been performed. The syndrome often resolves with time but, if it persists, the patient may require a subtotal gastrectomy. The degree of jejunal stasis contributing to this problem is unknown.[28]

ILEOSTOMY

Permanent ileostomy, although used less frequently than before, continues to be an important technique with which surgeons must be familiar. An ileostomy is used for patients in whom an ileoanal reconstruction is inappropriate. Positioning of the stoma is important for adequate long-term function. It should be placed in the outer third of the right rectus muscle at or just below a line between the umbilicus and anterior iliac spine. It must be sufficiently far from bony prominences or abdominal scars so that the appliance can be placed without difficulty. Ideally, an enterstomal therapist will mark out the ideal location prior to surgery after taking into consideration the patient's body habitus, clothing preferences, and any preexisting creases or scars. If possible, the terminal ileum should be passed through an extraperitoneal tunnel to the point where it emerges through the abdominal wall. This will prevent late obstructive complications resulting from the "maypole" effect that can occur when the terminal ileum is taken di-

rectly to the anterior abdominal wall. It is important to make the stoma at or slightly medial to the margin of the rectus to prevent eventration and parastomal hernias.

The terminal ileum should be divided at its junction with the cecum. The mesentery of the final 2.5 to 3 cm of the ileum should be completely excised and that of an additional 2.5 to 3 cm proximal to that partially removed. This will maintain adequate blood supply to the Brooke ileostomy. The entire 5 to 6 cm segment is brought through the abdominal wall and the most distal 2.5 to 3 cm is everted back on itself. Absorbable sutures are placed to create the final stoma. These absorbable sutures should be fine (4-0) and should include full thickness of the distal cut edge of the bowel and a seromuscular portion where the bowel exits the abdominal wall. A third portion of the suture is taken to the dermis and secured. This holds the everted segment of the Brooke ileostomy in place. Sutures are placed at all four quadrants and further reinforced as necessary.

Eversion can be made easier by use of a Guy rope technique[29] (Fig 43–19). In this technique, U stitches are placed 2.5 to 3 cm proximal to the cut edge of the ileum and retracted as demonstrated. This everts the mucosa and allows proper placement of the absorbable sutures through the full thickness wall, seromuscular layer and dermis.

When a permanent ileostomy is not necessary but temporary diversion is required, a loop ileostomy may provide an excellent method for decompressing the bowel and protecting distal anastomoses.[30] The loop is brought up to the abdominal wall without tunneling and a plastic rod to support the loop is placed under the loop, bridging the skin. The distal, nonfunctioning side is opened and a stoma is created by everting, with interrupted sutures, this portion of the bowel. Internal and external fixation sutures typically are not used. This stoma can be easily taken down through a local procedure in which the bowel eventually is divided, proximal and distal limbs are checked, a GIA stapler is run across the two antimesenteric margins, and the resulting confluent defect closed with one or two TA staplers.

APPENDECTOMY (FIG 43–20)

Appendectomy is performed whenever the diagnosis of appendicitis is proven or suspected. Typically, appendectomy is performed through one of two incisions. The first is a limited right paramedian incision made laterally on the right rectus muscle. This technique enjoys the strength and ease of a paramedian incision and provides efficient mobility for the surgeon to allow exploration of the remainder of the right lower quadrant and right pelvis. Nonetheless, it is a larger incision and for that reason may provide greater short-term postoperative morbidity for the patient. An alternative is the oblique

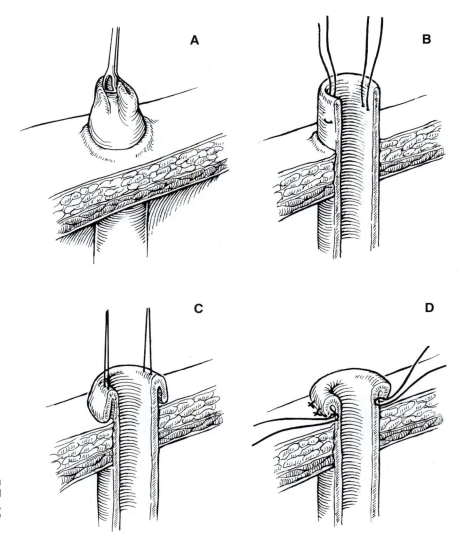

Figure 43–19. Ileostomy, Guy rope technique. **A.** Ileum brought through abdominal wall. **B.** Mattress sutures placed 3 cm from cut end of ileum. **C.** Mattress sutures held taut, everting distal 3 cm of ileum. **D.** Standard Brooke ileostomy sutures placed.

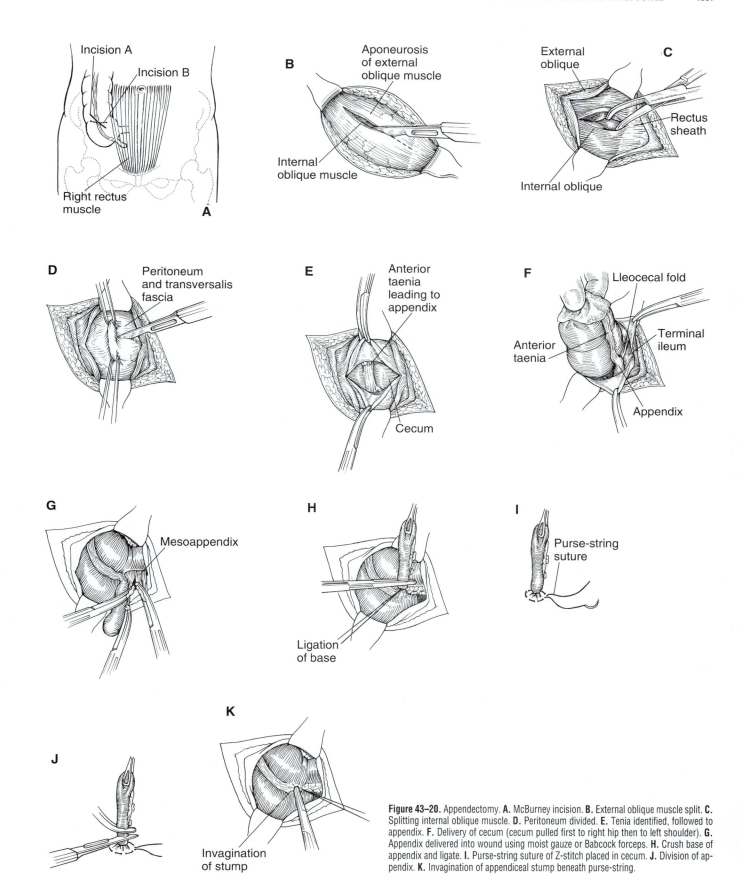

Figure 43–20. Appendectomy. **A.** McBurney incision. **B.** External oblique muscle split. **C.** Splitting internal oblique muscle. **D.** Peritoneum divided. **E.** Tenia identified, followed to appendix. **F.** Delivery of cecum (cecum pulled first to right hip then to left shoulder). **G.** Appendix delivered into wound using moist gauze or Babcock forceps. **H.** Crush base of appendix and ligate. **I.** Purse-string suture of Z-stitch placed in cecum. **J.** Division of appendix. **K.** Invagination of appendiceal stump beneath purse-string.

Rockey-Davis incision first described in 1905. This transverse or oblique transverse right lower quadrant muscle-splitting incision is placed at McBurney's point, lateral to the lateral extent of the rectus muscle. This is an important consideration when operating on young people because of the relatively larger width of the rectus muscle. In this approach, the external oblique muscle is spread along its fibers running in an oblique fashion under which the obliquely running fibers of the internal oblique will be identified. The thin areolar fascia overlying the internal oblique can be incised along its length and this muscle can be spread using narrow angled retractors such as an Army-Navy retractor. This will allow access to the transversus-abdominus and the peritoneum which can be incised sharply in an oblique fashion extending from lateral to medial.

Studies of various incisions has demonstrated that there is a significantly decreased wound infection when the Rockey-Davis right lower quadrant muscle-splitting incision is used, as compared to a vertical incision. Wound infections occur in <10% of patients after appendectomy.

Any fluid identified at this time is cultured for both aerobic and anaerobic bacteria and a limited manual examination is performed, usually with one or two fingers. In the case of an obvious appendicitis, the thickened, woody appendix often will be felt in the depths of the wound. Gentle, blunt dissection will allow mobilization of the appendix, which can be grasped with an atraumatic instrument such as a Babcock and gently teased from the companion structures and brought into the wound.

When the appendix has been fully elevated into the wound, the mesoappendix will be seen, generally somewhat foreshortened because of the inflammatory process. The mesentery can be taken between hemostatic clamps, dividing and ligating the vascular supply with 3-0 or 2-0 sutures. These sutures are generally of silk although absorbable sutures such as Vicryl or Dexon can be used. The dissection is taken to the base of the appendix and the mesoappendix is entirely cleared to this area. Occasionally small vascular tributaries may be coagulated with a brief application of a coagulating current.

In general, the base of the appendix will be relatively uninvolved in the inflammatory process and this will facilitate not only management of the stump but also inversion, should that be required.

A crushing clamp is applied to the base of the appendix, generally a right-angle clamp will suffice. This is released and slipped more distally on the appendix where it is once again clamped and left in place. The initially crushed area is encircled with a 2-0 or 3-0 absorbable suture which is tied with a single square knot. A hemostat is applied to the knot and left in place. The specimen then is removed. The freshly cut edge of the appendiceal base is cauterized with an electrocauterization current to obliterate the mucosa and prevent development of a mucoceal.

The appendiceal stump is dunked into the cecum; this is performed through either a Z stitch or a purse-string stitch. The dunking maneuver is facilitated with the use of the hemostat which is removed when the purse-string or Z stitch is tied. Prior to dividing the purse-string or Z stitch, which is typically fashioned using a 3-0 silk suture ligature, a segment of the epiploic fat around the cecum is placed over the purse-string and further secured with the tie to provide additional security in this closure. The cecum is replaced within the right lower quadrant and the abdomen is widely irrigated.

Drains are used at all times when there is a purulent collection, but also may be used at the discretion of the surgeon if there is free perforation. If there is a purulent collection, drainage should be placed into the abscess cavity or collection, extending into the right pelvis. Additionally, drains may be placed along the right gutter. These can be brought out through the incision. Drains may be either Penrose or latex drains or closed-suction drains, such as Jackson Pratt. Lau recommends use of drains if gangrene or perforation is identified.[31] The most common bacteria are *E coli*, *S viridans*, *pseudomonas* and group D strep. Also *B fragilis* is noted. Cefoxitin is felt to be the antibiotic of choice. Other antibiotics used are cefotetan or cefoperazone.

Wound closure is performed in anatomic layers using absorbable sutures. 0 Vicryl is preferred. The closure may be running or interrupted. The peritoneum should be closed and additionally, the loose fascia over the internal oblique also should be reapproximated. The external oblique fascia is closed in a running fashion. In the setting of frank purulence, the surgeon may choose to leave the skin and subcutaneous tissue open. Otherwise, it can be closed with either a running subcuticular stitch, interrupted nonabsorbable skin sutures, or staples. Perioperative antibiotics are administered to cover colonic flora. Second or third generation cephalosporins are appropriate. These antibiotics should be given preoperatively and for one dose postoperatively. When an appendiceal abscess has been found, a longer antibiotic course should be begun, based on intraoperative cultures.

RIGHT COLECTOMY (FIG 43–21)

Right colectomy is typically performed for cancer and large neoplastic lesions, inflammatory bowel disease, or hemorrhage. A variety of incisions may be used including midline, paramedian, or transverse (based slightly above the umbilicus). A formal right colectomy encompasses the terminal ileum, the entire right colon,

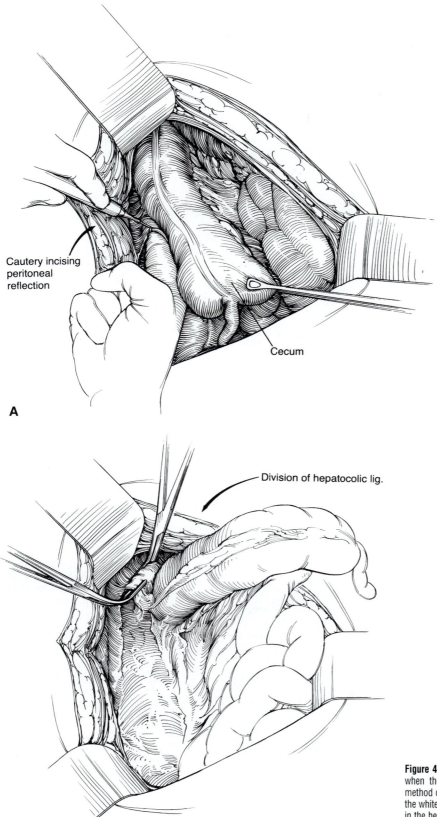

A

Cautery incising
peritoneal
reflection

Cecum

Division of hepatocolic lig.

B

Figure 43–21. Right colectomy. **A.** Except in the presence of cirrhosis when there is tremendous retroperitoneal hypervascularity, the best method of mobilization of the ascending colon is with the cautery along the white line of Toldt. **B.** A number of small vessels are usually present in the hepatocolic ligament, which is divided between Kelly clamps, and these vessels are ligated. Mobilization in this region should extend posteriorly to near the aorta. *Continued*

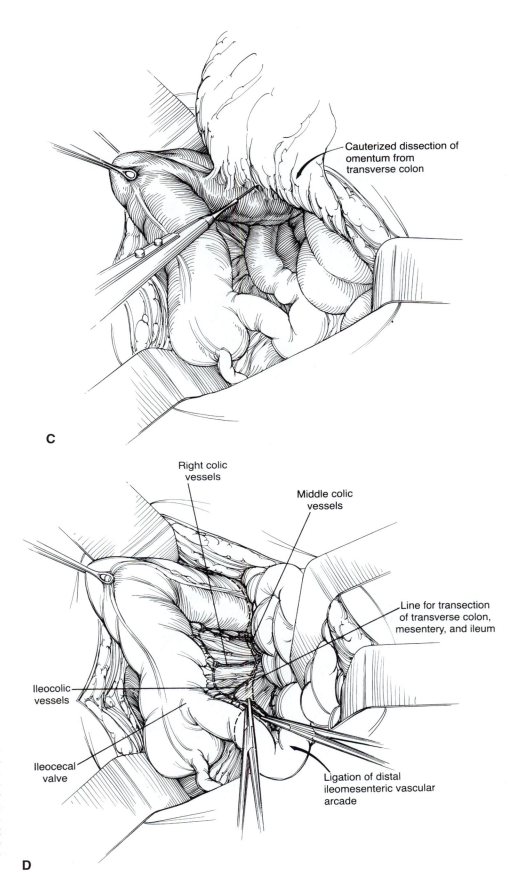

Cauterized dissection of
omentum from
transverse colon

C

Right colic
vessels

Middle colic
vessels

Line for transection
of transverse colon,
mesentery, and ileum

Ileocolic
vessels

Ileocecal
valve

Ligation of distal
ileomesenteric vascular
arcade

Figure 43–21, cont'd. C. The greater omentum is mobilized off the transverse colon by dissecting along the avascular plane next to the bowel wall. **D.** The sites for division of the bowel are selected, and an area of relatively little vascularity approximately 2 inches proximal to the ileocecal valve is chosen, as the mesenteric vessels are divided. These include the ileocolic artery and right trunk of the middle colic vessels The origin of the ileocolic artery is included, but branches are preserved to the left transverse colon. *Continued*

D

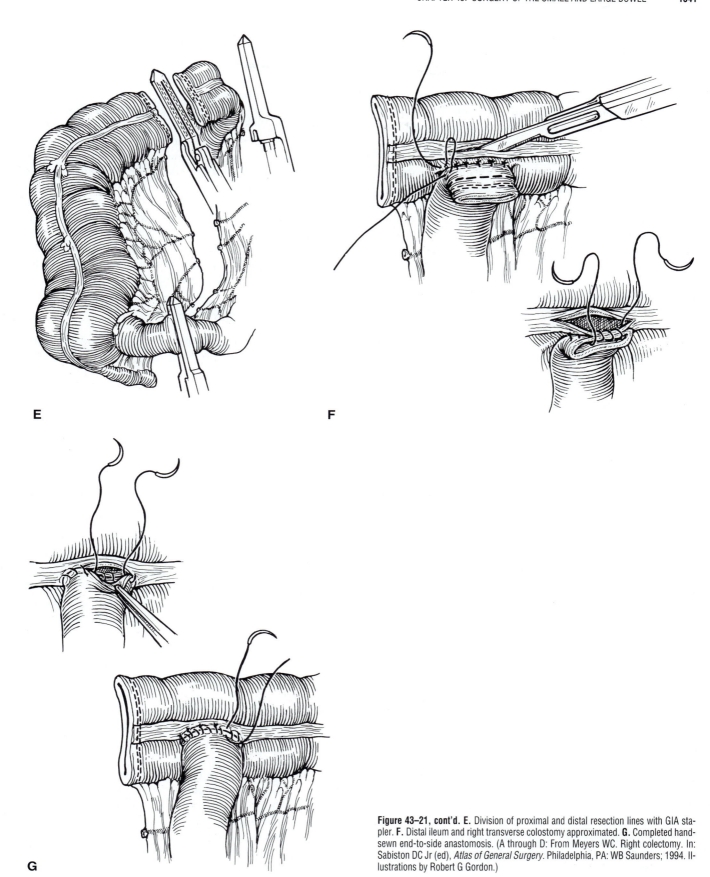

E

F

G

Figure 43–21, cont'd. E. Division of proximal and distal resection lines with GIA stapler. **F.** Distal ileum and right transverse colostomy approximated. **G.** Completed hand-sewn end-to-side anastomosis. (A through D: From Meyers WC. Right colectomy. In: Sabiston DC Jr (ed), *Atlas of General Surgery.* Philadelphia, PA: WB Saunders; 1994. Illustrations by Robert G Gordon.)

and the proximal portion of the right transverse colon. The subsequent establishment of intestinal continuity involves creation of an ileo-transverse colostomy. Although the bacterial flora of the right colon is less problematic than the left, a full mechanical and antibiotic bowel preparation is performed in the elective setting. This includes intravenous antibiotics at the time of induction of anesthesia.

Following the incision and a full manual and visual exploration of the abdomen, retractors are placed and uninvolved bowel is packed out of the operative field. The bowel is inspected and palpated, identifying the lesion and ensuring that there will be adequate margins following resection. The avascular attachments to the right gutter are sharply incised (the white line of Toldt) and the entire right colon is retracted to the left of the abdomen by the operator's nondominant hand. After the white line has been incised, avascular fatty tissue between the colon and the retroperitoneum will be encountered and should be bluntly separated from the bowel. This also will allow the surgeon to visualize the ureter in its abdominal course as the bowel is brought towards the midline. The dissection continues cranially until the vascular attachments of the hepatic flexure are encountered. These require specific isolation, clamping, division, and ligation and this must be performed close to the colon. The duodenum is just behind the hepatic flexure and must be guarded closely at this location to prevent injury.

After the entire right colon has been mobilized medially, proximal and distal resection lines are selected depending on the location of the lesion to be removed. Typically, a short segment of the terminal ileum will be included in the specimen. The ileocolic, the right colic and right-sided branches of the middle colic will be taken with the specimen. The peritoneal surface of the mesentery is incised with Metzenbaum scissors along the proposed resection line. This will be a fairly straight line extending from a point 4 to 6 cm proximal to the cecum to a point adjacent to the hepatic flexure. The colon is lifted and the mesentery is transilluminated to clarify the major vessels to be sacrificed. In years past, an early high ligation of the vascular pedicle was encouraged, but there is insufficient data to support the need for this maneuver, even in the malignant disease.

The mesenteric vessels are doubly clamped, divided, and ligated with 2-0 silk sutures for security and permanence. The small end-vessels at the mesenteric margin of the colon are controlled with fine sutures or electrocautery. The omental attachments to the right transverse colon must be resected with the specimen in order to clear a sufficient length of the distal bowel to accommodate the anastomosis. The specimen is removed and the bowel is prepared for reanastomosis. Reanastomosis can be performed with either staples or sutures. Stapled anastomoses are almost invariably created in a side-to-

side fashion using a 55- or 60-cm linear cutting apparatus. An end-to-side anastomosis can be fashioned using the circular stapler, but this offers no particular advantages over the side-to-side technique.

Hand-sewn anastomoses can be created as either end-to-end (the most common), as end-to-side, or as side-to-side. With the exception of end-to-end anastomosis, the ileum should be anastomosed into the anterior taenia of the colon. If a side-to-side anastomosis is used, the cut ends of both the large and small bowels must be closed. This should be accomplished in two layers, an inner running layer of chromic or some synthetic absorbable suture and an outer, interrupted layer employing Lembert-type sutures.

The mesenteric defect may be closed at the discretion of the surgeon with fine silk sutures. Alternatively, it can be left untouched without untoward outcome.

TRANSVERSE COLOSTOMY (FIG 43–22)

Transverse colostomies were once more common than at present. They were used regularly to decompress the large bowel and divert the fecal stream as the first stage of a three-stage approach for diverticulitis. They are of particular importance even now for the management of complete bowel obstruction secondary to large, bulky malignant lesions of the distal bowel.

In elderly, frail, and thin patients, diverting transverse colostomies can be performed under local anesthesia with adequate intravenous sedation but, in general, this is a less desirable technique. Rather, the patient should be anesthestized under general endotracheal anesthesia to provide sufficient relaxation for the surgeon and to protect the airway should there be any tendency towards vomiting or regurgitation brought on by traction on the bowel or general peritoneal irritation.

Transverse colostomies may be performed through a midline incision or a local incision in the right upper quadrant. The choice will depend, to a large degree, on the general state of the patient, the body habitus, and the preference of the surgeon. Additionally, transverse colostomies can be performed as either loop diversion or as double-barreled diversion. The latter is the more reliable for complete diversion but the former is simpler to perform and in general large amounts of stool do not traverse the ostomy into the distal segment.

Using an upper midline incision, the abdomen is entered and the right transverse colon is identified. The omentum, if present, is cleared and a small window is fashioned beneath the area to be used for the colostomy. If a loop is anticipated, umbilical tape is passed through the window and the cutaneous site is selected. A short transverse or oblique incision is made in the skin overlying this area, the abdomen entered and the umbilical tape passed externally through the incision. The

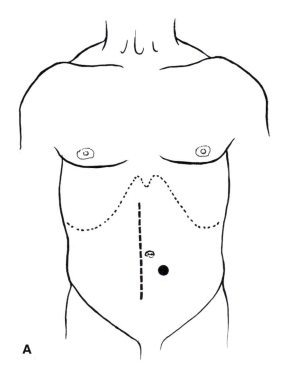

A

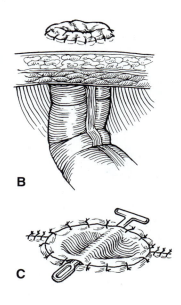

B

C

Figure 43–22. Colostomies. **A.** Site for end-sigmoid colostomy. **B.** End colostomy with primary maturation. **C.** Transverse loop colostomy placed over bar.

bowel loop is eviscerated, a glass or plastic rod passed through the window to hold the loop above the skin and the wounds closed. Following closure, the loop is opened and an appliance is placed. If the surgeon prefers a double-barreled colostomy, the bowel is divided with staplers, the mesentery further separated with clamps and ligatures, and proximal and distal stoma sites are selected. Typically, the mucus fistula may be placed at the upper margin of the midline incision and the end-colostomy at a point in the right upper quadrant away from the costal margin so that the appliance will fit easily. The wounds are closed and the stoma is matured with fine absorbable sutures. A DeMartel clamp may be left on the mucus fistula for 5 to 7 days to prevent contamination of the midline incision.

A short transverse or oblique incision is made in the right upper quadrant. The incision should be approximately 6 to 10 cm in length depending on the degree of abdominal wall thickness. Upon entering the abdomen, dilated large bowel will be identified at the hepatic flexure or right transverse colon. This should be teased away from the surrounding tissue and elevated into the wound. Sharp mobilization of mesenteric and omental tissue may be necessary in order to achieve adequate length to bring the colon above the level of the skin. Vascularized attachments should be controlled with fine sutures or electrocautery. After the bowel has been fully mobilized and brought above the level of the skin, a plastic or glass rod is placed under the loop, the fascia

is closed snugly around the afferent and efferent segments, and the skin beneath the bridge is loosely approximated. After the skin is closed the bowel is opened and an appliance positioned. The bowel should be opened close to the distal edge in order to minimize stool passing from the proximal to the distal limb.

LEFT COLECTOMY (FIG 43–23)

Left colectomy is required for neoplastic lesions, diverticular disease, and, occasionally, inflammatory lesions. The amount of colon resected is dependent on the pathologic process. The incision is either midline or left paramedian depending on the preference of the surgeon. Regardless, the incision should be of sufficient length to allow the operator full access to the splenic flexure and the liver to evaluate for metastases in cases of malignant disease.

The proximal bowel is packed out of the wound and held in place by a retractor over a moist gauze to prevent drying of the serosa. The avascular attachments between the colon and the left gutter are sharply incised and the colon is rolled medially. If the splenic flexure must be mobilized for a tension-free anastomosis, this must be done under direct vision, meticulously isolating the vascular attachments between clamps, dividing and ligating them with silk sutures. As this is sequentially performed, the colon may be mobilized medially and caudally. For elective resection of diverticular disease,

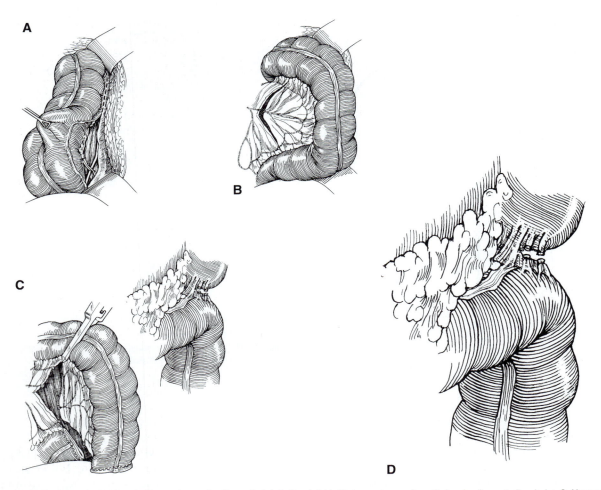

Figure 43–23. Sigmoid colectomy. **A.** Mesenteric resection lines selected. **B.** Bowel divided between clamps; alternatively using linear stapling device. **C.** Maneuver for mobilizing splenic flexure for higher lesions.

all involved colon must be taken to prevent recurrent attacks. As the colon is mobilized, attention is turned to the retroperitoneum just inside the pelvic brim where the ureter is identified and protected. The distal resection line is selected and the serosal surface of the bowel is prepared circumferentially. The mesenteric peritoneal surface is divided in preparation for taking the vascular supply to the distal left colon. On the right side, the ureter must be identified as well. This is accomplished by gently spreading the retroperitoneal tissues until the structure is seen, gently clamped, and its peristalsis recognized. As before, the mesenteric vessels are taken between clamps, divided and ligated with silk sutures. Proximally, the omentum must be sufficiently cleared from the anterior surface of the left transverse colon to allow a fresh anastomosis.

The middle colic is identified and its left-sided branches are taken, as are the vascular splenocolic ligaments attaching the splenic flexure to the spleen and the left upper quadrant. After the mesentery has been divided, the colon itself is divided, as before, using either staples or noncrushing clamps. The anastomosis between the residual proximal and distal bowel is performed either by hand or stapler. In order to maintain adequate length, an end-to-end anastomosis may be preferred when using the stapler. This can be accomplished by making a proximal colotomy through the anterior tenia and inserting the circular stapler. The anvil will be placed in the distal segment, secured with a manually or mechanically placed purse-string. The largest diameter device possible should be used but, in patients with significant diverticular thickening, devices larger than 30 mm may be difficult to insert into the colon lumen. The colotomy used to place the circular stapler is closed transversely using a 30 or 60 mm linear stapler.

Hand-sewn anastomoses may be performed in one or two layers depending on the preference of the surgeon. These are almost always fashioned end-to-end.

ANTERIOR RESECTION OF THE RECTOSIGMOID (FIG 43–24)

Anterior resection of the rectosigmoid, either high or low, is used in the management of neoplastic disease of the sigmoid colon or the rectum. It is differentiated from left colectomies by the need to incise the peritoneal reflection and mobilize the retroperitoneal portion of the rectosigmoid. The portion of the colon removed encompasses that part supplied by the left colic artery and extending inferiorly to that segment just proximal to the middle hemorrhoidal. Particularly low resections continue distal to the middle hemorrhoidals and are considered low anterior resections.

The principles of this resection are similar to those discussed in removal of more proximal portions of the colon. Of particular importance is identification of both the right and left ureter prior to dividing any tissue. The resection is begun at the site of the proximal resection line, usually at or slightly above the pelvic brim. The lateral avascular attachments are sharply incised, the retroperitoneum opened, and the ureter identified on the left side. The peritoneal incision is continued downwards into the pelvis, staying at least 6 to 8 cm from the bowel wall at the level of the base of the bladder. At this location, the incision in the peritoneum turns anteriorly and to the right until it is well lateral to the right side of the distal sigmoid colon. The peritoneal layer covering the mesentery is divided on each side and the right ureter is identified in a comparable location to the left. It is generally advantageous to divide the sigmoid colon at this time. This allows the operator a "handle" to control the bowel and maintain proximal, upward traction on the rectosigmoid. The surgeon should dissect until at least 2 cm distal to the neoplastic lesion, although a longer distal margin is desirable when there is sufficient length. Care must be taken when dividing the lateral at-

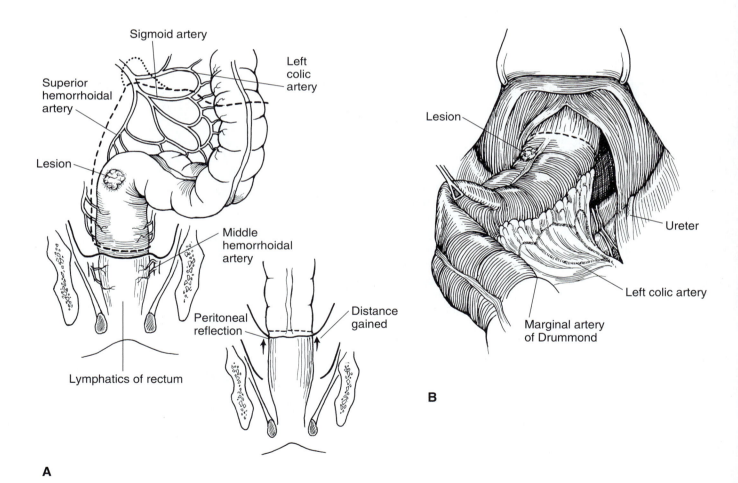

Figure 43–24. Low anterior resection (hand-sewn). **A.** Diagram of vascular supply and proposed resection segment. **B.** Peritoneal floor incised, tumor mobilized upwards. Resection lines selected.

tachments to the rectosigmoid at and below the peritoneal reflection. These attachments may be highly vascular and will require ligatures or clips to control. A
wide dissection is employed to clear sufficient adjacent
tissue that may harbor local extension of the disease
and/or lymph nodes which will be important in establishing accurate staging of the disease.

When the specimen is completely isolated it is divided, sent to pathology to determine margins and frequently returned to the operating suite so that the surgeon may more precisely gauge the proximity of the
margins. Reanastomosis is performed with either staplers or hand sewing. This resection is particularly
suited for the circular stapler. If this type of reanastomosis is anticipated, the patient must be placed in a
modified lithotomy position at the onset of the case in
order to gain access to the anus for placement of the stapling device. Alternatively, the circular stapler can be introduced from the proximal either as an end-to-end
(through a proximal colotomy) or side-to-end (through
the divided proximal bowel end). If circular staples are
to be inserted from the rectum, a triple staple technique
is used. The stapled distal resection line is traversed by
the pointed end of the circular stapling device introduced through the rectum and piercing the rectum just
anterior or posterior to the transversely placed staple
line.

Hand-sewn anastomoses can be either end-to-end or
side-to-side (Baker anastomosis). These are constructed
in either one or two layers. Side-to-end anastomoses will
require slightly more length in the proximal colon and
this can be achieved by incising the peritoneal covering
of the mesentery all the way to the right of the middle
colic vessels. The anastomosis should be placed in an anterior tenia on the proximal portion of bowel.

When circular stapled anastomoses are created it is
important to closely check the two "doughnuts" of tissue
that lie within the head of the stapler after being fired.
Confirmation that these rings are intact ensures that
there is no unsuspected hole in the anastomosis. Additionally, the anastomosis can be checked by filling the
pelvis with saline and instilling air into the rectum with
an Asepto syringe. If air bubbles are seen, the anastomosis must be checked and any defects reinforced with
sutures.

LOW ANTERIOR RESECTION OF RECTUM (FIGS 43–25 AND 43–26)

Low anterior resection of the rectum is performed for
malignant disease of the anorectum and should be confined to lesions no lower than 4 cm from the anus. Controversy continues as to whether a hand-sewn or a stapled anastomosis is better and which can provide a
lower approach. Goligher states that the circular sta-

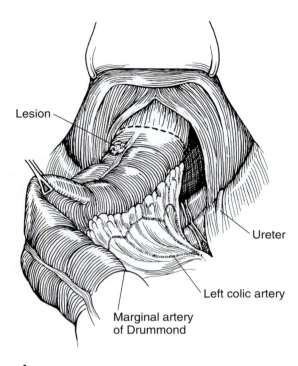

A

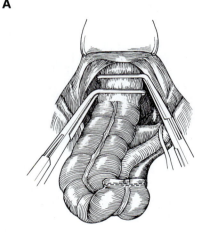

B

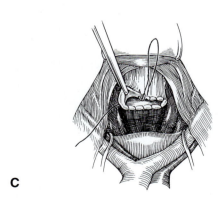

C

Figure 43–25. Low anterior resection (stapled). **A.** Proximal bowel divided; purse-string device placed. **B.** Distal resection site divided. **C.** Baseball-type purse-string suture placed on distal segment. *Continued*

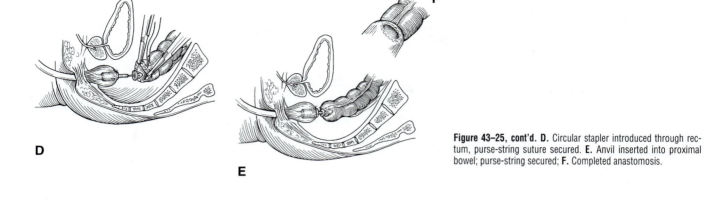

Figure 43–25, cont'd. D. Circular stapler introduced through rectum, purse-string suture secured. **E.** Anvil inserted into proximal bowel; purse-string secured; **F.** Completed anastomosis.

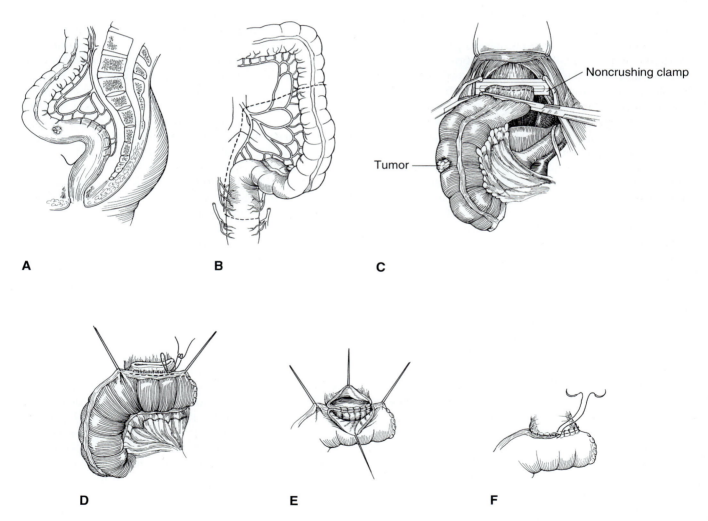

Figure 43–26. Low anterior resection (side-to-end Baker anastomosis). **A.** Tumor and vascular arcade. **B.** Resection lines. **C.** Distal bowel divided. **D.** Posterior row of sutures placed. **E.** Bowel opened for inner sutures. **F.** Completed anastomosis.

pling device allows a much lower resection than the hand anastomosis.[32] Others have found similar results and believe that the EEA stapler creates an anastomosis that is as secure as the hand-sewn and probably can be placed lower.[33]

The patient is placed in a dorsal lithotomy position and in Trendelenburg and the abdomen is opened either through a lower abdominal incision or through an oblique left lower quadrant incision. The sigmoid colon is identified at the pelvic brim and a point for proximal resection is selected and marked. The white line of Toldt in this area is taken down sharply and the retroperitoneum is entered bluntly. The left ureter is identified and the dissection continues in a manner designed to avoid compromising the ureter. The covering of the mesentery is sharply incised on the medial and lateral sides. The retroperitoneum on the right side is entered and the right ureter is identified in that location as well.

The peritoneum at the floor, extending anteriorly from the cul-de-sac, is incised, allowing complete mobility. The mesentery of the proximal bowel is taken between clamps and the bowel is divided using either noncrushing clamps or a GIA stapler of sufficient size to encompass the bowel. The distal bowel to be resected then can be maneuvered completely to facilitate dissection of the vascular structures. The lateral attachments are taken first, extending inferiorly, and identifying their vascular supply including the superior, middle, and inferior vessels that are clamped, divided, and ligated well away from the specimen. Alternatively, hemostatic clips can be used. Using blunt and sharp dissection and staying out of the presacral venous plexus, the dissection is taken down until a free margin approximately 3 to 4 cm distal to the tumor has been cleared circumferentially.

Two methods for dividing the bowel are available. A double-staple technique can be performed in which a TA stapler is passed across the rectum and fired. This may be compromised to some degree in males and thin women in whom the 55- or 60-mm TA cannot be easily placed into the narrow pelvis. Alternatively, with the bowel on tension, the rectum can be incised with electrocautery and a purse-string or whipped suture placed in segments as the bowel is divided.

Using the double-staple technique, when the bowel has been completely divided it is removed from the operative field. An EEA stapler, with the sharpened point retracted, is inserted into the rectum and brought up to the staple line. The sharpened midstrut of the EEA stapler is advanced through the stapled rectum just posterior to the transverse staple line.

The appropriate sized anvil is placed into the proximal colon through a purse-string after cutting the edges and using the purse-string applicator. The anvil is fitted to the head, the instrument is advanced and the anvil and head are brought into close approximation. When the suitable colors are evident, the instrument is fired, creating a circular anastomosis.

COLOSTOMY

Like the above mentioned ileostomy, a colostomy depends on close consultation between the surgeon, enterostomal therapist, and the patient prior to surgery. The comfort and ultimate funtionability of the stoma depend on appropriate placement. The stoma should be placed in the lower quadrant of the abdomen through the rectus muscle somewhat lateral to the midsection of the rectus. It should be below the umbilicus but well away from any bony prominences to allow proper fitting of the appliance. It must be easy for the patient to see and dress so that the appliance can be placed without difficulty.

At surgery after the bowel has been divided, a 2 cm diameter opening is made in the abdominal wall at the site selected. This can be done by grasping the tattoo or dot with a Kocher clamp, placing this on tension and amputating the skin. The fat in the subcutaneous space is excised down to the anterior rectus fascia, which is opened in a cruciate fashion with care being taken to not damage the underlying rectus or its vasculature. With blunt separation, the rectus fibers can be separated and the peritoneum entered sharply with a tonsil forceps or a Kelly clamp. Once the peritoneal opening has been made, two fingers are inserted to allow adequate diameter for the eventual stoma.

Like the ileostomy, colostomy should ideally be brought through a peritoneal tunnel up to the site of the stoma. This not only prevents postoperative obstructive phenomenon with loops of bowel kinking around the stoma but also may diminish the likelihood of parastomal hernias.

Temporary stomas can be created either as loop or right transverse colostomies or double-barrel colostomies depending on the mobility of the colon and the desires of the surgeon. Loop transverse colostomies are easy to create but because of their bulky size may be difficult for patients to manage in the interim before they are closed. Nonetheless, they are easy to close because of the proximity of the proximal and distal limbs. Double-barrel colostomies, in which a mucous fistula is created, may be somewhat easier for the patient to manage. It is important that the stoma sites be separated to facilitate placement of the appliance.

When creating an end colostomy, the bowel need not be matured and everted in the same manner as the ileostomy because a skin level colostomy will be easier to irrigate and will allow a patient to wear a stomal cap or plug after appropriate training. The historical place-

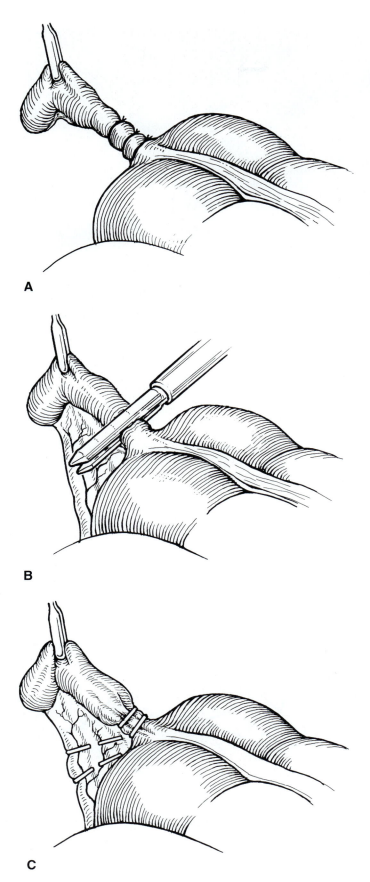

A

B

C

ment of a DeMartell clamp across the stoma and maturation of the stoma on the floor 5 to 6 days after surgery has been replaced with immediate creation of the stoma at the time of surgery, after the abdomen and skin have been closed. This will allow immediate placement of an appliance and also will allow the surgeon to closely inspect the viability of the stoma in the immediate postoperative period.

LAPAROSCOPIC PROCEDURES

Laparoscopic Diagnosis and Management of Appendicitis (Figs 43–27 through 43–30)

Misdiagnosis of appendicitis continues to be a significant problem particularly in women in the childbearing age with rates of misdiagnosis approaching 40%.[34] Laparoscopy offers the potential for improved diagnosis as well as the management of an acute appendicitis or atypical lower abdominal pain in both men and women. Ganz demonstrated the suitability of appendectomies done via the laparoscope.[35] In 431 cases, he was able to successfully perform appendectomy in 388, with an average operating time of 15 to 20 minutes. Only 3% required conversion to open. Nearly three-quarters of these case were acute. Importantly, in this series there were no wound infections and only two of the patients subsequently developed intra-abdominal abscesses after removal of a perforated appendix. The potential for laparoscopy to provide significant improvement in diagnostic accuracy has been demonstrated in a variety of series.[36,37] While many series demonstrate significant accuracy in males with right lower quadrant pain, the continued inability to differentiate pelvic from appendiceal pathology and the known impact of ruptured appendicitis on subsequent fertility has made this an important adjunct to the management of right lower quadrant pain.

The technique for laparoscopic appendectomy is straightforward and uncomplicated. The first report of this procedure was by Semm in 1983 using available equipment developed for therapeutic laparoscopy. All procedures are performed under general endotracheal anesthesia and administration of perioperative antibiotics, as mentioned above. Necessary equipment for the performance of laparoscopic appendectomy includes high-resolution video monitor, CCD camera chip attached to a 10-mm forward viewing laparoscope, high-flow insufflator, suction irrigation apparatus. Addition-

Figure 43–27. Laparoscopic appendectomy; methods for controlling appendiceal base. **A.** Pre-tied sutures. **B.** Linear stapler. **C.** Clips. (Redrawn from Brooks DC (ed). *Current Techniques in Laparoscopy,* 1st ed. Philadelphia, PA: Current Medicine; 1994)

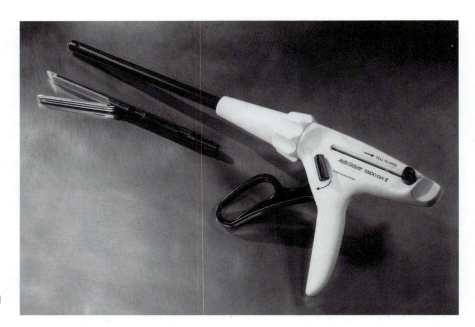

Figure 43–28. Endoscopic GIA (United States Surgical Corp, Norwalk, CT).

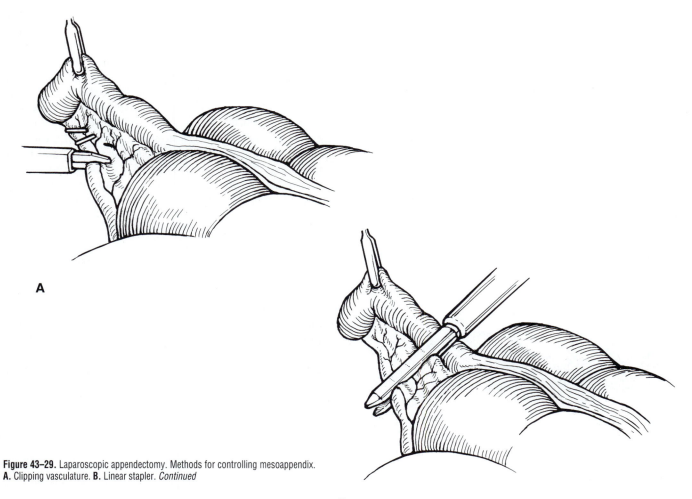

Figure 43–29. Laparoscopic appendectomy. Methods for controlling mesoappendix.
A. Clipping vasculature. **B.** Linear stapler. *Continued*

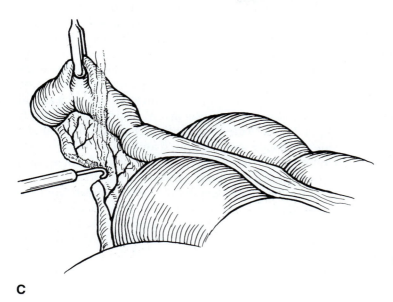

C

Figure 43–29, cont'd. C. Electrocautery. (Redrawn from Brooks DC (ed). *Current Techniques in Laparoscopy,* 1st ed. Philadelphia, PA: Current Medicine; 1994)

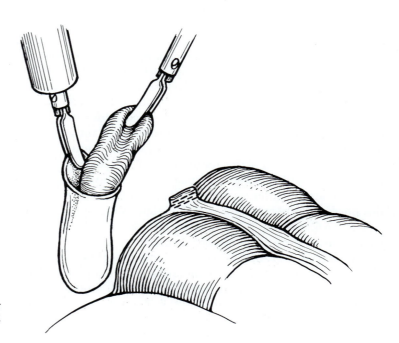

Figure 43–30. Laparoscopic appendectomy; specimen placed in plastic bag for removal. (Redrawn from Brooks DC (ed). *Current Techniques in Laparoscopy,* 1st ed. Philadelphia, PA: Current Medicine, 1994)

ally, necessary instruments include dissecting scissors and atraumatic bowel clamps. The surgeon should be proficient in laparoscopic dissection technique, use of the pretied surgical knots as well as rudimentary laparoscopic suturing techniques.

General endotracheal anesthesia is induced and the abdomen is prepared and draped as a sterile field. The video monitor is placed at the foot of the table. The patient's arms are tucked at his side. A Foley catheter is placed preoperatively for drainage of the urinary bladder to prevent inadvertent injury to the bladder during placement of the cannulas.

Under direct vision, an open technique is used to gain access to the peritoneum. This is performed through a 1.5 to 2 cm vertical incision located at the umbilicus and extending somewhat superiorly. Using blunt and sharp dissection, the midline fascia is identified, grasped, and incised over a distance of approximately 1 cm. The peritoneum is opened under direct vision. A purse-string suture or U stitch is placed using absorbable sutures such as 0 Dexon. The 10 mm cannula is placed and the purse-string suture is secured to prevent leakage. The high-flow insufflator is used at a setting between 2 and 4 L per minute and carbon dioxide is instilled. The laparoscope is inserted through the 10-mm cannula and the abdomen is inspected. The patient is placed in a steep Trendelenburg position and may be rolled slightly to the left. The operating surgeon stands on the left hand side of the patient. Two accessory ports are placed and, depending on the technique employed for control of the appendiceal stump, they will be either 5, 10, or 12 mm. The author prefers to place a 5 mm cannula at the lower midline and a 10 mm cannula at the right upper quadrant. These are placed under direct vision with care being taken not to damage intra-abdominal contents. Prior to placement of the cannulas, transillumination of the abdominal wall will prevent injury to epigastric vessels. After placement of the right upper quadrant cannula, the camera is transferred to this port and held by an assistant. This allows the operator to work with the lower midline and periumbilical instruments with ease. Grasping instruments and scissors are introduced and the right lower quadrant is gently inspected. The terminal ileum and distal ileum are moved gently out of the field. Any purulent fluid should be sampled and cultured and this may give inferential diagnosis of appendicitis.

Importantly, in women, the pelvic organs should be closely inspected. For this procedure, it is not necessary that the patient be placed in lithotomy or that a tenaculum be placed on the uterine cervix. The uterus and both tubes and ovaries can generally be bluntly manipulated to identify any unsuspected pathology in this area.

The cecum is gently grasped and reflected towards the midline allowing access to the retrocecal and infe-rior cecal margins. Appendicitis will be identified at this point through evidence of a thickened, woody mesoappendix and visualization of the inflamed appendix itself. When the appendix is identified, it is gently grasped with a noncrushing clamp and teased out of its loose inflammatory attachments to the pelvic brim. It is brought up under slight traction to tense the mesoappendix which is gently dissected with the right hand, establishing a small window through which clips can be placed and the mesoappendix divided. Care is taken to identify the appendiceal artery, which is also triply clipped and divided leaving two clips on the proximal side. With care and using judicious amounts of electrocautery, small accessory vessels can be coagulated moving towards the appendiceal base.

Once the mesoappendix has been stripped from the appendix itself and the appendix is ready for transection, there are several maneuvers available for control of the appendiceal stump. The initial technique employed was placement of two endoloops, pretied absorbable sutures that could be positioned over the appendix, snugged down at the base, secured and the appendix then divided between them.

This technique has certain advantages in that it does not require costly equipment but may, in certain cases, be difficult to employ because of thickening of the appendix. An alternative technique is to use a 12 mm cannula through which a stapling device such as the endo GIA can be inserted. This can be introduced through the periumbilical port and the appendix can be stapled and divided at its base. The endo GIA places six rows of staples and a knife fires between them such that there are three rows of staples on each side of the divided tissue. When the appendix is free and if it is only marginally thickened, it is gently grasped and removed without undo tension through either the 10- or 12-mm cannula. Should there be significant thickening, however, a specimen retrieval bag may be employed to minimize contamination of the port sites upon removal of the infected tissue.

A third technique involves placement of 2 pretied suture loops over the base of the appendix and division of the appendix between the 2 sutures. The appendix can be dunked within a hand-sutured purse-string similar to the technique used during open appendectomy. In most situations, however, this technique is cumbersome and is mentioned only for completeness sake. The facility with which the current 30-mm stapling device controls the appendiceal stump and the appendix makes this the preferred technique despite its somewhat increased cost. The speed and facility with which the procedure can be performed may outweigh any added costs that occur.

Following removal of the appendix, the right lower quadrant is widely irrigated and the wounds are closed in the usual fashion after being inspected for bleeding. The fascia of any port sites larger than 10 mm should be closed with interrupted absorbable sutures to prevent postoperative herniation.

Laparoscopic Colorectal Surgery

The introduction in the late 1980s and early 1990s of laparoscopic cholecystectomy sparked the interest of a number of investigator's in evaluating a variety of other intra-abdominal procedures that might theoretically be performed successfully using laparoscopic techniques. Among these has been laparoscopic colon resection which has been used since early 1990 and has achieved some enthusiasm albeit less so than for the laparoscopic cholecystectomy.

Preoperative evaluation of patients scheduled for laparoscopic colorectal surgery differs significantly from that of patients undergoing more typical open colectomy. This is necessary because of the complete absence of tactile feedback given to the operator when performing laparoscopic colectomy. For that reason, several important preoperative modifications must be undertaken prior to performing a laparoscopic colectomy. First and foremost, include a complete colonoscopy on all patients. The potential for overlooking or missing a small but potentially significant lesion is high and therefore, it is important that the entire colon be evaluated preoperatively. Secondly, because there is virtually no tactile feedback, it is important that lesions be marked with a tattoo of India ink during colonoscopy to assist the surgeon in subsequently identifying the lesion and recognizing the exact site of the pathology. Some authors prefer to perform intraoperative colonoscopy to assist in identifying lesions. This may be done with the assistance of a skilled endoscopist to perform the procedure at the time of surgery, bearing in mind the potential for obscuring vision by instilling air into the colon.

Of equally significant importance is the issue of patient positioning. The patient's position on the operating room table will depend to a large degree on the area of the colon to be resected. It is important for patients undergoing proposed sigmoid colectomy, low anterior resection or abdominoperineal resection to be placed in dorsolithotomy position with steep Trendelenburg. All laparoscopic colectomy procedures depend on table positioning and patient positioning to provide increased exposure and therefore, when possible, the operation should be performed on an electric table that facilitates position changes during the procedure. In Europe many laparoscopic surgeons prefer the dorsolithotomy position for all cases. This provides an extra standing space at the table and allows access to a variety of different portions of the abdomen and placement of the camera. If the patient is to be placed in a dorsolithotomy position, it is important that close periop-

erative monitoring of lower extremity profusion be performed either by pedal pulse oxymetry or compartment pressure monitoring. This is particularly so in extended cases. Femoral neuropathies also can develop. Additionally, the patients' arms should be placed at their sides to provide both surgeon and assistant with the maximal amount of mobility in operating.

Two important techniques are available for the performance of laparoscopic colectomies. These include laparoscopic-assisted colectomies and total intracorporeal laparoscopic colectomy. The differentiating features between the two procedures are whether or not a small incision is made over the specific segment to be removed and whether the specimen is removed at that site, the anastomosis done at skin level, and the bowel replaced within the abdomen. An alternative method, the totally intracorporeal method, involves resection, specimen retrieval through available orifices, and complete reanastomosis without a counter incision.

The later technique is of particular value when performing abdominoperineal resections or resections of the rectosigmoid. The experience of Franklin with the techniques for total intracorporeal colectomies suggest that this is a viable option, provides excellent exposure and significant opportunity to meticulously dissect the distal colon.[38] As in all forms of laparoscopic colon surgery, it requires significant experience and relies on important advanced techniques such as the two-handed technique, intracorporeal suturing, knot tying, and anastomotic techniques.

The laparoscopic-assisted technique is used more frequently largely because it requires less technical expertise and is appropriate for a variety of different procedures. This technique differs from the former in important ways. Although the initial dissection, mobilization, and isolation of the segment to be resected proceeds in a manner similar to that of the intracorporeal procedure, the bowel may be removed through a small incision made in the right lower quadrant measuring between 4 and 6 cm. This technique will allow extracorporeal anastomosis, and specimen retrieval.

Technical Aspects of Laparoscopic Colectomy. **(Figs 43–31, 43–32, and 43–33)** The access to the peritoneum is established through an open technique as described in the previous sections on laparoscopic appendectomy. Typically, a 10-mm cannula is placed at the umbilicus and accessory cannulus are placed in the four quadrants of the abdomen. The operating surgeon positions himself opposite the lesion and establishes his two operating hands in an isosceles triangle based on the object to be dissected. This provides the surgeon with sufficient mobility and lateral motion to control the operative field. The camera operator should be placed as unobtrusively as possible and this may be facilitated by use of

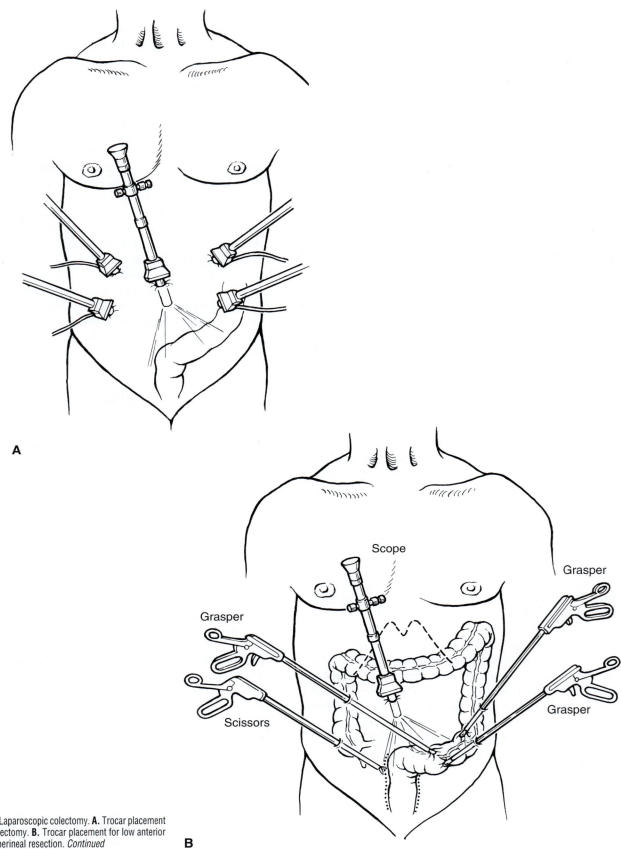

Figure 43–31. Laparoscopic colectomy. **A.** Trocar placement for sigmoid colectomy. **B.** Trocar placement for low anterior and abdominoperineal resection. *Continued*

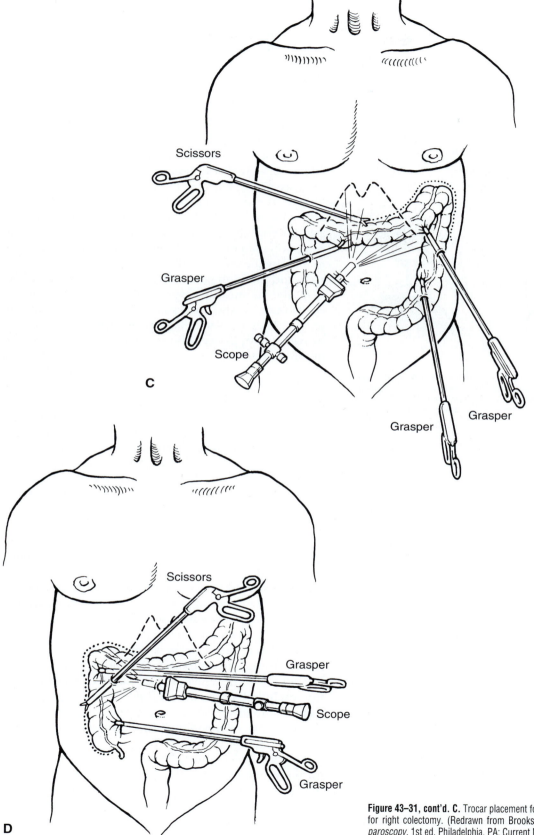

Figure 43–31, cont'd. C. Trocar placement for left colectomy. **D.** Trocar placement for right colectomy. (Redrawn from Brooks DC (ed). *Current Techniques in Laparoscopy,* 1st ed. Philadelphia, PA: Current Medicine; 1994)

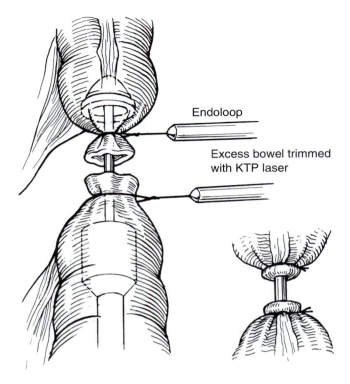

Endoloop

Excess bowel trimmed
with KTP laser

Figure 43–32. Laparoscopic colectomy. Bowel is mobilized, mesentery divided, and anvil inserted into proximal limb during sigmoid or left colectomy. (Note: endoloop placed around bowel end to secure closure). (Redrawn from Brooks DC (ed). *Current Techniques in Laparoscopy*, 1st ed. Philadelphia, PA: Current Medicine; 1994)

a mechanical apparatus to stabilize the camera. The first assistant should be placed in a location suitable for manipulating the bowel or the mesentery while the surgeon performs the dissection.

Right Colectomy. The amount of specimen removed during a right colectomy will include the terminal ileum, the cecum and the ascending colon up to and just beyond the hepatic flexure. The camera should be placed on the right side of the patient and the patient's arms should be tucked in to allow the operating surgeon and assistants to move without restriction. The operating surgeon stands on the left side of the patient, as does the camera operator. The first assistant is positioned to afford the best retraction and manipulation of the bowel. After the camera has been placed and the pneumoperitoneum established, the abdomen is thoroughly inspected. Additional trocars are placed to afford access of stapling devices and graspers. A total of 4 to 5 cannulas should be employed and the size of the cannula must be adequate to accept a variety of instruments. A 10-mm cannula allows the greatest variety of instruments. Additionally, a suprapubic 11- or 12-mm cannula is necessary for placement of the linear stapling devices.

The patient is placed in the Trendelenburg position and rotated to the left. The terminal ileum is identified and followed to the cecum using atraumatic bowel clamps such as Babcocks in a hand-over-hand technique. The lesion is identified either visually or by visualizing the tattoo placed preoperatively. The assistant retracts the cecum to the patient's left and the avascular attachments between the right colon and the abdominal wall are incised sharply. The colon is reflected medially sufficient to identify the right ureter and ensure that it is safely out of the way of the dissection. The distal and proximal resection lines are selected. Graspers then are placed adjacent to these areas and the colon is lifted to the abdominal wall, placing the mesentery under traction. Externally placed stabilizing devices such as sutures will markedly facilitate this. Tenting the right colon will splay out the mesentery and allow the surgeon to identify the major feeding vessels, including the ileocolic and the right colic. When these vessels are identified, the peritoneal covering over the mesentery is sharply incised and the vessels are circumferentially dissected. They are triply clipped with two clips on the proximal side. The vessels are divided and if there is any question as to the security of the clips, an endoloop is placed over the vessel for additional security.

The peritoneal surface of the mesentery is divided and the major vessels, including the ileocolic, are identified and triply clipped. Alternatively, energy sources such as the harmonic scalpel, or linear vascular stapling devices can be utilized to control the mesenteric vessels. A small window is created through the mesentery at the proximal and distal resection sites and a linear stapling device is passed across the bowel to divide it. If the bowel is particularly wide, several firings may be necessary. The remaining mesentery is divided with electrocoagulation or clips depending on the size of the vessel. For malignant disease, the specimen then is placed in a plastic bag to prevent dissemination of tumor cells. This will be removed at the completion of the procedure through the umbilical port, which can be extended superiorly a sufficient amount to allow removal of even a somewhat bulky lesion.

The ileum and transverse colon then are approximated so that the antimesenteric borders are in conjunction and the linear stapling device is introduced into each limb of bowel and fired twice to create a 5 to 6 cm anastomosis. The resulting defect is closed by suture or staplers depending on the preference of the surgeon.

For right colectomies, an easier alternative is to perform the anastomosis extracorporeally. After division of the bowel and mesentery, and after placing the specimen in a bag, a 4 to 5 cm incision is made in the midright abdomen. The specimen is removed and the proximal and distal ends of the bowel are brought into

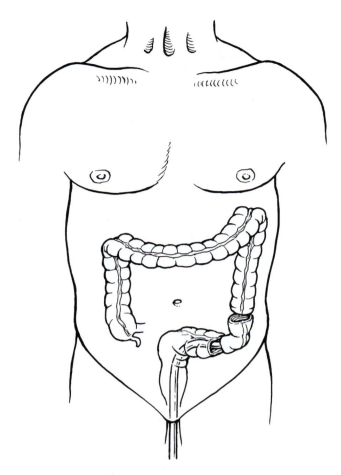

Figure 43–33. Laparoscopic colectomy. Bowel is retrieved through open end of rectal stump using colonoscope. (Redrawn from Brooks DC (ed). *Current Techniques in Laparoscopy,* 1st ed. Philadelphia, PA: Current Medicine; 1994)

the wound and an open sutured or stapled anastomosis is created. The bowel then is replaced into the abdomen, the incision is closed, and the pneumoperitoneum is reestablished. The anastomosis is inspected, the operative field irrigated, checked for hemostasis, and the ports are removed under direct vision.

Transverse Colectomy. Transverse colectomy can be particularly difficult because of the presence of the omentum and the interference this may cause in manipulating the bowel. The procedure is performed with the surgeon standing between the legs (lithotomy) or standing on the right side of the patient. A total of five cannulas are placed, located at the umbilicus (camera), the left lower quadrant, left upper quadrant, right midabdomen and right upper quadrant. After identifying the lesion the hepatic and splenic flexures are stabilized by the first assistant, allowing the operating surgeon to use a two-handed technique to divide the attachments at these locations. The lesser omentum is incised and di-

vided and the bowel is cleared at the proposed resection sites. Following division of the bowel by the linear stapling device, the greater omentum is flipped over the colon allowing the transverse mesocolon to be inspected. Reverse Trendelenburg positioning will allow the small bowel to fall towards the pelvis and will leave the upper abdomen relatively free of intestines. The peritoneal surface of the mesentery is incised and the middle colic vessels are identified and triply clipped. The mesentery then can be taken, using electrocautery or harmonic shears. The specimen is bagged for later retrieval and a small vertical midline incision is made sufficient to allow the two ends of the colon to be brought into the wound for reanastomosis. This is performed with either staplers or hand sewing.

Left and Sigmoid Colectomies

Five cannulas are employed. The operating surgeon stands on the right of the patient and the monitor is placed on the left of the patient at a position corresponding to the proposed segment to be resected. The first assistant is placed on the left side of the patient, with either 1 or 2 grasping/retracting instruments. After the lesion has been identified or, in the case of diverticular disease, after the involved segment has been delineated, the colon is reflected to the right and the patient is rolled to the right. Trendelenburg or reverse Trendelenburg positions are used as necessary. The white line of Toldt is identified and incised along the course of the resected segment and the bowel is further reflected to the right. The ureter must be identified and kept well away from the area to be resected. When the bowel has been sufficiently mobilized from its relatively avascular lateral attachments, it is tented up to the abdominal wall in order to allow identification of the left colic artery, which is divided at the base of the mesentery. The mesenteric resection line is marked and vessels are controlled with clips, harmonic shears, or coagulation, as appropriate. When the mesentery has been completely divided and the bowel cleared circumferentially at the proposed resection sites, it is divided without staplers, using either electrocautery or cold scissors. The specimen is bagged and retrieved through the open distal end of the colon using either a colonoscope or a long instrument clamp introduced through the rectum.

The circular stapling device is assembled and introduced through the rectum. Pretied ligature loops are placed around the proximal and distal segments and the anvil of the circular stapler is inserted into the proximal segment. The pretied knot is secured around the circumference of the proximal bowel 1 cm from its cut end and snugged down on the shaft of the anvil. The distal pretied loop is secured around the distal bowel segment in a similar fashion and the circular stapling is tightened, fired, and removed. The resected area is inspected for bleeding, irrigated, and the cannulas are removed under direct vision. As in the open technique using the circular stapler, the tissue doughnuts must be inspected.

Left colectomies performed through a laparoscopically assisted technique rather than a completely extracorporeal technique are also possible. After mobilization and division of the bowel, a small oblique incision is made in the left lower quadrant and the divided ends of the bowel are brought together for sutured or stapled anastomosis.

Other Colectomies

Modifications to the previously described dissections can be employed for creation of an end sigmoid colostomy, colostomy closure and abdominoperineal resection. The latter is suitable for laparoscopic approach and can be performed as a combined procedure, with two teams working simultaneously. The initial maneuver is to identify the proposed site of the sigmoid division, divided the colon intracorporeally and then dissect circumferentially into the pelvis on both sides of the colon. Both ureters are identified and maintained posterior and lateral to the dissection. The relatively avascular presacral space is cleared and the lateral attachments are divided between clips as the rectum is approached. The anterior peritoneum of the floor is divided and the rectum can be brought up under tension to allow the operator to visualize the lateral vascular attachments with precision. The dissection is continued circumferentially until the rectum dives under the pubis, at which point the perineal dissection should become evident. When the peritoneal portion of the dissection is opened into the abdomen the pneumoperitoneum is lost and all further dissection must be done from below.

The specimen is removed, the perineum closed, and the pneumoperitoneum reestablished. The pelvic floor is inspected for bleeding and closed with either staples of sutures and the colostomy is placed at a premarked position in the left lower quadrant. The cannulas are removed under direct vision and the colostomy is created after closure of the skin incisions.

REFERENCES

1. Pezim ME, Nicholls RJ. Survival after high or low ligation of the inferior mesenteric artery during curative surgery for rectal cancer. *Ann Surg* 1984;200:729–733
2. Stone HH. Antibiotics in colon surgery. *Surg Clin North Am* 1983;63:3–9
3. Clarke JS, Condon RE, Bartlett JG, et al. Preoperative oral antibiotics reduce septic complications of colon operations: results of a perspective randomized double blind clinical study. *Ann Surg* 1977;186:251–259
4. Barlett JG, Condon RE, Gorbach SL, Clarke JS, Nichols RL, Ochis. Veterans Administration Cooperative Study on Bowel Preparation for Elective Colorectal Operations: Impact of oral antibiotic regimen on colonic flora, wound irrigation cultures and bacteriology of septic complications. *Ann Surg* 1978;188:249–254
5. Keighly MR, Condon RE. A clinical and physiological evaluation of bowel preparation for elective colorectal surgery. *World J Surg* 1982;6:464–470
6. Polk HC, Lopez-Mayor JF. Postoperative wound infection: a prospective study of determinant factors in prevention. *Surgery* 1969;66:97–103
7. Wong-Beringer A, Corelli RL, Schrock TR, Guglielmo BJ. Influence of timing of antibiotic administration on tissue concentrations during surgery. *Am J Surg* 1995;169:379–381
8. Handelsman JC, Zeiler S, Coleman J, et al. Experience with ambulatory preoperative bowel preparation at the Johns Hopkins Hospital. *Arch Surg* 1993;128:441–444
9. Radcliff AG, Dudley HAF. Intraoperative antigrade irrigation of the large intestine. *Surg Gynecol Obstet* 1983;156:721–723
10. Guillou PJ, Hall TJ, Donaldson DR, et al. Vertical abdominal incisions—a choice? *Br J Surg* 1980;67:395–399
11. Bucknall TE, Ellis H. Abdominal wound closure: a comparison of monofilament nylon and polyglycolic acid. *Surgery* 1981;89:672–677
12. Greenall MJ, Evans M, Pollock AV. Midline or transverse laparotomy? a random controlled clinical trial, part II. influence on postoperative pulmonary complications. *Br J Surg* 1980;67:191–194
13. Cahalane MJ, Shapiro ME, Silen W. Abdominal incision: decision or indecision? *Lancet* 1989;146–148
14. Chung RS. Blood flow in colonic anastomoses: effect of stapling and suturing. *Ann Surg* 1987;206:335–339
15. Steichen FM, Ravitch MW. Contemporary stapling instruments in basic mechanical suture techniques. *Surg Clin North Am* 1984;64:425–440
16. Brolin RE, Ravitch MM. Studies in intestinal healing IV. effect of pharmacology induced peristalsis on fresh intestinal anastomoses in dogs. *Arch Surg* 1980;115:339–343
17. Goligher JC, Morris C, McAdam WAF, et al. A controlled trial of inverting vs. everting intestinal suture in clinical large bowel surgery. *Br J Surg* 1970;57:817–822
18. MacAdams AJ, Meikle G, Medina R. An experimental comparison of inversion and eversion colonic anastomoses. *Dis Colon Rectum* 1969;12:1–6
19. Chung RS. Blood flow and colonic anastomoses: effect of stapling and suturing. *Ann Surg* 1987;206:335–339
20. Weil PH, Scherz H. Comparison of stapled and hand sutured gastrectomies. *Arch Surg* 1981;116:14–16
21. Akyol AM, McGregor JR, Galloway DJ, et al. Recurrence of colorectal cancer after sutured and stapled large bowel anastomoses. *Br J Surg* 1991;78:1297–1300
22. Goligher JC, Graham NG, DeDombal FT. Anastomotic dehiscence after anterior resection of rectum and sigmoid *Br J Surg* 1970;57:109
23. Gingold BS, Jagelman DG. The value of pelvic suction-irrigation in reducing morbidity of low anterior resection of the rectum—a 10 year experience. *Surgery* 1982;91:394–398

24. Savassi-Rocha PR, Conceicao SA, Ferreira JT, et al. Evaluation of the routine use of the nasogastric tube in digestive operations by a perspective controlled study. *Surg Gynecol Obstet* 1992;174:317–320

25. Bickel A, Shtamler B, Mizrahi S. Early oral feeding following removal of nasogastric tube and gastrointestinal operations. *Arch Surg* 1992;127:287–289

26. Sitges-Serra A, Cabrol J, Gubern JM, Simo J. A randomized trial of gastric decompression after truncal vagotomy and anterior pylorectomy. *Surg Gynecol Obstet* 1984;158:557–560

27. Morris DL, Poxon V, Youngs D, Keighley M. Gastric juice factors after Roux-en-Y reconstruction compared to Billroth II gastrectomy. *Am J Surg* 1988;156:21–25

28. Ikard RW. The Y anastomosis of Caesar Roux. *Surg Gynecol Obstet* 1989;169:559–567

29. Kittur DS, Talamini M, Smith GW. Eversion of difficult ileostomies by Guy rope suture technique. *Am J Surg* 1989;157:593–594

30. Fasth S, Hulten L. Loop ileostomy: a superior diverting stoma in colorectal surgery. *World J Surg* 1984;8:401–407

31. Lau WY, Teoh-Chan CH, Fan SI, et al. The bacteriology and septic complication of patients with appendicities. *Ann Surg* 1984;200:576–581

32. Goligher JC, Lee PWR, MacFie J, et al. Experience with the Russian model 249 suture gun for anastomosis of the rectum. *Surg Gynecol Obstet* 1979;148:516–524

33. Ragins H, DeLuca FR. Technique for using the EEA stapler for low anterior resection of the rectum entirely from the abdominal approach. *Am J Surg* 1981;142:388–390

34. Whitworth CM, Whitworth PW, Sanfillipo J, Polk HC Jr. Value of diagnostic laparoscopy in young women with possible appendicitis. *Surg Gynecol Obstet* 1988;167:187–190

35. Gotz F, Pier A, Bacher C. Laparoscopic appendectomy: alternative therapy in all stages of appendicitis. *Langenbecks Arch Chir* 1990;(suppl II)1351–1353

36. McAnena OJ, Austin O, O'Connell PR, et al. Laparoscopic versus open appendicectomy: a prospective evaluation. *Br J Surg* 1992;79:818–820

37. Scott-Conner CEH, Hall TJ, Anglin BL, Muakkassa FF. Laparoscopic appendectomy. Initial experience in a teaching program. *Ann Surg* 1992;215:660–668

38. Franklin ME Jr. Laparoscopic colon and small bowel surgery. In: Brooks DC (ed), *Current Review of Laparoscopy*. Philadelphia, PA: Current Medicine; 1995

44

Ileal Pouch—Anal Canal Anastomosis: Operative Procedures

Santhat Nivatvongs ▪ *Keith A. Kelly*

The ileal pouch–anal anastomosis (IPAA) involves the removal of the cecum, the colon, the rectum, and the mucosa of the upper anal canal, and the creation of an ileal pouch. The pelvic floor muscles and the anal sphincter muscles are preserved. The ileal pouch or ileal reservoir, constructed for the storage of feces, then is brought down and anastomosed to the anal canal at the dentate line. The procedure eliminates mucosal diseases of the colon and rectum, and yet preserves fecal continence. IPAA has become the operation of choice for most patients with chronic ulcerative colitis and familial adenomatous polyposis.

▪ HISTORICAL

The concept of preserving the anal sphincter and maintaining bowel continuity after resection of colon and rectum is not new. In 1888, Julius Von Hochenegg in Vienna performed a coloanal pull-through. In 1910, Vignolo of Pisa interposed an isolated segment of ileum to bridge the gap between the sigmoid colon and the anus after an abdominosacral resection of a rectal malignancy. The first ileoanal anastomosis is attributed to Rudolph Nissen of Berlin, who, in 1933, performed a total proctocolectomy with ileoanal anastomosis in a child, 10 years of age, with polyposis. The early postoperative results were gratifying.[1]

After discovering that total proctocolectomy, anorectal mucosectomy, and the ileoanal anastomosis was feasible in dogs,[2] Ravitch,[3] in 1948, performed this operation successfully in two patients with longstanding ulcerative colitis. Both patients withstood the operation well and had excellent fecal continence. However, the operation never became popular. Review of the literature by Best in 1952 revealed overall satisfactory results in approximately 50% of cases, but there were numerous complications, particularly sepsis and anastomotic leaks.[4] He was pessimistic about the operation and stated, "I have difficulty in convincing myself that facing the issues described is worth the sweat and tears of both patients and surgeons." Goligher[5] shared the same opinion after having performed such an operation in two patients: "I certainly would not presume to condemn an operation on such a limited experience, but these results as they stand are discouraging and indicate quite clearly that the functional condition after this operation is not always satisfactory. Nevertheless, I propose to experiment further with this procedure."

To solve the problems of frequent bowel movements, fluid and electrolyte imbalances, fistulas and abscesses, Valiente and Bacon, in 1955,[6] created a pouch similar to the S pouch of today which they called the "pantaloon pouch." They applied the concept in dogs and found it to be successful. In discussing Valiente and Bacon's paper, the late Rupert Turnbull stated, "I think this is in the dream stage, however, at the present time;—I believe that somewhere in the future someone may perhaps solve this problem." Indeed, "someone" has solved this problem.

In 1977, Martin, LeCoultre, and Schubert reported on a proctocolectomy with anorectal mucosectomy to 1 cm above the mucocutaneous junction.[7] The terminal ileum (without reservoir or pouch) was anastomosed to the anal canal. A complementary loop ileostomy also was performed. Seventeen patients with ulcerative colitis who were between 11 and 20 years of age underwent this procedure. The results in 15 patients were successful, with good fecal continence. Overall, complications were significant, particularly pelvic infection and cuff abscess.

Ileoanal anastomosis enjoyed its place briefly in the late 1970s and early 1980s.[8,9] It was soon obvious that some kind of reservoir would be needed to reduce the intolerable number of bowel movements in most patients, particularly in adults.[10]

In 1978, Parks and Nicholls were the first to show that proctocolectomy, stripping of the anorectal mucosa, and the pouch-anal anastomosis were feasible for patients with ulcerative colitis.[11] They subsequently reported their experience with this operation in 21 patients (17 with ulcerative colitis, 4 with polyposis). Continence was good and the average number of bowel movements was four per day.[12] This report convinced others that a breakthrough in the new operative treatment of ulcerative colitis and polyposis had been achieved.

■ INDICATIONS FOR ILEOANAL POUCH PROCEDURE

The IPAA procedure thus far is reserved for patients with chronic ulcerative colitis and familial adenomatous polyposis. A few patients with colorectal inertia have also received the operation.[13]

■ SELECTION OF PATIENTS

Proctocolectomy with IPAA is a major operation with a potentially high complication rate if not performed properly. The functional results are not perfect, particularly if the patients are not properly selected physically and mentally. Crohn's disease is an absolute contraindication to this procedure.

The stool in the pouch is watery or at best, semisolid, and good anal sphincter control is required to achieve reasonable continence. Patients with known poor anal continence should not be considered for IPAA. Although patients >50 years of age have more frequent bowel movements and have less satisfactory sphincter control,[14] age per se should not necessarily be the determining factor. If the patient is fit, understands the less-than-perfect outcome, and still desires to have the procedure, it should be considered.

Patients with fulminant colitis and those with colitis and toxic megacolon should not have a simultaneous IPAA because of the high risk of intra-abdominal sepsis. Instead, a colectomy with oversewing of the upper rectum and an ileostomy should be done first. The IPAA can be postponed. Overweight males face a higher risk of anastomotic stricture, reflecting the difficulty of the operation; consequently, markedly obese patients should not have an IPAA. Anastomotic stricture may result in tension in the anastomosis with disruption, ischemia, and stricture as potential complications.[14]

Patients who plan to have an IPAA should have a preliminary diagnosis of ulcerative colitis, based on clinical diagnosis, including history, physical examination, endoscopy, and often, a biopsy. In a number of patients the diagnosis cannot be ascertained even at the time of proctocolectomy and even after frozen section of the operative specimen. In this group, the unusual distribution of inflammation, deep linear ulcers, neural proliferation, transmural inflammation, fissures, creeping fat, and retention of the goblet-cell population will make diagnosis difficult. This "indeterminate" colitis was found in 10% of 514 consecutive patients who underwent IPAA for ulcerative colitis at the Mayo Clinic.[15] In half of these patients (5% of total), the surgeon proceeded with an IPAA, as planned. In a retrospective study of this group of patients, with a mean follow-up of 38 ($\pm$18) months, no significant difference in complication rate, pouch function, incidence of pouchitis, or requirement of pouch excision was detected, as compared with the group of patients with IPAA with a definitive diagnosis of ulcerative colitis. These results indicate that, if the final diagnosis is not obviously Crohn's disease, IPAA can be performed with reasonable confidence.

Patients with familial adenomatous polyposis who have significant desmoid tumors or fibromatosis of the small bowel mesentery should not have the IPAA procedure. The disease usually progresses and may eventually cause small bowel obstruction.

Occasionally, the surgeon encounters a patient who is a candidate for proctocolectomy with IPAA, but who also has an associated carcinoma of the colon or rectum. Experience at the Mayo Clinic suggested that proctocolectomy with IPAA can be performed, provided the operation does not compromise a curative resection, and the predicted prognosis is good. IPAA should be avoided in patients with carcinoma of the middle and lower rectum, because proctocolectomy with IPAA is not an adequate operation for carcinoma. Moreover, radiation therapy, which may be needed postoperatively, is likely to damage the ileoanal pouch.[16,17]

The most satisfied patients are those who are highly motivated to have the procedure. The surgeon should keep in mind that "the Brooke ileostomy remains the benchmark against which other options must be compared."[10]

■ VARIOUS METHODS OF POUCH CONSTRUCTION

The single most important function of an ileal pouch is as a reservoir to hold gastrointestinal contents. Whether it is an isoperistaltic or an antiperistaltic pouch does not seem to matter significantly. The pouch should be large enough to hold ileal contents, but small enough to fit in the pelvis. The original type of reservoir, reported by Parks and Nicholls, in 1978, is called an S pouch and uses three segments of the terminal ileum.[11] In 1980, Utsunomiya and associates described a two-loop segment called a J pouch.[18] In 1980, Fonkalsrud introduced a side-to-side pouch.[19] In 1985, Nicholls and Pezim modified a double J pouch to expand the capacity; the result is called a W pouch.[20] Soon it was evident that configuration of the pouch is not the determining factor in predicting long-term functional outcome. At present, the J pouch and the S pouch are the most commonly used. The surgeon should know how to construct at least two types of reservoirs and use them appropriately, as dictated by the technical necessity in each patient.

TECHNIQUE OF J POUCH CONSTRUCTION

Abdominal Proctocolectomy

The patient is positioned to allow access to the abdomen and perineum. Mobilization of the colon and rectum is exactly the same as that described for proctocolectomy and ileostomy for ulcerative colitis or familial adenomatous polyposis. The terminal ileum is transected flush with the cecum, using a linear stapler. The ileal branch of the ileocolic vessels must be preserved at this point. The rectum is transected just above the levator ani muscle, using a linear stapler. The root of the small bowel mesentery is mobilized to the level of the pancreas.

Preparation of Terminal Ileum and its Mesentery

A site 15 to 20 cm proximal to the stapled cut end of the terminal ileum is chosen as the base of the pouch. It will reach the anus if this point extends 6 cm beyond the symphysis pubis.[21] The most important and, frequently, the most difficult part of the pouch procedure is to obtain adequate length of the mesentery to reach the anus. It is usually necessary to release tension by trans-

versely incising the peritoneum of the stretched mesentery of the small bowel.

The mesentery is transluminated to delineate the arcade of the blood vessels formed by the ileocolic artery and terminal ileal branch of the superior mesenteric artery. As traction is placed on the small bowel, the vessels between the first and the second arcade that are under tension are identified and divided.[22] This maneuver will gain small amounts of length. If 1.5 to 2 cm additional length is required, the superior mesenteric vessel, in its midportion, can be sacrificed, provided the ileocolic vessels are the ones that need to be taken. If the surgeon is not certain about the blood supply to the pouch, it is wise first to clamp them with bulldog clamps for 10 to 15 minutes to ensure adequate collateral blood supply to the terminal ileum before their division (Fig 44–1).

Construction of the Pouch

The J pouch is made from the distal 30 to 40 cm of ileum folded in half. Two small enterotomies are made approximately 7 cm from the base of the future reser-

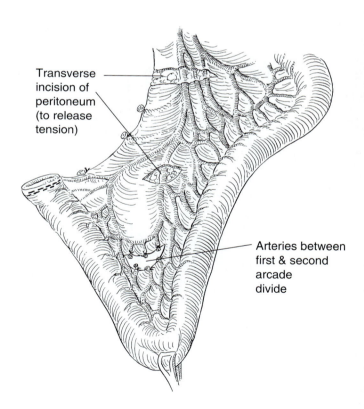

Figure 44–1. Technique of lengthening the mesentery in the J pouch construction. Transverse incisions of peritoneum release tension. Vessels between first and second arcade that are under tension are identified and divided. Additional length can be obtained by dividing superior mesenteric vessels in their mid portion. (Redrawn from Gordon PH, Nivatvongs S. *Principles and Practice of Surgery for the Colon, Rectum, and Anus.* St. Louis, MO: Quality Medical; 1992)

Transverse incision of peritoneum (to release tension)

Arteries between first & second arcade divide

voir. An anastomosing linear stapler is introduced and activated in the direction of the base, then in the opposite direction (Fig 44–2A). Two to three firings of the stapler are needed, depending on the length of the stapler chosen. With this technique, the ridge at the base of the pouch is everted through the enterotomies and transected with the stapler to prevent obstruction of the outlet of the pouch (Fig 44–2B). The enterotomies are closed longitudinally with one or two layers, running 3-0 synthetic absorbable suture.

An alternative technique is to staple the pouch through its base. A purse-string suture is placed at the base to prevent excessive stretching and an enterotomy is made within the purse-string suture. Multiple firings of the stapler are needed to complete the entire length of the pouch (Fig 44–3). In this way, no bridge is created and the opening at the base is used later in an anastomosis with the anus. This technique is preferred by some surgeons because it eliminates the need for enterotomy, and the distal bridge is eliminated automatically.

TECHNIQUE OF S POUCH CONSTRUCTION

Preparation of Terminal Ileum and its Mesentery

Unlike the J pouch, the S pouch reservoir reaches the anal canal with its efferent limb, the end of the terminal ileum. The ileal branch of the ileocolic artery is ligated and divided near its origin. The last vascular arcade near the tip of the terminal ileum must not be injured (Fig 44–4). Additional incisions on the peritoneum of the mesentery usually will provide extra length.

Construction of the Pouch

The terminal ileum with 10 to 12 cm in each limb is folded twice with a 2-cm projection that will be an outlet of the pouch for anastomosis to the anus. Originally, Parks, Nicholls, and Belliveau used 15 cm for each limb and a 5-cm projection.[12] However, a pouch that size with a long efferent limb resulted in an incidence of evacuation difficulties as high as 50%. The ileum is opened on its antimesenteric border, and the posterior wall is sutured, using running one or two layers of 3-0 synthetic

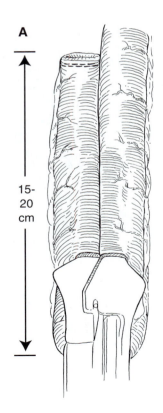

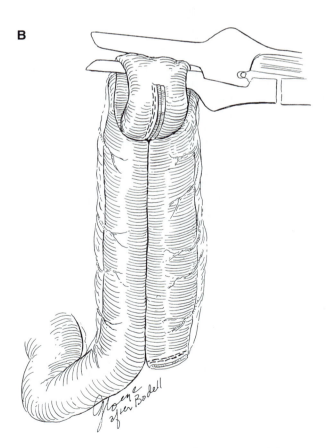

Figure 44–2. Construction of the J pouch. **A.** A 15- to 20-cm segment of terminal ileum is folded into the shape of a J. An enterotomy is made 6 to 7 cm from the base of the J. Multiple firings are required. **B.** Septum at base of pouch is everted and divided. (Redrawn from Gordon PH, Nivatvongs S. *Principles and Practice of Surgery for the Colon, Rectum, and Anus.* St. Louis, MO: Quality Medical; 1992)

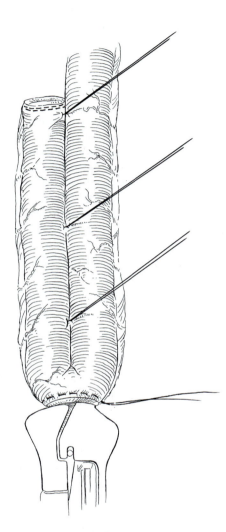

Figure 44–3. Construction of the J pouch through base. A purse-string suture is placed around base where enterotomy will be made. This suture will prevent tearing. Anastomosing stapler is inserted and activated. Multiple firings may be needed. (Redrawn from Gordon PH, Nivatvongs S. *Principles and Practice of Surgery for the Colon, Rectum, and Anus.* St. Louis, MO: Quality Medical; 1992)

A

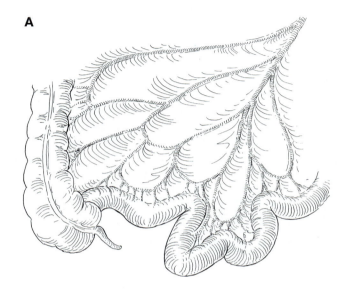

B

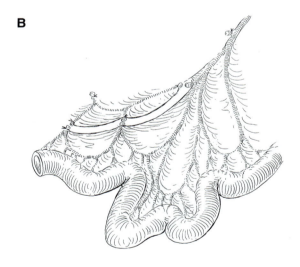

Figure 44–4. Technique of lengthening the mesentery in the S pouch. **A**. Identification of right colic and ileocolic vessels. **B**. Ileocolic vessels are ligated and divided near their origin. Last arterial arcade to terminal ileum must be preserved. (Redrawn from Gordon PH, Nivatvongs S. *Principles and Practice of Surgery for the Colon, Rectum, and Anus.* St. Louis, MO: Quality Medical; 1992)

absorbable suture. Finally, the anterior wall of the pouch is approximated in the same manner (Fig 44–5).

OTHER TYPES OF POUCH

Fonkalsrud preferred to use a lateral reservoir.[19] The ability of this type of pouch to reach the anus is similar to that of the S pouch. It is constructed by forming a side-to-side anastomosis between two 15-cm limbs of terminal ileum, with a 2-cm projection for the pouch-anal anastomosis (Fig 44–6).

To increase the capacity of the pouch, hoping to improve the functional results, Nicholls and Lubowski developed a four-loop reservoir (W pouch).[23] The terminal ileum is folded into two U shaped configurations with each limb 12-cm long. The antimesenteric border in each limb is incised. The posterior wall is sewn together with one or two running layers of 3-0 synthetic absorbable suture. The cut edges of the anterior wall are approximated in the same manner (Fig 44–7).

ANORECTAL MUCOSECTOMY

The technique and the concept of mucosectomy have changed during the past years. It now is known that the rectum can be transected at the level of the levator ani muscle without compromising the anal sphincter func-

tion. The shorter stripping procedure reduces the time of operation, bleeding, contamination, and the risk of infection and favors better expansion of the neorectum.[24] Traditionally, two Gelpi retractors are placed at right angles at the anus for exposure. Recently, Roberts and associates introduced the disposable Lone Star self-retaining retractor (Lone Star Medical Products, Houston, TX), which further facilitates the dissection.[25] The anus is effaced circumferentially by eight elastic adjustable stays (Fig 44–8), thereby eliminating the need for anal dilation.

Using electrocautery, mucosa is dissected circumferentially in the submucosal plane, starting at the dentate line. Dissection is carried up to the stapled rectum, where it is removed en bloc with a submucosal tube. Alternatively, the anorectal mucosa is stripped in four or five separate pieces. The anorectum is exposed with a Pratt anal speculum. The submucosa at each quadrant is injected with diluted epinephrine solution. The mucosa-submucosa at each quadrant is then stripped off the internal sphincter muscle, using scissors, starting at the dentate line. Bleeding is usually minimal and can be controlled easily by electrocautery. Using this technique, the rectum, just above the levator ani muscle, is transected without need of a linear stapler.

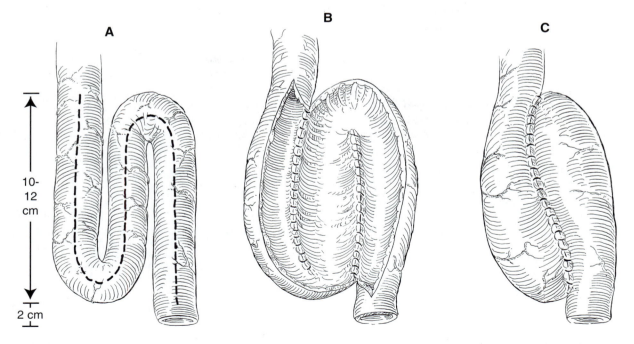

Figure 44–5. Construction of the S pouch. **A.** Terminal ileum is folded (10- to 12-cm for each limb) to make three segments, with a 2-cm projection remaining. **B.** Incision is made on antimesenteric border of bowel. Posterior walls are closed with one continuous layer of 3-0 synthetic absorbable sutures. **C.** Pouch is completed with one-layer closure of anterior wall using one continuous layer of absorbable sutures. (Redrawn from Gordon PH, Nivatvongs S. *Principles and Practice of Surgery for the Colon, Rectum, and Anus.* St. Louis, MO: Quality Medical; 1992)

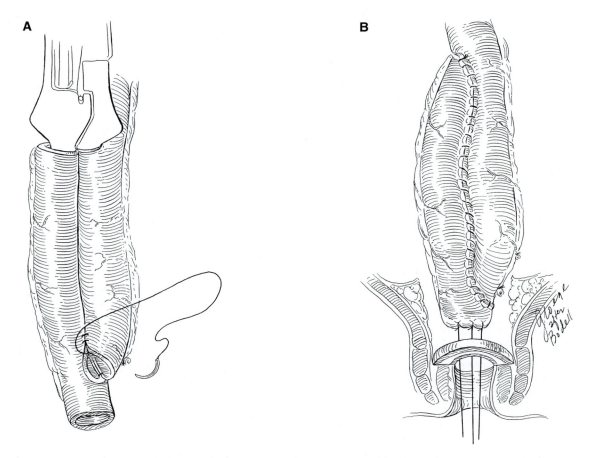

Figure 44–6. Lateral reservoir. **A.** A 15-cm segment of terminal ileum is divided. With an anastomosing stapler, the segment is anastomosed side-to-side with a proximal part of ileum. **B.** Enterotomies for stapler are closed with continuous sutures. Entire reservoir anastomosis is oversewn with a second layer of continuous absorbable sutures. (Redrawn from Gordon PH, Nivatvongs S. *Principles and Practice of Surgery for the Colon, Rectum, and Anus.* St. Louis, MO: Quality Medical; 1992)

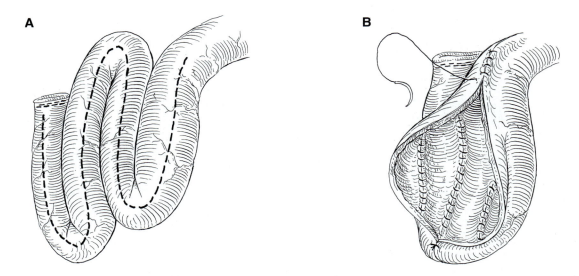

Figure 44–7. Construction of W pouch. **A.** Four segments of terminal ileum are folded in two U configurations. Antimesenteric border is incised. **B.** Posterior walls are closed with one layer of continuous 3-0 absorbable sutures. Anterior wall is closed with one layer of continuous 3-0 absorbable sutures. (Redrawn from Gordon PH, Nivatvongs S. *Principles and Practice of Surgery for the Colon, Rectum, and Anus.* St. Louis, MO: Quality Medical; 1992)

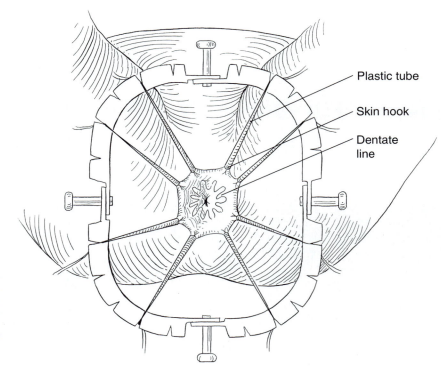

Plastic tube

Skin hook

Dentate line

Figure 44–8. Technique of anorectal mucosectomy with patient in lithotomy position in stirrups. The Lone Star, a self-retaining retractor, is used to efface anal canal. Its eight elastic stays can be adjusted to facilitate mucosectomy and anastomosis of the pouch to the dentate line. (Redrawn from Gordon PH, Nivatvongs S. *Principles and Practice of Surgery for the Colon, Rectum, and Anus.* St. Louis, MO: Quality Medical; 1992)

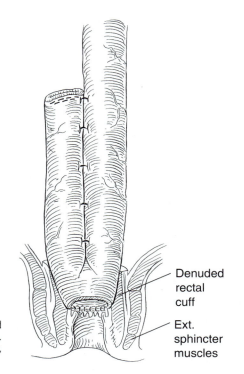

Denuded rectal cuff

Ext. sphincter muscles

Figure 44–9. Pouch-anal anastomosis. Pouch is delivered through denuded anorectum and is anastomosed to dentate line with one layer of interrupted 4-0 synthetic absorbable suture. (Redrawn from Gordon PH, Nivatvongs S. *Principles and Practice of Surgery for the Colon, Rectum, and Anus.* St. Louis, MO: Quality Medical; 1992)

ILEAL POUCH—ANAL CANAL ANASTOMOSIS

The pouch is delivered to the denuded anorectal cuff using a Babcock clamp. The base of the pouch is anastomosed to the anus at the dentate line, using interrupted 4-0 synthetic absorbable sutures (Fig 44–9). A closed-suction drain is placed in the presacral space behind the pouch and is brought out through a separate stab wound in the left lower quadrant.

LOOP ILEOSTOMY

A loop ileostomy is recommended for IPAA in patients with ulcerative colitis. It allows the reservoir and the anastomosis to heal and to regain their functions. The loop ileostomy is closed two months after the operation, provided the pouchogram shows no leak or pelvic abscess. Approximately 80% of loop ileostomy closures can be performed with a local incision around the ileostomy without the need to reopen the previous abdomen incision.[26] IPAA without a diverting ileostomy, however, has been performed successfully in a few carefully selected patients who are in good health, who are not on chronic steroid therapy, and in whom IPAA is constructed absolutely without tension.[27]

A loop of ileum as close to the pouch as possible (usually 45 to 60 cm from the apex of the pouch) is brought out through the aperture, which is premarked in the right lower quadrant. This loop of bowel should not be turned or twisted. The proximal limb of the bowel is anchored to the anterior abdominal wall with one stitch of 3-0 synthetic absorbable suture. The ileostomy is opened transversely closer to the distal limb. The longer proximal limb is everted with one stitch of 3-point anchoring suture of 3-0 chromic catgut, catching the stoma-seromuscular-dermis. A similar stitch is performed in the lower distal limb. The edges of the rest of the stoma then are sutured to the dermis all around, using running 3-0 chromic catgut. No rod is needed to support the ileostomy. A loop ileostomy must be constructed with care and absolutely without tension. Although we seldom have problems, other series reported a high incidence of complications, especially stoma retraction and small bowel obstruction.[28]

■ RESULTS

The IPAA was used in 1500 patients at the Mayo Clinic between January 1, 1981 and August 16, 1993. The ages of the patients ranged from 12 to 64 years, with a mean ± SD of 32 ± 10 years. Among the patients, 53% were males and 47% were females. Ulcerative colitis led to the operation in 88% of the patients and familial adenomatous polyposis in 12%. The operation was safe. Three

postoperative deaths occurred. One patient died from steroid-induced perforated gastric ulcer; one patient died from pulmonary embolism; the third patient died from ruptured cerebral aneurysm three hours after the operation. The main early complications were intestinal obstruction in 15% of patients, two-thirds of whom could be managed nonoperatively, and pelvic sepsis in 5% of patients, one-half of whom could be managed nonoperatively. Early and late complications led to excision of the pouch and permanent ileostomy in 81 patients, 5% of the total, from 6 months to 10 years after operation.

The outcome of operation was assessed at follow-up, which ranged from 1 year to more than 10 years after operation, with a mean follow-up of five years. The patients enjoyed an excellent quality of life, with fewer restrictions in areas such as sports, sexual activity, and travel than did patients with Brooke ileostomy or continent ileostomy.[29] The median number of bowel movements was 4.5 stools per day and 0.5 stools per night. Perfect continence was present in 75% of patients during the day, while 25% had occasional fecal spotting. In contrast, perfect continence was present in only 45% of patients during the night, with 55% having occasional nocturnal fecal spotting. Nocturnal spotting, however, improved with time; only 25% of patients followed 4 or more years continued to experience nocturnal spotting.[26] Urinary dysfunction occurred in <1% of patients and was transient. Among 43 women who became pregnant after operation, all delivered healthy, viable infants, except for one whose premature baby died of hyaline membrane disease of the lung. Pregnancy and childbirth are well tolerated in women who have undergone the IPAA procedure.[30,31] Comparing functional outcome 1 and 10 years following IPAA for ulcerative colitis, in terms of stool frequency and incontinence, neither appeared to deteriorate with time.[32]

Pouch inflammation (pouchitis) appeared symptomatically in 28% of the patients during follow-up. The onset of pouchitis was heralded by symptoms of "rectal" cramping, diarrhea, and sometimes, hematochezia. Malaise, fever, anorexia, and even extraintestinal manifestations of colitis, such as arthritis, uveitis, or erythema nodosum sometimes accompanied pouchitis. Treatment with metronidazole usually resulted in prompt resolution of symptoms, but recurrence and repeated treatments were required in more than half of affected patients. When metronidazole failed, sulfasalazine, corticosteroids, and other antibiotics and anti-inflammatory agents were used.[33]

■ COMPLICATIONS

Vast experience has been accumulated in terms of understanding the function of the pouch, patient preparation, patient selection, and particularly, operative techniques. The use of a short mucosectomy and rectal cuff has made the operation much easier, and consequently, has decreased the number of pelvic complications.

SMALL BOWEL OBSTRUCTION

A survey of the literature reveals an overall frequency of intestinal obstruction after IPAA ranging from 15% to as high as 44%. The incidence of obstruction requiring operative intervention is between 5% and 20%.[34] Two-thirds of the patients with small bowel obstructions—stomal stenosis, volvulus, internal hernia, and adhesive bands—have the temporary loop ileostomy as their cause. After closure of the ileostomy, most obstructions were the result of adhesions and anastomotic strictures.[34]

PELVIC ABSCESS

Most recent series cite the incidence of pelvic abscess as 4% to 6%.[35–37] A pelvic abscess most likely results from contamination of the presacral space, either during the operation or postoperatively, if there is partial disruption of the pouch-anal anastomosis. The latter may or may not be apparent radiologically. On occasion, a pelvic abscess will become evident clinically only after the ileostomy has been closed and intestinal continuity restored. The patient usually has a fever, pelvic or low-back pain sometimes radiating into the lower extremities and leukocytosis. A pouchogram or computed tomographic (CT) scan may demonstrate a leak communicating with an abscess cavity or distortion and anterior displacement of the ileal reservoir. A CT scan of the pelvic area often not only is diagnostic but also may help to determine the operative approach or may guide treatment.[38] However, not all pelvic abscesses are catastrophic or require major abdominal operations.

In the initial series of 188 patients who had an IPAA at the Mayo Clinic, 9 of 21 patients in whom a pelvic abscess developed could be treated by local drainage and antibiotics.[39] In some situations, CT-guided drainage also was successful. In approximately half of the patients, transabdominal exploration with evacuation of the purulent collection and placement of drains was required to overcome the septic process. If the ileostomy had been closed, it was reestablished. In some instances, the ileal reservoir was excised because of the insurmountable pelvic sepsis, despite one or even multiple revisional operations. Pelvic sepsis was responsible for about half of the reservoirs that required excision.

LEAKAGE OF POUCH AND POUCH–ANAL ANASTOMOSIS

Leakage of the pouch and pouch-anal anastomosis occurs in 2% to 10%.[14,26,36] Asymptomatic leaks revealed by x-ray studies most often are diagnosed when the pa-

tients return to have the ileostomy closed and intestinal continuity restored. Such leaks represent incomplete healing of the anastomosis or the ileal reservoir, and the only treatment needed is to defer closure of the ileostomy, usually for two months. The patient is restudied after this period. In most instances, the leak will have disappeared by then, and the ileostomy can be closed. In a few cases, a perianastomotic leak persists for 9 or even 12 months without causing any symptoms. If the leak is small and asymptomatic, the ileostomy can be closed without adverse sequelae.[38] Patients with symptomatic leaks may present with low-grade fever, perineal or low-back (sacral) pain, and intermittent perianal purulent discharge. A preoperative pouchogram may show a small fistulous track starting in the vicinity of the anastomosis and extending for a variable length, most often behind the pouch. The pouch should be examined with the patient under anesthesia, the track curetted, and the patient placed on an antibiotic such as metronidazole. Usually the symptoms will resolve rapidly and the fistulous track will heal. The temporary ileostomy may be closed later. Failure to heal should suggest Crohn's disease, and the ileostomy should be left in place.[38]

VAGINAL FISTULA

Ileal pouch-vaginal fistula is uncommon, but it presents a difficult management problem. A multicenter survey conducted by Wexner and associates revealed 22 pouch-vaginal fistulas among 304 females who underwent IPAA (7%).[40] Ninety-two percent of the fistulas were recognized clinically, and the rest were asymptomatic. The mean time of presentation of the pouch-vaginal fistula was 21 weeks after the IPAA (range 1 to 130 weeks). In approximately one-third of the patients, the diagnosis was made before the ileostomy closure, and two-thirds appeared after the ileostomy had been closed.

Pelvic sepsis, particularly rectal cuff abscess, apparently played an important role in the development of pouch-vaginal fistula. Approximately 75% of patients had the colectomy for acute fulminant ulcerative colitis, and the pouch was constructed either simultaneously or later as a three-stage procedure. Another high-risk group includes patients in whom IPAA was performed without a temporary diverting ileostomy (one stage).[40] In any case, Crohn's disease must be ruled out.

The basic principle in the management of the pouch-vaginal fistula is delaying the closure of the diverting ileostomy for two to three months. If the ileostomy has been closed already, it should be re-established. This step alone will heal the majority of cases. If the fistula persists, a transvaginal or transanal repair of the fistula should be done.[38,40]

ANAL STRICTURE

Some degree of narrowing of the anal canal at the anastomosis is common and presents no problem. A lumen that admits the distal interphalangeal joint of the index finger or admits a 1.5-cm diameter proctoscope is satisfactory. Anastomotic strictures can occur after pelvic sepsis. Other factors such as undue tension on the IPAA, inadequate blood supply, and poor technique may play important roles.[38]

Significant stricture of the pouch-anal anastomosis occurs in 5% to 8% of cases.[14,26,36] The stricture is usually apparent on postoperative examination before closure of the ileostomy. Mild strictures can be dilated with Hegar dilators in the office or clinic, preferably gradually graduating to a #13 Hegar dilator. A tight stricture (5 mm or smaller) should be dilated with the patient under anesthesia, and repeated dilation will be required. Occasionally a tight band in the anoderm or internal sphincter muscle requires incision.

REOPERATION FOR POUCH-RELATED COMPLICATIONS

Pouch-related complications occur in 12% to 22% of patients. They include anastomotic stricture, perianal fistula or abscess, intra-abdominal fistula or abscess, residual septum in a J pouch, long efferent limb in an S pouch, and unsatisfactory pouch function.[38,41] What is the outcome of these patients? Galandiuk and associates reviewed their experience with 114 patients at the Mayo Clinic.[41] Complications prevented initial ileostomy closure in 25% of these patients. The salvage procedures performed included anal dilation for stricture with the patient under anesthesia, placement of a Seton and/or fistulotomy for perianal fistula, unroofing anastomotic sinuses, simple drainage and antibiotic administration for perianal abscess, abdominal exploration with drainage of intra-abdominal abscess with or without establishment of ileostomy, and a complete or partial reconstruction of the reservoir for patients with inadequate emptying. None of the reoperated patients died, and reoperation led to restoration of pouch function in two-thirds of the patients. However, 20% of 114 pouches required excision. Excision was especially common among patients who had pelvic sepsis.

SEXUAL DYSFUNCTION

The impact of ileal pouch-anal canal anastomosis on sexual function is important, because patients are generally young and in their reproductive years. Despite using an operative technique that spares presacral nerves and preserves the pelvic floor and anal canal, sexual dysfunction still occurs. In the series from the Mayo Clinic in which 670 IPAA were performed for ulcerative colitis, impotence occurred in 1% and retrograde ejacula-

TABLE 44–1. CAUSES OF COMPLETE FAILURE OF IPAA.

	Wexner et al[37]	Pescatori & Mattana[44]	Dozois et al[42]
Patients	180[a]	207[a]	670[b]
Failures	14 (8%)	12 (6%)	25 (4%)
Functional Failures	36%	Yes	44% (incontinence, diarrhea)
Crohn's Disease	36%	Not Specified	12%
Intractable Pouchitis	14%	Not Specified	Not Specified
Pelvic Sepsis	7%	Not Specified	Not Specified
Other Causes	7%	Yes	44%

[a]Includes polyposis; [b]ulcerative colitis only.

tion in 3%.[42] In females, dyspareunia occurred in 7%. A prospective study of 100 male patients with IPAA from Goteborg, Sweden, revealed impotence in 2% (excluding preoperative impotence) and retrograde ejaculation in 2%.[43] The sexual dysfunction in females was greater: dyspareunia in 7% (excluding preoperative dyspareunia) and fecal leaks during intercourse in 2% (excluding preoperative leaks).

COMPLETE FAILURE OF IPAA

Despite a complex operation and the relatively high complication rate after proctocolectomy with IPAA, the incidence of total failure requiring excision of the pouch and the establishment of a permanent ileostomy is relatively low, 4 to 8% (Table 44–1).[37,42,44]

■ DRAWBACKS

The three main drawbacks of ileal pouch-anal anastomosis are frequent stools, fecal spotting, especially at night, and pouchitis.

FREQUENT STOOLS

Frequent stools likely relate to the increased fecal output after IPAA. Healthy persons produce about 150 gm of stool per day that is passed with a frequency that ranges from three motions per day to one motion every three days. In contrast, IPAA patients who have lost their colons expel a mean of 650 gm of stool per day passed as five semisolid motions per 24 hours. The four-fold increase in fecal output likely accounts for the four-fold increase in frequency of defecation.[45] The greater the fecal output, the more the number of stools per day (Fig 44–10).

Decreasing the fecal volume could be of great benefit to IPAA patients. A small volume of thicker stool would decrease the frequency of stooling and likely also

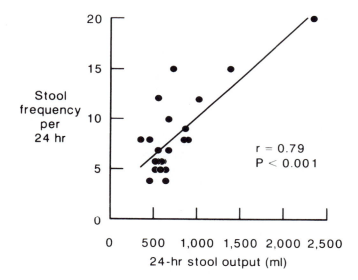

Figure 44–10. Graph plotting volume of stool against frequency of stooling in patients after ileal pouch–anal anastomosis. (From O'Connell PR, Pemberton JH, Brown ML, et al. Determinants of stool frequency after ileal pouch–anal anastomosis. *Am J Surg* 1987;153:157)

improve continence. The volume of fecal output can be decreased by about one-third by the use of loperamide hydrochloride,[46] but the chronic use of this medication is expensive and unattractive to many patients. Bulking agents also have been used to thicken the stool but, unfortunately, do not decrease fecal output.

Efforts are being made to develop new methods of decreasing enteric output. A somatostatin analogue might diminish fecal output in IPAA patients, as it has done in patients with conventional ileostomies.[47] However, a careful trial in IPAA patients has not yet been reported. Calcium per os also may have a role.[48] Slowing small intestinal transit to allow more time for absorption is an attractive hypothesis, but reversing intestinal segments in an attempt to do so has not been successful, at least not in dogs.[49] Electrically pacing the small intestine backwards to slow transit and improve absorption has been successful in dogs with jejunal loops,[50] but not in dogs with ileostomy.[51] The human small intestine also has been paced, but so far, improved human small bowel absorption with pacing has not yet been achieved. Decreasing fecal output below a minimal volume may, in fact, impair digestion and absorption.

FECAL INCONTINENCE

Two major prerequisites must be present to achieve fecal continence: a compliant, receptive fecal reservoir of adequate size that empties well and a competent barricade to fecal outflow provided by an intact pelvic floor and a strong anal sphincter.

The ileal J pouch does provide a compliant reservoir of adequate volume. Measurements of J pouches have shown a rate of distensibility of 15 mL per mm Hg intrapouch pressure, a maximum tolerable volume of 320 mL, and a voluntary emptying rate of 11 mL of stool per minute.[45,52,53] The patients empty 84% of pouch content spontaneously at will.[54] These values are similar to those of patients with a healthy rectum.

Other motor features of the pouch, however, do not mimic the motility of the healthy rectum. The healthy rectum exhibits few, if any, contractions when distended to 350 mL. In contrast, large amplitude, phasic contractions appear in most ileal pouches at a threshold of distention of about 100 mL (Fig 44–11). The contractions increase intrapouch pressure to a value near anal sphincter pressure. The increases in pouch pressure usually are accompanied by increases in anal sphincter pressure,[55] but sometimes pouch contractile strength exceeds anal sphincter strength. When this happens, leakage may result.[56]

A method of decreasing the strength of pouch contractions as the pouch fills has not yet been devised. Anticholinergics have been used with anecdotal success, but large enough doses to inhibit pouch contraction have undesirable side effects, secondary to the inhibition of contraction in smooth muscle elsewhere. The contractile response of most pouches seems to depend mainly on the size of the pouch, rather than the particular style of pouch. Excessively large pouches, however, are not recommended, since they do not empty well and may predispose the patient to pouchitis.

The anal sphincters are reasonably well, but not perfectly, preserved by the operation. Resting anal sphincteric strength, largely a function of internal anal sphincter, is decreased about 15% after the procedure (Fig 44–12).[57] Among 50 IPAA patients we studied, resting sphincter pressure was 56 mm Hg, while resting pressure in healthy controls was 65 mm Hg.[58] Moreover, anal small waves superimposed on the resting pressure had a slower frequency and a larger amplitude in pouch patients than in controls. Additionally, the resting pressure in some patients decreased more at night, as sleep deepened, than it did in healthy controls.[59] There were periods during which pressures in patients decreased during rapid eye–movement sleep to near zero.

The decrease in resting anal sphincter pressure may be due to mechanical damage from dilation of the sphincter during the anal mucosal stripping or from direct injury to the sphincter during the stripping. It is also possible that partial extrinsic denervation of the sphincter occurs when the distal rectal wall and its adjacent vasculature are transected. Adrenergic fibers that accompany the vessels are known to augment anal sphincter strength, at least in the dog.[60] Clearly, careful mucosal dissection, minimal dilation of the sphincter

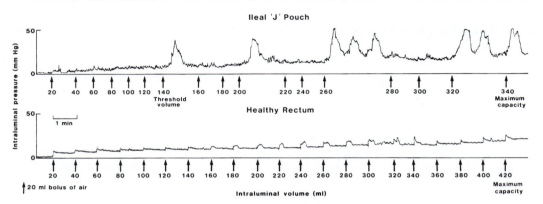

Figure 44–11. Motor response of healthy rectum (lower) and ileal pouch (upper) to gradual distention. (From O'Connell PR, Pemberton JH, Brown ML, et al. Determinants of stool frequency after ileal pouch–anal anastomosis *Am J Surg* 1987;153:157)

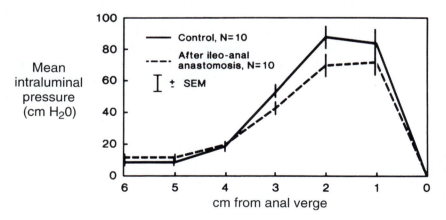

Figure 44–12. Anal sphincteric resting pressure profile from 10 patients with ileoanal anastomosis and 10 healthy nonoperated controls. (From Heppell J, Kelly KA, Phillips SF, et al. Physiologic aspects of continence after colectomy, mucosal proctectomy and endorectal ileo-anal anastomosis. (From *Ann Surg* 1982;195:435)

during operation, and the protection of sphincter innervation are keys to maintaining a well-functioning anal sphincter postoperatively.

New methods of augmenting resting anal sphincter strength after surgery would be welcomed. Anal sphincter resting pressure can be increased by loperamide hydrochloride[46] and valproate sodium,[61] and perhaps by biofeedback. Whether the strength can be further augmented with adrenergic drugs is unknown. In contrast to anal sphincter resting pressure, anal sphincter squeeze pressure, a function of the external anal sphincter, is usually well maintained by operation (Fig 44–13).[57,58] While we documented damage to the striated muscle of the external anal sphincter or its innervation in some patients who had episodic fecal leakage after operation,[62] overall in our series,[57,58] as in others,[63] anal squeeze pressure after operation was similar to that found in healthy controls. The anorectal angle and the pelvic floor dynamics also are maintained well by operation.[64]

POUCHITIS

The cause of pouchitis is unknown, although it is believed to be disease-related. Thus for example, colitis patients have a much greater incidence of pouchitis than do patients undergoing the operation for familial adenomatous polyposis. Additionally, colitis patients who have extraintestinal manifestations of the disease are more likely to get pouchitis than are those patients without extraintestinal manifestations.[65] Patients with backwash ileitis are not particularly predisposed to the condition.[66] Although mechanical causes such as anastomotic stricture and excessively large pouches that empty poorly sometimes cause pouchitis, in most patients such a mechanical problem cannot be identified. Pouchitis seems to be related to stasis in the pouch, with subsequent proliferation of bacteria in the lumen, especially anaerobes. The bacteria or their exotoxins appear to damage the mucosa of the pouch. Erosions, ulcerations, and an acute inflammatory response then appear. One supporting fact for the stasis-bacterial overgrowth theory is that metronidazole, an antibiotic directed primarily at anaerobic bacteria, decreases bacterial counts and improves inflammation and symptoms. However, this theory does not explain why colitis patients are more susceptible to pouchitis than are polyposis patients.

The ileal pouch develops an altered mucosal anatomy when compared with the anatomy of a healthy ileum. The pouch mucosa has shortened, blunted villi and elongated crypts that show an increased rate of crypt-cell production. Mucous cells of the colonic type appear in the mucosa. In fact, the mucosal histology of the ileal pouch resembles the mucosal histology of the colon.

Our colleagues at the Mayo Clinic found that total fecal concentrations of short-chain fatty acids in patients with pouchitis were significantly lower ($P<.01$) than those in asymptomatic control patients.[67] Specifically, acetic acid and butyric acid concentrations were significantly decreased, whereas those of propionate were not. This finding has led to the hypothesis that pouchitis may be caused by a deficiency of nutrients for the ileal or colonic epithelium. Accordingly, a deficiency of butyric acid (a primary nutrient of colonocytes) or of glutamine (a major nutrient of enterocytes) may contribute to the syndrome of pouchitis, similar to the pathophysiologic basis for diversion colitis. Treatment of pouchitis with butyrate suppositories was disappointing. Only three of nine patients responded favorably. Treatment with glutamine suppositories yielded encouraging results. Six of ten patients so treated developed no recurrent symptoms. Further studies of glutamine in the treatment of pouchitis seem warranted. Mucosal ischemia that results in the production of oxygen-free radicals, which in turn incite inflammation, also may have a role in the development of pouchitis. Treatment with Allopurinol, an oxygen-free radical "scavenger," caused improvement

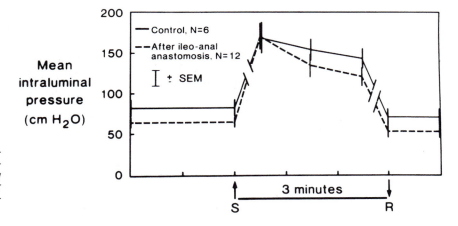

Figure 44–13. Anal sphincteric squeeze pressure from 12 patients with ileoanal anastomosis and 6 healthy nonoperated controls. S=squeeze, R=release. (Redrawn from Heppell J, Kelly KA, Phillips SF, et al. Physiologic aspects of continence after colectomy, mucosal proctectomy and endorectal ileo-anal anastomosis. *Ann Surg* 1982;195:435)

in 50% of patients in a preliminary pilot trial at the Mayo Clinic.[68]

Identifying the exact cause of pouchitis remains a major challenge for the future. Further, pouchitis and the other problems associated with IPAA have caused surgeons to seek an alternative to this operation. Recently, the ileal pouch–distal rectal anastomosis has emerged as a viable alternative.[69,70]

■ ILEAL POUCH–DISTAL RECTAL ANASTOMOSIS TECHNIQUE

The abdominal colectomy is performed in the same manner as for the IPAA with mucosectomy. The rectum is transected 2 cm proximal to the dentate line, using a linear stapler (Fig 44–14). The level of transection must be verified precisely by checking (with a finger through the anus) the level of the stapler before preparing the anorectal stump.

The J pouch is constructed using an anastomosing stapler through the base of the pouch. A 28- or 29-mm

circular stapler is used for anastomosing the J pouch to the anorectal stump (Fig 44–14). At completion, the anastomosis should be approximately 1 to 2 cm proximal to the dentate line and should be palpated with the index finger through the anus to detect any defect. The pelvis then is filled with saline solution. The ileum above the pouch is clamped and a small amount of air is introduced via the anal canal to check for air leaks. A diverting loop ileostomy is performed. Some authors eliminated the covering loop ileostomy altogether.[28,71] The operation is thought to be faster than the IPAA and less technically demanding. The likelihood of constructing a precise anastomosis under no tension and with good blood supply may be better with ileal pouch–distal rectal anastomosis than with ileal pouch–anal canal anastomosis.

Proponents of this procedure state that ileal pouch–distal rectal anastomosis results in better anal sensation and better anal sphincteric function than IPAA.[70,72] However, retention of the mucosa of the distal rectum and upper anal canal may pose some risk to the patient since colitis, dysplasia, and carcinoma can develop.

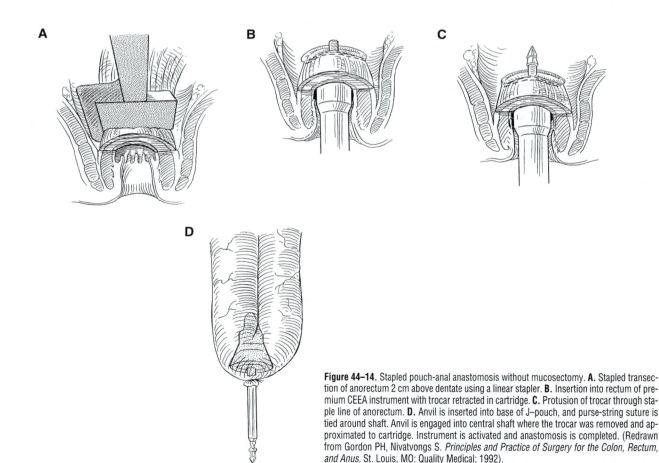

Figure 44–14. Stapled pouch-anal anastomosis without mucosectomy. **A.** Stapled transection of anorectum 2 cm above dentate using a linear stapler. **B.** Insertion into rectum of premium CEEA instrument with trocar retracted in cartridge. **C.** Protusion of trocar through staple line of anorectum. **D.** Anvil is inserted into base of J–pouch, and purse-string suture is tied around shaft. Anvil is engaged into central shaft where the trocar was removed and approximated to cartridge. Instrument is activated and anastomosis is completed. (Redrawn from Gordon PH, Nivatvongs S. *Principles and Practice of Surgery for the Colon, Rectum, and Anus.* St. Louis, MO: Quality Medical; 1992).

RESULTS

To date, this operation has not been used much at the Mayo Clinic. Others report that the operation is faster than IPAA and that anal sensation and anal sampling are better preserved.[70,72,73] Anal sphincter strength, however, may not be any better maintained than with the IPAA. While some surgeons have found better preservation of the sphincter when the proximal anal canal is left intact,[70,72,74] others have noted a similar strength of sphincter in patients, whether the proximal anal canal has been removed or not.[63,75] Also, although some authors report that the frequency of stooling has been less, and nocturnal continence better, with the ileal pouch–distal rectal anastomosis,[70,72–74,76] others report that preservation of the proximal rectal mucosa resulted in a pattern of stooling and nocturnal continence similar to that following IPAA.[63,75,77] A well-controlled prospective clinical trial published recently revealed no clear-cut differences in postoperative complications or functional outcome between the two operations.[63,78]

DRAWBACKS

The main drawback of the ileal pouch–distal rectal anastomosis is the lack of complete excision of the disease. A study of 50 proctocolectomy specimens from 50 ulcerative colitis patients at the Mayo Clinic showed that the columnar epithelium of the rectal mucosa formed digitations within 1 cm of the dentate line, in 89% of the specimens. Although the transitional epithelium does not become inflamed in ulcerative colitis, the columnar epithelium that extends past the transitional epithelium causes inflammation of the anal canal. In 9% of the specimens, the columnar epithelium was in direct apposition to the dentate line.[79] The retention of the distal rectal and proximal anal mucosa leaves the patient at risk for the development of dysplasia and carcinoma in this area. In fact, dysplasia and adenocarcinoma have been described in the mucosa of the proximal anal canal, in patients with ulcerative colitis.[80,81] Even surgeons who advocate the ileal pouch–distal rectal operation do not recommend it for patients who have dysplasia in other parts of the large intestine, or who have already developed a carcinoma of the large intestine. One must keep in mind that many of these young patients may live 50 more years.

Another concern is that continuing inflammation of the mucosa of the proximal anal canal will demand continuing and costly surveillance, which patients dislike. Strictures or other proximal anal inflammatory complications may develop in future years. Such complications may require treatment or even reoperation, a procedure that can be technically difficult.

Whether the ease of operation and the possible improvement in continence with ileal pouch–distal rectal anastomosis will offset the risk of continuing inflammation and carcinoma in the residual diseased mucosa requires further testing. Continence may be better, but stool output and, therefore, frequency of stooling after ileal pouch–distal rectal anastomosis will likely be similar to that after the IPAA. Also, the threat of pouchitis, perhaps the most serious complication of the ileal pouch operation, will continue after ileal pouch–distal rectal anastomosis.

REFERENCES

1. Stryker SJ, Dozois RR. The ileoanal anastomosis: historical perspectives. In: Dozois RR (ed), *Alternatives to Conventional Ileostomy*. Chicago, IL: Yearbook Medical; 1985:255
2. Ravitch MM, Sabiston DC. Anal ileostomy with preservation of the sphincter: a proposed operation in patients requiring total colectomy for benign lesions. *Surg Gynecol Obstet* 1947;84:1095
3. Ravitch MM. Anal ileostomy with sphincter preservation in patients requiring total colectomy for benign conditions. *Surgery* 1948;24:170
4. Best R. Evaluation of ileoproctostomy to avoid ileostomy in various colon lesions. *JAMA* 1952;150:637
5. Goligher JC. The functional results after sphincter-saving resections of the rectum. *Ann R Coll Surg Engl* 1951;8:421
6. Valiente MA, Bacon HE. Construction of pouch using "pantaloon" technique for pull-through of ileum following total colectomy. *Am J Surg* 1955;90:742
7. Martin LW, LeCoultre C, Schubert WK. Total colectomy and mucosal proctectomy with preservation of continence in ulcerative colitis. *Ann Surg* 1977;186:477
8. Telander RL, Smith SL, Marcinek HM, et al. Surgical treatment of ulcerative colitis in children. *Surgery* 1981;90: 787
9. Beart RW Jr, Dozois RR, Kelly KA. Ileoanal anastomosis in the adult. *Surg Gynecol Obstet* 1982;154:826
10. Beart RW Jr. Surgical management of chronic ulcerative colitis. *Semin Colon Rectal Surg* 1990;1:186
11. Parks AG, Nicholls RJ. Proctocolectomy without ileostomy for ulcerative colitis. *Br Med J* 1978;2:85
12. Parks AG, Nicholls RJ, Belliveau P. Proctocolectomy with ileal reservoir and anal anastomosis. *Br J Surg* 1980;67:533
13. Nicholls RJ, Kamm MA. Proctocolectomy with restorative ileoanal reservoir for severe idiopathic constipation. *Dis Colon Rectum* 1988;31:968
14. Fleshman JW, Cohen Z, McLeod RS, et al. The ileal reservoir and ileoanal anastomosis procedure: factors affecting technical and functional outcome. *Dis Colon Rectum* 1988; 31:10
15. Pezim ME, Pemberton JH, Beart RW Jr, et al. Outcome of "indeterminant" colitis following ileal pouch–anal anastomosis. *Dis Colon Rectum* 1989;32:653
16. Taylor BA, Wolff BG, Dozois RR, et al. Ileal pouch–anal anastomosis for chronic ulcerative colitis and familial polyposis coli complicated by adenocarcinoma. *Dis Colon Rectum* 1988;31:358
17. Fozard JBJ, Nelson H, Pemberton JH, et al. Primary ileal

pouch–anal anastomosis and colorectal cancer—results and contraindications. *Dis Colon Rectum* 1992;35:P22

18. Utsunomiya J, Iwama T, Imajo M, et al. Total colectomy, mucosal proctectomy and ileoanal anastomosis. *Dis Colon Rectum* 1980;23:459

19. Fonkalsrud EW. Total colectomy and endorectal ileal pullthrough with internal ileal reservoir for ulcerative colitis. *Surg Gynecol Obstet* 1980;150:1

20. Nicholls RJ, Pezim ME. Restorative proctocolectomy with ileal reservoir for ulcerative colitis and familial adenomatous polyposis: a comparison of three reservoir designs. *Br J Surg* 1985;72:470

21. Smith L, Friend WG, Medwell SJ. The superior mesenteric artery. The critical factor in the pouch pull–through procedure. *Dis Colon Rectum* 1984;27:741

22. Burnstein MJ, Schoetz DJ Jr, Coller JA, et al. Technique of mesenteric lengthening in ileal reservoir–anal anastomosis. *Dis Colon Rectum* 1987;30:863

23. Nicholls RJ, Lubowski DZ. Restorative proctocolectomy: the four loop (W) reservoir. *Br J Surg* 1987;74:564

24. Dozois RR. Technique of ileal pouch–anal anastomosis. *Perspect Colon Rectal Surg* 1989;2:85

25. Roberts PL, Schoetz DJ Jr, Murray JJ, et al. Use of new retractor to facilitate mucosal proctectomy. *Dis Colon Rectum* 1990;33:1063

26. Pemberton JH, Kelly KA, Beart RW Jr, et al. Ileal pouch–anal anastomosis to facilitate mucosal proctectomy. *Dis Colon Rectum* 1990;33:1063

27. Galandiuk S, Wolff BG, Dozois RR, et al. Ileal pouch–anal anastomosis without ileostomy. *Dis Colon Rectum* 1991;34:870

28. Winslet MC, Barsoum G, Pringle W, et al. Loop ileostomy after ileal pouch–anal anastomosis—is it necessary? *Dis Colon Rectum* 1991;34:267

29. Köhler L, Pemberton JH, Zinsmeister AR, et al. Quality of life after proctocolectomy: a comparison of Brooke ileostomy, Kock pouch, and ileal pouch–anal anastomosis. *Gastroenterology* 1991;101:679

30. Nelson H, Dozois RR, Kelly KA, et al. The effect of pregnancy and delivery on the ileal pouch–anal anastomosis functions. *Dis Colon Rectum* 1989;32:384

31. Fozard JBL, Nelson H, Dozois RR. Pregnancy, birth and ileal pouch–anal anastomosis. *Dis Colon Rectum* 1992;35:P14

32. McIntyre PB, Pemberton JH, Wolff BG, et al. Comparing functional outcome 1 and 10 years following ileo–anal anastomosis for chronic ulcerative colitis. *Dis Colon Rectum* 1992;36:P2

33. Kelly KA. Anal sphincter-saving operations for chronic ulcerative colitis. *Am J Surg* 1992;163:5

34. Francois Y, Dozois RR, Kelly KA, et al. Small intestinal obstruction complicating ileal pouch–anal anastomosis. *Ann Surg* 1989;209:46

35. Scott NA, Dozois RR, Beart RW Jr, et al. Postoperative intra-abdominal and pelvic sepsis complicating ileal pouch–anal anastomosis. *Int J Colorectal Dis* 1988;3:149

36. Schoetz DJ Jr, Coller JA, Veidenheimer MC. Can the pouch be saved? *Dis Colon Rectum* 1988;31:671

37. Wexner SD, Wong WD, Rothenberger DA, et al. The ileoanal reservoir. *Am J Surg* 1990;159:178

38. Dozois RR. Pelvic and perianastomotic complications after ileoanal anastomosis. *Perspect Colon Rectal Surg* 1988;1:113

39. Metcalf AM, Dozois RR, Kelly KA, et al. Ileal J pouch-anal anastomosis: clinical outcome. *Ann Surg* 1985;202:735

40. Wexner SD, Rothenberger DA, Jensen L, et al. Ileal pouch vaginal fistulas: incidence, etiology, and management. *Dis Colon Rectum* 1989;32:460

41. Galandiuk S, Scott NA, Dozois RR, et al. Ileal pouch–anal anastomosis. reoperation for pouch-related complications. *Ann Surg* 1990;212:446

42. Dozois RR, Kelly KA, Welling DR, et al. Ileal pouch–anal anastomosis: comparison of results in familial adenomatous polyposis and chronic ulcerative colitis. *Ann Surg* 1989;210:268

43. Oresland T, Fasth S, Nordgren S, et al. The clinical and functional outcome after restorative proctocolectomy: a prospective study in 100 patients. *Int J Colorectal Dis* 1989;4:50

44. Pescatori M, Mattana C. Factors affecting anal continence after restorative proctocolectomy. *Int J Colorectal Dis* 1990;5:213

45. O'Connell PR, Pemberton JH, Brown ML, et al. Determinants of stool frequency after ileal pouch–anal anastomosis. *Am J Surg* 1987;153:157

46. Emblem R, Stein R, Morkrid L. The effect of loperamide on bowel habits and anal sphincter function in patients with ileoanal anastomosis. *Scand J Gastroenterol* 1989;24:1019

47. Williams NS, Cooper JC, Axon ATR, et al. Use of a long acting somatostatin analogue in controlling life threatening ileostomy diarrhea. *BMJ* 1984;289:1027

48. Barsoum G, Winslet M, Kappas A, et al. Influence of dietary calcium supplementation on ileoanal pouch function. *Gut* 1990;31:A1170

49. Williams NS, King RFGJ. The effect of a reversed ileal segment and artificial valve on intestinal transit and absorption following colectomy and low ileorectal anastomosis in the dog. *Br J Surg* 1985;72:169

50. Collin J, Kelly KA, Phillips SF. Enhancement of absorption from the intact and transected canine small intestine by electrical pacing. *Gastroenterology* 1979;76:1422

51. O'Connell PR, Kelly KA. Enteric transit and absorption after canine ileostomy: effect of pacing. *Arch Surg* 1987;122:1011

52. Taylor BM, Cranley B, Kelly KA, et al. A clinical physiologic comparison of ileal pouch–anal and straight ileoanal anastomosis. *Ann Surg* 1983;198:462

53. O'Connell PR, Kelly KA, Brown ML. Scintigraphic assessment of neorectal function. *J Nucl Med* 1986;27:422

54. Soper NJ, Chapman NJ, Kelly KA, et al. The ileal brake after ileal pouch–anal anastomosis. *Gastroenterology* 1990;98:111

55. Ferrara A, Pemberton JH, Hanson RB. Preservation of continence after ileoanal anastomosis by the coordination of ileal pouch and anal canal motor activity. *Am J Surg* 1992;163:83

56. Stryker SJ, Kelly KA, Phillips SF, et al. Anal and neorectal function after ileal pouch–anal anastomosis. *Ann Surg* 1986;203:55

57. Heppell J, Kelly KA, Phillips SF, et al. Physiologic aspects of continence after colectomy, mucosal proctectomy and endorectal ileo-anal anastomosis. *Ann Surg* 1982;195:435

58. O'Connell PR, Stryker SJ, Metcalf AM, et al. Anal canal pressure and motility after ileoanal anastomosis. *Surg Gynecol Obstet* 1988;166:47

59. Orkin BA, Soper NJ, Kelly KA, et al. The influence of sleep on anal sphincteric pressure in health and after ileal pouch-anal anastomosis. *Dis Colon Rectum* 1992;35:137

60. Kubota M, Szurszewski JH. Innervation of the canine internal anal sphincter. *Gastroenterology* 1984;86:1146

61. Shoji Y, Kusunoki M, Sakanoue Y, et al. Effects of sodium valproate on various intestinal motor functions after ileal J pouch–anal anastomosis. *Surgery* 1993;113:360

62. Stryker SJ, Daube JR, Kelly KA, et al. Anal sphincter electromyography after colectomy, mucosal rectectomy, and ileoanal anastomosis. *Arch Surg* 1985;120:713

63. Hallgren T, Fasth S, Nordgren S, et al. The stapled ileal pouch–anal anastomosis: a randomized study comparing two different pouch designs. *Scand J Gastroenterol* 1990; 25:1161

64. Barkel DC, Pemberton JH, Pezim ME, et al. Scintigraphic assessment of the anorectal angle in health and after ileal pouch–anal anastomosis. *Ann Surg* 1988;208:42

65. Lohmuller JL, Pemberton JH, Dozois RR, et al. Pouchitis and extraintestinal manifestations of inflammatory bowel disease after ileal pouch–anal anastomosis. *Ann Surg* 1990; 211:622

66. Gustavsson S, Weiland LH, Kelly KA. Relationship of backwash ileitis to ileal pouchitis after ileal pouch–anal anastomosis. *Dis Colon Rectum* 1987;30:25

67. Wischmeyer P, Pemberton JH, Phillips SF. Chronic pouchitis after ileal pouch-anal anastomosis: responses to butyrate and glutamine suppositories in the pilot study. *Mayo Clin Proc* 1993;68:978

68. Levin KE, Pemberton JH, Phillips SF, et al. Effect of a xanthine oxidase inhibitor (allopurinol) in patients with pouchitis after ileal pouch–anal anastomosis. *Gut* 1990;31: A1168

69. Heald RJ, Allen DR. Stapled ileoanal anastomosis: a technique to avoid mucosal proctectomy in the ileal pouch operation. *Br J Surg* 1986;73:571

70. Johnston D, Holdsworth DJ, Nasymth DG. Preservation of the entire anal canal in conservative proctocolectomy for ulcerative colitis: a pilot study comparing end-to-end ileo-anal anastomosis without mucosal resection with mucosal proctectomy and endoanal anastomosis. *Br J Surg* 1987; 74:940

71. Sagar PM, Lewis W, Holdsworth PJ, et al. One-stage restorative proctocolectomy without temporary defunctioning ileostomy. *Dis Colon Rectum* 1992;35:582

72. Sagar PM, Holdsworth PJ, Johnston D. Correlation between laboratory findings and clinical outcome after restorative proctocolectomy: serial studies in 20 patients with end-to-end pouch–anal anastomosis. *Br J Surg* 1991; 78:67

73. Martin LW, Torres AM, Fischer JE, et al. The critical level for preservation of continence in the ileoanal anastomosis. *J Pediatr Surg* 1985;20:664

74. Tuckson W, Lavery I, Fazio V, et al. Manometric and functional comparison of ileal pouch–anal anastomosis with and without anal manipulation. *Am J Surg* 1991;161:90

75. Williams NS, Marzouk DEMM, Hallan RI, et al. Function after ileal pouch and stapled pouch–anal anastomosis for ulcerative colitis. *Br J Surg* 1989;76:1168

76. Lavery IC, Tuckson WB, Fazio VW, et al. Pouch surgery—the importance of the transitional zone. *Can J Gastroenterol* 1990;4:428

77. Keighley MRB, Winslet MC, Yoshioka K, et al. Discrimination is not impaired by excision of the anal transition zone after restorative proctocolectomy. *Br J Surg* 1987;74:1118

78. Seow-Choen F, Tsunoda A, Nicholls RJ. Prospective randomized trial comparing anal function after hand sewn ileoanal anastomosis with mucosectomy versus stapled ileoanal anastomosis without mucosectomy in restorative proctocolectomy. *Br J Surg* 1991;78:430

79. Ambroze WL, Pemberton JH, Dozois RR, et al. Does retaining the anal transition zone (ATZ) fail to extirpate chronic ulcerative colitis (CUC) after ileal pouch–anal anastomosis (IPAA)? *Dis Colon Rectum* 1991;34:A20

80. King DW, Lubowski DZ, Cook TA. Anal mucosa in restorative proctocolectomy for ulcerative colitis. *Br J Surg* 1989; 76:970

81. Tsunoda A, Talbot IC, Nicholls RJ. Incidence of dysplasia in the colorectal mucosa in patients having restorative proctocolectomy. *Br J Surg* 1990;77:506

45

Continent Ileostomy

Steven L. Glorsky ▪ *Robert W. Beart*

Many patients require total proctocolectomy in the surgical management of inflammatory or neoplastic colorectal diseases that are complicated or medically intractable. The pathologic entities of ulcerative colitis, Crohn's colitis, and familial adenomatous polyposis are most frequently the indication. Preoperatively and at the time of surgery, the appropriate choice of an alternate modality for fecal evacuation is an important management priority. Consideration must be given to the identity, severity, and extent of the specific disease involved, as well as patient factors such as age, personality, employment, state of acute and chronic health, previous surgical history, and prior state of gastrointestinal function.

There are a number of surgical options that one must consider when an extensive colorectal resection is indicated. Historically, total proctocolectomy with end ileostomy was the first procedure to be established in this setting. The earliest end ileostomies were not primarily matured and were frequently plaqued by dysfunction, secondary to serositis. This problem was obviated by Brooke, in 1952, who first suggested immediate maturation of the exteriorized ileum, by eversion.[1]

Subsequently, total proctocolectomy with Brooke ileostomy became, for many, the standard by which all other operations for this indication would be judged. Authors have cited its simplicity and, therefore, safe accomplishment by virtually all well-trained general surgeons.[2] The operation is often curative of the diseases to which it is applied, mitigating the future risks of recurrent inflammation or malignant degeneration. Subsequent improvements in ostomy appliance technology and enterostomal therapy have enhanced the abilities of ileostomates to accommodate to this alternative. Roy and associates reported that approximately 90% of individuals after total proctocolectomy with end ileostomy described their general health as excellent or good.[3] Moreover, 96% of these patients had returned to gainful employment.

There remain, however, significant morbidities associated with the Brooke ileostomy. Series have revealed an approximate 14% subsequent reoperation rate, including required ileostomy revisions and procedures relating to perineal and abdominal wound complications.[4] There remains a finite risk of sexual and bladder dysfunction, secondary to pelvic nerve injury, during the course of proctectomy. Many patients suffer from chronic peristomal skin irritation, associated with appliance products and leakage. Odor and excessive noise remain troublesome. Additionally, a significant number of patients have found the alteration in body image and loss of fecal continence associated with an ileostomy to be psychologically problematic, inhibiting their choice of clothing, participation in leisure activities, and sexual function.[5]

These problems have inspired subsequent efforts to recreate fecal continence after proctocolectomy. A number of mechanical occlusion devices have been introduced, to be implemented in concert with end ileostomies. These include the Erlangen magnetic ring closing device[6] and a balloon device for chronic intermittent ileostomy occlusion.[7] These techniques, although theoretically attractive, have failed to achieve popularity.

Proctocolectomy with Brook ileostomy retains a role today for a significant subset of patients. Older individuals, with multiple medical problems, benefit from the relative simplicity of this procedure. It is further indicated for individuals who have sustained anal sphincter damage or dysfunction. Additionally, it is most appropriate for patients with extensive Crohn's proctocolitis or low rectal cancer.[8]

Total colectomy with ileorectal anastomosis, first popularized in the 1960s by Aylett,[9] retains a limited and controversial role in the surgical treatment of inflammatory bowel disease.[10–12] Currently, the best defined role for ileorectostomy is in patients with Crohn's disease, without significant proctitis or perianal involvement, and in individuals with indeterminate colitis.[13]

In the late 1960s, Professor Nils Kock introduced the continent ileal reservoir, as an alternative for patients facing total proctocolectomy,[14] extending the indications for a procedure originally devised as a urinary bladder substitute after total cystectomy. Kock hypothesized that the aboral peristaltic forces at the ileostomy site could be neutralized by folding the terminal ileum upon itself. After incising the adjacent antimesenteric borders and suturing these common walls together, the remaining ileal defect would be approximated in a transverse manner. This would constitute a capacious, low-pressure aperistaltic reservoir, which could be intubated on an interval basis, allowing the patient discretion over the time and setting of fecal evacuation. Theoretically, the patient would not require an external appliance or be subject to the additional difficulties inherent in conventional ileostomy management.

In the original Kock continent ileostomy, the efferent conduit was passed, obliquely, through the rectus abdominus muscle, based upon the theory that rectus muscular contractions would assist continence by occluding the conduit below skin level. This concept was flawed, however, and a significant number of patients experienced leakage between catheterizations.[8] Kock addressed this problem in 1972 by designing a one-way nipple valve, constructed by intussuscepting the efferent conduit, retrograde, into the reservoir.[15] Through a significant improvement in reservoir continence, the nipple valve has become the technical essense of this procedure. Unfortunately, it also constitutes its greatest vulnerability, with complications related to nipple valve failure constituting the most common indications for the relatively frequent reoperation rate after construction of the Kock pouch.[16] Despite effective efforts in valve stabilization, attention has broadly turned away from this procedure.

Today, variations of the ileoanal anastomotic procedure,[17–19] offering a more physiologic mode of fecal evacuation as well as freedom from an ostomy, are most prevalently requested by and offered to patients with ulcerative colitis and familial adenomatous polyposis. Although the indications for the continent ileostomy have largely been supplanted by the ileoanal procedures, there remains a subset of patients for whom the Kock pouch provides the most appropriate alternative. Surgeons treating patients with these diseases must maintain facility with patient selection criteria and techniques relevant to continent ileostomy construction.

■ PATIENT SELECTION

The indications for continent ileostomy are least controversial for patients who have already undergone total proctocolectomy with end ileostomy. These patients, who have suffered anatomic loss of the anal sphincter apparatus, usually seek the Kock pouch as a means to improve their lifestyle.[2] Similarly, patients who will require total proctocolectomy in the near future, usually for ulcerative colitis or familial adenomatous polyposis, but who are not candidates for an ileoanal reservoir, may best retain continence in this manner. Examples are patients with poor anal sphincter function, secondary to neurogenic disease or previous surgery, patients with a history of severe perianal suppurative or fistulous disease, and those with low rectal cancer.[20] Some patients opt for the continent ileostomy because their employment or leisure activities preclude frequent access to lavatory facilities.[21] Additionally, the continent ileostomy has provided an alternative for patients who have experienced failure of a previous ileoanal reservoir anastomosis. In these situations, the former pelvic reservoir may be used in the construction of a Kock pouch, adding a nipple valve through intussusception of the immediately afferent ileum.[22] There is a very unique indication in the pediatric population for patients with Hirschsprung's disease, when attempts at surgical reconstruction have failed.[23]

Patients who suffer severe acute complications of their colonic disease (such as toxic megacolon or massive hemorrhage), who require emergent colectomy, should not be offered the continent ileostomy as a primary procedure. It would be performed best in a staged fashion subsequent to physiologic stabilization, after the specific pathology is histologically confirmed and following a full discussion with the patient of their therapeutic options.[2]

Patients with Crohn's disease generally are not considered candidates for this procedure. These patients are at high risk for recurrent disease, either in the reservoir or proximally. Should the Kock pouch fail, these patients could potentially lose enough functional small intestine to develop short bowel syndrome.[24] Similarly, patients who have previously undergone significant small bowel resections also should be excluded from eligibility for this procedure. Bloom and associates have retrospectively identified, within a larger group of indeterminate colitis patients, a subpopulation of patients with Crohn's disease who were not receiving systemic steroids at the time of surgery or who had been asymptomatic for five years before continent ileostomy construction.[25] Although the outcome for this small group of patients was similar to that of other patients who had previously received a Kock pouch, such a population is difficult to identify prospectively and thus does not justify altering the accepted contraindications to this procedure.

Older age is considered a contraindication to continent ileostomy construction. Dozois and associates determined a 50% required revision rate, within 6 months, for patients more than 50 years of age who underwent this operation. Additionally, it is the older population that is most likely to harbor coincident medical conditions which would render them intolerant of multiple operations. Obese patients see a higher incidence of nipple valve failures, thus constituting another contraindication with respect to the continent ileostomy.[27]

Patients who lack the cognitive, visual, or motor capacities to reliably perform interval self-catheterization or to recognize the signs of pouch complications should not be offered this procedure. Moreover, the best candidates for this procedure have an emotional constitution that allows them to accept these potential complications and any necessary surgical revisions that might ensue without undue psychologic strain.[2]

■ PREOPERATIVE PREPARATION

Preoperative preparation properly begins with patient education and full informed consent. The patient should understand the relative risks and benefits of all procedures for which he or she is a candidate, including the simpler Brooke ileostomy (Table 45–1). With the assistance of their surgeon, an enterostomal therapist and, ideally, a volunteer patient with a functioning Kock pouch, the patient should develop an appreciation for the appearance, physiology, potential complications, daily management, and lifestyle impact of the continent ileostomy.

The demands with respect to stoma marking are less rigid than for a conventional end ileostomy. The stoma usually is situated inferiorly and more medially than the standard ileal stoma, still within the borders of the rectus sheath, but immediately above the pubic escutcheon.[28] This location provides better cosmesis. The patient receives a standard mechanical and antibiotic bowel preparation. Broad-spectrum preoperative antibiotics are infused. Patients who have recently been

TABLE 45–1. ALTERNATIVES TO CONVENTIONAL ILEOSTOMY

Procedure	Conventional Ileostomy	Continent Ileostomy	Ileoanal Anastomosis
Advantages and Disadvantages			
Stoma	Yes (protruding)	Yes (flush)	No
Continence	No	Yes	Yes[a]
Bag	Yes	No	No
Diarrhea	Rare	Rare[b]	
Drugs	No	No	Yes[c]
Reoperation Rate (%)	5–14	22	?

[a]Nocturnal incontinence common; [b]Average intubations: 2 to 4 per day; [c]First 6 to 12 months.

maintained with corticosteroids, at risk for perioperative adrenal insufficiency, receive augmented perioperative dosing but may anticipate rapid corticosteroid weaning postoperatively.

■ OPERATIVE TECHNIQUE

The procedure is performed under general endotracheal anesthesia, in the supine position, through a midline celiotomy. A mechanical retractor enhances operative exposure. Adjunct procedures, such as total proctocolectomy or ileostomy takedown are performed first, if indicated. The meticulous preservation of ileal length and of the vascular arcades perfusing the terminal ileum constitutes a high priority at all stages of this operation.[21]

The terminal 45 cms of the ileum are used to construct the continent ileostomy. The first temporal sequence of the procedure involves the fashioning of an ileal reservoir from the more proximal 30 cm of this segment. As classically described, two 15-cm lengths of afferent terminal ileum are folded into approximation, assuming the configuration of the letter U (Fig 45–1).[29] These limbs then may be affixed, adjacent to their antimesenteric borders, with continuous 3-0 absorbable sutures.[21] The antimesenteric aspect of each adjacent limb is incised with an electrocautery in a continuous manner. The incision in the more proximal of the two limbs extends approximately 2 cm longer than that of the more distal limb, in order to correct any subsequent tendency towards kinking, as the two limbs are further approximated (Fig 45–2).[30] The posterior wall of the reservoir then is completed by affixing the full thickness of the adjacent, antimesenteric ileal borders with a continuous 2-0 absorbable seromucosal suture. The reservoir should be oriented with the ileal terminus posi-

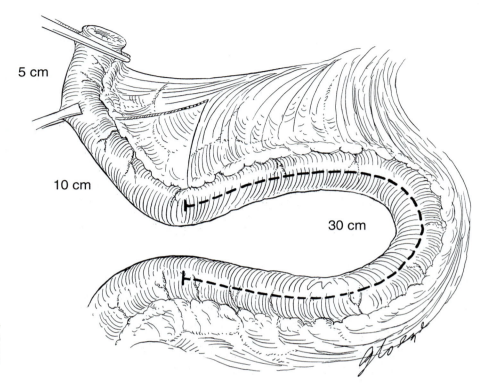

Figure 45–1. The terminal 45 cm of the ileum is configured to create a distalmost exit conduit (5 cm), an intermediate intussusception-valve segment (10 cm) and a proximal reservoir, constructed from two 15 cm segments.

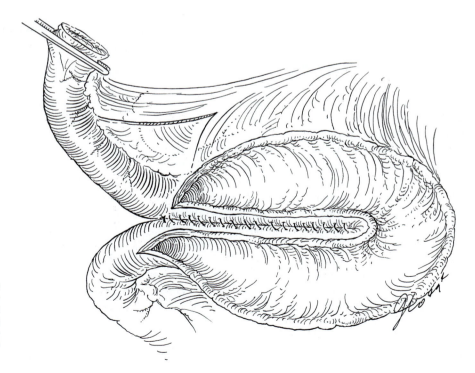

Figure 45–2. The reservoir is created by affixing the two constituent ileal limbs at their antimesenteric borders before incising the antimesenteric aspect of each limb in a longitudinal fashion. Note the different length of these incisions as well as the denuded, visceral peritoneum at the mesentery supplying the intussusception-valve segment.

tioned craniad and the curve of the "U" towards the patient's left side.[30]

Attention then is turned towards the creation of the continent nipple valve and exit conduit from the terminal 15 cm of ileum. The proximal 10 cm of this segment are used to construct the valve. The mesentery supplying this ileal segment is denuded of visceral peritoneum and adipose, in a triangular configuration, with care to preserve the ileal vascular arcades.[30] This maneuver effectively reduces mesenteric bulk in an effort to later assure the positional integrity of the valve. This is augmented through the use of electrocautery to scarify the serosa of the valve segment, in order to induce firm adhesions between the valve components following its establishment.[28] A one-way nipple then is created by the insertion of a Babcock clamp, through the open lumen of the reservoir into the efferent limb. The full thickness of the ileal wall is grasped from its mucosal aspect, 5 cm distally, and gently reduced, retrograde, into the lumen of the future reservoir, thus achieving intussusception.[31] This technique additionally assures the optimum valve length of 5 cm, retaining a 5-cm exit conduit. Interrupted 3-0 nonabsorbable sutures are placed through the full thickness of the valve walls, in order to enhance the maintenance of intussusception (Fig 45–3). Further positional stabilization of the valve is achieved within the reservoir lumen through three applications of a noncutting (bariatric) linear stapling instrument across the full thickness of the valve, with one stapled row on either side of the ileal mesentery.[28] Great care is taken in both of these maneuvers not to incorporate the mesenteric vascular supply. Additional fixation is achieved by the placement of multiple 2-0 absorbable seromuscular sutures between the fundus of the reservoir and the efferent conduit site at its exit point from the pouch (Fig 45–4).[28]

The anterior wall of the reservoir is completed by approximating the curved apex of the U shaped ileal configuration to the pouch wall, adjacent to the base of the valve. These are sutured in continuous inverting fashion, using the same 2-0 absorbable suture initially used to create the posterior wall (Fig 45–5). Following this, the earlike lateral corners of the reservoir are pushed downwards to lay between the adjacent mesenteric leaves.[29] This rotates the posterior aspect of the reservoir anteriorly and give it a globular shape (Fig 45–6).

A 28-Fr ileostomy catheter then is inserted through the exit conduit and valve into the reservoir. Ease of intubation must be insured. The reservoir is filled with air, through the catheter, which then is removed temporarily. It should remain completely inflated, assuring nipple valve competence and suture line integrity.[24] The reservoir then is emptied via the catheter.

The stomal orifice is created at the previously marked site on the anterior abdominal wall. A 2-cm diameter disk of skin is excised, along with a limited quantity of subcutaneous fat. The anterior rectus sheath is incised in a cruciate manner, exposing the rectus musculature, which then is bluntly distracted, parallel to its fibers. The exposed parietal peritoneum is incised sharply. The ileal stomal orifice then is dilated digitally, to the point at which it easily admits two of the surgeon's fingers.

Multiple anchoring sutures of 2-0 nonabsorbable material are placed circumferentially between the fundus of the pouch and the musculofascial elements of the stomal orifice (Fig 45–6).[30] The exist conduit is brought through the stomal orifice and the reservoir properly seated within the abdomen before the anchoring su-

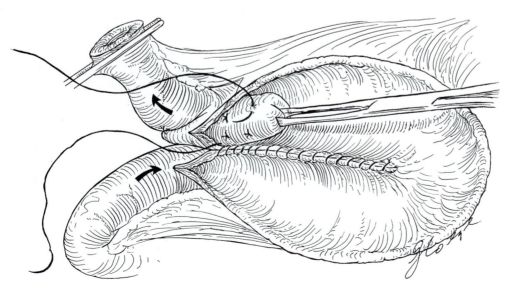

Figure 45–3. The posterior wall of the reservoir has been completed by suturing together the approximated walls of the constituent ileal segments. The nipple-valve segment is intussuscepted into the ileal reservoir and initially stabilized with full-thickness sutures. Positioning of the exit conduit has been established.

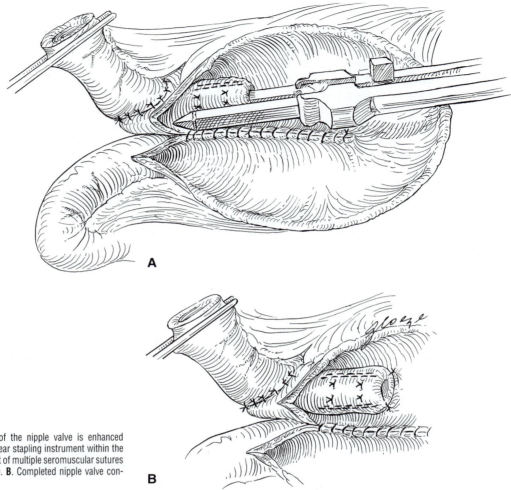

Figure 45–4. A. Positional stabilization of the nipple valve is enhanced through three applications of a bariatric linear stapling instrument within the reservoir lumen, as well as by the placement of multiple seromuscular sutures where the efferent conduit exits the pouch. **B.** Completed nipple valve construction and stabilization.

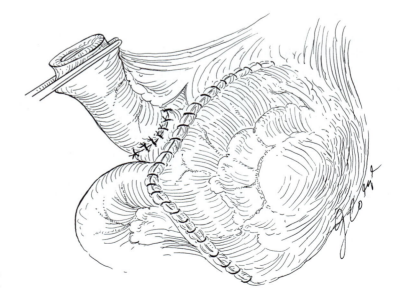

Figure 45–5. The anterior wall of the reservoir is completed by suture, approximating the apex of the U shaped ileal configuration to the pouch wall, adjacent to the base of the valve.

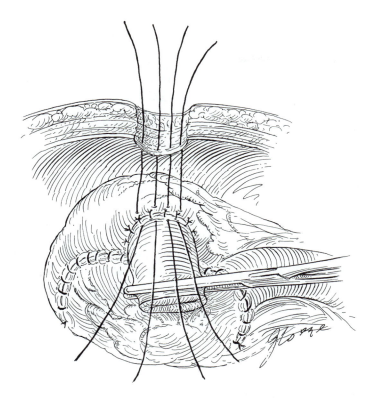

Figure 45–6. The lateral corners of the reservoir are pushed downwards to lie between the mesenteric leaves, rotating the posterior aspect of the reservoir anteriorly and conferring a globular shape. Seromuscular to myofascial approximation of the pouch to the margins of the stomal aperture is initiated with interrupted sutures.

susception in order to promote fibrotic stabilization of the nipple valve.[21,33] The use of prosthetic collars in continent ileostomy construction has been largely abandoned because of the significant incidence of mesh erosion and pouch fistulization.[20] Fazio and Tjandra have sought to further stabilize the nipple valve by stapling its antimesenteric aspect to the anterior wall of the reservoir with a noncutting stapler.[34] This is introduced through a limited enterotomy in the anterior wall of the pouch, immediately proximal to the valve site.

Barnett has developed a continent ileostomy that combines an isoperistaltic nipple valve, created from the ileum immediately afferent to the reservoir, and an intestinal collar.[35] This collar is constructed from the most distal ileum and designed to wrap around the exit conduit, much like the fascial sling. Theoretically, an isoperistaltic nipple valve follows the direction of naturally-occurring ileal intussusceptions. Thus, in this case, peristaltic forces exist which resist valve extrusion. The intestinal collar maintains continuity with the lumen of the reservoir. Pressure increases within the reservoir, which occur during progressive filling, are transmitted to the collar which, when wrapped around the exit conduit, exerts extrinsic closing pressure about it. This additional mechanism for reservoir continence is similar

tures are tied. Whenever possible, the ileal mesenteric edge is affixed to the adjacent parietal peritoneum with interrupted 3-0 nonabsorbable sutures, in order to obliterate any lateral potential space. Excess ileum, projecting above the peristomal skin level, is excised. The flush ileostomy then is matured by suturing the full thickness of the ileum to the stomal dermis with 3-0 absorbable sutures in interrupted fashion. The ileostomy catheter is replaced within the reservoir and secured to the peristomal skin with sutures (Fig 45–7). The celiotomy wound is then closed and dressed in the usual manner.

A number of technical modifications subsequently have been introduced to continent ileostomy construction, mainly to address the most vulnerable point within its design, the loss of nipple valve competence, usually through dessusception. Bokey and Fazio mobilized adjacent abdominal wall fascia, placing a single strip through the ileal mesentery, adjacent to the egress point of the exit conduit from the fundus of the pouch.[32] This "mesenteric sling" was designed to stabilize the nipple valve at the point where it is most likely to initiate extrusion. Others have used prosthetic mesh in a similar manner, or have wrapped it around the point of ileal intus-

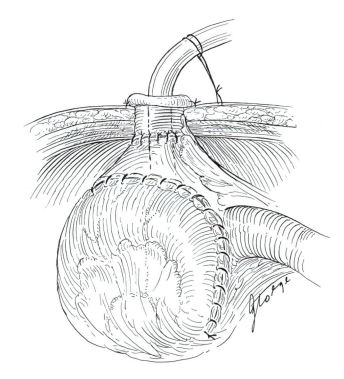

Figure 45–7. Completed continent ileostomy construction. A 28-Fr ileostomy catheter decompresses the pouch lumen. Anterior myofascial pouch approximation has been fully achieved. The exit conduit has been brought through the stomal aperture and sutured to the peristomal skin with full-thickness interrupted sutures.

to the pinchcock mechanism which supports the success of the Nissen fundoplication. A resultant salutory effect upon the incidence of required reoperation has been claimed in Barnett's series, albeit with limited follow-up.[35]

Others have sought to completely redesign the valve mechanism. Orangio and associates have adapted a mucosal valve to the continent ileostomy, which is not dependent upon intussusception to maintain its functional integrity.[36] Immediately distal to the reservoir, the efferent ileal seromuscular layer is stripped for 50% of its antimesenteric circumference, exposing an area of submucosa. After the modified efferent limb is sutured to the afferent limb (proximal to the reservoir), its mucosa invaginates into its lumen, thus occluding the exit conduit. As the reservoir fills and the afferent limb distends, it further transmits the increased intraluminal pressure, extrinsically, to the more compliant exit conduit, further enhancing continence. This valve mechanism, although elegantly demonstrated in an animal model, has not yet been adopted for clinical use.

■ POSTOPERATIVE CARE

In the immediate postoperative period, the patient receives parenteral fluid therapy as well as all other components of standard postceliotomy care. The ileostomy catheter is maintained to gravity drainage and is irrigated three times daily with 30 mL of normal saline, to prevent its obstruction by blood and ileal debris. The ileal stoma is frequently evaluated in the early postoperative period for signs of ischemia. The passage of small bowel effluent through the catheter indicates resolution of the postoperative ileus and oral intake is advanced as tolerated. Diets including undigestable residue, such as nuts and fibrous vegetables, should be avoided to prevent their interference with catheter drainage.[21] Continuous gravity drainage, with frequent irrigation, is maintained for 1 week, allowing the suture lines of the adequately decompressed reservoir and valve to heal without interference.

At 1 week, intermittent occlusion of the catheter ensues for 2 hour periods during the day. Continuous gravity drainage is reinstituted at night. After 2 weeks, the occlusion schedule is advanced to every 3 hours. Each subsequent week, the occlusion interval is advanced by 1 hour until the patient is able to tolerate ileostomy catheter clamping for 8 hour periods. The catheter then is removed. This schedule promotes the gradual expansion of reservoir capacity so that eventually an average of 3 to 4 daily catheterizations are required.[29] Between catheterizations, the patient wears a light gauze dressing over the stoma. The patient should maintain access to an ileostomy catheter at all times.

Patients are encouraged to irrigate the reservoir daily if the ileal effluent is particularly thick. Especially during the first 6 postoperative months, patients are warned to avoid abdominal straining or pushing, in attempts to hasten reservoir emptying.[21] With demonstrated good reservoir function eventually, patients usually will tolerate the limited reintroduction of fiber back into their diet. Interval outpatient follow-up is provided at 2 weeks, 1 month, and every 3 months thereafter, for the first postoperative year, followed by yearly visits thereafter. This is important in the monitoring of continent ileostomy function and its effect upon the well being of the patient, in addition to the early identification of complications.

ENTERIC MORPHOLOGIC, HISTOLOGIC, PHYSIOLOGIC AND BACTERIOLOGIC ALTERATIONS ASSOCIATED WITH THE CONTINENT ILEOSTOMY

The average capacity of a newly constructed Kock pouch approximates 50 mL.[37] These reservoirs undergo dilation during the ensuing months, initially stimulated by scheduled advancements in the interval of time between emptying and later, by the daily physiologic requirements of the individual patient. With time, the reservoir achieves an average capacity of approximately 670 mL,[38] ranging between approximately 500 to 1000 mL.[37] It has been demonstrated that patients averaging larger daily outputs of ileal effluent tend to increase the capacitance of their reservoir rather than to require more frequent catheterizations.

Brevinge and associates have demonstrated that the daily output of gas and feces from a continent ileostomy does not differ significantly from that of a conventional ileostomy. Accordingly, it has been shown that the absorptive capabilities of the Kock pouch, with respect to sodium, chloride and water, are similar to those of normal ileum.[39] Thus, no greater burden is placed upon tendencies of the ileostomate towards dehydration. The physiologic functions of the continent ileostomy are otherwise similar to those of the normal ileum, with respect to bicarbonate secretion and the absorptions of vitamin B_{12} and bile acids.[39,40] The Kock pouch, therefore, does not increase the risks of cholelithiasis, urolithiasis, or macrocytic anemia over those incurred by the patient with a Brooke ileostomy.[41]

Motility studies of the continent ileostomy reservoir demonstrate phasic alterations in contractility and pressure that are minimal when the pouch is empty, increasing in amplitude with progressive filling.[39] Stimulated by this higher range of intrapouch pressures is an afferent neural impulse mediating conscious sensation of the need to empty the pouch. In the average individual, this occurs approximately three times on a daily basis. Some patients, however, are required to catheterize their pouch only once daily, contrasting with others who range up to 17 daily evacuations.[40] Myenteric contractions within the Kock pouch progress sequentially from the base towards the fundus of the reservoir, finally terminating through the nipple valve. A high-pressure zone is maintained by phasic contractions within the nipple valve, both at rest and during active pouch contractions. Increases in pouch contractility and intraluminal pressure during incremental filling stimulate motility within the nipple valve, maintaining a gradient of pressure between the valve and reservoir that enhances continence.[42]

In time, the quality and quantity of bacterial colonization within the Kock pouch, approximates that within the normal colon.[43] Histologic studies upon ileal reservoir mucosa, in comparison to that of normal ileum, reveal an attenuation in villus height, associated with an increased crypt cell density and mucosal volume. There is no tendency towards atrophy or dysplasia.[44] A mild chronic inflammatory infiltrate may be manifest within the lamina propria; however, this does not correlate with pouch dysfunction.[43]

COMPLICATIONS OF THE CONTINENT ILEOSTOMY AND THEIR MANAGEMENT

The specific operative mortality associated with the construction of a continent ileostomy is very low.[15] The complication rate is significant, however, secondary to its technical complexity and has been considered by many to limit the overall efficacy of this procedure.[5,16,24] The incidence of these complications has declined through constructional modifications and the extensive experience of those surgeons who have sustained great interest in the procedure.

Dozois and associates compared the outcomes of patients in the early Mayo Clinic experience with patients who later benefited from modifications in patient selection, nipple valve length, mode of valve stabilization, and postoperative management. The requirement of reoperation and pouch revision descended from 43% to 22%. Complete long-term continence rose from 60% to 75%. The need for pouch excision fell from 10% to 3%. Fazio and Church were able to decrease their first year reoperation rate to 6.5% and increase the long-term continence rate to 91%.[20] Kock's own series reflects these improvements.[41]

Because the creation of a continent ileostomy involves significant intraperitoneal dissection, this procedure shares a subset of potential complications in common with other intra-abdominal, gastrointestinal operations. No relative increase is noted, with respect to the Kock pouch, in the incidence of complications such as bowel obstruction, wound and intra-abdominal sepsis, or postoperative hemorrhage.[20] However, there are

a number of both early and late complications that are unique to the procedure, requiring particular surveillance and therapy.

The specific, early postoperative complications include intraluminal hemorrhage, pouch leakage, with sepsis or fistulization, and necrosis of the exit conduit and valve.[21] Hemorrhage within the pouch lumen may occur during the first week after surgery and is usually related to its recent suture lines. Hemodynamically compromised patients may require emergent pouch exploration or excision. In others, the cessation of intraluminal hemorrhage may be achieved through gentle, frequent saline irrigation to remove old blood and promote spontaneous hemostasis. Adding norepinephrine to the irrigant may improve its efficacy. Systemic vasopressin has been successfully used in difficult cases. Endoscopic diagnosis or treatment in such circumstances is discouraged because of the risk of pouch perforation.[21]

Perforation of the reservoir, secondary to suture line dehiscence, has been reported at an incidence of approximately 1% to 4% in large patient series.[20,46] Early, postoperative leakage often is localized poorly and may manifest as generalized peritonitis, requiring reexploration for repair, diversion, or excision of the reservoir. Suture line leakage, occurring after two postoperative weeks, is more likely to result in a peripouch abscess or controlled pouch-cutaneous fistula,[21] amenable to nonoperative therapy. Peripouch sepsis may require systemic antibiotics, percutaneous abscess drainage, and defunctionalization of the reservoir by continuous catheter drainage.

Fistulas, both internal and external, occur with an incidence of 1% to 7%.[20] Pouch cutaneous or external fistulas often arise from suture line confluences, near the base of the nipple valve, the exit conduit, or the afferent ileum.[20] They may occur secondary to technical complications, such as a localized tissue ischemia related to necrosis by sutures or staples. The use of prosthetic mesh in pouch construction and the previously unrecognized presence of Crohn's disease are additional known etiologies.[20] External fistulas may be manifest within the first postoperative weeks or occur late, depending on their source.

They may be heralded by peristomal inflammation, which resolves spontaneously or, on incision and drainage, as a fistula.[21] Treatment for controlled fistulas is as noted above for delayed suture line dehiscence, with the addition of local skin care measures, including pouching. Failure of resolution after 6 weeks, or the presence of Crohn's disease, may mandate reservoir excision with conversion to an end ileostomy, although certain non-Crohn's related fistulas may be amenable to direct repair.[20] Pouch-nipple valve or internal fistulas share similarities in etiology and treatment with external fistulas but manifest as either frank incontinence or by the leakage of ileal effluent around the catheter during drainage maneuvers.[20,21] Nonhealing may dictate valve excision with pouch rotation.[20,47] Direct repair is rarely successful and associated prosthetic mesh should be excised.

Similar to end ileostomies, the continent ileostomy may manifest ischemia, secondary to failure in attempted preservation of the ileal vascular arcades during pouch construction, or by mesenteric compression during nipple valve creation and stabilization maneuvers. This may present in the initial postoperative period with typical dark stomal discoloration, mucosal friability, and bleeding.[21] Pain and constitutional symptoms may herald extension below the fascial level, for which close surveillance is necessary to avoid perforation and peritonitis. Chronic ischemia is variously manifested and treated. Stenosis and stricturing of the exit conduit and stoma may present as difficulty in intubation.[47] Separation and retraction of the ileal stoma may be readily visible.[21] Continuous catheter drainage, local skin protection, and antibiotics will assist patient function and speed the resolution of peristomal inflammation. After the stabilization of this process, stomal revision by scar excision, Z-plasty or local skin flap rotation may be necessary only if patients are unable to insert an ileostomy catheter through the stenotic area.[47]

Nipple valve necrosis is a manifestation of local ischemia, usually an untoward result of attempts at valve stabilization with transfixing sutures or staples.[20,45] Reported in approximately 2% of patients[20,46] this complication may be announced by the drainage of necrotic or sanguinous material and sutures or staples from the Kock pouch, followed by the onset of incontinence secondary to valve shortening.[21] This eventually may result in the need for revision, which may be accomplished through pouch rotation.

In the pouch rotation procedure,[15,21] initiated via celiotomy, the stoma, exit conduit and reservoir are dissected from the anterior abdominal wall. The nipple valve and exit conduit then are excised. The ileum, directly afferent to the pouch, is divided 15 cm proximally and used as a new nipple valve and exit conduit, after isoperistaltic intussusception and stabilization by standard means. The reservoir then is rotated and a new anastomosis created between it and the neoterminal ileum. Pouch fixation and stomal maturation then proceed in the previously described manner.

Valve extrusion, secondary to dessusception, is the most common late complication following continent ileostomy construction. The incidence of revisional surgery related to this problem is highest in postoperative year 1, gradually declining and becoming uncommon after year 3.[41,46] This is exemplified in the series of Sjodahl and associates in which the comparative valve revision rates for postoperative years 1 and 3 were 16%

and 5%, respectfully.[46] As noted previously, the majority of technical modifications that have been applied to Kock pouch construction throughout the history of the procedure have sought to address this specific complication.

The etiology of nipple valve extrusion has been attributed to peristaltic activity within the continent ileostomy[42] and to the intermittent development of high intrapouch pressures, secondary to coughing, abdominal wall straining,[21] or pouch distention by overfilling. The process usually is initiated at the mesenteric aspect of the nipple valve, with the antimesenteric walls, early on, remaining stationary. This "unrolling" of the valve commences in its acute angulation, with respect to the reservoir.[21] Clinically, this is manifest by difficulty in intubation and partial incontinence. The total inability to intubate the pouch may result in complete small bowel obstruction, necessitating endoscopically directed catheterization, with a rigid pediatric proctoscope, on an urgent basis.[48] Complete nipple valve dessusception results in frank incontinence.[20]

Confirmation of nipple valve extrusion can be made endoscopically or through contrast radiography.[15,49] Initial treatment is by continuous intubation, which both prevents the sequelae of small bowel obstruction and stents the valve. Stenting, over several weeks, maintains the nipple valve in a position of function, where, hopefully, it will heal. Failure of such management necessitates surgical revision. This commonly involves valve reintussusception and stabilization or valve excision and pouch rotation. Both of these approaches require abdominal reexploration and pouch mobilization. Thompson and Williams have modified the latter technique, using the original valve-exit conduit segment as an intestinal collar to stabilize the new nipple valve, created from afferent ileum, in the fashion of Barnett.[50]

Stomal prolapse is an uncommon complication, presenting in a similar manner to that occurring in association with end stomas. It usually is ascribed to a fascial orifice that is too large[15] but sustained increases to intra-abdominal pressure, such as during late pregnancy[47], may also contribute to a stomal prolapse. Continuous intubation may be required in such temporary situations.[51] Operative correction of prolapse ranges from local plasty of the fascial orifice to stomal relocation.[21] Gottlieb and Handelsman describe a technique for "stiffening" of the exit conduit, using scarification of the mucocutaneous junction with an electrocautery and the use of reefing sutures within the lumen of the stoma.[47]

Pouch ileitis is an episodic, often recurrent mucosal inflammatory condition that specifically is associated with ileal reservoir procedures. The reported incidence, ranging from 7% to 43% in the literature, credits its variability to the number of definitions that are held for this condition.[52] The etiology of pouchitis has popularly been ascribed to the overgrowth of anaerobic bacteria within the pouch lumen. This is because of the known therapeutic response to antibiotics. Alternatively theorized are mucosal alterations related to other idiopathic inflammatory bowel diseases.[52,53] Neither of these mechanisms has been consistently supported by bacteriologic or histologic studies.[43,52] It is remarkable that the syndrome is much more frequent in those patients with a history of ulcerative colitis.[21,52,53]

The clinical features of pouchitis include fevers, colicky abdominal pain, and high volume (1000 mL/day), occasionally hemorrhagic, ileostomy drainage. Extraintestinal manifestations, such as malaise, dermatitis, and arthralgias, may ensue.[53] In patients who present with this syndrome for the first time, mimicking conditions such as infectious enteritis, Crohn's disease, and mechanical pouch dysfunction should be ruled out by appropriate cultures, ileoscopy, and mucosal biopsies.[21,49] Fiberoptic ileoscopic findings such as mucosal erythema, edema, friability, and ulceration are variable; however, the absence of ulcerations has been correlated with an improved response to treatment.[52] The mainstay of therapy for this condition is oral metronidazole. Other antibiotic agents also have proven efficacious. More recalcitrant cases may require the addition of sulfasalazine or corticosteroid therapy.[52] On rare occasions, pouch ileitis is so recurrent and severe as to mandate excision of the continent ileostomy.[15]

The occurrence of tubulovillous adenomata in the continent ileostomy of a patient with documented Gardner's syndrome has been described.[54] This has prompted the recommendation for careful clinical and endoscopic surveillance of Kock pouches in patients who have a history of familial polyposis. Pouch excision is considered appropriate if adenomas are subsequently discovered.[54]

■ FUNCTIONAL OUTCOME AND PATIENT SATISFACTION

In testimony to the success of the continent ileostomy, when properly selected and executed, retrospective patient surveys have revealed high rates of general lifestyle satisfaction.[41,55,56] McLeod and associates found that all of their patients would choose retrospectively to undergo the procedure and that 97% would submit to revisional surgery, rather than return to a Brooke ileostomy.[55] These lifestyle improvements have been reflected, mainly, in employment activities, sports and leisure activities, travel, clothing selection,[41,46,55,56] and sexual function.[51] Normal pregnancy and successful vaginal delivery should be expected following continent ileostomy construction, with an acceptable incidence of temporary pouch dysfunction and few requirements for revisional surgery.[57]

Definite indications remain for the continent ileostomy, among well-selected patients who have undergone total proctocolectomy. The successful candidate must be mature, well-informed, highly motivated, and able to accept the risk of postoperative complications. Surgeons with a special interest in the treatment of colorectal disease should maintain the continent ileostomy in their armamentarium. Skills in candidate selection, patient preparation, and technical execution, with respect to this procedure, should be fostered. A thorough knowledge of potential postoperative complications and their treatment, as well as the willingness to provide follow-up adequate to assure their prompt recognition, is requisite. Through this proper combination of patient and surgeon cooperation, a gratifying outcome can result, insuring a complete and satisfying recovery from what was once a chronically debilitating or potentially life-threatening disease.

REFERENCES

1. Brooke BN. Management of ileostomy including its complications. *Lancet* 1952;2:102
2. Dozois RR, O'Rourke JS. New operations for ulcerative colitis and Crohn's disease. *Surg Clin North Am* 1988; 68:1339
3. Roy PH, Sauer WG, Beahrs OH, et al. Experience with ileostomies: evaluation of long-term rehabilitation in 497 patients. *Am J Surg* 1970;119:77
4. Watts J McK, DeDombal FT, Goligher JC. Long-term complications and prognosis following major surgery for ulcerative colitis. *Br J Surg* 1966;53:1014
5. Sackier JM, Wood CB. Ulcerative colitis and polyposis coli: surgical options. *Surg Clin North Am* 1988;68:1319
6. Hager J, Schellerer M. Botticher D, et al. The Erlangen magnetic closure system for colostomies and ileostomies. Sixth International Meeting of the Society of University Colon and Rectal Surgeons, Salzburg, Austria, 1976.
7. Pemberton JH, Van Heerden JA, Beart RW, et al. A continent ileostomy device. *Ann Surg* 1983;197:618
8. Mcleod RS. Chronic ulcerative colitis: traditional surgical techniques. *Surg Clin North Am* 1993;73:891
9. Aylett SO. Diffuse chronic ulcerative colitis and its treatment by ileorectal anastomosis. *Ann R Coll Surg Engl* 1960; 27:260
10. Mowschenson PM. Inflammatory bowel disease, part I. new surgical approaches. *Sem Colon Rectal Surg* 1993;4:25
11. Hawley P. Ileorectal anastomosis. *Br J Surg* 1985;72:S75
12. Oakly Jr, Jagelman DG, Fazio VW. Complications and quality of life after ileorectal anastomosis for ulcerative colitis. *Am J Surg* 1985;149:23
13. Khubchandani IT. Ileorectal anastomosis for inflammatory bowel disease in 1993. *Perspect Colon Rectal Surg* 1993; 6:79
14. Kock NG. Intra-abdominal "reservoir" in patients with permanent ileostomy. *Arch Surg* 1969;99:223
15. Kock NG. Continent ileostomy. *Prog Surg* 1993;12:180

16. Goligher JC. Procedures conserving continence in the surgical management of ulcerative colitis. *Surg Clin North Am* 1983;63:49

17. Nissen R. Sitzuagsberichte aus chirugischen Gesell-schaften: Berlinger Gesellschaft für chirugie: *Sitzung 14 Zentralbl Chir* 1933;15:888

18. Ravitch MM, Sabiston DC. Anal ileostomy with preservation of the sphincter: a proposed operation in patients requiring total colectomy for benign lesions. *Surg Gynecol Obstet* 1947;84:1095

19. Martin LW, Lecoultre C, Schubert WK. Total colectomy and mucosal proctectomy with preservation of continence in ulcerative colitis. *Ann Surg* 1977;86:477

20. Fazio VW, Church JM. Complications and function of the continent ileostomy at the Cleveland Clinic. *World J Surg* 1988;12:148

21. Gorfine SR, Bauer JJ, Gelernt IM. Continent Stomas. In: MacKeigan JM, Cataldo PA (eds), *Intestinal Stomas: Principles, Techniques and Management.* St. Louis, MO: Quality Medical; 1993: 154–187

22. Kusunoki M, Sakanoue Y, et al. Conversion of malfunctioning J pouch to Kock's pouch. *Acta Chir Scand* 1990;156:179

23. Ein SH. A ten-year experience with the pediatric Kock pouch. *J Pediatric Surg* 1987;22:764

24. Schoetz DJ, Coller JA, Veidenheimer MC. Alternatives to conventional ileostomy in chronic ulcerative colitis. *Surg Clin North Am* 1985;65:21

25. Bloom RJ, Larsen CP, Watt R, Oberhelman HA. A reappraisal of the Kock continent ileostomy in patients with Crohn's disease. *Surg Gynecol Obstet* 1986;162:105

26. Dozois RR, Kelly KA, Illstrup D, et al. Factors affecting revision rate after continent ileostomy. *Arch Surg* 1981;116:610

27. Schrock TR. Complications of continent ileostomy. *Am J Surg* 1979;138:162

28. Beart RW. Ileostomy and its alternatives. In: Zeidema GD (ed), *Shackelford's Surgery of the Alimentary Tract,* 3rd ed. Philadelphia, PA: WB Saunders; 1991:172–178

29. Kock NG. Continent ileostomy. In: Nyhus LM, Baker RJ (eds), *Mastery of Surgery,* 2nd Ed. Boston, MA: Little, Brown; 1992:1176–1182

30. Nivatvongs S. Ulcerative colitis: operative options. In: Gordon PH, Nivatvongs S (eds), *Principles and Practice of Surgery for the Colon, Rectum and Anus.* St. Louis, MO: Quality Medical; 1992:688–904

31. Kodner IJ, Fleshman JW, Fry RD. Intestinal stomas. In: Schwartz SI, Ellis H (eds), *Maingot's Abdominal Operations,* 9th Ed., Stamford, CT: Appleton and Lange; 1990: 1164–1172

32. Bokey L, Fazio VW. The mesenteric sling technique: new method for constructing an intestinal nipple valve for continent ileostomy. *Clev Clin Q* 1978;45:231

33. Cohen Z. Evolution of the Kock continent reservoir ileostomy. *Can J Surg* 1982;25:509

34. Fazio VW, Tjandra JJ. Technique for nipple valve fixation to prevent valve slippage in continent ileostomy. *Dis Colon Rectum* 1992;35:1177

35. Barnett WO. Current experience with the continent intestinal reservoir. *Surg Gynecol Obstet* 1989;168:1

36. Orangio GR, Bronsther B, Abrams M, et al. A new type of continent ileostomy: results of an animal study. *Dis Colon Rectum* 1984;27:238

37. Beahrs OH. Present status of the continent ileostomy; ileal reservoir with ileostomy, rather than ileostomy alone. *Dis Colon Rectum* 1976;19:192

38. Brevinge H, Berglund B, Kock NG. Ileostomy output of gas and feces before and after conversion from conventional to reservoir ileostomy. *Dis Colon Rectum* 1992;35:662–669

39. Gadacz TR, Kelly KA, Phillips SF. The continent ileal pouch: absorptive and motor features. *Gastroenterology* 1977;72:1287

40. Jagenburg, Kock NG, Philipson B. Vitamin B_{12} absorption in patients with continent ileostomy. *Scand J Gastroenterol* 1975;10:141

41. Ojerskog B, Kock NG, Nilsson LO, et al. Long-term follow-up of patients with continent ileostomies. *Dis Colon Rectum* 1990;33:184

42. Nordgren S, Cohen Z, Greig PD, et al. Pressure studies on the continent reservoir ileostomy. *Surg Gynecol Obstet* 1982;155:646.

43. Kelly DG, Phillips SF, Kelly KA, et al. Dysfunction of the continent ileostomy: clinical features and bacteriology. *Gut* 1983;24:193

44. Nilsson LO, Kock NG, Lindgen I, et al. Morphological and histochemical changes in the mucosa of the continent ileostomy reservoir 6–10 years after its construction. *Scand J Gastroenterol* 1980;15:737

45. Dozois RR, Kelly KA, Beart RW, et al. Improved results with continent ileostomy. *Ann Surg* 1980;192:319

46. Sjodahl R, Lemon E, Nystrom P-E, et al. Complications, surgical revision and quality of life with conventional and continent ileostomy. *Acta Chir Scand* 1990;156:403

47. Gottlieb LM, Handelsman JC. Treatment of outflow tract problems associated with continent ileostomy (Kock pouch): report of six cases. *Dis Colon Rectum* 1991; 34:936

48. Tichenor GA, Orkin BA, Lavery IC. A technique for decompression of the obstructed Kock continent ileostomy. *Surg Gynecol Obstet* 1990;170:75

49. Church JM, Fazio VW, Lavery IC. The role of fiberoptic endoscopy in the management of continent ileostomy. *Gastrointest Endosc* 1987;33:203

50. Thompson JS, Williams SM. Technique for revision of continent ileostomy. *Dis Colon Rectum* 1992;35:87

51. Nilsson LO, Kock NG, Krylberg F, et al. Sexual adjustment in ileostomy patients before and after conversion to continent ileostomy. *Dis Colon Rectum* 1981;24:287

52. Zuccaro G, Fazio VW, Church JM, et al. Pouch ileitis. *Dig Dis Sci* 1989;34:1505

53. Madden MV, Farthing MJG, Nicholls RJ. Inflammation in ileal reservoirs: "pouchitis". *Gut* 1990;31:247

54. Beart RW, Fleming CR, Banks PM. Tubulovillous adenomas in a continent ileostomy after proctocolectomy for familial polyposis. *Dig Dis Sci* 1982;27:553

55. McLeod RS, Fazio VW. Quality of life with the continent ileostomy. *World J Surg* 1984;8:90

56. Kohler LW, Pemberton JH, Zinsmeister AR, et al. Quality of life after proctocolectomy: a comparison of Brooke ileostomy, Kock pouch and ileal pouch-anal anstomosis. *Gastroenterology* 1991;101:679

57. Ojerskog B, Kock NG, Philipson BM, et al. Pregnancy and delivery in patients with a continent ileostomy. *Surg Gynecol Obstet* 1988;167:61

46

Large Bowel Obstruction: Operative Procedures

Mika N. Sinanan   ▪   *Carlos A. Pellegrini*

Acute obstruction of the large bowel is an important cause of the surgical acute abdomen. Although the obstruction may be the result of mechanical, inflammatory, or neoplastic processes, diagnosis often is made and treatment initiated on clinical grounds with limited radiographic or other information. Nonoperative interventions are possible for some types of large bowel obstruction, but most eventually will require surgical treatment. At operation, options for treatment are dictated by the nature of the disease, patient status, and the experience of the operating surgeon. Traditional techniques of proximal diverting ileostomy or colostomy limit anesthesia and the risk of anastomotic disruption in the severely ill patient, but the morbidity associated with the ostomy and a second and perhaps third operation often can be safely avoided. Increasingly, definitive treatment, using one of several techniques to protect the new anastomosis, appears to be a reasonable alternative in healthier patients. Although an understanding of the physiological consequences of obstruction to the patient and to anastomotic wound healing may allow safer and more effective early intervention, colonic obstruction owing to cancer remains a grave prognostic sign.

▪ PHYSIOLOGICAL CONSEQUENCES OF COLONIC OBSTRUCTION

Colonic obstruction has both generalized systemic effects and important local effects on the obstructed bowel.

Depending on the competence of the ileocecal valve[1,2] and the location, degree, and chronicity of obstruction, a distally-obstructed colon also prevents normal small bowel function.[3] These effects on both large and small bowels eventually result in third-space fluid and electrolyte losses with hypovolemia,[4] bacterial overgrowth,[5] and malnutrition[6] that contribute to the morbidity of the condition and the risk of treatment. Obstruction in one part of the bowel also may have remote effects on motility[1,7] and blood flow[8] elsewhere in the gastrointestinal (GI) tract. In patients with chronic lung disease, progressive abdominal distention due to a colonic obstruction limits respiratory excursion and increases the difficulty of ventilation under anesthesia until the abdomen is opened. Correction of these problems is an important part of the early resuscitation of patients with large bowel obstruction and may provide the impetus for urgent operative treatment.

Local effects of obstruction on the colon also have become increasingly clear. Obstruction transforms the net normal absorption of the bowel to a secretory state[9,10] perhaps through the effects of bacterial products or other circulating factors,[11,12] although obstruction does not apparently increase luminal bacterial content.[13] As the degree of obstruction increases, colon motility becomes disordered, with an increased range of amplitudes,[14] the onset of nonperistaltic high-amplitude contractions,[15] and eventually, hypomotility that may persist for an extended period after relief of the obstruction.[14,16]

Experimental studies and clinical reports suggest that normal autoregulation of blood flow[17] also is disrupted in the colon above an obstruction. Acute obstruction of the colon has been associated with a high luminal pressure (>35 mm Hg[18]), in contrast to the small increases in luminal pressure found proximal to a small bowel obstruction.[19] Reasons for this difference between the large and small bowel include competence of the ileocecal valve[2] and the poor distensibility of the colon leading to a more rapid onset of a closed-loop obstruction. Under conditions of increased intraluminal pressure (>20 to 30 mm Hg), total colonic-wall blood flow is *decreased* and what flow persists is shunted away from the mucosa to the muscularis propria, compromising mucosal integrity.[20,21] Indeed, the effects of high luminal pressure added to an already injured, chronically obstructed segment of bowel may markedly potentiate the ischemic effects of obstruction.[22] In patients with prolonged obstruction and distention of the bowel, these effects may predispose to ulceration or ischemic perforation.[23–25] The combined effects of venous, or both arterial and venous, compromise and high luminal pressure on colon blood flow may accelerate development of a full-thickness necrosis within the strangulated bowel. Mucosal ulceration,[26] a necrotizing colitis,[24] stricture formation,[27] and the failure of anastomotic healing[28] in previously obstructed colon, presumably owing to the ischemic effects of a high luminal pressure, also have been reported.

In experiments designed to simulate a more gradual chronic obstruction of the colon, such as might occur with a distal cancer, blood flow to the obstructed segment has been shown to *increase*.[28,29] This correlates with the hyperemic inflamed appearance of the colon during operations for chronic obstructive lesions. Control of this vascular response has been variously attributed to autonomic reflexes[17] or bacterial products.[30] There is no evidence for direct bacterial invasion of the obstructed but viable colon wall.[31,32] Although the hyperemic response occurs largely in the muscular elements of the bowel wall rather than the mucosa,[28] these findings emphasize the importance of mechanical factors and the nature of the obstruction to blood flow in the colon wall. Thus, while the proximal bowel may be sufficiently healthy to consider primary anastomosis in patients treated for a distal, incomplete chronic obstruction, the only safe course is some form of fecal diversion in those patients who present with an acute obstruction, high luminal pressures, and ischemic injury of the proximal colon.

■ FACTORS THAT INFLUENCE HEALING IN COLONIC ANASTOMOSES

Basic principles of wound healing dating from Halsted require that anastomoses be constructed with proper technique that joins well-vascularized, apparently healthy bowel segments in a watertight fashion and without tension.[33,34] But even in anastomoses constructed according to these principles, clinically evident anastomotic dehiscence occurs in up to 11% of patients,[35] with a resulting mortality that may reach 4%.[36,37] Radiographic studies are more sensitive and indicate some degree of anastomotic disruption in up to 50% of patients,[36] regardless of the anastomotic technique employed.[38,39] To minimize the risk of this complication, a decision to proceed with immediate anastomosis in the emergency setting should be made only after careful consideration of all factors that might adversely affect anastomotic healing.

Patients with colonic obstruction are at increased risk for anastomotic disruption,[37,40] a risk that is influenced by several factors.[41,42] Local conditions about the healing wound are probably of greatest importance. These include perianastomotic infection due to perforation or gross fecal spillage and the condition of the bowel, especially with respect to ischemia, radiation change, or other secondary consequences of chronic obstruction.[33,43] Experimental and clinical studies suggest that healing in any surgical wound also may be impaired in patients with anemia, recent significant blood loss, or perioperative transfusion, malnutrition, and chronic steroid therapy.[33,35,44] Both local and systemic factors seem to influence outcome by altering collagen content and turnover in the healing wound.[45–47] The role of luminal bacterial count and fecal loading remains uncertain. Some studies suggest that the unprepared bowel increases anastomotic leaks[36,48] while others have found no effect[33] or emphasize the salutory role of bacteria and other luminal growth factors and nutrients on anastomotic healing.[32,43,49–52] In the individual patient, no ready formula for assessing multifactoral risk has been described. Nevertheless, the benefits of correcting systemic illness when possible, minimizing intraoperative contamination, and finding healthy bowel for anastomosis seem well justified. In addition, mechanical and antibiotic bowel preparation appear important enough in a number of clinical and experimental studies that, in the acute setting of colonic obstruction and a large fecal load, patients considered for primary anastomosis also should have measures taken to reduce the fecal load or otherwise protect the anastomosis.[43,53,54] Wide variations in surgeon-to-surgeon complications[55] emphasize the importance of surgical judgment and technical expertise in deciding which patients might be candidates for such anastomosis and in guiding the strategy and surgical technique employed.[56]

■ EPIDEMIOLOGY

Obstruction of the large bowel accounts for 6.3% of all intestinal obstruction.[57] The causes of colorectal obstruction are listed in Table 46–1, in order of decreasing incidence. Primary and occasionally, metastatic carcinoma are responsible for >90% of all large bowel obstruction,[58] yet only 10% to 30% of all colorectal carcinomas cause obstruction.[59,60] Other common causes of large bowel obstruction include volvulus (4% to 5%) and diverticulitis (3%).[61] Adhesions,[4] carcinomatosis,[62] pancreatitis,[63,64] endometriosis,[65,66] inflammatory bowel disease,[4] foreign bodies,[67] strictures from nonsteroidal medication,[68] and other benign strictures from various causes are rare, each making up <1% of the group. Diet and lifestyle have been shown to alter the distribution of lesions so that, in developing nations with a higher fiber diet, up to 50% of large bowel obstruction is the result of volvulus, while the incidence of cancer and diverticular diseases are proportionally decreased.[69,70]

TABLE 46–1. ETIOLOGIES OF LARGE BOWEL OBSTRUCTION[4,61]

Cancer
   Colon/rectal cancer
   Extraluminal, metastatic cancer (ie, ovarian cancer, breast cancer, etc.)
Volvulus
Diverticular disease with obstruction
Inflammatory bowel disease
Foreign body obturation (ie, impacted feces, gallstone, other)
Stricture (ie, radiation, anastomotic)
Adhesions
Hernia
Intussusception
Other
   Pancreatitis
   Abdominal aortic aneurysm
   Endometriosis

■ CLINICAL PRESENTATION

Large bowel obstruction from all causes appears to affect males and females with nearly equal frequency.[61] Most large bowel obstruction occurs in older people (mean age, 64 years), although the congenitally mobile cecum may predispose to cecal volvulus at any age.[61,71,72] Certainly, obstructing cancers occur more often in an older population. Sigmoid volvulus appears to be more common in institutional patients, those with a history of psychosis, and those with colonic dysmotility and chronic laxative use.[69,73] Acute symptoms and a prior history of volvulus strongly suggest recurrence of the volvulus, if prior treatment has consisted of detorsion alone.[74] A gradual change in bowel habits and progressive problems with constipation during weeks or months raise suspicion for benign or malignant strictures, while long-term relapsing symptoms are more commonly linked to recurrent volvulus, hernias, or inflammatory lesions. Prior laparotomy with adhesions, anastomosis in the colon, or pelvic irradiation each suggest a potential cause for the obstruction, but these and other clues derived from the history of the patient are rarely definitive. New colonic obstruction in the debilitated patient hospitalized for other reasons may indicate colonic pseudoobstruction, a diagnosis confirmed radiographically or endoscopically that usually responds to conservative measures.[75–77]

Clinical-pathological correlation suggests that the colon adapts remarkably well to chronically constricting lesions.[78] Not infrequently, a patient will have no or minimal symptoms despite marked luminal narrowing until compensatory mechanisms fail, usually at a critical luminal diameter of several millimeters.[3,79,80] The presentation of large bowel obstruction may, therefore, be subtle and the location and cause, even the fact of obstruction itself, may be obscure until radiographic, endoscopic, or surgical investigations are carried out. Nevertheless, large bowel obstruction remains a *clinical* diagnosis. Patients selected for retrospective inclusion in clinical studies of large bowel obstruction are, for the most part, only included because they meet *clinical criteria* of acute obstruction: pain, distention, obstipation, typical plain radiographic findings, and subsequently undergo emergency surgery.[61,81,82] Few prospective studies of large bowel obstruction are available (the *UK Large Bowel Cancer Project,* 1976 to 1980, is the best exception[59,82,83]) and there do not appear to be any recent studies that specifically correlate clinical presentation with the size or degree of luminal narrowing. Thus, data on the signs and symptoms of obstruction are influenced by the patient selection criteria employed in the literature.

Signs and symptoms of colorectal obstruction without concomitant perforation depend on the degree and

TABLE 46–2. CLINICAL PRESENTATION OF COMMON CAUSES FOR LARGE BOWEL OBSTRUCTION

	Cancer[3,59,84,195]	Volvulus[69,71,212] (%)	Diverticulitis[a]
SYMPTOMS			
Pain	81–85	67–100	97
Nausea/Vomiting	65	50–87	78
Hx of Constipation	35	43–66	80
Obstipation	47	**[b]	**[b]
Diarrhea	**[b]	24	52
SIGNS			
Abdominal Distention	69–80	80–100	**[b]
Abdominal Tenderness	44	70	100[c]
Fever	rare	11	78
Peritonitis	30	10–19	73

[a]Values based on all diverticulitis patients, not just those presenting with concomitant obstruction[216,221]
[b]Figures not available
[c]Tenderness is often focal rather than diffuse

acuity of the obstruction, whether the obstructing lesion is inflammatory in nature (ie, diverticulitis), and how the blood supply to the obstructed bowel is affected. Clinical findings for the most common causes of large bowel obstruction are listed in Table 46–2.

Essentially all patients with nonperforated large bowel obstruction have or, without treatment, will develop abdominal pain, constipation, and distention, perhaps after a period of diarrhea. Colicky pain derives from increased wall tension in the distended obstructed colon, while continuous progressive pain suggests the more serious problems of strangulation and ischemic injury. Distention may be the most prominent initial finding in patients with volvulus but untreated, pain and other signs of obstruction eventually become apparent. Fever is common, but not invariably present, in those with acute diverticulitis, perforation (which may occur either at the site of obstruction or more proximally in the cecum[3]), or in patients with ischemic injury to the proximal colon. Blood in the stool is worrisome for a mucosal process such as inflammatory bowel disease but is a rare finding in obstructing carcinoma of the colon.[84] In the appropriately ill patient, passage of blood may serve as further evidence for an ischemic injury to the colon, although the absence of blood does not exclude injured bowel above a complete obstruction.

In the 20% to 30% of obstructed cancer patients who present with perforation, the signs of peritonitis often obscure other findings and the obstruction may only become apparent at laparotomy.[59] A pattern of acute abdominal symptoms together with a history of constipation or obstipation and abdominal distention should alert the clinician to the possibility of large bowel obstruction and prompt, urgent evaluation and treatment.

■ DIAGNOSTIC STUDIES

Laboratory investigations in the patient with acute abdominal symptoms are designed to assess the extent of systemic illness, identify metabolic derangements that must be corrected, and support diagnostic efforts directed at the underlying illness.[4] Measurement of the serum electrolytes, serum amylase and bilirubin, and urinalysis help identify upper GI derangement, renal dysfunction, and the consequences of vomiting and third-space fluid losses. Significant anemia in the acutely hypovolemic patient should prompt investigation for active bleeding while microcytic changes often accompany chronic blood loss from an ulcerating lesion of the GI tract. Leukocytosis is an important indication of acute inflammation. As further investigation proceeds, initial steps at correcting these metabolic problems should be undertaken, especially if operative treatment is planned.

The goals of radiographic or endoscopic investigation in patients suspected of large bowel obstruction include (1) distinguishing psuedoobstruction or ileus from mechanical obstruction, (2) localizing the level or site of the obstruction, (3) establishing the cause of obstruction, and (4) determining if strangulation is present.[1,57,85] Radiographic contrast studies and endoscopy also may be therapeutic. Barium reduction of an intussusception and both endoscopic and contrast reductions of sigmoid and cecal volvulus have been described.[57,86] Radiographic and other studies useful in elucidating the causes of large bowel are listed in Table 46–3. Often, several studies complement each other and aid in the diagnosis or treatment of obstructive lesions.

The initial diagnostic study, in most patients, is an upright chest X-ray and a set of upright and supine radiographs of the abdomen. Characteristic findings of obstruction on abdominal radiographs include abnormal gas and fluid distending the proximal colon (>5 cm) to a fixed cutoff, distal to which no gas is visible.[87,88] Depending on ileocecal competence and the severity of obstruction, small bowel dilation and air-fluid levels may also be present.[89] Dilated loops of small bowel may

TABLE 46–3. DIAGNOSTIC STUDIES FOR LARGE BOWEL OBSTRUCTION

Abdominal radiograph (Supine)
Upright/decubitus abdominal radiograph
Chest radiograph (upright)
Contrast enema (barium or water soluble agent)
Small bowel contrast study
CT scan
Endoscopy

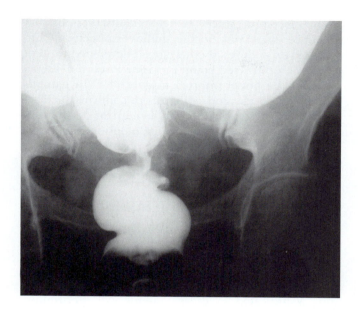

Figure 46–1. Barium enema in a patient with chronic progressive obstructive symptoms. The proximal rectum is obstructed and the sigmoid colon dilated by a rectal adenocarcinoma that gives an "apple-core" appearance.

be the only finding in patients with ileocolic intussusception or cecal obstruction[90] while the distended, "bent inner–tube" appearance of sigmoid or cecal volvulus is often readily apparent on an abdominal radiograph.[91,92] Free intra-abdominal air should be sought on the upright chest X-ray, but even in its absence, cecal dilation beyond 10 to 14 cm raises concern for impending cecal perforation.[93] Although several radiographic findings in patients with large bowel obstruction may direct attention to the correct diagnosis, plain abdominal films are only accurate in about half of all patients.[59] When compared with retrograde contrast studies, plain radiographs are sensitive in 60% to 84%, specific for the diagnosis of large bowel obstruction in 72%, and have a false-positive rate of 35% to 40%.[87,88]

Once the question of a large bowel obstruction has been raised, several options for further investigation exist. In most cases, patients with free intra-abdominal air or diffuse peritonitis should have further definition of the lesion at laparotomy. Rigid or flexible sigmoidoscopic examination, to exclude obstructing rectal cancers, is an important maneuver in the rest.[59] If a large bowel obstruction is suspected on clinical grounds, the surgeon must decide whether a contrast study of the bowel, a computed tomography (CT) scan, or a more extensive colonoscopic investigation is warranted. Although more than one of these studies may be required, choosing the best sequence of examinations can improve the efficiency and safety of the diagnostic evaluation.

Retrograde contrast studies have proven useful in distinguishing true obstruction from pseudoobstruction, identifying the level, type, and degree of the obstruction, and evaluating the proximal colon for synchronous disease.[57,94] Sensitivity and specificity of these studies for obstruction approach 100%.[57,87] Characteristic radiographic images such as the "apple-core" narrowing of a near obstructing rectal cancer (Fig 46–1) or the "beak-like" appearance of the torsed colon in sigmoid volvulus (Fig 46–2) essentially make the diagnosis. Retrograde contrast studies are also useful in patients with an atypical presentation and as previously noted, have a potential therapeutic role in patients with intussusception or cecal volvulus.[86] Barium without air as a single contrast agent provides all the necessary information and is more readily obtained in an emergency setting than double-contrast studies.[88] Apparently complete obstruction to *retrograde* flow during such a study must be evaluated in the clinical context and viewed skeptically in the patient with mild or chronic symptoms. Only 50% of patients obstructed on retrograde contrast studies will also have prograde obstruction.[59] In such patients, a barium small bowel follow-through is safe and, if the information is important for planning treatment, distinguishes partial from complete obstruction.[95]

Contraindications to a retrograde contrast examination include suspected perforation, peritonitis, and gross cecal dilation ($\geq$10 cm) worrisome for impending perforation.[57] Although barium provides better definition

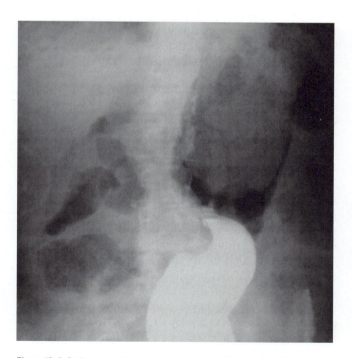

Figure 46–2. Barium enema in a nursing home patient with obstipation. The column of barium ends in a sharp "beak" with the suggestion of spiraled folds. The sigmoid volvulus is evident proximally.

of the lesion than water soluble agents, leakage of barium from a perforation has been associated with an increased risk of infection and septic mortality. In patients with acute abdominal symptoms, but no bowel dilation on abdominal radiographs, a retrograde contrast study is rarely helpful.[87]

CT of the abdomen is useful in patients with subacute obstructive symptoms suspected of having a cancer. It has also proven useful in patients with early postoperative obstruction of the large bowel and in those with obstruction associated with clinical signs of infection, bowel infarction, or an abdominal mass. In one large retrospective study of intestinal obstruction, CT accurately predicted mechanical obstruction in 95% of patients,[85] but only provided clues as to the cause of the obstruction in 73%. Other parameters that may be determined from the CT scan include bowel wall thickness, soft-tissue edema associated with inflammation or infection, intramural or extraintestinal gas, abnormal fluid collections, and abnormalities of the retroperitoneum.

In patients with cancer, CT has become indispensible to staging the disease, with regard to adenopathy, retroperitoneal involvement, and metastatic spread to other organs including the liver. CT also has become increasingly important in the early management of complicated diverticulitis, accurately demonstrating pericolonic inflammation or abscesses requiring percutaneous or radiographically assisted drainage.[96] Fluid-filled bowel is difficult to identifying on plain radiographs[97] but is readily identified with CT. A single prominent fluid-filled loop may indicate a closed-loop obstruction and, in the appropriate clinical setting, should be treated emergently.[85,98] CT findings of mucosal edema and enhancement giving a "target" appearance to the bowel and, particularly the finding of gas within the bowel wall (pneumatosis), are strongly suggestive of ischemic injury or infarction.[99–101] The CT "whirl" sign of a volvulus is characteristic but rarely achieved.[102] Conversely, adhesive obstruction and Crohn's disease of the colon are difficult to distinguish from ileus by CT. Although proximally dilated and distally decompressed bowel are readily identified, the point of obstruction in these disease processes is often obscure, and endoscopy or a contrast study may be necessary to further define the process.[85]

Diagnostic colonoscopy should be considered in patients suspected of nonstrangulated sigmoid volvulus, those with a distal colonic stricture that might be malignant, and chronically ill patients with cecal dilation suggesting pseudoobstruction. In each of these situations, colonoscopy offers therapeutic as well as diagnostic benefits. The finding of a corkscrew-tapered luminal narrowing at endoscopy suggests a volvulus and often, detorsion using the endoscope is possible.[70,76] Inspection and biopsy of colonic strictures helps identify lesions that should be staged with further studies or resected.[103] Endoscopic procedures also have been developed to stent or reopen obstructed bowel for palliation or for preparation of the bowel prior to surgery.[104,105] In patients with pseudoobstruction, colonoscopy confirms the diagnosis and offers the additional benefit of decompression.[106] Direct mucosal inspection, biopsy, and perhaps temporary correction of the obstruction during colonoscopy may simplify later surgical intervention.

■ INDICATIONS FOR SURGICAL TREATMENT

Most patients with mechanical large bowel obstruction require surgical treatment. The goals of surgery in these patients are (1) relief of the obstruction and (2) treatment of the primary obstructing lesion. Urgent laparotomy is indicated in those patients with peritonitis, those with proximal colonic dilation (>10 cm) and acute abdominal symptoms that threaten perforation,[2,25] and those with clinical and radiographic evidence for high-grade obstruction and bowel ischemia. Rarely, decompressing the obstructed bowel is all that is possible and definitive treatment of the lesion causing the obstruction must be deferred. With advances in preoperative resuscitation and anesthetic management, resection with or without primary anastomosis to reestablish intestinal continuity has become an increasingly reasonable option.

Surgical maneuvers to definitively treat obstructing lesions depend on the nature of the obstructive lesion, the severity of obstruction, and the status of the obstructed proximal colon. In patients with a malignant obstruction, surgery is indicated for relief of the obstruction and, if possible, resection of the cancer for cure. Patients with volvulus that cannot be reduced nonoperatively, those with a recurrent volvulus, or those with accompanying signs of bowel ischemia also require urgent surgical treatment. In patients with acute diverticulitis and obstruction, diversion of the fecal stream and drainage of pericolonic infection is often necessary, but resection is indicated less frequently. Those considered for resection usually will have evidence for perforation, chronic scar and stricture, proximal ischemic injury, or a persisting suspicion for occult malignancy. Radiation strictures, fixed adhesions, or other mural or extrinsic causes of large bowel obstruction usually require surgical treatment although some delay may be useful in preparing the patient and cleansing the bowel. In the absence of progressive abdominal symptoms, emergent surgical decompression often can be avoided by nasogastric suction and intensive supportive therapy for patients with an inflammatory obstruction owing to otherwise uncomplicated diverticulitis or Crohn's disease.

■ TECHNIQUES

PATIENT PREPARATION

Patients with large bowel obstruction and an *acute abdomen* must be resuscitated with fluid, electrolyte, and if necessary, transfusion support to improve the safety of anesthesia. Careful monitoring in this group of elderly, often chronically ill patients avoids iatrogenic over-resuscitation.[59] Nasogastric drainage may reduce the risk of aspiration during anesthetic induction and ameliorates the effects of concomitant small bowel distention, present in up to 50% of patients with a malignant obstruction.[107] Rarely is any preoperative attempt at bowel preparation in these acutely ill patients either possible or justified. Broad-spectrum antibiotics, including coverage for gram-negative organisms and anaerobes, reduces infectious morbidity[108–110] and should be administered prior to the incision. In patients with chronic cardiopulmonary or endocrine disease, further specific interventions may be optimal, but the benefits of such treatment must be weighed against the risk of further delay. Often, careful intraoperative monitoring and intensive-care support in the postoperative period are sufficient.

In patients presenting with more indolent symptoms of partial obstruction or those in whom nonoperative measures (vide infra) have been successful at reopening the bowel lumen, preparation for elective, definitive treatment also should include correcting nutritional deficits and, when possible, mechanical bowel preparation. Although the necessity of preoperative mechanical bowel preparation has been debated in the literature,[111] retrospective studies suggest that reducing the fecal load may reduce the risks of wound infection and postoperative anastomotic disruption.[3,83] Following these measures, elective surgical treatment can be carried out with increased safety.

MANAGEMENT OF MALIGNANT LARGE BOWEL OBSTRUCTION

Malignant obstruction is the most common cause of large bowel obstruction and methods developed to deal with this problem have been used to treat obstruction from all causes. Trends in the management of colorectal malignant obstruction have been reviewed by Wangensteen[112] and, more recently, Matheson.[59] From these accounts and other reviews of malignant obstruction,[3,4,49,113] it is evident that patient age and physical condition, the location and extent of the obstructive lesion, and the experience of the surgical team are all key factors in determining operative strategy.

Younger patients are generally healthier and more tolerant of potential complications. They have the most to gain from the improved long-term survival associated with early resection,[83] while even the simplest procedures in an elderly or chronically ill population are associated with increased mortality.[3] Despite improvements in preoperative resuscitation and anesthesia, the combination of acute and chronic illness in these elderly patients with large bowel obstruction often limits treatment to fecal diversion alone or limited resection and diversion.

Tumor extent also has a profound effect on surgical treatment. Obstructive cancer that is unresectable must be managed with diversion of the fecal stream to relieve the obstruction. The palliative benefit of internal diversion (ie, cecosigmoidostomy) must be balanced against the risk of an anastomosis under these conditions and the morbidity of the alternative, external diversion with a colostomy. Short survival time and the prospect for early postoperative chemotherapy in patients with widely metastatic disease suggest that extensive procedures and a prolonged recovery are ill-advised in this group.

Under conditions where curative resection is possible, the location of the lesion largely determines the extent of resection and what options are available for a primary repair. For example, right colon cancers are routinely treated by resection and ileocolic anastomosis in a single stage, whereas a variety of options with varying indications, risks, and benefits exist for obstructing lesions of the left colon. During the past 30 years, operative strategy in patients with a distal obstruction has shifted from a three-stage process marked by proximal diversion of the fecal stream (stage I), interval resection of the cancer with anastomosis (stage II), and later closure of the diverting stoma (stage III),[1,3,114–116] to a more aggressive approach of primary resection and in many cases, immediate anastomosis. An important reason for this change is the repeated observation that staged resection does not improve survival but rather promotes an excessive morbidity and operative mortality, in spite of the apparent conservatism of the approach. The largest prospective study to address this problem, the *UK Large Bowel Cancer Project,* showed that immediate resection could be achieved with a degree of safety at least equivalent to staged treatment,[83] and these findings have been validated by other studies.[117–119] As a result, most surgeons in the current era approach the problem of obstructing left-sided colon cancer with the intention to perform an immediate resection of the lesion.

Primary anastomosis is also increasingly common in these patients, but is dependent on other factors and requires both specialized techniques and experience.[81,120,121] The presence of synchronous polyps or cancer should prompt consideration for subtotal resection, but often the status of the remaining large bowel is unknown. In patients with severe bowel injury from obstruction, resection back to healthy bowel and/or diversion are the only reasonable options, since any attempt at anastomosis under these conditions is fraught with a high risk of failure. Similarly, although experimental anastomoses heal in the presence of infection,[122] major fecal soilage or established peritonitis usually should prompt diversion rather than anastomosis.[123,124] Finally, a large or liquid fecal load often prevents simple decompression of the proximal colon because of the increased risk of spillage. Fortunately, newer techniques, such as on-table lavage, offer means of protecting an anastomosis and preventing colostomy in the majority of such patients.

Diversion

Diversion Alone. Despite the trend to more aggressive primary resection for obstructing left-colon cancer, proximal diversion alone remains a useful technique for some patients.[60,125,126] The principle indication for diversion as a primary treatment is severe comorbid illness that renders any but the most cursory anesthesia hazardous.[84,119] Other indications for diversion alone include locally invasive, unresectable cancer or an obstructing rectal carcinoma (Table 46–4).

In the hands of a less experienced surgical team dealing with a fragile patient, a proximal-loop colostomy is an effective and easily achieved therapy.[126] Minimizing the immediate surgical trauma may be life-saving, but the benefits of this option must be weighed against the increased morbidity and mortality of a planned, multistage procedure.[81,114,118,127] For patients with an unresectable obstruction of the splenic flexure or left colon, external diversion is the only alternative or cecosigmoidostomy. The merits of each palliative procedure must be determined for the individual. Proximal diversion affords the patient with obstructing rectal cancer a safe interval for preparation of the bowel or other therapy (ie, radiation). However, regardless of the operative risk, no diversion procedure alone can be justified if the colon is ischemic and questionably viable or when perforation and peritonitis are present. With the risk of potentially lethal septic consequences, resection of such compromised colon is essential.

Techniques for Diversion of the Fecal Stream. Options for proximal diversion without resection include (1) tube cecostomy, (2) loop-right or transverse colostomy positioned proximal to the site of obstruction, and (3) internal bypass by a cecal-sigmoid anastomosis. It should be noted that since the obstruction is still present in these patients, all three techniques drain the colon proximally and distally, down to the level of the obstruction. Because of a potentially competent ileocecal valve, loop ileostomy is an unreliable method for decompressing the obstructed large bowel.

Cecostomy. Cecostomy can be achieved by bringing the cecum to the skin surface in the right lower abdomen, but the term more commonly implies placement of a tube through the abdominal wall into the cecum. Tube cecostomy involves placement of one or preferably, two concentric purse-strings centered on a tenae on the lateral surface of the mobilized cecum. They are used to secure a balloon or mushroom-tipped catheter in the lumen of the cecum (Fig 46–3). In selected patients, this procedure even can be performed under local anesthesia via a muscle splitting, right lower quadrant incision while others require laparoscopy or laparotomy. A Witzel tunnel is optional but may reduce morbidity.[128] The catheter is passed through the abdominal wall and the adjacent cecum is secured to the parietal peritoneum around the tube, sealing the catheter tract. Frequent saline irrigation and gravity drainage of the cecostomy, rather than suction, prevents obstruction of the tube with fecal matter.

Tube cecostomy is most useful at decompressing a gas-filled colon due to distal obstruction or pseudoobstruction. It also has been used as a means of anchoring the cecum in patients with a history of cecal volvulus.[129,130] With careful management, some report it to be an effective means of decompressing and cleansing the proximal bowel[128]; however most reports emphasize the difficulty of maintaining patency and the temporary nature of the technique.[131] Recent reviews show a mortality rate of up to 30% and complications in 60% that include leakage, wound infection, and persistent fecal fistula after catheter removal.[131,132] Given these results, tube cecostomy should probably be reserved for tempo-

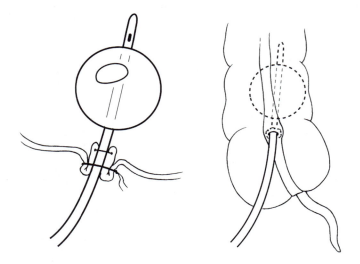

Figure 46–3. The balloon-tipped catheter is secured by a double purse-string placed through a tenae or the base of the appendix. Alternatively, a Witzel tunnel may be constructed to prevent leakage.

TABLE 46–4. INDICATIONS FOR DIVERSION PROCEDURES

ILEOSTOMY	Obstructing right colon cancer
	Cecal volvulus
	Following emergency subtotal colectomy
CECOSTOMY	Massive right colon distention (>10 cm)
	(Fixation of cecal volvulus)[a]
	(Temporary proximal diversion)[a]
COLOSTOMY	Surgeon's judgment of unacceptable anastomotic risk
	Multiple risk factors for anastomotic disruption
	Obstruction with perforation
	Generalized peritonitis
	Viable but diffusely injured bowel

[a]Indications for which cecostomy may be less effective than other methods (see text)

rary decompression and used only in patients for whom technical considerations preclude a diverting loop colostomy.

Loop Colostomy. The historical basis of this procedure has been reviewed by Corman.[133] In patients with distal colonic obstruction, loop colostomy diverts the fecal stream completely[134] and traditionally forms the first part of a staged resection.[114] As previously noted, loop colostomy is effective palliation for unresectable lesions and also has been used to protect a distal anastomosis although, in reality, the nature of this protection is an attempt to limit the infectious complications of anastomotic disruption rather than influencing healing.[36] Unfortunately, even in patients with a planned, temporary colostomy, up to one in three patients will never have the colostomy reversed owing to chronic illness or the anticipated morbidity of the procedure.[117]

The transverse colon usually is used to form the loop colostomy.[135] Preserving the marginal vasculature, the colon is mobilized from omental attachments and any adhesions. At a site that is optimally chosen before surgery to avoid clothing or the waist crease, an abdominal aperature is fashioned that will admit three or more fingers, depending on the bowel thickness. The ostomy site usually is positioned in the right upper abdomen to keep the bowel away from the midline incision and a left-sided malignancy. However, under rare conditions of a foreshortened mesentery, severe obesity, or marked abdominal distention, the loop may only reach the surface through the midline incision.[136] Once exteriorized, the colon is draped over a rod or bar passed through the mesocolon, elevating the back wall of the ostomy to skin level until fixation has occurred.[133,137] Alternatively, a small fascial bridge may be constructed posteriorly behind the loop. Special integrated ostomy devices that have a built-in bar have been developed for this application. After closure of the abdominal wound, the loop is opened and matured to adjacent skin margins, except over the rod. An extra-large ostomy appliance is usually necessary to accommodate the rod and oval extent of the looped colon. This maneuver anchors the colon and completely diverts both lumens to the skin surface (Fig 46–4).

Internal Bypass (Cecosigmoidostomy). Internal bypass is an important technique for avoiding a colostomy in some of the 20% to 30% of patients with malignant colonic obstruction who are found to have locally extensive, unresectable disease.[119] For this procedure to be considered, the obstructing lesion must be located between the cecum and the sigmoid colon and the operative findings must be favorable for anastomotic healing. The principle advantage of this procedure is avoiding the burden of a colostomy in these often elderly patients with a terminal illness.

After appropriate maneuvers to confirm and stage the diagnosis of unresectable left colon cancer, the cecum and sigmoid colon are mobilized as necessary and a side-to-side, cecosigmoid anastomosis is constructed, using standard techniques. Care must be taken to control adverse risks to anastomotic healing such as tension, ischemia, or spillage. Usually, the two loops of bowel join over the pelvic promontory below the retroperitoneal attachment of the small bowel mesentery. Tacking of the mesentery and colon posteriorly avoids

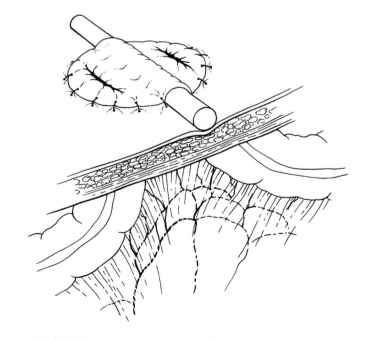

Figure 46–4. The colon is supported, until mature, by a rod placed under the loop. A loop constructed in this fashion is completely diverting.

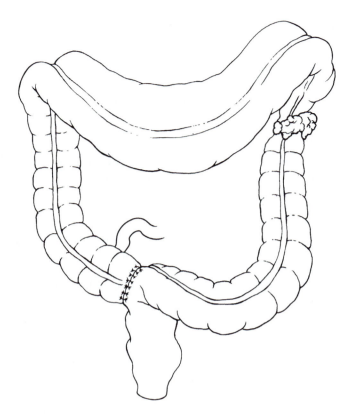

Figure 46–5. Palliative anastomosis between the cecum and the loop of the sigmoid colon is distant from the locally unresectable disease and avoids colostomy.

small bowel herniation behind the new anastomosis (Fig 46–5).

Resection with Proximal Diversion (Hartmann's Procedure). The Hartmann's procedure with a proximal-end colostomy or ileostomy is the most common operation carried out by general surgeons for management of malignant obstruction of the distal colon.[138,139] During this procedure, the lesion is removed, the distal bowel closed intraperitoneally, and the proximal bowel diverted with a stoma. In the current era, indications for this procedure include (1) localized or generalized peritonitis owing to perforation of the cancer and (2) viable but injured proximal bowel that, in the opinion of the operating surgeon, precludes safe anastomosis. Use of the Hartmann's procedure has been associated with a low perioperative mortality of 9%, but at the cost of a colostomy that, in up to two-thirds of patients, is never reversed.[3,125,140]

Complications of Colostomy. Two-thirds of all colostomies are created in patients with obstruction owing to colorectal malignancy or perforated diverticulitis.[141] The relative risks associated with colostomy formation and closure have been extensively debated in the literature, but it is generally agreed that colostomy formation and closure are major abdominal procedures with significant perioperative morbidity.[139,141,142] Complications occur in 5% to 49% of patients undergoing colostomy closure, with a resulting mortality that may reach 3%.[143,144] Complications associated with the colostomy itself include prolapse, paracolostomy abscess, necrosis, retraction, and peritonitis, although most occur rarely.[141] Complications of colostomy closure include wound infection (5% to 20%), anastomotic leaks (0% to 23%),[143] bowel obstruction, incisional hernia, and other cardiopulmonary problems associated with anesthesia and an operative procedure in elderly, debilitated patients.[145] Possible risk factors for these complications have been analyzed. Perioperative antibiotic therapy and the experience of the operative team,[143] as well as the timing of colostomy closure, influence outcome while age, pathology, type of colostomy, site, and drain placement appear to be less important.[127,143]

Primary Resection with Anastomosis

Emergency procedures on the unprepared colon are associated with increased septic and other complications.[146,147] This is especially true for patients with obstructing cancers of the colon or rectum.[148] The advantages of a one-stage procedure for these patients are obvious but in a given patient, the decision to perform a primary anastomosis using previously obstructed bowel is often difficult.[125] In the *right colon,* resection and primary ileocolostomy are standard therapy and are supported by numerous studies.[59,82,120] However, even as late as 1974, primary anastomosis for *left colon* lesions was associated with a high complication rate and mortality approaching 60%.[3,149] Several studies have emphasized the importance of an experienced team in making this important decision and achieving a good outcome.[56,150] Problems associated with diverting colostomy and colostomy closure have been emphasized and, together with several favorable reports of primary anastomosis, have prompted further interest in the single-stage approach.

A number of parallel developments have contributed to the increased use of primary anastomosis in the unprepared colon. Experimental and clinical studies of anastomotic healing have shown that while fecal loading may be associated with an increase in anastomotic disruption,[36,43] the exact cause of this complication remains unclear. More liberal application of extended resection as well as new techniques of on-table lavage and variations on the intracolonic sleeve (vide infra) have been developed to protect the anastomotic wound. Broad-spectrum antibiotics and perioperative intensive care management also have contributed to reducing the complications of elective and emergency colon surgery, previously among the greatest deterrents to primary anastomosis. In the stable patient with no diffuse peritonitis, severe bowel injury, or unresectable malignancy, primary resection and anastomosis by an experienced surgeon has become an increasingly attractive option.

Subtotal Colectomy.

Partial colectomy with ileocolic anastomosis is safe and is the treatment of choice for right colon cancers regardless of whether the colon is prepared or not.[114] Anastomosis after right colectomy in the presence of peritonitis must be carefully considered since, under these conditions, an increased risk of septic complications and anastomotic failure has been reported.[123] Extended resection and ileocolic anastomosis also has been applied to obstructing cancers of the left colon, most commonly for treatment of frank or impending cecal perforation.[138] Good anastomotic healing generally has been observed[151–154] despite an 11% 30 day operative mortality.[155] Further analysis has shown that less than half of this mortality is the result of anastomotic failure.

The benefits of subtotal colectomy include potentially better healing when small bowel, with its richer blood supply, higher collagen content, and more rapid collagen deposition forms half of the anastomosis.[46,156] By carrying the resection from the cecum beyond the obstructing lesion, all dilated, injured colon and most of the associated fecal load are excised and discarded, minimizing the risk of intraoperative wound soilage.[152] Subtotal resection also reduces the area of colonic epithelium at risk for other cancers. Synchronous malignant polyps or cancers have been reported in up to 50% of patients with obstructing colorectal cancer.[79,157] In younger patients with a history of colorectal carcinoma, the incidence of metachronous cancer ranges from 0.35% per year to 0.75% per year depending on patient age.[158,159] Since a high proportion of metachronous lesions occur in the right colon, this risk is markedly reduced after subtotal colectomy, and follow-up is simplified for these patients.[160]

Unfortunately, subtotal colectomy also has several disadvantages. Subtotal resection is a more extensive operation, with the necessity for a larger incision, longer anesthetic and operative period, and an increased lifetime risk for adhesive bowel obstruction due to the extent of the dissection.[152] Beneficial functions of the colon such as water absorption and storage also are lost. Bowel movements are looser and the increased stool frequency in these often elderly patients with reduced sphincter tone may lead to incontinence, especially if the resection is carried beyond the proximal sigmoid colon. Although most series indicate that stool frequency eventually stabilizes at 2 to 3/day with good control,[157] many patients require supplemental antidiarrheal agents for an extended period.[151]

Left Colon Anastomosis in the Unprepared Bowel.

Segmental resection of obstructing left-colon lesions with immediate anastomosis in the unprepared bowel is a controversial, but increasingly employed, alternative that requires careful patient selection. As previously discussed, anastomotic integrity and healing appear to be more dependent on the character of the bowel wall and blood supply than luminal contents.[161] Indeed, bacterial density within the lumen is not changed by mechanical bowel preparation.[162] In the emergency setting, resection with immediate anastomosis preserves colon length and avoids the morbidity of a colostomy. However, a long clinical experience dating to the 1950s suggests that this procedure, especially in patients with sepsis (ie, perforated, obstructing diverticulitis), is associated with a mortality of up to 50%.[140] In reviewing this experience, the contribution of fecal load from among many other risk factors to patient outcome remains unclear, as previously discussed. What is evident is that with careful selection of patients, along with excellent control of the bowel to avoid spillage and technical precision, primary anastomosis in the unprepared colon can be achieved with results comparable to any alternative form of treatment.[163]

Clinical support for anastomosis in the unprepared colon comes from a growing experience with primary repair of penetrating colon injuries in trauma patients.[161,164] In these reports, patients were selected carefully with isolated, intraperitoneal colon injuries (rectum excluded), minimal or no peritoneal contamination, and an otherwise healthy colon. Under these conditions, primary repair resulted in a mortality of 1% to 2% and a morbidity less than that associated with colostomy formation.[165]

Several small series also report the results of this technique in the obstructed left colon. Goodall and associates restricted the procedure to otherwise healthy patients without significant systemic (steroids, malnutrition, inflammatory bowel disease) or local (diffuse metastatic disease, diverticulitis, radiation injury, ischemia, or necrosis) disease.[166] Liquid stool was emptied from the colon proximal to the obstruction using a double purse-string and tube inserted just above the obstruction. Antegrade irrigation was not employed. Goodall reported a reduced length of stay, with a 5% mortality rate and a 40% complication rate, primarily from wound complications. Dorudi and associates used a similar technique in 18 patients, but decompressed the obstructed proximal colon via a tube advanced through a small bowel enterotomy and the ileocecal valve.[111] In their series, there were no anastomotic complications. Analysis from the *UK Large Bowel Cancer Project* by Phillips and associates showed that anastomotic leakage occurred in 18% of patients after primary resection and anastomosis, with a 23% overall mortality in this group.[83] McMillan and Bell developed a stapling technique for the anastomosis that simplified management of differences in colonic diameter,[167] whereas Amsterdam and associates emphasized the fragile nature of this population, demonstrating the feasibility of primary anastomosis despite a 60% incidence of other complications.[168] Thus although primary anastomosis can be effective, the highly septic consequences of even rare anastomotic failures in these patients suggest that this option should be employed by an experienced team and reserved for those with a distal sigmoid obstruction, no infection, and an otherwise healthy bowel.

On-table Lavage. On-table lavage of the colon was first described by Muir, in 1968,[169] but the current technique is based on modifications suggested by Dudley and associates.[124] In patients unable to achieve an adequate preoperative mechanical preparation, on-table lavage reduces the fecal load that is a persisting concern in patients considered for primary anastomosis. Lavage also has been shown, experimentally, to increase anastomotic and perianastomotic collagen content in the colon.[54] A colostomy is avoided and bowel length preserved, thereby reducing the diarrhea risk of subtotal colectomy. However the procedure necessitates a longer operation, some specialized equipment, and familiarity with the technique. Only those patients with a proximally viable bowel, who are able to tolerate the longer anesthetic, should be considered for this procedure.

After mobilization of the sigmoid colon, enteric contents are milked back into the descending colon and noncrushing bowel clamps are applied to the colon distally but above the site of obstruction. Using care to avoid spillage, one end of a sterile evacuation drain (commonly gas-sterilized anesthesia gas evacuation tubing) is inserted into the descending colon and secured with cotton tape. The other end of the drain is passed off the field and drained into a floor bag or bucket. Proximally, a Foley catheter is inserted into the cecum via an enterotomy[124] or the base of the appendix.[170] Sterile saline via sterile irrigation tubing is flushed through the Foley catheter while massaging the bowel to break up solid stool (Fig 46–6). A total of 10 L of irrigant may be necessary to achieve clear effluent. Upon completion of the procedure, the irrigation catheter may be removed and the colon oversewn or converted into a cecostomy for postoperative radiographic study of the anastomosis.[124] Converting an ileal catheter into a tube enterostomy has been associated with enteric leakage and sepsis and is not advised.[171] The effluent tube and involved segment of colon are removed together after milking residual contents distally, and a primary anastomosis is constructed using standard techniques.

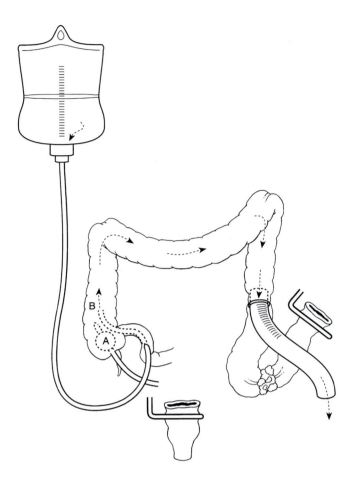

Figure 46–6. Saline irrigation through a catheter placed via the appendiceal stump (A) or distal ileum (B) flushes the colon distally and is vented off the operative field.

Koruth and associates reported a 7% anastomotic leak rate and 13% mortality in 15 patients with on-table lavage for distal colonic lesions.[120] In their series, mortality was unrelated to the anastomosis, and they advocated broader use of the technique. Thompson and Carter detected anastomotic leakage in 6 of 122 patients (4.8%) with rectal or rectosigmoid lesions treated with on-table lavage,[172] and Pollock and associates reported a 17% operative mortality in 44 patients (none anastomosis related) treated similarly.[171] Radcliff and Dudley had two clinically significant anastomotic leaks (3%) and two deaths (3%, one related to anastomotic dehiscence) in 64 patients treated with on-table lavage for distal colonic or rectal lesions.[173] Allen-Mersh compared anastomosis after lavage to colostomy and found no difference in perioperative morbidity or mortality.[174] A number of other studies[170,175,176] confirm these findings and suggest that the risk of primary anastomosis after on-table lavage is reasonable and comparable to the risks associated with other methods of managing distally obstructing lesions. With employment of this technique, >80% of all patients presenting with distal large bowel obstruction should be candidates for resection and primary anastomosis.

Intraluminal Shield Devices. The various forms of intraluminal shield device (produced commercially as the Coloshield intracolonic bypass tube by Deknatel, Fall River, MA) provides another option for protection of a new anastomosis in the unprepared colon. In a review of anastomotic healing, Ravo suggested that anastomotic dehiscence for other than strictly technical factors, occurs during the period of maximal weakness between 3 and 5 days after the operation.[177] For anastomoses protected by proximal diversion, intraoperative lavage, or a luminal shield, such a dehiscence usually is controlled by normal peritoneal defenses and may be asymptomatic. By his analysis, the benefits of luminal shield devices derive from *limiting* the consequences of anastomotic dehiscence rather than *preventing* dehiscence. This protection against disruption of the healing anastomosis has experimental support.[178]

The shield is placed after resection of the diseased segment.[177] After appropriate packing of the abdominal space, the proximal colon is occluded with a noncrushing clamp 3 to 5 cm from the cut end of the bowel, which is everted for a distance of 2 cm using stay sutures. Povodone-iodine is used to prepare the exposed mucosa. An appropriate-sized sleeve is introduced and sutured to the everted mucosa and submucosa using a polyglycolic acid suture in an interlocking, running technique. The proximal colon then is inverted back into its normal position and the posterior aspect of the anastomosis achieved, using standard techniques. Prior to completion of the anterior row, the sleeve is attached to a previously placed rectal tube and advanced through the anus. The anterior anastomosis is completed and the sleeve divided at the anus (Fig 46–7). Techniques for use of the sleeve with a stapled anastomosis[179] and more proximal colonic anastomosis[180] also have been described. In the postoperative period, sleeve position can be checked radiographically and the sleeve should pass within 2 to 3 weeks.

The intracolonic shield has been used as a means of avoiding colostomy in patients with colorectal trauma,[181,182] perforated diverticulitis,[183] volvulus, and obstructing cancers.[179,184] In this series of small reports, anastomotic healing generally has been successful, although the contribution of the shield remains unclear since no prospective randomized comparison with simple anastomosis or intraoperative lavage has been published. Erosion by the stiff supporting ring of the Coloshield through the bowel wall has been reported.[185]

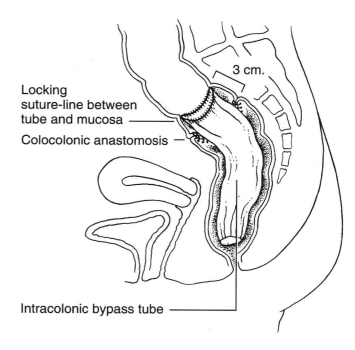

Figure 46–7. The intracolonic bypass is secured circumferentially with absorbable suture within the proximal bowel and is brought through the anastomosis to the anus. Stool passes through the sleeve and the anastomosis is protected.

Exteriorization of Anastomosis. In trauma patients, colotomies and, in some cases, entire anastomoses exteriorized onto the anterior abdominal wall heal in 70% of patients.[153,186] Morbidity and mortality of the procedure in this population are similar to colostomy, with the principle advantage of avoiding an ostomy appliance.[187] To be considered for this operation, patients should have an anastomosis at least 20 cm proximal to the peritoneal reflection, potentially compromised anastomotic healing, and must be able to tolerate a longer operation. Exteriorizing an anastomosis requires sufficient mobilization of the colon to reach the anterior abdominal wall without tension. Once brought through the incision, a fascial bridge is constructed behind the exteriorized segment, which then is protected with appropriate dressings. A second operation is necessary to return the colon to the abdomen. Although apparently effective in the trauma population, there is no published experience with this technique in other conditions. With the range of alternative options for primary intraperitoneal repair available, it seems unlikely that this technique will find much application in the patient with large bowel obstruction.

Protective Proximal Colostomy. Construction of a proximal, diverting loop colostomy is another technique that has been historically employed to protect a new anastomosis in patients undergoing emergency colectomy for obstruction, complications of diverticulitis,[115,116,125] or penetrating trauma.[161] Loop ileostomy for similar indications also has been described.[188] The ostomy is created using the same techniques as previously described.[137] Closure of the ostomy usually is delayed until the patient has recovered and anastomotic healing is confirmed by radiographic studies, usually after an interval of several months.

Experimental studies of the anastomotic wound suggest that proximal diverting colostomy may slow collagen accumulation at the suture line, but diverting the fecal stream does not otherwise adversely affect healing.[189,190] Conversely, clinical studies suggest that proximal fecal diversion does not prevent anastomotic dehiscence and may not limit the septic consequences of this complication.[117,191,192] No recent experience detailing outcome from loop colostomy has been published. In series dating from more than 14 years ago, clinically significant anastomotic leakage occurred in 14% to 22% of patients with a proximal diverting colostomy,[117,193] half of which required surgical treatment to survive. In the current era, probably the major indication for a proximal-loop colostomy is a tenuous low anterior anastomosis or coloanal anastomosis where the risk of anastomotic dehiscence is increased owing to infection, weakness of the tissues, or the anatomical constraints of the pelvis, but delaying formation of the anastomosis is not a safe or anatomically feasible option.

SURVIVAL AFTER TREATMENT FOR MALIGNANT LARGE BOWEL OBSTRUCTION

Patients undergoing emergent surgical treatment for malignant large bowel obstruction have a poorer immediate and 5 year, cancer-specific survival than others undergoing elective colorectal procedures. Operative mortality for both palliative and curative procedures in obstructed patients ranges from 7% to 23%,[58,83,194] one-half or more of which is related to septic events.[147] Preoperative factors linked to an increase in operative mortality include patient age, cardiovascular disease, poor nutrition, compromised physiological status, and the presence of perforation or sepsis.[84,147,194] These data contrast with a mortality of 5% to 7% following elective colorectal resection.[58] Resection for cure is possible in only 50% to 70% of obstructed patients, about 20% less than for patients without obstruction.[195] Overall, the crude 5 year survival for patients presenting with obstruction is half that of nonobstructed patients, 22% versus 49%.[58] In patients who are candidates for curative resection, some studies suggest that long-term survival is not influenced by the presence of obstruction.[3] However, most report a persistent adverse effect of the obstruction with a 5 year survival of 30% to 55% *with ob-*

struction versus 50% to 75% *without obstruction,* when comparing these two groups.[58,195,196]

Reasons for the reduced long-term survival after curative resection of patients with obstructing cancer have been analyzed. Increased operative mortality and a bias toward higher-stage disease as compared to patients without obstruction provide part of the explanation.[58,197] Multivariant analysis suggests that, in addition to these factors, many patients with obstruction have a biologically more aggressive tumor with a greater propensity to infiltrate, metastasize, and recur.[83,195,198] For this reason, earlier detection before obstruction and spread of the tumor may be necessary to achieve results comparable to the elective experience with colorectal malignancy.

MANAGEMENT OF VOLVULUS

Volvulus is a mechanical obstruction of the large bowel that occurs because of an anatomical torsion of bowel around a narrow mesenteric pedicle. Complete luminal obstruction occurs, and the torsion also may involve the vascular supply to the bowel, resulting in a strangulated obstruction. Volvulus has been described in all parts of the colon that have a mobile mesentery. Most episodes of volvulus occur in the sigmoid colon (45% to 80%), the right colon (15% to 30%), and transverse colon or splenic flexure (2% to 5%).[69,71,73,199,200] Mobility of the cecum is usually on a congenital basis owing to incomplete bowel rotation or fixation,[201] while lengthening of the sigmoid mesentery is an acquired phenomenon, usually occurring after years of high fiber intake or laxative use.[188,199] Abnormal patterns of motility are also frequently present in patients with all types of volvulus.[71,73] The goals of therapy are to resolve the obstruction, remove any perforated, necrotic, or otherwise severely injured bowel, and to prevent recurrence with a minimum of morbidity. In most cases, surgical treatment is eventually required. Overall mortality for all patients treated for volvulus is 11% to 15%.[72,200]

Sigmoid Volvulus
Sigmoid volvulus occurs most commonly in debilitated patients who are nonambulatory and patients who have a history of chronic illness, previous abdominal surgery, laxative use, and dementia.[69] Patients with sigmoid volvulus often come from a nursing home or other institutional setting. Their median age is 60 to 70 years and the frailty of this elderly population is an important restraint on the options for surgical treatment.[71,200] During development of the volvulus, the sigmoid colon develops a clockwise twist of >200° that creates a proximal obstruction and the closed loop of the involved segment, as well (Fig 46–8). Only 7% to 10% of patients

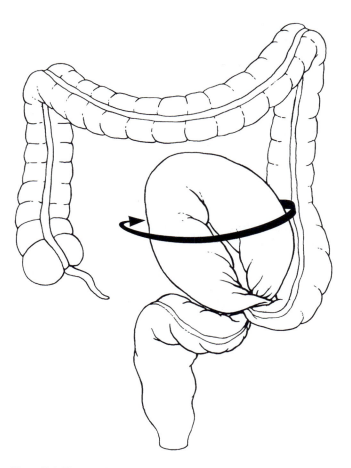

Figure 46–8. The axial, clockwise twist of the mobile sigmoid colon leads to a closed-loop obstruction and vascular compromise. Reasons for the "bent inner tube" radiographic appearance of a volvulus are evident.

with sigmoid obstruction will have colonic infarction or perforation at presentation.[71,200]

Patients with sigmoid volvulus present with nausea, vomiting, abdominal distention, pain, and obstipation. On clinical grounds, simple obstruction may be difficult to distinguish from strangulated obstruction since nonperforated ischemic injury may not alter the clinical picture.[72] Over half will have acute rather than chronic symptoms[71] and up to one-third will have had previous episodes of volvulus treated nonoperatively.[202] The history and abdominal radiographs are usually suggestive and barium enema is highly accurate at confirming the diagnosis. Diagnostic maneuvers and the accuracy of radiographic investigations have been reviewed previously.

Management of patients with sigmoid volvulus depends on the acuity of presentation, whether an ischemic injury has occurred, and the initial success of nonoperative techniques at detorsing the colon. In otherwise stable patients, rigid proctosigmoidoscopy is ef-

fective in reducing sigmoid volvulus, in 80% of patients.[71,200,203–205] The scope is passed above 25 cm to derotate the colon and drain the closed loop. A rectal tube is used to stent the colon as the scope is withdrawn. Increasing experience with flexible sigmoidoscopy or colonoscopy suggests that these instruments are also highly effective.[70,76,206,207] Unfortunately, recurrence after endoscopic detorsion occurs in 50% to 90% of patients, often during the same admission.[69,71] While a majority of the torsion in these patients can be reduced successfully a second and perhaps third time,[69] multiple recurrent volvulus is associated with an increased mortality.[200] In the patient who can tolerate bowel preparation and presents an acceptable anesthetic risk, most authors recommend laparotomy, with definitive treatment after the first or second recurrence of sigmoid volvulus. Surgical detorsion alone is associated with a recurrence rate of up to 30%[73,200] and attempts at colopexy have not apparently reduced the rate of recurrence.[202,208] Resection of the redundant sigmoid colon is curative,[73,200] even though operative mortality in this group has historically been as high as 30%.[69,73] In retrospective studies that likely select sicker patients for diversion, Hartmann's procedure has been associated with greater morbidity and mortality than primary anastomosis.

Patients in whom nonoperative endoscopic measures fail generally require urgent laparotomy. The utility of therapeutic barium enema to reduce a sigmoid volvulus in these patients is not known. If the colon is viable, options for surgical treatment range from simple detorsion in the frailest patients to more definitive treatment.[209] Just as in patients with an obstructing left colon cancer, patient and bowel status, prior surgery, fecal loading, and the experience of the surgical team are some of the factors that must be considered in planning management for patients with an obstructing volvulus. The various options of diversion or anastomosis, with or without ancillary measures to protect the anastomotic wound, apply and the reader is referred to the prior discussion.

Those patients with clinical, endoscopic, or radiographic evidence for severe ischemic injury or perforation of the involved sigmoid require emergent exploration and, depending on the severity of the injury, immediate sigmoid colectomy. Given the characteristics of this population, most patients are treated with diverting colostomy. Mortality in patients with colonic gangrene owing to volvulus is increased by a factor of 4 over those with viable bowel, up to 80% in some reviews.[69,74] Although primary anastomosis may be considered in highly selected patients, the morbidity and mortality of an extended procedure in these patients must be balanced against the increased risk of anastomosis in a septic field.[43]

CECAL VOLVULUS

An anatomically mobile cecum occurs in 11% of the population, an incidence 400 times greater than the reported incidence of cecal volvulus.[188] This suggests that other, possibly acquired, factors such as dietary fiber also may be important in cecal volvulus. The most common form of cecal volvulus (85%) involves an axial clockwise twist in the right colon that rotates the terminal ileum to the right of the cecum[210] (Fig 46–9). Another type of cecal volvulus, the *cecal bascule* (15%), occurs when the mobile cecum becomes folded on itself without twisting, pointing the appendix at the diaphragm but retaining the ileocolic junction to the left of the cecum (Fig 46–9, inset). The mean age of patients developing cecal volvulus is 50 to 60 years, with a female preponderance.[211] Most patients present with clinical findings of a distal closed-loop obstruction: nausea, vomiting, abdominal distention and pain, and altered bowel function that might initially include diarrhea.[210,212] While abdominal films suggest the diagnosis in half of all patients and barium enema is highly accurate and safe, 50% of patients are diagnosed during emergency laparotomy for an acute abdomen.[188,210] Cecal infarction is present in 17% to 21% of patients at pre-

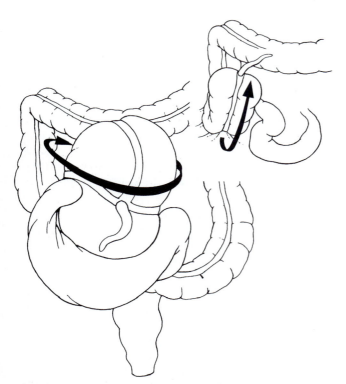

Figure 46–9. The clockwise twist of cecal volvulus rotates the ileocecal junction laterally and superiorly while the ileocecal junction remains medial with formation of a cecal bascule (inset).

sentation[200,210] and contributes to the 17% perioperative mortality in these patients.[71]

Most patients with cecal volvulus require urgent surgical treatment. Several reports indicate occasional success with colonoscopic or barium enema detorsion of a cecal volvulus,[72,213] but in most patients, nonoperative measures have not been successful.[71] In patients with severe ischemic injury or perforation of the cecum, resection is necessary for survival but is associated with a 15% incidence of complications and a 22% to 45% mortality.[188,200,210] Diversion with an ileostomy and mucus fistula should be strongly considered in patients with diffuse bowel injury and peritonitis because of the severe risks of anastomosis in this group.[73]

In patients with a viable cecum, options include detorsion alone, cecopexy, cecostomy, and right colectomy. Recurrence after detorsion is 13% and several studies suggest that cecopexy does not alter this recurrence rate.[188,210] Right colectomy is definitive treatment with the best long-term control of symptoms[211] but there is wide variation in the reported mortality, ranging from 5% to 25%.[200,210,211] The Mayo Clinic experience with cecostomy for decompressing and fixing the cecum is favorable[200] but seems unique. Most other series report a high rate of complications (50%), mortality (22% to 100%) and recurrence (14%) with this technique.[69,210] Thus, in the fragile patient with limited tolerance for an anesthetic, detorsion alone is fast, safe, and effective in more than 85% of patients. However, resection with primary anastomosis can probably be carried out with an acceptable risk in patients who are stable and in whom the bowel appears reasonably healthy. In the current era, cecostomy should rarely be necessary for the treatment of cecal volvulus.

MANAGEMENT OF OBSTRUCTING DIVERTICULITIS

Colonic obstruction requiring surgical treatment occurs in 1.5% of all patients with diverticulitis[214] and must be distinguished clinically from ileus due to the inflammatory disease. Radiological criteria for obstructed diverticulitis include an inflammatory mass with wall thickening, obstruction to retrograde flow, and proximal colonic dilatation.[215] Obstruction is the indication for surgical intervention in 10% of all diverticulitis patients who come to surgery, usually for disease involving the sigmoid colon (Fig 46–10).[216–218] In some patients, distinguishing an inflammatory obstruction from cancer may be difficult and, until the diagnosis is established, measures appropriate to a cancer resection must be followed.

Proximal diversion or resection, with or without anastomosis, are the only options available for treatment of diverticular obstruction.[219] In nonperforated patients, comparison of diversion without resection and the Hart-

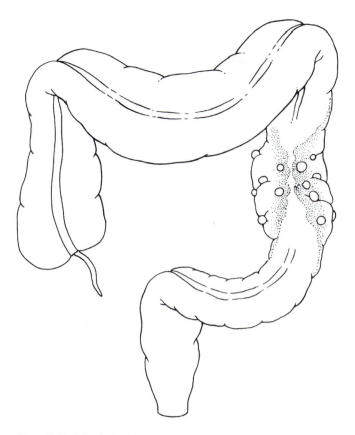

Figure 46–10. A diverticular phlegmon involves the sigmoid colon and results in proximal colonic obstruction.

mann's procedure shows that patients achieve benefit from removal of the inflammatory mass. Recovery occurs faster and patients generally have a shorter hospitalization.[217] This difference is even more pronounced in patients with concomitant perforation and peritonitis or severe proximal bowel injury where removal of the septic focus may be life saving.[220] Under these conditions, Hartmann's procedure remains the best option. Unfortunately, morbidity may still exceed 70% with a mortality of 2% to 28%, depending on the severity of sepsis and concomitant chronic illness of the population.[216,218,220–222] Anastomosis in patients with diverticulitis and peritonitis has been associated previously with a prohibitive anastomotic failure rate,[223,224] but in selected patients without diffuse peritonitis or abscess formation, a single-stage procedure can be performed with reasonable safety.[214,225]

RADIATION STRICTURE

Chronic radiation enteritis requiring surgical treatment occurs in up to 5% of patients receiving abdominal or pelvic radiation treatment for malignancy.[113] The principle radiation effect is a chronic, obliterative vasculitis that leads to ischemic damage, scarring, and the late complications of stricture, bleeding, and fistula formation.[226,227] Radiation doses to the large bowel that exceed 65 to 80 Gray are associated with a 50% chance of significant radiation injury but may take 10 to 15 years to develop, depending on the dose, fractionation, and type of bowel involved.[228] Evaluation of chronic obstructive symptoms in this population should include the possibility of recurrent cancer, malnutrition, and the extent of involved bowel.[229] Management is directed to optimizing physiological status, precisely defining the radiation field, and resecting, bypassing, or diverting the fecal stream away from the injured area using unirradiated, well-vascularized bowel.[113,227,230] Historically, anastomosis in irradiated colon has been associated with a 50% failure rate and similar, associated mortality,[113] but several more recent reports indicate successful treatment of distal radiation strictures.[228,231,232] Surgical palliation in these patients is often possible when skillful technique is employed to achieve modest goals.

INDICATIONS FOR LAPAROSCOPIC TREATMENT

Diagnostic and therapeutic laparoscopy are new fields that may eventually find application in large bowel obstruction. However, because of the dilated, often fragile nature of the colon and small bowel and frequent history of prior surgery, large bowel obstruction has been considered a relative contraindication to laparoscopic treatment. Laparoscopic procedures for fixation of the sigmoid colon have been described[233] as have techniques for colostomy formation, intracorporeal bowel resection, and anastomosis.[234–236]

■ NONOPERATIVE TREATMENT

Recently, several nonoperative techniques have been developed to avoid emergent surgery in patients with acute large bowel obstruction. Transendoscopic balloon dilatation has been successfully used as a definitive treatment for benign anastomotic stenosis[237,238] and as a temporary measure for obstructing colorectal malignancy.[239] Similar to the experience in sigmoid volvulus, endoscopically placed tubes[105,240] or stents[241] through an obstructing cancer allows decompression and semielective preparation of the bowel, reducing the risks of subsequent surgery. Numerous reports attest to the value of endoscopic laser photoablation for both colon and rectal lesions,[242] especially for palliation of otherwise unresectable tumors.[243–245] Photoablation also has been employed to unobstruct the bowel temporarily so that preoperative radiation treatment and later, elective bowel preparation can be achieved.[104] All patients considered for nonoperative interventions must be stable

without evidence for perforation, sepsis, or severe ischemic bowel injury. Although effective in anecdotal
experience, these nonoperative techniques require
careful patient selection, specialized equipment and
skills, and are not without risk. Their appropriate role
in the management of patients with large bowel obstruction remains to be defined.

REFERENCES

1. Horwitz A, Smith DF, Rosensweig J. The acutely obstructed colon. *Am J Surg* 1962;104:474
2. Lowman RM, Davis L. An evaluation of cecal size in impending perforation of the cecum. *Surg Gynecol Obstet*
1956;103:711
3. Welch JP, Donaldson GA. Management of severe obstruction of the large bowel due to malignant disease. *Am J Surg*
1974;127:492
4. Farmer KCR, Phillips RKS. True and false large bowel obstruction. *Baillieres Clin Gastroenterol* 1991;5:563
5. Deitch EA, Bridges WM, Ma JW, et al. Obstructed intestine
as a reservoir for systemic infection. *Am J Surg*
1990;159:394
6. Sarr MG, Bulkley GB, Zuidema GD. Preoperative recognition of intestinal strangulation obstruction. *Am J Surg*
1983;145:176
7. Hunter TB, Fajardo LL, Jarvis JL, Villar HV. Altered gastric and duodenal motility in intestinal obstruction. *Gastrointest Radiol* 1990;15:193
8. Nikas D, Ahn Y, Fielding LP. Sensitivity of colon blood
flow to changing hemodynamic events. *Curr Surg* 1985;20
9. Shields R. The absorption and secretion of fluid and electrolytes by the obstructed bowel. *Br J Surg* 1965;52:774
10. Wright HK, O'Brien JJ, Tilson MD. Water absorption in
experimental closed segment obstruction of the ileum in
man. *Am J Surg* 1971;121:96
11. Revhaug A, Lygren I, Lundgren T-I, et al. Release of gastrointestinal peptides during *E. coli* endotoxinaemia. *Acta
Chir Scand* 1984;150:535
12. Revhaug A, Lygren I, Lundgren TI, et al. Increased
plasma levels of vasoactive intestinal polypeptide in pigs
during endotoxinaemia. *Eur Surg Res* 1985;17:75
13. Arabi Y, Dimock F, Burdon DW, et al. Influence of bowel
preparation and antimicrobials on colonic microflora. *Br
J Surg* 1978;65:555
14. Yoshino H, Abe Y, Yousen T, Ohsato K. Clinical application of spectral analysis of bowel sounds in intestinal obstruction. *Dis Colon Rectum* 1990;33:753
15. Fraser ID, Condon RE, Schulte WJ, et al. Intestinal motility changes in experimental large bowel obstruction.
Surgery 1980;87:677
16. Coxon JE, Dickson C, Taylor I. Changes in colonic motility during the development of chronic large bowel obstruction. *Br J Surg* 1985;72:690
17. Kvietys PR, Granger DN. Regulation of colonic blood
flow. *Fed Proc* 1982;41:2106
18. Wangensteen OH. *Intestinal Obstructions; Physiological,
Pathological, and Clinical Considerations with Emphasis on
Therapy, Including Description of Operative Procedures*. Springfield, IL: Charles C Thomas; 1955.
19. Shikata CI, Shida T, Amino K, Ishioka K. Experimental
studies on the hemodynamics of the small intestine following increased intraluminal pressure. *Surg Gynecol Obstet*
1983;156:155
20. Boley JJ, Agralwal GP, Warren AR. Pathophysiologic effects of bowel distension on intestinal blood flow. *Am J
Surg* 1969;117:228
21. Ruf W, Suchiro GT, Suehiro A, et al. Intestinal blood flow
at various intraluminal pressures in the piglet with closed
abdomen. *Ann Surg* 1980;191:157
22. Enochsson L, Nylander G, Ohman U. Effects of intraluminal pressure on regional blood flow in obstructed and
unobstructed small intestines in the rat. *Am J Surg* 1982;
144:558
23. Chiche B, Dupin P, Louvel A, Leger L. Colectomie
presque totale d'urgence pour occlusion par tumeur col-
ique. *Chirurgie* 1981;107:275
24. Teasdale C, McC Mortensen NJ. Acute necrotizing colitis
and obstruction. *Br J Surg* 1983;70:44
25. Johnson CD, Rice RP, Kelvin FM, et al. The radiologic
evaluation of gross cecal distension: emphasis on cecal
ileus. *AJR Am J Roentgenol* 1985;145:1211
26. Toner M, Condell D, O'Brian DS. Obstructive colitis: ul-
ceroinflammatory lesions occurring proximal to colonic
obstruction. *Am J Surg Pathol* 1990;14:719
27. Scott B, Isbister WH. Ischemic colitis as a complication of
left-sided large bowel obstruction: a case report. *Aust NZJ
Surg* 1991;61:73
28. Coxon JE, Dickson C, Taylor I. Changes in intestinal
blood flow during the development of chronic large
bowel obstruction. *Br J Surg* 1985;71:795
29. Papanicolaou G, Ahn YK, Nikas DJ, Fielding LP. Effect of
large-bowel obstruction on colonic blood flow: an experimental study. *Dis Colon Rectum* 1989;32:673
30. Osborne DL, Seidel ER. Microflora-derived polyamines
modulate obstruction-induced colonic mucosal hypertrophy. *Am J Physiol* 1989;256:G1049
31. Tornqvst A, Forsgren A, Faldt K, et al. Bacterial load and
inflammatory reaction in the bowel wall after colonic obstruction: an experimental study in rats. *Eur J Surg* 1991;
157:539
32. Roediger WE. Role of anaerobic bacteria in the metabolic welfare of the colonic mucosa in man. *Gut* 1980;21:
793
33. Schrock TR, Deveney CW, Dunphy JE. Factors contributing to leakage of colonic anastomosis. *Ann Surg* 1973;
177:513
34. Hawley PR. Causes and prevention of colonic anastomotic
breakdown. *Dis Colon Rectum* 1973;16:272
35. Curley SA, Allison DC, Smith DE, Doberneck RC. Analysis of techniques and results in 347 consecutive colon
anastomoses. *Am J Surg* 1988;155:597
36. Irvin TT, Goligher JC. Etology of disruption of intestinal
anastomosis. *Br J Surg* 1973;60:461
37. Jex RK, van Heerden JA, Wolff BG, et al. Gastrointestinal
anastomoses: factors affecting early complications. *Ann
Surg* 1987;206:138
38. Polglase AL, Hughes ESR, McDermott FT, et al. A com-

parison of end-to-end staple and suture colorectal anastomosis in the dog. *Surg Gynecol Obstet* 1981;152:792

39. Waxman BP. Large bowel anastomoses, II. the circular staplers. *Br J Surg* 1983;70:64

40. Khoury GA, Waxman BP. Large bowel anastomoses, I. the healing process and sutured anastomoses: a review. *Br J Surg* 1983;70:61

41. Koruda MJ, Rolandelli RH. Experimental studies on the healing of colonic anastomoses. *J Surg Res* 1990;48:504

42. Brasken P. Healing of experimental colon anastomosis. *Eur J Surg Suppl* 1991;566:1

43. Smith SRG, Connolly JC, Gilmore OJA. The effect of faecal loading on colonic anastomotic healing. *Br J Surg* 1983;70:49

44. Ehrlich HP, Hunt TK. Effects of cortisone and vitamin A on wound healing. *Ann Surg* 1968;167:324

45. Cronin K, Jackson DS, Dunphy JE. Changing bursting strength and collagen content of the healing colon. *Surg Gynecol Obstet* 1968;126:747

46. Wise L, Mcalister W, Stein T, Schuck P. Studies on the healing of anastomosis of small and large intestine. *Surg Gynecol Obstet* 1975;141:190

47. Agrez MV. Control of collagen strength in bowel anastomoses: correct status and future prospects. *Aust NZ J Surg* 1991;61:179

48. Irvin TT, Bostock T. The effects of mechanical preparation and acidification of the colon on the healing of colonic anastomoses. *Surg Gynecol Obstet* 1976;143:443

49. MacKenzie S, Thomson SR, Baker LW. Management options in malignant obstruction of the left colon. *Surg Gynecol Obstet* 1992;174:337

50. Stueland D. The acute presentation of intestinal nonrotation. *Am J Emerg Med* 1989;7:235

51. Blomquist P, Jiborn H, Zederfeldt B. Effect of diverting colostomy on collagen metabolism in the colonic wall. *Am J Surg* 1985;149:330

52. Blomquist P, Jiborn J, Zederfeldt B. Effect of diverting colostomy on breaking strength of anastomosis after resection of the left side of the colon: studies in the rat. *Am J Surg* 1985;149:712

53. Tornqvist A, Blomquist P, Jiborn H, Zederfeldt B. Anastomotic healing after resection of left-colon stenosis: effect on collagen metabolism and anastomotic strength. An experimental study in the rat. *Dis Colon Rectum* 1990;33:217

54. Foster ME, Johnson CD, Billings PJ, et al. Intraoperative antegrade lavage and anastomotic healing in acute colonic obstruction. *Dis Colon Rectum* 1986;29:255

55. Tucson JRD, Everett WG. A retrospective study of colostomies, leaks and stricures after colorectal anastomosis. *Int J Colorectal Dis* 1990;5:44

56. Fielding LP, Stewart-Brown S, Blesovsky L, Kearney G. Anastomotic integrity in patients treated for large bowel cancer: a multicentre study. *Br Med J* 1980;281:411

57. Ericksen AS, Krasna MJ, Mast BA, et al. Use of gastrointestinal contrast studies in obstruction of the small and large bowel. *Dis Colon Rectum* 1990;33:56

58. Kaufman Z, Eiltch E, Dinbar A. Completely obstructive colorectal cancer. *J Surg Oncol* 1989;41:230

59. Matheson NA. Management of obstructed and perforated large bowel carcinoma. *Baillieres Clin Gastroenterol* 1989;3:671

60. Myrvold HE. Surgical procedures in colorectal cancer emergencies. *Scand J Gastroenterol* 1988;23(suppl 149):120

61. Buechter KJ, Boustany C, Caillouette R, Cohn IJ. Surgical management of the acutely obstructed colon: a review of 127 cases. *Am J Surg* 1988;156:163

62. Feller E, Schiffman FJ. Colonic obstruction as the first manifestation of ovarian carcinoma. *Am J Gastroenterol* 1987;82:25

63. Macerollo P, Segal I, Epstein B, et al. Total obstruction of the ascending colon complicating acute pancreatitis. *Am J Gastroenterol* 1983;78:28

64. Hudson DA, de Beer JD. Acute large bowel obstruction complicating acute pancreatitis. *South Med J* 1988;81:804

65. Graham B, Mazier WP. Diagnosis and management of endometriosis of the colon and rectum. *Dis Colon Rectum* 1988;31:952

66. Petros JG, Spirito N, Gosshein R. Endometriosis causing colon obstruction in two postmenopausal women. *Mt Sinai J Med* 1992;59:362

67. Fisher WE, Holden CR, Salt WB. Gallstone obstruction of the colon: thorough treatment prevents serious complications. *Postgrad Med* 1992;91:249

68. Fellows IW, Clarke JM, Roberts PF. Nonsteroidal antiinflammatory drug-induced jejunal and colonic diaphragm disease: a report of two cases. *Gut* 1992;33:1424

69. Theuer C, Cheadle WG. Volvulus of the colon. *Am Surg* 1991;57:145

70. Arigbabu AO, Badejo OA, Akinola DO. Colonoscopy in the emergency treatment of colonic volvulus in Nigeria. *Dis Colon Rectum* 1985;28:795

71. Friedman JD, Odland MD, Bubrick MP. Experience with colonic volvulus. *Dis Colon Rectum* 1989;32:409

72. Hiltunen KM, Syrja H, Matikainen M. Colonic volvulus. Diagnosis and results of treatment in 82 patients. *Eur J Surg* 1992;158:607

73. Jones IT, Fazio VW. Colonic volvulus. Etiology and management. *Dig Dis* 1989;7:203

74. Ballantyne GH. Review of sigmoid volvulus: history and results of treatment. *Dis Colon Rectum* 1982;25:494

75. Vanek VW, Al Salti M. Acute pseudo-obstruction of the colon (Ogilvie's syndrome). An analysis of 400 cases. *Dis Colon Rectum* 1986;29:203

76. Strodel WE, Brothers T. Colonoscopic decompression of pseudo-obstruction and volvulus. *Surg Clin North Am* 1989;69:1327

77. Bode WE, Beart RWJ, Spencer RJ, et al. Colonoscopic decompression for acute pseudo-obstruction of the colon (Ogilvie's syndrome). *Am J Surg* 1984;147:243

78. Sjodahl R, Franz'en T, Nystrom PO. Primary versus staged resection for acute obstructing colorectal carcinoma. *Br J Surg* 1992;79:685

79. Bat L, Neumann G, Shemesh E. The association of synchronous neoplasms with occluding colorectal cancer. *Dis Colon Rectum* 1985;28:149

80. Irvin TT, Greaney MG. Duration of symptoms and prognosis of carcinoma of the colon and rectum. *Surg Gynecol Obstet* 1977;144:883

81. Huddy SP, Shorthouse AJ, Marks CG. The surgical treatment of intestinal obstruction due to left sided carcinoma of the colon. *Ann R Coll Surg Engl* 1988;70:40

82. Aldridge MC, Phillips RKS, Hittinger R, et al. Influence of tumor site on presentation, management and subsequent outcome in large bowel cancer. *Br J Surg* 1986;73:663

83. Phillips RKS, Hittinger R, Fry JS, Fielding LP. Malignant large bowel obstruction. *Br J Surg* 1985;72:296

84. Leitman IM, Sullivan JD, Brams D, DeCosse JJ. Multivariate analysis of morbidity and mortality from the initial surgical management of obstructing carcinoma of the colon. *Surg Gynecol Obstet* 1992;174:513

85. Megibow AJ, Balthazar EJ, Cho KC, et al. Bowel obstruction: evaluation with CT. *Radiology* 1991;180:313

86. Schwab FJ, Glick SN, Teplick SK. Reduction of cecal volvulus by multiple barium enemas. *Gastrointest Radiol* 1985;10:185

87. Chapman AH, McNamara M, Porter G. The acute contrast enema in suspected large bowel obstruction: value and technique. *Clin Radiol* 1992;46:273

88. Stewart J, Finan PJ, Courtney DF, Brennan TG. Does a water soluble contrast enema assist in the management of acute large bowel obstruction: a prospective study of 117 cases. *Br J Surg* 1984;71:799

89. Siebert TL, Finby N. Roetgenographic appraisal of large bowel obstruction in adults. *Am J Surg* 1962;104:490

90. Coleman MJ, Hugh TB, May RE, Jensen MJ. Intussusception in the adult. *Aust NZ J Surg* 1981;51:179

91. Young WS, Engelbrecht HE, Stoker A. Plain film analysis in sigmoid volvulus. *Clin Radiol* 1978;29:553

92. Gilbeau JP, Vanhaudenarde C, Sergent H, Pringot J. Volvulus of the caecum. *J Belge Radiol* 1988;71:726

93. Levine MS. Plain film diagnosis of the acute abdomen. *Emerg Med Clin North Am* 1985;3:541

94. Doris PE, Strauss RW. The expanded role of the barium enema in the evaluation of patients presenting with acute abdominal pain. *J Emerg Med* 1985;3:93

95. Gotta C, Palau GA, Demos TC, et al. Colonic stenoses: use of oral barium when retrograde flow is completely obstructed on barium enema studies. *Radiology* 1990; 177:703

96. Hachigian MP, Honickman S, Eisenstat TE, et al. Computed tomography in the initial management of acute left-sided diverticulitis. *Dis Colon Rectum* 1992;35:1123

97. Maglinte DD, Herlinger H, Nolan DJ. Radiologic features of closed-loop obstruction: analysis of 25 confirmed cases. *Radiology* 1991;179:383

98. Balthazar EJ, Birnbaum BA, Megibow AJ, et al. Closed-loop and strangulating intestinal obstruction: CT signs. *Radiology* 1992;185:769

99. Alpern MB, Glazer GM, Francis IR. Ischemic or infarcted bowel: CT findings. *Radiology* 1988;166:149

100. Smerud MJ, Johnson CD, Stephens DH. Diagnosis of bowel infarction: a comparison of plain films and CT scans in 23 cases. *AJR Am J Roentgenol* 1990;154:99

101. Knechtle SJ, Davidoff AM, Rice RP. Pneumatosis intestinalis. Surgical management and clinical outcome. *Ann Surg* 1990;212:160

102. Shaff MI, Himmelfarb E, Sacks GA, et al. The whirl sign: a CT finding in volvulus of the large bowel. *J Comput Assist Tomogr* 1985;9:410

103. King DW, Lubowski DZ, Armstrong AS. Sigmoid stricture at colonoscopy—an indication for surgery. *Int J Colorectal Dis* 1990;5:161

104. Kiefhaber P, Kiefhaber K, Huber F. Preoperative neodymium-YAG:laser treatment of obstructive colon cancer. *Endoscopy* 1986;18(suppl 1):44

105. Lelcuk S, Ratan J, Klausner JM, et al. Endoscopic decompression of acute colonic obstruction: avoiding staged surgery. *Ann Surg* 1986;203:292

106. Munro A, Youngson GG. Colonoscopy in the diagnosis and treatment of colonic pseudo-obstruction. *J R Coll Surg Edinb* 1983;28:391

107. Gandrup P, Lund L, Balslev I. Surgical treatment of acute malignant large bowel obstruction. *Eur J Surg* 1992;158:427

108. Gorbach SL. Antimicrobial prophylaxis for appendectomy and colorectal surgery. *Rev Infect Dis* 1991;13(suppl 10):S815

109. Coppa GF, Eng K. Factors involved in antibiotic selection in elective colon and rectal surgery. *Surgery* 1988;104:853

110. Tartter PI. Determinants of postoperative stay in patients with colorectal cancer: implications for diagnostic-related groups. *Dis Colon Rectum* 1988;31:694

111. Dorudi S, Wilson NM, Heddle RM. Primary restorative colectomy in malignant left-sided large bowel obstruction. *Ann R Coll Surg Engl* 1990;72:393

112. Wangensteen OH. Evolution of surgery for large-intestinal obstruction. *Dis Colon Rectum* 1978;21:135

113. Galland RB, Spencer J. Natural history and surgical management of radiation enteritis. *Br J Surg* 1987;74:742

114. Goligher JC, Smiddy FG. The treatment of acute obstruction or perforation with carcinoma of the colon and rectum. *Br J Surg* 1957;45:270

115. Becker WF. Acute obstruction of the colon. *Surg Gynecol Obstet* 1953;96:677

116. Ulin AW, Ehrlich EW. Current views related to management of large bowel obstruction caused by carcinoma of the colon. *Am J Surg* 1962;104:463

117. Wara P, Sorenson K, Berg V. Proximal fecal diversion: review of ten years experience. *Dis Colon Rectum* 1981; 24:114

118. Fielding LP, Wells BW. Survival after primary and after staged resection for large bowel obstruction caused by cancer. *Br J Surg* 1974;61:16

119. Irvin TT, Greany MG. The treatment of colonic cancer presenting with intestinal obstruction. *Br J Surg* 1977; 64:741

120. Koruth NM, Hunter DC, Krukowski ZH, Matheson NA. Immediate resection in emergency large bowel surgery: a 7 year audit. *Br J Surg* 1985;72:703

121. Valerio D, Jones PF. Immediate resection in the treatment of large bowel emergencies. *Br J Surg* 1978;65:712

122. Ryan P. The effect of surrounding infection upon the healing of colonic wounds: experimental studies and clinical experience. *Dis Colon Rectum* 1970;13:124

123. Debas HT, Thomson FB. A critical review of colectomy with anastomosis. *Surg Gynecol Obstet* 1972;135:747

124. Dudley HAF, Radcliff AG, McGeehan D. Intraoperative

irrigation of the colon to permit primary anastomosis. *Br J Surg* 1980;67:80

125. Carty NJ, Corder AP, Johnson CD. Colostomy is no longer appropriate in the management of uncomplicated large bowel obstruction: true of false? *Ann R Coll Surg Engl* 1993;75:46

126. Gutman M, Kaplan O, Skornick Y, et al. Proximal colostomy: still an effective emergency measure in obstructing carcinoma of the large bowel. *J Surg Oncol* 1989;41:210

127. Mileski WJ, Rege RV, Joehl RJ, Nahrwold DL. Rates of morbidity and mortality after closure of loop and end colostomy. *Surg Gynecol Obstet* 1990;171:17

128. Brewer MS, Brewer RJ. Tube cecostomy for obstructing cancer of the left colon. *J Ky Med Assoc* 1993;91:14

129. Avots-Avotins KV, Waugh DE. Colon volvulus and the geriatric patient. *Surg Clin North Am* 1982;62:249

130. Howard RS, Catto J. Cecal volvulus. *Arch Surg* 1980;115:274

131. Rosenberg L, Gordon PH. Tube cecostomy revisited. *Can J Surg* 1986;29:38

132. Hoffmann J, Jensen HE. Tube cecostomy and staged resection for obstructing carcinoma of the left colon. *Dis Colon Rectum* 1984;27:24

133. Corman JM, Odenheimer DB. Securing the loop—historic review of the methods used for creating a loop colostomy. *Dis Colon Rectum* 1991;34:1014

134. Morris DM, Rayburn D. Loop colostomies are totally diverting in adults. *Am J Surg* 1991;161:669

135. Doberneck RC. Revision and closure of the colostomy. *Surg Clin North Am* 1991;71:193

136. Porter JA, Salvati EP, Rubin RJ, Eisenstat TE. Complications of colostomies. *Dis Colon Rectum* 1989;32:299

137. Hines JR, Harris GD. Colostomy and colostomy closure. *Surg Clin North Am* 1977;57:1379

138. Pain J, Cahill J. Surgical options for left-sided large bowel emergencies. *Ann R Coll Surg Engl* 1991;73:394

139. Mosdell DM, Doberneck RC. Morbidity and mortality of ostomy closure. *Am J Surg* 1991;162:633

140. Koruth NM, Krukowski ZH, Youngson GG, et al. Intraoperative colonic irrigation in the management of left-sided large bowel emergencies. *Br J Surg* 1985;72:708

141. Mirelman D, Corman ML, Veidenheimer MC, Coller JA. Colostomies—indications and contraindications. *Dis Colon Rectum* 1978;21:172

142. Livingston DH, Miller FB, Richardson JD. Are the risks after colostomy closure exaggerated? *Am J Surg* 1989;158:17

143. Demetriades D, Pezikis A, Melissas J, et al. Factors influencing the morbidity of colostomy closure. *Am J Surg* 1988;155:594

144. Mitchell WH, Kovalcik PJ, Cross GH. Complications of colostomy closure. *Dis Colon Rectum* 1978;21:180

145. Morgenstern L, Yamakawa T, Ben-Shoshan M, Lippman H. Anastomotic leakage after low colonic anastomosis. *Am J Surg* 1972;123:104

146. Runkel NS, Schlag P, Schwarz V, Herfarth C. Outcome after emergency surgery for cancer of the large intestine. *Br J Surg* 1991;78:183

147. Irvin GL, Horsley JS, Caruana JAJ. The morbidity and

148. Waldron RP, Donovan IA. Mortality in patients with obstructing colorectal cancer. *Ann R Coll Surg Engl* 1986;68:219

149. McSherry CK, Grafe WRJ, Perry HS, Glenn F. Surgery of the large bowel for emergent conditions. *Arch Surg* 1969;98:749

150. Hunt TK, Hawley PR. Surgical judgment and colonic anastomoses. *Dis Colon Rectum* 1969;12:167

151. Morgan WP, Jenkins N, Lewis P, Aubrey DA. Management of obstructing carcinoma of the left colon by extended right hemicolectomy. *Am J Surg* 1985;149:327

152. Antal SC, Kovacs ZG, Feigenbaum V, Engelberg M. Obstructing carcinoma of the left colon: treatment by extended right hemicolectomy. *Int Surg* 1991;76:161

153. Hughes ESR. Mortality of acute large bowel obstruction. *Br J Surg* 1966;53:593

154. Arnspiger RC, Helling TS. An evaluation of results of colon anastomosis in prepared and unprepared bowel. *J Clin Gastroenterol* 1988;10:638

155. Wilson RG, Gollock JM. Obstructing carcinoma of the left colon managed by subtotal colectomy. *J R Coll Surg Edinb* 1989;34:25

156. Hesp FLEM, Hendriks T, Lubbers EC, DeBoer HHM. Wound healing in the intestinal wall. A comparison between experimental ileal and colonic anastomoses. *Dis Colon Rectum* 1984;27:99

157. Brief DK, Brener BJ, Goldenkranz R, et al. Defining the role of subtotal colectomy in the treatment of carcinoma of the colon. *Ann Surg* 1991;213:248

158. Bussey HJR, Wallace MH, Morson BC. Metachronous carcinoma of the large intestinal and intestinal polyps. *Proc R Soc Med* 1967;60:208

159. Bulow S, Svendsen LB, Mellemgaard A. Metachronous colorectal carcinoma. *Br J Surg* 1990;77:502

160. Demeter JG, Freeark RJ. The role of prophylactic subtotal colectomy in metachronous carcinoma of the colon and rectum. *Surg Gynecol Obstet* 1992;175:1

161. Burch JM, Martin RR, Richardson RJ, et al. Evolution of the treatment of the injured colon in the 1980s. *Arch Surg* 1991;126:979

162. Keighley MRB, Taylor EW, Hares MM, et al. Influence of oral mannitol bowel preparation on colonic microflora and the risk of explosion during endoscopic diathermy. *Br J Surg* 1981;68:554

163. Duthie GS, Foster ME, Price Thomas JM, Leaper DJ. Bowel preparation or not for elective colorectal surgery. *J R Coll Surg Edinb* 1990;35:169

164. Schultz SC, Magnant CM, Richman MF, et al. Identifying the low-risk patient with penetrating colonic injury for selective use of primary repair. *Surg Gynecol Obstet* 1993;177:237

165. Shannon FL, Moore EE. Primary repair of the colon: when is it a safe alternative? *Surgery* 1985;98:851

166. Goodall RG. Park M. Primary resection and anastomosis of lesions obstructing the left colon. *Can J Surg* 1988;31:167

167. McMillan I, Bell G. Resection and immediate anastomosis in large bowel obstruction using a stapling technique. *J R Coll Surg Edinb* 1984;29:377

168. Amsterdam E, Krispin M. Primary resection with coloco-lostomy for obstructive carcinoma of the left side of the colon. *Am J Surg* 1985;150:558

169. Muir EG. Safety in colonic resection. *Proc R Soc Med* 1968;61:401

170. Tan SG, Nambiar R, Rauff A, et al. Primary resection and anastomosis in obstructed descending colon due to cancer. *Arch Surg* 1991;126:748

171. Pollock AV, Playforth MJ, Evans M. Preoperative lavage of the obstructed left colon to allow safe primary anastomosis. *Dis Colon Rectum* 1987;30:171

172. Thomson WHF, Carter SSC. On-table lavage to achieve safe restorative rectal and emergency left colonic resection without covering colostomy. *Br J Surg* 1986;73:61

173. Radcliffe AG, Dudley HAF. Intraoperative antegrade irrigation of the large intestine. *Surg Gynecol Obstet* 1983; 156:721

174. Allen-Mersh TG. Should primary anastomosis and on-table colonic lavage be standard treatment for left colon emergencies? *Ann R Coll Surg Engl* 1993;75:195

175. Murray JJ, Schoetz DJJ, Coller JA, et al. Intraoperative colonic lavage and primary anastomosis in nonelective colon resection. *Dis Colon Rectum* 1991;34:527

176. Konishi F, Kanazawa K, Morioka Y. Intraoperative irrigation and primary resection for obstructing lesions of the left colon. *Int J Colorectal Dis* 1988;3:204

177. Ravo B. Colorectal anastomotic healing and intracolonic bypass procedure. *Surg Clin North Am* 1988;68:1267

178. Goldman G, Aladgem D, Kahn PJ, Wiznitzer T. Intrarectal bypass graft in low anterior resection and sigmoid obstruction—an experimental study. *Eur Surg Res* 1988;20:238

179. Ravo B, Ger R. Temporary colostomy—an outmoded procedure? *Dis Colon Rectum* 1985;28:904

180. Ravo B, Reggio D, Frattaroli FM. Insertion of the Colo-shield through a colotomy after completion of a colonic anastomosis. *Int J Colorectal Dis* 1991;6:46

181. Carpenter D, Bello J, Sokol TP, et al. The intracolonic bypass tube for left colon and rectal trauma. *Am Surg* 1990;56:769

182. Falcone RE, Wanamaker SR, Santanello SA, Carey LC. Colorectal trauma: primary repair or anastomosis with intracolonic bypass vs. ostomy. *Dis Colon Rectum* 1992; 35:957

183. Rosati C, Smith L, Deitel M, et al. Primary colorectal anastomosis with the intracolonic bypass tube. *Surgery* 1992;112:618

184. Keane PF, Ohri SK, Wood CB, Sackier JM. Management of the obstructed left colon by the one-stage intracolonic bypass procedure. *Dis Colon Rectum* 1988;31:948

185. Egozi L, Sorrento JJ, Golub R, Schultz EH. Complication of the intracolonic bypass: report of a case. *Dis Colon Rectum* 1993;36:191

186. Irvin TT, Hunt TK. Reappraisal of the healing process an anastomosis of the colon. *Surg Gynecol Obstet* 1974; 138:741

187. Hawley PR. Infection the cause of anastomotic breakdown: an experimental study. *Proc R Soc Med* 1970;63:752

188. Tejler G, Jiborn H. Volvulus of the cecum: report of 26 cases and review of the literature. *Dis Colon Rectum* 1988; 31:445

189. Senagore A, Milsom JW, Walshaw RK, et al. Does a proximal colostomy affect colorectal anastomotic healing? *Dis Colon Rectum* 1992;35:182

190. Tornqvist A, Blomquist P, Jiborn H, Zederfeldt B. The effect of diverting colostomy on anastomotic healing after resection of left colon obstruction: an experimental study in the rat. *Int J Colorectal Dis* 1990;5:167

191. Garnjobst W, Hardwick C. Further criteria for anastomosis in diverticulitis of the sigmoid colon. *Am J Surg* 1970;120:264

192. Yamakawa T, Patin CS, Sobel S, Morgenstern L. Healing of colonic anastomoses following resection for experimental diverticulitis. *Arch Surg* 1971;103:17

193. Hoier-Madsen K, Hansen JB, Lindenberg J. Anastomotic leakage following resection for cancer of the colon and rectum. *Acta Chir Scand* 1975;141:304

194. Brown SCW, Abraham JS, Walsh S, Sykes PA. Risk factors and operative mortality in surgery for colorectal cancer. *Ann R Coll Surg Engl* 1991;73:269

195. Serpell JW, McDermott FT, Katrivessis H, Hughes ES. Obstructing carcinomas of the colon. *Br J Surg* 1989; 76:965

196. Ohman U. Prognosis in patients with obstructing colorectal carcinoma. *Am J Surg* 1982;143:742

197. Datta S, Welch JP. Obstructing cancers of the right and left colon: critical analysis of perioperative risk factors, morbidity, and mortality. *Conn Med* 1991;55:453

198. Steinberg SM, Barkin JS, Kaplan RS, Stablein DM. Prognostic indicators of colon tumors: the Gastrointestinal Tumor Study Group experience. *Cancer* 1986;57:1866

199. Ballantyne GH. Review of sigmoid volvulus. Clinical patterns and pathogenesis. *Dis Colon Rectum* 1982;25:823

200. Ballantyne GH, Brandner MD, Beart RWJ, Ilstrup DM. Volvulus of the colon. Incidence and mortality. *Ann Surg* 1985;202:83

201. Sawyer RB, Sawyer KCJ, Sawyer KC. Volvulus of the colon. *Am J Surg* 1962;104:468

202. Pahlman L, Enblad P, Rudberg C, Krog M. Volvulus of the colon: a review of 93 cases and current aspects of treatment. *Acta Chir Scand* 1989;155:53

203. Arnold GJ, Nance. Volvulus of the sigmoid colon. *Ann Surg* 1973;177:527

204. Drapanas T, Stewart JD. Acute sigmoid volvulus. *Am J Surg* 1961;101:70

205. Bruusgaard C. Volvulus of the sigmoid colon and its treatment. *Surgery* 1947;22:466

206. Orchard JL, Mehta R, Khan AH. The use of colonoscopy in the treatment of colonic volvulus: three cases and review of the literature. *Am J Gastroenterol* 1984;79:864

207. Brothers TE, Strodel WE, Eckhauser FE. Endoscopy in colonic volvulus. *Ann Surg* 1987;206:1

208. Wertkin MG, Aufses AHJ. Management of volvulus of the colon. *Dis Colon Rectum* 1978;21:40

209. Shepherd JJ. Treatment of volvulus of sigmoid colon: a review of 425 cases. *Brit Med J* 1968;1:280

210. Rabinovici R, Simansky DA, Kaplan O, et al. Cecal volvulus. *Dis Colon Rectum* 1990;33:765

211. Ostergaard E, Halvorsen JF. Volvulus of the cecum: an evaluation of various surgical procedures. *Acta Chir Scand* 1990;156:629

212. Geer DA, Arnaud G, Beitler A, et al. Colonic volvulus: the Army Medical Center experience 1983–1987. *Am Surg* 1991;57:295

213. Janardhanan R, Bowman D, Brodmerkel GJ Jr, et al. Cecal volvulus: decompression and detorsion with a colonoscopically placed drainage tube. *Am J Gastroenterol* 1987; 82:912

214. Alexander J, Karl RC, Skinner DB. Results of changing trends in the surgical management of complications of diverticular disease. *Surgery* 1983;94:690

215. McKee RF, Deignan RW, Krukowksi ZH. Radiological investigation in acute diverticulitis. *Br J Surg* 1993;80:560

216. Mortensen NJ, Kettlewell MGW. Emergency surgery for complicated diverticular disease. *Dis Colon Rectum* 1989; 32:849

217. Sarin S, Boulos PB. Evaluation of current surgical management of acute inflammatory diverticular disease. *Ann R Coll Surg Engl* 1991;73:278

218. Rodkey GV, Welch CE. Changing patterns in the surgical treatment of diverticular disease. *Ann Surg* 1984; 200:466

219. Rothenberger DA, Wiltz O. Surgery for complicated diverticulitis. *Surg Clin North Am* 1993;73:975

220. Eisenstat TE, Rubin RJ, Salvati EP. Surgical management of diverticulitis: the role of the Hartmann procedure. *Dis Colon Rectum* 1983;26:429

221. Alanis A, Papanicolaou GK, Tadros RR, Fielding LP. Primary resection and anastomosis for treatment of acute diverticulitis. *Dis Colon Rectum* 1989;32:933

222. Krukowski ZH, Matheson NA. Emergency surgery for diverticular disease complicated by generalized and fecal peritonitis: a review. *Br J Surg* 1984;71:921

223. Botsford TW, Zollinger RMJ. Diverticulitis of the colon. *Surg Gynecol Obstet* 1969;128:1209

224. Botsford TW, Zollinger RMJ, Hicks R. Mortality of the surgical treatment of diverticulitis. *Am J Surg* 1971; 121:702

225. Krukowski ZH, Koruth NM, Matheson NA. Evolving practice in acute diverticulitis. *Br J Surg* 1985;72:684

226. Milsom JW, Senagore A, Walshaw RK, et al. Preoperative radiation therapy produces and early and persistent reduction in colorectal anastomotic blood flow. *J Surg Res* 1992;53:646

227. Mann WJ. Surgical management of radiation enteropathy. *Surg Clin North Am* 1991;71:977

228. Cross MJ, Frazee RC. Surgical treatment of radiation enteritis. *Am Surg* 1992;58:132

229. Russell JC, Welch JP. Operative management of radiation injuries of the intestinal tract. *Am J Surg* 1979; 137:433

230. Morgenstern L, Thompson R, Friedman NB. The modern enigma of radiation enteropathy: sequalae and solutions. *Am J Surg* 1977;134:166

231. Palmer JA, Bush RS. Radiation injuries to the bowel associated with the treatment of carcinoma of the cervix. *Surgery* 1976;80:458

232. Marks G, Mohiudden M. The surgical management of the radiation-injured intestine. *Surg Clin North Am* 1978; 63:81

233. Miller R, Roe AM, Eltringham WK, Espiner HJ. Laparoscopic fixation of sigmoid volvulus. *Br J Surg* 1992;79:435

234. Paterson Brown S. The acute abdomen: the role of laparoscopy. *Baillieres Clin Gastroenterol* 1991;5:691

235. Elftmann TD, Nelson H, Ota DM, et al. Laparoscopic-assisted segmental colectomy: surgical techniques. *Mayo Clin Proc* 1994;69:825

236. Ambroze WL, Orangio GR, Tucker JG, et al. Laparoscopic assisted proctosigmoidectomy with extracorporeal transanal anastomosis. *Surg Endosc* 1993;7:29

237. Aston NO, Owen WJ, Irving JD. Endoscopic balloon dilatation of colonic anastomotic strictures. *Br J Surg* 1989; 76:780

238. Karukurichi S, Venkatesh S, Ramanujam PS, McGee S. Hydrostatic balloon dilatation of benign colonic anastomotic strictures. *Dis Colon Rectum* 1992;35:789

239. Stone JM, Bloom RJ. Transendoscopic balloon dilatation of complete colonic obstruction. An adjunct in the treatment of colorectal cancer: report of three cases. *Dis Colon Rectum* 1989;32:429

240. Rattan J, Klausner JM, Rozen P, et al. Acute left colonic obstruction: a new nonsurgical treatment. *J Clin Gastroenterol* 1989;11:331

241. Keen RR, Orsay CP. Rectosigmoid stent for obstructing colonic neoplasms. *Dis Colon Rectum* 1992;35:912

242. Low DE, Kozarek RA, Ball TJ, et al. Colorectal neodynium-YAG photoablative therapy. Comparing applications and complications on both sides of the peritoneal reflection. *Arch Surg* 1989;124:684

243. Mathus Vliegen EM, Tytgat GN. Laser ablation and palliation in colorectal malignancy. Results of a multicenter inquiry. *Gastrointest Endosc* 1986;32:393

244. Bown SG, Barr H, Matthewson K, et al. Endoscopic treatment of inoperable colorectal cancers with the Nd YAG laser. *Br J Surg* 1986;73:949

245. Tranberg KG, Moller PH. Palliation of colorectal carcinoma with the Nd-YAG laser. *Eur J Surg* 1991;157:57

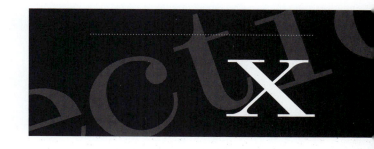

RECTOSIGMOID, RECTUM, AND ANAL CANAL

47

Pelvic Floor Abnormalities and Disordered Defecation

James W. Fleshman ▪ *Han C. Kuijpers*

Pelvic floor abnormalities and disordered defecation include conditions such as anal incontinence, rectal prolapse, internal intussusception, rectocele, enterocele, cystocele, nonrelaxing puborectalis muscle, and constipation owing to outlet obstruction. Disordered defecation implies dysfunctional and discoordinated relationships between the rectum, muscles of the pelvic floor, and anal sphincter mechanism. The anatomic abnormalities involved in these syndromes include anatomic disruption of the anal sphincter mechanism, a redundant mesorectum, inadequate fixation of the rectum to the sacrum, infolding of the rectum into itself in a funnel-shaped formation, and bulge of the anterior rectal wall into the rectovaginal septum.

▪ HISTORY

The history of these syndromes is very confusing. The overall problem reflects a spectrum of diseases, which have been given various names including amismus, levator syndrome, proctalgia fugax, idiopathic anal incontinence, solitary rectal ulcer syndrome, and descending perineum syndrome (Table 47–1). Numerous operations have been developed for some of these problems that often were poorly conceived and have not been completely successful. As seen in Table 47–1, most of the old classifications can be fitted into four major headings.

Amismus, levator syndrome, proctalgia fugax, and descending perineum syndrome can be explained by pelvic floor outlet obstruction and discoordination of defecation. Intussusception, rectal prolapse, and solitary rectal ulcer syndrome are all the result of the same problem of infolding of the rectum and funnel formation. The new classifications simplify and characterize the problems in terms of their underlying physiologic abnormalities, making them easier to understand, diagnose and treat.

▪ EPIDEMIOLOGY

The incidence of anal incontinence, prolapse and constipation is unknown. In our clinical experience, it is estimated that 30% of colorectal practice is related to pelvic floor problems. However, only a small percentage of patients who are evaluated will be found to have significant problems that require surgical therapy. Individuals complain to their physicians at different stages of the problem and relate varying degrees of symptoms for both mild and severe abnormalities. Objective evaluation using defecography, balloon expulsion, and anal manometry is necessary to identify the true incidence of these problems. Even so, abnormal findings on defecography are seen in normal asymptomatic patients and the true significance of these findings remains unclear.

TABLE 47–1. PELVIC FLOOR ABNORMALITIES AND DISORDERS OF DEFECATION

Old Classification	New Classification
Anismus Levator ani syndrome Proctalgia fugax Descending perineum syndrome Rectocele	Pelvic floor outlet obstruction
Internal rectal prolapse Solitary rectal ulcer syndrome Colitis cystica profunda	Internal intussusception of the rectum
Procidentia Rectal prolapse Solitary rectal ulcer syndrome	Rectal prolapse
Idiopathic anal incontinence	Neurogenic anal incontinence

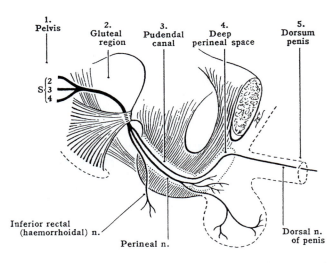

Figure 47–1. Diagram of the pudendal nerve. Note the five regions in which it runs, and the three divisions into which it divides. (From Anderson JE. *Grant's Atlas of Anatomy*, 8th ed, Baltimore, MD: Williams & Wilkin; 1983)

Anal incontinence in women is most commonly caused by mechanical sphincter injury during childbirth. Less than 2% of patients undergoing midline episiotomy at the time of vaginal delivery develop anal incontinence. However, this is a higher incidence than found in patients undergoing mediolateral episiotomy.

The high incidence of constipation and pelvic floor abnormalities in the Western industrialized countries may be related to a lack of fiber. There is no data available to suggest that fiber can prevent these problems. However, fiber is a major component of the treatment of these problems in the early stage.

■ ANATOMY

The normal anatomic relationships of the rectum and pelvis are important in understanding pelvic floor abnormalities. The rectum lies attached by its mesorectum within the curve of the sacrum. The junction of the rectosigmoid is found at the sacral promontory and descends only 2 to 3 cm during a valsalva maneuver. The rectum exists the pelvis surrounded by a sling of muscle from the pubis through a slit in the pelvic floor. The sling is created by the horseshoe-shaped puborectalis muscle that circles behind the rectum and reinserts on the pubis anteriorly. Contraction of the muscle pulls the rectum forward creating a more acute angle at the anal outlet. The anal canal itself measures 3 to 4 cm and is a funnel-shaped extension of the pelvic floor musculature. The pressure generated by this voluntary muscle prevents egress of rectal contents. The internal sphincter muscle is a continuation of thick-

ened circular muscle of the rectum. As such, it is an autonomic muscle and has no voluntary control. The innervation of the voluntary muscles of the pelvic floor is via direct fibers from S2, 3, 4 in the pelvis from the sacrum (Fig 47–1). The nerves of the external sphincter are derived from S2, 3, 4 nerve roots from the sacral plexus and arrive at the external sphincter via the pudendal nerve around the ischial spine at Alcock's canal. The uterus and vagina are closely approximated to the anterior surface of the rectum, but not attached. There is no ligamentous suspension of the rectum or the uterus at the lower aspect of the pelvis. The slit-like defect in the pelvic floor through which the rectum passes also provides an outlet for the vagina and the urinary bladder.

■ ANAL INCONTINENCE

PATHOPHYSIOLOGY

The etiology of anal incontinence can be divided into three major categories: mechanical, neurogenic, and idiopathic. Muscular or mechanical injury usually is the result of obstetric injury, trauma, or fistula disease where the external muscle is divided or damaged (Table 47–2). Neurogenic incontinence may be caused by stretch of the pudendal nerves during prolonged labor, descent of the perineum and nerve stretch during straining at stool, or systemic diseases such as multiple sclerosis, scleroderma, or spinal cord injury. Idiopathic incontinence may be the result of medical disease such as diarrhea in a patient with limited rectal capacity, irri-

TABLE 47–2. ANAL INCONTINENCE ETIOLOGY

Mechanical	Neurogenic	Idiopathic
Obstetric injury	Pudendal nerve stretch	No clear etiology
Fistula disease	Strain	Medical illness
Trauma	Prolonged labor	
Iatrogenic	Trauma	
	Systemic disease	
	MS, DM, scleroderma	

table bowel syndrome, or sedatives that cause poor anal canal sensation in patients with no evidence of neurogenic or mechanical incontinence.

The normal continence mechanism has several components, and normal rectal capacity and compliance are essential. The rectum normally holds between 200 to 250 cc. It distends readily with filling and has limited muscular activity intrinsically. The sampling reflex is a function of rectal distension allowing anal sphincter relaxation via an intramural neural reflex to the internal sphincter. The rectal contents descend and can be sensed in the sensory nerve-rich transitional zone and anoderm to discriminate the true nature of the rectal contents. This sampling reflex occurs frequently throughout the day to provide continence and also serves to initiate the defecation process. The voluntary external sphincter muscle contraction in response to this sampling reflex provides the final active component of anal continence. The subconscious voluntary contraction of the external sphincter, puborectalis, and pelvic floor muscle provide complete control of rectal contents. The pelvic floor muscles maintain a continual activity even during sleep to provide anal continence. This situation also seems to be a learned response, since infants and children require one to two years prior to achieving control.

It is important to realize that the degree of incontinence affects the lifestyle of the patient. The frequency of incontinence may vary and the loss of control may involve solid stool, liquid stool, or gas only. Frequent episodes of incontinence of gas may be as incapacitating as infrequent episodes of solid stool. It is essential to document the exact type of incontinence before planning treatment. It is especially important to define clearly the incontinence before attempting to report a series of patients who undergo a specific treatment.

DIAGNOSIS AND EVALUATION

Signs of anal incontinence seen during office examination include a thin scarred perineal body and a poor squeeze on command. There is controversy regarding the adequacy of digital assessment of the anal sphincter mechanism. It is possible that an experienced examiner

may be able to determine the adequacy of resting tone but it is difficult to quantitate and accurately evaluate the voluntary squeeze pressure generated by an anal sphincter mechanism. The digital and anoscopic examinations are essential to document the presence of a rectovaginal fistula in the setting of an anterior sphincter injury.

Anal manometry is useful to document reduced resting and squeeze pressure as well as sphincter length in individual quadrants. Three-dimensional vectorgrams (three-dimensional pressure volume curves) may be more useful in research settings or for the very complicated patient who has confounded the examiner. Normal resting pressure is at least 40 mm of mercury, normal squeeze pressure, 80 mm of mercury, and sphincter length, 3 cm. Normal sensation should allow detection of a balloon inflated with 10 to 20 cc of air. Hydraulic capillary perfusion of a flexible polyvinyl catheter with multiple radial ports allows a profile of the sphincter pressure to be developed (Fig 47–2). The microballoon and solid state transducer methods only yield global pressures, since there is only one point of measurement. These may be more accurate, however,

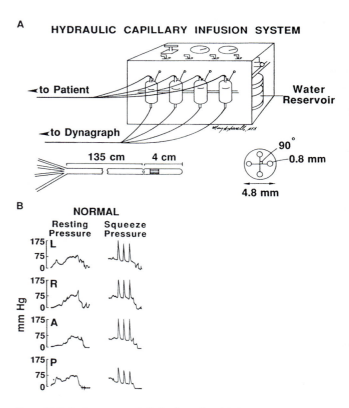

Figure 47–2. Anal manometry. **A.** Hydraulic capillary infusion system and multiport polyvinyl catheter. **B.** Sphincter pressures, resting and maximal squeeze. (From Fleshman JW, Kodner IJ, Fry RD. Anal Incontinence. In: Zuidema GD (ed), *Shackelford's Surgery of the Alimentary Tract*, 3rd ed, vol. 1, Philadelphia, PA: WB Saunders; 1991:349–361)

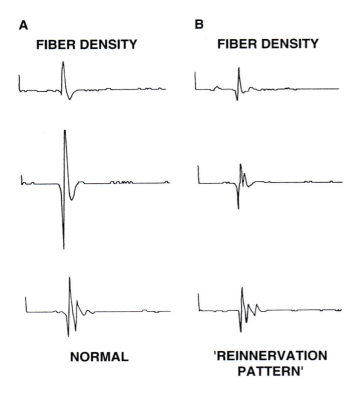

A

FIBER DENSITY

B

FIBER DENSITY

NORMAL

'REINNERVATION PATTERN'

Figure 47–3. Single-fiber needle electromyography. **A**. Normal pattern of motor unit potentials. **B**. Nerve injury patterns of motor unit potentials. (From Fleshman JW, Kodner IJ, Fry RD. Anal Incontinence, In: Zuidema GD (ed), *Shackelford's Surgery of the Alimentary Tract*, 3rd ed, vol. 1, Philadelphia, PA: WB Saunders; 1991:349–361)

since they measure true pressures rather than resistance to water flow, as measured in capillary perfusion techniques.

Electromyography

Single-fiber density determination measures the number of phases in the spontaneous motor unit potential of the resting external sphincter muscle. An increase in the number of phases in each motor unit potential reflects evidence of injury to the terminal branches of the pudendal nerve and reinnervation by adjacent terminal fibers of the pudendal nerve (normal single-fiber density = 1.5 ± 0.16) (Fig 47–3). This is a very sensitive method of detecting pudendal nerve injury but requires a degree of examiner experience. It is also extremely painful to the patient.

Pudendal nerve terminal motor latency determination measures the conduction velocity of the action potential through the terminal 4 cm of the pudendal nerve between Alcock's canal and the external sphincter (Fig 47–4). A delay in conduction reflects injury to the fast-conducting fibers of the nerve. This injury usually is the result of stretch, direct trauma, or systemic disease. The normal terminal motor latency is 2.2 ± 0.2 milliseconds. Any delay in conduction velocity greater than this indicates nerve injury.

Transrectal Ultrasound

The most sensitive method for documenting sphincter injury may be the use of anal ultrasound using a 360° rotating 10 megahertz transducer inserted into the anal canal. The focal length of the anal probe transducer is approximately 1 to 2 cm. A cross-section

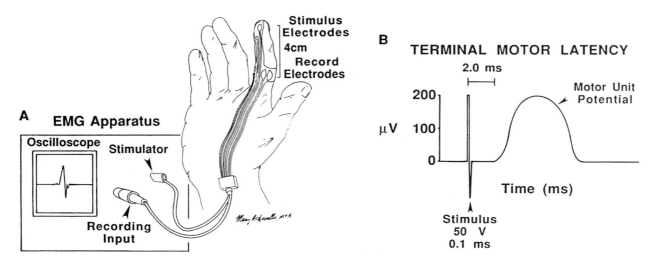

A **EMG Apparatus**

Oscilloscope Stimulator Recording Input

Stimulus Electrodes 4cm Record Electrodes

B **TERMINAL MOTOR LATENCY**

2.0 ms

200

μV 100

0

Motor Unit Potential

Time (ms)

Stimulus 50 V 0.1 ms

Figure 47–4. Pudendal nerve terminal motor latency. **A**. Equipment. **B**. Normal tracing. (From Fleshman JW, Kodner IJ, Fry RD. Anal Incontinence. In: Zuidema GD (ed), *Shackelford's Surgery of the Alimentary Tract*, 3rd ed, vol. 1, Philadelphia, PA: WB Saunders; 1991:349–361)

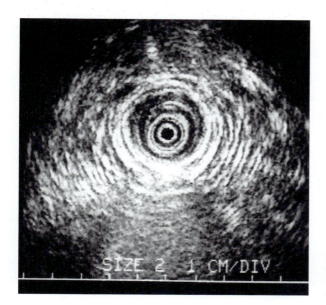

Figure 47–5. Transrectal ultrasound of a normal male sphincter reveals internal (I) and external (E) sphincter muscles. An anal cap covers the 7.5- or 10-MHz rotating transducer of the Bruel and Kjaer ultrasound probe. The innermost dark layer is the mucosa of the anal canal (M). (From Fleshman JW. Anorectal motor physiology and pathophysiology. *Surg Clin North Am* 1993;73:1256.)

image of the sphincter is obtained on each rotation of the transducer and allows evaluation of the anal sphincter muscles in three dimensions as the probe is withdrawn from the rectum (Fig 47–5). Scarring at the site of an injury is documented by the ultrasound. A rectovaginal fistula can also be detected. An algorithm for the evaluation and management of anal incontinence can be produced using these diagnostic techniques (Fig 47–6).

TREATMENT

Anal Sphincter Reconstruction

The injured anal sphincter can be reconstructed successfully in most patients who have an isolated mechanical sphincter defect. The patient requires complete bowel preparation in order to avoid a colostomy at the time of the procedure. The ends of the injured sphincter are identified in the anterior perineum, in patients with obstetric injury, overlapped and secured or reefed in the midline to reconstruct the circular muscle (Fig 47–7). Control of solid and liquid stool will be adequate in 90% of patients after this type of repair. Complete continence usually is achieved only in 75% of patients. Leakage of liquid, mucus and gas may continue to affect the patient after repair. Restoration of normal squeeze pressures are essential to achieve complete control. The presence of at least one normal pudendal nerve is necessary for an improvement after sphincter reconstruction. Complications of wound infection, fistula formation, and breakdown of the sphincter repair are reduced by leaving a drain in the

perineal body after the repair. A repeat procedure is usually successful in those cases where the sphincter repair is disrupted.

Muscle Sensory Retraining or Biofeedback

Operant conditioning, using manometric and balloon sensation techniques, is possible in patients with a mechanical sphincter defect. Electromyographic anal plugs also provide biofeedback for conditioning. Much of the literature suggests a benefit to biofeedback, but does not indicate which patients benefit from a particular technique. Obviously, patients with extremely poor pudendal nerve function or complete disruption of the anal sphincter will not benefit at all.

Neosphincter/Artificial Sphincter

New techniques are being developed to implant an artificial sphincter of silicone or a stimulator that provides constant activity in a muscle transferred to the anal canal. However, the techniques are still highly investigational. As the techniques mature, however, patients with severe neuromuscular damage and even those who have had the sphincter mechanism removed may benefit from replacement of the anal sphincter. The Parks posterior sphincter repair has been shown to give poor results in patients with severe anal incontinence. The only indication at present for a posterior sphincter reefing is in patients with remain incontinent after an abdominal repair of rectal prolapse. The perineal proctosigmoidectomy described by Prasad for rectal prolapse and anal incontinence offers both a posterior and an an-

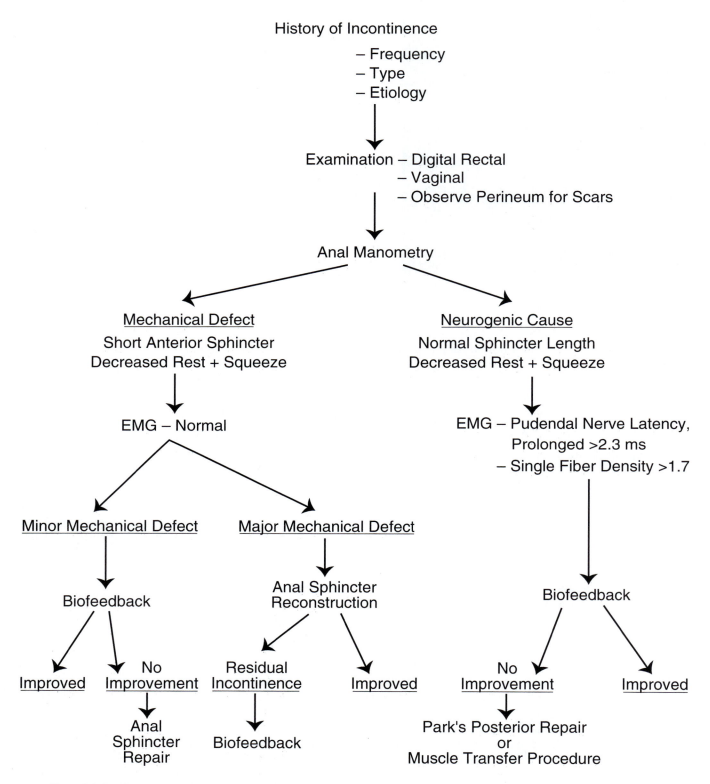

Figure 47–6. Algorithm for evaluation and management of anal incontinence. (From Kodner IJ, Fry RD, Fleshman JW, Birnbaum EH. Colon, Rectum and Anus. In: Schwartz SI (ed), *Principles of Surgery,* 6th ed, New York, NY: McGraw-Hill; 1993:1216)

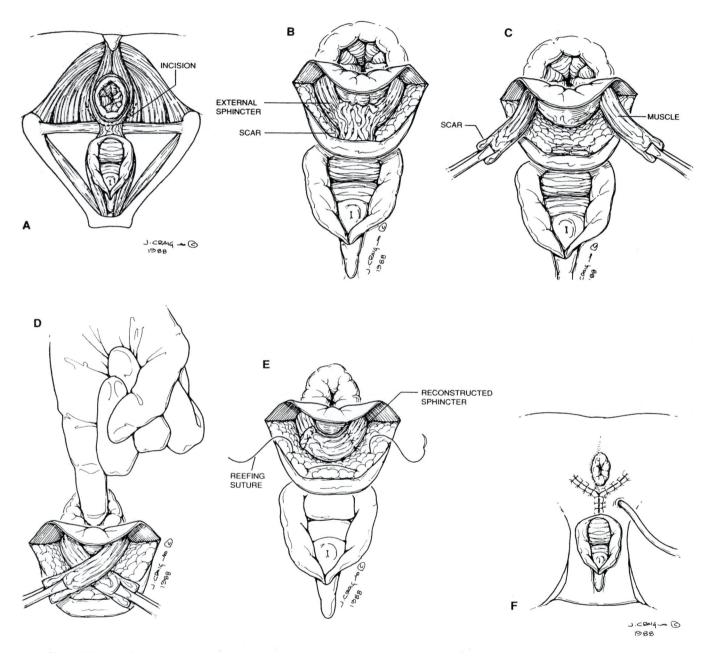

Figure 47–7. Anal sphincter overlapping muscle repair. **A.** Anterior incision and perineal view of muscles. **B.** Rectal flap is created and sphincter muscles are isolated. **C.** Muscle flaps are fully mobilized. **D.** Muscle flaps are overlapped around a 15-mm rubber dilator or fingertip. **E.** Muscle flaps are sutured in place and perineal body repaired. **F.** Drain is placed behind vaginal wall and closed. (From Fleshman JW, Fry RD, Kodner IJ. Anal Incontinence. In: Zuidema GD (ed), *Shackelford's Surgery of the Alimentary Tract,* 3rd ed, vol. 1, Philadelphia, PA: WB Saunders; 1991:349–361)

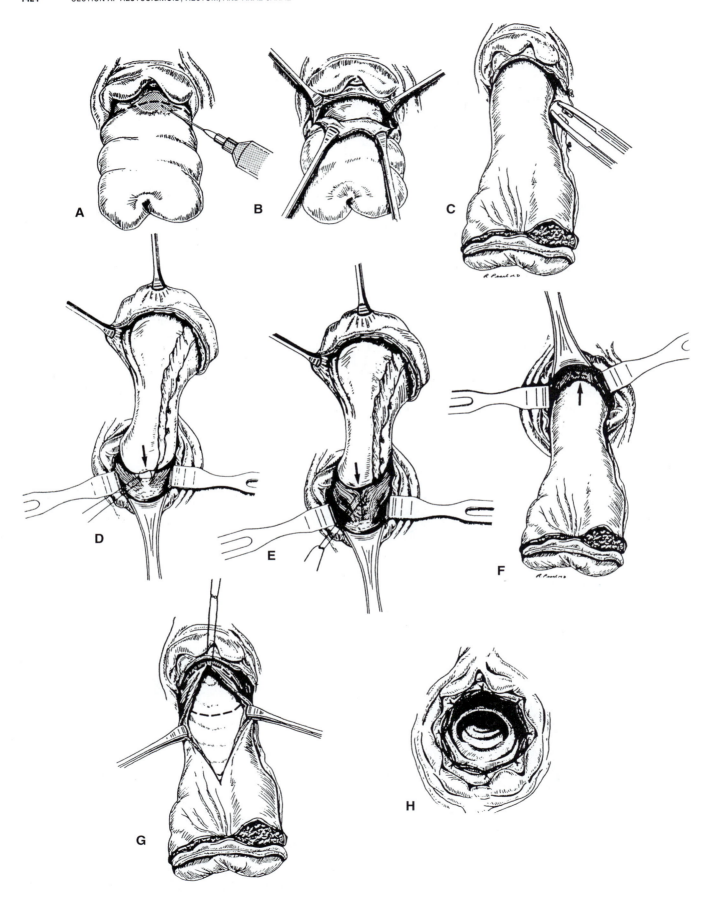

Figure 47–8. Perineal proctectomy. **A.** Patient in the lithotomy position: after applying gentle traction on the rectal wall, a diluted epinephrine solution is injected into the outer layer of the prolapsed rectal wall. **B.** A circular incision is made through the full thickness of the outer layer of the prolapsed segment just proximal to the everted dentate line. **C.** The rectal prolapse has been completely unfolded. The mesenteric vessels are carefully ligated close to the bowel wall. **D.** The rectum is elevated anteriorly to expose the presacral space. A posterior rectopexy is performed (*arrow*) by approximating the seromuscular layers of the bowel wall to the precoccygeal fascia above the levator ani muscles. **E.** The levator ani muscles are approximated posteriorly (*arrow*). This repair pushes the bowel anteriorly to help recreate the anorectal angle. **F.** One or two sutures are used to approximate the levators anterior to the rectum to reinforce the pelvic floor. **G.** The prolapse is amputed and the colon is sutured to the dentate line in a circumferential fashion (*dotted line*). **H.** Completed anastomosis. (From Prasad ML, Pearl RK, Abcarian H, Orsay CP, Nelson RL. Perineal proctectomy, posterior rectopexy, and postanal levator repair for the treatment of rectal prolapse. *Dis Colon Rectum* 1986;29:547)

terior reefing at the end of the repair to improve the tone in the anal canal (Fig 47–8).

■ RECTAL PROLAPSE AND INTERNAL INTUSSUSCEPTION

PATHOPHYSIOLOGY

Etiology and Physiology

The true etiology of rectal prolapse and intussusception is unknown. There are three components that require attention in both diagnosis and repair of rectal prolapse and internal intussusception. The rectum and rectosigmoid junction are unusually mobile from the sacrum. Descent of the rectosigmoid junction into the pelvis allows a funnel-shaped intussusception in the rectum as the rectum attempts to expel itself (Fig 47–9). Poor relaxation of the pelvic floor and external sphincter mechanism also occurs during straining. This outlet obstruction eventually is overcome by continued straining, resulting in descent of the per-

ineum, expulsion of the rectum and true rectal prolapse. There is no long-term data to document the progression of internal intussusception (funnel formation) to full rectal prolapse. However, there are anecdotal incidences in most practices that suggest this possibility. The anal canal is injured during rectal prolapse by stretch of the internal sphincter and/or injury to the pudendal nerve during descent of the perineum. The classic defecographic picture of rectal prolapse and severe intussusception is a funnel that descends into the deep pelvis as the rectosigmoid junction descends (Fig 47–10). This situation causes a ball-valve type obstruction at the level of the anal canal before being pushed through to the outside (Fig 47–11).

Distal mucosal prolapse is occasionally mistaken for full rectal prolapse. The typical appearance is that of mucosa separated by radial lines around the anus (Fig 47–12). Concentric rings of mucosa are seen in true rectal prolapse (Fig 47–12). Defecography is helpful to differentiate between these two entities, which are treated

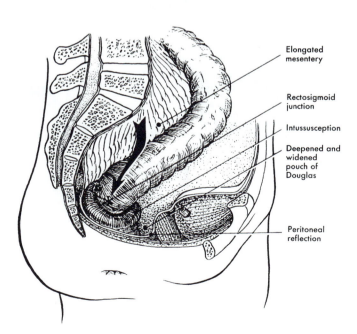

Elongated mesentery

Rectosigmoid junction

Intussusception

Deepened and widened pouch of Douglas

Peritoneal reflection

Figure 47–9. Rectum with internal intussusception. (From Hoffman MJ, Kodner IJ, Fry RD. Internal intussusception of the rectum: diagnosis and surgical management. *Dis Colon Rectum* 1984;27:435)

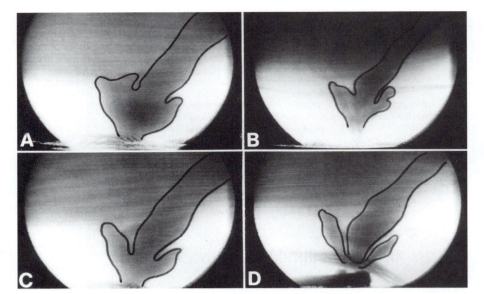

Figure 47–10. Defecogram showing the progression of severe intussusception of the rectum. (From Kodner IJ, Fry RD, Fleshman JW. Rectal prolapse and other pelvic floor abnormalities. In: Nyhus LM (ed) *Surg Annu*, part 2. 1992;24:157)

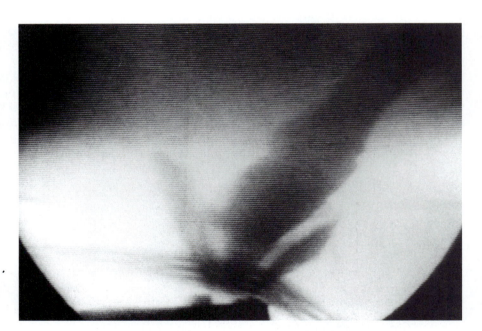

Figure 47–11. Defecogram showing rectal prolapse. (From Kodner IJ, Fry RD, Fleshman JW. Rectal prolapse and other pelvic floor abnormalities. In: Nyhus LM (ed) *Surg Annu* part 2. 1992;24:157)

Figure 47–12. Rectal prolapse. (From Kodner IJ, Fry RD. Anorectal Disorders. CIBA Foundation Symposium 37, 1985. Copyright 1985 CIBA-GEIGY Corporation. Reprinted with permission from CLINICAL SYMPOSIA. (Redrawn from illustrations by John A Craig, MD All rights reserved.)

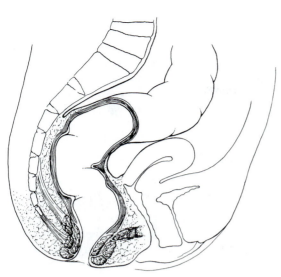

Normal anatomic position
of rectum in sacral hollow

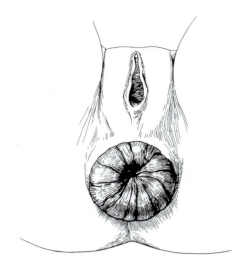

Folds in mucosal prolapse
usually radial in orientation

Loss of normal rectal fixation in sacral
hollow allows lower bowel to form straight
tube, which allows rectum to intussuscept
and prolapse. Deep pouch of Douglas
present; condition may be aggravated by
weak pelvic musculature and lax sphincters.

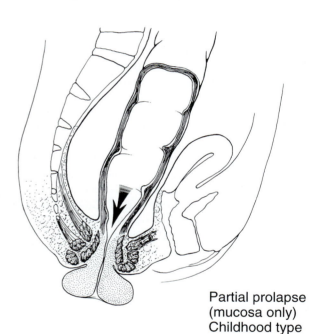

Partial prolapse
(mucosa only)
Childhood type

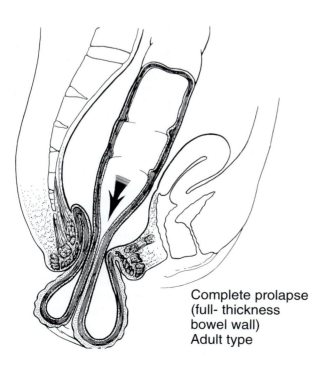

Complete prolapse
(full- thickness
bowel wall)
Adult type

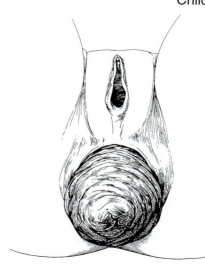

differently. Thickened barium simulates stool and allows reconstruction of the defecating process during cinedefecography.

DIAGNOSIS AND EVALUATION

Symptoms of rectal prolapse include rectal pressure and pain, incomplete evacuation, constipation, and prolonged straining. Mucus discharge and bleeding from the fully prolapsed tissue also may be present. Examination most often reveals prolapsing concentric rings of rectal tissue with a patulous anal canal, poor voluntary tone, and a very mobile rectum within the vault. Proctosigmoidoscopy reveals descent of tissue during straining and, occasionally, an ulcer on the anterior wall. Defecography reveals severe mobility of the rectum from its point of fixation to the sacrum, redundancy of the mesorectum, and the funnel formation as the rectum prepares to descend through the pelvic floor opening at the anal canal. Defecography is not necessary in obvious instances of rectal prolapse. It is most useful in occult cases that cannot be documented or visualized in the office. It is also helpful in cases in which mucosal prolapse is suspected and the intent is to rule out full rectal prolapse.

A grading system of intussusception has been developed to assist in planning management (Table 47–3). Mild to moderate intussusception with some mobility, some funnel formation, and descent of the rectum usually can be treated conservatively. However, grade IV intussusception with severe outlet obstruction may require treatment using operative resection of the redundant rectum or rectopexy, to fix the rectum to the sacrum.

Anal manometry and electromyogram (EMG) is sometimes useful to document the true function of the sphincter. The pudendal nerve latencies provide objective evidence of pudendal nerve injury and allow some prediction of outcome after repair; nerve injury indicates poor recovery of sphincter function.

TABLE 47–3. DEFECOGRAPHY GRADING SYSTEM[a]

Grade	Description
N	Rectum remains fixed to sacrum, sphincter relaxes, and rectum empties
1	Nonrelaxation of puborectalis
2	Mild intussusception or mobility from sacrum
3	Moderate intussusception
4	Severe intussusception
5	Prolapse
R	Rectocele

[a]Lateral view on videofluoroscopy unit of patient in sitting position, passing thickened barium.
(From Kodner IJ, Fry RD, Fleshman JW. Rectal prolapse and other pelvic floor abnormalities. Surg Ann 1992;24:157–190)

MANAGEMENT

Rectal Prolapse

There are numerous techniques for management of rectal prolapse. More than 100 procedures have been described in the past. The procedures can be broken down into basic types which include: rectopexy, low anterior resection, perineal proctectomy, or anal encirclement procedures.

Rectopexy uses some means to fix the rectum to the sacrum without removing a portion of the rectum. Foreign material or sutures attach the rectum to the sacrum. All of these procedures require complete mobilization of the rectum all the way to the pelvic floor and stretching the rectum out of the pelvis to fit into the curve of the sacrum. A modification of the Ripstein method wraps the rectum with enough Marlex mesh to allow passage of sterile proctoscope adjacent to the rectum to prevent obstruction (Fig 47–13). The mesh is stapled using a transverse stapler behind the rectum and leaving 4 cm–long wings of mesh. The wings of the mesh are fixed to the sacrum at the S2, 3 level. The mesh is tacked to the anterior surface of the rectum with sutures. The success rate of this procedure in repair of the prolapse is approximately 90%. An approximately 50% decrease in incontinence has been reported using this procedure. Postoperatively, patients will occasionally complain of constipation owing to acute angulation of the rectum at the sacral promontory. A potential complication has been erosion of the mesh through the rectal wall and subsequent infection and fistula formation.

The *low anterior resection* technique uses the standard technique for removal of the middle and upper portions of the rectum and redundant sigmoid colon. The left colon is reattached to the middle to lower third of the rectum by using either a double-staple or hand-sewn technique (Fig 47–14). The rectum is mobilized to the level of the pelvic floor circumferentially and the left colon and rectum, now in continuity, are returned to the curve of the sacrum. The incidence of anal incontinence may be higher after this procedure because the rectal capacity is reduced. However, in patients who report constipation preoperatively, this is an excellent procedure. Preoperative and physiologic testing may assist in the selection of patients who are candidates for the low anterior resection (ie, those patients with no evidence of sphincter injury or dysfunction).

The use of a perineal proctectomy with anterior and posterior reefing of the sphincter muscle is becoming more popular for the treatment of rectal prolapse. This procedure is a revival of the Altmeyer perineal resection technique. The entire prolapsing rectum and redundant sigmoid are removed through

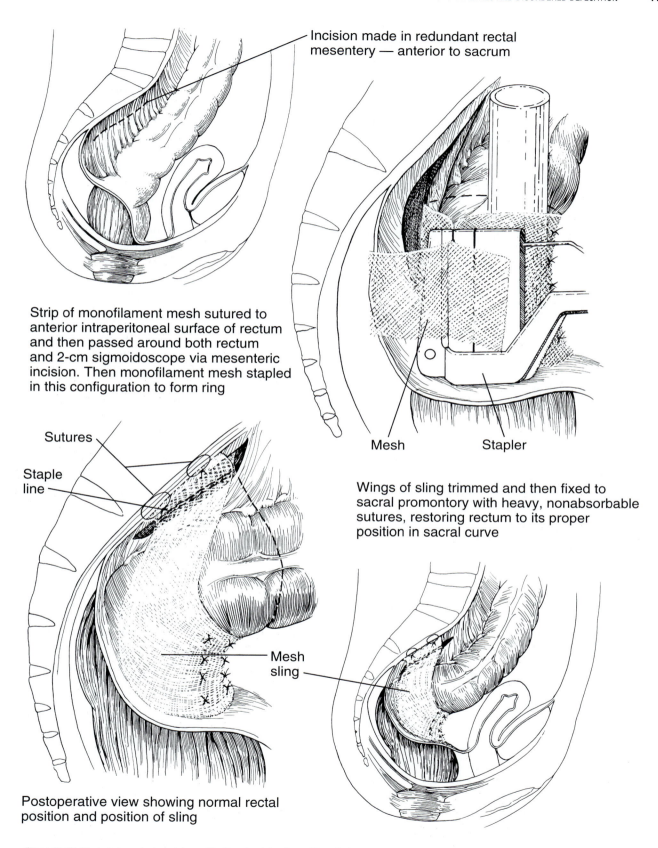

Incision made in redundant rectal mesentery — anterior to sacrum

Strip of monofilament mesh sutured to anterior intraperitoneal surface of rectum and then passed around both rectum and 2-cm sigmoidoscope via mesenteric incision. Then monofilament mesh stapled in this configuration to form ring

Mesh   Stapler

Sutures

Staple line

Wings of sling trimmed and then fixed to sacral promontory with heavy, nonabsorbable sutures, restoring rectum to its proper position in sacral curve

Mesh sling

Postoperative view showing normal rectal position and position of sling

Figure 47–13. The technique of retrorectal sacral fixation of rectal prolapse. (From Kodner IJ, Fry RD. Anorectal Disorders. CIBA Foundation Symposium 37, 1985. Copyright 1985 CIBA-GEIGY Corporation. Reprinted with permission from CLINICAL SYMPOSIA. (Redrawn from illustration by John A Craig, MD All rights reserved.)

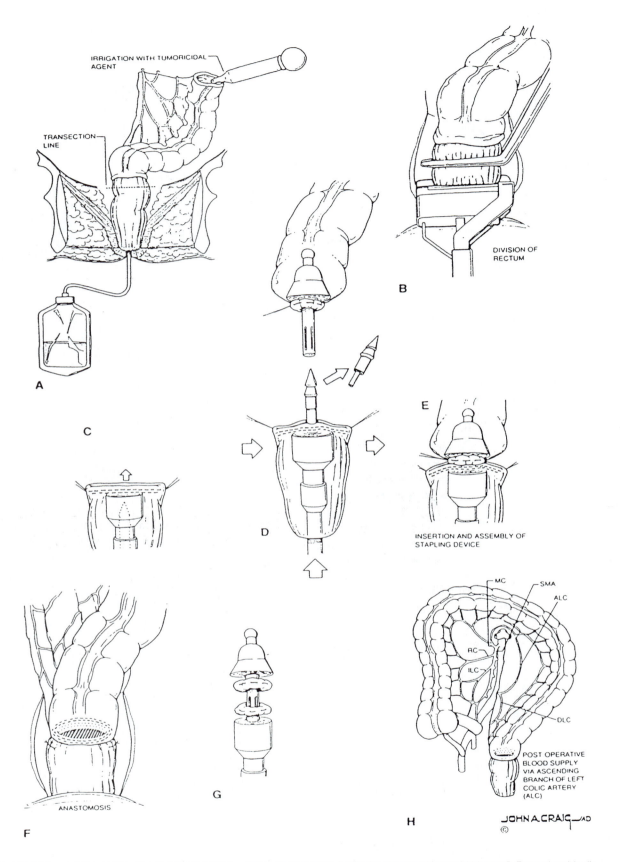

Figure 47–14. Low anterior resection with colorectal anastomosis —double-staple technique. **A.** Irrigation of rectum with tumoricidal agent. **B.** Transection of the distal rectum with linear stapler. **C.** Stay sutures placed in corners of rectal staple line and stapling instrument introduced through rectum. **D.** Trocar of stapling instrument penetrating through staple line: descending colon purse-string suture is tied around shaft of anvil. Trocar is removed before reconnecting anvil to shaft. **E.** Instrument reconnected, reapproximated, and fired. **F.** Completed anastomosis. **G.** Inner donuts containing purse-string sutures and center of staple line. **H.** Completed

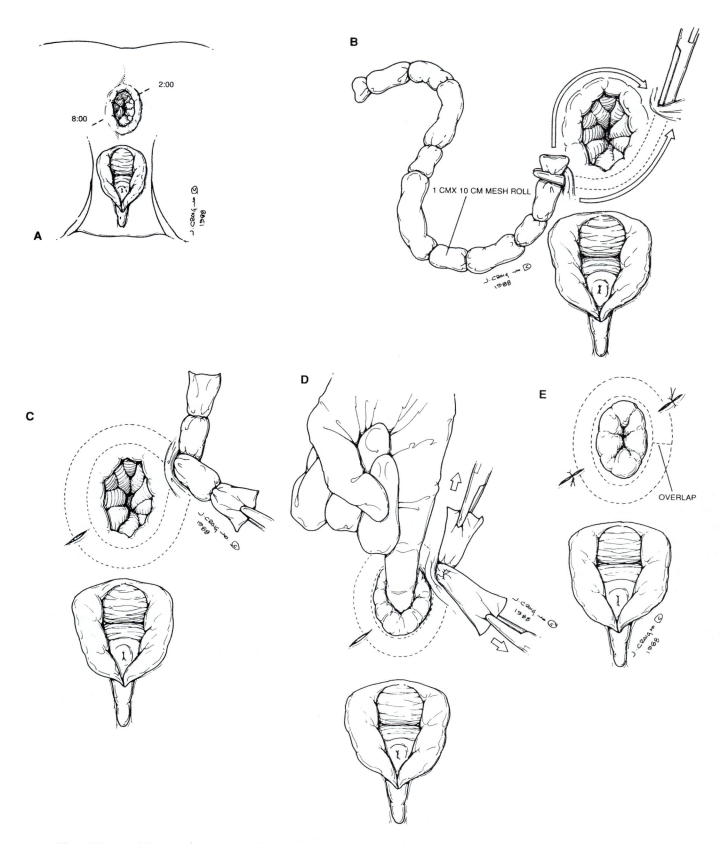

Figure 47–15. Anal sphincter encircling procedure. **A.** Perineal skin incisions placed at the 2 o'clock and 8 o'clock positions outside external sphincter. **B.** Mesh roll tunneled outside of external sphincter through posterior wound. **C.** Mesh is overlapped and tightened to draw in external sphincter muscle. **D.** Anal opening is calibrated and sutured with mesh. **E.** Mesh is trimmed and rotated to protect suture line. (From Fleshman JW, Fry RD, Kodner IJ. Anal incontinence. In: Zvidema GD (ed), Shackelford's Surgery of the Alimentary Tract, 3rd ed., vol. 1, Philadelphia, PA; WB Saunders; 1991: 349–361. Courtesy of John Craig, MD)

a perineal approach beginning at the top of the transitional zone columns (Fig 47–8). The left colon or proximal sigmoid is sutured to the transitional zone 1 to 2 cm above the dentate line. The external anal sphincter and pelvic floor muscles can be reefed in the anterior and posterior midline to restore anal tone in patients with incontinence. The incidence of recurrence of prolapse is approximately 10% and the sphincter function has been adequate. There have been no long-term studies. Even though the operation has been recommended for elderly patients, it may be indicated for patients of all ages with severe compromise of sphincter tone and pronounced procidentia. This procedure is not possible, technically, in patients who do not evert the entire anal canal with the rectum.

Anal encirclement procedures are useful in only the most debilitated patient who has very short survival. The anal canal at the level of the pelvic floor is encircled with a foreign material such as a silicone drain or a 1-cm roll of nylon mesh to create an outlet obstruction (Fig 47–15). The risks of erosion of the mesh, infection, and constipation/complete impaction requiring maneuvers to clear the rectum may outweigh the benefits of controlling the prolapse.

INTERNAL INTUSSUSCEPTION OF THE RECTUM

The treatment of internal intussusception of the rectum should start with a high fiber diet and patient counseling. Once the patient is assured that there is no cancer, high doses of psyllium may prevent formation of the funnel and outlet obstruction. The bowel function is normalized and the need for operation is obviated. If the intussusception is severe or causes bleeding or incontinence, an operation may be the only satisfactory course of action. A low anterior resection or rectopexy is appropriate for these patients, depending on whether they have constipation or incontinence, respectively. The use of perineal proctectomy is not recommended since the sphincter mechanism is intact and the resection of redundant rectum will be extremely difficult in patients with an incomplete prolapse. Prior to operation for internal intussusception, colonic transit times are essential to document normal colonic transit. Defecography will show the surgeon the level of the funnel formation within the rectum as he/she plans the operation. A balloon expulsion test is necessary to eliminate the possibility that the patient has pelvic floor outlet obstruction causing excessive straining and thereby exacerbating the rectal intussusception. This situation also may be the cause of postoperative constipation and persistent symptoms in a small number of patients.

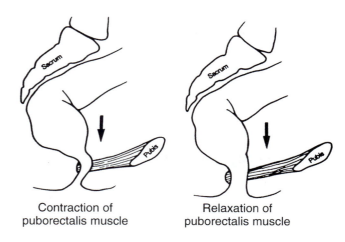

Contraction of puborectalis muscle   Relaxation of puborectalis muscle

Figure 47–16. Normal defecation occurs when the puborectalis muscle relaxes. This normal mechanism may fail in the case of a nonrelaxing puborectalis muscle. (From Kodner IJ, Fry RD, Fleshman JW. Rectal prolapse and other pelvic floor abnormalities. In: Nyhus LM (ed) *Surg Annu* part 2. 1992;24:157)

■ PELVIC FLOOR OUTLET OBSTRUCTION AND SOLITARY RECTAL ULCER SYNDROME

PATHOPHYSIOLOGY

The presenting complaints of patients with pelvic floor outlet obstruction usually include constipation and straining. Defecation is a learned process and pelvic floor outlet obstruction may be either a change in the defecating mechanism or a failure to learn an appropriate series of events to allow normal function. The muscle of the pelvic floor is completely normal but the function and control are abnormal. Patients who have been sexually abused or who have suffered severe psychological trauma may develop this outlet obstruction. A need to dominate and control has also been documented in most patients. The syndrome results from inappropriate contraction of the puborectalis muscle, pelvic floor, and external sphincter during straining to defecate which obstructs the anal canal (Fig 47–16). Attempts to defecate against a closed pelvic floor result in chronic funnel formation of the rectum and descent of the anterior rectal wall into the anal canal. This chronic trauma and ischemia may lead to the formation of an ulcer on the anterior wall of the rectum. The stimulus to defecate is often forgotten. The end result is a discoordinated effort at defecation that causes the pelvic floor to obstruct the outlet even when the rectum begins to distend and the autonomic muscles begin to relax.

It is possible that pelvic floor outlet obstruction is etiologically related to rectal prolapse and intussusception. However, no long-term studies have provided data as conclusive evidence. Patients also may present with megarectum from outlet obstruction, anal incontinence owing to nerve injury from chronic straining, or severe mucosal prolapse/hemorrhoids.

The solitary rectal ulcer is assumed to be the result of ischemia of an isolated portion of the anterior rectal wall, approximately 10 cm above the anal verge, that prolapses partially into the anal canal and becomes ischemic during prolonged straining. The healing process occasionally may incorporate mucosal glands beneath the new mucosal surface and form a localized area of colitis cystica profunda. These entrapped glands continue to produce mucus and occasionally are mistaken for an early neoplasm of the rectum.

DIAGNOSIS AND EVALUATION

Patients with pelvic floor outlet obstruction complain of a number of problems, including constipation and straining at defecation, the need for digital maneuvers to evacuate the rectum, bleeding, mucosal prolapse, and hemorrhoids. They occasionally complain of chronic pain of the anal canal and symptoms that have been designated in the past as amismus, proctalgia fugax, or levator ani syndrome. On examination, they have a normal resting sphincter. However, a paradoxical motion, anteriorly, of the puborectalis muscle is noted during attempts to expel the finger. Defecography generally shows a persistent puborectalis impression on the posterior rectum as the patient attempts to evacuate the rectal contents (Fig 47–17). Defecography tends to overdiagnose the problem of nonrelaxing puborectalis. This situation may be caused by the embarrassment of the patient of the unnatural setting in a cold radiology suite. The presence of nonrelaxing puborectalis muscle therefore must be confirmed using expulsion of a rectal balloon. The method best suited to our practice has been to have the patient expel a 60 cc air-filled soft latex balloon on the end of a soft catheter while sitting in a private bathroom. Some centers add weights to the catheter to document and quantitate the amount of effort required to remove the balloon. However, a simple technique such as expulsion of the balloon within the confines of a private bathroom seems to be adequate. Electromyography using concentric needle EMG may be inaccurate because of the pain of the needle in the muscle and the inability of the patient to relax the sphincter during the pain. Surface EMG may also be inaccurate because of irritation and lack of patient cooperation. However, surface EMG is useful in the treatment of nonrelaxing puborectalis muscle, since it documents decreased electrical activity during proper straining techniques. A colonic transit time is essential to document outlet obstruction. The findings in this circumstance would be a rapid accumulation of all of the administered radiopaque markers

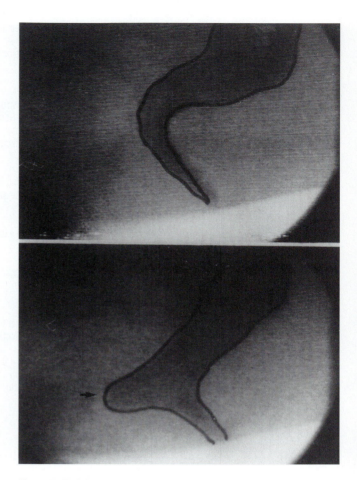

Figure 47–17. Defecogram shows a nonrelaxing puborectalis muscle during straining to defecate. *Arrow* indicates rectocele. (From Kodner IJ, Fry RD, Fleshman JW. Rectal prolapse and other pelvic floor abnormalities. In: Nyhus LM (ed) *Surg Annu* part 2. 1992;24:157)

within the rectum and retention of the markers after an elapsed period of time adequate for clearance (>7 days). An algorithm can be constructed to differentiate between and plan treatment for isolated nonrelaxing puborectalis muscle, nonrelaxing puborectalis muscle and intussusception, and colonic transit delay in conjunction with intussusception or puborectalis dysfunction (Fig 47–18).

TREATMENT AND MANAGEMENT

The initial steps in the treatment of outlet obstruction problems include high doses of fiber and establishment of a normal bowel routine with counseling. Outpatient biofeedback using surface electromyography, balloon expulsion, sensation techniques, and a simulated stool also are effective in severe cases of nonrelaxing puborectalis muscle. Psychological counseling and relaxation techniques may be of help in patients who have a stress component or a psychological component to

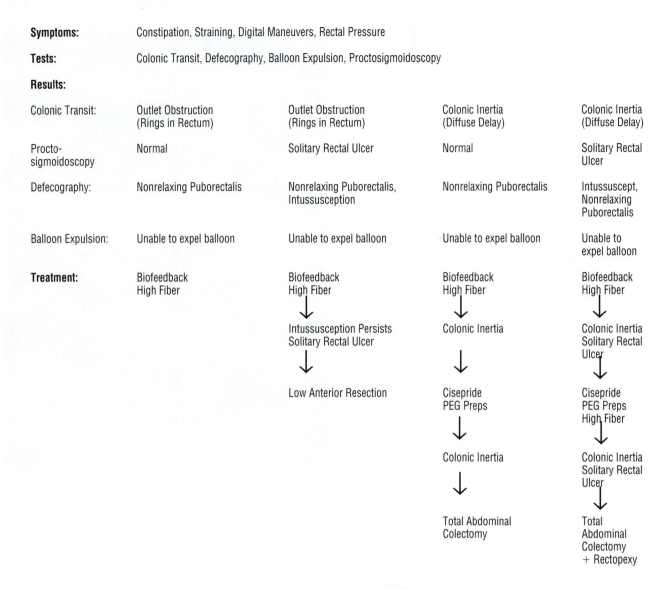

Figure 47–18. Algorithm for diagnosis and treatment of pelvic floor outlet obstruction.

their problem. Inpatient biofeedback has been used effectively but requires a prolonged hospital stay. Operative treatment of nonrelaxing puborectalis muscle is ineffective and results in total incontinence if the puborectalis muscle is divided laterally. Injection of *Botulinum* toxin into the puborectalis muscle essentially paralyzes the puborectalis muscle but does not treat the underlying problem of discoordinated defecation. Additionally, it may result in anal incontinence.

SUMMARY

Pelvic floor disorders are sometimes difficult to diagnose but, once the diagnosis is made, they are fairly straightforward to treat. Rectal prolapse and severe in-

ternal intussusception with incontinence or a persistent solitary rectal ulcer require operative approach. Nonrelaxing puborectalis muscle causing outlet obstruction and solitary rectal ulcer syndrome owing to mild to moderate intussusception and straining are best treated with medical regimens that include high doses of fiber, biofeedback, and psychological counseling.

SELECTED READINGS

Barnes PRH, Hawley PR, Preston DM, et al. Experience of posterior division of the puborectalis muscle in the management of chronic constipation. *Br J Surg* 1985;72:475

Bleijenberg G, Kuijpers HC. Treatment of the spastic pelvic

floor syndrome with biofeedback. *Dis Colon Rectum* 1987; 30:108

Broden G, Dolk A, Holmstrom B. Evacuation difficulties and other characteristics of rectal function associated with procidentia and the Ripstein operation. *Dis Colon Rectum* 1988; 31:283

Felt-Bersma RJF, Cuesta MA, Koorevaar M, et al. Anal endosonography: Relationship with anal manometry and neurophysiologic tests. *Dis Colon Rectum* 1992;35:944

Fleshman JW, Dreznik Z, Cohen E, et al. Balloon expulsion test facilitates diagnosis of pelvic floor outlet obstruction due to nonrelaxing puborectalis muscle. *Dis Colon Rectum* 1992;35:1019

Fleshman JW, Dreznik Z, Fry RD, et al. Anal sphincter repair for obstetrical injury: manometric evaluation of functional results. *Dis Colon Rectum* 1991;34:1061

Fleshman JW, Dreznik Z, Meyer K, et al. Outpatient protocol for biofeedback therapy of pelvic floor outlet obstruction. *Dis Colon Rectum* 1992;35:1

Fleshman JW, Fry RD, Kodner IJ. The surgical management of constipation. In: Henry MM (ed), *Anorectal Disorders. Bailliere's Clinical Gastroenterology*, vol 6, no 1. London, England: Bailliere/Tindall; 1992

Fleshman JW, Kodner IJ, Fry RD. Internal intussusception of the rectum: a changing perspective. *Neth J Surg* 1989;41:145–148

Fleshman JW, Peters WR, Shemesh EI, et al. Anal sphincter reconstruction: anterior overlapping muscle repair. *Dis Colon Rectum* 1991;34:739

Goei R. Anorectal function in patients with defecation disorders and asymptomatic subjects: evaluation with defecography. *Radiology* 1990;174:121

Hoffman MJ, Kodner IJ, Fry RD. Internal intussusception of the rectum: diagnosis and surgical management. *Dis Colon Rectum* 1984;27:435

Holmstrom B, Broden G, Dolk A. Results of the Ripstein operation in the treatment of rectal prolapse and internal rectal procidentia. *Dis Colon Rectum* 1986;29:845

Johansen OB, Wexner SD, Daniel N, et al. Perineal rectosigmoidectomy in the elderly. *Dis Colon Rectum* 1993;36:767

Jones PN, Lubowski DZ, Swash M, et al. Is paradoxical contraction of puborectalis muscle of functional importance? *Dis Colon Rectum* 1987;30:667

Kamm MA, Hawley PR, Lennard-Jones JE. Lateral division of the puborectalis muscle in the management of severe constipation. *Br J Surg* 1988;75:661

Keighley MRB, Matheson DM. Results of treatment for rectal prolapse and fecal incontinence. *Dis Colon Rectum* 1981; 24:449

Kiff ES, Swash M. Slowed conduction in the pudendal nerves in idiopathic (neurogenic) fecal incontinence. *Br J Surg* 1984;71:614

Kodner IJ, Fry RD, Fleshman JW. Rectal prolapse and other pelvic floor abnormalities. *Surg Ann* 1992;24:157

Kuijpers HC. Application of the colorectal laboratory in diagnosis and treatment of functional constipation. *Dis Colon Rectum* 1990;33:35

Kuijpers HC, Bleijenberg G. The spastic pelvic floor syndrome: a cause of constipation. *Dis Colon Rectum* 1985; 28:669

Kuijpers HC, Bleijenberg G. deMorree H. The spastic pelvic floor syndrome. Large bowel outlet obstruction caused by pelvic floor obstruction: a radiological study. *Int J Colorectal Dis* 1986;1:44

Lubowski DZ, Jones PN, Swash M, et al. Asymmetrical pudendal nerve damage in pelvic floor disorders. *Int J Colorectal Dis* 1988;3:158

MacLeod JH. Biofeedback in the management of partial anal incontinence: a preliminary report. *Dis Colon Rectum* 1979; 22:169

Orrom WJ, Wong WD, Rothenberger DA, et al. Evaluation of an air-filled microballoon and mini-transducer in the clinical practice of anorectal manometry: preliminary communication. *Dis Colon Rectum* 1990;33:594

Selvaggi F, Pesce G, Scotto Di Carlo E, et al. Evaluation of normal subjects by defecographic technique. *Dis Colon Rectum* 1990;33:698

Simmang C, Birnbaum EH, Kodner IJ, et al. Anal sphincter reconstruction in the elderly: Does advancing age affect outcome? *Dis Colon Rectum* (1994;37:1065–1069).

Snooks SJ, Barnes PRH, Swash M, et al. Damage to the innervation of the pelvic floor musculature in chronic constipation. *Gastroenterology* 1985;89:977

Tjandra JJ, Milsom JW, Stolfi VM, et al. Endoluminal ultrasound defines anatomy of the anal canal and pelvic floor. *Dis Colon Rectum* 1992;35:465

Watts JD, Rothenberger DA, Buls JG, et al. The management of procidentia: 30 years' experience. *Dis Colon Rectum* 1985; 28:96

Wexner SD, Cheape JD, Jorge JMN, et al. Prospective assessment of biofeedback for the treatment of paradoxical puborectalis contraction. *Dis Colon Rectum* 1992;35:145

Williams NS, Hallan RI, Koeze TH, et al. Restoration of gastrointestinal continuity and continence after abdominoperineal excision of the rectum using an electrically stimulated neoanal sphincter. *Dis Colon Rectum* 1990;33:561

48

Benign Diseases of the Anorectum

Robert D. Fry

Mankind has been plagued by anal disease since the beginning of recorded history. In 1686, the French royal surgeon Felix cured King Louis XIV of an anal fistula. Fifteen generations later, surgeons still treat anal fistulas with an operation very similar to the fistulotomy performed by Felix. Benign diseases of the anus range from relatively simple disorders such as hemorrhoids to extremely complex problems such as extrasphincteric or horseshoe fistulas. An adequate understanding of the pertinent anatomy is essential for satisfactory diagnosis and treatment of these anal diseases.

■ ANATOMY

The alimentary tract terminates at the anus, which provides continence of flatus and feces. The anus is only about 3 cm in length, and is completely collapsed in the normal patient owing to the tonic contraction of the anal sphincters (Fig 48–1). The anus more closely resembles an anterior-posterior aperture rather than the commonly conceived circular orifice. Posteriorly, it resides in close proximity to the coccyx, separated only by small amounts of fibrous, fatty, and muscular tissue. The ischiorectal fossae are located laterally, and the inferior rectal vessels and nerves that enter the wall of the anal canal traverse through these fat-filled spaces. Anteriorly, the anal canal lies in close proximity to the bulb of the urethra and the membranous urethra in the male, or the perineal body and distal posterior vagina in the female.

It is useful to consider the anus and surrounding structures as a single unit, the anorectum. The anorectum includes the perianal skin, the anal canal, the anal sphincters, and the distal rectum. The three main anatomic points of reference are the anal verge, the dentate line, and the anorectal ring. The distal, external boundary of the anal canal is the anal verge, which is also the junction between the anal and perianal skin. Anal epithelium (anoderm) is devoid of the hair follicles, sebaceous glands, or apocrine glands that are present in the perianal skin, a fact worth remembering when attempting to distinguish between hidradenitis (inflammation of the apocrine glands in the perianal skin) and cryptoglandular anal disease.

The cephalad border of the anal canal is a true mucocutaneous junction, the dentate line. This union of the embryonic ectoderm with the entodermal gut resides approximately 1.0 to 1.5 cm above the anal verge. In a transitional zone of 6 to 12 mm in length, the columnar epithelium of the rectum changes to cuboidal epithelium, which joins the squamous epithelium at the dentate line.

The upper border of the anal sphincteric complex is the anorectal ring. It may be palpated by digital examination about 1.0 to 1.5 cm above the dentate line.

Anatomists consider the anal canal to begin at the dentate line and end at the anal verge. However, most surgeons consider the anal canal to start at the anorectal ring and terminate at the anal verge. This latter conception of the anal canal will be used throughout this chapter.

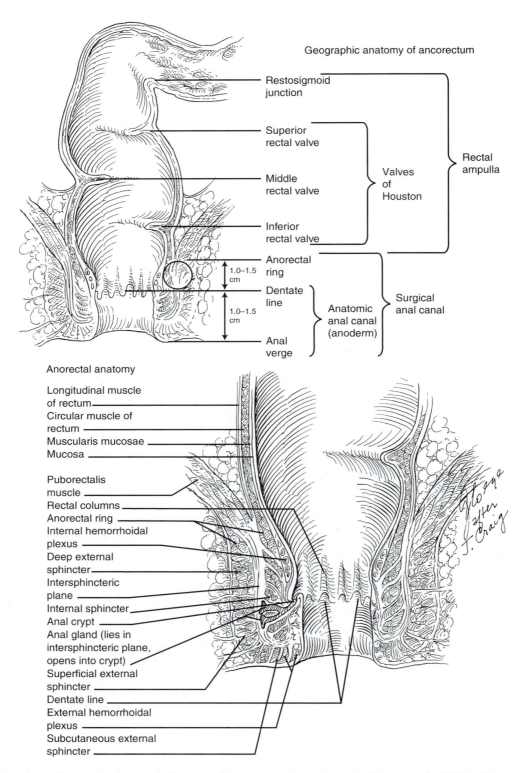

Figure 48–1. Anatomy of the anus and rectum: geographic anatomy of the anorectum and anorectal anatomy. (Redrawn from Fry RD, Kodner IJ. Anorectal Diseases. *Clin Symp* 1985;37:3. Copyright 1985, CIBA-GEIGY; originally illustrated by John Craig, MD)

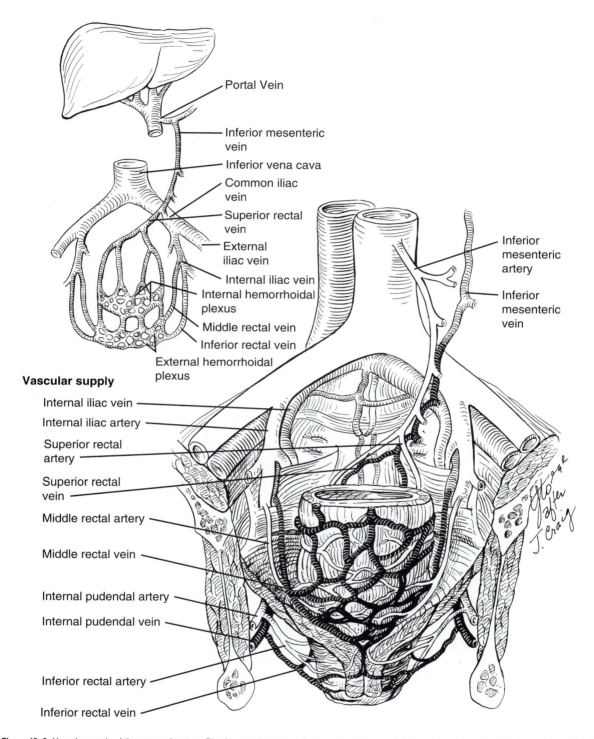

Portal Vein

Inferior mesenteric vein

Inferior vena cava

Common iliac vein

Superior rectal vein

External iliac vein

Internal iliac vein

Internal hemorrhoidal plexus

Middle rectal vein

Inferior rectal vein

External hemorrhoidal plexus

Inferior mesenteric artery

Inferior mesenteric vein

Vascular supply

Internal iliac vein

Internal iliac artery

Superior rectal artery

Superior rectal vein

Middle rectal artery

Middle rectal vein

Internal pudendal artery

Internal pudendal vein

Inferior rectal artery

Inferior rectal vein

Figure 48–2. Vascular supply of the anus and rectum. Blood returns from anus via two routes. Below dentate line, external hemorrhoidal plexus drains into inferior vena cava via inferior pudendal veins. Above dentate line, internal hemorrhoidal plexus drains into portal system via superior rectal vein. (Redrawn from Fry RD, Kodner IJ. Anorectal Diseases. *Clin Symp* 1985;37:6. Copyright 1985, CIBA-GEIGY; originally illustrated by John Craig, MD)

Just above the dentate line, the rectal mucosa forms from 8 to 14 longitudinal folds known as the rectal columns. Between each two columns at the dentate line is a small pocket termed an anal crypt. Small, rudimentary anal glands open into some, but not all, of these anal crypts. The glands may extend through the internal sphincter as far as the intersphincteric plane, but they do not extend into the external sphincter.

The capacious rectal ampulla is located immediately above the anorectal ring. Prominent mucosal folds, the rectal valves of Houston, are found within the rectum. It is often stated that the lower and upper valves lie on the left side of the rectum, while the middle valve lies on the right. However, there are actually a variable number of rectal valves, with variable locations. Since these valves are not composed of the full thickness of the rectal wall, they afford an excellent site for rectal mucosal biopsy.

Two muscular sphincters surround the anus. The internal sphincter, approximately 2.5 cm in length, is composed of involuntary smooth muscle. It is actually a thickened continuation of the circular smooth muscle of the rectum. The internal sphincter is enveloped by the external sphincter, which is a voluntary muscle comprised of striated muscle. The external sphincter is actually a downward extension of the puborectalis and extends slightly below the distal internal sphincter. The internal and external anal sphincters are separated by the intersphincteric plane, a fibrous continuation of the longitudinal smooth muscle layer of the rectum.

The puborectalis, a component of the levator ani, forms a muscular sling originating at the pubis and joining posterior to the rectum. The anorectal ring that is palpable by digital anorectal examination is actually a combination of the puborectalis, the upper external sphincter, and the internal sphincter.

The striated fibers of the external sphincter and levator ani are innervated by the inferior rectal branch of the internal pudendal nerve (S2, S3, S4). The anorectum receives both sympathetic and parasympathetic nerves. The sympathetic nerves originate from thoracolumbar segments, and unite below the inferior mesenteric artery to form the inferior mesenteric plexus. These fibers then descend to the superior hypogastric plexus located just inferior to the aortic bifurcation. These purely sympathetic fibers bifurcate and descend as the hypogastric nerves. Parasympathetic fibers from S2, S3, and S4 (the nervi erigentes) join the hypogastric nerves anterolateral to the rectum to form the inferior hypogastric plexi. Mixed fibers from the plexi innervate the prostate, rectum, bladder, penis, and internal anal sphincter. The sympathetic innervation of the internal sphincter is motor, while the parasympathetic innervation is inhibitory. Injury to the pelvic autonomic nerves during pelvic surgery may result in bladder dysfunction, impotence, or both.

Below the dentate line, cutaneous sensations of heat, cold, touch, and pain are conveyed by afferent fibers in the inferior rectal nerves. Cephalad to the dentate line, poorly defined dull sensations, elicited when the mucosa is pinched or internal hemorrhoids are ligated, are probably carried by parasympathetic fibers.

The superior rectal artery, the terminal branch of the inferior mesenteric artery, descends to the upper rectum where it divides into lateral branches. Subsequent smaller divisions penetrate the rectal wall. The middle rectal arteries arise from the internal iliac arteries and supply the distal rectum and upper anal canal. The inferior rectal arteries, branches from the internal pudendal arteries, cross the ischiorectal fossae to supply the anal sphincters (Fig 48–2).

There are two paths for venous blood return from the anorectum. Above the dentate line venous blood flows into the portal system through the superior rectal vein and inferior mesenteric vein. Below the dentate line, the external hemorrhoidal plexus drains into the internal iliac vein, via the middle rectal vein or via the pudendal vein, which receives blood from the inferior rectal vein.

The lymphatic channels from the anorectum generally follow the paths of the arteries. Lymph from the upper two-thirds of the rectum drains into the inferior mesenteric lymph nodes. Lymph from the distal rectum also can flow to the inferior mesenteric nodes, or laterally, parallel to the middle rectal arteries, to the internal iliac nodes.

Lymphatic channels from the anal canal above the dentate line extend to the inferior mesenteric nodes, but there are also channels that cross the ischiorectal fossa and carry lymph to the internal iliac nodes. Lymph from the anal canal below the dentate line usually flows to the inguinal nodes.

■ HEMORRHOIDS

Hemorrhoids have long been considered to be varicosities of the hemorrhoidal veins. However, their nature is more complex. Current theories of the development of hemorrhoids consider the nature of anal "cushions." Such cushions are aggregations of blood vessels (arterioles, venules, and arteriolar-venular communication), smooth muscle, and elastic connective tissue in the submucosa that normally reside in the left lateral, right posterolateral, and right anterolateral anal canal.[1] Smaller discreet secondary cushions may reside between the main cushions. Hemorrhoids are likely the result of a sliding downward of these anal cushions. It appears that anchoring and supporting connective tissue above the hemorrhoids disintegrates, thereby allowing these structures to slide distally.[2,3]

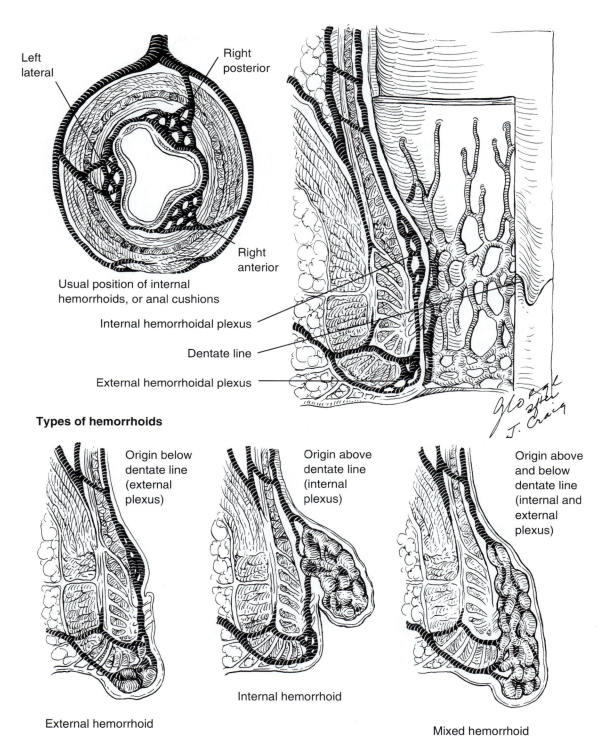

Types of hemorrhoids

Figure 48–3. Types of hemorrhoids. (Redrawn from Fry RD, Kodner IJ. Anorectal Diseases. *Clin Symp* 1985;37:7. Copyright 1985, CIBA-GEIGY; originally illustrated by John Craig, MD)

CLASSIFICATION

Anal skin tags are discrete folds of skin located at the anal verge. These may be the result of thrombosed external hemorrhoids, or, more rarely, may be associated with inflammatory bowel disease.

Internal hemorrhoids reside above the dentate line and are covered by transitional and columnar epithelium (Fig 48–3). Internal hemorrhoids can be classified according to symptoms. First-degree internal hemorrhoids cause painless bleeding, usually associated with defecation. Second-degree hemorrhoids protrude through the anal canal at the time of defecation, but spontaneously reduce. Third-degree internal hemorrhoids protrude with defecation, but must be manually reduced. Fourth-degree internal hemorrhoids are permanently prolapsed and cannot be manually reduced. All four degrees may be associated with bleeding.

External hemorrhoids consist of the dilated vascular plexus located below the dentate line and are covered by squamous epithelium. Mixed hemorrhoids are composed of elements of both internal and external hemorrhoids.

Internal Hemorrhoids

It is important to recognize that the mere presence of hemorrhoids is not necessarily an indication for treatment. Hemorrhoids should be treated only to alleviate symptoms; the best treatment is the least intervention possible to achieve this goal.

Even though internal hemorrhoids are the most common source of rectal bleeding, it is imperative that other causes be excluded. Since internal hemorrhoids cannot be detected by digital examination, diagnosis can only be made by anoscopy. It is mandatory that proctosigmoidoscopy be performed to exclude other sources of bleeding, such as carcinoma or proctitis. For patients more than 45 years of age with rectal bleeding, a colonoscopic examination generally is recommended to exclude a more proximal site of bleeding.

Treatment. Regulation of diet, bowel movement, and avoidance of prolonged straining at the time of defecation comprise the initial treatment of mild symptoms of bleeding and protrusion. Increasing the fiber content of the diet with raw vegetables, fruits, whole grain cere-

Elastic ligation technique

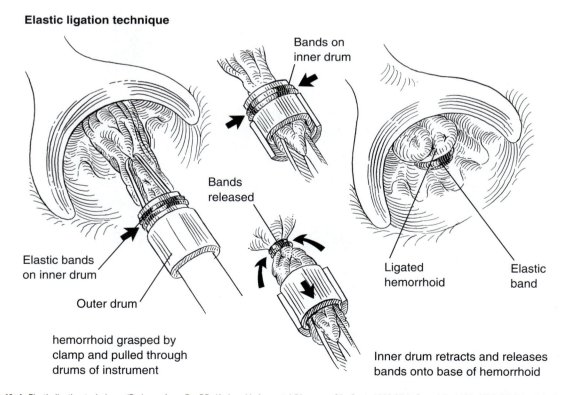

Figure 48–4. Elastic ligation technique. (Redrawn from Fry RD, Kodner IJ. Anorectal Diseases. *Clin Symp* 1995;37:9. Copyright 1985, CIBA-GEIGY; originally illustrated by John Craig, MD)

als, and hydrophilic bulk-forming agents can reduce and often alleviate all symptoms. If bleeding and protrusion persist, however, the hemorrhoids should be treated surgically.

Elastic ligation of the friable redundant hemorrhoidal tissue is quite satisfactory, in most instances. The procedure is quite simple. The hemorrhoid is visualized with the aid of an anoscope and grasped with forceps. The redundant tissue is pulled into a double-sleeved cylinder on which there are two latex bands. The bands are discharged from the cylinder, and the hemorrhoidal bundle thus is ligated. The necrotic redundant tissue sloughs in 5 to 10 days (Fig 48–4).

Certain precautions, however, must be taken with this form of treatment. The ligatures must be placed at least 5 mm above the dentate line to avoid extreme discomfort. Ideally, the ligatures should be placed at the level of the anorectal ring. About 25% of patients experience mild, dull anorectal discomfort, lasting for 2 to 3 days following the procedure. Mild analgesics and warm baths usually suffice to relieve the discomfort. In about 1% of patients, brisk bleeding occurs when the necrotic tissue sloughs off; electrocautery is then necessary to stop the hemorrhage. A suction cautery can be very useful in this instance. About 2% of patients treated with

ligation of the internal hemorrhoid develop thrombosis of an external hemorrhoid, which may cause considerable discomfort.

Hemorrhoidal ligation is an office procedure, and no special preparation is required. Patients with a bleeding diathesis or with portal hypertension are not good candidates for ligation. Usually only one hemorrhoid is ligated per visit. Further ligations can be performed every 4 weeks until all symptoms of bleeding or prolapse are alleviated.

Although diet, bowel regulation, or elastic ligation will alleviate most symptoms of internal hemorrhoids, occasionally, an excisional hemorrhoidectomy will be necessary. This treatment is indicated for large mixed (combined internal/external) hemorrhoids that are not amenable to ligation because the ligature would have to incorporate pain-sensitive tissue at or below the dentate line.

Occasionally the entire ring of internal hemorrhoidal tissue may be incarcerated outside the anal canal, resulting in spasm of the anal sphincter, massive local edema, and severe pain. In such circumstances, the edematous tissue may be injected with a local anesthetic containing epinephrine and hyaluronidase. Dissipation of the edema by manual compression then can be

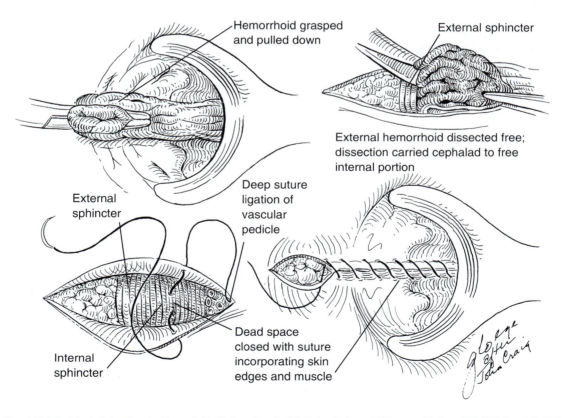

Hemorrhoid grasped and pulled down

External sphincter

External hemorrhoid dissected free; dissection carried cephalad to free internal portion

External sphincter

Deep suture ligation of vascular pedicle

Internal sphincter

Dead space closed with suture incorporating skin edges and muscle

Figure 48–5. Excision technique for mixed hemorrhoids (Redrawn from Fry RD, Kodner IJ. Anorectal Diseases. *Clin Symp* 1985;37:9. Copyright 1985, CIBA-GEIGY; originally illustrated by John Craig, MD)

achieved, allowing reduction of the prolapsed tissue. A three quadrant hemorrhoidectomy then should be performed. The patient should be kept in the hospital after the procedure until the pain is minimal or until spontaneous voiding is possible.

Mixed hemorrhoids

The mucosal component of mixed hemorrhoids occasionally can be treated by elastic ligation. Large symptomatic mixed hemorrhoids generally are treated best by excisional hemorrhoidectomy. The patient is placed in the prone flexed position under local anesthesia. An elliptical excision incorporates the external and internal hemorrhoids from the perianal skin to the anorectal ring. The hemorrhoidal tissue is dissected from the underlying internal sphincter (Fig 48–5). The entire wound is closed with a running 3-0 chromic catgut suture. The largest hemorrhoid initially is excised, with care taken not to excise excessive tissue that may result in a stricture. If there is any question of leaving an adequate anal aperture covered by normal anoderm, it is best to modify a planned three quadrant hemorrhoidectomy to a two-quadrant hemorrhoidectomy.

Thrombosed External Hemorrhoids

These are caused by a perianal intravascular thrombus. The thrombus is confined to the anoderm and perianal skin and does not extend above the dentate line. The problem presents as a painful perianal mass. The overlying skin may be stretched to 2 cm or greater. Pain usually peaks within 48 hours, and generally becomes minimal after the fourth day. If untreated, the thrombus is absorbed within a few weeks. Occasionally, the pressure of the underlying clot will cause the adjacent skin to become necrotic, and the clot will be extruded through the area of necrosis. Generally, this is noted by the patient as rectal bleeding followed by relief of the anal pain.

Treatment of thrombosed hemorrhoids is aimed at relief of the pain. If symptoms are minimal, mild analgesics, sitz baths, proper anal hygiene, and bulk-producing agents will suffice. However, if pain is severe, excision of the thrombosed hemorrhoid may be beneficial. Since numerous vessels usually are involved, it is necessary to excise the entire mass along with the overlying skin and subcutaneous tissue. The wound is left open, and packing is unnecessary. Postoperative care consists of mild analgesics and warm sitz baths or showers.

■ ANAL FISSURE

An anal fissure is an elliptical ulcer in the anal canal that may extend from the dentate line to the anal verge, overlying the lower half of the internal sphincter (Fig 48–6). The fissure is almost always located close to the midline of the anal canal; in men, 95% are close to the posterior midline, and 5% near the anterior midline, whereas in women, about 80% will be located posteriorly and 20% anteriorly. The precise cause of an anal fissure has yet to be determined. However, fissures probably are related to tearing of the anoderm at the time of defecation. A recent study has suggested that the increased anal canal pressure that accompanies an anal fissure is associated with ischemia in the area of the fissure.[4]

CLINICAL FEATURES AND DIAGNOSIS

Most fissures are superficial and heal rapidly with no specific treatment. Occasionally, the fissure may extend deeply through the anoderm to expose the fibers of the internal sphincter. The skin adjacent to such a fissure may become edematous, forming a "sentinel tag," which should not be mistaken for an external hemorrhoid. In addition, the associated anal valve may become enlarged, forming a hypertrophied anal papilla. Surprisingly, secondary infection rarely occurs.

Fissures that are aberrantly located may be caused by previous anal operations that result in scarring, stenosis, and loss of anoderm. Individuals with chronic diarrhea may develop anal stenosis associated with a fissure. Crohn's disease often is complicated by anal fissures, which may be a primary manifestation of the disease. These fissures usually are associated with the shiny anal skin tags typical of anal Crohn's disease, and may lie laterally instead of close to the midline of the anus.

Patients with an anal fissure usually complain of anal pain accompanying and following defecation. Bright-red bleeding may accompany a bowel movement, although it is usually minimal. A slight discharge also may be present.

An anal fissure is detected by gently separating the buttocks to reveal the lower edge of the fissure at the anal verge, where a sentinel tag also may be seen. A deep gluteal cleft or tight spasm of the sphincter may sometimes obscure the fissure, and examination with a small anoscope may be required.

If the fissure is located laterally instead of close to the midline, less common etiologies of fissures must be considered. These include Crohn's disease, leukemia, tuberculosis, and syphilis. If the fissure does not heal after adequate treatment, a biopsy is necessary to exclude carcinoma.

TREATMENT

Treatment depends upon the severity of the pain and the chronicity of the symptoms. Most anal fissures heal spontaneously, and treatment with topical ointments or suppositories is of little value. Thus, insertion of a suppository will only abrade the fissure, is painful, and can have no possible beneficial effect upon healing since

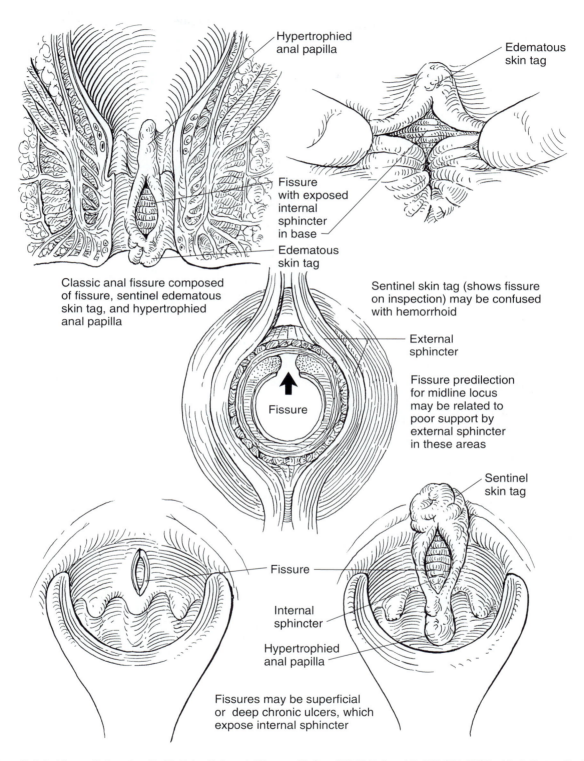

Hypertrophied anal papilla

Edematous skin tag

Fissure with exposed internal sphincter in base

Edematous skin tag

Classic anal fissure composed of fissure, sentinel edematous skin tag, and hypertrophied anal papilla

Sentinel skin tag (shows fissure on inspection) may be confused with hemorrhoid

External sphincter

Fissure

Fissure predilection for midline locus may be related to poor support by external sphincter in these areas

Sentinel skin tag

Fissure

Internal sphincter

Hypertrophied anal papilla

Fissures may be superficial or deep chronic ulcers, which expose internal sphincter

Figure 48–6. Anal fissure. (Redrawn from Fry RD, Kodner IJ. Anorectal Diseases. *Clin Symp* 1985;37:12. Copyright 1985, CIBA-GEIGY; originally illustrated by John Craig, MD)

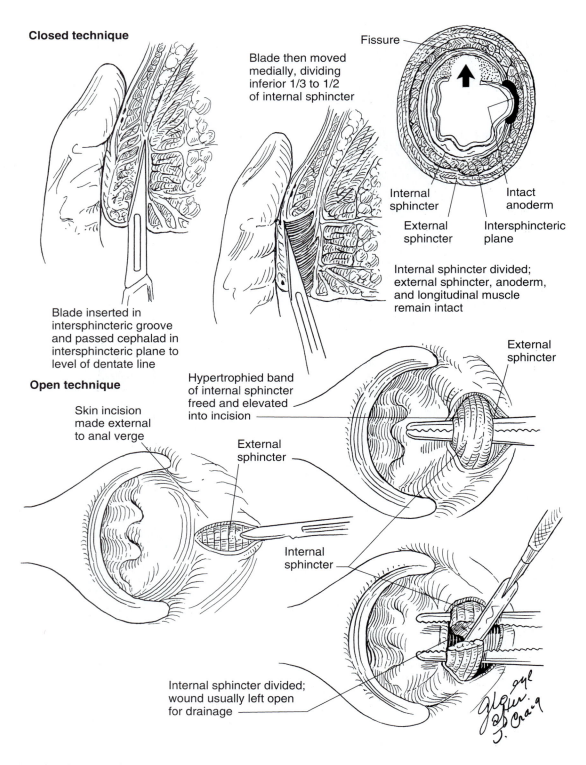

Closed technique

Blade then moved medially, dividing inferior 1/3 to 1/2 of internal sphincter

Fissure

Internal sphincter

External sphincter

Intact anoderm

Intersphincteric plane

Internal sphincter divided; external sphincter, anoderm, and longitudinal muscle remain intact

Blade inserted in intersphincteric groove and passed cephalad in intersphincteric plane to level of dentate line

Open technique

Skin incision made external to anal verge

Hypertrophied band of internal sphincter freed and elevated into incision

External sphincter

External sphincter

Internal sphincter

Internal sphincter divided; wound usually left open for drainage

Figure 48–7. Lateral internal sphincterotomy. (Redrawn from Fry RD, Kodner IJ. Anorectal Diseases. *Clin Symp* 1985;37:14. Copyright 1985, CIBA-GEIGY; originally illustrated by John Craig, MD)

the suppository will reside in the rectum. Dietary recommendations and appropriate prescription of bulk agents to promote a soft stool are beneficial, and warm soaks may provide comfort. The great majority of fissures will heal with this type of conservative treatment. However, deep, chronic fissures associated with a sentinel skin tag and, occasionally, hypertrophied anal papilla require surgical treatment.

Early in this century, excision of the fissure was the recommended surgical treatment. While this approach usually results in healing, an incision in the anoderm of the anterior or posterior anal canal can be quite painful. In addition, incisions in the anteroposterior axis of the anus may cause a "keyhole deformity" that results in anal incontinence. The base of an anal fissure is composed of the exposed internal sphincter; thus, excising the fissure is actually tantamount to dividing a portion of the internal sphincter (sphincterotomy). Excellent results can be achieved if the internal sphincter is divided laterally rather than in the midline. Furthermore, lateral sphincterotomy is not associated with keyhole deformity.

Sphincterotomy can be performed under local anesthesia, using either an open or closed technique (Fig 48–7). The open technique consists of incision of the anoderm and division of the internal sphincter under direct vision. The closed method entails dividing the internal sphincter by a subcutaneous approach. Either technique may be used in the outpatient setting, and both operations afford rapid pain relief. Approximately 98% of fissures heal following sphincterotomy. However, there is a small incidence of minor anal incontinence following the procedure, so careful patient selection is mandatory. Elderly patients with decreased anorectal sensation are generally not ideal candidates for internal sphincterotomy because of this risk.

■ ANORECTAL ABSCESS AND ANAL FISTULA

More than 95% of all anorectal abscesses are caused by infections arising in the anal glands that communicate with the anal crypts (cryptoglandular disease). The acute phase of the infection causes an anorectal abscess, while the chronic stage is recognized as an anal fistula. The anal glands lie in the intersphincteric space between the internal and external anal sphincters. Inflammation of an anal gland leads to the formation of a local abscess in the intersphincteric plane. The clinical presentation, natural history, and proper treatment of anorectal abscess and fistula are understood easily if it is recognized that the disease originates as an intersphincteric abscess.

As the abscess enlarges, it escapes the confines of the intersphincteric plane and spreads in one of several possible directions to form a perianal abscess or ischiorectal abscess (Fig 48–8). The most common of all anorectal abscesses is a perianal abscess, which presents as a tender, erythematous bulge at the anal verge. An ischiorectal abscess is formed when a growing intersphincteric abscess penetrates the skeletal muscle of the external sphincter below the level of the puborectalis and expands into the fat of the isochiorectal fossa. These abscesses can become quite large, because the levator ani (the upper border of the ischiorectal fossa) slopes upward. Thus, an ischiorectal abscess may be palpated as a bulge above the puborectalis, although it actually lies below the levator ani musculature. In contrast to the perianal abscess, this abscess seldom presents as a visible bulge because of the large potential space in the ischiorectal fossa. Thus, the abscess preferentially expands upward rather than protruding through the skin of the buttock. Rarely, an intersphincteric abscess may expand upward between the circular internal sphincter and the external sphincter, forming a supralevator abscess.

TREATMENT

Perirectal abscesses should be drained immediately, before fluctuance or erythema develop. Antibiotics are not indicated and should be used only in the presence of specific disorders—extensive cellulitis, valvular heart disease, diabetes, or states of compromised immunity. If the diagnosis is suspected but in doubt, examination under regional anesthesia should be performed.

With adequate anesthesia, the abscess can be detected and localized by digital examination. An intersphincteric abscess is treated definitively by excising the infected crypt and performing an internal sphincterotomy, which serves to unroof and drain the abscess. However, if the infection has developed into a perianal or an ischiorectal abscess, adequate drainage of the abscess cavity first must be done by making a cruciate incision in the skin overlying the abscess, or excising a small disc of overlying skin to permit complete evacuation of the contents of the abscess cavity. Incision and drainage alone will result in complete resolution of the infection in about half the patients. Unfortunately, in the other half, an anal fistula will develop. This fistula results in a localized chronic infection that is characterized by intermittent tenderness and drainage. The fistula consists of a chronically infected tract with an internal opening located in a crypt at the level of the dentate line and an external opening located at the drainage site of the earlier abscess. It is important to drain the abscess as close as possible to the anus to avoid a long fistula tract.

The appropriate treatment for an anal fistula is dependent upon the anatomy and the location of the fistula tract. Goodsall's rule states that if the anus is bi-

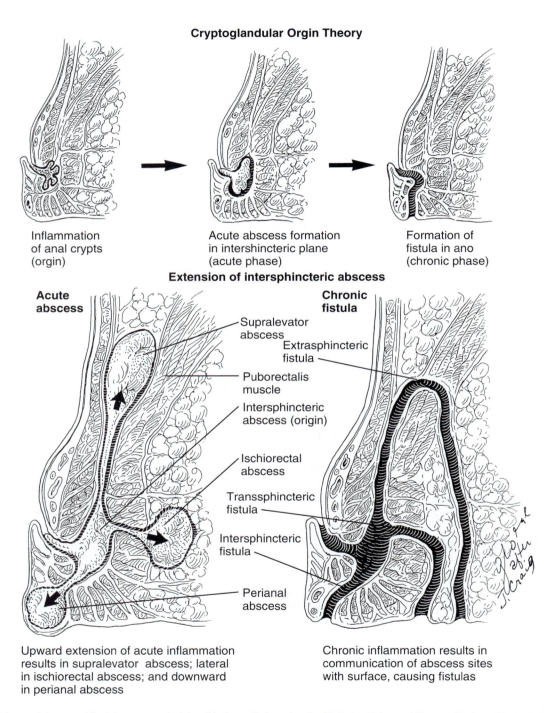

Cryptoglandular Orgin Theory

Inflammation of anal crypts (orgin)

Acute abscess formation in intershincteric plane (acute phase)

Formation of fistula in ano (chronic phase)

Extension of intersphincteric abscess

Acute abscess

Chronic fistula

Supralevator abscess

Extrasphincteric fistula

Puborectalis muscle

Intersphincteric abscess (origin)

Ischiorectal abscess

Transsphincteric fistula

Intersphincteric fistula

Perianal abscess

Upward extension of acute inflammation results in supralevator abscess; lateral in ischiorectal abscess; and downward in perianal abscess

Chronic inflammation results in communication of abscess sites with surface, causing fistulas

Figure 48–8. Anorectal abscess and fistula in ano crpytoglandular origin theory. (Redrawn from Fry RD, Kodner IJ. Anorectal Diseases. *Clin Symp* 1985;37:15. Copyright 1985, CIBA-GEIGY; originally illustrated by John Craig, MD)

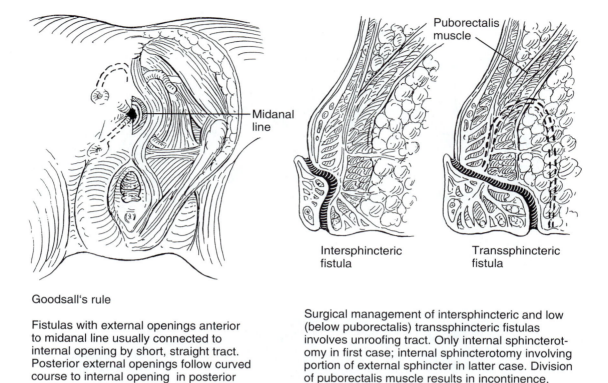

Puborectalis
muscle

Midanal
line

Intersphincteric
fistula

Transsphincteric
fistula

Goodsall's rule

Fistulas with external openings anterior
to midanal line usually connected to
internal opening by short, straight tract.
Posterior external openings follow curved
course to internal opening in posterior
midline

Surgical management of intersphincteric and low
(below puborectalis) transsphincteric fistulas
involves unroofing tract. Only internal sphincter-
omy in first case; internal sphincterotomy involving
portion of external sphincter in latter case. Division
of puborectalis muscle results in incontinence,
so high fistulas not treated by sphincterotomy

Figure 48–9. Surgical management of fistula in ano. (Redrawn from Fry RD, Kodner IJ. Anorectal Diseases. *Clin Symp* 1985;37:21. Copyright 1985, CIBA-GEIGY; originally illustrated by John Craig, MD)

sected by a line in the frontal plane, an external opening, anterior to the line, will connect to an internal opening by a short, direct fistula tract (Fig 48–9). However, if
the external opening is located posterior to this imaginary line, the fistula tract follows a curved course to the
crypt in the posterior midline. This rule, while useful, is
not infallible. Occasionally, an external opening anterior to the imaginary bisecting line connects to an internal opening in the posterior midline. Because of its
shape, this fistula is usually called a "horseshoe fistula."

Horseshoe fistulas usually have an internal opening
in the posterior midline of the anus and may extend anteriorly and laterally to both ischiorectal spaces by way
of the deep space. The anterior extensions of the horseshoe tracts then can be drained by a secondary opening,
avoiding a long skin incision that would unroof the entire tract (Fig 48–10).

If a perianal abscess develops into a fistula, the condition is appropriately treated by simple fistulotomy,
which divides a portion of the internal sphincter and
unroofs the tract entirely.

An anorectal fistula that persists after drainage of an
ischiorectal fossa abscess is usually a transphincteric fistula, since the tract crosses the lower portion of the ex-

ternal sphincter. The fistulotomy required to unroof
this tract results in division of a portion of the internal
sphincter as well as a portion of the lower external
sphincter. If the tract lies below the puborectalis, the external sphincter usually can be divided at the site of the
fistula tract without loss of continence. However, the puborectalis must not be divided, or incontinence will invariably ensue.

The anal sphincter is much less prominent in the anterior midline. Thus, fistulotomy as treatment for an anterior midline anal fistula is associated with an increased
risk of anal incontinence, particularly in women. Consequently, treatment of such fistulas often involves eradicating the internal opening of the fistula at the level of
the dentate line by advancing a flap of rectal mucosa.[5]
It is important to ensure adequate drainage of the fistula through the external opening until the suture line
of the advancement flap is well healed; otherwise, an abscess can reform and disrupt the suture line, causing a
recurrence of the fistula (Fig 48–11).

Although most anorectal abscesses originate in the
anal crypts, other disease entities must be considered if
the pathology appears atypical. Crohn's disease should
be suspected if there are numerous complex fistula

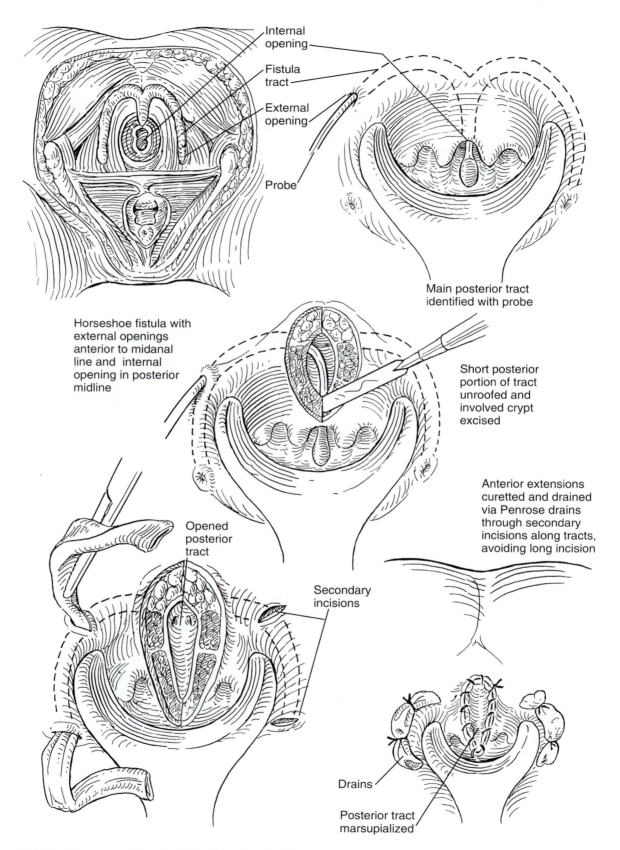

Internal opening

Fistula tract

External opening

Probe

Main posterior tract identified with probe

Horseshoe fistula with external openings anterior to midanal line and internal opening in posterior midline

Short posterior portion of tract unroofed and involved crypt excised

Anterior extensions curetted and drained via Penrose drains through secondary incisions along tracts, avoiding long incision

Opened posterior tract

Secondary incisions

Drains

Posterior tract marsupialized

Figure 48–10. Surgical management of horseshoe fistula. (Redrawn from Fry RD, Kodner IJ. Anorectal Diseases. *Clin Symp* 1985;37:18. Copyright 1985, CIBA-GEIGY; originally illustrated by John Craig, MD)

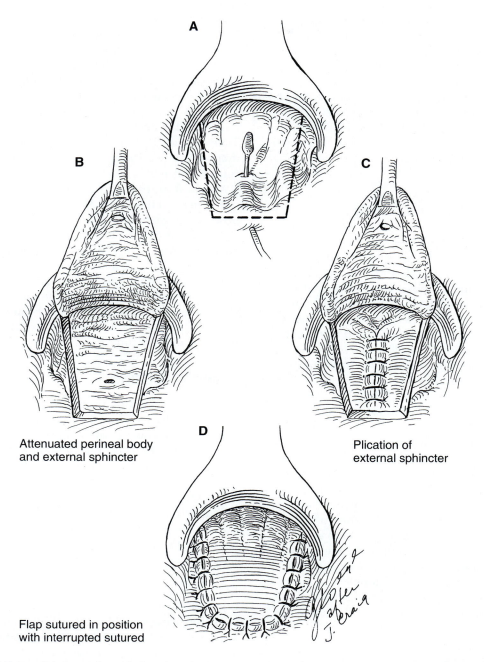

Figure 48–11. Endorectal advancement flap repair of complex anal-perineal or low rectal-perineal fistula. (Redrawn from Kodner IJ, Mazor A, Shemesh EI, et al. *Surgery* 1993;114:682–690)

tracts associated with edematous skin tags, or if there is inflammation of the rectal mucosa. Tuberculosis is now a rare cause of anal abscesses and fistulas, but has recently been observed in immigrants to America. Hidradenitis suppurativa also may mimic cryptoglandular suppurative disease. However, close examination will reveal that the disease arises from the area of the perianal skin and not the anal crypts. Actinomycosis should be suspected if typical "sulphur granules" are seen in the abscess cavity or fistula tract.[6] Pilonidal disease sometimes can be confused with a posterior perirectal abscess, but careful examination should reveal that there is no communication with the anus. Hair obtained from the abscess cavity when the pilonidal abscess is drained will indicate the true nature of the disease.

■ SEXUALLY TRANSMITTED ANAL DISEASE

During recent years there has been a profound change in the prevalence and types of sexually transmitted diseases. Genital-anal, oral-anal, and other anal-based erotic practices among homosexual or bisexual men and among women who engage in anal-receptive intercourse account for the transmission of most of these diseases. The promiscuous lifestyle attributed to many homosexual men has undoubtedly played a major role in the epidemic increase of these infections. It has been estimated that the average homosexual has about 1000 sexual partners during his life.[7,8] While the term "gay bowel syndrome" has been used to include all sexually transmitted diseases of the colon, rectum and anus,[9] it should be recognized that these diseases also can occur in heterosexual women who practice anal intercourse.

The liberalization of sexual mores that occurred during the past two decades has now been tempered by the recognition of the acquired immunodeficiency syndrome (AIDS), which has led to public concern over the transmission of the causative agent, the human immunodeficiency virus (HIV). Surprisingly, the incidence of other venereal diseases appears to be increasing. While a detailed discussion of these infections is beyond the scope of this textbook, the surgeon will often be consulted for evaluation of complications of these diseases.

HUMAN PAPILLOMA VIRUS (HPV)

HPV is the etiologic agent causing venereal warts. These lesions are common in homosexual men, and can have a varied appearance, including (1) discrete warts: papillary or acuminate white lesions, usually occurring singly or in clusters at or below the dentate line, (2) circumferential wart ring lesions located at the dentate line and encompassing 60% to 100% of the anal canal, and (3) flat white epithelium: pale areas of smooth opaque

epithelium that often extends cephalad to the dentate line.[10] These later lesions may be detected more easily by using a colposcope to magnify the anal canal. A recent study has found a high prevalence of histologically confirmed dysplasia in these internal lesions detected in asymptomatic homosexual men.[10] Dysplasia was found in 70% of HIV-seronegative men and 85% and 90% of nonimmunosuppressed and immunosuppressed HIV-seropositive men, respectively. Biopsy of the lesions was necessary for detection, since it could not be predicted by the gross appearance of the warts.

The association of dysplasia with HPV is now well recognized. There are at least 60 different HPV types. Types 6 and 11 are associated with warts and low-grade dysplasia. Types 16 and 18 have been found in cervical cancer and high-grade cervical dysplasia, and type 16 has been found in high-grade anal dysplasia and invasive cancers. HPV types 31, 33, and 35 are thought to pose an intermediate cancer risk.

While it is clear that HPV is implicated in the pathogenesis of anal cancer in homosexual men, the rates of progression from dysplasia to cancer in the anal canal are unknown. It is likely that the progression is low, but further study is needed for documentation. At present the appropriate therapy seems to be ablation of the lesions, either by excision, cautery or laser. It is still not known if such treatment will reduce the cancer risk.

CHLAMYDIAL INFECTIONS

Chlamydial infections are now the most common sexually transmitted disease in the United States and account for increasing numbers of cases of proctitis in patients who practice receptive anal intercourse.[11,12] There are 15 recognized immunotypes of *Chlamydia trachomatis,* but for practical purposes it should be recognized that there are nonlymphogranulomatous (non-LGV) and lymphogranulomatous (LGV) types. The non-LGV organisms are a common cause of urethritis, epididymitis, and pelvic inflammatory disease. At least half of the genital infections previously diagnosed as "nonspecific" or "nongonococcal" are caused by non-LGV chlamydia. Chlamydial proctitis may coexist with other rectal infections, especially gonorrhea. Several serotypes are responsible for proctitis, and serotypes L_1, L_2, and L_3 are responsible for lymphogranuloma venereum.[13] The pathogen is introduced by either genital-anal or oral-anal intercourse. The non-LGV organisms are obligate intracellular parasites that can penetrate only columnar or transitional epithelium. The LGV organisms also can penetrate mononuclear cells, which may account for the prominent lymphadenopathy in patients with lymphogranuloma venereum.

Infection may be asymptomatic, or may consist of nonspecific symptoms such as anal pain, pruritus, purulent discharge, and bleeding. More severe forms of infection, especially severe proctitis, usually indicate the presence of one of the LGV serotypes. Perianal fistulas and rectovaginal fistulas may develop, with untreated cases progressing to severe rectal stricture. Two weeks after the initial symptoms, inguinal lymphadenopathy becomes predominant and the inguinal nodes may fuse together in a large mass.

The organism is an obligate intracellular organism, and rectal cultures are usually inconclusive. A biopsy of the rectal mucosa is probably the most commonly used method to confirm the diagnosis. The diagnosis of chlamydial infections used to be difficult because satisfactory culture techniques were not widely available. Diagnosis usually required the detection of rising antibody titers. However, the organism now can be identified by using tissue culture techniques or DNA probes.

Chlamydial infections should be treated as soon as the diagnosis is suspected. The recommended treatment for non-LGV chlamydial infection is tetracycline or, alternatively, erythromycin for 7 to 14 days. LGV chlamydial infection should be treated with tetracycline and sulfamides for a minimum of 21 days.[13]

HERPES SIMPLEX VIRUS

Anorectal herpes is usually caused by the type II herpes simplex virus (HVS-2), although the HSV-1 virus is responsible for approximately 10% of anal infections. Patients who have been previously infected have virus-specific antibodies. The first symptoms of infection are perianal pruritus or paraesthesia, followed by intense anal pain. Small vesicles surrounded by red areolas may appear. These vesicles subsequently rupture, leaving small ulcers which appear on the perianal skin, in the anal canal, or even on the rectal mucosa. Fever and malaise are frequently present. The ulcerated lesions may become secondarily infected, with increased pain and discharge.[14,15]

The lesions usually heal in about two weeks. Unfortunately, a chronic relapsing course is common, although recurrent lesions are usually much less painful.

Scrapings from the base of a ruptured vesicle can be stained to show typical intranuclear inclusion bodies, but the diagnosis is most expeditiously made by viral culture.

There is no known cure for herpes. Acyclovir applied as a topical ointment may reduce the duration of symptoms. Oral acyclovir is more effective than topical acyclovir; taken at the onset of symptoms, oral acyclovir can reduce the formation of new vesicles.[16–18] Patients with AIDS may suffer from frequent recurrent herpetic infections. Suppressive therapy with acyclovir is helpful in such circumstances.[19] AIDS patients with perianal herpes resistant to acyclovir may benefit from two new compounds, foscarnet or vidarabine.[20,21]

Patients are contagious while the lesions are present and should abstain from sexual activity until all lesions are completely healed. Even after the lesions have completely healed, a condom should be used during sexual intercourse.

GONORRHEA

Anorectal infection caused by the bacterium *Neisseria gonorrhoeae* are common in the male homosexual population and frequently accompany other venereal diseases. Over half of homosexual men seen in screening clinics have been found to be infected,[22,23] with the rectum being the only site infected in about half of cases. The majority of these infections are asymptomatic.

Symptoms vary from none to intense anorectal pain and tenesmus accompanied by a viscid, yellow anal discharge. Anoscopy may reveal anusitis or distal proctitis. Diagnosis is confirmed by obtaining cultures from the rectal mucosa, or more recently, by DNA probes.

Treatment should be initiated if the disease is suspected. Untreated rectal gonorrhea can lead to septic arthritis, endocarditis, perihepatitis, and meningitis, as well as infection of sexual partners. Several drugs (penicillin, tetracycline, ampicillin, and spectinomycin) may be used for treatment, although increasing numbers of resistant strains are being recognized. Cultures should be repeated after treatment is completed, since antibiotic therapy may fail in as many as a third of the patients. All sexual contacts also must be treated. All patients with confirmed rectal gonorrhea should have a serologic test for syphilis three months after treatment is completed.

SYPHILIS

The classic lesion of primary syphilis is a chancre on the genitalia, but in homosexual males the chancre usually presents in the anal canal or at the anal verge. These ulcerated lesions may mimic an anal fissure, but an aberrant location of the lesion (eg, lateral anus instead of midline) should arouse suspicion. Classic descriptions indicate that the syphilitic chancre is a painless lesion, but anal chancres may be extremely painful. The causative organism is the spirochete, *Treponema pallidum,* which may occasionally cause severe proctitis without an accompanying chancre. Inguinal adenopathy is common.

Early syphilis can be diagnosed by examining scrapings from the base of the chancre with dark-field microscopy; these lesions are teeming with spirochetes that can be seen as cork-screw shaped motile fluorescent yellowish-green organisms. Serology is also very helpful in establishing the diagnosis. In untreated primary syphilis, the Venereal Disease Research Laboratory (VDRL) assay is reactive in about 75% of cases; in early latent syphilis, about 95%; and in the secondary state, it is 100% reactive. The fluorescent treponemal antibody (FTA) absorption test usually becomes positive in about 4 to 6 weeks after the initial infection.[13] The rapid plasma reagin (RPR) becomes positive later than the FTA. Therefore, the FTA and dark-field microscopy are the appropriate tests for suspected early syphilis.

The second stage of anal syphilis appears 6 to 8 weeks after the chancre has healed in untreated patients. It may present as condyloma latum, a pale-brown or flesh-colored flat verrucous lesion, or as a mucocutaneous rash. All three serologic tests for syphilis will be positive at this stage. Skin lesions are highly contagious.

Benzathine penicillin is the treatment of choice for syphilis. Alternate treatments include aqueous penicillin G, tetracycline, or erythromycin. Patients with syphilis must abstain from sexual contact until treatment is complete. All sexual contacts should be prophylactically treated.

REFERENCES

1. Thomson WHF. The nature of hemorrhoids. *Br J Surg* 1975;62:542–552
2. Bernstein WC. What are hemorrhoids and what is their relationship to the portal venous system? *Dis Colon Rectum* 1983;26:829–834
3. Haas PA, Fox TA Jr, Haas GP. The pathogenesis of hemorrhoids. *Dis Colon Rectum* 1984;27:442–450
4. Schouten W, Briel J, Auwerda J. Relationship between anal pressure and anodermal bloodflow: the vascular pathogenesis of anal fissure. Presented at the 92nd Annual Convention of the American Society of Colon and Rectal Surgeons. Chicago, Il: May 4, 1993
5. Kodner IJ, Mazor A, Shemesh EK, et al. Endorectal advancement flap repair of rectovaginal and other complicated anorectal fistulas. *Surgery* 1993;114:682–690
6. Fry RD, Birnbaum EH, Lacey DL. Actinomyces as a cause of recurrent perianal fistula in the immunocompromised patient. *Surgery* 1992;111:591–594
7. Kinsey AC, Pomeroy WB, Martin LE. Sexual behavior in the human male. Philadelphia, PA: WB Saunders; 1948:610
8. Darrow WW, Barret D, Jay K, et al. The gay report on sexually transmitted diseases. *Am J Public Health* 1981;71:1004–1011
9. Weller IV. The gay bowel. *Gut* 1985;26:869–875
10. Surawicz CM, Kirby P, Critchlow C, et al. Anal dysplasia in homosexual men: role of anoscopy and biopsy. *Gastroenterology* 1993;105:658–666
11. Holmes K. The chlamydia epidemic. *JAMA* 1981;245:1718–1723
12. Quinn TC, Goodell SE, Mkrtichian EE, et al. Chlamydia trachomatic proctitis. *N Engl J Med* 1981;305:195–200
13. Wexner SD. Sexually transmitted diseases of the colon, rectum and anus: the challenge of the nineties. *Dis Colon Rectum* 1990;33:1048–1062
14. Goodell SE, Quinn TC, Mkritchian EE, et al. Herpes simplex virus: an important cause of acute proctitis in homosexual men. *Gastroenterology* 1981;80:1159 (abstract)
15. Jacobs E. Anal infections caused by herpes simplex virus. *Dis Colon Rectum* 1976;19:151–157
16. Corey L. The diagnosis and treatment of genital herpes. *JAMA* 1982;248:1041–1949
17. Bryson YJ, Dillon M, Lovett M, et al. Treatment of first episodes of genital herpes simplex virus infection with oral acyclovir: a randomized controlled trial in normal subjects. *N Engl J Med* 1983;308:916–921
18. Reichman RC, Badger GJ, Mertz GJ, et al. Treatment of recurrent genital herpes simplex infections with oral acyclovir. *JAMA* 1984;251:2103–2107
19. Mertz GJ, Jones CC, Mills J, et al. Long-term acyclovir suppression of frequently recurring genital herpes simplex virus infection. *JAMA* 1988;260:201–206
20. Chatis PA, Miller CH, Schrager LE, et al. Successful treatment with Foscarnet of an acyclovir-resistant mucocutaneous infection with herpes simplex virus in a patient with acquired immunodeficiency syndrome *N Engl J Med* 1989;320:297–300
21. Wexner SD. Treatment of AIDS patients with herpes simplex virus infections resistant to acyclovir. *CR Surg Outlook* 1989;2:1–2
22. Janda WM, Bonhoff M, Morgello JA, et al. Prevalence and site pathogen studies of Neisseria meningitides and Neisseria gonorrhea in homosexual men. *JAMA* 1980;244:2060–2064
23. Knapp JS, Zenilman JM, Thompson SE. Gonorrhea. In: Morse Sa, Moreland AA, Thompson SE (eds), *Sexually Transmitted Diseases*. Philadelphia, PA: JB Lippincott; 1990:512–522

49

Rectal Cancer

Ira J. Kodner

■ PATHOPHYSIOLOGY, ETIOLOGY, ANATOMY

PATHOPHYSIOLOGY

Rectal cancer is similar to colon cancer in that the majority of malignant neoplasms of the rectum are adenocarcinomas, and the significant premalignant conditions (adenomatous and villous polyps, familial adenomatous polyposis, and ulcerative colitis) are the same. The management of squamous cell cancer of the anal cancer differs significantly from the management of adenocarcinomas. Malignant melanoma, which is rarely found in the rectum, must be managed differently from adenocarcinoma because the poor prognosis for rectal malignant melanoma often contraindicates resective surgery.

The surgical management of rectal cancer is very different from that for colon cancer because of the anatomic location and configuration of the rectum. Wide excision of the cancer and surrounding structures, possible with colon cancer, is impossible because the rectum resides within the confines of the pelvis. The proximity of the anal sphincter mechanism to the rectum presents another difficult challenge to successful surgical management. In attempting to achieve a curative distal margin beyond the cancer, the surgeon must consider the function of the sphincter mechanism. If the risk for injury is so great that the sphincter will not function perfectly, it should be removed, which necessitates a colostomy. The construction and care of the colostomy are described elsewhere, but the critical fac-

tor to consider is the cure of the cancer. The patient, who often assumes that a colostomy indicates a hopelessly incurable cancer, must understand that the colostomy is necessary because of the anatomic location, not the severity, of the rectal cancer and that removal of the sphincter means the cancer may be cured.

The surgical management of rectal cancer is also unique owing to the close proximity of the organs of the urogenital tract and the innervation of the urogenital system (Fig 49–1). Radical treatment of rectal cancer results in a high impotency rate in men; the rate in women is unknown owing to the lack of accurate definitions of female impotency. The specific surgical procedure may be determined by the proximity of the urogenital system. The posterior wall of the vagina can be resected in continuity with an invasive rectal cancer, but a cancer invading the prostate or bladder base in a man requires a much more extensive and complicated surgical procedure. Special consideration during surgery also must be given to the dual arterial blood supply of the rectum (Fig 49–2) and to the lymphatic channels of cancer metastasis that follow the arterial routes (Fig 49–3).

Another main consideration in treating rectal cancer is the primary physiologic function of the rectum to serve as a reservoir, storing fecal material until the individual decides to evacuate it. Any surgical disturbance of the reservoir or continence mechanism can cause significant handicap to the individual. The distensible capacity of the rectal reservoir can allow cancers to grow to considerable size before causing any symptoms, which makes screening for rectal as well as colon can-

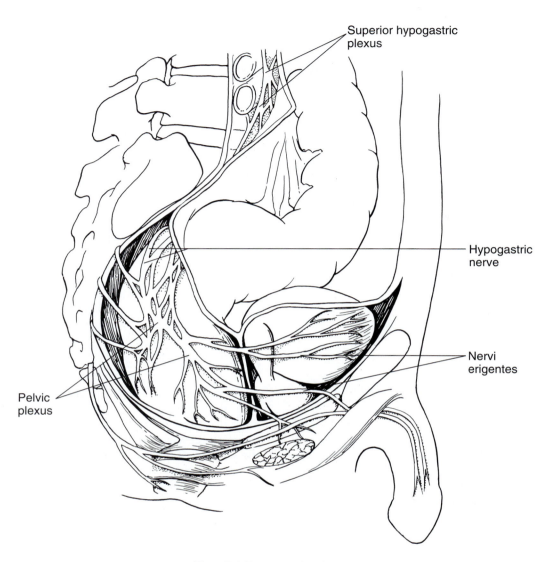

Figure 49–1. Nerve supply of pelvic organs.

cers mandatory. Routine screenings, especially for individuals known to be at significant risk, can detect asymptomatic cancers in their more curable stages.

Perhaps the most unique aspect of the anatomy of the rectum is its easy accessibility through the anus for several therapeutic and diagnostic modalities, including the physician's finger. This easy access has resulted in consideration of tumor treatment less than the radical resection procedures that often require removal of the rectum and anus, necessitating construction of a colostomy.

These unique features of the rectum must be considered for the screening, diagnosis, and treatment of patients known to have, or suspected of having, rectal cancer. One must consider the *local* factors related to the rectum itself. The next level of consideration involves the relationship of the cancer to the structures *adjacent* to the rectum, such as lymph nodes, sphincter mechanism, and surrounding organs. Perhaps the most important prognostic consideration lies in the status of the cancer with respect to *distant* metastasis. Rectal cancer can spread through the lymphatics of the mesenteric or iliac systems. It can metastasize to the liver via the portal venous system or to the lungs or, rarely, to the brain or bones via other hematogenous routes.

MODE OF METASTASIS AND DEATH

Cancer of the rectum spreads locally via lymphatics and by direct invasion. The lymphatic spread of rectal cancer is mainly in an upward direction along the superior hemorrhoidal vessels, with little extension below the

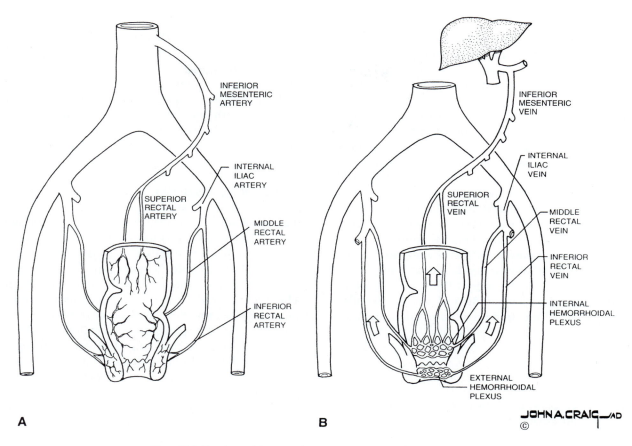

Figure 49–2. Vasculature of the anus and rectum. **A**. Arterial supply. **B**. Venous drainage.

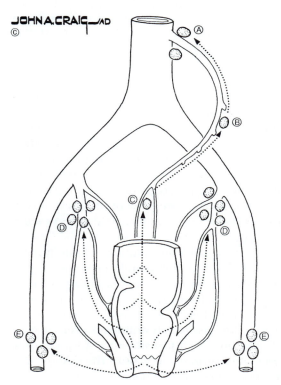

Figure 49–3. Lymphatic drainage of the rectum and anus. A: nodes at origin of inferior mesenteric artery. B: nodes at origin of sigmoid branches. C: sacral nodes. D: internal iliac nodes. E: inguinal nodes.

level of the tumor. Resection of the inferior zone of lymphatic drainage does not prevent regional metastasis of rectal cancer. Thus, it is possible to conserve the anal sphincter in the treatment of cancer of the upper and middle rectum.

Hematogenous spread to the liver through the portal system occurs in 30% to 50% of patients dying of rectal cancer. Other sites of distant hematogenous spread include the lung, bone, brain, spleen, adrenal gland, and ovaries. Local recurrence in the pelvis after surgical resection is common and can occur with and without distant metastatic disease. Death in patients with pelvic recurrence is characterized by extreme discomfort and poor quality of life. This situation has stimulated efforts to eliminate pelvic recurrence and has led to the use of such adjunctive modalities as preoperative radiation therapy. Any treatment that eliminates local recurrence allows patients to die with much less suffering, and palliative resection is recommended whenever possible.

ETIOLOGY

Although the exact cause of colon and rectal cancer is not known precisely, it seems that there is both an inherited and an environmental component. There are some cancers that are caused by known genetic disorders, some that have very strong familial tendencies, and others that seem to be related to specific premalignant diseases.

Genetic Predisposition

It has been estimated that approximately 15% of colorectal cancers occur in patients with a genetic predisposition.

Hereditary Nonpolyposis Colon Cancer (Lynch's Syndromes).

Lynch and associates described two different forms of hereditary, nonpolyposis colon cancer. These cancers arise from adenomas and may account for 4% to 6% of colorectal malignancies. Lynch's syndrome I is a hereditary cancer that usually occurs in the proximal colon, is site-specific within an affected family, and is usually the only type of tumor these patients exhibit. Metachronous colorectal cancer may develop in 40% of patients followed for at least 10 years. The syndrome appears to be autosomal dominant and is not associated with the presence of a large number of colonic polyps. Lynch's syndrome II, or "the family cancer syndrome," exhibits colorectal, endometrial, gastric, and other types of cancer. This cancer is also an autosomal dominant syndrome and may have a possible link to deletion of a "mismatch repair" gene. Members of families with these syndromes should be screened at an early age for the presence of polyps or colon can-

cer. If polyps are found, a subtotal colectomy with an ileorectal anastomosis is recommended, especially in patients with Lynch's syndrome I. A subgroup of patients present as young adults with multiple polyps or multiple cancers. These patients should have subtotal colectomy with ileorectal anastomosis, since they are at high risk for development of cancer or polyps in the future, and their families should be screened for colorectal polyps.

Familial Adenomatous Polyposis.

Familial adenomatous polyposis (FAP) is an autosomal dominant syndrome diagnosed when a patient has more than 100 adenomatous polyps in the colon or when a member of an FAP family has any number of colonic adenomas discovered. FAP includes a spectrum of syndromes formerly defined by various extraintestinal manifestations. The genetic defect responsible for familial adenomatous polyposis was described on chromosome 5, near the q 21 locus. The gene has been called the APC (adenomatous polyposis coli) gene. FAP occurs in anywhere from 1 in 8000 to 1 in 29 000 individuals. The common expression of the syndrome is the presence of multiple polyps in the colon and the associated extraintestinal manifestations, including epidermoid cysts, desmoid tumors in the abdomen, osteomas of the bones, and brain tumors (usually gliomas or medulloblastomas). The gene expression occurs in 100% of patients with the defect. Ten to twenty percent of all patients with FAP appear to acquire the genetic defect as a result of spontaneous mutation. All patients with the defective gene will develop cancer of the colon if left untreated. The average age of discovery of a new patient with FAP is 29 years. The average age of a patient who is newly discovered to have colorectal cancer related to FAP is 39 years.

Screening by detection of the chromosome 5q 21 APC gene or the protein products of the gene may soon be available for clinical use. Currently, recommendations for screening include endoscopy after 10 years of age, since family members of known FAP patients often will develop polyps around puberty. Early screening can be performed with proctoscopy or flexible sigmoidoscopy. If no rectal polyps are present, it is very rare to have cancer even though more proximal polyps eventually may develop.

Current recommendations state that all family members of a propositus with FAP should be screened periodically with colonoscopy from ten years of age until the age of forty. The syndrome has been reported to occur as late as age thirty-five. Upper endoscopy should be used to screen for gastric and duodenal adenomas beginning at age thirty. This surveillance must continue for life, even after surgery, because of the risk of upper gastrointestinal cancer in FAP patients.

Surgical Management. In patients with polyposis in whom there are fewer than 50 polyps in the rectum and no rectal cancer, a total abdominal colectomy with ileorectal anastomosis is a good choice. This method requires biannual proctoscopic examination to monitor the rectum for polyps and cancer.

Another method for management of FAP, which maintains intestinal continuity, is total proctocolectomy with ileal reservoir and ileoanal anastomosis. This procedure removes all tissue at risk for developing colorectal cancer. Poorly compliant patients who refuse periodic proctoscopic examination may also be candidates for the pouch procedure.

Acquired Somatic Defects

The chromosome defect in FAP is a germ cell line defect and is present from birth. The majority of patients with colorectal cancer have no inherited component and the initiating genetic mutation that causes neoplastic growth occurs in a single cell or in a group of mucosal cells. These tumors are not inherited, but there may be a familial predisposition to their development. Lynch has shown that the risk for developing colorectal cancer is increased anywhere from three- to nine-fold if one or more first-degree relatives have had colorectal cancer.

Available evidence suggests that adenomas of the colon develop after such a gene mutation. The adenomatous tissue contains crypt cells with atypical genetic expression. Tumor formation may be the result of more than one mutation. A *somatic* mutation, associated with an *inherited* mutation, may be expressed as the adenoma or tumor progresses. The inherited mutation is felt to be tumorigenic but may not be expressed or detectable in the tumor. Once the adenoma has developed, Fearon and Vogelstein have proposed that a second mutation may be required to change the adenoma to a cancer. A progression of mutations actually can occur in the course of development of a malignancy. *Oncogenes* function by initiating events that result in abnormal cellular growth and the development of tumors. For example, the *ras* gene family has been found in 50% of colorectal cancers and in adenomas >1 cm, but it has been found in <10% of adenomas <1 cm.

As a tumor develops, subsequent mutation can result in the deletion of *suppressor genes*. This loss usually occurs on chromosomes 17, 18, and 5. For example, the p53 gene is absent from chromosome 17 in 85% of colorectal cancers. The chromosome 5 MCC gene (mutated in colorectal cancer) is found in some tumors in patients with nonpolyposis cancers. The chromosome 18 DCC gene (deleted in colorectal cancer) is found in more than 70 percent of colorectal cancers. These mutations are postulated to affect cell-to-cell relationships in all tumors and thereby also affect the development of metastasis.

Fearon and Vogelstein have proposed a model for genetic changes leading to colorectal cancer (Fig 49–4). First, a mutational *activation* is initiated by oncogenes. This mutational activation is accompanied by a mutational *inactivation* of multiple suppressor genes. The mutations allow uncontrolled growth in varying degrees. More mutations are required for the development of cancer than for the development of benign polyps. The progression of cellular changes from normal mucosa, to adenoma, to cancer could be related to a progression of mutations during the course of time.

Environmental Factors

Diet. Diet has been proposed as a significant etiologic factor in the development of colorectal cancer. Fats have been suggested to be toxic to the colonic mucosa. Diets high in oleic acid (found in olive oil, coconut oil, and fish oil) cause no increase in cancer in animals. The monounsaturated fatty acids (omega-3 and omega-6 fatty acids) appear to be less carcinogenic than polyunsaturated or saturated fats. Epidemiologic studies of populations that consume <5% of their diet as fat have shown a lower incidence of colorectal cancer, whereas those having diets with 20% of their fat as either corn oil or safflower oil have an increase in cancer. Therefore, it appears that unsaturated animal fats and highly saturated vegetable oils may cause some event to occur in the colonic mucosa that stimulates the development of colorectal cancer.

Exposure to Carcinogens. No clear relationship has been established between specific carcinogens and colorectal cancer, but potential agents currently under investigation include bile acids (such as chenodeoxycholic acid), food additives, alcohol, and ionizing radiation. Each of these may function as a promoter of mutational changes in the colonic mucosa, but none have been clearly shown to have a carcinogenic effect. Oxygen radicals, which are unstable by-products of oxygen metabolism, may serve as promoters or chemical stimulants to the development of altered gene expressions. This effect is not a true carcinogenic effect but the creation of a milieu that predisposes to the development of mutations.

Premalignant Conditions

Ulcerative Colitis. The overall incidence of neoplasia in patients with pancolitis is 1% per year after 10 years; so that the cumulative risk of a cancer is 10% by 20 years' duration of disease. Dysplasia identified in the colonic mucosa by repeated colonoscopic biopsies has been

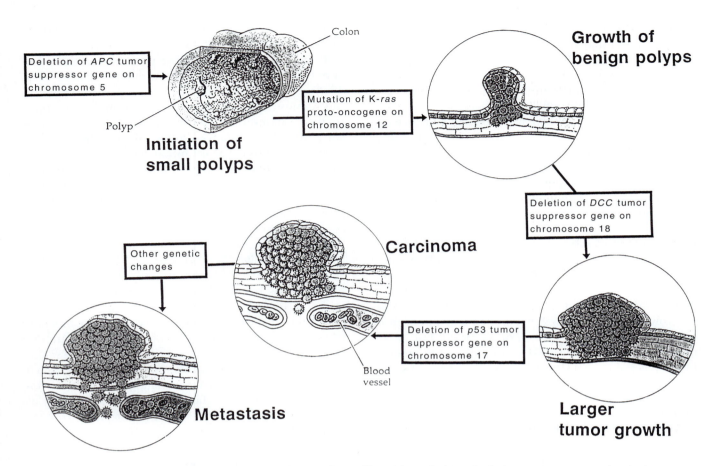

Figure 49–4. Stepwise changes in the development of sporadic colorectal cancer. Three of the genetic changes involve tumor suppressor genes and one involves a mutation to an oncogene. APC = adenomatous polyposis coli; DDC = deleted in colon cancer.

shown to be a precursor of cancer. The cancers tend to be more advanced because they are difficult to detect at an early stage. Approximately 35% are Dukes' C or D lesions. There is controversy over the implication of adenomatous polyps found in patients with chronic ulcerative colitis. The question arises whether this represents dysplasia and is an indication for total colectomy or whether this is a benign polyp arising from inflamed mucosa.

The most effective method for preventing colon cancer in patients with ulcerative colitis is to remove the colon once dysplasia has been identified. The risk of cancer in the setting of dysplasia is approximately 30%.

Crohn's Disease. The overall incidence of cancer occurring in patients who have Crohn's disease for more than 20 years is approximately 7%. Most of the intestinal cancers were found in the excluded segments in pa-

tients treated by segmental bypass. This procedure is no longer recommended because of a 20% incidence of adenocarcinoma and persistent disease in these bypassed segments. Patients with colonic strictures have a slightly higher incidence of adenocarcinoma at the site of the fibrotic narrowing. Reports of adenocarcinoma arising at the site of stricturoplasty in the small intestine have made it apparent that there is a risk of adenocarcinoma in these lesions. For this reason, a biopsy of the intestinal wall should be performed at the time of stricturoplasty. There also have been reports of squamous cell cancer and adenocarcinoma arising in chronic fistulas (especially of the anus and perineum) in patients with Crohn's disease. Overall, the risk for neoplasia in patients with Crohn's disease is only slightly higher than that of the general population and is certainly lower than in patients with ulcerative colitis or familial adenomatous polyposis.

■ RELATIONSHIP OF POLYPS TO CANCER

Most adenocarcinomas of the large intestine originate in adenomatous epithelium found in both pedunculated and sessile polyps. A large body of data confirms the transition through a spectrum of histologic changes, from benign adenomatous epithelium to intraepithelial carcinoma, to intramucosal carcinoma, and finally to invasive cancer. Long-term clinical studies have suggested that colorectal cancer can be reduced in a population that undergoes sigmoidoscopy, colonoscopy, and removal of all polyps. Evaluation of cancers of the rectum at each level of invasiveness has shown that exclusively intramucosal cancer is not capable of metastasizing. Only when the cancerous glands come into apposition with the muscularis mucosae can they truly be considered invasive cancer. The malignancy, at that stage, has access to lymphatics and occasionally can metastasize. The development of rectal cancer is uncommon in individuals under the age of 40, unless they have predisposing conditions such as ulcerative colitis or one of the polyposis syndromes. The earliest sign of rectal cancer is bleeding, either occult or visible.

Clinically, there are two types of polyps: pedunculated and sessile (Figs 49–5 and 49–6). Controversy exists as to whether a pedunculated polyp with invasive carcinoma should be treated differently from the sessile type. Frequently both pathologists and surgeons incor-

rectly identify the anatomy of the polyp, especially the pedunculated type. A sessile polyp attaches itself flush on the mucosa; a pedunculated polyp attaches itself on a stalk of varying length. The stalk is covered on both sides by normal mucosa and a center core of submucosa. A line drawn across the section of the transition between normal and adenomatous epithelium is the boundary line between the stalk and the head of the polyp. The junction is called the neck of the polyp (Fig 49–5). The most common mistake made by pathologists and surgeons is to refer to the center core of the muscularis mucosae and submucosa in the head of the polyp as the stalk.

The incidence of lymph node metastasis in polyps containing invasive cancer, including all types of polyps, is 9%. Generally speaking, the risk of lymph node metastasis is higher in sessile polyps than it is in pedunculated polyps, but the pedunculated lesions must be further divided into those in which the invasion is limited to the head of the polyp and those in which the invasion has reached the neck or stalk of the polyp. The significant risk of metastatic disease belongs to the latter group.

In sessile polyps with invasive carcinoma (Fig 49–6), the incidence of lymph node metastasis is 15%, and the incidence of residual tumor after snare removal is 6%. A local recurrence rate of 21% can be anticipated if further treatment is not done. Bowel resection is clearly indicated in these lesions. Pedunculated polyps with inva-

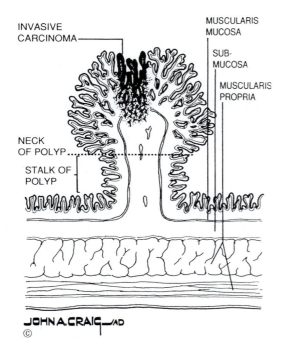

Figure 49–5. Pedunculated polyp containing an invasive cancer.

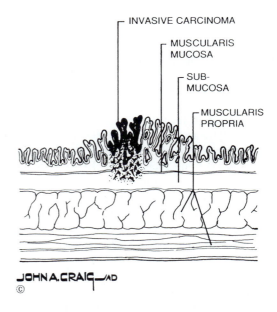

Figure 49–6. Sessile polyp containing an invasive cancer.

sive cancer have incidences of lymph node metastasis and residual tumor of 8% and 2%, respectively. This incidence represents a failure rate of 10% if further treatment is not undertaken. If these lesions are divided further into those in which the carcinomas are limited to the head of the polyp and those in which the carcinomas have invaded into the neck or stalk, it becomes apparent that the risk is much higher in the latter group. Evidence suggests that pedunculated polyps with invasive cancer limited to the head of the polyp infrequently require bowel resection, since the overall risk of lymph node metastasis is only 3%. The risks of surgery must be carefully weighed against the risk of metastasis, in each individual. The incidence of cancer spreading is higher if the cancer is poorly differentiated or has invaded the lymphatic channels or venules in the head of the polyp, as shown by microscopic examination. In these cases, bowel resection should be performed.

Once a cancer has been found in the large intestine, the incidence of synchronous cancer is 5% and the incidence of a synchronous neoplastic polyp is 28%. Therefore, a total colonoscopy should be done in patients who have an invasive carcinoma of the large bowel. Unlike carcinoma of the breast or malignant melanoma, colorectal cancer is rather predictable. A long latent period with recurrence after 10 or more years is rare, and 5 year survival figures are meaningful. The risk of local recurrence should be minimal after the 5th year. Patients should continue to be followed every 3 years, ideally by total colonoscopy. Additionally, patients with polyps without evidence of invasion should be followed until the colon is completely cleared of polyps and then every 2 to 3 years thereafter. The rate of finding metachronous lesions is 44% for polyps and 10% for cancers.

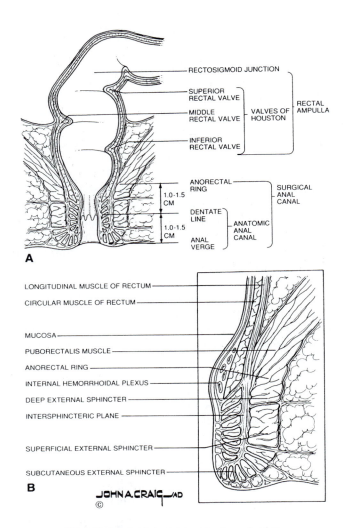

Figure 49–7. Anatomic landmarks of the anus and rectum.

■ ANATOMY OF THE ANUS AND RECTUM

BASIC ANATOMIC LANDMARKS

The alimentary tract terminates at the funnel-shaped anorectum. The anorectum includes the skin of the surrounding perianal region, the anal canal, and the rectum (Fig 49–7). The anal verge, the dentate line, and the anorectal ring are the three main anatomic points of reference. The anal verge, the external boundary of the anal canal, is the junction between the anal and perianal skin. Although the precise border is often indistinct, anal epithelium lacks hair follicles, sebaceous glands, or sweat glands found in perianal skin.

The dentate line (anorectal line), the cephalad border of the anatomic anal canal, is a true mucocutaneous junction. It represents the union of the embryonic ectoderm with the entodermal gut, and lies approximately 1.0 to 1.5 cm above the anal verge. In a transitional zone (6- to 12-mm in length), the columnar epithelium of the rectum changes to cuboidal epithelium, which joins the squamous epithelium at the dentate line.

The anorectal ring, 1.0 to 1.5 cm above the dentate line, is the upper border of the anal sphincteric complex and the surgical anal canal and is easily palpable by digital examination of the anus.

For anatomists, the anal canal begins at the dentate line and ends at the anal verge. Surgeons, however, view the anal canal as starting at the anorectal ring and terminating at the anal verge. In this chapter, the surgeon's concept of the anal canal prevails.

Above the anorectal ring, the lower intestine dilates to form the rectal ampulla. Prominent mucosal folds, the rectal valves of Houston, are found within the rectum. The lower and upper valves lie on the left side of the rectum, and the middle valve lies on the right side.

The middle rectal valve usually lies at the level of the anterior peritoneal reflection. Since these valves are not as thick as the rectal wall, they are excellent biopsy sites.

VASCULAR SUPPLY

The terminal branch of the inferior mesenteric artery, the superior rectal artery, descends to the upper rectum in the sigmoid mesentery. It then divides into right and left branches, with subsequent smaller branches penetrating the muscular coat of the rectum (Fig 49–2A). The middle rectal arteries arise from the internal iliac arteries and supply the lower rectum and the upper anal canal. The inferior rectal arteries arise from the internal pudendal arteries and cross the ischiorectal fossae to supply the anal sphincter muscles.

Blood returns from the anus by two routes. Above the dentate line, the internal hemorrhoidal plexus drains into the superior rectal vein and subsequently into the inferior mesenteric vein and portal system (Fig 49–2B). Below the dentate line, the external hemorrhoidal plexus drains into the internal iliac vein via the middle rectal vein or via the pudendal vein, which receives blood from the inferior rectal vein.

LYMPHATIC DRAINAGE

The lymph channels follow the arterial routes (Fig 49–3). Lymph from the upper and middle rectum drains into the inferior mesenteric lymph nodes. Lymph from the lower rectum also can flow to the inferior mesenteric nodes, or it can flow laterally, close to the middle rectal arteries, to the internal iliac nodes.

Lymphatics from the anal canal above the dentate line flow to the inferior mesenteric nodes, as well as laterally to the internal iliac nodes, traversing the is-chiorectal fossa. Lymph from the anal canal below the dentate line usually flows to the inguinal nodes.

■ DIAGNOSIS, CLASSIFICATION, AND SURVEILLANCE

GENERAL CONCEPTS

The important aspects of complete evaluation of rectal cancer are related to the *local, regional,* and *systemic* manifestations of the cancer (Fig 49–8).

Local Aspects

Local evaluation of a rectal cancer helps determine the proper modality of management and gives some insight into the prognosis of the cancer. Careful digital rectal exam must be performed to evaluate size, fixation, and ulceration of the cancer, as well as any suggestion of extension of the cancer to pararectal lymph nodes or adjacent organs. The rectal cancer needs to be visualized by the surgeon. Using a rigid sigmoidoscope, adequate biopsy is taken, degree of fixation to surrounding tissue is evaluated, risk of obstruction is predicted, size and ulceration of lesions is determined, and the distance from the distal edge of the tumor to the dentate line is measured carefully. Flexible fiberoptic instruments are not totally reliable, because only tiny biopsies can be taken, and the flexibility of the instrument can give a false sense of security relative to the distance between the cancer and the mucocutaneous junction (dentate line). It is this distance that ultimately determines if a surgeon can preserve the anal sphincter mechanism.

Cancers that have an adequate "clinical" classification system allow the treating physicians to plan securely a course of treatment before operation. So far this cannot be fully accomplished with rectal cancer, because

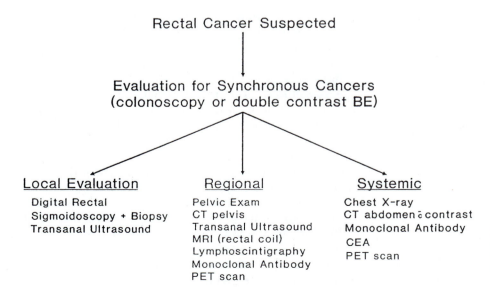

Figure 49–8. Evaluation of suspected rectal cancer. (From Kodner IJ, Fry RD, Fleshman JW, et al: Colon, rectum and anus. In: Schwartz SI (ed), *Principles of Surgery,* 6th ed. New York, NY: McGraw-Hill; 1993:1279)

the important variables either have not been completely defined or cannot be determined before initiating treatment. Classification systems (Figs 49–9 and 49–10) describe the depth of cancer invasion and the status of cancer spread to surrounding lymph nodes. These are histologic classifications that require removal of the rectum and pararectal tissue before their application.

The biologic behavior of rectal cancer cannot be predicted by its location or size. Poorly differentiated cancers have a worse long-term prognosis than those that are well differentiated. Some very aggressive histologic patterns such as "signet-ring" cell and mucinous cancers carry an especially poor prognosis. Attempts are being made to predict further the biologic aggressiveness of rectal cancers by evaluation of various tumor markers from biopsies of the cancers. These biologic predictors become important when local nonresective techniques are described for small, favorable-appearing cancers. If the cancers that look favorable but have aggressive biologic behavior can be identified, they should be treated by nothing less than radical resection.

The *depth of invasion* of a rectal cancer is known to be an important variable. In order for a rectal cancer to be classified as invasive, it must extend at least into the muscularis mucosae, since at this level it has first access to the vascular and lymphatic systems and metastasis becomes a possibility. Morson demonstrated that even a small mobile cancer, confined to the rectal wall but extending into the muscularis mucosae, will have a 10% incidence of metastasis to pararectal lymph nodes. A major unfulfilled challenge in evaluating rectal cancer is the pretreatment determination of lymph node involvement by cancer.

The depth of cancer invasion can be accurately determined by use of *transanal ultrasound* (Fig 49–11). Each layer of the rectal wall can be identified and its penetration by cancer described. Although lymph nodes can be visualized by ultrasound, the presence of cancer within these nodes cannot be accurately predicted. Computed tomography (CT) scanning of the rectum has been extremely helpful for the evaluation of the cancer itself, but nuclear magnetic imaging, especially with the use of newly available transrectal positioned coils, should be very helpful in predicting depth of invasion and involvement of lymph nodes and other pararectal structures by the primary cancer.

The advantages of these accurate descriptions of the cancer become evident when the treatment is chosen and decisions must be made regarding extent of operation and use of adjuvant modalities such as chemotherapy or radiation therapy.

Regional Aspects

Regional evaluation of pararectal structures involves transanal ultrasound and CT or magnetic resonance imaging (MRI) scanning, as described, plus some special considerations. A major factor early in the evaluation of a patient with rectal cancer involves determination of the possibility and extent of resectability. After a cancer grows through the wall of the rectum, it can invade any of the surrounding structures. This is usually determined by evaluation of the *fixation* or tethering of the tumor to these structures. This makes complete examination of these structures necessary. A woman should have a complete pelvic examination with care to determine if the tumor is suspected of invading the

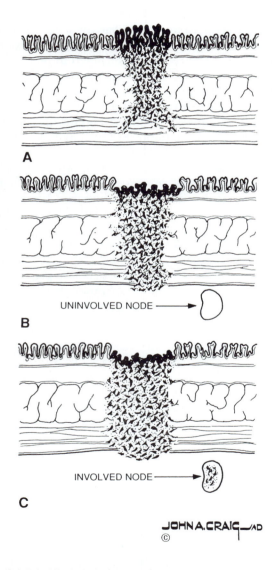

Figure 49–9. Dukes' histologic classification system for rectal cancer. **A.** Cancer growth limited to the wall of the rectum. **B.** Cancer growth extended through the wall of the rectum, but not involving adjacent lymph nodes. **C.** Cancer metastatic to regional lymph nodes.

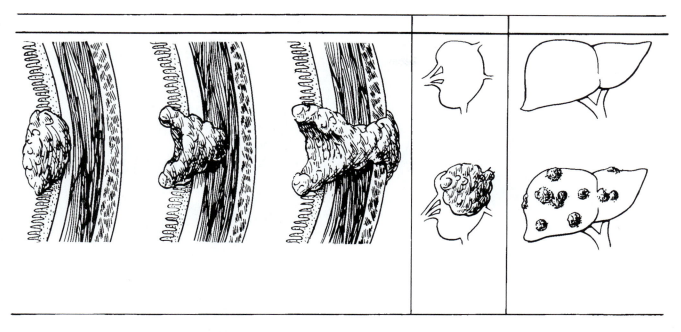

Figure 49–10. TNM staging system for colorectal cancer. (Redrawn from John A Craig, MD in Fry RD, Fleshman JW, Kodner IJ: Cancer of colon and rectum. *CIBA Clinical Symposia* 1989;41:5) Copyright 1989 CIBA-Geigy Corp. Reprinted with permission from Clinical Symposia.

vagina or has spread to the ovaries. In a man, evaluation of extension into the prostate or bladder is important. This could require transanal ultrasound, CT, MRI, or even cystoscopy and biopsy.

The degree of *fixation* of the tumor is important. It is also a major factor in determining the need for adjuvant radiation therapy, sometimes coupled with chemotherapy. Even if the cancer shrinks with preoperative adjuvant therapy, consideration must be given to resection of the involved structures originally suspected of invasion by the cancer. The performance of very extensive resective procedures must be tempered by the age and general health of the patient. The determination of extent of fixation of the cancer is complicated by the fact that many invasive cancers are surrounded by an intense inflammatory reaction that creates the sensation of fixation, rather than actual invasion by the cancer.

The surgeon also should know the status of the upper urinary tract. If, for example, one of the ureters is involved with the invasive cancer, a determination should be made before operation that the contralateral kidney is functioning. Specific plans may need to be made for a urologist to deal with the bladder and ureter at the time of surgery. Our own preference is to use intravenous contrast at the time of CT scanning for liver metastases to evaluate kidney size and function, as well as position and possible involvement of the ureters.

One of the most frustrating aspects of regional evaluation of rectal cancer is the inability to determine cancer involvement of the adjacent or regional lymph nodes. This one fact would be most helpful in determining need for adjuvant treatment preoperatively. CT and transanal ultrasound, as well as digital palpation, have allowed determination of the presence of enlarged nodes, but have not been helpful in determining presence of cancer within these nodes. There is hope that improved MRI techniques, PET scanning, and utilization of monoclonal antibodies will be helpful in this important aspect of staging. Most studies have shown the involvement of lymph nodes in the resected specimen to be the most influential predictor of prognosis. Recently, more credence is being placed on the involvement of the "tangential" margin of resection (Fig 49–12). This is the peripheral margin, including the extent of clearance of the cancer from surrounding tissue. Interestingly, this margin is not reported by the pathologist unless special effort is made to "ink" the tissue immediately after the resection. A great deal of discussion exists in the surgical literature regarding what represents an adequate *distal* margin, the range being 2 to 5 cm. This is based on studies to evaluate the extent of microscopic spread of cancer distal to the palpable edge of the tumor. What difference does it make if the distal margin is 2 or 5 cm, when the tangential margin is minimal or nonexistent? Many surgeons believe that this nonreported regional margin is the major cause of local recurrence of rectal cancer. Although the cure of primary rectal cancer can be very high, the cure of *locally recurrent* rectal cancer is

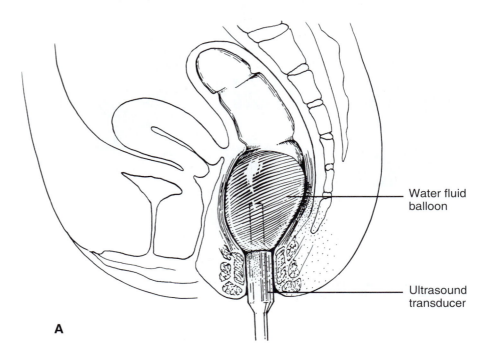

A

Water fluid balloon

Ultrasound transducer

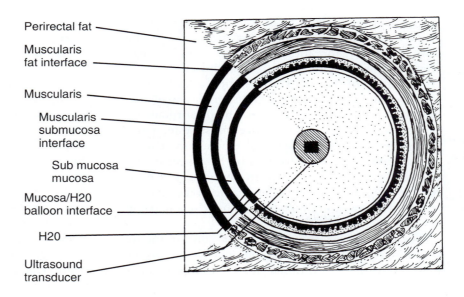

Perirectal fat

Muscularis fat interface

Muscularis

Muscularis submucosa interface

Sub mucosa mucosa

Mucosa/H20 balloon interface

H20

Ultrasound transducer

B

Figure 49–11. A. Endorectal ultrasonography assesses depth of tumor penetration and degree of perirectal involvement. **B.** Intact rectum typically shows five-banded echoic pattern on ultrasound examination. (Redrawn from John A Craig, MD in Fry RD, Fleshman JW, Kodner IJ: Cancer of colon and rectum. CIBA Clinical Symposia 1989;41:5) Copyright 1989 CIBA-Geigy. Reprinted with permission of Clinical Symposia. All rights reserved.

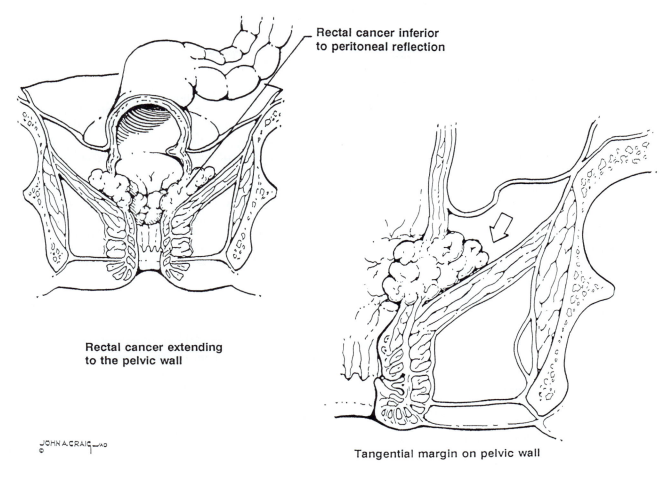

Rectal cancer inferior
to peritoneal reflection

Rectal cancer extending
to the pelvic wall

Tangential margin on pelvic wall

JOHN A.CRAIG___AD

Figure 49–12. Tangential margins in rectal cancer. (Courtesy of John Craig, MD)

exceedingly small and often requires devastatingly radical surgery. Thus, the complicated evaluation of regional spread is critical.

Distant Spread

Determination of *distant spread* of rectal cancer is important, because these patients generally are considered to be incurable. The knowledge of metastasis to
the liver or lungs may significantly modify the surgical
management of the primary cancer. Routine evaluation
for distant metastatic disease consists of a chest x-ray, determination of CEA level, and a CT scan, with contrast,
of the upper and lower abdomen. The latter also allows
evaluation of the urinary tract, as previously described.
Suspicious lesions in the liver may need further evaluation by MRI or angio-CT. CT will also help in determining metastasis to the ovaries or dissemination within the
peritoneal cavity. Rectal cancer rarely metastasizes to
the bones or to the brain, and without symptoms, these
two areas are not included in routine surveillance. The
liver must be extensively involved with cancer before

liver function tests become abnormal, and most authors
find these tests to be of limited use.

CLASSIFICATION

In the absence of obvious metastatic disease, the precise
stage of colorectal cancer can be determined only after
surgical resection and histopathologic analysis. Unlike
other solid tumors, the size of the primary lesion has little influence on prognosis of colon cancer. The factors
that are most clearly related to outcome are (1) the depth
of tumor penetration into the bowel wall, (2) the involvement of regional lymph nodes, and (3) the presence
of distant metastases. Numerous staging systems have
been developed during the past several decades, but the
system proposed by Dukes in 1932 for description of rectal cancer has continued to be widely used because of its
simplicity (Fig 49–9). The classification scheme proposed
by Dukes concerned only rectal cancer and recognized
three stages; however, the most often used variant of this
system recognizes a fourth stage (distant metastases) and

has been extended to include colon cancers. This system fails to include important prognostic information such as vascular invasion, perineural invasion, histologic differentiation, or DNA content of tumor cells. Nevertheless, the simplicity of the Dukes' classification system and its consistent correlation with prognosis suggest that it will continue to be in use for some time.

The American College of Surgeons' Commission on Cancer has urged adoption of the TNM (tumor-node-metastasis) staging system (Fig 49–10). This system separately identifies the depth of invasion of the tumor (T), the regional lymph node status (N), and the presence of distant metastases (M):

Primary Tumor (T)

TX–Primary tumor cannot be assessed

T0–No evidence of primary tumor

Tis–Carcinoma in situ

T1–Tumor invades submucosa

T2–Tumor invades muscularis propria

T3–Tumor invades through the muscularis propria into the subserosa or into nonperitonealized pericolic or perirectal tissues

T4–Tumor perforates the visceral peritoneum or directly invades other organs or structures

Regional Lymph Nodes (N)

NX–Regional lymph nodes cannot be assessed

N0–No regional lymph node metastasis

N1–Metastasis in 1 to 3 pericolic or perirectal lymph nodes

N2–Metastasis in 4 or more pericolic or perirectal lymph nodes

N3–Metastasis in any lymph node along the course of a named vascular trunk

Distant Metastasis (M)

MX–Presence of distant metastasis cannot be assessed

M0–No distant metastasis

M1–Distant metastasis

The *stage* of the TNM system is as follows:

Stage 0	Tis	N0	M0
Stage I	T1	N0	M0
	T2	N0	M0
Stage II	T3	N0	M0
	T4	N0	M0
Stage III	Any T	N1	M0
	Any T	N2, N3	M0
Stage IV	Any T	Any N	M1

The TNM system provides more detailed pathologic information and easily can be converted to the simpler Dukes' system. Stage I is equivalent to Dukes' stage A,

stage II to Dukes' stage B, stage III to Dukes' stage C, stage IV to Dukes' stage D.

The 5 year survival rates clearly demonstrate the prognostic importance of disease staging. The best outcome is associated with stage I disease, with more than 90% of patients surviving at 5 years. For stage II disease, this figure drops to between 60% and 80%, and for patients with lymph node metastasis (stage III), 5 year survival rates range from 20% to 50%. When distant metastases are present, fewer than 5% of patients survive for 5 years.

For all but stage IV disease, survival rates have improved since the 1940s and 1950s. Whether this improvement is attributable to diagnostic or treatment advances is not clear. More thorough and precise staging procedures may now be responsible for eliminating or reducing the misclassification of patients, which can artificially and adversely affect the observed response to treatment.

Other disease factors that have a negative prognostic influence include poor histologic differentiation of the tumor (mucin-producing tumors and signet-ring cell tumors have a poor prognosis), venous or perineural invasion by the cancer, bowel perforation, elevated CEA level, and aneuploid nuclei. The latter factor has recently generated interest as it appears that the DNA distribution pattern in the nuclei of cancer cells may help predict treatment failure. Flow cytometry can evaluate the DNA content of the cancer cells. It appears that tumors with predominantly diploid nuclei are less likely to metastasize than tumors with aneuploid nuclei. Some preliminary studies suggest that the DNA content of cancer cells may provide prognostic information independent of the clinicopathologic stage of the disease. Currently, specific abnormalities of the tumor DNA are proving to be more accurate in predicting long-term survival.

SURVEILLANCE

There is some controversy about the frequency of follow-up examinations for tumor recurrence in patients treated for rectal cancer. Some physicians have adopted a nihilistic approach (because of poor prognosis once recurrent cancer is detected), and recommend that once a patient is discharged following surgery, further treatment should be given only if symptoms of recurrent disease develop.

A small group of patients, however, definitely benefit from detection and aggressive treatment of recurrent cancer. About 70% of recurrent cancers become detectable within 2 years of initial treatment and 90% within 4 years. Patients who have been successfully treated for colon or rectal cancer have a higher incidence of metachronous colorectal cancer, and early detection and treatment of these cancers can improve the prognosis for these patients. This fact alone should provide sufficient rationale for long-term follow-up of all patients treated for colorectal cancer.

Follow-up evaluation may include physical examination, sigmoidoscopy, colonoscopy, liver function tests, carcinoembryonic antigen assay, chest radiography, barium enema, liver scan, CT, and MRI.

Physical examinations following surgical treatment for colorectal cancer may assuage both patient and physician, but they are of little value in the early detection of recurrent disease. By the time a recurrent cancer has become palpable by abdominal examination, it is invariably unresectable.

Sigmoidoscopy is of some value when following patients treated with low anterior resection and anastomosis for rectal or sigmoid cancer because it allows direct inspection of the anastomosis. *Colonoscopy* is most useful for the detection of metachronous polyps or cancers in patients with previously treated colorectal cancer. A special problem exists in the patient who presents with an obstructing rectal cancer because complete evaluation of the colon cannot be performed before treatment is begun. Such patients should have colonoscopy or contrast study accomplished soon after access is available. These patients should have careful evaluation of the residual colon at the time of rectal resection.

Both *liver function tests* and *CEA assay* can indicate the presence of liver metastases from colorectal cancer. A significant elevation of any of the liver function tests or a rising CEA level calls for a CT scan of the abdomen and a chest X-ray.

The principles of managing metastatic disease are similar for cancer of the colon and the rectum and have been discussed in the section on colon cancer.

■ MANAGEMENT OF RECTAL CANCER

GENERAL CONCEPTS OF SURGICAL TREATMENT

The ideal goal of treatment for any patient afflicted with cancer is the eradication of the malignancy with preservation of anatomic and physiologic function. Unfortunately, the surgical treatment of rectal carcinoma may require concomitant resection of the anal sphincter, resulting in the need for colostomy (Fig 49–13). Most surgeons agree that carcinoma of the upper rectum should be treated by resection of the proximal rectum through an abdominal incision, with reestablishment of intestinal continuity by colorectal anastomosis. This operation generally is referred to as *anterior resection*. Resection of the rectosigmoid colon performed above the pelvic peritoneum is called a *high anterior resection*, whereas an operation in which it is necessary to open the pelvic

peritoneum to resect the cancer is called a *low anterior resection*. When performing these operations, it has been our practice to resect the sigmoid colon in continuity with the rectum, assuming that after the inferior mesenteric artery has been divided, the more constant collateral circulation to the descending colon will provide a safer colorectal anastomosis. Thus, the correct terminology for the operation described in detail in this section is *anterior proctosigmoidectomy with colorectal anastomosis or restorative proctectomy*.

For many years it was believed that cancer of the rectum was most appropriately treated by abdominal perineal proctectomy and permanent colostomy (Fig 49–14). The technical challenge of fashioning an anastomosis deep in the pelvis, the assumption that the distal 5 or 6 cm of rectal mucosa was a necessary component of anal continence, and the belief that an adequate operation for cancer required a margin of normal bowel at least 5 cm distal to the visible tumor prohibited general use of anterior resection for carcinoma of the rectum within 10 cm of the anal verge. However, factors that include increased knowledge of the biologic behavior of rectal carcinoma, a greater understanding of the determinants of anorectal continence, and the introduction and widespread acceptance of circular stapling instruments that facilitate the fashioning of a bowel anastomosis deep in the pelvis have resulted in increasing use of low anterior resection for carcinoma of the rectum.

Although anterior resection is frequently considered a more conservative approach to the treatment of rectal cancer than abdominal perineal proctectomy, the experienced surgeon realizes that a properly performed anterior resection is every bit as "radical" a cancer operation: there is no compromise in the dissection of the lymphatic drainage or the extent of the tangential margins. In fact, anterior resection may be a considerably more difficult operation because of the challenge of fashioning a colorectal anastomosis deep in the pelvis. Nevertheless, the benefits of preserving anorectal continence and avoiding a colostomy without compromising the principles of cancer surgery should be obvious to both patient and surgeon. In 1982, Goligher estimated that 70% of patients being treated with rectal excision for cancer could have been treated with a sphincter-saving resection.

BIOLOGICAL BEHAVIOR OF RECTAL CANCER

The lymphatic spread of rectal cancers located higher than 5 cm from the anal verge follows a cephalad course parallel to the inferior mesenteric vascular supply. One problem facing the surgeon concerns the determination of an adequate margin of tissue distal to the cancer to assure complete eradication of the disease. Until re-

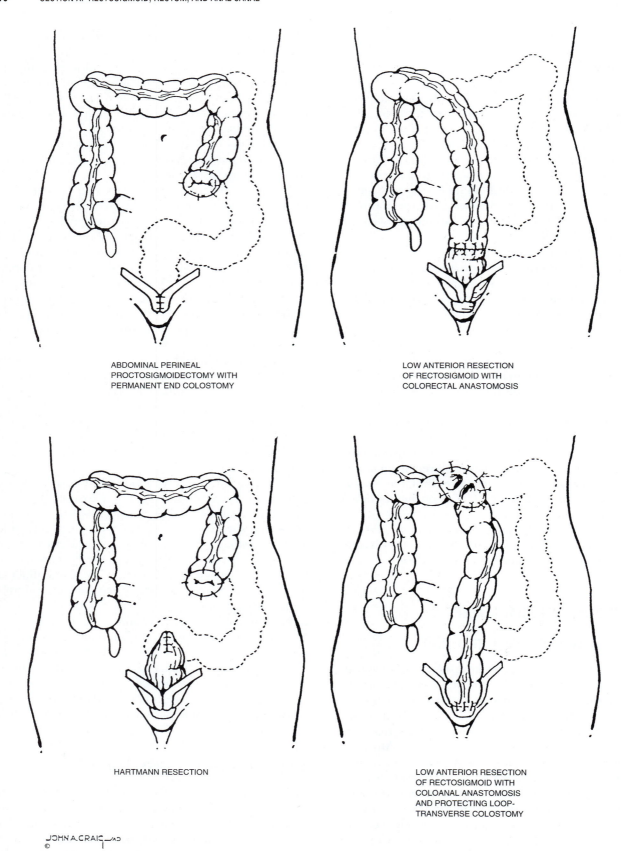

ABDOMINAL PERINEAL
PROCTOSIGMOIDECTOMY WITH
PERMANENT END COLOSTOMY

LOW ANTERIOR RESECTION
OF RECTOSIGMOID WITH
COLORECTAL ANASTOMOSIS

HARTMANN RESECTION

LOW ANTERIOR RESECTION
OF RECTOSIGMOID WITH
COLOANAL ANASTOMOSIS
AND PROTECTING LOOP-
TRANSVERSE COLOSTOMY

Figure 49–13. Options in the surgical management of rectal cancer. (Courtesy of John Craig, MD)

MAJOR RESECTIONS

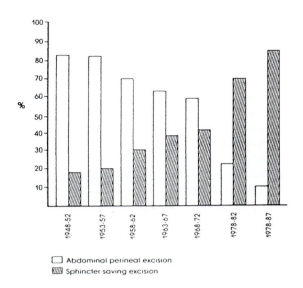

Figure 49–14. Trends in surgery for rectal carcinoma, 1948 to 1988. (From Hackford AW. The extent of major resections for rectal cancer. Seminar in Colon & Rectal Surg 1990;1(1):17)

cently it was believed that 5 cm of normal tissue distal to the grossly visible lesion provided a necessary margin. This conclusion was based on the advice of Dukes who, after a study of a large number of specimens, failed to detect downward submucosal or lymphatic spread greater than a distance of 4.5 cm from the tumor. However, grade of malignancy, as determined by the differentiation of the tumor, was not evaluated in that study. More recent studies have clearly demonstrated that for well-differentiated or moderately differentiated rectal cancer, a margin of 2 cm is adequate clearance. Poorly differentiated carcinomas probably require a distal margin of at least 5 cm, but these tumors represent a small percentage of all tumors treated.

Although many studies have been concerned with what constitutes an adequate distal margin for surgically treated rectal carcinoma, there has been relatively little appreciation for the importance of the lateral or tangential margins of resection. These margins are seldom measured or reported by the pathologist, but failure to completely eradicate the lateral extension of the cancer probably accounts for most instances of local recurrence following proctectomy. The lateral extent of resection during either abdominal perineal proctectomy or low anterior resection is restricted by the pelvic walls. However, the goal should be to achieve as wide a lateral margin as possible, and the lateral extent of the dissection should be exactly the same for low anterior resection as for an abdominal perineal proctectomy.

CHOICE OF PROCEDURES AND PRINCIPLES OF TREATMENT

The management of rectal cancer has been based on the assumption that the ideal goal of treatment for any patient with cancer would be eradication of the malignancy, preserving as much anatomic and physiologic function as possible. The choice of treatment has been confused by the fact that an accurate clinical staging system does not exist. In addition, the rectum lies deep within the pelvis and is surrounded by the musculature and bony structures of the pelvis, thus making access difficult. The use of high-dose radiation therapy from external sources also has been limited, because it is necessary to traverse normal tissue before the damaging radiation can affect the malignant cells.

The important factors in determining prognosis and selection of therapy for rectal cancer also have not been clearly defined. It became evident from the work of Crile, Turnbull, and Madden that there were certain small favorable rectal cancers that could be managed without radical surgical removal of the rectum. A detailed study of patients with rectal cancer treated at Washington University, St. Louis, revealed the important variables in determining prognosis to be degree of fixation of the cancer, the involvement of pararectal lymph nodes, and the degree of histologic dedifferentiation. The size of the tumor and the distance of the tumor from the dentate line have not been shown to affect survival or recurrence.

Cancers felt to be invading through the rectal wall or that show evidence of an aggressive histologic nature should be removed surgically, with preservation of anal sphincter function, if possible, and with consideration for the use of adjuvant radiation or chemotherapy (to be discussed later). The choice of surgical procedure should not be affected by the use of adjuvant therapy. Details of why one operative procedure is chosen over another are covered in the following discussion of the procedures—either complete removal of the rectum and sphincter mechanism or preservation of the sphincter function.

PROGNOSIS FOR RECTAL CANCER

Local recurrence of rectal cancer after proctectomy has been found in 3% to 32% of patients. Distance of tumor from the dentate line, wall penetration, lymph node involvement, rectal perforation during dissection, and tumor differentiation have all be suggested as factors influencing local recurrence. Recently, preoperative radiation has been shown to reduce local recurrence significantly (<3% in our series). This would suggest that control of lateral margins may be the most important factor in preventing local recurrence. Preoperative radiation also has been shown to increase the resectability of large rectal tumors. Controversy still exists about the effect of adjuvant radiation on survival of patient with rectal cancer. Survival at 5 years after surgery without adjuvant radiation has been reported as high as 95% for Dukes' A cancer, 71% for Dukes' B, and 45% for Dukes' C. In a recent update of our series of patients with rectal cancer, 5 year survival after preoperative radiation and resection was 100% for Dukes' A lesions, 85% for Dukes' B, and 73% for Dukes' C. The evidence supporting adjuvant radiation of rectal cancer is growing.

RESTORATIVE PROCTECTOMY (LOW ANTERIOR RESECTION)

Determinants of Anorectal Continence

Knowledge of the components of anorectal continence has recently accumulated as a result of increased interest in sphincter-saving procedures used for the surgical treatment of ulcerative colitis. These procedures involve extirpation of the entire rectal mucosa and creation of an ileal reservoir that is anastomosed to the anus. Evaluation of continence in these patients has provided information directly applicable to patients requiring proctectomy for rectal carcinoma. Factors contributing to anorectal continence include the structural integrity of the anal sphincter, the anorectal angle, innervation of the sphincter and anus, distensibility and capacity of the rectum, colonic transit time, stool consistency, and stool volume. Although all of these factors are pertinent to a patient who has rectal cancer that is amenable to treatment by low anterior resection, the loss of rectal capacity following this operation results in a change in bowel habit that is of immediate concern. As much as two-thirds of the rectum and all of the sigmoid colon are excised, with the descending colon anastomosed to the distal rectum. In addition to the loss of the physiologically capacious rectum, the inflammation and induration characteristic of a healing intestinal anastomosis result in loss of distensibility of the intestine immediately above the anus. It is common for patients treated by low anterior resection to suffer from the frequent passage of small volumes of stool. If the patient is warned prior to the operation that this problem may occur and almost always will resolve with the passage of time, the symptoms are usually well tolerated.

Preoperative Evaluation and Management

The general health of the patient is obviously important when considering any operation. Although advanced age is not a definite contraindication to low anterior resection, the physiologic status of the patient must be evaluated carefully. The cardiac, pulmonary, and renal systems must be assessed, and steps must taken to correct any physiologic abnormalities prior to the operation.

If the patient is believed to be a candidate for proctectomy, the indication for low anterior resection depends on the assessment of the rectal cancer. The location of the tumor is important for obvious reasons. Using a rigid proctoscope, the surgeon measures the exact site of the carcinoma from the dentate line. A cancer residing within 5 cm usually cannot be treated by low anterior resection. Such a lesion is located in the anal canal or immediately adjacent to the sphincter, and resection with adequate tangential margins requires excision of the sphincter, with inevitable incontinence. However, a carcinoma residing exactly 5 cm above the dentate line may be amenable to low anterior resection after mobilization of the rectum straightens the contours and lengthens the extraperitoneal bowel. With adequate mobilization of the rectum, a tumor measured at 5 cm by rigid proctoscopy can actually be moved 7 or 8 cm from the dentate line, a distance that permits satisfactory margins with sphincter preservation (Fig 49–15 A, B). Although sphincter preservation is anticipated, before embarking on any of the resective procedures for rectal cancer, the surgeon should assure that a site is chosen on the abdominal wall for a colostomy. It compounds the difficulty for the patient if an unanticipated colostomy is placed in an unfavorable location (see Chapter 12).

We have found it helpful during endoscopy to inject 0.1 mL of India ink into the subserosa on the anterior rectal wall adjacent to tumors in the middle or upper rectum (Fig 49–15C) to allow visualization of the tumor site at the time of the operation. The India ink will cause a dark discoloration of the bowel wall at the tumor site, a marker that facilitates determining the level of transection of the bowel to obtain a satisfactorily distal margin (Fig 49–15D). The injection of India ink can be done several days prior to the operation, since the dye remains at the local site for many months.

SURGICAL ALTERNATIVES TO ANTERIOR PROCTOSIGMOIDECTOMY FOR SPHINCTER PRESERVATION

Hartmann Operation

The Hartmann procedure (Fig 49–13) entails excision of the middle or upper rectum in continuity with the sigmoid colon, closure of the rectal stump with sutures or staples, and creation of a descending colostomy. Although used more frequently in the treatment of diverticulitis, it is occasionally a suitable operation for a patient with rectal cancer in whom a pelvic anastomosis cannot be safely achieved. Patients with impending obstruction as the result of rectal cancer that has invaded the pelvic wall can be treated by this approach, leaving the tumor in situ to be treated by radiation. In such cases, the rectal stump should be brought up as a mucous fistula to avoid perforation should the distal tumor cause complete obstruction. If there is a good response to the radiation, consideration can be given to curative resection. Elderly patients with rectal cancer who are in-

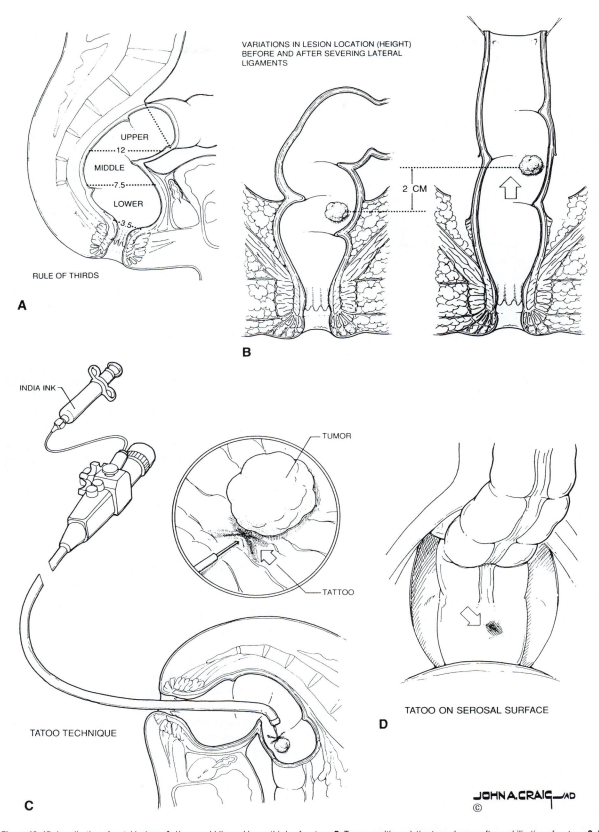

Figure 49–15. Localization of rectal lesions. **A**. Upper, middle, and lower thirds of rectum. **B**. Tumor position relative to anal verge after mobilization of rectum. **C**. Injection of 0.1 mL of India ink adjacent to tumor in rectum. **D**. India ink shadow on rectal surface.

continent may best be served by anterior resection of the rectal tumor, closure of the rectal stump, and formation of a permanent colostomy. This operation would be preferred to abdominal perineal proctosigmoidectomy in such cases, since it avoids the problems associated with a perineal wound.

Pull-through Procedure and Coloanal Anastomosis

Pull-through procedures were popular in some centers about two decades ago. The operation usually was used for treating cancer of the midrectum. The distal rectal stump was everted and the proximal sigmoid colon was "pulled through" the transected anus and allowed to adhere to the bowel. A transverse colostomy protected the anastomosis, which was made approximately 7 days after the first stage of the operation. The everted rectum was replaced in the pelvis after the anastomosis was completed, and the colostomy was closed approximately 10 weeks later. The results of this operation were usually satisfactory, and most patients preferred the procedure to a colostomy. However, patients often experienced some degree of incontinence, which was probably the result of damage to the sphincter caused by everting the distal rectum. An alternative to this approach has been the peranal anastomosis described by Parks in 1982. In this procedure, the colon is approximated to the dentate line through an anal retractor, and the problem of sphincter damage is eliminated, theoretically. The use of circular stapling instruments has allowed low anterior resection to be used in instances amenable to the pull-through procedures, and the latter operations are seldom used today.

Coloanal Anastomosis

We reserve coloanal anastomosis (Fig 49–13) for the patient with a large villous adenoma when deep invasion is not suspected or for the patient with a radiation injury (fistula) who still has enough sphincter function to allow restorative reconstruction. Currently, we do not use the procedure for deeply invasive cancers, although there comes a point at which the difference between a very low colorectal anastomosis and a coloanal anastomosis becomes academic. The classic procedure described by Parks and Percy involves leaving a significant muscular sleeve after mucosal dissection, construction of the hand-sewn anastomosis, and protection using a temporary diverting-loop colostomy.

TECHNIQUE OF ANTERIOR PROCTOSIGMOIDECTOMY WITH COLORECTAL ANASTOMOSIS

Anterior resection as treatment for carcinoma of the upper and middle rectum has increased significantly in the past few years, probably as a result of general acceptance of the circular stapling device. Numerous studies have shown that there is no difference in survival of patients treated by low anterior resection when compared with patients treated by abdominal perineal proctectomy with colostomy. There is also sufficient experience to conclude that stapled anastomoses can be accomplished with equal or superior patient survival when compared with hand-sewn colorectal anastomoses. The operative procedure should be essentially the same for hand-sewn and stapled techniques. Since the stapled technique facilitates the construction of an anastomosis deep in the pelvis and is quite easy to use for an anastomosis above the peritoneal reflection, we routinely use this method for all colorectal anastomoses. However, a sutured anastomosis, with either one or two rows of inverting sutures, is still favored by some surgeons.

Preoperative Bowel Preparation

Patients who are to undergo resection of the rectum require complete bowel preparation. Good results have been obtained using cathartics such as mannitol, magnesium citrate, or phospho-soda, or volume washout using polyethylene glycol compounds (Colyte, Golytely), or saline lavage. Varying degrees of fluid loss and electrolyte imbalance occur after such a preparation and must be corrected by intravenous replacement prior to surgery. Mechanical preparation reduces the number of bacteria present in the colon. Oral or parenteral antibiotics reduce pelvic and wound infection by reducing intraluminal bacteria. Selection of coverage that has a spectrum including gram-negative aerobes and anaerobes as well as gram-positive surface bacteria is preferred. As new antibiotics become available, the choices will change, but the bacteria to be covered will not. Our method of bowel preparation is to prescribe 2 days of clear liquids and a cathartic mechanical preparation. Oral neomycin is given. Intravenous cephalosporin and metronidazole are administered preoperatively.

Position of the Patient

The patient is placed in the modified lithotomy-Trendelenburg position, with the lower extremities supported by special leg rests designed by Allen or Lloyd-Davies. The perineum is allowed to project over the end of the table, providing adequate exposure of the anus to the perineal surgeon (Fig 49–16).

After the patient is anesthetized, a catheter is placed in the bladder via the urethra and is connected to a closed gravity drainage system. A large mushroom catheter is inserted through the anus into the rectum, and the lower bowel is irrigated with warm saline solution until the effluent returns clear. A bactericidal agent (povidone iodine) then is instilled in the rectum through the mushroom catheter, and the rectal catheter is connected to a gravity drainage system.

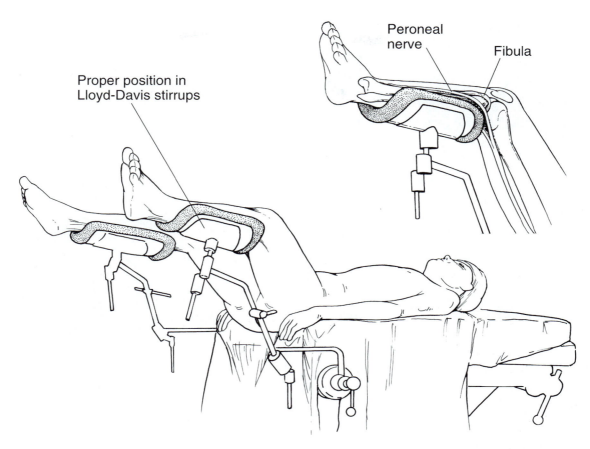

Figure 49–16. Position of patient for surgical treatment of rectal cancer allows access to both the abdomen and the perineum. (Redrawn from Goldberg SM, Gordon PH, Nivatvongs S. *Essentials of Anorectal Surgery.* Philadelphia, PA: Lippincott; 1980)

Operative Technique

Preparation of the Intra-Abdominal Colon. The abdomen is explored through a long midline incision that extends upward from the pubis. The sigmoid and descending colon are mobilized by dividing the embryonic fusion planes and peritoneum on the lateral side of the mesocolon (Fig 49–17A). The blood supply to the proximal component of the colorectal anastomosis will depend on collateral flow from the middle colic artery once the inferior mesenteric artery is divided. We believe that the collateral circulation to the descending colon is more constant than that of the sigmoid colon, and for this reason we routinely include the sigmoid in the resected specimen during an anterior resection. Thus, it is almost always necessary to mobilize the descending colon completely by dividing the peritoneal attachments inferior to the spleen (the splenic flexure is dissected from the greater omentum, which is left attached to the splenic capsule), and by reflection of the colon anteriorly and medially off Gerota's fascia overlying the left kidney (Fig 49–17A, B). The left ureter and gonadal vessels are identified and left laterally in situ.

The peritoneum at the base of the mesosigmoid is incised anterior to the aorta, exposing the origin of the inferior mesenteric artery. The inferior mesenteric artery is then doubly ligated and divided close to the aorta. Dividing this artery adjacent to the aorta preserves the arterial arcade in the mesosigmoid, permitting collateral flow to the distal descending colon from the middle colic artery (Fig 49–17C, D). The mesentery is divided to the junction of descending colon and sigmoid, and then the colon is divided at that point (Fig 49–17C). Downward traction on the descending colon will indicate if there is sufficient length to reach the rectal component of the anastomosis. If the length appears inadequate, the point of fixation prohibiting further mobility will be the inferior mesenteric vein just below the duodenum. Dividing the inferior mesenteric vein at this point will allow the descending colon to reach the deep pelvis (Fig 49–17D).

MOBILIZATION OF THE LEFT COLON

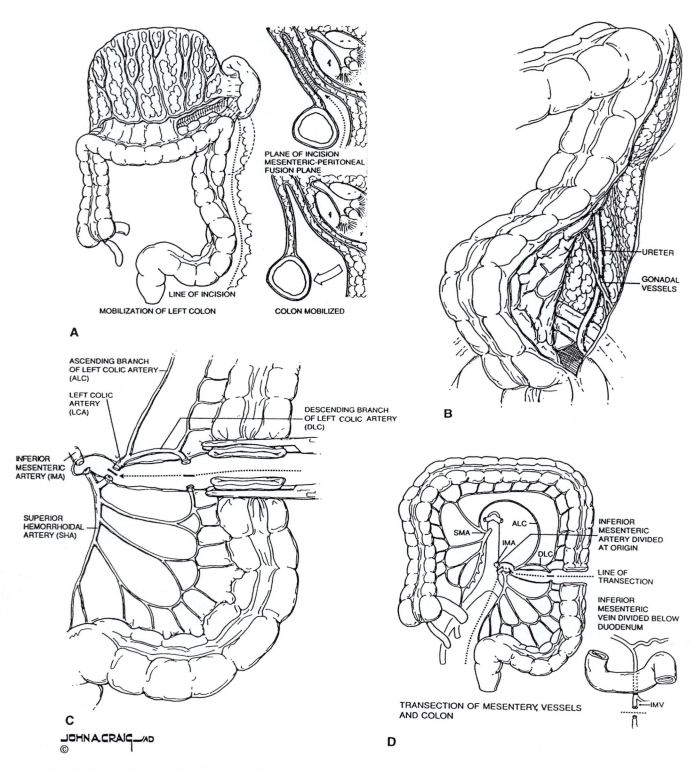

Figure 49–17. Mobilization of the left colon. **A.** Incision line around left colon and avascular fusion plane between mesentery and retroperitoneum. **B.** Left colon reflected medially, exposing retroperitoneum. **C.** Inferior mesentery artery divided close to aorta; arcade of Riolan is preserved, and left colon and mesentery are divided at junction of descending and sigmoid colon. **D.** Proximal ligation of inferior mesenteric vein for extra mobility.

Mobilization of the Rectum. The incisions in the peritoneum are extended downward on both sides of the rectum and around the brim of the pelvis to meet in the midline at the deepest part of the peritoneal cul-de-sac (Fig 49–18A). The rectosigmoid is reflected anteriorly, and the avascular presacral space is developed by a combination of blunt and sharp dissection (Fig 49–18B through D). Dissection is continued in this plane until the tip of the coccyx is reached.

Next, the bladder, seminal vesicles, and prostate (or posterior vaginal wall) are separated from the anterior rectal wall by sharp dissection under direct vision (Fig 49–18B). The lateral ligaments that contain branches of the hypogastric artery are defined and transected (Fig 49–18C). As a result of this dissection, the rectum can be lifted out of the pelvis, a maneuver that straightens the anatomic curvatures and often provides additional length distal to the tumor for an acceptable distal margin (Fig 49–18D).

The pelvic autonomic nerves are subject to injury during this operation, and adequate pararectal lymphadenectomy often will render the male impotent. The anatomic location of the nerves is illustrated in Figure 49–18E. The hypogastric plexus is located at the aortic bifurcation at the level of the fifth lumbar vertebra. Dissection of all soft tissue from the aortic bifurcation will interrupt this sympathetic plexus. An isolated sympathetic injury will result in absence of emission, or a "dry orgasm." The hypogastric nerve unites the hypogastric plexus with the pelvic plexus and contains only sympathetic fibers. These nerves reside 1 to 2 cm medial to the ureter, descending in the pelvis. The pelvic plexus receives the sympathetic fibers from the hypogastric nerves, as well as parasympathetic fibers from the pelvic splanchnic nerves. This plexus is superior to the levators, anterior and lateral to the rectum, and between the peritoneum and endopelvic fascia. Injury to the pelvic plexus can occur at the time of division of the lateral stalks or during the dissection of the rectum from the region of the seminal vesicles. Injury to both of the pelvic plexuses will result in complete impotence in the male.

In summary, during resection of the rectum, the innervation of the genitalia and bladder can be injured at five points (Fig 49–18E). The first is at the point of ligating the inferior mesenteric artery at the aorta. The preaortic sympathetic plexus can be drawn up into the resected specimen while the inferior mesenteric artery is encircled. Second, the presacral sympathetic plexus (hypogastric plexus) is vulnerable to injury during mobilization of the mesorectum from the sacral promontory. Entering the avascular plane between the fascia propria of the rectum and presacral fascia affords protection to these strands of nerve. Third, the hypogastric nerve and plexus carrying both sympathetic and parasympathetic fibers are susceptible to injury during

wide lateral dissection along the lateral pelvic wall. The fourth point of injury occurs during division of the lateral ligaments at an extremely lateral point, which may injure the nervi erigentes. The final point of injury is to the nervi erigentes, which are found within the prostatic capsule and around the seminal vesicles and are thus at risk during the anterior perineal dissection.

Colorectal Anastomosis with Circular Stapler. Before the rectum is divided at the selected site distal to the cancer, a tumoricidal agent (40% ethanol) is instilled into the devascularized sigmoid colon and is allowed to drain through the mushroom catheter exiting the anus (Fig 49–19A). This procedure theoretically kills viable intraluminal cancer cells and prevents their implantation in the suture or staple line.

The rectum is divided with a scalpel below an anterior resection clamp. Monofilament purse-string sutures are placed around the descending colon and rectal stump. Rectal stay sutures facilitate placement of the rectal purse-string suture deep in the pelvis. Various closed or open techniques can be used for placement of the purse-string sutures (Fig 49–19B).

The anvil head of the circular stapler is inserted into the lumen of the descending colon, and the purse-string suture is tied firmly around the central shaft (Fig 49–19C). The base of the stapling instrument is inserted into the rectum through the anus, and the purse-string suture is secured around the extended post of this instrument (Fig 49–19C). This phase can be facilitated by doing preliminary sigmoidoscopy to empty the rectum and to determine the course which the stapling instrument must follow. The stapling gun is closed and activated, creating a stapled anastomosis (Fig 49–19D, E). The instrument then is opened, rotated, and withdrawn. The excised fragments of the colon and rectum should be intact and resemble donuts (Fig 49–19F). The staple line is inspected by the abdominal surgeon, who fills the pelvis with saline. The perineal surgeon inserts a proctoscope through the anus to inspect the intraluminal aspect of the anastomosis. Air is insufflated through the proctoscope to distend the bowel in the region of the anastomosis, and the abdominal surgeon watches for bubbles arising in the saline solution, which would indicate a defect in the anastomosis. If an anastomotic leak is detected, it is repaired with seromuscular sutures. The completed anastomosis derives its blood supply from the superior mesenteric artery via the ascending left colic artery or the so-called arch of Riolan (Fig 49–20H).

Colorectal Anastomosis—Double-Stapling Technique. Another technique for achieving a colorectal anastomosis deep in the pelvis utilizes two stapling devices: a linear stapler to close the rectal stump and a circular, intraluminal

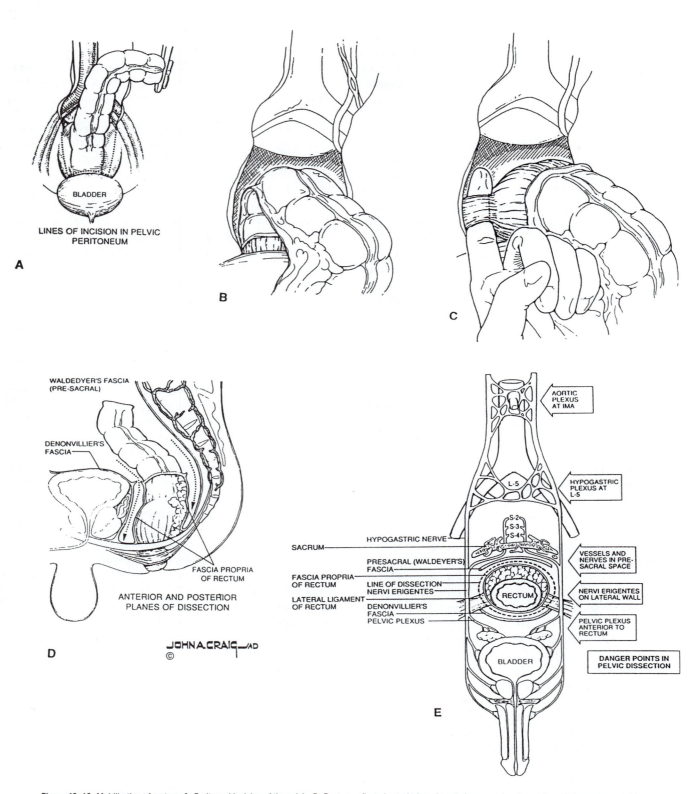

Figure 49–18. Mobilization of rectum. **A.** Peritoneal incision of the pelvis. **B.** Rectum reflected anteriorly and posterior avascular plane entered between presacral fascia of Waldeyer and fascia propria of rectum. **C.** Division of lateral stalks. **D.** Projected line of dissection in pelvis, vertical plane. **E.** Pelvic autonomic nerves and points of injury.

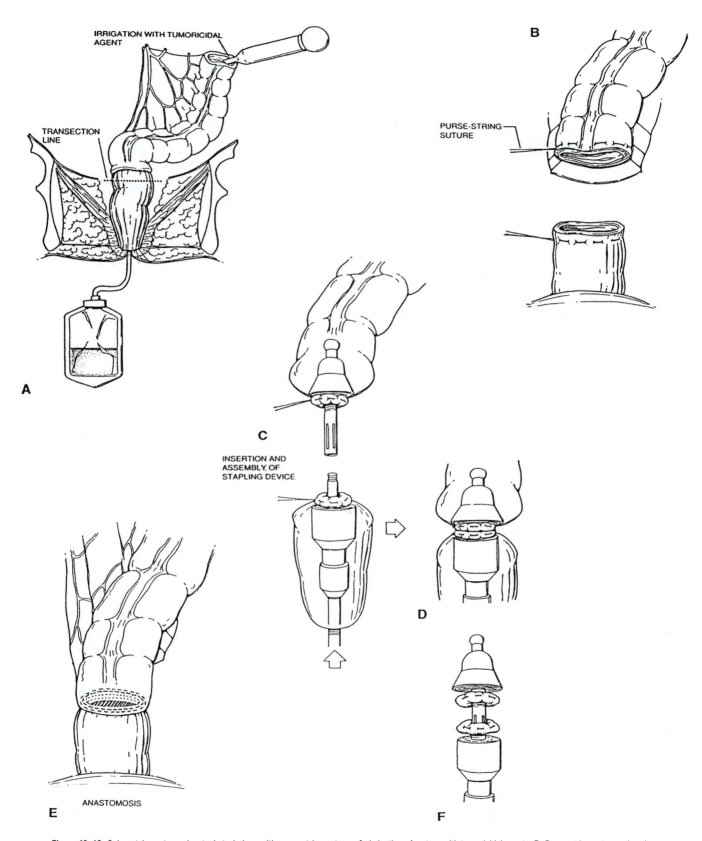

Figure 49–19. Colorectal anastomosis: staple technique with purse-string sutures. **A.** Irrigation of rectum with tumoricidal agents. **B.** Purse-string sutures placed on rectum and descending colon. **C.** Purse-string suture tied around anvil and proximal stapler shaft inserted via anus. **D.** Instrument is reconnected, reapproximated, and fired. **E.** Completed anastomosis. **F.** Inner donuts containing purse-string sutures.

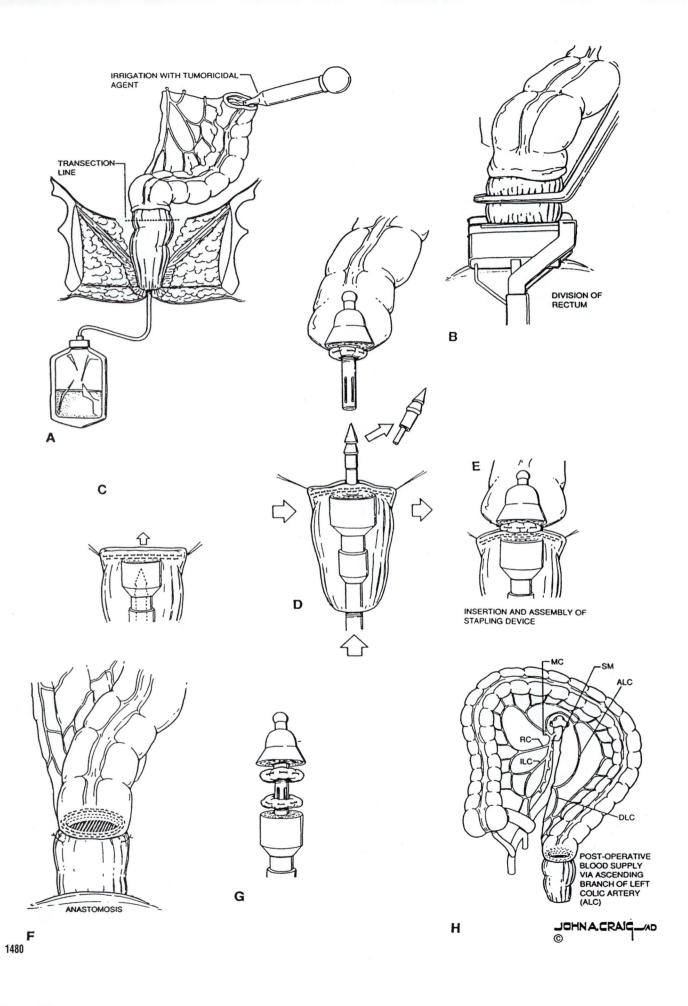

IRRIGATION WITH TUMORICIDAL AGENT

TRANSECTION LINE

A

DIVISION OF RECTUM

B

C

D

E

INSERTION AND ASSEMBLY OF STAPLING DEVICE

ANASTOMOSIS

F

G

MC

SM

ALC

RC

ILC

DLC

POST-OPERATIVE BLOOD SUPPLY VIA ASCENDING BRANCH OF LEFT COLIC ARTERY (ALC)

H

JOHN A. CRAIG—AD ©

1480

Figure 49–20. Colorectal anastomosis: double staple technique. **A.** Irrigation of rectum with tumoricidal agent. **B.** Transection of the distal rectum with linear stapler. **C.** Stay sutures placed in corners of rectal staple line and stapling instrument introduced through rectum. **D.** Trocar of stapling instrument penetrating through staple line; descending colon purse-string suture is tied around shaft of anvil. Trocar is removed before reconnecting anvil to shaft. **E.** Instrument reconnected, reapproximated, and fired. **F.** Completed anastomosis. **G.** Inner donuts containing pursestring sutures and center of staple line. **H.** Completed low anterior resection; arterial blood supply after low anterior resection. ILC = ileocolic; RC = right colic; MC = middle colic; SM = superior mesenteric; ALC = ascending left colic; DLC = descending left colic.

stapler to construct the anastomosis; hence, the term "double-stapling technique." The mobilization of the rectum is carried out exactly as described previously. However, after the tumoricidal agent has been instilled into the devascularized sigmoid (Fig 49–20A), a linear stapler is applied across the rectum at the site selected for transection (Fig 49–20B). An anterior resection clamp is used to occlude the lumen proximal to the linear stapler. The stapling instrument is fired, closing the rectal stump with two rows of staples, and the rectum is transected with a scalpel immediately proximal to the stapler, which is then released and removed. Two stay sutures or Allis clamps are placed at the corners of the rectal staple line to allow upward traction on the rectum (Fig 49–20C).

The anvil head of the circular stapler is secured in the descending colon as described previously. The proximal portion of the stapling instrument is introduced through the anus and is directed upward until the base of the instrument abuts on the staple line of the rectal stump. The upward traction of the stay sutures placed on the corners of the rectal stump helps to straighten any curvatures of the distal rectum and facilitates insertion of the instrument (Fig 49–20C). The trocar of the instrument then is extended and allowed to penetrate the rectal wall immediately adjacent to the staple line. It is anticipated that the central portion of the rectal staple line will be resected by the circular stapling instrument (Fig 49–20D). The components of the instrument are coupled and the stapling instrument is closed and activated, forming the anastomosis (Fig 49–20E,F). Remnants of the linear staple line will remain at both corners of the rectal stump and may be inverted with sutures. The donuts of tissue within the stapling instrument are examined to verify their integrity (Fig 49–20G). The anastomosis is inspected with a proctoscope, and the integrity is proven by insufflating air into the rectum with saline solution in the pelvis, as described previously. The completed anastomosis with its blood supply is illustrated in Fig 49–20H.

Drainage of the Pelvis. If the colorectal anastomosis is made entirely below the peritoneal reflection, we routinely drain the pelvis with suction catheters in the manner to be described for abdominal perineal proctectomy. Fluid which accumulates in the extraperitoneal area of dissection will not be absorbed as readily as intraperitoneal fluid. This fluid serves as an excellent culture medium and may permit formation of an abscess in the area adjacent to the anastomosis, resulting in an anastomotic leak. Although this premise is theoretic rather than proven, there has been wide experience with the use of suction catheters following low anterior resection, and it appears that there may be some benefit to this practice. We remove the catheters when the drainage is minimal, usually between postoperative day 4 to 7.

COMPLETE REMOVAL OF THE RECTUM AND ANUS (ABDOMINOPERINEAL PROCTOSIGMOIDECTOMY)

History of Abdominoperineal Resection

Czerny described a *perineal* approach for resection of rectal carcinoma in 1884, but survival following this treatment was dismal. Ernest Miles observed lymph node metastases along the mesorectum and the vessels as far as the inferior mesenteric artery and aorta in patients with rectal cancer. He was convinced that removal of the upward spread of rectal cancer affected the cure rate after resection of a rectal cancer as much as removal of the tumor itself. In 1908, Miles described the combined *abdominal* and *perineal* approach for resection of the rectum for malignancy. The mortality rate in his first 12 patients was 42%, but Miles justified the treatment with the knowledge that perineal proctectomy alone resulted in 90% mortality from local recurrence. The technique he described involved a one-team approach, with repositioning of the patient to perform the perineal procedure. The coccyx was removed, the rectum was pulled through from below to complete the anterior dissection, and the perineal wound was left open.

Lockhart-Mummery first described the perineal dissection performed with the patient in the lithotomy position. Rhoads described a two-team, simultaneous abdominoperineal approach in 1965. While other modifications have been introduced concerning peritoneal floor closure, perineal wound closure, omental pedicle slings, pelvic drains, adjuvant radiation, and stoma construction, the basic principle of resection of the rectum in continuity with its vascular and lymphatic supply remains unchanged.

The number of patients treated by total proctectomy for cancer of the rectum has decreased in recent years. This is not due to a drop in the number of patients with rectal cancer. Improved techniques have allowed anastomosis of the colon to the distal rectum after anterior resection of the middle or upper rectum. As recently as 1979, Butcher commented that unless a tumor of the rectum, when fully mobilized, could be delivered to the level of the abdominal wound, a total proctectomy should be performed. However, it has become obvious that a shorter distal margin will not compromise the cure rate in patients with well-differentiated or moderately differentiated cancers.

The introduction of the circular intraluminal stapler has reduced the requirement for perineal proctectomy by enabling the surgeon to achieve an anastomosis deep in the pelvis. The percentage of patients with rectal cancer requiring abdominoperineal resection has fallen markedly in the past decade. In some cases the anastomosis has been made close to the dentate line, with no compromise in cure (Fig 49–14).

Special Considerations

Pararectal Cancers Extending into the Rectum. Rarely do nonrectal cancers extend into the rectum and require total proctectomy for removal. The most common tumors with this presentation are those classified as presacral tumors. This group includes malignant teratomas and chordomas that occasionally invade the rectum. To obtain adequate margins, it may be necessary to remove a portion of the rectum with the specimen. If the anal sphincter is involved, a total proctectomy will be required. Other tumors such as prostatic, ovarian, and cervical cancers may invade directly or implant on the rectum and require a total proctectomy for cure. These are rare situations, and the chance for cure must be very low.

Anal Sphincter. The external anal sphincter is separated from the internal sphincter only by the intersphincteric plane formed by the distal longitudinal fibers of the rectum. If a cancer is present in the anal canal and invades the muscularis propria of the rectum, the external sphincter must be resected to obtain an adequate margin of clearance. The lateral margin of dissection is important in achieving local control of a rectal cancer. The lateral extent of pelvic dissection is the same for abdominoperineal proctectomy as for low anterior resection. In most circumstances, a portion of levator muscles can be retained to facilitate perineal wound closure and to reduce the incidence of perineal hernia (Fig 49–21).

Selection of Colostomy Site. The colostomy site should be marked preoperatively as described in Chapter 12. If the left lower quadrant site is chosen, the stoma should be brought through the rectus muscle. A midline stoma site is an alternative choice. A full discussion of the stoma and its implications should be carried out with the patient and family prior to surgery.

Operative Technique

The patient is positioned in the modified lithotomy-Trendelenburg position (Fig 49–16). The lower bowel is cleansed by rectal irrigation after induction of anesthesia.

The incision most suitable for abdominal excision of the rectum is a midline incision from the pubis to the upper abdomen. Should the splenic flexure of the colon need to be mobilized, the incision may be extended to the xiphoid. A self-retaining retractor allows adequate lateral exposure. Care must be used when opening the peritoneum at the pubis to avoid injury to the dome of the bladder. The fascial incision should first be carried to the pubic symphysis, and the peritoneum should be incised to one side or the other of the bladder. A pelvic retractor with a lip placed over the bladder or uterus allows full exposure of the anterior cul-de-sac in the majority of cases.

Abdominal Dissection. The abdominal dissection is performed in the same manner as described for low anterior resection (Figs 49–17 and 49–18). The colon is divided at the descending colon-sigmoid colon junction. The distal limb of the colon can be irrigated with 40% ethanol to prevent cancer cell implantation during the rectal dissection should perforation occur. The sigmoid mesentery is freed from the anterior surface of the aorta to the sacral promontory. The sigmoid colon may be removed for convenience. In the one-team approach, a metal ring is tied to the proximal stump of the rectum with a tracheostomy tape to allow retrieval of the rectum through the perineal wound when the patient is in the prone position (Fig 49–22).

Pelvic Dissection. The pelvic dissection for the abdominoperineal proctectomy is the same as for a low anterior resection of the rectum and has been described. Several details specific to this procedure follow.

Posterior Dissection. The posterior dissection is extended to the pelvic floor, while the rectum is held anteriorly with a retractor. The dissection is accomplished in the avascular plane between Waldeyer's fascia and the thin, but definite, enveloping fascia of the rectum (Fig 49–21F). Waldeyer's fascia is encountered as it reflects forward from the presacral fascia onto the fascia propria of the rectum, and it is incised anterior to the coccyx. If the presacral fascia is disrupted during the posterior dissection, the vertebral venous system may be torn, resulting in exsanguinating hemorrhage. Should this oc-

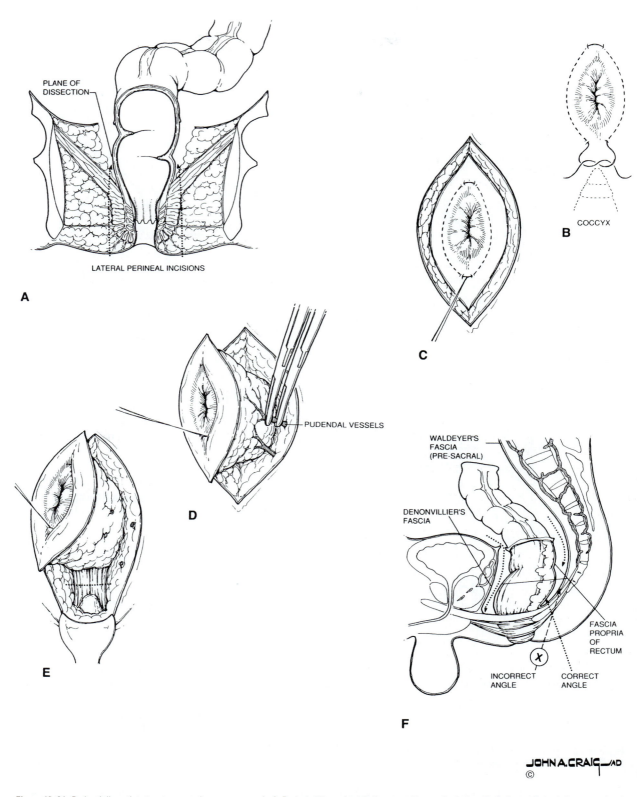

Figure 49–21. Perineal dissection: two team synchronous approach. **A.** Projected lines of pelvic floor resection, vertical plane. **B, C, D,** and **E.** Anal closure, perineal incision, and dissection. Incision line in front of coccyx through anococcygeal ligament. **F.** Planes of pelvic dissection and posterior plane of entry into pelvis through pelvic floor.

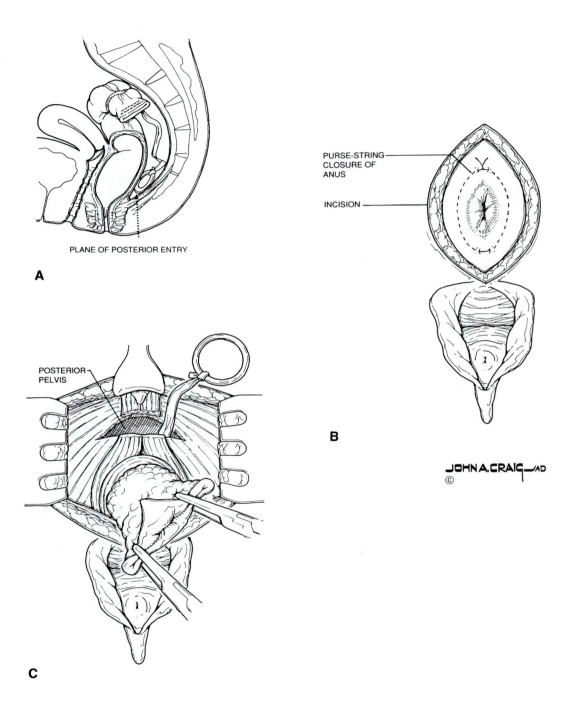

PLANE OF POSTERIOR ENTRY

A

PURSE-STRING
CLOSURE OF
ANUS

INCISION

B

JOHN A. CRAIG
©

POSTERIOR
PELVIS

C

Figure 49–22. Perineal dissection: single-team approach. **A.** Line of pelvic entry; the rectum is tucked posteriorly, with a traction ring secured to the stump. **B.** Anal purse-string suture in place and perineal incision to posterior vagina. **C.** Pelvis is entered posteriorly in front of the coccyx, and the traction ring is delivered. *Continued*

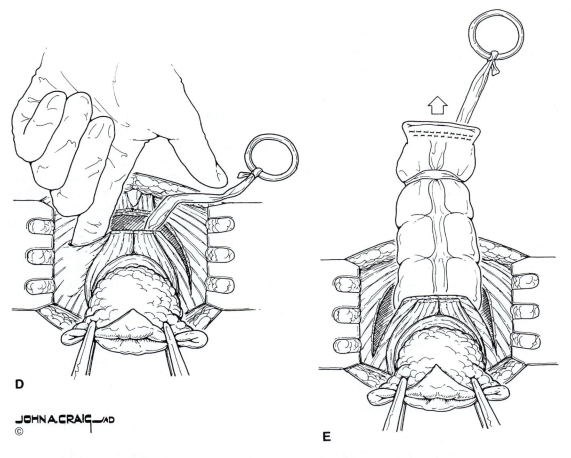

D

JOHN A.CRAIG—AD
©

E

Figure 49–22, cont'd. D. Levator ani muscles are divided. **E**. Rectum is pulled through the perineal wound.

cur, careful inspection of the sacrum to identify the bleeding point and insertion of a sterile thumbtack into the sacrum, a technique described by Wang and associates will stem the flow.

Lateral Dissection. The lateral ligaments of the rectum consist of fat and connective tissue superiorly. The middle hemorrhoidal artery crosses inferiorly and anteriorly at the distal aspect of the tissue mass. However, there may be multiple vessels scattered through the tissue that require individual control. Some authors (including Miles) have proposed that these vessels can be divided without taking measures to control their bleeding, other than to pack the pelvis. This greatly increases the blood lost during the procedure and would seem unjustified today.

Anterior Dissection. The anatomy seen during this part of the procedure depends on the sex of the patient. In a woman, the avascular rectovaginal septum is encoun-

tered after incising the peritoneum across the pouch of Douglas. If the rectal cancer is located on the anterior wall, the posterior wall of the vagina should be resected. The rectovaginal septum is entered only if the lesion is not located on the anterior wall of the rectum. In a man, it is not necessary to expose the posterior wall of the bladder and seminal vesicles, especially in the patient who has received preoperative radiation. This prevents injury to the nervi erigentes around the seminal vesicles and prostate. The plane posterior to Denonvilliers fascia and anterior to the rectum is followed to avoid injury to the prostatic capsule. A retractor is used to reflect the bladder and prostate anteriorly, and the rectum is dissected from the posterior aspect of the prostate.

When the abdominal dissection is completed, drains are placed into the pelvis through the abdominal wall. Soft-suction drains or alternating suction and irrigation through sump drains has been used successfully to reduce the complications of pelvic sepsis. Serum and blood accumulation in the pelvis can serve as a culture medium and should be removed. When drains are used from above, there is no need for "reperitonealizing" the pelvis; and the pelvic floor can be closed securely from below.

In an ovulating woman, the ovaries may fall into the pelvis and become covered by mesothelial growth, placing them in a retroperitoneal, rather than intraperitoneal, location. The resulting "trapped ovary" has required reoperation for symptoms of pain, obstruction, and an expanding pelvic mass. This is prevented easily by tacking the ovaries to the lateral pelvic wall with a nonabsorbable suture. If preoperative radiation has been used, the ovaries should be removed because they will have been rendered nonfunctional by the radiation and may theoretically represent a locus of metastatic or primary malignant disease.

Construction of Colostomy. The colostomy is brought through the left lower quadrant abdominal wall through the rectus muscle sheath at the previously marked site. The mesentery of the colon is sutured to the lateral abdominal wall to prevent tension and internal hernia formation. The abdominal wall is closed, and attention is directed to constructing the colostomy (see Chapter 12). A flush stoma is created, using interrupted sutures of absorbable material that include the full thickness of bowel and skin.

Perineal Dissection: Combined Synchronous Approach

General. The perineal portion of the procedure can be performed at the same time as the pelvic dissection from above, using a combined synchronous approach. A second team of surgeons stationed between the legs of the patient begins the perineal portion of the proctectomy when the abdominal team of surgeons has begun the deep pelvic dissection. The patient is already in the lithotomy position, with buttocks taped apart. The table is placed in maximal Trendelenburg position, and the rectal catheter is removed before the perineum is prepared again.

The entire sphincter mechanism should be removed, with the rectum and a cuff of adjacent levator ani muscle spared (Fig 49–21). This will allow closure of the pelvic floor and does not compromise margins in the usual case, especially when combined with preoperative radiation.

Technique. The anal canal is closed first, with a heavy purse-string suture placed around the circumference of the anus just outside the intersphincteric groove (Fig 49–21B). The ends of the suture are left long, after they are tied to allow traction. An elliptical incision is made from the midpoint of the perineal body, in the male, or the posterior aspect of the vaginal introitus, in the female, to a point over the coccyx. The incision is extended laterally to include the entire sphincter mechanism (Fig 49–21C, D). The incision is deepened into the ischiorectal fossa to the level of the levator ani muscles just external to the external sphincter muscles. The inferior hemorrhoidal (pudendal) vessels and nerves must be controlled for hemostasis by ligation or electrocautery. This portion of the dissection is facilitated by the placement of a deep rake retractor to separate the ischiorectal fat from the sphincter mechanism.

Posterior Dissection. The incision is carried posteriorly to expose the anococcygeal ligament or raphe. The superficial postanal space is entered by incising sharply the anococcygeal ligament anterior to the coccyx (Fig 49–21E). The fibers of the external sphincter are separated bluntly in the midline posteriorly until the levator muscles are traversed, and the pelvis is entered posteriorly in the line indicated in Fig 49–21F. The total distance between the anococcygeal ligament and the pelvis may be <2 cm. The maneuver usually requires sharp dissection with scissors or electrocautery. It should prevent lifting the presacral fascia from the sacrum and entering the presacral venous plexus, which may occur if blunt finger dissection is used. The abdominal operator can direct the perineal operator during this maneuver by retracting the rectum anteriorly and palpating the direction of the scissors as they are advanced into the pelvis. Once the pelvis is entered, the opening is widened to allow the perineal operator to place a finger into the pelvis.

Lateral Dissection. The intended transection of the muscles of the pelvic floor for the entire operation is depicted in Figure 49–23A. The levator muscles are divided laterally over the finger placed into the pelvis and on either side, lateral to the rectum along the pelvic floor (Fig 49–23B). The levator muscles are divided lateral to the puborectalis band to leave an adequate cuff to close the pelvic floor (Fig 49–23C, D). This margin is adequate in patients who have had preoperative radiation and does not increase the risk of local recurrence. A lateral margin that includes all gross tumor must be ob-

Figure 49–23. Perineal dissection: two-team synchronous approach. **A.** Projected lines of pelvic floor transection. **B.** Lateral transection of levator ani muscle. **C.** Anterior transection of rectourethralis, puborectalis, and pubococcygeus. **D.** Completion of anterior dissection and removal of the rectum through the perineal wound. **E.** Pelvic floor closed and drains in place.

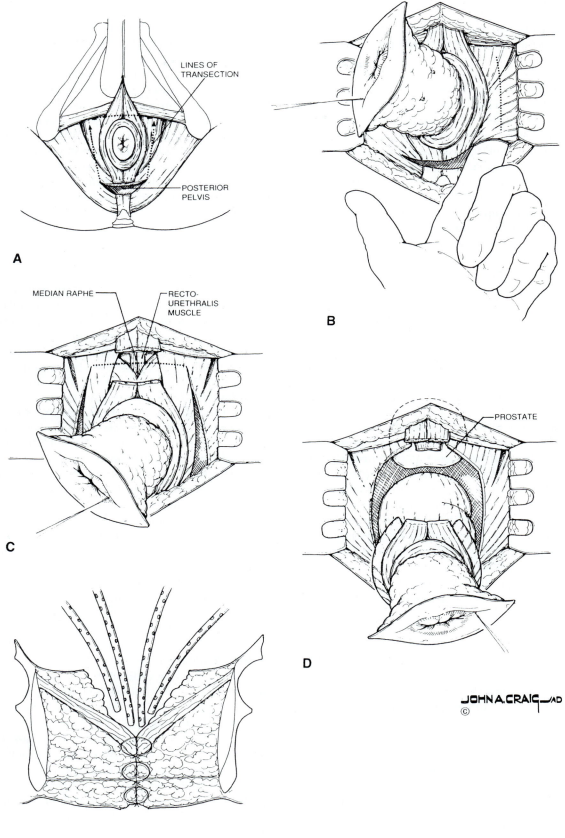

A

LINES OF
TRANSECTION

POSTERIOR
PELVIS

B

MEDIAN RAPHE

RECTO-
URETHRALIS
MUSCLE

C

D

PROSTATE

JOHN A. CRAIG ᴀᴅ
©

E

1487

tained. The advantage of this technique is to allow adequate pelvic floor closure and to avoid perineal wound herniation.

Anterior Dissection. The perineal operator should now have a clear view of the posterior pelvis. The dissection can be continued anteriorly in one of two ways. The first is to pull the rectum through the perineal wound, to use the rectum itself to provide traction, and to expose the anterior aspect for dissection. The second method is to continue with the rectum in situ. Either method must be performed with care to avoid the urethra and prostatic capsule anteriorly. The posterior fibers of the superficial and deep transverse perineal muscles are first exposed through a transverse incision in the anterior decussating fibers of the external sphincter (Fig 49–23C). Deep to the transverse perineal muscles, the median raphe in the rectourethralis and puborectalis muscles is identified. The median raphe is followed with blunt scissor dissection into the pelvis, aiming at the apex of the prostate and using either a finger placed into the pelvis from the abdomen or the perineum as a guide. The rectum is retracted posteriorly by pulling downward on the rectum, which is drawn through the wound, or by pulling posteriorly, using the same guiding finger wrapped around the rectum. Thus, a communication is established between the perineum and pelvis anteriorly. The medial fibers of the puborectalis and pubococcygeus muscles, rectourethralis muscle, visceral fascia, and remaining lateral ligaments on either side are divided from the lateral aspect by using a finger hooked around the tissue as a guide. If the rectum has been pulled through, this procedure is facilitated by rotational countertraction on the rectum. When it is completed, the rectum can be removed (Fig 49–23D). The pelvis is irrigated from above through the perineal wound with 1% kanamycin in saline solution, and drains are placed in the depths of the pelvis (Fig 49–23E).

Closure of the Perineum. The peritoneum is left open, and the perineal wound is closed in layers (Fig 49–23E). The levator muscles are approximated in the midline with interrupted synthetic absorbable sutures. The fibrofatty tissue of the ischiorectal fossa is approximated, subcutaneous sutures are placed, and the skin edges are left open.

Perineal Dissection: Single-Team Approach

Indications. The single-team approach should be considered when there is a large anteriorly placed lesion or when a posterior vaginectomy is required. The exposure afforded by the prone, flexed position greatly facilitates the anterior dissection in these circumstances.

There will be less blood loss with the absence of venous engorgement caused by the lithotomy position.

General. During the abdominal portion of the procedure, the rectum is transected at the sacral promontory, and a metal ring is secured to the stump with a tracheostomy tape. The stump and ring are then tucked posteriorly before closing the abdomen (Fig 49–22A). The perineal dissection is performed after the abdomen is closed, the pelvic drains are placed, and the colostomy is constructed. The patient is turned to the prone flexed position, with a large roll under the hips, and chest rolls to allow lung expansion and prevent brachial plexus injury. The buttocks are taped apart. The rectum remains tucked into the presacral space, with a ring in place for easy retrieval. Suction is maintained on the pelvic drains.

Technique. The anus is first closed with a purse-string suture. The incision is elliptical from the coccyx to the perineal body or the posterior vagina, including the sphincters (Fig 49–22B). The majority of the dissection is the same as for the two-team approach. The pelvis is entered posteriorly between the coccyx and the rectum (Fig 49–22C). The lateral pelvic floor muscles are divided lateral to the puborectalis over a guiding finger placed through the posterior incision (Fig 49–22D). The ring and rectal stump are retrieved and are pulled through the perineal wound (Fig 49–22E). In a man, the dissection anteriorly can be continued from a lateral approach, with upward and lateral countertraction to expose the rectourethralis, puborectalis, and pubococcygeus muscles during division (Fig 49–24A). The prostate and membranous urethra are avoided more easily because the visibility is excellent. In a woman, this approach also allows easy visualization of the rectovaginal septum and therefore facilitates complete hemostasis (Fig 49–24B). The wound is irrigated with 1% kanamycin solution, and the perineal wound is closed, as previously described, after the pelvic drains have been repositioned from below.

Posterior Vaginectomy. A low anterior rectal cancer in a woman is always an indication for a posterior vaginectomy when an abdominoperineal proctectomy is necessary. The posterior wall of the vagina should be removed as the anterior margin of the resection (Fig 49–24C). The simplest method of performing this portion of the procedure is to use the single-team approach, with the patient in the prone, flexed position. The circumanal incision includes the posterior introitus (Fig 49–24D). After completing the posterior and lateral dissections, the surgeon delivers the rectum through the wound by grasping the ring at the stump of the rectum (Fig 49–24E). As the rectum is pulled upward and inferiorly, the posterior vaginal wall is tented up. An incision is

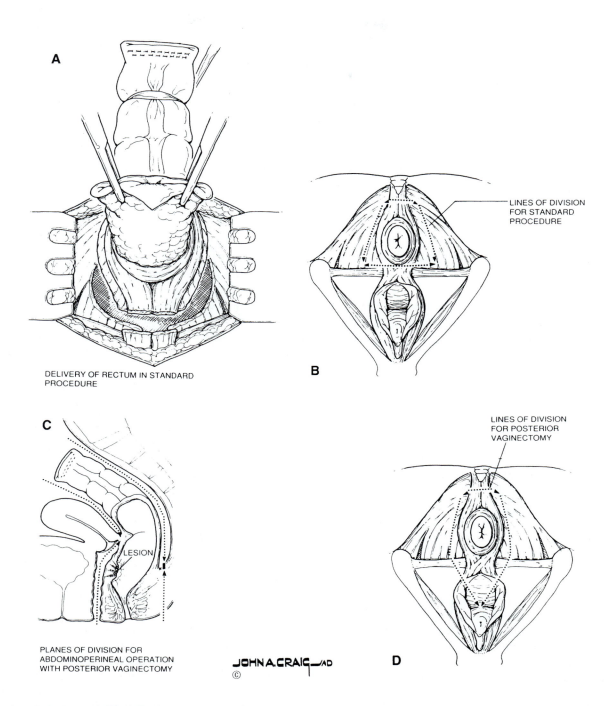

A

DELIVERY OF RECTUM IN STANDARD
PROCEDURE

B

LINES OF DIVISION
FOR STANDARD
PROCEDURE

C

LESION

PLANES OF DIVISION FOR
ABDOMINOPERINEAL OPERATION
WITH POSTERIOR VAGINECTOMY

JOHN A. CRAIG—AD
©

D

LINES OF DIVISION
FOR POSTERIOR
VAGINECTOMY

Figure 49–24. Perineal dissection: single-team approach and posterior vaginectomy. **A.** Anterior dissection is completed. **B.** Lines of muscle transection in female *not* having vaginectomy. **C.** Line of dissection, including posterior wall of vagina for low anterior rectal cancer. **D.** Lines of transection, including posterior wall of vagina. *Continued*

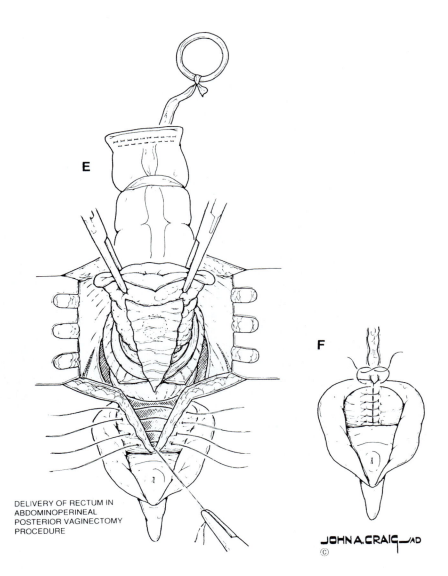

DELIVERY OF RECTUM IN
ABDOMINOPERINEAL
POSTERIOR VAGINECTOMY
PROCEDURE

JOHN A. CRAIG—AD
©

Figure 49–24, cont'd. E. Posterior vaginal wall is resected in continuity with the rectum, beginning at the cervix; the vaginal wall defect is closed with simple sutures placed as the incision is made. **F**. Closure of the vagina and reconstruction of the perineum.

made in the vagina to allow an adequate margin of resection. The incision is extended only around the posterior one-third to one-half of the vagina to avoid denervation of the urethra. As the incision is directed toward the perineum, interrupted 2-0 absorbable sutures are placed through the full thickness of the vagina from either side, starting at the apex of resection, and are tied. In this way, the opening is closed as the specimen is excised, and hemostasis is complete throughout the procedure. The incisions are extended to the vaginal introitus, which is reconstructed (Fig 49–24F). The specimen can be removed as this final point of connection is divided, and the vaginal closure is completed. The perineal wound then should be closed after irrigation and placement of drains, as described previously.

■ COMPLICATIONS OF PROCTECTOMY

Complications resulting from the surgical management of rectal cancer overlap with those of any major abdominal procedure, including sepsis, myocardial infarction, pulmonary embolus, and wound problems.

There are some specific problems related to rectal cancer. One is risk of injury to sexual function. The sites of these injuries have been described. It is not known how to completely avoid these injuries and still do an adequate cancer operation. There is at least a 50% incidence of significant impotence in men following resection of the rectum for cancer. For this reason, it is critical to discuss the situation with the patient before surgery and to record the pretreatment status of sexual function. It is prudent to include this risk of sexual impairment as part of a preoperative informed-consent note. This safeguard and mention of possible need for a colostomy are the two most important elements of such a note for the patient with rectal cancer.

If a man is rendered impotent by treatment of a rectal cancer, it is advisable to wait a year before seeking consultation for implantation of some type of penile prosthetic device. The wait is important to be sure that the malignant growth has been cleared from the pelvis and to give the patient a chance to overcome functional and psychological impediments to normal sexual function which can result from pelvic surgery and the change in body image caused by the colostomy.

Leakage from colorectal anastomosis has been reported in up to 20% of cases using current techniques. This complication can be avoided by constructing the anastomosis with well-vascularized bowel under no tension and by draining the pelvis from above. Most leaks are believed to result from sepsis in the pelvis that dissects into the anastomosis rather than from primary defects in the anastomosis. Young, muscular men have a higher incidence of anastomotic leaks. This may be the result of the technical difficulty of operating within a muscular pelvis, or it may be the result of the power of their sphincter mechanism, which acts as a postoperative obstruction and stresses the anastomosis. Such patients should probably have dilation of the anal sphincter in the operating room, at the conclusion of the procedure.

A leaked colorectal anastomosis usually presents between 4 and 7 days postoperatively. The symptoms range from mild temperature elevation, to fecal fistula in the wound, to diffuse peritonitis. When such a problem is suspected, feeding is discontinued and radiologic studies are performed (supine and upright films of the abdomen and chest, at first), looking for extraluminal gas. CT scan can be helpful to show abscess formation, inflammation, or extraluminal gas; water soluble contrast study can demonstrate the actual leak. Barium should be avoided, because leakage of barium, especially when mixed with stool, creates a severely destructive form of peritonitis.

The management of a leaking colorectal anastomosis depends on the severity of the problem. The majority cause minimal symptoms of sepsis and are demonstrated only with water soluble contrast studies of the rectum. Antibiotics and bowel rest usually suffice for treatment. If the leakage has caused an abscess that drains into the rectum or a fistula that drains to the wound, the patient should be placed on antibiotics, complete bowel rest, and total parenteral nutrition for at least 2 weeks. If a large leak is demonstrated, or if the patient has symptoms of diffuse peritonitis, laparotomy should be performed with the intention of constructing a completely diverting colostomy, and mucous fistula, if necessary. Rarely, the anastomosis and the proximal component used for the colostomy are taken down. However, the anastomosis should never be reconstructed in the presence of significant sepsis.

A special problem can occur intraoperatively during the performance of the rectal dissection: *massive venous bleeding* from the presacral space. This type of bleeding has been notoriously difficult to control because it actually comes from venous structures within the bone. The older control maneuvers of ligating the iliac vessels are ineffective and may be hazardous. The specimen should be removed and the pelvis packed for 24 to 48 hours, or preferably, a surgical metal "tack" is driven into the sacrum to compress the venous space.

Malfunction of the urinary system is also common after resection of the rectum. This is especially true in men, in whom prostatic hypertrophy may coexist with the rectal cancer. The perineal dissection of the rectum comes very close to the membranous urethra. Foley catheters should be left in place at least one week after proctectomy. If urinary symptoms exist preoperatively, urologic consultation should be obtained. Rarely, a patient must be discharged from the hospital with an indwelling urinary catheter, or have prostatic resection performed before discharge. Some patients also may have problems with bladder function postoperatively. One of the most serious is that of urinary incontinence resulting from resection of the anterior aspect of the vagina, which contains the neurologic control of the urethra. The other problem is distortion of the vagina, which impairs sexual function in the postoperative period.

■ STOMA COMPLICATIONS

Complications arising after formation of a stoma include ischemia, retraction, hernia, stenosis, prolapse and fistula. Data collected in the United Ostomy Association's registry from 6612 patients with an end colostomy for cancer reveal that 3.5% of people who replied had stomal retraction, 4% had stricture, 1% had a fistula, and 12.5% had developed a peristomal hernia. The construction of a good colostomy can afford a patient a good quality of life after this procedure. Every effort should be made in this regard.

Stoma care is important in the immediate postoperative period. Early education of the patient is useful in the process of adjusting to life with a stoma. As the stoma loses edema and shrinks to its final size, a change of appliance will be necessary (usually 2 to 3 weeks postoperatively). An end colostomy can be irrigated to establish a bowel control regimen and to allow more freedom and an improved quality of life for the patients.

■ MORTALITY

The operative mortality after an abdominoperineal resection should be <2%. As with all forms of major abdominal surgery, improved anesthesia techniques and invasive perioperative monitoring have allowed the reduction in mortality from the 42% reported by Miles in 1908.

■ SPECIAL PROBLEMS OF RECTAL CANCER

OBSTRUCTING CANCER OF THE RECTUM

Unfortunately, some rectal cancers still present at a late stage with complete obstruction. The new concepts of managing rectal cancer still can be employed and the guiding principle should be to do the procedure that gives the best chance of cure. For cancers residing above the level for considering preoperative external radiation (higher than 15 cm from the mucocutaneous junction), the following choices are available:

1. Decompressing colostomy, followed by bowel preparation and single-stage resection with restoration of intestinal continuity.
2. Hartmann resection of the obstructing cancer with subsequent restoration of continuity, made easier by the use of new stapling instruments.
3. On-table colonic washout followed by primary resection and anastomosis. We have not used this latter technique frequently, but others report good results using it.
4. Total abdominal colectomy with ileal rectal anastomosis. This allows the surgeon to deal with a nonfecal-filled ileum, in which case some dilation actually makes the anastomosis easier. The functional results are acceptable, and the procedure removes most of the at-risk colonic tissue, reducing the risk of subsequent cancer and simplifying long-term follow-up.

For obstructing cancers of the true rectum (0 to 15 cm from the mucocutaneous junction), our preference is not to compromise the chance for cure or effective palliation. Even if limited metastatic disease is found at the time of presentation of these advanced lesions, we believe everything should be done to provide local control in the pelvis. To accomplish this, a decompressing colostomy or loop ileostomy is constructed. External radiation (4500 cGy) is administered over 5 weeks, and after a 6- to 7-week waiting period, the cancer is resected and the diverting stoma is closed. For the rare patient who has an obstructing or perforating rectal cancer, in whom, because of previous surgery, the small intestine is fixed in the pelvis, the same staged procedure is used that we advise for recurrent rectal cancer.

■ INCURABLE AND RECURRENT RECTAL CANCER

INCURABLE CANCER

The management of hepatic and pulmonary metastases is described elsewhere in this text. The question arises: what to do with the rectal cancer itself in the patient who presents with incurable, massive metastatic disease? If the life expectancy is >6 months, it is probably appropriate to give 4500 cGy external radiation (perhaps combined with systemic chemotherapy), to shrink the tumor, and then perform a palliative resection. This takes away a significant amount of "out-of-hospital" time from the patient whose time has become precious, but it is clearly the best form of palliation, even if it requires a colostomy. An alternative recently described is to give a course of external radiation, with or without chemotherapy, and maintain a lumen through the cancer by laser destruction, thus avoiding resective surgery and need for a colostomy. This choice must be used in highly selected patients. Since both plans start with external radiation therapy, the ultimate choice of treatment can be delayed until response to the external radiation is observed. It also allows the surgeon to better understand the patient, his desires, and his general state of health during the process.

RECURRENT CANCER

A special and complicated problem exists for local recurrence of rectal cancer. It was previously believed that

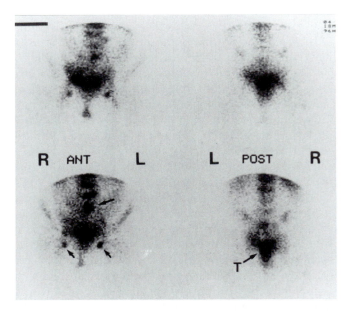

Figure 49–25. Anterior and posterior scintigrams of a patient with recurrent rectal cancer. T is recurrent cancer; *arrows* are cancer metastases in lymph nodes. (From Philpott GW, Siegel BA, Schwarz, SW, et al. Immunoscintigraphy with a new ¹¹¹In-labeled monoclonal antibody (MAb 1A3) in patients with colorectal cancer. *Dis Colon Rectum* 1994;37:782–92)

the cancers recurred at the distal margin of the anastomosis and grew into the lumen. This surely happens with an inadequate margin, but most surgeons now believe that there is residual cancer on the pelvic wall at the time of initial resection. It takes approximately 18 months for this cancer to grow large enough to present through the anastomosis. These cancers, by their nature, are fixed to the pelvic wall and surrounding viscera. They cause significant symptoms and are difficult to palliate and almost impossible to cure. This low salvage for locally recurrent rectal cancer has been the major impetus for investigating adjuvant modalities of treatment, such as preoperative radiation therapy.

Locally recurrent disease can be detected by biopsy after a low anterior resection and, in women, after an abdominoperineal resection. A more difficult problem exists in men after an abdominoperineal resection, when no orifice exists to allow access to the suspicious area. Any postoperative patient with symptoms in the pelvis or a rising CEA should be suspected of recurrent disease. MRI along with monoclonal antibody and PET scanning is becoming helpful in the diagnosis of these patients (Fig 49–25). Once the suspicious area is identified, CT-guided biopsy becomes helpful in confirming the diagnosis.

Once the diagnosis is made, therapy must be planned carefully. External radiation is especially important, if it has not been used before. The tissue damage from radiation is cumulative, and repeat courses are impossible. Resection should plan to include all involved organs, such as the vagina, bladder, sacrum, or adherent small intestine. Preoperative cystocopy with biopsy and careful pelvic examination are mandatory. Removal of the rectum and urinary bladder with surrounding lymphatic tissue is called a "pelvic exenteration" (Fig 49–26). This requires the patient to have two permanent stomas, one for feces and one for urine. Some, but not all, of the sacrum can be removed without impairing ambulation.

Consideration has been given for intraoperative radiation therapy to the tumor using a linear accelerator; this requires a combined operating room–radiation therapy suite, and the results so far have not been convincing. Techniques currently are being developed for implanting high-dose, afterload radiation therapy catheters to the areas suspicious for unclear margins.

Despite such heroic measures, the palliation and salvage rate of recurrent rectal cancer is very low (10% to 20%). The mode of death from locally recurrent rectal cancer involves much more intense suffering than that which results from the progressive malnutrition of distant metastatic disease. For these reasons, it is important that the surgeon managing rectal cancer knows all the management options, and that the first therapy applied be the best "curative" procedure for a given patient.

■ OTHER RECTAL TUMORS

VILLOUS ADENOMA OF THE RECTUM

Villous adenomas of the rectum are typically flat, velvety, and soft sessile polyps within the rectum. They occasionally present with watery diarrhea and hypokalemia. The finding of a large (>4 cm) villous adenoma in the rectum, with areas of ulceration, indicates a very high risk for cancer (90%). Transrectal ultrasound of the villous lesion is helpful to determine the thickness and depth of invasion of the lesion. Ultrasound, however, is unable to distinguish between carcinoma in situ and invasive cancer. Because of the risk of sampling error in these large, exuberant lesions, the only adequate biopsy is complete excision, preferably transanally, if possible. If cancer is present, the patient should be treated with appropriate resection. The transanal excision should include adequate peripheral margins for complete cure, if cancer is not present. It is helpful to inject the submucosal layer with epinephrine to both elevate the lesion from the underlying muscle and to reduce blood loss. The defect should be closed with suture to provide primary healing and to mark the site. There is a high risk of recurrence if inadequate excision is performed.

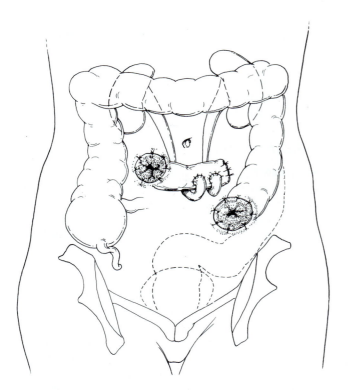

Figure 49–26. Pelvic exenteration. (Redrawn from John A Craig MD in Kodner IJ, Fry RD, Fleshman JW, et al. Colon, rectum and anus. In: Schwartz SI (ed), *Principles of Surgery,* 6th ed. New York, NY: McGraw-Hill; 1993:1296)

Occasionally, a villous tumor will cover the entire mucosal surface of the distal rectum. If the polyp appears to be benign, a coloanal anastomosis after mucosal proctectomy and full-thickness proximal proctectomy is the preferred treatment. The coloanal anastomosis allows preservation of the anal sphincter and removes all the mucosa at risk in the rectum. It is important to document, by frozen section, the absence of cancer in this situation, unless the tumor is well above the anal canal and there is very little risk of invasion into the levator or external sphincter muscles.

Laser ablation of the villous adenoma has been used in some cases where local excision is not possible. The disadvantages of laser ablation include the risk of undiagnosed cancer or cancer developing in the base of a repeatedly lasered, scarred segment. If the villous adenoma recurs after several laser treatments, the patient should be referred for surgical treatment.

In the past, transsphincteric (York-Mason) and transsacral (Kraske) approaches to the rectum were used to remove villous adenomas and allow sphincter preservation. These methods currently are used infrequently because the colonal anastomosis and low stapled anastomotic techniques allow preservation of anorectal function and appear to be more effective in treatment of the disease.

LYMPHOMA

Most gastrointestinal lymphomas represent metastatic disease. Primary, non-Hodgkin's, colonic lymphomas account for approximately 10% of all gastrointestinal lymphomas. For the diagnosis of primary lymphoma of the gastrointestinal tract to be made, there should be no palpable peripheral adenopathy, no involvement of the liver or spleen, a normal white blood cell count, and no involvement of other sites. The cecum and rectum are the most common sites of colonic involvement.

Lymphoma of the intestinal tract may appear as annular thickening, bulky exophytic growth, or thickened aneurysmal dilations of the bowel wall. The cut surface has the appearance of "fish flesh." Colonic lymphomas are classified by cell type and, in order of frequency, are histiocytic, lymphocytic, mixed cell, or Hodgkin's disease.

Diagnosis

Patients are typically between 50 to 60 years of age, with colonic lymphoma more common in men, and rectal involvement more common in women. Abdominal or rectal pain, altered bowel habits, weight loss, and rectal bleeding are the most common presenting symptoms. Approximately 20% of patients will present with obstructive symptoms.

Most rectal lymphomas are palpable by digital examination or visible by sigmoidoscopy; patients with colonic lymphoma may have tender, palpable abdominal masses. Barium enema examination may reveal multiple lesions consisting of filling defects and infiltrating or ulcerating lesions. The appearance of a lymphoma on barium enema examination can be similar to that of a carcinoma. The lesions are often submucosal; consequently, superficial colonoscopic biopsies are not diagnostic. An accurate history and physical examination, as well as complete blood work, chest x-ray, barium enema, abdominal CT scan, and bone marrow biopsy are used for preoperative staging.

Treatment

Complete excision is the treatment of choice for these tumors. Resection of primary gastrointestinal lymphomas permits accurate staging, better local control of the tumor, and decreased complications of bleeding and perforation. Liver and lymph node biopsies, as well as splenectomies, have been recommended for complete operative staging.

Postoperative radiation therapy and chemotherapy are given according to the stage of the tumor. Radiation therapy is indicated for palliation of unresectable disease and in cases when the surgical resection is not complete. Chemotherapy is recommended for treatment of systemic disease.

Prognosis depends on the stage of the disease at diagnosis. Regional nodal involvement is not related to prognosis. The 5 year survival following curative resection is 50%. The best prognosis exists in patients with intraluminal lymphomas <5 cm in diameter with no lymph node metastases. Patient with AIDS and those with widespread disease have a poor prognosis.

RETRORECTAL TUMORS

Pathophysiology

The retrorectal space is bound anteriorly by the rectum, posteriorly by the presacral fascia, superiorly by the peritoneal reflection, inferiorly by the rectosacral fascia, and laterally by the lateral ligaments, ureters, and iliac vessels.

More than 50% of these lesions are congenital. The remainder are classified as neurogenic, osseous, or miscellaneous lesions. Inflammatory lesions and metastatic carcinoma should also be considered in the differential diagnosis of lesions in this space. Malignancy is more common in lesions found in the postnatal pediatric population than in adults. In the adult population, 10% of cystic lesions are malignant, whereas solid lesions have a 60% malignancy rate.

Developmental cysts constitute the majority of congenital lesions and may arise from any of the germ cell layers. Dermoid and epidermoid cysts are benign lesions that have an ectodermal origin. When these cysts communicate with the skin surface, a postanal dimple is found. These cysts can become infected and may be misdiagnosed as a fistula-in-ano. Enterogenous cysts are entodermal in origin and are benign, thin-walled, and lined by columnar epithelium. They are usually asymptomatic but have a tendency to become infected. Teratomas are true neoplasms and contain tissue from each germ cell layer. They are more common in women and are considered tumors of infancy and childhood. Teratomas are uncommon in adults, but when they occur, 30% become malignant.

Chordomas are the most common malignant tumors found in this region and are believed to arise from remnants of the notochord. These cancers are slow-growing, invasive lesions that destroy adjacent bone. Plain radiographs show the expansion and destruction of bone, trabeculation, and calcification.

Anterior sacral *meningoceles* contain cerebrospinal fluid. Patients present with headaches, often associated with constipation and low back pain. The "scimitar" sign (a sacrum with a rounded, concave border without bony destruction) is the pathognomonic x-ray appearance of anterior sacral meningoceles. Meningitis can occur, and aspiration of these lesions should be avoided to prevent this complication.

Diagnosis

Patients with retrorectal tumors often complain of postural pain in the lower back, perianal, or rectal region, with the pain often referred to the legs or buttocks. Other complaints include recurrent infections, constipation, diarrhea, urinary symptoms, or obstructed labor. More than 90% of these lesions are palpable by digital rectal examination.

Plain x-ray or CT scans are used to confirm the diagnosis and to aid in surgical planning. CT scans help to define the limits of the lesion and to determine whether it is cystic or solid. Bony destruction indicates malignancy. Barium enema will show anterior displacement of the rectum. Myelograms may be indicated if central nervous system involvement is suspected. Biopsy is not recommended if the lesion is deemed operable, since tumor seeding along biopsy tracts and septic complications after needle biopsies have been reported.

Treatment

Surgical resction is the treatment of choice, even in asymptomatic patients, because of the risk that the lesion may become infected, cause dystocia, be malignant, or have malignant potential. The abdominal approach is recommended for high retrorectal and extraspinal neurogenic lesions. The posterior (transsacral) approach is recommended for low lesions and infected cysts. For large lesions, an abdominal-sacral approach has been most useful. The coccyx needs to be removed to gain better exposure and to decrease the risk of recurrence, as it is frequently the source of the cysts. If needle biopsy was performed, the tract must be included in the resection to prevent tumor implantation in the needle tract. En bloc resections of sacrum, neural structures, and rectum are sometimes needed for curative resection of chordomas. Anterior sacral meningoceles can be treated by posterior laminectomy, anterior transabdominal, or a combination anterior-posterior approach.

Benign tumors and cysts have a good prognosis and are adequately treated by surgical excision. Chordomas have a high local recurrence rate. They are slow-growing tumors, and 10 year survival rates vary from 20% to 70%. High-dose radiotherapy may provide palliation in inoperable or inadequately resected chordomas. Chemotherapy has no role in the management of tumors in this region.

RECTAL CARCINOID

Diagnosis

Rectal carcinoids are yellow-gray submucosal nodules covered by intact mucosa. They are usually small and asymptomatic and may be seen on proctosigmoidoscopy. Larger lesions can ulcerate, causing rectal bleeding and pain. Malignancy correlates with the size of the lesion and is based on invasion into the muscularis propria, not histologic differentiation. There is a 4% chance of malignancy in lesions <2 cm, but it is unsafe to presume that a lesion is benign based solely on its size. More than 60% of rectal carcinoids >2 cm have liver metastases, and 90% have local lymph node metastases at the time of diagnosis.

Treatment

Transanal excision is indicated for small, asymptomatic rectal lesions. The depth of invasion should be evaluated, and a more extensive cancer operation should be performed for those lesions with invasion of the muscularis propria. Malignant lesions should be treated by anterior resection or abdominoperineal resection. Radical surgery, however, has not been beneficial for rectal carcinoids with evidence of distant metastatic disease. The 5 year survival among persons with no metastases is 92%. The 5 year survival is 44%, if there are local lymph node metastases, and <10%, if distant metastases are present.

POSTOPERATIVE MANAGEMENT OF SYSTEMIC DISEASE

If curative resection was done, then long-term follow-up should consist of routine screening for metachronous colonic and rectal neoplasms, assuming the entire colon and rectum have been cleared of synchronous lesions at some time in the perioperative period. This is best done by colonoscopy 1 year after resection, unless adenomatous polyps were present prior to resection. In such cases, an examination at 6 months would be reasonable. If the colonoscopy is clear at 1 year, then examinations every 2 to 3 years would be appropriate. The advantages of routine chest x-ray, CT scan, and CEA determination in the postoperative period are not clear. Closer observation is indicated for patients at high risk for subsequent cancer such as those with ulcerative colitis, multiple polyposis, or a strong family history of cancer.

■ ADJUVANT CHEMOTHERAPY

Consideration should be given to adjuvant systemic therapy if the primary lesion was unfavorable in that it was deeply invasive, had spread to adjacent lymph nodes, or displayed an aggressive histologic pattern (mucin-production or the presence of signet-ring cells). Until very recently, little justification for adjuvant chemotherapy existed. Recent reports from the National Surgical Adjuvant Breast Project (NSABP) suggest that leucovorin plus 5-fluorouracil (5-FU) may be advantageous in certain situations, and a current multiple institutional report suggests an advantage in long-term survival and diminished local recurrence by the use of levamisole plus fluorouracil in patients with Dukes' C lesions.

If a palliative resection was done because the primary lesion was incurable, aggressive management of liver and lung metastasis should not be undertaken. The use of systemic chemotherapy may alleviate some symptoms by diminishing tumor mass, but no change in survival has been reported. If the primary lesion can be completely resected, surgery should be considered for the potential resectablity of distant metastatic lesions such as those of the lung or liver. Management of these lesions depends on the patient's general status of age and health. Unresectable liver metastases may be considered for arterial perfusion. New protocols are being evaluated that may offer some advantage over the previous ones in which the slight advantage was not compensated by the high risk of complications from the techniques and agents utilized.

■ ADJUVANT RADIATION THERAPY

Control of tumor deposits in the pararectal tissue has been one of the goals of using adjuvant radiation therapy for the management of rectal cancer. Various forms of this administration have been suggested: preoperative, postoperative, or a combination of the two that has come to be known as the "sandwich technique." Most radiation oncologists now agree that the early study on the use of radiation therapy at Sloan-Kettering that showed no advantage has been invalidated by newer techniques of administration. Many groups who have reported on the use of adjuvant radiation have shown an improvement in local control, and some have shown a significant improvement in long-term survival. In none of the studies have more radical surgical procedures been used to explain the improved results; in single-institution studies, the surgical variable in the management of rectal cancer has been controlled, while various other aspects of combined modality have been varied. Since a pretreatment clinical staging system does not exist, a prospective randomized trial is impossible for a single institution. This is because the local recurrence rate becomes so low that the number of patients necessary to truly test any variables would have to be enormously high. Multicenter studies have shown at least improved local control by use of adjuvant therapy with radiation alone or combined with chemotherapy.

Postoperative radiation is advantageous in that by not treating the most favorable lesions that have such a high cure rate, no adjuvant treatment is needed. The disadvantages of waiting until after surgery include the risk of violating potential tumor-containing margins in the lymphatics or at the tangential margin of resection. We believe that this compromises a major principle of cancer surgery. An additional hazard results if the small intestine becomes fixed to the postoperative adhesions in the pelvis. Although the rectum seems to tolerate radiation well, fixed loops of small intestine do not. Our early experiences and those of others have shown a significant incidence of postoperative complications (perforation and obstruction) from radiated small intestine. We believe this so strongly that we will make major efforts to protect the small intestine that we think may already be adherent in the pelvis. For patients who have had previous pelvic surgery, we will operate to remove the small intestine from the pelvis and suspend it by a polyglycolic acid sling before administering significant preoperative radiation therapy for a rectal cancer. Recent reports have shown improved survival and decreased local recurrence rates for selected aggressive rectal cancers, as determined after resection and evaluation of the specimen. With increased precautions, the serious complication rate is reduced from that of earlier studies.

For the reasons just described and our long experience using preoperative radiation therapy without significant complications, we have found no advantage to the concept of the "sandwich technique." We understand that preoperative radiation therapy has the disadvantage of treating some patients with favorable lesions who will not benefit from the costly and sometimes inconvenient radiation, but it must be remembered that the most favorable lesions in our series have always been treated with something less than proctectomy. Because of the disaster that postoperative local recurrence of rectal cancer represents, we are currently content to recommend preoperative radiation therapy even though this may represent over-treatment in a significant number of cases. We look forward to more effective pretreatment clinical staging that will sharpen our management choices and suggest the need for adjuvant preoperative radiation therapy in only those cases in which it will be known to be advantageous.

PREOPERATIVE EXTERNAL ADJUVANT RADIATION

Initial results with preoperative external radiation suggested that reduction in local recurrence, but no change in long-term survival, could be achieved. The only prospective randomized trial was a European study that verified such findings. Later reports from the University of Florida showed not only marked reduction in local recurrence, but also improved long-term survival.

Patients in our institution entered a protocol developed 15 years ago that involved combining preoperative external radiation with definitive resection for suspected deeply invasive lesions. It is important to understand that those lesions that were clinically invasive (by biopsy) yet favorable were culled out to be treated with something less than proctectomy; first by excision and deep coagulation, then by endocavitary radiation, and most recently, by a combination of external and endocavitary radiation (to be discussed in a later section).

In our extensive experience using preoperative radiation therapy, no complications have been attributed to the use of radiation therapy. In particular, no colostomies have been needed and no leaked anastomoses have occurred that could be attributed to the radiation. One component of the anastomosis, however, must not have been irradiated. This is accomplished by resecting the entire sigmoid colon and using descending colon for the proximal component of the anastomosis or for the colostomy. We currently use two treatment regimens, each with similar biologic dosage, but one of which gives the advantage of tumor shrinkage.

Rectal cancers that are suspected of being deeply invasive but are not significantly tethered to the surrounding tissue and are not histologically poorly differentiated receive 2000 cGy of external radiation during a 5 day period and are then resected early the following week. To understand the biologic effectiveness of this, one must remember the importance of the time factor in determining the biologic dose of the radiation. Those cancers that are even more aggressive, in that they are poorly differentiated or are significantly fixed to the surrounding tissue (clinically not thought to be clearly resectable), are treated with a regimen that we believe not only controls tumor deposits in the pararectal tissue, but also allows tumor shrinkage and increases the chances of definitive resectability. This regimen consists of 4500 cGy

TABLE 49–1. SURVIVAL AND LOCAL RECURRENCE OF RECTAL CANCER TREATED BY PREOPERATIVE RADIATION AND SURGICAL RESECTION

Results	Number of Patients (%)	
	2000 cGy + surgery	*4500 cGy + surgery*
5 year survival	81	73
5 year survival (excluding initially incurable lesions)	85	86
Local recurrence	0	1.8

(From Kodner IJ, Shemesh EI, Fry RD, et al. Preoperative irradiation for rectal cancer: Improved local control and long-term survival. Ann Surg 1989;209:196)

administered during a 5 week period (25 treatments), a 6 to 7 week waiting period, and then resection. This latter regimen allows maximum tumor shrinkage, without waiting so long that the cancer cells begin to repopulate. It also is chosen, somewhat arbitrarily, as a schedule that allows the acute inflammatory changes of the radiation to subside; yet it allows the surgery to be performed before the chronic fibrotic changes of the radiation occur. It has long been feared that these fibrotic changes might complicate the surgery; however, in the few cases in which surgery has been significantly more delayed, they have not been of major consequence. The long-term results of this series are presented in Table 49–1. They show that the use of combined preoperative external radiation followed by definitive surgery significantly increases the long-term survival as compared to many reports in the literature, and local recurrence of rectal cancer essentially was eliminated. Of most interest was the fact that the survival of the B and C lesions was very similar (Fig 49–27), perhaps indicating that if this modality is used, the importance of determining lymph node involvement pretreatment becomes less critical. The statistics also revealed that the 2000-cGy regimen was very effective and could be used for invasive cancers, unless the tumor is fixed, poorly differentiated, or extremely large.

Since more radical surgery was not performed in this series, it may be concluded that preoperative radiation therapy controls the cancer at the peripheral or tangential margin of resection, and that it destroyed tumor deposits in pararectal lymph nodes. The series has been ongoing for 15 years. The standard surgical techniques are not extremely efficient for clearing lymph nodes; therefore, it must be assumed that involved pelvic nodes were left in some patients, but disease did not recur because of the effect of the radiation therapy. Analysis of all variables showed only histologic differentiation and fixation to be of importance (Fig 49–28). In particular, lymph node involvement was not a major variable.

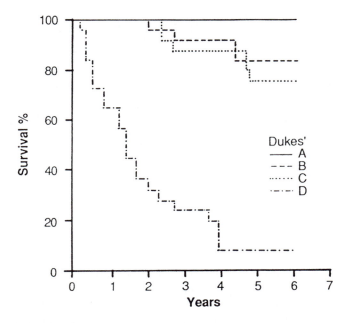

Figure 49–27. Survival of patients with rectal cancer treated with preoperative radiation, followed by excisional surgery according to the Dukes' classification of the resected specimen and to findings made at surgery. (From Kodner IJ, Shemesh EI, Walz BJ, et al. Preoperative irradiation for rectal cancer: improved local control and long-term survival. *Ann Surg* 1989;209:194–199)

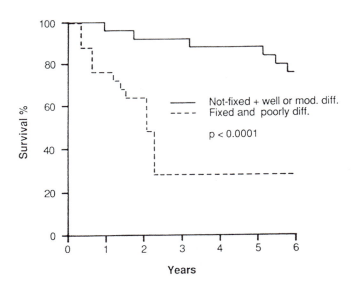

Figure 49–28. Survival of patients with rectal cancer treated with preoperative radiation, followed by excisional surgery according to the combined variables of tumor fixation and histologic differentiation. Initially incurable patients have been excluded. (From Kodner IJ, Shemesh EI, Walz BJ, et al. Preoperative irradiation for rectal cancer: improved local control and long-term survival. *Ann Surg* 1989;209:194–199)

Therefore, if preoperative radiation therapy is used, a clinical staging system may become possible.

AFTER ADJUVANT TREATMENT AND IMMEDIATELY PRIOR TO RESECTION

We repeat the tumor evaluation just prior to resection in those patients who have had the longer course of adjuvant radiation therapy. For the administration of 4500 cGy and completion of the waiting period, it will be approximately 3 months from the time of diagnosis to the time of surgical resection. During that time, the tumor should shrink (some disappear completely) and become less fixed. Should the cancer remain fixed, special arrangements should be made to resect the adherent structure or to administer postresection adjuvant treatment, either in the form of intraoperative radiation therapy or interstitial radiation therapy. If these options are not available, the patient should be sent to a center where they are available, because leaving residual cancer on the pelvic wall will render the patient incurable and subject to a painful death without good means of palliation. If the cancer is fixed to resectable structures, plans should be made for extensive resection even if this involves exenteration, hysterectomy, or sacrectomy. Some, unfortunately few, long-term survivors are reported, but the morbidity of such procedures is significant.

THE VERY FAVORABLE, YET INVASIVE, RECTAL CANCER

For many years authors such as Crile and Turnbull, Madden and Kandalaft, Papillon, and Sischy, have suggested that something less than the radical surgery of proctectomy could be curative for favorable, yet invasive, rectal cancers (Fig 49–29). Morson and associates reported that 10% of such patients would have lymphatic involvement even in the face of a favorable local tumor and, in these, cure could not be achieved by local destruction alone. The French radiation oncologist Jean Papillon described a technique of applying high-dose, superficially effective, radiation directly to a rectal cancer via a transanal route, using a device that fits within a large proctoscope. We began using this technique, called endocavitary radiation, in 1981 (Fig 49–29), and found it to be of value in treating very favorable lesions, usually in poor-risk patients. We attempted its use for palliation in extremely poor-risk patients with more aggressive cancers and found it to be of no help. The very high-risk patients continued to be sent for less than proctectomy. Out of desperation, in an attempt to treat these patients, we combined our experience using preoperative external radiation with the new endocavitary modality for intended palliation, and found that we cured many of these patients and achieved local control in most (Table 49–2).

Excision

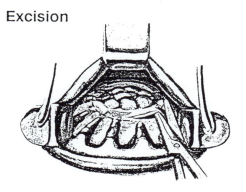

Contraindications

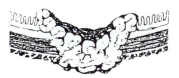

Endophytic ulcerated, undifferentiated lesion (>3 cm diameter) with radial penetration located more than 12 cm above anal verge

Indications

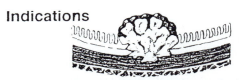

Exophytic, well-differentiated intramural lesion (<3 cm diameter) located less than 12 cm above anal verge

Fulguration

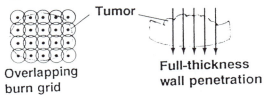

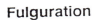 Tumor

Overlapping burn grid

Full-thickness wall penetration

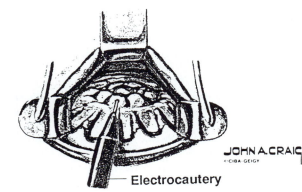

JOHN A. CRAIG AD
CIBA GEIGY

Electrocautery

Endocavitary radiation

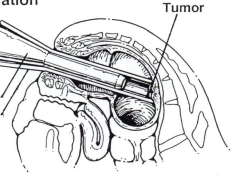

Tumor

Radiation probe

Speculum

Figure 49–29. Local therapy for rectal cancer. (From Kodner IJ, Fry RD, Fleshman JW, et al. Colon, rectum and anus. In: Schwartz SI (ed), *Principles of Surgery,* 6th ed. New York, NY: McGraw-Hill; 1993:1296)

TABLE 49–2. SUMMARY OF RESULTS FOR LOCAL CONTROL OF RECTAL CANCER USING RADIATION THERAPY AS DEFINITIVE TREATMENT

	Ideal and nonideal but potentially curable (%)	Nonideal or aggressive (%)
Endocavitary alone (19 patients)	62	0
Endocavitary + salvage resection	86 (62 disease free)	
External + endocavitary (65 patients)	95	14
External + endocavitary + salvage resection	100 (84 disease free)	50

(From Kodner IJ, Gilley MT, Shemesh EI, et al. Radiation therapy as definitive treatment for selected invasive rectal cancer. Surgery 1993;114:850–857)

TABLE 49–3. TREATMENT RECOMMENDATIONS FOR INVASIVE RECTAL CANCER

Favorable (yet invasive)	4500 cGy external radiation (5 weeks) + 6000 cGy endocavitary radiation
Suspected transmural invasion (nonfixed; favorable histologic findings)	2000 cGy external radiation (5 weeks) + surgical resection
Suspected transmural invasion (fixed; unfavorable histologic findings)	4500 cGy external radiation (5 weeks) + surgical resection
Poor operative risk or extensive metastatic disease	4500 cGy external radiation (5 weeks) + reevaluation for endocavitary radiation or resection

(From Kodner IJ, Gilley MT, Shemesh EI, et al. Radiation therapy as definitive treatment for selected invasive rectal cancer. Surgery 1993;114:850–857)

The protocol for treating good operative–risk patients with favorable, yet invasive, rectal cancers consists of a combination of external radiation (4500 cGy in 5 weeks), followed by a 6 to 7 week waiting period, and then 6000 cGy of endocavitary radiation to the tumor bed (3000 cGy per application, with the treatment 2 weeks apart).

The challenge for the future will be the selection of patients for each mode of treatment. If we can control the tangential margin and the lymphatics using external radiation, and can control the local tumor using various nonresective techniques, then it leaves us with needing to define only the deeply invasive or biologically aggressive lesions for radical surgical resection. Our current concept in the overall management of the patient with rectal cancer is summarized in Table 49–3.

SELECTED READINGS

Amato A, Pescatori M, et al. Local recurrence following abdominoperineal excision and anterior resection for rectal carcinoma. *Dis Colon Rectum* 1991;34:317

Beart RW. Prevention and management of recurrent rectal cancer. *World J Surg* 1991;15:589

Birnkrant A, Sampson J, Sugarbaker PH. Ovarian metastasis from colorectal cancer. *Dis Colon Rectum* 1986;29:767

Broders AC, Buie LA, Laird DR. Prognosis in carcinoma of the rectum: a comparison of the Broders and Dukes methods of classification. *Dis Colon Rectum* 1985;28:687

Brunschwig A, Barber HRK. Pelvic exenteration combined with resection of segments of bony pelvis. *Surgery* 1969; 65:417

Butcher HR Jr. Carcinoma of the rectum: choice between anterior resection and abdominal perineal resection of the rectum. *Cancer* 1971;28:204

Cohen AM, Enker WE, et al. Proctectomy and coloanal reconstruction for rectal cancer. *Dis Colon Rectum* 1990;33:40

Corman ML. Carcinoma of the rectum. In: Corman ML (ed), *Colon and Rectal Surgery.* Philadelphia, PA: JB Lippincott; 1989:469–578

Corman ML. Classic articles in colonic and rectal surgery: (Lithotomy-Trendelenburg position for resection of rectum and lower pelvic colon by Lloyd-Davies OV). *Dis Colon Rectum* 1989;32:172

Crile G, Turnbull RB Jr. The role of electrocoagulation in the treatment of carcinoma of the rectum. *Surg Gynecol Obstet* 1972;135:391

Daneker GW Jr, Carlson GW, et al. Endoscopic laser recanalization is effective for prevention and treatment of obstruction in sigmoid and rectal cancer. *Arch Surg* 1991;126:1348

Dukes CE: The surgical pathology of rectal cancer. *J Clin Pathol* 1949;2:95

Dukes CE, Bussey HJR. The spread of rectal cancer and its effect on prognosis. *Br J Cancer* 1958;12:309

Fazio VW. Cancer of the rectum: sphincter-saving operation: stapling techniques. *Surg Clin North Am* 1988;68:1367

Fearon ER, Vogelstein B. A genetic model for colorectal tumorigenesis. *Cell* 1990;61:759

Fleshman JW, Kodner IJ, Fry RD. Total proctectomy for malignancy. In: Schwartz SI, Ellis H (eds), *Maingot's Abdominal Operations,* vol II, 9th ed, Stamford, CT: Appleton & Lange; 1989:1131–1141

Fleshman JW, Myerson RJ, Fry RD, et al. Accuracy of transrectal ultrasound in predicting pathologic stage of rectal cancer before and after preoperative radiation therapy. *Dis Colon Rectum* 1992;35:823

Fry RD, Fleshman JW, Kodner IJ. Cancer of colon and rectum. *Clin Symp* 1989;41(5)

Fry RD, Fleshman JW, Kodner IJ. Sphincter-saving procedures for rectal cancer. In: Schwartz SI, Ellis H (eds), *Maingot's Abdominal Operations,* vol II, 9th ed. Stamford, CT: Appleton & Lange; 1989:1119–1130

Fry RD, Kodner IJ. Colon, rectum and anus. In: Davis JH (ed), *Clinical Surgery.* St. Louis, MO: CV Mosby; 1987:1519–1567

Gastrointestinal Tumor Study Group. Prolongation of the disease-free interval in surgically treated rectal carcinoma. *N Engl J Med* 1985;312:1465

Gazet J. Parks' coloanal pull-through anastomosis for severe, complicated radiation proctitis. *Dis Colon Rectum* 1985;28:110

Grinnell RS. Distal intramural spread of carcinoma of the rectum and rectosigmoid. *Surg Gynecol Obstet* 1954;99:421

Gunderson LL, Martin JK, Beart RW, et al. Intraoperative and external beam irradiation for locally advanced colorectal cancer. *Ann Surg* 1988;207:52

Heald RJ. The "holy plane" of rectal surgery. *J R Soc Med* 1988;81:503

Jao SW, Beart RW Jr, et al. Retrorectal tumors: Mayo Clinic experience, 1960–1979. *Dis Colon Rectum* 1985;28:644

Kodner IJ. Colostomy and ileostomy. *Clin Symp* 1978;30:5

Kodner IJ. Preoperative irradiation for rectal cancer: improved local control and long-term survival. *Ann Surg* 1989;209(2):194

Kodner IJ, Fleshman JW, Fry RD. Anal and rectal cancer: principles of management. In: Schwartz SI, Ellis H (eds), *Maingot's Abdominal Operations*, vol. II, 9th ed. Stamford, CT: Appleton & Lange; 1989:1107–1117

Kodner IJ, Fleshman JW, Fry RD. Intestinal stomas. In: Schwartz SI, Ellis H (eds), *Maingot's Abdominal Operations*, vol. II, 9th ed. Stamford, CT: Appleton & Lange; 1989:1143–1172

Kodner IJ, Fry RD, Fleshman JW. Current options in the management of rectal cancer. In: Cameron JL (ed), *Advances in Surgery*, 4th ed. St. Louis, MO: Mosby Year Book; 1990:1

Kodner IJ, Fry RD, Fleshman JW, et al. Colon, rectum and anus. In: Schwartz SI (ed), *Principles of Surgery*, 6th ed. New York, NY: McGraw-Hill; 1993:1191–1306

Kodner IJ, Gilley MT, Shemesh EI, et al. Radiation therapy as definitive treatment for selected invasive rectal cancer. *Surgery* 1993;114:850–857

Kraybill WG, Lopez MJ, Bricker EM. Total pelvic exenteration as a therapeutic option in advanced malignant disease of the pelvis. *Surg Gynecol Obstet* 1988;166:259

Krook JE, Moertel CG, et al. Effective surgical adjuvant therapy for high-risk rectal carcinoma. *N Engl J Med* 1991;324:709

Lee JF, Maurer VM, Block GE. Anatomic relations of pelvic autonomic nerves to pelvic operations. *Arch Surg* 1973;107:324

McAnena OJ, Heald RJ, et al. Operative and functional results of total mesorectal excision with ultra-low anterior resection in the management of carcinoma of the lower one-third of the rectum. *Surg Gynecol Obstet* 1990;170:517

Miles WE. A method of performing abdomino-perineal excision for carcinoma of the rectum and of the terminal portion of the pelvic colon. *Lancet* 1908;ii:1812

Morson BC. Factors in influencing the prognosis of early cancer of the rectum. *Proc R Soc Med* 1966;59:607

Morson BC, Bussey HJR, Samoorian S. Policy of local excision for early cancer of the colorectum. Gut 1977;18:1045

Papillon J. Intracavitary irradiation for cure of early rectal cancer. *Medicamundi* 1976;21(3):184

Philpott GW, Siegel BA, Schwarz SW, et al. Immunoscintigraphy with a new ^{111}In-labled monoclonal antibody (MAb 1A3) in patients with colorectal cancer. *Dis Colon Rectum* 1994;37:782–92

Stockholm Rectal Cancer Study Group. Preoperative short-term radiation therapy in operable rectal cancer: a prospective randomized trial. *Cancer* 1990;66:49

Qinyao W, Weijin S, et al. New concepts in severe presacral hemorrhage during proctectomy. *Arch Surg* 1985;120:1013

Quirke P, Durdey P, Dixon MF, et al. Local recurrence of rectal adenocarcinoma due to inadequate surgical resection: Histopathological study of lateral tumor spread and surgical excison. *Lancet* 1986;ii:996

Rhoads JE, Schwegman CW. Surgical techniques: one-stage combined abdominoperineal resection of the rectum (Miles) performed by two surgical teams. *Surgery* 1965;58(3):600

Schoetz DJ Jr. *Controversies in the Management of Rectal Cancer.* Philadelphia, PA: WB Saunders; 1990

Stahle E, Pahlman L, Enblad P. Double stapling technique in the management of rectal tumours. *Acta Chir Scand* 1986;152:743

Uhlig BE, Johnson RL. Presacral tumors and cysts in adults. *Dis Colon Rectum* 1975;18:581

Willett CG, Shellito PC, et al. Intraoperative electron beam radiation therapy for recurrent locally advanced rectal or rectosigmoid carcinoma. *Cancer* 1991;67:1504

Wolmark N, Fisher B. An analysis of survival and treatment failure following abdominoperineal and sphincter-saving resection in Dukes' B and C rectal carcinoma. *Ann Surg* 1986;204:480

50

Carcinoma of the Anus

Elisa Birnbaum ■ *Robert J. Myerson*

Malignancies of the anal canal and margin are uncommon and account for <5% of all anorectal carcinomas.[1] The most common histology is epidermoid carcinoma, which is further subdivided into keratinizing squamous carcinoma, nonkeratinizing epidermoid carcinoma with basaloid (cloacogenic) features, and undifferentiated carcinoma. Other less common histologies include melanoma, primary adenocarcinoma of the anus, Paget's disease, and Bowen's disease. The differential diagnosis includes leukoplakia, lichen sclerosis et atrophicus, psoriasis and condylomata acuminata.

There is a slight female predominance in anal canal tumors in contrast to a slight male predominance in carcinomas at the anal margin.[1–5] Recently, there has been an increase in the percentage of males with anal canal cancers who are homosexual, bisexual, or who have a history of anal condyloma.[3] There have been increasing reports in the literature of malignant transformation of anal condyloma. Anal and genital squamous carcinomas appear to be associated with HPV (subtypes 16 or 18) and sustained viral infection in these areas may be a precursor of malignancy.[6–8] Anal cancer also has been reported in association with prior radiation therapy and chronic draining sinus tracts from Crohn's disease.[9]

Neoplasms of the anal canal generally present with local or locoregional disease and usually are detected at a fairly early stage.[2,10] Occasionally, a patient presents with an advanced T4 lesion or distant metastases.

Pretreatment evaluation of patients with anal carcinoma should include a careful history and physical examination. Biopsy of suspicious lesions should be performed for diagnosis. Four-quadrant mapping is necessary if there is evidence of premalignant changes in the perianal skin.[11] A computed tomography (CT) scan of the abdomen and pelvis with contrast should be obtained to screen for inguinal and pelvic nodal metastases as well as distant metastatic disease. The patient should undergo a chest X-ray to screen for metastatic disease. In addition, the full length of the large intestine should be evaluated by colonoscopy or barium enemia to rule out additional pathology. The use of transrectal ultrasound in staging anal cancers generally is limited.

The current American Joint Commission on Cancer staging system is a clinical system (Table 50–1).[12] The depth of invasion into the anal sphincter is not included in this staging system since many of these lesions are now treated nonsurgically. Boman and associates reviewed case reports of patients treated surgically for epidermoid carcinoma of the anal canal and demonstrated that a clinical staging system similar to the current AJC system was comparable to the Dukes' staging system for determining prognosis.[10] The treatment of the anal carcinomas is dictated by histology, anatomic location, and patient morbidity. In general, these lesions tend to have a cure rate that compares favorably with other neoplasms of the gastrointestinal tract.

TABLE 50–1. CLASSIFICATION AND STAGING OF CARCINOMA OF THE ANAL CANAL[a]

PRIMARY TUMOR (T)

TX	Primary tumor cannot be assessed
T0	No evidence of primary tumor
Tis	Carcinoma *in situ*
T1	Tumor ≤2 cm in greatest dimension
T2	Tumor >2 cm but <5 cm in greatest dimension
T3	Tumor >5 cm in greatest dimension
T4	Tumor of any size invades adjacent organ(s), which should be specified (eg, vagina, urethra, bladder); involvement of the sphincter muscle(s) *alone* is not classified as T4

REGIONAL LYMPH NODES (N)

NX	Regional lymph nodes cannot be assessed
N0	No regional lymph node metastasis
N1	Metastasis in perirectal lymph node(s)
N2	Metastasis in unilateral internal iliac or inguinal lymph node(s)
N3	Metastasis in perirectal and inguinal lymph nodes and/or bilateral internal iliac and/or inguinal lymph nodes

DISTANT METASTASIS (M)

MX	Presence of distant metastasis cannot be assessed
M0	No distant metastasis
M1	Distant metastasis

STAGE GROUPING

Stage 0	TIS	N0	M0
Stage I	T1	N0	M0
Stage II	T2	N0	M0
	T3	N0	M0
Stage IIIA	T1	N1	M0
	T2	N1	M0
	T3	N1	M0
	T4	N0	M0
Stage IIIB	T4	N1	M0
	Any T	N2, N3	M0
Stage IV	Any T	Any N	M1

[a]The TNM classification is for the staging of cancers that arise in the anal canal only. Cancers that arise in the anal margin are staged according to cancers of the skin. (Beahrs OH, Hensen DE, Hutter RVP, Kennedy BJ [eds], *Manual for Staging of Cancer,* 4th ed. Philadelphia, PA: JB Lippincott; 1992)

■ ANATOMY

Although there are several definitions of the anal canal, the definition utilized in the AJC and UICC staging systems is the most practical for treatment of anal carcinomas.[12] These systems define the anal canal as extending from the distal rectum to the anal verge (Fig 50–1). The anal verge marks the junction between hair-bearing perianal skin and the anal canal. The AJC system defines the anal margin as the junction between the perianal skin and the anal canal. This is in distinction to the definition proposed by Morson in which the anal margin extends from the dentate line to the verge.[5] The latter definition, while perhaps more histologically appropriate, is less so from a treatment standpoint.

There are several different histologic regions within the anal canal. The transitional zone comes from the same embryonic cloacogenic membrane as does the cervical and vaginal epithelium. Columnar, cloacogenic, transitional, and squamous epithelium are present 6 to 12 mm above the dentate line. Distal to the dentate line, nonkeratinized squamous epithelium merges with keratinized squamous epithelium of the perianal skin.

Deep to the anal canal lie the muscles of the anal sphincter. The internal sphincter is an extension of the inner circular smooth muscle layer, and the external sphincter is an outer layer of striated muscle. The vascular supply is complex. Branches of the superior rectal artery and vein supply the most cephalad aspects of the anus. The middle and inferior rectal system provides blood supply throughout the anus. Lymphatic drainage

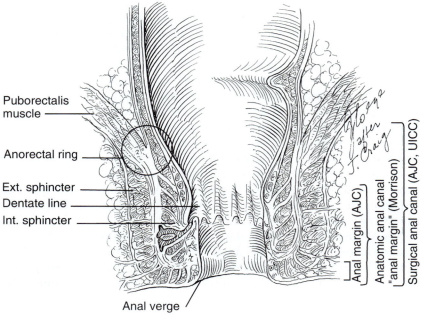

Figure 50–1. Normal anatomy of anal canal. (Redrawn from Fry RD, Kodner IJ. Anorectal Disorders. *Clin Symp* 1985;37:3. Copyright 1985, CIBA-GEIGY; originally illustrated by John Craig, MD)

parallels the vascular supply. Thus, lymphatic drainage from the anus can extend to the inguinal, external iliac, perirectal, and internal iliac lymph nodes. Lymphatic drainage at the anal margin is to the superficial inguinal nodes.

■ CARCINOMAS OF THE ANAL CANAL

EPIDERMOID CARCINOMA

Epidermoid carcinomas of the anal canal are referred to as squamous, basaloid, cloacogenic, or transitional carcinomas. Cloacogenic carcinomas have a histologic appearance of palisading nuclei and eosinophilic necrosis.[1,13] Squamous carcinomas in this region are generally nonkeratinizing, as compared to squamous cancers of the anal margin.[1,4] Although these cancers have different histologic features, they exhibit similar biologic behavior and are grouped together as epidermoid carcinomas of the anal canal.

Diagnosis

Many patients with epidermoid carcinoma of the anal canal have a long history of minor anorectal symptoms and are frequently misdiagnosed as having benign anorectal disease. These lesions can present as indurated, bleeding masses that itch, cause discomfort, or a mild discharge. It is not uncommon, however, for patients to present with painless anal masses. Malignancy should be considered in patients with continual anal pain and nonhealing perineal ulcers.

Biopsy of anal lesions and chronic sinus tracts may be diagnostic. Proctoscopy is important to determine the full local extent of disease, while colonoscopy or barium enema should be done to rule out additional sources of rectal bleeding. Other recommended studies include chest x-ray and CT scan to screen for enlarged regional lymph nodes (inguinal or pelvic) and distance metastasis.

Treatment

Until the early 1980s the mainstay of treatment for epidermoid carcinomas of the anal canal was surgical resection. Approximately 20% of tumors were found to have metastasized to perirectal lymph nodes and an additional 15% had metastasized to inguinal lymph nodes at presentation.[10,14–16] The earliest stage lesions (those without nodal metastases and without invasion of the anal sphincter) had a cure rate of about 90%, in most series.[10,16,17] The overall cure rate after surgery was about 60% to 70%.[4,10,14–16,18]

Nigro and associates began studying a preoperative regimen consisting of low-dose radiation therapy (3000 cGy), infusional 5-FU, and Mitomycin-C.[19–21] This regimen was based on in vitro and early clinical studies in-

dicating a marked synergism between the radiation and 5-FU chemotherapy.[22] The preoperative regimen was quite successful with the majority of patients achieving a complete remission. Therefore, in the 1970s and early 1980s, a number of institutions began to utilize chemoradiotherapy as a primary treatment modality. Initially, biopsies were performed 4 to 6 weeks following completion of chemoradiotherapy.[21,23] More recent evidence from institutions, such as the Princess Margaret Hospital in Canada, indicates that the majority of lesions that eventually achieve a complete response require more than a month to do so.[24,25] Thus, routine posttreatment biopsy is no longer performed except in protocol settings, unless there is evidence of residual disease. Surgery for epidermoid carcinomas of the anal canal is reserved for those cases that do not respond to nonsurgical treatment.

How best to combine chemotherapy and radiation is still somewhat open to debate. Most reported series utilize two courses of infusional 5-FU separated by at least 3 weeks.[21,24–28] Generally, 1 gm/m² per day is administered for 96 hours by continuous IV infusion in each of the two cycles. Some series have utilized lower concentrations of 5-FU and appear to have reduced rates of local control, unless high doses of radiation are utilized.[29] The recently completed study by the Radiation Therapy Oncology Group (RTOG) evaluated the use of Mitomycin-C.[30] Preliminary reports indicate that the colostomy-free survival rate is improved if 10 mg/m² of Mitomycin-C is delivered on day 1 of each cycle of 5-FU. The dose of radiation therapy is also somewhat controversial. It is well established that 3000 cGy delivered in 180 to 200 cGy daily fractions is highly effective in controlling subclinical disease. Metachronous nodal failure occurs in <5% of patients treated with chemoradiotherapy,[21,25,26,28] whereas approximately 20% of patients in the surgical series subsequently failed in either the inguinal or pelvic nodes.[4,10,14,18] Some authors have advocated limiting radiation to 3000 cGy.[23] However, a boost of 1500 cGy in 1.5 weeks to sites of gross disease does not increase morbidity and may reduce the need for salvage surgery. At Washington University, St. Louis, the need for salvage surgery was reduced by 15% when the moderate-boost dose was added to the treatment regimen.[28]

A typical portal encompassing the pelvic lymph nodes, inguinal lymph nodes, and anal region is shown in Figure 50–2. Boost portals are highly individualized. Typically, patients develop acute skin reactions in the perianal area and in skin folds of the inguinal and genital areas. Meticulous local hygiene is mandatory. These acute skin reactions sometimes mandate a treatment break midway through the course of chemoradiotherapy. Patients must be informed that these acute skin reactions will be marked but temporary and that long-term functional re-

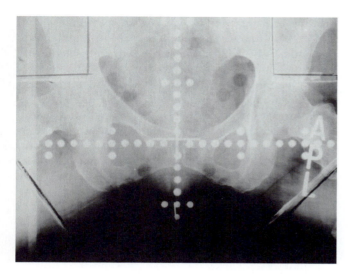

Figure 50–2. Radiation portal for treatment of the primary tumor with elective coverage of the pelvic and inguinal lymph nodes. For patients receiving concurrent chemotherapy, this portal should be treated to 3000 cGy. Boost techniques after the first 3000 cGy are discussed in the text. (From Myerson RJ, Shapiro SJ, Lacey D, et al: Carcinoma of the anal canal. *Am J Clin Oncol* 1995;18:32–39)

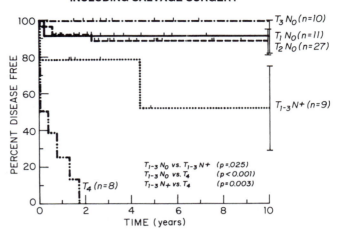

Figure 50–3. Disease-free survival (Kaplan-Meier) vs. clinical stage. Tumors successfully salvaged by surgery are scored as NED in this figure. (From Myerson RJ, Shapiro SJ, Lacey D, et al: Carcinoma of the anal canal. *Am J Clin Oncol* 1995;18:32–39)

sults will be excellent. Other reported morbidities of treatment include acute hematologic and gastrointestinal toxicities that are generally controlled with conservative outpatient management. Long-term results are favorable, with <5% of patients experiencing significant genitourinary or gastrointestinal morbidity.[28]

About 80% of tumors will be cured by chemoradiotherapy alone. Results at Washington University, St. Louis, are displayed in Fig 50–3. The 10 year actuarial survival, including salvage surgery, for T1 to T3, N0 epidermoid carcinomas of the anal canal is 90%; 100% of T1 lesions were locally controlled with chemoradiotherapy alone. Although 20% of T2 and T3 lesions required surgery for salvage, the ultimate cure rate for T2 and T3, N0 carcinomas was equal to that of the T1, N0 carcinomas. Patients who presented with involved lymph nodes had a poorer prognosis. The disease-free survival for this group (52% at 10 years), however, compares favorably with historical controls treated with primary surgery. In the prechemoradiotherapy era, only about one-third of patients who presented with clinically involved lymph nodes were cured of their disease.[14,31,32]

Several issues with regard to the treatment of epidermoid carcinoma of the anal canal currently are being investigated. The EORTC is conducting a randomized trial comparing radiation therapy alone with radiation therapy plus chemotherapy. In the United States several groups are investigating the utility of higher doses of radiation therapy. This may conceivably reduce the need for salvage surgery for T2 and T3 lesions and improve the cure rate for T4 lesions. On the other hand, higher

doses of radiation also may lead to greater complications and may render salvage surgery less feasible. Currently, the standard of care for epidermoid carcinoma of the anal canal consists of low to moderate doses of radiation therapy (3000 cGy or less to areas of subclinical involvement and about 4500 cGy to areas of gross tumor) in conjunction with infusional 5-FU-based chemotherapy.

ADENOCARCINOMA

Adenocarcinoma of the anal canal is usually a downward extension of a primary rectal carcinoma. Primary adenocarcinoma of the anal canal, however, may arise from the columnar epithelium of the anal glands or in a long-standing anorectal fistula. Patients are usually elderly and female. Perianal pain, swelling, and bleeding are frequent presenting symptoms and many patients have an associated abscess or fistula in ano. Since the symptoms mimic benign disease, correct diagnosis is frequently delayed, by which time most tumors have destroyed the primary site. Biopsy is needed to confirm the diagnosis. Abdominal perineal resection is indicated for treatment of these carcinomas, although most patients have distant metastasis to regional lymph nodes, liver or lung by the time of diagnosis.[33] The long-term outlook is poor, and mortality approaches 100% within two years after diagnosis.

MELANOMA

Melanoma of the anal canal occurs in 1% to 3% of all patients with melanoma. The anal canal is the third most common site for melanoma, following skin and eye. Most anal melanomas arise from the epidermoid lining of the anal canal adjacent to the dentate line and spread submucosally. By the time they cause symptoms, the level of invasion usually precludes surgical cure. The lesions range from sessile to exophytic polypoid masses and approximately 70% of melanomas reported in the literature have gross evidence of pigmentation.[34]

Diagnosis

The average age at presentation is between 50 and 60 years, equally distributed between men and women. The majority of patients reported in the literature are Caucasian. Patients frequently have nonspecific symptoms and may complain of bleeding, pain, or an anal mass. Many patients are initially misdiagnosed as having a thrombosed hemorrhoid or anorectal polyp. Biopsy is necessary for diagnosis.

Approximately 60% of patients have metastatic disease at the time of diagnosis.[34] Metastases occur via lymphatic and hematogenous routes. Metastases to the mesenteric lymph nodes are more frequent than to the inguinal lymph nodes. Lung, liver and bone are the most frequent sites of hematogenous spread.

Treatment

These tumors are resistant to chemotherapy and radiation therapy. Immunotherapy has been proven to be ineffective. Abdominal perineal resection controls local disease and is the only procedure that removes clinically undetected mesenteric lymph nodes. There appears to be no difference, however, in survival between patients treated by wide local excision or those treated by abdominal perineal resection.[34,35] Prophylactic lymph node dissection is of no value. Therapeutic lymph node dissection is advised for patients with positive inguinal lymph nodes. The average length of survival is <2 years, with the average length of survival after proven distal metastasis <6 months. Overall, 5 year survival is <20%, with few reported long-term survivors.[35,36]

CARCINOMA OF THE ANAL MARGIN

Squamous Carcinoma

Squamous cell carcinomas of the anal margin are well-differentiated keratinizing lesions similar to squamous cell carcinoma of the skin. These cancers grow slowly, invade locally, and metastasize late.

Diagnosis. There is a slight male predominance and an increased incidence of associated conditions, for instance, condylomata, fistula, abscess, and prior radiation therapy.[4] Patients frequently present with complaints of bleeding, itching, pain or tenesmus. The lesions have rolled, everted edges and central ulceration. Biopsy is necessary for diagnosis.

Treatment. Small lesions are treated by wide local excision with a 2 cm margin, if possible. Combined chemotherapy and radiation has been used with some success to induce regression of large lesions. Likewise tumors involving the anal sphincter that are not responsive to chemoradiation require abdominal perineal resection. Synchronous metastasis to the inguinal nodes are included in the radiation portals and, if unresponsive, are treated by groin dissections. Visceral metastases are uncommon. Local recurrence in the perianal skin can be treated by local excision with success rates approaching 90%.[37]

The overall 5 year survival rate is 60% to 80%. Prognosis is related to the extent of infiltration. Patients with lesions >5 cm, or positive inguinal nodes at the time of diagnosis, have a poorer prognosis.

BASAL CELL CARCINOMA

Basal cell carcinomas are rare tumors of the anal margin. They arise from basal cells at the dermoepidermal junction and behave like basal cell carcinoma elsewhere in the skin. Basal cell carcinomas should not be confused with basaloid carcinomas of the anal canal, which behave differently and are discussed separately.

Diagnosis

These lesions are more common in men and present as an anal mass with raised edges and central ulcerations. Pruritus, bleeding, and pain are frequent symptoms, if ulceration is present. The average duration of symptoms is 5 years, with an incorrect initial diagnosis rate of approximately 25%.[38]

Treatment

Basal cell carcinoma is treated by wide local excision and primary closure or skin grafting. These cancers rarely metastasize. Local recurrences are treated by re-excision.

BOWEN'S DISEASE

Bowen's disease was initially described by Bowen in 1912 as a precancerous dermatosis.[39] It is a rare, slow-growing intraepidermal squamous cell carcinoma (carcinoma in situ). Bowen's disease progresses to invasive carcinoma in <5% of cases.

Diagnosis

Bowen's disease usually presents in the elderly, but has been reported in association with anal condyloma in young, sexually active patients. Patients often complain of perianal itching, burning or bleeding. The typical lesion is a dull brownish plaque, although nonpigmented lesions also are seen. Irregular erythematous, scaly plaques are found on examination and may have the appearance of eczema or chronic irritation owing to pruritus ani. Many lesions go unnoticed or are found incidentally during histologic examination of tissues removed during minor anal procedures. Multinucleated giant cells with vacuolated halos (Bowenoid cells) may be seen on microscopic examination. These lesions are slowly progressive and the presence of ulceration may indicate the development of an invasive carcinoma. Associated malignancies have been reported in up to 70% to 80% of patients with Bowen's disease, although many groups feel this finding is speculative.[40]

Treatment

Treatment consists of wide local excision with clear margins confirmed microscopically. Skin grafts may be necessary for coverage, if the excision is large. Recurrences can be treated by reexcision, if there is no evidence of invasion.

PAGET'S DISEASE

Extramammary perianal Paget's disease is a rare clinic pathologic entity first reported in 1893 by Darier and Coulillaud.[41] Paget's disease arises from intraepidermal apocrine glands and, if left untreated, adenocarcinoma of the apocrine glands may develop after a long, preinvasive phase. Typical Paget's cells are large faintly basophilic or vacuolated cells found in the epidermis. The nuclei are vesicular and there is little mitotic activity. High mucin content causes these cells to stain positive with the periodic acid Schiff stain. These cells also stain positively with CEA immunofluorescent stain.[42]

Diagnosis

Patients are usually 60 to 70 years of age, and there is an equal sex distribution.[11] Severe intractable pruritus is characteristic of this disease. Examination usually reveals a well-demarcated eczematoid plaque that may show whitish-grey ulcerations. A mass or indurated skin suggests an underlying carcinoma.

Any eczematoid lesion of the perianal region that does not improve with local medical therapy should be biopsied to exclude this diagnosis. A full-thickness biopsy into the subcutaneous tissue must be done to rule out invasive carcinoma. Multiple biopsies in all four quadrants of the anal canal are taken to assure complete resection. A complete bowel workup should be performed to exclude associated malignancies.

Treatment

Wide local excision with multiple biopsies of the anal canal to assess completeness of resection is the treatment of choice. Clear margins should be confirmed by frozen section since Paget's cells extend beyond the gross margins of the lesions.[43] Abdominal perineal resection may be necessary for advanced lesions associated with carcinoma. Lymph node dissection is indicated only for patients with positive inguinal nodes.

The most frequent sites of metastatic disease are the inguinal and pelvic lymph nodes followed by liver, bone, lung, brain, bladder, prostate, and adrenal glands. Patients with invasive carcinoma at the time of diagnosis have a poor prognosis, and those with metastatic disease do poorly despite aggressive treatment. Local recurrence is as high as 40% at 5 years; therefore, long-term follow-up is necessary.[44] Reexcision for local recurrence is usually adequate, if there is no evidence of invasion.

REFERENCES

1. Klotz RG, Jr, Pamukcoglu T, Souilliard DH. Transitional cloacogenic carcinoma of the anal canal. *Cancer* 1967; 20:1727–1745
2. Pintor MP, Northover JMA, Nicholls RJ. Squamous cell carcinoma of the anus at one hospital from 1948 to 1984. *Br J Surg* 1989;76:806–810
3. Wexner SD, Milsom JW, Dailey TH. The demographics of anal cancers are changing: identification of a high-risk population. *Dis Colon Rectum* 1987;30:942–946
4. Greenall MJ, Quan SH, Stearns MW, et al. Epidermoid cancer of the anal margin: pathologic features, treatment, and clinical results. *Am J Surg* 1985;149:95–101
5. Morson BC. The pathology and results of treatment of squamous cell carcinoma of the anal canal and anal margin. *J R Soc Med* 1960;53:416–420
6. Palmer JG, Scholefield JH, Coates PJ, et al. Anal cancer and human papillomaviruses. *Dis Colon Rectum* 1989;32: 1016–1022
7. Croxson T, Chabon AB, Rorat E, et al. Intraepithelial carcinoma of the anus in homosexual men. *Dis Colon Rectum* 1984;27:325–330
8. Aparicio-Duque R, Mittal KR, Chan W, et al. Cloacogenic carcinoma of the anal canal and associated viral lesions: an in situ hybridization study for human papilloma virus. *Cancer* 1991;68:2422–2425
9. Buchman AL, Ament ME, Doty J. Development of squamous cell carcinoma in chronic perineal sinus and wounds in Crohn's disease. *Am J Gastroenterol* 1991; 86:1829–1832
10. Boman BM, Moertel CG, O'Connell MJ, et al. Carcinoma of the anal canal: a clinical and pathologic study of 188 cases. *Cancer* 1984;54:114–125
11. Beck DE, Fazio VW: Perianal Paget's disease. *Dis Colon Rectum* 1987;30:263–266
12. Beahrs OH, Henson DE, Hutter RV, Kennedy BJ (eds). *American Joint Commission on Cancer Manual for Staging of Cancer*, 4th ed. Philadelphia, PA: JB Lippincott; 1992
13. Fenger C. Anal neoplasia and its precursors: facts and controversies. *Semin Diag Path* 1991;3:190–201
14. Kuehn PG, Beckett R, Eisenberg H, et al. Epidermoid carcinoma of the perianal skin and anal canal. *N Engl J Med* 1964;270:614–616

15. Salmon RJ, Zafrani B, Labib A, et al. Prognosis of cloaco-genic and squamous cancers of the anal canal. *Dis Colon Rectum* 1986;29:336–340

16. Golden GT, Horsley JS III. Surgical management of epidermoid carcinoma of the anus. *Am J Surg* 1976;131: 275–280

17. Shepherd NA, Scholefield JH, Love SB, et al. Prognostic factors in anal squamous carcinoma: a multivariate analysis of clinical, pathological and flow cytometric parameters in 235 cases. *Histopathology* 1990;16:545–555

18. Dillard BM, Spratt JS Jr, Ackerman LV. Epidermoid cancer of the anal margin and canal: review of 79 cases. *Arch Surg* 1963;86:772–777

19. Nigro ND, Vaitkevicus VK, Buroker T, et al: Combined therapy for cancer of the anal canal. *Dis Colon Rectum* 1981;24:73–75

20. Nigro ND, Seydel HG, Considine B, et al. Combined preoperative radiation and chemotherapy for squamous cell carcinoma of the anal canal. *Cancer* 1983;54:1826–1829

21. Nigro ND. An evaluation of combined therapy for squamous cell cancer of the anal canal. *Dis Colon Rectum* 1984;27:763–766

22. Byfield JE. Theoretical basis and clinical applications of 5-Fluorouracil as a radiosensitizer: an overview. In: Rotman M, Rosenthal CJ (eds), *Medical Radiology*. New York, NY: Springer-Verlag; 1991:115–128

23. Nigro ND. The force of change in the management of squamous cell cancer of the anal canal. *Dis Colon Rectum* 1991;34:482–486

24. Cummings BJ, Rider WD, Harwood AR, et al. Combined radical radiation therapy and chemotherapy for primary squamous cell carcinoma of the anal canal. *Cancer Treat Rep* 1982;66:489–492

25. Cummings BJ, Keane TJ, O'Sullivan B, et al. Epidermoid anal cancer: treatment by radiation alone or by radiation and 5-Fluorouracil with and without Mitomycin C. *Int J Radiat Oncol Biol Phys* 1991;21:1115–1125

26. John MJ, Flam M, Lovalvo L, et al. Feasibility of non-surgical definitive management of anal canal carcinoma. *Int J Radiat Oncol Biol Phys* 1987;13:299–303

27. Sischy B, Doggett RL, Krall JM, et al. Definitive irradiation and chemotherapy for radiosensitization in management of anal carcinoma: interim report on Radiation Therapy Oncology Group Study No. 8314. *J Natl Cancer Inst* 1989; 81:850–856

28. Myerson RJ, Shapiro SJ, Lacey D, et al. Carcinoma of the anal canal. *Am J Clin Oncol* 1995;18:32–39

29. Hughes LL, Rich TA, Delclos L, et al. Radiotherapy for anal cancer: experience from 1979 to 1987. *Int J Radiat Oncol Biol Phys* 1989;17:1153–1160

30. Flam MS, John MJ, Peters T, et al. Radiation and 5-Fluorouracil (5FU) vs radiation, 5FU, Mitomycin C (MMC) in the treatment of anal canal carcinoma: preliminary results of a Phase III randomized RTOG/ECOG intergroup trial. RTOG Philadelphia, PA & ECOG, Madison, WI.

31. Papillon J, Mayer M, Montbarbon JF, et al. A new approach to the management of epidermoid carcinoma of the anal canal. *Cancer* 1983;51:1830–1837

32. Frost DB, Richards PC, Mantague ED, et al. Epidermoid cancer of the anorectum. *Cancer* 1984;53:1285–1293

33. Jensen SL, Shokouh-Amiri MH, Hagen K, et al. Adenocarcinoma of the anal ducts: a series of 21 cases. *Dis Colon Rectum* 1988;31:268–272

34. Cooper PH, Mills SE, Allen MS. Malignant melanoma of the anus: report of 12 patients and analysis of 255 additional cases. *Dis Colon Rectum* 1982;25:693–703

35. Wanebo HJ, Woodruff JM, Quan SH. Anorectal melanoma. *Cancer* 1981;47:1891–1900

36. Chiu YS, Unni KK, Beart RW Jr. Malignant melanoma of the anorectum. *Dis Colon Rectum* 1980;23:122–124

37. Greenall MJ, Magill GB, Quan SH, et al. Recurrent epidermoid cancer of the anus. *Cancer* 1986;57: 1437–1441

38. Nielsen OV, Jensen SL. Basal cell carcinoma of the anus - a clinical study of 34 cases. *Br J Surg* 1981;68:856–857

39. Bowen JT: Precancerous dermatoses: a study of two cases of chronic atypical epithelial proliferation. *J Cutan Dis* 1912;30:241–255

40. Arbesman H, Ransohoff DF. Is Bowen's disease a predictor for the development of internal malignancy? a methodological critique of the literature. *JAMA* 1987;257: 516–518

41. Darier J, Couillard P. Sur un cas de maladie de Paget de la region perineo-anale et scrotale. *Ann Dermatol Syph* 1893;4:25–31

42. Nadji M, Morales AR, Girtanner RE, et al. Paget's disease of the skin: a unifying concept of histogenesis. *Cancer* 1982;50:2203–2206

43. Grodsky L. Extramammary Paget's disease of the perianal region. *Dis Colon Rectum* 1960;3:502–509

44. Besa P, Rich TA, Delclos L, et al. Extramammary Paget's disease of the perineal skin: role of radiotherapy. *Int J Radiation Oncology Biol Phys* 1992;24:73–78

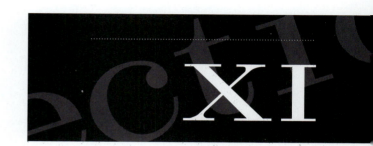

LIVER

51

Liver Abscess and Hydatid Cyst Disease

Stephen A. Barnes ▪ *Keith D. Lillemoe*

Pyogenic and amebic abscesses, and hydatid cysts are all uncommon entities that share the clinical characteristics of a space-occupying cavitary hepatic lesion of infectious origin. Yet each diagnosis has a unique clinical presentation, patient population, and most importantly, a specific treatment. In past decades, difficulty in diagnosis and inadequate treatment regimens have led to significant morbidity and mortality for hepatic abscesses and hydatid cysts. Fortunately, earlier clinical recognition, advances in diagnostic and therapeutic radiology, and recent improvements in treatment regimens have dramatically improved patient outcomes.

▪ PYOGENIC LIVER ABSCESS

Descriptions of liver abscesses date back to Hippocrates in approximately 4000 BC. John Bright provided the first description of the disease in modern medicine in his 1836 discourse on jaundice. Waller and later, Dieulafoy, both are credited with recognizing the association of hepatic abscesses in patients with appendicitis and pylephlebitis. In 1938, Ochsner and associates provided a landmark collective review of pyogenic liver abscesses in the preantibiotic era.[1] In this study, appendicitis was established as the most common site of origin of infection in patients with liver abscesses. Since the beginning of the modern era of antibiotic therapy, however, a fun-

damental shift has occurred in both the etiology of pyogenic liver abscesses and the patient population involved.[2] The biliary tract now surpasses all other locations as the most common source of pyogenic liver abscesses. Presently, liver abscesses rarely complicate appendicitis. Most patients are now elderly and debilitated, and many have a coexisting malignancy. Yet, despite more complicated comorbid pathology and an older patient population, the mortality rates from pyogenic liver abscesses have slowly decreased, owing to earlier diagnoses and improved therapeutic intervention.

ETIOLOGY

In the liver, the Kupffer cell functions as a primary barrier and filter for the clearance of microorganisms from arterial, venous, biliary, and local sources. Pyogenic liver abscesses are believed to occur when this normal hepatic clearance fails or is overwhelmed. Distant infectious sites may seed the liver with pathogenic bacteria via the portal vein or the hepatic artery. Hepatic necrosis from trauma or embolic events, obstruction of the biliary tree, and malignancy all produce favorable conditions for the invasion and growth of microorganisms. Optimal treatment, therefore, includes discovering and treating not only the abscess, but also the source responsible for seeding the abscess. Traditionally, the etiologies of pyogenic liver abscesses are divided into six categories: biliary, portal, arterial, direct extension,

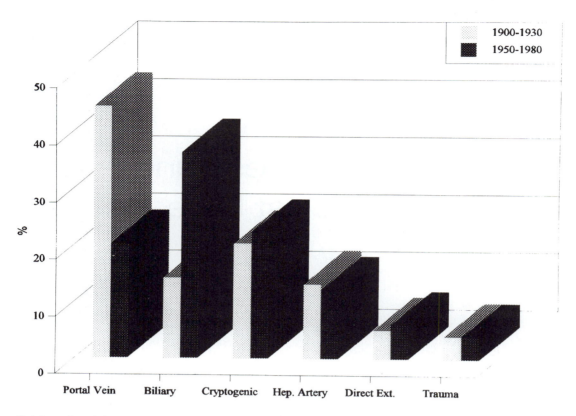

Figure 51–1. Comparison of etiology of pyogenic liver abscess treated before 1930 and between 1950 and 1980. (From Pitt HA. Liver abscess. In: Zuidema GD, Turcotte JG (eds), *Shackelford's Surgery of the Alimentary Tract,* 3rd ed. Philadelphia, PA: WB Saunders; 1991:444

traumatic, and cryptogenic. Although the portal venous route was the most common etiology before the widespread use of antibiotics, biliary diseases now produce more pyogenic abscesses than any other category. In contrast, antibiotic therapy has not significantly altered the number of abscesses originating from arterial, local, traumatic, or cryptogenic sources (Fig 51–1).

Diseases of the biliary system currently account for approximately 40% of pyogenic liver abscesses. Most cases involve a partial or complete obstruction of the biliary tract, with ascending cholangitis occurring in one-third of these patients. Benign conditions such as acute cholecystitis, choledocholithiasis, and benign strictures may lead to hepatic abscesses. However, malignant biliary obstruction owing to pancreatic carcinoma, cholangiocarcinoma, and metastatic adenocarcinoma account for 20% to 40% of patients with liver abscesses secondary to biliary sources.[3] Biliary manipulations, including cholangiography, percutaneous transhepatic biliary stents, endoprostheses, and bilioenteric anastomoses, predispose many patients to bacterial growth within the biliary tract. Therefore, as performance of these procedures has increased in frequency in the treatment of hepatobiliary disease, it is likely that in the current setting, this etiology will account for an even greater percentage of liver abscesses. Finally, patients

with advanced malignant conditions often are immunosuppressed and malnourished, which decreases their resistance to bacterial invasion of the biliary tree.

A portal venous source arising from intestinal pathology is found in 20% of patients with pyogenic liver abscesses. Transient portal bacteremia has been found to occur in many gastrointestinal disease states by means of bacterial translocation.[4] Intestinal perforation may lead to overwhelming numbers of microorganisms traversing the portal venous system, resulting in a liver abscess. Appendicitis with concomitant pylephlebitis, the primary etiology of pyogenic hepatic abscesses in the pre-antibiotic era, now accounts for only 2% of bacterial liver abscesses. Perforated colon cancers and diverticulitis, however, continue to be common causes of pyogenic hepatic abscesses. Purulent collections or abscesses in the spleen, pancreas, pelvis, and ischiorectal fossa also produce liver abscesses through this mechanism. In addition to normal liver parenchyma, primary and metastatic hepatic tumors show a propensity to become colonized by enteric flora.

Embolization of bacteria via the hepatic artery produces approximately 12% of pyogenic liver abscesses. Today, intravenous drug abuse and its complications account for most of these cases. Arterial embolization also may occur from many other sources of systemic bacteremia including endocarditis, otitis media, dental abscesses, pneumonia, pyelonephritis, and osteomyelitis. Umbilical artery catheterization and hepatic artery chemoembolization also have been reported to cause bacterial liver abscesses.

Approximately 4% of pyogenic liver abscesses result from traumatic injuries to the liver. Penetrating trauma causes the majority of these abscesses, most commonly from skin flora seeding necrotic liver tissue. Recently, hepatic abscesses have been reported to complicate cryosurgical ablation of liver tumors.[5] The abscess forms within the necrotic tumor cavity, with possible etiologies including intraoperative contamination, ascending transport of bacteria from concurrent bilioenteric anastomoses after liver or biliary tract resection, and skin flora traversing external drainage devices placed within the biliary tract or near the site of ablation. Finally, direct extension and suppurative invasion of liver tissue by subphrenic abscesses, perforated peptic ulcers, and gangrenous cholecystitis are the antecedent processes in 6% of pyogenic hepatic abscesses.

The number of patients presenting with cryptogenic abscesses, that is, those of unknown etiology, has remained constant for decades despite improvements in diagnosis. Most series find that 20% of patients with a pyogenic liver abscess will have no definable source for their disease. Recent data would suggest that aggressive investigation, using imaging studies as well as upper and lower endoscopy in the evaluation of patients, may decrease the number of cryptogenic abscesses to approximately 10%.[6] Typically, patients with cryptogenic abscesses have coexisting disease or are otherwise ill. Diabetes, malignancy, and other immunosuppressed states have been associated with cryptogenic abscesses, with many patients manifesting a degree of reticuloendothelial dysfunction.[7] Interestingly, however, the majority are solitary and contain a single species of anaerobic organism.

INCIDENCE

The incidence of pyogenic liver abscesses has remained constant for the last 100 years, in both autopsy series and hospital admissions. Pyogenic hepatic abscesses have been reported to occur in 0.008% to 0.035% of hospitalized patients in the United States, with an average incidence of 0.016%.[8] Clinically silent abscesses may occur more frequently, since in series of postmortem examinations, the prevalence of bacterial liver abscesses ranges from 0.2% to 1.5%. Although the actual incidence of pyogenic abscesses has remained stable, the affected patient population has changed dramatically since the onset of the modern antibiotic era. Ochsner and associates, in their review, reported a peak incidence of bacterial abscesses in the third and fourth decades of life, reflecting the role of appendicitis as the primary site of origin during this era.[1] Presently, however, the elderly are at

highest risk for developing a pyogenic abscess, with the peak incidence of the disease in the seventh decade. Historically, pyogenic liver abscesses occurred more frequently in men. Whereas children and young adults continue to manifest this male predominance, the overall ratio of men to women is now about equal. The rising incidence of bacterial abscesses in women reflects the expanding role of biliary pathology in the development of the disease. Contrary to its role in amebic abscesses, race does not appear to correlate with the occurrence of pyogenic hepatic abscesses.

PREDISPOSING FACTORS

Comorbid conditions associated with pyogenic liver abscesses differ by age group (Table 51–1). Younger children manifesting host-defense abnormalities or immunological disorders such as chronic granulomatous disease, complement deficiencies, acquired immunodeficiency syndrome (AIDS), leukemia, and other malignancies are at an increased risk of developing pyogenic hepatic abscesses. Liver abscesses also may complicate polycystic liver disease, congenital hepatic fibrosis, posttransplant liver failure, and sickle cell anemia. In contrast, traumatic injury to the liver causes most pyogenic hepatic abscesses in older children and young adults.

Chronic diseases and immunocompromise occur in many adult patients with bacterial liver abscesses, as well. Liver abscesses arise more frequently in adult patients with jaundice, diabetes mellitus, hepatic cirrhosis, chronic pancreatitis, peptic ulcer disease, chronic pyelonephritis, and inflammatory bowel disease. Solid organ cancers, leukemias, and lymphomas occur in 17% to 36% of patients with pyogenic liver abscesses. Abscesses also may develop in transplant recipients and patients with collagen vascular diseases. The use of chemotherapeutic agents, steroids and other immunosuppressive medications may be partially responsible for this association.[9] The human immunodeficiency virus

TABLE 51–1. COMORBID DISEASES ASSOCIATED WITH PYOGENIC LIVER ABSCESSES

Children	Adults
Chronic granulomatous disease	Diabetes mellitus
Complement deficiencies	Cirrhosis
Leukemia	Chronic pancreatitis
Malignancy	Peptic ulcer disease
Sickle cell anemia	Inflammatory bowel disease
Polycystic liver disease	Jaundice
Congenital hepatic fibrosis	Pyelonephritis
Posttransplant liver failure	Malignancy
Necrotizing enterocolitis	Leukemia and lymphoma
Chemotherapy and steroid therapy	Chemotherapy and steroid therapy
Acquired immunodeficiency syndrome	Acquired immunodeficiency syndrome

TABLE 51–2. PATHOGENESIS OF PYOGENIC LIVER ABSCESS BY ETIOLOGY

Etiology	Source of infection	Distribution	Primary microorganisms
Biliary system	Cholangitis, biliary obstruction	Both lobes, multiple	Single species, gram (-) aerobes and anaerobes *E coli*
Portal circulation	Intra-abdominal infection	Right lobe > left multiple or single	Polymicrobial, enteric aerobes and anaerobes *E faecalis, E coli, B fragilis*
	Liver metastasis	Area of metastasis	Single species, anaerobic *B fragilis*
Arterial circulation	Bacteremia, systemic infection	Both lobes, multiple	Single species, gram (+) aerobes *S aureus, S pyogenes*
Trauma	Direct exposure, necrosis	Area of injury	Single species gram (+) aerobes *S aureus, S pyogenes*
Direct extension	Cholecystitis, perforated ulcer	Adjacent area	Single species, gram (-) aerobes *E coli*
Cryptogenic	Unknown	Right lobe > left	Single species, anaerobic *B fragilis*

Modified from Garrison, RN, Polk, HC: Liver abscess and subphrenic abscess, In: Blumgart, LH (ed), Surgery of the Liver and Biliary Tract, 2 ed. New York, NY: Churchill Livingston 1994;1092.

also has been associated with an increasing number of adult patients with pyogenic liver abscesses.

PATHOLOGY

The etiology of a liver abscess serves as the best predictor of the size, number, and location of abscesses affecting a given patient (Table 51–2). Generally, portal, traumatic, and cryptogenic hepatic abscesses are solitary and large, while biliary and arterial abscesses are multiple and small. In the review by Gyorffy and colleagues, 40% of pyogenic hepatic abscesses were found to be 1.5 to 5 cm in diameter, 40% were 5 to 8 cm, and 20% were 8 cm or larger.[2] Overall, pyogenic liver abscesses localize to the right hepatic lobe in 65% of cases, with the majority of these being solitary. The left lobe is solely involved in 12% of cases, with 23% of patients having bilateral abscesses. The number of bilateral and multiple abscesses has increased as more patients present with a biliary etiology. Bilateral disease occurs in 90% of cases with a biliary or arterial source of infection, distributing along the terminal branches of the portal triad. In contrast, liver abscesses resulting from intra-abdominal infectious sources have a propensity to develop in the right hepatic lobe, a process that may be explained by the preferential blood flow from the superior mesenteric vein to this location. Fungal hepatic abscesses are most often multiple, bilateral, and miliary in nature.

BACTERIOLOGY

Improved isolation and culture techniques have resulted in greater recovery and better definition of the bacteria causing pyogenic liver abscesses (Table 51–3). Gram-negative enteric bacteria, including *Escherichia coli, Klebsiella, Enterobacter,* and *Proteus* species are isolated from 50% to 75% of liver abscesses. Anaerobic bacteria such as *Bacteroides, Clostridium, Fusobacterium, Actinomyces,* and *Peptostreptococcus* can be cultured from 40% to 50% of patients, if appropriate handling protocols are used. Gram-positive aerobes, mostly *Staphylococcus* and *Streptococcus* species, occur in 30% of abscesses.[10] Fungal species currently are being isolated at an increased frequency. Approximately 25% of hepatic liver abscesses occurring in tertiary health care centers may have fungal infection as their etiology.

The species of microorganisms found in a hepatic abscess are related to the source of the abscess (Table 51–2). If a disease of the biliary tract gives rise to a hepatic abscess, gram-negative rods such as *E. coli* and *Klebsiella* species predominate, since these bacteria commonly occur in infected bile. Similarly, enteric pathogens such as *E. coli, Enterococcus,* and anaerobic organisms frequently are recovered from liver abscesses resulting from a disorder of the intestinal tract. Cryptogenic bacterial abscesses often contain anaerobic bacteria. Patients with liver metastases may develop cryptogenic abscesses in both normal hepatic parenchyma and in the metastatic tumors themselves.

The majority of pyogenic hepatic abscesses contain multiple organisms, with three or more species of bacteria existing in one-third of cases. Polymicrobial abscesses occur most commonly in adults and are typically solitary. Liver abscesses harboring a single species of gram-positive aerobic bacteria are seen with a relatively high frequency in children, diabetics, intravenous drug users, and trauma victims. The most common organisms in such cases are *Staphylococcus aureus* and *Streptococcus pyogenes,* which spread to the liver from direct extension or by the arterial system. These bacteria are quite virulent and the host often is immunocompromised, both of which explain the high mortality rate associated with these abscesses.

TABLE 51–3. ORGANISMS ISOLATED FROM PYOGENIC LIVER ABSCESSES

Category of Organism	% of Patients
GRAM-NEGATIVE AEROBES	50–70
Escherichia coli	35–45
Klebsiella	18
Proteus	10
Enterobacter	15
Serratia	rare
Morganella	rare
Actinobacter	rare
GRAM-POSITIVE AEROBES	30
Streptococcal species	20
Enterococcus faecalis	10
B-Streptococci	
A-Streptococci	
Staphylococcal species	15
ANAEROBES	40–50
Bacteroides species	24
Bacteroides fragilis	15
Fusobacterium	10
Peptostreptococcus	10
Clostridium	5
Antinomyces	rare
FUNGAL	26
STERILE	7

Fungal hepatic abscesses usually arise in patients with leukemia and lymphoma, or patients with other malignancies receiving chemotherapy.[11] Mycotic colonization of the biliary tract is also quite common in patients with biliary stents who are receiving prolonged courses of antibiotics. *Candida albicans* and *Aspergillus* species are the most common fungal isolates. Mycobacteria species, including tubercular infections, occasionally infect the liver and, through caseous necrosis, cause a hepatic abscess. Identification of fungi and mycobacteria requires special staining procedures and selected culture media. When evaluating abscess fluid from an individual with a malignant disorder or an immunodeficiency syndrome, these isolation techniques are particularly important.

Sterile hepatic abscesses, those which behave like microbial infections but which fail to grow organisms on culture, were once quite common. Proper isolation, rapid handling, and selective culture techniques, particularly for anaerobic bacteria, have decreased the incidence of sterile hepatic abscesses to approximately 7%.[12] Amebic and parasitic organisms are difficult to identify with either standard or selective bacterial staining and culture techniques. Thus, these infections should be suspected if bacterial cultures are repeatedly negative.

DIAGNOSIS

Because pyogenic liver abscesses are rare, and their presentation is often nonspecific, a delay in diagnosis is common. Furthermore, once suspected, the diagnosis also may be delayed while laboratory values, culture data, and radiological studies are obtained. Despite the advances in bacteriology and imaging techniques, clinical acumen is the foundation for diagnosing liver abscesses in a timely fashion. Presently, up to one-third of patients suffer delayed evaluation and therapy; therefore, in those clinical situations with a high index of suspicion for the disease, treatment should not be withheld until the diagnosis is confirmed.

Clinical Presentation

The clinical presentation of pyogenic liver abscesses has changed little since Ochsner's review in 1938.[1] Symptoms and signs of a hepatic abscess are frequently vague and nonspecific (Table 51–4). Most patients manifest symptoms for less than 2 weeks, but a more indolent course occurs in approximately one third of individuals. Patients with such chronic courses typically have solitary hepatic abscesses. Fever is the most common symptom, present in greater than 80% of patients, and is typically of a sustained nature. Less than 25% of patients report

TABLE 51–4. CLINICAL MANIFESTATIONS OF PYOGENIC LIVER ABSCESSES IN ADULT PATIENTS

	% Pyogenic Abscesses
SYMPTOM	
Fever	83
Weight loss	60
Pain	55
Nausea and vomiting	50
Malaise	50
Chills	37
Anorexia	34
Cough, pleurisy	30
Pruritus	17
Diarrhea	12
SIGN	
Right upper quadrant tenderness	52
Hepatomegaly	40
Jaundice	31
Right upper quadrant	25
Ascites	25
Pleural effusion, rub	20
LABORATORY	
Increased alkaline phosphatase	87
WBC >10 000/mm^3	71
Albumin <3 g/dL	55
Hematocrit <36%	53
Bilirubin >2 g/dL	24

the classic spiking fever pattern associated with other abdominal abscesses, and 10% are afebrile when evaluated. Right upper quadrant pain, malaise, nausea, and vomiting occur in slightly more than half of individuals. Pruritus, secondary to obstructive jaundice, and diarrhea are rare but important manifestations of bacterial liver abscesses. Hepatomegaly and right upper quadrant tenderness are the only consistent physical findings. Other less common signs include a right upper quadrant mass, ascites, jaundice, and a right pleural effusion. These processes occur in only approximately 25% patients.

Laboratory Evaluation

As with most bacterial infections, a number of laboratory abnormalities may be seen in patients with pyogenic liver abscesses (Table 51–4). There is, however, no specific laboratory test that can invariably diagnose the disease. Markedly abnormal laboratory studies are usually indicative of a systemic involvement of the bacterial infection. In uncomplicated cases, leukocytosis with a left shift is present in two-thirds of patients. Anemia and hypoalbuminemia are also quite common, particularly in more chronic presentations, occurring in about half of individuals. Abnormal liver function tests exist in most patients with pyogenic hepatic abscesses and are the most sensitive markers for the disease. Elevations of alkaline phosphatase and gamma-glutamyl transpeptidase occur in approximately 90% of individuals. Hyperbilirubinemia, usually associated with underlying biliary tract disease as an etiology, exists in greater than 25% of patients. Pitt and Zuidema have reported several laboratory abnormalities associated with poor outcomes in patients with pyogenic liver abscesses.[13] These include an increased serum glutamic-oxalacetic transaminase (SGOT), hyperbilirubinemia, elevated white count with left shift, and hypoalbuminemia (<2 gm/dL).

Aseptically obtained peripheral blood cultures are useful in diagnosing, treating, and predicting the outcome of patients with bacterial liver abscesses. If obtained before the initiation of antibiotic therapy, peripheral blood cultures are positive in more than half of patients. Blood cultures turning positive in the first twenty-four hours usually indicate a staphylococcal, streptococcal, or gram-negative aerobic infection. As opposed to the abscess cavity itself, blood cultures typically yield a single microorganism. Polymicrobial bacteremia, although uncommon, is associated with an increased mortality rate.

Radiology

The diagnosis of a liver abscess in most patients is based on noninvasive radiologic imaging studies. Ultrasonography and computerized tomography (CT) are both useful examinations capable of establishing the diagnosis of pyogenic liver abscesses. Currently, these studies are used to not only image the liver lesion, but also to guide aspiration of the abscess cavity, which greatly improves the diagnosis and management of these lesions. In addition, percutaneous drainage catheters also can be placed, using either imaging modality. Finally, CT and ultrasound are useful in documenting abscess resolution during therapy.

CT is probably the most effective study in diagnosing patients with liver abscesses (Fig 51–2). Thus, CT is the procedure of choice for the initial assessment of a suspected pyogenic liver abscess and should be performed routinely in virtually all patients when this diagnosis is considered. Compared to ultrasound, CT offers several advantages, including better diagnosis of concurrent and causative pathology. If contrast-enhanced, CT has a reported sensitivity in detecting liver abscesses approaching 95%.[14] While CT typically detects abscesses greater than 0.5 cm in diameter, even smaller lesions may be visualized with either simultaneous administration of arterial contrast or newer contrast-enhanced spiral techniques. Furthermore, compared to ultrasound, CT better delineates small abscesses near the diaphragm and abscesses in fatty livers. Finally, CT also visualizes coexisting intra-abdominal pathology including pancreatic masses, colon cancers, diverticulitis, appendicitis, and intraperitoneal abscesses.

Ultrasonography is also an excellent imaging modality for the initial evaluation of hepatic abscesses, with sensitivities reported between 85% to 95% (Fig 51–3). Ultrasound often is used as a preliminary screen to confirm the presence of a suspected space-occupying liver lesion. Further diagnostic tests or radiological studies, such as CT, however, often are required to delineate the source of the abscess. Because of resolution limitations, ultrasound can only identify lesions >2 cm in diameter. As noted above, ultrasound is also inferior to CT in locating abscesses that are multiple, small, in the liver dome, or in fatty livers. Compared to CT, ultrasound does have the advantages of being less expensive, not using nonionizing radiation, and being portable for imaging critically ill patients. In addition, ultrasound is more useful in differentiating cystic from solid masses, and is more sensitive than CT for diagnosing gallstones.

Early results with magnetic resonance imaging (MRI) in defining hepatic abscesses appear promising (Fig 51–4). In animal models, MRI can identify hepatic abscesses as small as 0.3 cm in diameter, with abscesses appearing as high-intensity signals on T2-weighted images.[15] Edema surrounding the abscess varies with the severity of infection and may be useful in documenting an early response to therapy. MRI is also superior to other radiographic techniques in defining hepatic venous anatomy. Therefore, this study may prove useful for those patients requiring a liver resection to treat the abscess.

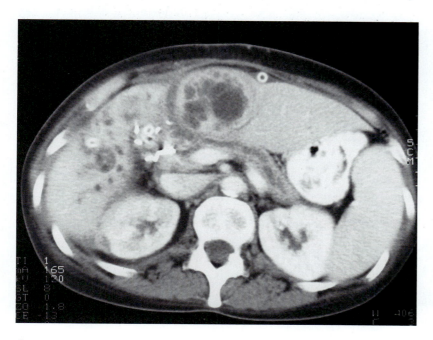

A

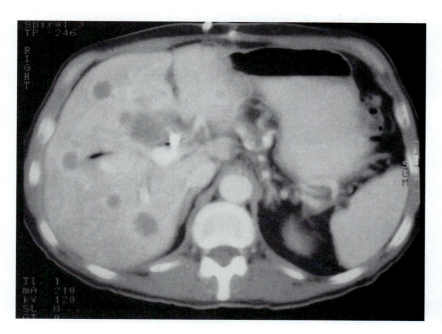

B

Figure 51–2. A. CT of a large, multiseptated pyogenic liver abscess in the medial portion of the left hepatic lobe. Note surgical clips in hilum and surgical drains. **B**. CT revealing multiple low-density lesions within the liver and characteristic peripheral rim enhancement. The biliary tract was the source of these pyogenic abscesses.

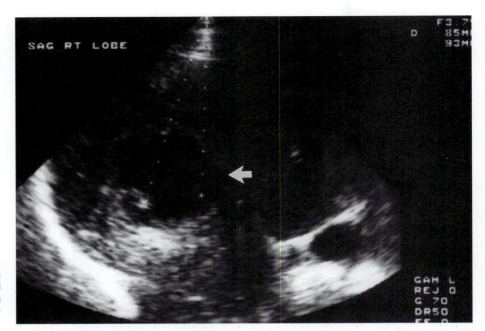

Figure 51–3. Sagittal abdominal ultrasound demonstrating a pyogenic liver abscess (*arrow*). The lesion appears as a low-density collection with small internal echoes and through-transmission characteristic of a fluid-filled mass. The abscess was later aspirated under sonographic guidance.

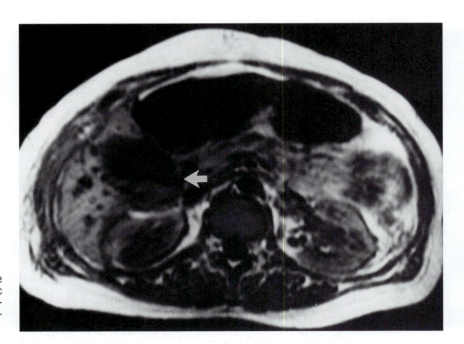

Figure 51–4. T1-weighted magnetic resonance image revealing a pyogenic liver abscess in the right hepatic lobe (*arrow*). The enhanced area in the dependant portion of the abscess is consistent with debris or hemorrhage.

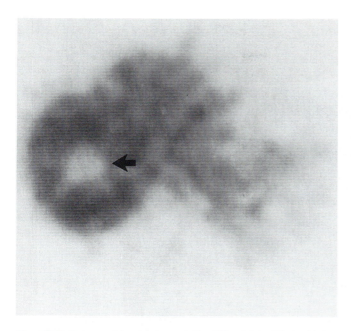

Figure 51–5. Nuclear medicine scan demonstrating a filling defect within the right hepatic lobe (*arrow*), consistent with a liver abscess.

Nuclear medicine liver scans, once a valuable method of imaging liver abscesses, have been replaced largely by ultrasound and CT (Fig 51–5). Although the sensitivity of liver scans varies from 80% to 97%, these studies have the disadvantages of being nonspecific as to the etiology of the liver image filling defect and providing little information concerning the possible source of the abscess.

There are limited roles for other imaging modalities in the diagnosis of liver abscesses. Plain films of the chest are abnormal in approximately 50% of patients, revealing nonspecific findings of a right pleural effusion, atelectasis or an elevated hemidiaphragm. Less frequently, abdominal films disclose such nonspecific findings as right upper-quadrant gas, air-fluid levels within the abscess, or ileus (Fig 51–6). In cases in which gastrointestinal pathology is suspected as a cause of a liver abscess, barium contrast studies of the upper and lower gastrointestinal tract may delineate the lesion. Invasive biliary studies, including endoscopic retrograde cholangiography (ERC) or percutaneous cholangiography (PTC), may be indicated for patients in which clinical, laboratory, or microbiologic data, in conjunction with CT or ultrasound, suggest the biliary system as the source of a pyogenic liver abscess (Fig 51–7). Cholangiography will reveal an abnormality in as many as 60% of these patients.[16] Although these procedures are valuable for defining biliary causes of the liver ab-

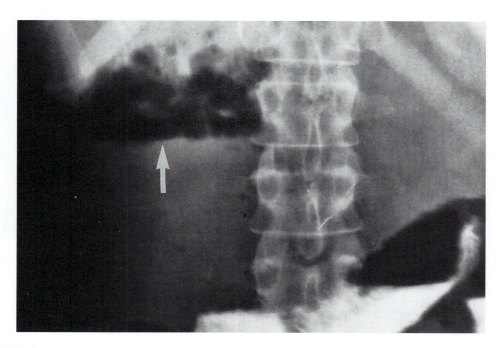

Figure 51–6. Plain film of a barium enema performed on a patient with a large gas-filled abscess located in the right hepatic lobe (*arrow*). (From Pitt HA. Liver abscess. In: Zuidema GD, Turcotte JG (eds), *Shackelford's Surgery of the Alimentary Tract,* 3rd ed. Philadelphia, PA: WB Saunders; 1991:447)

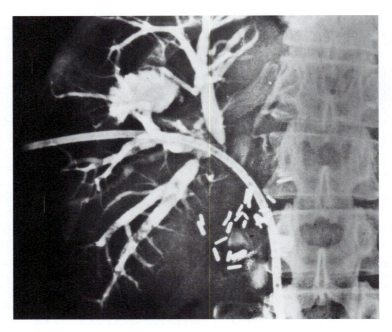

A

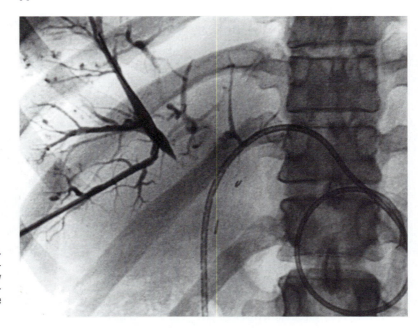

Figure 51–7. A. PTC demonstrating a large abscess cavity in communication with the biliary tree in a patient with stenosis and cutoff of the proximal hepatic duct. A transhepatic catheter is decompressing the biliary system. **B**. PTC of the right hepatic lobe revealing multiple small abscesses communicating with the peripheral biliary tract and cutoff of the right hepatic bile duct.

B

scess, they can be associated with complications, including severe cholangitis in patients with bacterial colonization of the biliary system.

TREATMENT

The cornerstone for management of a pyogenic liver abscess is appropriate antibiotic therapy and prompt drainage of the purulent collection. Furthermore, discovering and treating the source of the abscess is imperative for successful cure. Currently, the traditional role of surgical drainage of pyogenic abscesses is being challenged by percutaneous techniques, which appear safe and have acceptable success rates. Surgery now is reserved primarily for treatment failures of percutaneous drainage or for patients with coexisting intra-abdominal pathology.

Antibiotics

Although the identification of the specific microorganisms involved in pyogenic liver abscess requires appropriate culture information, initial empiric treatment with antibiotics is prudent in most cases. The etiology of the abscess, if known, may suggest appropriate antibiotic regimens; however, broad-spectrum coverage with antibiotics effective against gram-negative rods, streptococcal species, and anaerobes should be initiated and continued until definitive organisms are isolated and their sensitivities established. Antifungal therapy should be initiated only in those patients with positive fungal identification under microscopic examination or when fungi are isolated from appropriate cultures.

Several combinations of antibiotics are effective against the variety of bacteria found in hepatic abscesses. Regimens consisting of a broad-spectrum synthetic penicillin (ampicillin), an aminoglycoside (gentamicin or tobramycin), and metronidazole will cover the organisms found in the majority of pyogenic liver abscesses. Metronidazole should be the primary choice for anaerobic coverage, since this drug offers the advantage of also treating what may prove to be an amebic abscess. Renal function and aminoglycoside levels should be monitored closely, particularly in elderly or septic patients, and an appropriate substitute for the aminoglycoside, such as aztreonam, should be instituted if toxicity occurs. Imipenem is also useful in this situation, as well as with those patients with penicillin allergies. Newer broad-spectrum synthetic penicillins and cephalosporins are available for treating pyogenic liver abscesses, and combination antibiotics such as ampicillin/sulbactam, ticarcillin/clavulanate, and piperacillin/clavulanate also appear efficacious for the early management of such abscesses. For confirmed fungal infections, both amphotericin B and fluconazole are effective agents.[17] Once culture and sensitivity data are available, the an-

tibiotic regimen can be modified to optimize treatment of the abscess. Antibiotics initially should be administered intravenously, but patients that show clinical improvement with appropriate therapy can be discharged on an oral regimen.

Conventionally, a prolonged course of antibiotics, lasting 4 to 6 weeks, is required for patients with a pyogenic liver abscess. The justification for long-term antibiotic therapy has been the perceived avascularity of both the intact and decompressed abscess cavities and the concern for concurrent, but undiagnosed, purulent collections within the liver. Recent studies suggest, however, that in adequately drained abscesses, only 2 weeks of antibiotic administration are necessary.[18–19] Northover has reported acceptable cure rates for pyogenic abscesses when antibiotics are discontinued 1 week after imaging studies such as CT or sinogram reveal resolution of the abscess cavity.[20] However, prolonged antibiotic therapy does remain necessary in patients with multiple or fungal hepatic abscesses, and, in general, the length of treatment must be individualized for each patient with a pyogenic liver abscess.

In most patients, antibiotic treatment must be accompanied by adequate drainage of the abscess cavity. However, in certain clinical settings, successful treatment of pyogenic liver abscesses with antibiotics alone has been reported.[21,22] Patients with multiple, small (<1.5 cm diameter) abscesses, uncomplicated by concurrent surgical disease, are best treated with several weeks of antibiotic administration. Aspiration of a representative abscess is performed primarily to obtain culture material to direct therapy. However, since most patients presenting with multiple small abscesses have coexisting biliary tract disease, a careful and detailed evaluation for such disorders is essential before following this course of therapy. Many of these patients will require some form of biliary drainage procedure to relieve the biliary obstruction and source of infection. Finally, most fungal abscesses are miliary; therefore, they are not amenable to percutaneous or surgical drainage. Prolonged therapy with a systemic antifungal agent is appropriate.

Aspiration

Aspiration of a liver abscess provides valuable diagnostic and bacteriologic data. Controversy remains, however, as to whether the treatment of pyogenic liver abscesses should be undertaken with antibiotics and aspiration alone. Aspiration with concurrent antibiotic therapy may be useful in young, otherwise healthy patients with a solitary abscess and no coexisting intra-abdominal pathology. McFadzean and colleagues treated 108 of such patients in this manner with only one death, and other series document comparable survival rates when selected patients undergo this form of management.[23] There appears to be no role for simple aspiration of pyogenic liver abscesses in elderly, debilitated patients or those with underlying malignancy or biliary tract disease. Such patients have higher morbidity and mortality rates when treated solely with aspiration than do their younger counterparts and often require more aggressive management.[24]

Percutaneous Drainage

Advances in radiology since the 1970s, including both imaging and interventional techniques, resulted in the introduction of radiologically guided aspiration and drainage of intra-abdominal abscesses. The application of such procedures to pyogenic liver abscesses has revolutionized their management. Indeed, most authors now recommend percutaneous drainage as the initial management for essentially all patients with pyogenic liver abscesses. The role of percutaneous drainage has been most useful for those critically ill patients who cannot undergo surgery. However, despite the widespread availability and applicability of percutaneous techniques, it should be recognized that no randomized trials exist comparing percutaneous drainage of pyogenic liver abscesses to operative interventions.

The highest success rates for percutaneous drainage have been reported in patients with solitary, uniseptate abscesses (Fig 51–8). The procedure is successful in 70% to 90% of individuals, with the length of catheter drainage lasting from 11 to 19 days. Catheter placement in experienced hands causes little discomfort to the patient and is tolerated well. Inadequate drainage and subsequent treatment failure most commonly results from catheter obstruction with purulent material or untreated loculations within the abscess. Percutaneous drainage is also frequently unsuccessful in immunocompromised patients. In one series, 50% of patients with comorbid malignancy, diabetes, chronic renal failure, or other immunosuppressed states required further surgical therapy after initial percutaneous decompression of the abscess.[25]

There are a number of absolute and relative contraindications to percutaneous drainage of liver abscesses. Absolute contraindications include associated biliary or intra-abdominal pathology requiring simultaneous operative intervention. In addition, coagulopathy and anatomic inaccessibility preclude percutaneous catheter placement, owing to the increased risk of life-threatening hemorrhage or violation of hollow organs such as the bowel. Multiple abscesses and generalized ascites are relative contraindications for percutaneous catheterization. A mutiloculated or septated abscess is not a contraindication for percutaneous drainage, but this factor should be kept in mind as a potential reason for failed drainage. Finally, one of the limitations of percutaneous drainage lies in failure to identify the abscess source. Because exploratory laparotomy is not performed, clinical judgment and imaging studies alone are used to determine the antecedent pathology. Theoretically, then, the incidence of what appear to be "cryptogenic" abscesses may increase as percutaneous management becomes more common, although no published data presently exist to support this concept. It is also unknown whether the widespread use of these procedures will result in cases of missed malignancies or other sites of abdominal infection.

Procedure-related morbidity and mortality associated with interventional procedures is low, and current reviews describe overall patient mortality between 3% to 4%. Most of these patients were critically ill at the time of the drainage procedure and had concurrent immunosuppressive disease. Complications associated with percutaneous drainage of liver abscesses include sepsis, hemorrhage, contamination of the pleural or peritoneal spaces, and bowel perforation. These occur in less than 5% of patients. Many of these complications are themselves life-threatening, and potentially devastating for critically ill patients. Fortunately, the majority are amenable to aggressive antibiotic therapy, intensive care resuscitation, and further nonoperative interventions. Nevertheless, complications such as bowel perforation often require operative management which again results in an increased risk to the patient. More frequent but relatively minor complications include catheter-related pain and catheter displacement, which may be prevented by proper and timely administration of analgesics and catheter suturing techniques, respectively.

Surgical Drainage

As a result of the success of aspiration and percutaneous drainage of pyogenic abscesses, surgical drainage procedures now are performed less frequently than in the past. Nonetheless, surgery is indicated in several circumstances. Laparotomy, with careful exploration, is superior to current imaging techniques in delineating intra-abdominal pathology and providing concurrent treatment of both the abscess and its source. Thus, strong clinical suspicion of an abdominal infectious etiology may warrant surgical intervention, even when radiologic scans are negative for bowel pathology. Patients with loculated or multiple abscesses and abscesses inaccessible to percutaneous drainage, or involving an entire hepatic lobe, are also candidates for surgical treatment. Operative intervention also is indicated for patients with coexisting biliary pathology, such as biliary stones or strictures. Finally, surgical drainage remains the treatment of choice for abscesses recalcitrant to less invasive procedures.

Prior to the current availability of antibiotics, an extraperitoneal approach for drainage of pyogenic liver abscesses was commonplace. During this era, peritoneal

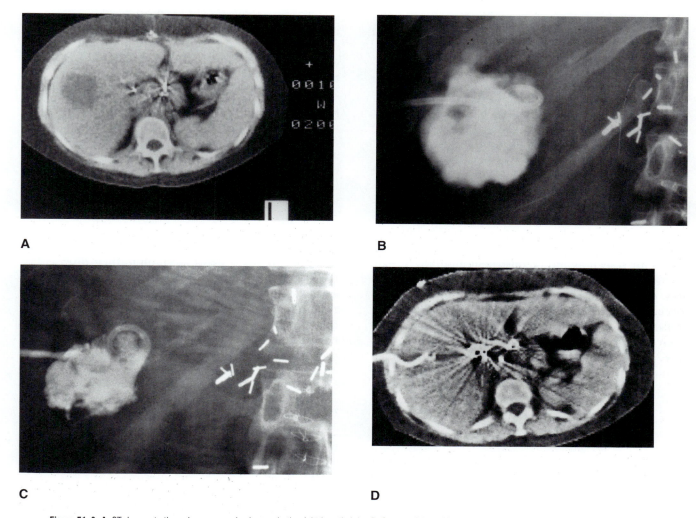

Figure 51–8. A. CT demonstrating a large pyogenic abscess in the right hepatic lobe. **B**. Contrast injected into the abscess cavity through a percutaneously placed catheter. **C**. Sinogram performed 2 weeks later revealing a decrease in the size of the abscess cavity. **D**. CT after 4 weeks, demonstrating complete resolution of the abscess. (From Pitt HA. Liver abscess. In: Zuidema GD, Turcotte JG (eds), *Shackelford's Surgery of the Alimentary Tract*, 3rd ed. Philadelphia, PA: WB Saunders; 1991:449–451)

contamination resulted in a 90% mortality rate, thus intra-abdominal operations were avoided. Subcostal, transpleural, and retroperitoneal procedures, which avoided the free peritoneal cavity by following a plane defined by perihepatic adhesions to the abdominal wall or diaphragm, were frequently utilized to gain access to the abscess. Presently, such extraperitoneal procedures are rarely undertaken, as they do not permit exploration of the abdomen or exposure of the biliary tree. This approach remains useful only for selected abscesses located superiorly in the liver dome.

Transperitoneal operative drainage is now the standard treatment for most patients with pyogenic liver abscesses requiring surgical drainage. A midline incision usually is preferred in that it permits full evaluation of the liver and abdominal contents as well as facilitating

bowel resection, biliary surgery, and drain placement, as indicated. Once the abdomen has been explored and any infectious source managed, surgical drainage of a pyogenic liver abscess is straightforward. Bimanual examination of the liver and judicious use of intraoperative ultrasound both localize the abscess and decrease the possibility of missing synchronous hepatic lesions.[26] After the abscess is isolated from the surgical field, it is aspirated for culture and then opened with cautery. Loculations are commonly present and are carefully broken down with finger dissection. Biopsies of the abscess wall as well as normal liver should be obtained to rule out concurrent amebic disease, tumor, or microabscesses. After the abscess site is irrigated, soft, closed-suction drains are placed within the abscess cavity in dependent locations.

Rarely, the treatment of pyogenic abscesses requires hepatic resection. Typically, isolated lobar involvement with single or multiple nonhealing abscesses is an indication for wedge resection or formal lobectomy, depending on the size of the lesion. Patients with infected hepatic malignancies, hemobilia, and chronic granulomatous disease also may be candidates for hepatic resection. The actual extent of hepatic resection depends on the magnitude of disease involvement and the physiologic reserve of the patient.

The role of laparoscopic surgery in the management of pyogenic liver abscesses is presently limited. Extensive perihepatic adhesions often hinder attempts at laparoscopic abscess drainage, and controlled evaluation and isolation of the abscess is often more difficult than with an open procedure. Moreover, laparoscopic techniques for resection and reconstruction of biliary, pancreatic, or colonic disorders that may give rise to the liver abscess are presently unavailable or limited to specialized centers. Nevertheless, laparoscopy may be useful in diagnosing concurrent abdominal pathology when disease is suspected but radiological scans are negative. In addition, the use of laparoscopically guided liver biopsies has proven beneficial in diagnosing cryptogenic fungal hepatic abscesses in patients with fever of unknown origin, and successful resolution of abscesses with catheters placed under laparoscopic guidance has been reported.

COMPLICATIONS

Approximately 40% of patients with pyogenic liver abscesses develop complications, which increase both morbidity and mortality rates. Young and otherwise healthy patients can tolerate most complications, but when complications develop in elderly, moribund, or immunosuppressed patients, the results are often catastrophic. Generalized sepsis is the most common systemic complication of a liver abscess. Approximately 85% of patients who develop sepsis succumb to their disease. Pulmonary complications such as pleural effusion, empyema, and pneumonia also frequently occur. Intraperitoneal rupture of a pyogenic hepatic abscess, although rare, is frequently fatal. More commonly, a controlled leak results in a perihepatic abscess. Rarely, pyogenic abscesses may cause hemobilia or hepatic vein thrombosis.

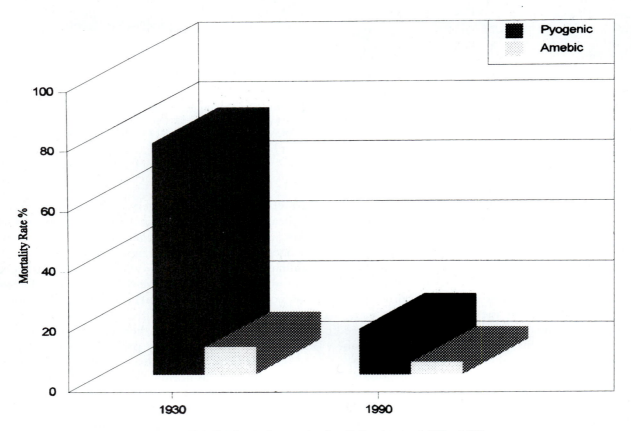

Figure 51–9. Mortality rates for pyogenic and amebic liver abscesses in 1930 and 1990.

TABLE 51–5. FACTORS ASSOCIATED WITH POOR PROGNOSIS IN PATIENTS WITH PYOGENIC LIVER ABSCESS

Age >70	WBC >20 000
Diabetes mellitus	Increasing bilirubin
Associated malignancy	Increasing SGOT
Biliary etiology	Albumin <2 gm/dL
Multiple abscesses	Aerobic abscess
Septicemia	Significant complication
Polymicrobial bacteremia	

PROGNOSIS

If untreated, nearly all pyogenic liver abscesses prove fatal. In the preantibiotic era, 75% of patients succumbed to their illness despite timely surgical management. Despite the institution of combined antibiotic and surgical therapy, mortality rates remained approximately 50%, owing primarily to delays in diagnosis. With modern diagnostic imaging, antibiotics, and early percutaneous decompression, 80% to 90% of patients presently survive (Fig 51–9). When uncomplicated, both solitary and anaerobic liver abscesses have mortality rates of <5%, but the incidence of such abscesses is falling.

Several factors are associated with a poor prognosis in patients with pyogenic hepatic abscesses (Table 51–5).[13,27] Delayed diagnosis, undrained or improperly drained abscesses, and untreated primary infectious sites frequently result in patient mortality. Elderly patients, as well as those with concurrent diabetes, major trauma, AIDS, endocarditis, or other immunosuppressive states also have increased mortality rates. The development of a pyogenic liver abscess in a patient with advanced hepatic or biliary malignancy is often a terminal event. Other factors associated with a poor prognosis are multiple abscesses, such as those occurring with biliary tract disease, abscesses containing more than three species of microorganisms, and abscesses containing strictly aerobic bacteria. These presentations all have reported mortality rates approaching 75%. Septicemia, polymicrobial bacteremia, marked leukocytosis, and severe hepatic dysfunction are grave signs of systemic involvement of the liver abscess, and a minority of patients with these abnormalities survive. Complications such as pleural effusions, empyemas, and intra-abdominal ruptures also are associated with poor outcomes.

■ AMEBIC ABSCESS

In many countries, amebiasis and amebic dysentery continue to be common health problems. Amebic infections of the colon, liver, and other organs are common in areas of poor sanitation and particularly in de-

veloping nations with contaminated water supplies and poor public hygiene. Typically, these endemic areas of amebiasis are located in tropical and subtropical areas of the world. Worldwide, complications of amebiasis such as amebic liver abscesses are quite common; thus, even though such abscesses are rare in industrialized areas such as Western Europe and North America, on a global basis, amebic abscesses exceed pyogenic abscesses in overall frequency.

The early descriptions of amebic disease, including amebiasis and amebic liver abscesses, came from India. In the United States, Sir William Osler first reported coexistent hepatic and colonic amebiasis in 1890. Councilman and LaFleur, working at the Johns Hopkins Hospital, in Baltimore, characterized the pathogenic role of amebas in the affected liver, first using the term "amebic liver abscess" in 1891. The management of amebic liver abscesses has evolved with the recognition of colonic amebiasis as the antecedent source of the liver infection. Early treatment by open surgical drainage alone had met with only limited success. Efforts to treat both the liver abscess and the colonic infestation improved the response rates. Eventually, the development of systemic amebicidal agents coupled with closed aspiration became the treatment of choice for amebic abscesses, with the majority of patients cured. Today, most amebic liver abscesses are managed successfully with amebicidal agents alone, with interventional procedures directed at the abscess itself reserved for resistant or complicated cases.

ETIOLOGY

Of the many species of ameba, only *Entamoeba histolytica* is pathogenic in man. As definitive hosts, asymptomatic individuals shed trophozoites and cysts in their stool. Infection with the organism usually occurs after ingestion of contaminated water or vegetables, although sexual transmission of the parasite also may occur. Cysts are the infective form of amebic disease, surviving in feces, soil, and even chlorinated water supplies. After ingestion of the cysts, the small intestine digests the cyst wall, releasing immature trophozoites. Adult trophozoites reside in the large intestine, predominantly in the cecum. Most trophozoites are small and noninvasive, and infected individuals may be asymptomatic or proceed to develop amebic dysentery. However, certain strains of *E histolytica* can invade the colonic wall. These strains are manifested by large trophozoites that, under light microscopy, appear to ingest red blood cells and polymorphonucleocytes. Host resistance also may play a role in the development of invasive amebiasis, since invasive disease occurs more commonly in immunosuppressed patients.

Locally invasive amebiasis can cause colonic hemorrhage, perforation, and fistula formation. In some cases, an inflammatory mass known as an ameboma may arise within the cecum, and appendicitis also may develop as a result of parasitic obstruction of the appendiceal lumen. Distant sites of invasive amebic infection include the lung, brain, and, most commonly, the liver. This wide distribution of target tissues suggests that ameba may invade other organs either by local extension or by gaining access to the circulatory system. Liver abscesses have been hypothesized to arise from invasion of the portal venous system, mesenteric lymphatic channels, or by intraperitoneal spread of microorganisms. Once within the liver parenchyma, microscopic sites of thrombosis, cytolysis, and liquefaction develop, a process termed amebic hepatitis. If these sites coalesce, an amebic abscess is formed.

The generation of amebic liver abscesses appears to require a deficit in cell-mediated immunity. Lymphocytes cytotoxic to amebic parasites have been isolated from patients who have recovered from liver infestation. Evaluation of individuals recently acquiring invasive amebiasis reveals that these lymphocytes decrease in number during the first 2 weeks of infection.[28] In animal infection models, experimentally induced deficits in cell-mediated immunity such as splenectomy, thymectomy, and administration of macrophage or lymphocyte antisera all result in greater numbers of amebic liver abscesses in treated animals when compared to control groups.

INCIDENCE

The incidence of amebiasis and amebic liver abscesses has remained stable in the tropical and subtropical areas of the globe, where the disease is often endemic. In contrast, the overall incidence of amebic disease is decreasing in the Western world. In the United States, amebic hepatic abscesses occur in 0.0013% of hospital inpatients and constitute only 5% of all liver abscesses. However, even within developed nations, amebiasis and amebic abscesses may develop more frequently in specific regions and in certain subpopulations (Table 51–6). The southern portions of the United States continue to report an equal incidence of pyogenic and amebic liver abscesses, and amebic abscesses actually may

TABLE 51–6. POPULATIONS WITH INCREASED INCIDENCE OF AMEBIC LIVER ABSCESS IN THE UNITED STATES

Southern United States
American Indians
Lower socioeconomic strata
Military personnel
Immigrants from endemic areas
Travelers to endemic areas
Homosexual men

predominate in cities with high immigrant populations. Amebic liver abscesses occur more commonly in individuals from lower socioeconomic strata, probably because of poor sanitation. Other high-risk groups include institutionalized patients, military personnel, American Indians living on reservations, and immigrants from and travelers to such endemic areas as Mexico, Central America, and Southeast Asia. Nationwide, less than 1% of individuals living in the United States have amebic infestation of the colon, compared to 15% to 30% of persons inhabiting endemic areas of the world.[29] Fortunately, only 7% of patients with amebiasis develop hepatic abscesses, with children being at a higher risk for developing this complication. Although amebiasis occurs frequently in homosexual men, the organisms involved are less virulent, and hepatic abscesses develop in a disproportionately lower number of these individuals.

Unlike pyogenic abscesses, the age and gender distributions of amebic liver abscesses have remained constant throughout the 20th century. Amebic liver abscesses occur most frequently during the third and fourth decades of life. Although men and women develop amebic dysentery in equal numbers, 90% of amebic hepatic abscesses develop in men. These gender differences may be the result of differences in iron availability and storage.[30] Invasive amebiasis appears to be somewhat dependent on the availability of free iron. Therefore, since many women in the third and fourth decade of life have chronic depletion of iron stores owing to menstruation, they may be at a decreased risk of developing an amebic liver abscess. Moreover, a greater incidence of invasive disease also is seen in individuals receiving exogenous iron supplementation.

PATHOLOGY

The structure of an amebic liver abscess consists of a fluid interior, an inner wall, and a connective tissue capsule. Classically, abscess fluid resembles "anchovy paste" and is reddish-brown in color, a result of digested liver tissue and red blood cells. Abscesses also may contain green or yellow fluid. Unlike bacterial abscesses, amebic abscess fluid is typically sterile and odorless. The evaluation of abscess fluid for various cell counts and enzymatic levels is generally unhelpful in diagnosing an amebic etiology. The inner abscess wall is an ill-defined layer of necrotic liver tissue and viable trophozoites. Consequently, a biopsy of this layer often can confirm the diagnosis of an amebic liver infestation. In larger, older abscesses, a surrounding connective tissue capsule created by host fibroblasts develops. In contrast to pyogenic abscesses, leukocytes and other inflammatory cells are absent from the capsule of an amebic liver abscess.

Compared to pyogenic abscesses, amebic liver abscesses more often are located in the right lobe of the liver and are often superficial and solitary. Current data reveal involvement of the right hepatic lobe in 70% to 90% of cases. As with pyogenic liver abscesses, preferential portal blood flow to the right side of the liver may account for the greater number of amebic abscesses occurring in this area. The left hepatic lobe is involved in 13% of patients. Amebic abscesses usually grow from within the liver and by the time of diagnosis commonly about the liver capsule, which serves as a barrier to their growth. This superficial location explains the propensity for amebic abscesses to rupture or extend to contiguous structures. Over 85% of amebic liver abscesses are solitary. This trend has been hypothesized to result from early coalescence of multiple, microscopic infectious sites. Amebic abscesses vary in size from 1 to 25 cm in diameter, with growth continuing in an uninterrupted fashion by active necrosis of surrounding liver tissue. Thus, an untreated abscess invariably will rupture.

DIAGNOSIS

Because amebic liver abscesses require less invasive treatment, discriminating them from pyogenic abscesses is vital. Both processes may have similar clinical presentations and standard laboratory findings. Although a careful history, including epidemiological data, as well as certain radiologic findings, may suggest an amebic liver abscess as the likely diagnosis (Table 51–7), serology is the cornerstone for differentiating between the two diseases.

Clinical Presentation

Acute presentations are more common with amebic liver abscesses than with their pyogenic counterparts, although indolent cases can occur. Rarely, an individual with a ruptured amebic abscess may present in shock. Most adult patients have symptoms similar to, but more severe than, pyogenic abscesses (Table 51–8). However, several symptoms and signs exist that clinically may dif-

TABLE 51–7. DISTINGUISHING CLINICAL CHARACTERISTICS IN PATIENTS WITH HEPATIC ABSCESS

Amebic	Pyogenic
Age <50 years	Age >50 years
Male:Female=10:1	Males=Females
Hispanic descent	No ethnic predisposition
Recent travel to endemic area	Malignancy
Pulmonary dysfunction	High fevers
Abdominal pain	Pruritus
Diarrhea	Jaundice
Abdominal tenderness	Septic shock
Hepatomegaly	Palpable mass

TABLE 51–8. CLINICAL MANIFESTATIONS OF AMEBIC LIVER ABSCESSES IN ADULT PATIENTS

	% Amebic Abscesses
SYMPTOM	
Pain	90
Fever	87
Nausea and vomiting	85
Anorexia	50
Weight loss	45
Malaise	25
Diarrhea	25
Cough, pleurisy	25
Pruritis	<1
SIGN	
Hepatomegaly	85
Right upper quadrant tenderness	84
Pleural effusion, rub	40
Right upper quadrant mass	12
Ascites	10
Jaundice	5
LABORATORY	
Increased alkaline phosphatase	80
WBC >10 000/mm^3	70
Hematocrit <36%	49
Albumin <3g/dL	44
Bilirubin >2 g/dL	10

ferentiate amebic from pyogenic liver abscesses.[31,32] Patients with amebic liver abscesses frequently will report a history of antecedent diarrhea. Presentations with severe pain, pulmonary symptoms, and hepatomegaly are also more common with amebic liver abscesses than with pyogenic abscesses. Fevers and jaundice occur less frequently in amebic disease than in bacterial infections. In contrast to adult patients, children with amebic hepatic abscesses usually have more indolent presentations and fewer symptoms.

Laboratory Evaluation

In contrast to the often dramatic clinical presentation, many patients with amebic liver abscesses have only mild alterations in laboratory parameters. As with pyogenic liver abscesses, leukocytosis occurs in 70% of patients, whereas anemia is found approximately 50% of the time. Although the SGOT and serum bilirubin correlate with acuity, morbidity, and mortality in amebic abscesses, liver function test abnormalities are less common and less severe than in pyogenic abscesses. Hyperbilirubinemia, for example, is found in only 10% of patients with amebic liver abscesses, even when the abscess cavity is large. Because amebic abscesses involve active destruction of liver parenchyma, and are often larger on presentation than pyogenic liver abscesses, elevations in the plasma prothrombin time may develop. Stool analy-

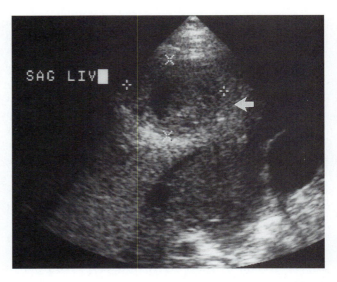

A

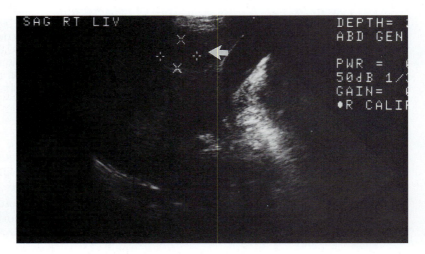

Figure 51–10. A. Sagittal abdominal ultrasound of an amebic abscess located in the right hepatic lobe demonstrating a complex, predominantly cystic fluid collection (*arrow*). **B**. Follow-up ultrasound after 2 weeks of treatment with metronidazole revealing a decrease in the size of the abscess (*arrow*).

B

sis, even when the sample is obtained with a proctoscope, is an unreliable method for diagnosing amebic infestation. Stool cysts and trophozoites are identified in only 15% to 50% of patients with amebic liver abscesses, because the colonic infection often has resolved by the time the patient presents with a hepatic abscess.

Radiology

Amebic liver abscesses are usually solitary and large, and unlike pyogenic abscesses, concurrent intra-abdominal pathology rarely exists. Ultrasound has a sensitivity equal to CT in identifying amebic liver lesions, and the lower cost and the absence of ionizing radiation theoretically make ultrasound the imaging modality of choice for diagnosing amebic liver disease. However, since radiologic scans often are obtained prior to sero-

logical data and a definitive diagnosis, CT remains an important radiologic tool in the work-up of amebic liver abscesses.

Ultrasonography detects 90% to 95% of amebic liver abscesses, and several sonographic criteria actually may allow preliminary differentiation of amebic from pyogenic abscesses (Fig 51–10). Boultbee and Ralls described sonographic characteristics typical of an amebic abscess, including cyst homogeneity, decreased internal echoes, and a smooth wall.[33,34] Unfortunately, these properties are found in only 40% of amebic abscesses. The sensitivity of CT in diagnosing amebic hepatic abscesses approaches 100% (Fig 51–11). CT characteristics also can differentiate abscesses from necrotic tumors and echinococcal cysts. Presently, CT should be performed on those patients in whom a potential diag-

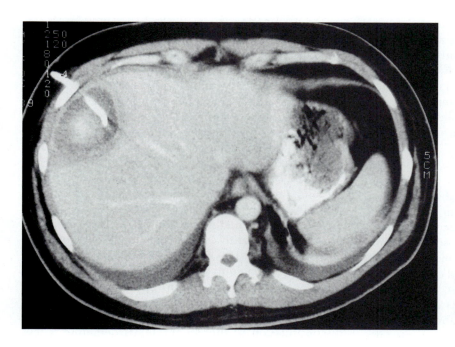

Figure 51–11. CT of an amebic abscess in the right hepatic lobe demonstrating a complex cystic mass in the typical peripheral location with peripheral rim enhancement. Percutaneous drainage of this abscess was performed owing to concerns for secondary infection.

nosis of pyogenic liver abscess remains, or when positive amebic serologies exist but a hepatic sonogram is negative. Although there are no criteria that differentiate amebic from pyogenic liver abscesses by CT, an acceptable preliminary diagnosis often can be obtained, based on the size and location of the lesion within the liver parenchyma, as well as the patient presentation. Experience with MRI of amebic liver abscesses is limited. It would appear that MRI is quite sensitive at detecting amebic abscesses and may visualize early responses to therapy; however, the cost is higher compared to ultrasound and CT. Nuclear medicine liver scans may demonstrate a nonspecific hepatic filling defect in 90% of amebic abscesses, but ultrasound and CT have largely supplanted their use. Reports differentiating amebic from pyogenic liver abscesses by combined technetium and indium scans exist[35] but, with modern serological testing, this technique saves little time and adds additional cost to the treatment of the patient. Plain films of the chest are abnormal in two-thirds of patients with an amebic liver abscess, reflecting the increased frequency of pulmonary complications associated with this disease. Chest radiographs commonly reveal a pleural effusion, pulmonary infiltrate, or elevated hemidiaphragm.

Serology

Differentiating pyogenic from amebic liver abscesses is often impossible using clinical criteria, routine laboratory tests, and radiologic scans. Therefore, serological procedures are necessary to confirm the presence of amebic disease. Serological studies should be obtained

as soon as the diagnosis of a liver abscess is entertained. Currently available serological tests include indirect hemagglutination (IHA), gel diffusion precipitin (GDP), the enzyme-linked immunosorbent assay (ELISA), counterimmunelectrophoresis, indirect immunofluorescence, and complement fixation. Currently, IHA and GDP are the most frequently used procedures. Both tests are readily available at most hospitals, and results are often available to the physician within 24 hours. IHA is considered positive if dilutions exceed 1:128, which occurs in 95% of patients with an amebic liver abscess. The sensitivity may reach 100% if the test is repeated. IHA is also highly specific for invasive amebic disease. However, positive results may occur up to 20 years after the infection resolves. Furthermore, 5% of asymptomatic, noninfected, Hispanic males have positive IHA titers. GDP, although also capable of detecting approximately 95% of amebic hepatic abscesses, detects patients with noninvasive amebic colitis as well. Thus, this test is sensitive but not specific for amebic liver disease. Nevertheless, GDP is inexpensive, simple to perform, and rarely remains positive 6 months after abscess resolution. Therefore, in the setting of a space-occupying lesion within the liver on radiologic scan, GDP is quite helpful in confirming an amebic origin to the pathology.

ELISA, counterimmunelectrophoresis, and indirect immunofluorescence are also very sensitive and rapid procedures for diagnosing invasive amebic disease. Furthermore, the results of these tests often are obtainable within several hours. However, the availability of these tests is not as widespread as IHA or GDP, and their cost is often greater. Further development of rapid, inexpensive ELISA procedures is underway, and these tests, in kit form, may replace the IHA and GDP in the future. Complement fixation procedures, the first serologic tests developed for diagnosing invasive amebiasis, remain difficult to perform and are less sensitive than the aforementioned studies. Therefore, they are rarely used at the present time.

Diagnostic Aspiration

The need to aspirate a suspected amebic abscess for diagnosis is questionable, as serological data are usually available after 1 or 2 days. Most diagnostic aspirations are performed to rule out pyogenic liver abscesses when amebic serologies are negative. With amebic abscesses, the aspirate is odorless and gram stain and cultures are negative. Recovery of amebic organisms occurs in 33% to 90% of aspirates. The addition of wall scrapings, containing viable trophozoites, can increase the sensitivity of aspiration. Diagnostic aspiration is contraindicated if a hepatic neoplasm or echinococcal cyst is suspected, since the malignancy may spread along the aspiration tract, and systemic or peritoneal exposure to hydatid cyst fluid may result in fatal anaphylactic shock.

TREATMENT

With the introduction of metronidazole in the 1960s, surgical drainage of most amebic liver abscesses has become unnecessary. The majority of amebic liver abscesses are now successfully treated with metronidazole alone. Aspiration, or percutaneous or surgical drainage, remain valuable when the diagnosis of an amebic liver abscess is questionable or if complications arise. When successfully treated, amebic abscesses rarely recur.

Antibiotics

Imidazole antibiotics, including metronidazole, tinidazole, and niridazole, will eradicate both intestinal and hepatic amebic organisms. An oral course of metronidazole, 750 mg, 3 times a day for 10 days, cures approximately 95% of patients with amebic liver abscesses.[36] Metronidazole is equally effective when delivered intravenously, which may be necessary in the nauseated or critically ill patient. A positive response to empirically administered metronidazole may confirm the diagnosis of an amebic liver abscess. Symptomatic improvement occurs within days, and imaging studies reveal a decrease in abscess size within 7 to 10 days. Metronidazole is inexpensive and safe, although the drug is contraindicated during pregnancy. Minor side effects include nausea, a metallic taste, and intolerance to alcoholic beverages. Major neurological effects, such as peripheral neuropathies, rarely occur. Patients unre-

sponsive to imidazole antibiotics may have resistant amebic organisms or an undiagnosed bacterial infection, and further interventions such as multidrug therapy or diagnostic aspiration often prove helpful.

Emetine, dehydroemetine, and chloroquine are useful for complicated amebic liver abscesses or when metronidazole therapy fails. Because these drugs eliminate invasive organisms only, simultaneous administration of an intestinal amebicidal agent is necessary. Continuation of metronidazole usually fulfills this role, although diiodohydroxyquin, iodoquinol, diloxanide furoate, carbarsone, and tetracycline are effective as well. Unlike the imidazoles, emetine and its structural analog, dehydroemetine, require intramuscular administration. Importantly, emetine has a rather narrow therapeutic range, producing a proarrhythmic, cardiotoxic effect that is related to the cumulative dose of the drug. Bed rest and frequent monitoring of vital signs are necessary for patients receiving this drug, and development of an arrhythmia warrants critical care supervision and discontinuation of the agent. Dehydroemetine is less toxic than emetine and therefore, rarely requires such labor-intensive management. However, dehydroemetine is a less potent compound and requires longer periods of administration to effect a cure. Emetine and dehydroemetine are indicated primarily when patients develop pulmonary complications from amebic liver abscesses, as these individuals are usually quite ill and require multidrug therapy for rapid symptom resolution. Fortunately, lower, less toxic doses of these compounds are effective if given concurrently with metronidazole.

Chloroquine is an orally administered compound. Successful treatment of an amebic liver abscess requires a prolonged course of therapy, typically lasting 4 to 6 weeks. Although it produces fewer side effects than emetine or dehydroemetine, chloroquine is also less potent than these agents and relapses occur frequently when it is used alone. Currently, chloroquine is administered in combination with low-dose emetine for metronidazole-resistant amebic strains. Together, combined administration of chloroquine and emetine cures 90% to 100% of patients with resistant extracolonic amebic disease.

Therapeutic Aspiration

With the wide availability of serological tests, diagnostic aspirations of amebic liver abscesses are performed infrequently. Certain indications remain, however, for therapeutic aspiration.[36] Patients receiving systemic amebicidal agents, yet with symptoms persisting for greater than 72 hours after drug initiation, appear to benefit from aspiration of the abscess cavity. Aspiration in this setting is useful as it not only relieves pressure symptoms, but also rules out secondary bacterial infection of the amebic abscess. In addition, aspiration decreases the risk of rupture in abscesses greater than

250 mL in volume, those located in the left hepatic lobe, or lesions associated with marked tenderness and diaphragmatic elevation. Aspiration also appears valuable when metronidazole therapy is contraindicated, such as during pregnancy. Both prospective and retrospective studies confirm that routine aspiration of amebic liver abscesses does not affect disease resolution time.[38,39] Furthermore, several recent studies have confirmed an increase in secondary bacterial infection rates when amebic abscesses are aspirated routinely.

Percutaneous Drainage

Percutaneous drainage of amebic liver abscesses has been extensively reported in the medical literature, and good results usually are obtained with this approach (Fig 51–11).[40] Similar to aspiration, however, routine percutaneous drainage of amebic liver abscesses is seldom necessary, since neither interventional procedure has a cure rate greater than that obtained with amebicidal agents alone. Percutaneous drainage remains most useful for the management of pulmonary, peritoneal, and pericardial complications, since catheter drainage often eliminates the need for operative intervention. The high viscosity of amebic abscess fluid requires a large diameter catheter for adequate drainage, which can be quite bothersome to the patient unless proper drain care is undertaken and analgesics prescribed. Secondary infection of the cavity following percutaneous drainage procedures also occurs.

Surgical Drainage

The surgical treatment of amebic liver abscesses has largely been replaced by antibiotic therapy. Furthermore, the majority of complications of amebic liver abscesses can be successfully managed by either aspiration or percutaneous drainage. Presently, the most common indication for surgery is in the management of abscesses that have failed to respond to more conservative therapy. Laparotomy also is indicated in the rare event of life-threatening hemorrhage, with or without concomitant abscess rupture. Operative intervention is also mandatory when an amebic abscess erodes into a neighboring viscus, as partial resection and closure of the involved organ is necessary. Finally, patients with septicemia from secondarily infected amebic abscesses are candidates for surgical management, particularly if percutaneous decompression attempts are unsuccessful. As with pyogenic liver abscesses, limited experience is available concerning laparoscopic evaluation and treatment of patients with amebic liver abscesses. Laparoscopy has been forwarded as a possible means of assessment after intraperitoneal amebic abscess rupture. During this procedure, percutaneous catheters placed under laparoscopic guidance may successfully drain the amebic phlegmon and prevent the need for a formal laparotomy.[41]

COMPLICATIONS

Approximately 10% of individuals with amebic liver abscesses will develop complications. As with pyogenic abscesses, mortality rates are increased for these patients. Fortunately, the majority of complications from amebic abscesses are not fatal and often can be managed nonoperatively. The most common complication is rupture of the abscess into the peritoneum or the thorax (Fig 51–12). Abscesses also may erode into other contiguous organs or become infected secondarily with bacteria. Rarely, hemobilia and hepatic replacement with subsequent liver failure can occur as the result of the erosive growth of the amebic liver abscess.

The pleuropulmonary system is the most frequent site affected when an amebic hepatic abscess ruptures. Typically, such cases originate from lesions located in the right hepatic lobe. The abscess perforates the diaphragm, and patients may subsequently develop a pleural effusion, empyema, pulmonary abscess, or pneumonia. Bronchopleural, biliopleural, and biliobronchial fistulas also may arise from ruptured amebic abscesses. Patients with these fistulas may present with expectoration of chocolate-colored sputum containing viable amebas. Most pleuropulmonary complications respond to antibiotics and postural drainage alone. Pa-

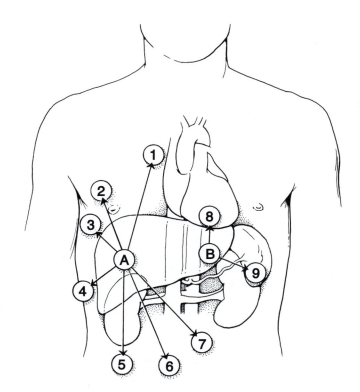

Figure 51–12. Paths of extension of amebic liver abscesses located within the right hepatic lobe (A) and the left hepatic lobe (B). **Right Lobe Abscess (A)** 1. Tracheo-bronchial 2. Pulmonary 3. Pleural/Subphrenic 4. Cutaneous 5. Free Intraperitoneal 6. Mesenteric 7. Enteric **Left Lobe Abscess (B)** 8. Pericardial 9. Splenic

tients with amebic empyemas, however, frequently develop severe dyspnea and hemithoracic opacification, and will require multidrug therapy, tube thoracostomy, and often thoracotomy with decortication.[42] Thoracotomy may also be necessary in patients with nonhealing biliobronchial fistulas.

Thirty percent of amebic abscess complications involve peritoneal contamination, commonly from a right hepatic abscess. Although most intraperitoneal ruptures are contained within the right upper quadrant, the mortality rate for these patients may approach 20%, despite aggressive management. Occasionally, amebic liver abscesses erode through the abdominal wall or into the intestinal tract. The treatment of amebic intraperitoneal rupture is controversial. Certain authors recommend systemic antibiotic therapy alone, while others advocate percutaneous drainage of the amebic phlegmon.[40,43] Patients with a coexisting life-threatening hemorrhage or who fail conservative treatment, however, require laparotomy, abscess drainage, and amebicidal irrigation. Systemic amebicidal therapy is the initial treatment for hepatocutaneous fistulas, while erosions into the bowel mandate the addition of broad-spectrum antibacterial agents and prompt surgical exploration.

In less than 2% of patients, a left hepatic abscess may rupture into the pericardium. This complication is catastrophic, with mortality rates ranging from 30% to 73%. Most patients will present with indolent congestive heart failure, although fulminant cardiovascular collapse may occur also. Rarely, hepatic symptoms resulting from venous congestion predominate. The management of amebic pericardial disease is nonoperative, with lower mortality rates reported with treatment by needle aspiration and systemic amebicidal agents rather than an open drainage procedure.[44]

PROGNOSIS

Unlike pyogenic abscesses, the mortality rates for individuals with amebic liver abscesses have been historically low (Fig 51–9). In Ochsner's 1935 report, 9% of patients with amebic abscesses died of their disease.[45] Currently, this number is <4%. Furthermore, patients with amebic liver abscesses have similar outcomes despite different treatment strategies. Investigators evaluating treatment with antibiotics alone, antibiotics coupled with needle aspiration, and antibiotics and open drainage all have reported similar mortality rates of 2% to 3%.[42,46,47] Several clinical factors have been associated with a worse prognosis in patients with amebic liver abscesses[48] (Table 51–9). Increased age, delayed presentation, and complications such as intrapericardial rupture or extensive pulmonary involvement more than triple mortality rates. Hyperbilirubinemia is also a risk factor, with rupture occurring more frequently in jaundiced patients. Nevertheless, the majority of patients with amebic liver abscesses, with or without complications, respond favorably to medical management and survive their disease.

TABLE 51–9. FACTORS ASSOCIATED WITH POOR PROGNOSIS IN PATIENTS WITH AMEBIC LIVER ABSCESSES

↑Age
↑Bilirubin
Pulmonary involvement
Rupture or extension
Late presentation

■ HYDATID LIVER CYSTS

Hydatidosis, also known as echinococcosis, is a parasitic infection of the liver and other organs by the flatworm, echinococcus. *Echinococcis granulosus* is the causative organism in classic hydatid cysts, while infection with *Echinococcis multilocularis* results in alveolar hydatid disease, a more aggressive, less localized affliction. Hydatid disease has a worldwide distribution and has been recognized since ancient times. Presently, infection with echinococcal organisms is the most common cause of liver cysts in the world. Hydatid cysts are characterized by indolent yet unremittent growth in the majority of infected patients, with the potential for cyst metastases to the peritoneal surface or lung. Thus, despite its benign, infectious etiology, hydatid cysts may exhibit malignant behavior. Unlike pyogenic and amebic liver abscesses, the treatment of hydatid cysts of the liver has remained primarily surgical, with medical or percutaneous management assuming an adjuvant role.

ETIOLOGY

Echinococcal parasites are members of the order Cestoda (flatworms) and the family *Taenia*. The propensity for these organisms to cause infection in pastoral and other rural settings is best explained by their life cycle (Fig 51–13). The adult form of echinococcus is a 5 mm long, hermaphroditic tapeworm which infests the small intestine of carnivorous animals, typically dogs, foxes, coyotes, and in the case of *E. multilocularis,* small rodents. Eggs are shed in the feces of these animals and are incidentally consumed by grazing animals such as cows, sheep, buffalo, zebras, moose, and caribou. In the duodenum, enzymatic digestion of the eggshell releases embryonic forms of the organism, which then pass through the mucosa of the small intestine and enter the portal circulation. Once filtered by the liver or lung, the embryo transforms into a microscopic, larval

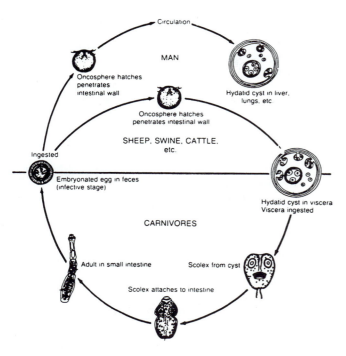

Figure 51–13. Life cycle of Echinococcus granulosus. (From McGreevy PB, Nelson GS. Larval cestode infections. In: Strickland GT (ed), *Hunter's Tropical Medicine.* Toronto, Canada: WB Saunders; 1984:771)

stage, the protoscolex or scolex, which is capable of multiplying asexually within the affected organ. When the host animal dies or is slaughtered, ingestion of organs infested with larva completes the life cycle, and the larva mature into adult parasites within the small intestine of the carnivore.

Man is an accidental, intermediate host in the echinococcal life cycle, as infection of human beings represents a terminal event for the parasite. Typically, man is exposed to the organism by ingestion of contaminated vegetables or meat, which cannot be washed or scrubbed free of eggs. Infection also may occur when playing with dogs harboring the tapeworm, as eggs cling to their fur. This is the most common means by which children acquire the disease. The larval form of echinococcus can invade any organ system, and the distribution of infection is limited only by bloodflow and filtration. Thus, hydatid cysts can occur in the liver, spleen, lungs, brain, muscle, and even bone. In humans, approximately 65% to 75% of hydatid cysts occur in the liver, 25% are found in the lungs, and 5% to 10% distribute along the peripheral arterial system.[49]

INCIDENCE

Hydatid cysts occur throughout the world, but are endemic in pastoral and farming regions of the Mediterranean, Eastern Europe, the Middle East, South Amer-

ica, Australia, and South Africa. Alveolar hydatid disease is limited to the Northern hemisphere and endemic in Alaska and portions of Canada. With both forms of hydatid infection, the treatment of infected patients has a major impact on the health care economy of the endemic area. In Western Europe and the United States, echinococcal cysts are rare. Currently, the incidence of hydatid liver cysts in the United States is approximately 200 cases per year, with an increased frequency in immigrant populations. Hydatid liver disease afflicts all age groups and both sexes with equal frequency, and there are no predisposing pathological conditions associated with infection. The incidence of hydatid cysts has decreased in endemic areas when public health measures and proper livestock handling procedures have been enacted. Public education about the disease and its transmission, including recommendations for vigorous handwashing after contact with canine species, elimination of vegetables grown at ground level from the diet, and discontinuation of the practice of feeding the entrails of slaughtered animals to dogs, has proven to be of value in decreasing the occurrence of hydatid cyst disease.

PATHOLOGY

Hydatid liver cysts expand slowly and asymptomatically and thus tend to be quite large at presentation. A single liver lesion is present in 75% of patients, with the right and left hepatic lobes affected in 80% and 20% of cases, respectively. Despite this singularity, half of these lesions contain daughter cysts and are multilocular in nature. Hydatid cysts typically are composed of a three-layered cyst wall surrounding a fluid cavity. The outer layer, known as the pericyst, is a thin, indistinct, host-derived layer of fibrous tissue present in hydatid cysts of the liver and spleen, but absent in cysts of the lung or brain. It represents an adventitial reaction to the parasitic infection. The pericyst provides mechanical support to the hydatid cyst and serves as the metabolic interface between the host and the parasite. As the cyst grows within the liver, bile ducts and blood vessels stretch and finally become incorporated within this structure, explaining the propensity for biliary and hemorrhagic complications of cyst growth or resection. With time, portions of the pericyst may calcify. Complete calcification of the pericyst interrupts the nutrient and oxygen supply to the parasites and thus represents the death of the hydatid cyst. It is unknown why this process occurs in only a minority of cysts.

The other layers of a hydatid cyst are derived from the parasite itself. A 1 to 2 mm thick layer of proteinaceous material known as the laminated membrane is found abutting the pericyst. Lining the inside of the laminated membrane is a single-cell layer termed the germinal membrane, which is the location of the actual parasites. The germinal membrane may remain as a uniform spherical structure, but it also may invaginate spontaneously or with trauma, forming daughter cysts. Aggregates of scolices termed brood capsules also are generated from the germinal membrane. These structures, like daughter cysts, have no pericyst of their own and float freely within the cyst fluid, appearing as fine, granular particles termed hydatid sand. Hydatid cyst fluid is secreted actively by the infecting parasites. Thus, a tense cyst wall indicates a living hydatid cyst, while a flaccid but intact wall is typical of an involuted, nonviable cyst. Fluid pressure within a living hydatid cyst can reach 70 cm of water, and explosive rupture of a cyst can occur if it is subjected to trauma or unnecessary manipulation. Typically, hydatid cyst fluid is thick, clear, and slightly alkaline. However, opaque fluid may be obtained from dead cysts as well as those secondarily infected with bacteria. Bile-stained fluid may occur as a result of cyst erosion into an intrahepatic bile duct.

The alveolar cysts resulting from infection with *E multilocularis* are atypical from other hydatid cysts, being smaller, thin walled, and lacking a definitive capsule. These cysts appear as a spongy or jelly-like mass, often at the liver hilum. Because of the poor delineation of individual cysts, the mass often extends and branches within the liver parenchyma in a fashion not unlike a malignant disease. As opposed to the incorporation of hepatic structures within an expansatile cyst wall, alveolar hydatid disease causes liver pathology by a simple space-occupying process or by local encasement or invasion of vascular, lymphatic, and biliary structures. In addition, the high fluid pressure found in classic hydatid cysts is absent from alveolar cysts, since the wall structure is insufficiently strong to support such a force.

DIAGNOSIS

A primary diagnosis of hydatid liver pathology is quite uncommon in Western nations due to the rarity of the disease and the indolent and often asymptomatic nature of the affliction. Often, hydatid cysts are discovered incidentally during a diagnostic work-up for an unrelated complaint. Nevertheless, a thoughtful history and thorough physical examination prove quite useful in diagnosing the disease. When evaluating a patient with a liver mass, a history, even remote, of travel to or immigration from a region in which the disease is endemic warrants suspicion of echinococcal infestation. The majority of symptoms, signs, and laboratory tests are nonspecific for hydatid cysts. Fortunately, a unique appearance on radiologic scan often verifies the existence of hydatid liver disease, and serological tests also can confirm the diagnosis.

TABLE 51–10. CLINICAL MANIFESTATIONS OF HYDATID LIVER CYSTS

	% Hydatid Cysts
ASYMPTOMATIC	75
Symptoms	25
Abdominal pain	(79)
Dyspepsia	(50)
Fever and chills	(30)
Jaundice	(25)
Arthritis	(5)
SIGNS	
Right upper quadrant mass	70
Right upper quadrant tenderness	20
LABORATORY	
Eosinophilia	35
Bilirubin >2 mg/dL	20
WBC <10 000/mm^3	10

Clinical Presentation

Hydatid cysts have slow growth rates and rarely cause systemic symptoms. Thus, the majority of patients with hydatid liver disease have indolent presentations and are otherwise healthy. Approximately 75% of cases present as an asymptomatic abdominal mass or a suspicious calcification on a routine chest x-ray. The cyst is usually quite large (>5 cm) when symptoms do occur. Symptomatic patients most commonly complain of mild to moderate right upper quadrant pain or dyspepsia, and a firm hepatic mass can often be palpated (Table 51–10). However, acute, severe abdominal pain does occasionally occur and usually indicates rupture, biliary complications, or secondary bacterial infection. Rupture and extrusion of cyst contents into the biliary tree may result in extrahepatic biliary obstruction and subsequent cholangitis, with resultant fevers, chills, and jaundice. Urticaria is an uncommon finding in echinococcal disease. However, a fall or other patient trauma may cause limited leakage of cyst contents, and a resulting allergic reaction to the cyst fluid may ensue. Thus, urticaria in the setting of recent trauma can be quite diagnostic for hydatidosis, particularly if the individual has travelled from an area with endemic hydatid disease. Rarely, patients with hydatid liver cysts develop polyarthritis secondary to increased levels of circulating IgE and immune complexes. Bronchobilia is also an uncommon presentation.

Laboratory Evaluation

As with pyogenic and amebic liver abscesses, laboratory evaluation of patients with hydatid liver disease often yields nonspecific data. Because the disease is localized in the majority of patients, the white blood count is usually within normal limits, although it may be elevated if the cyst has become secondarily infected. Similarly, liver function tests, which are typically normal or mildly elevated in uncomplicated cases, may become quite abnormal if involvement of the biliary tree occurs. Eosinophilia (>3%) occurs in 25% to 45% of patients with hydatid cysts in Western countries, but is a nonspecific finding in endemic areas.[50] Serum immunoglobulin levels also may be abnormal in patients with hydatid liver cysts. Elevated IgE levels are a nonspecific indicator of prior sensitization or active infection with parasitic organisms, while elevation of IgM classes specific to echinococcal organisms may be a sensitive indicator for recurrent disease.

Serology

Several serological tests are available that are specific to hydatid disease, and they are often necessary to confirm the diagnosis. Because hydatid cysts often are localized infections, however, the absence of a positive echinococcal serology does not rule out the disease. Serum immunoelectrophoresis is currently the most reliable procedure, detecting approximately 90% of individuals infected with *E granulosus*. This test remains positive for 1 year after eradication of the organism. The indirect hemagglutination test has a sensitivity of 85%, yet remains positive for several years, decreasing its usefulness in endemic areas. Complement fixation procedures have an estimated sensitivity of 70%, but revert to negative after only 6 months. ELISA appear to be quite sensitive for detecting echinococcal infection, and the low cost and ability to automate the procedures are distinct advantages. Serological tests for *E multilocularis* are typically not as sensitive or specific as for *E granulosus*. However, excellent preliminary results have been obtained with Western Blot analysis.[51]

The Casoni skin test has been used extensively in the past to evaluate patients for echinococcal infection. The skin test consists of a subcutaneous injection of sterilized hydatid cyst fluid, and patients sensitized to echinococcal antigens develop a wheal and flare reaction at the injection site. The Casoni skin test has a sensitivity and specificity of 80% and 70%, respectively, but may remain positive for years after the initial hydatid cyst has been eradicated. False-positive results occur frequently owing to poor standardization of the protein antigens within the test kits. Furthermore, the test may actually sensitize the patient to echinococcal antigens and cause anaphylaxis in those individuals with high levels of circulating echinococcal IgE. These disadvantages, coupled with the development of alternative serological tests, have limited the usefulness of Casoni skin testing.

Radiology

Radiologic evaluation of patients with hydatid liver disease is the cornerstone of diagnosis. Indeed, the asymptomatic patient often is diagnosed with a hydatid cyst only after an abnormality is detected on x-rays or scans performed for unrelated purposes. Distinct calcifications in the right upper quadrant are visualized by plain films in over 50% of patients with hydatid liver cysts. Abdominal plain films reveal no other pathology. Plain films of the chest, however, are quite helpful as they may not only detect calcifications within the liver, but also may reveal concurrent hydatid cysts of the lung or involvement with the pleural space. As with pyogenic and amebic abscesses of the liver, ultrasound and CT are both excellent imaging modalities for hydatid cysts. These procedures can identify daughter cysts and hydatid sand, both of which are specific to echinococcal infestation. Ultrasound detects approximately 90% of hydatid liver cysts (Fig 51–14). Sonography is cost-effective in endemic areas and when the diagnosis of hydatidosis is quite certain. However, ultrasound is less accurate than CT in localizing and delineating the extent of the cyst. The sensitivity of CT in detecting hydatid liver cysts approaches 100% (Fig 51–15). CT is useful when the diagnosis of hydatid disease is uncertain or when complications such as cyst rupture or infection are suspected, since differentiation between these complicated cysts and amebic or pyogenic abscesses is often difficult. Liver radionucleotide scans are seldom used to diagnose hydatid cysts.

If a complication involving the biliary tree is suspected, ERC or PTC should be performed, although ERC results in less complications when the cyst is very large. Cholangiography allows delineation of biliary connections within the hydatid cyst wall, the presence of which may alter the operative management of the cyst (Fig 51–16). These procedures are particularly useful in the jaundiced patient, since visualization of the common bile duct allows differentiation of obstructive jaundice from nonobstructive cholangitis. If the common duct indeed is obstructed with hydatid material on preoperative cholangiography, an endoscopic sphincterotomy may clear the duct of debris and eliminate the need for an intraoperative common bile duct exploration and/or open sphincterotomy.[52]

TREATMENT

Surgery remains the treatment of choice for the majority of individuals infected with *E granulosus* and is presently the only available treatment for alveolar hydatid disease. However, considerable controversy exists as to the extent of operation performed. Advances in medical management of hydatidosis with newer antihelminthic medications have been made, and limited experience with percutaneous aspiration and drainage of hydatid cysts has been reported. Despite these advances, however, medical and percutaneous management of hy-

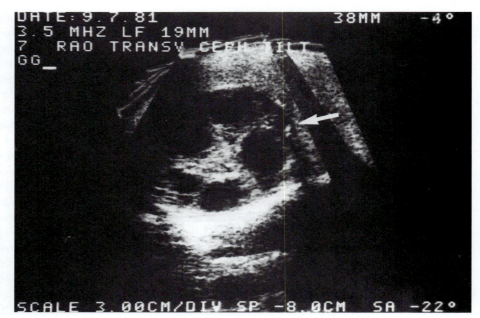

Figure 51–14. Transverse abdominal ultrasound of the right hepatic lobe revealing a large hydatid cyst (*arrow*) with internal reflections created by daughter cysts characteristic of echinococcal liver lesions. (From Kune, GA, Morris DL. Hydatid disease. In: Schwartz, SI, Ellis H (eds), *Maingot's Abdominal Operations*, 9th ed. Stamford, CT: Appleton and Lange; 1989:1231)

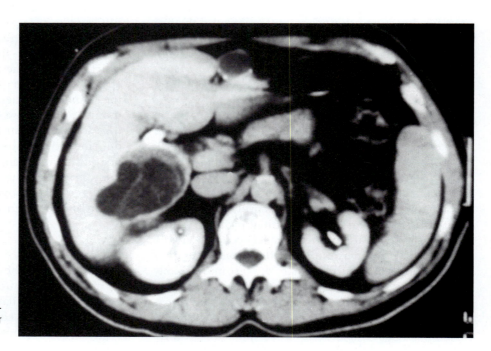

Figure 51–15. CT demonstrating a large, exophytic hydatid cyst with internal septations located in the inferior right hepatic lobe.

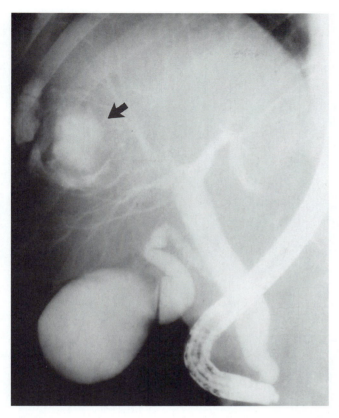

Figure 51-16. Endoscopic retrograde cholangiogram of a hydatid cyst in the right hepatic lobe revealing incorporation and communication of the biliary tree with the cyst cavity (*arrow*). The common bile duct is free of cyst debris.

datid liver cysts remain primarily adjuncts to surgical intervention. Fortunately, the majority of patients with echinococcal cysts are otherwise healthy and thus have low perioperative morbidity and mortality rates.

Antihelminthics

Presently, the use of antihelminthic medications complement surgical management but do not replace it, since poor results have been reported when hydatid liver cysts are managed with systemic antihelminthics alone. Most of these drugs are poorly absorbed from the gastrointestinal tract and are incapable of concentrating within the cyst cavity at levels necessary to kill the parasites. A newer class of antihelminthics, benzimidazolecarbamates, have produced higher response rates. Mebendazole and its structural analogues, albendazole and flubendazole, are orally administered benzimidazoles that require long-term dosing for positive effects to occur. These drugs have been used both systemically and locally, by percutaneous instillation, for attempted sterilization of hydatid cysts. Antihelminthics work best when given for small, unilocular hydatid cysts. Successful treatment of such cysts has been reported in 30% of

patients treated with mebendazole and 40% of those treated with albendazole.[53] The success rates are generally higher when treating pulmonary hydatid cysts with these medications. Antihelminthic treatment of hydatid disease secondary to *E multilocularis* is less successful than with classic hydatid cysts. Although the drug praziquantel occasionally may arrest the growth and metastases of *E multilocularis,* the prognosis for the majority of patients so treated remains poor. Current indications for systemic antihelminthic therapy include concurrent pulmonary or disseminated hydatid disease, multiple, recurrent, or inaccessible hydatid liver cysts, spontaneous intraperitoneal or intrathoracic rupture, accidental contamination of the peritoneum with cyst contents during operative cystectomy, and when the patient is unfit for a definitive surgical procedure. Mebendazole typically is administered at 60 mg/kg per day for 6 to 24 months. Its side effects include granulocytopenia, neurotoxicity, gastrointestinal ulcers, and hepatic dysfunction. Albendazole is dosed at 10 mg/kg per day for 6 months, and is associated with fewer and less severe side effects than mebendazole.

Percutaneous Aspiration and Drainage

Traditionally, the uncontrolled percutaneous aspiration of a hydatid liver cyst was absolutely contraindicated because of the perceived risk of intraperitoneal cyst rupture, parasitic spread, and subsequent anaphylaxis. Controversy presently exists, however, concerning the validity of this risk with modern percutaneous transhepatic aspiration techniques. Reports of successful management of hydatid liver cysts with percutaneous drainage are available on a limited number of patients, with the risk of inducing anaphylaxis or uncontrolled cyst rupture appearing to be quite low.[54,55] Hypertonic saline and other benign pharmacologic agents are used as scolicidal agents for these procedures, as traditional scolicides, including ethanol solutions and formalin, can cause cholangitis, peritonitis, or systemic toxicity, if they enter the bile ducts, peritoneum, or bloodsteam during percutaneous instillation. When percutaneous drainage is coupled with both local and systemic administration of albendazole, approximately 70% of patients have been cured of their disease. The number of patients treated in this fashion are quite small, however, and no controlled trials exist comparing surgical and percutaneous management of hydatid liver disease. Moreover, follow-up periods in these reports typically average only 1 year. Nevertheless, percutaneous aspiration or drainage may prove beneficial for patients with uncomplicated unilocular cysts, poor surgical candidates, and patients with multiple previous operations. The procedure is contraindicated in patients with multilocular cysts, secondarily infected cysts, or suspected biliary communication (bile-stained aspirate), owing to the increased risk of complications.

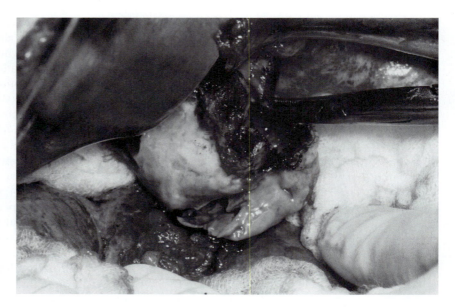

A

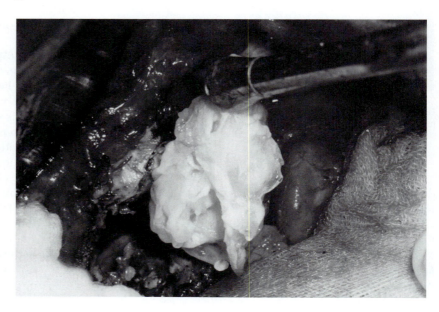

Figure 51–17. Partial pericystectomy. **A.** The cyst has been isolated from the remainder of the operative field and unroofed. **B.** After removal of the cyst contents, the laminated membrane and adherent germinal membrane are stripped free from the pericyst and removed.

B

Surgery

The growth of hydatid cysts secondary to *E granulosus* is slow, localized, and predictable. Thus, surgical intervention preferably is undertaken when the patient is otherwise healthy and has a readily accessible cyst. Most authors agree that all patients with symptoms related to their cyst should undergo some form of surgical intervention. In addition, asymptomatic patients with cysts greater than 5 cm in diameter, particularly if superficial, should be considered surgical candidates. With multiple cysts, surgical excision should be performed only on the accessible lesions, as reoperation for the remaining cysts may be delayed safely until their growth places them in a more superficial location. Expectant management is prudent in cases where the patient is asymptomatic and the cyst is less than 4 cm in size or lies deep within the liver. These patients should be followed with sonograms every 6 months to document cyst growth. Hydatid cysts that have completely calcified are no longer viable and should not be resected, since the remaining cavity is difficult to obliterate surgically and thus, often becomes secondarily infected.

Preparation for surgery consists of preoperative administration of an antihistamine to the patient and ensuring the availability of intravenous corticosteroids and epinephrine in the event of intraoperative anaphylactic shock. After entering the abdominal or thoracic cavity, the cyst first is isolated from the remainder of the operative field and the peritoneum to prevent soilage, spread, and possible anaphylaxis, should the cyst unexpectedly rupture (Fig 51–17). Controversy lies within the various techniques available for resecting a hydatid liver cyst, and whether the site of resection should be drained. One should realize, however, that different procedures may need to be performed under varying circumstances. Thus, the definitive operation needs to be tailored to the age of the patient and fitness for surgery, presence of coexisting extrahepatic disease, involvement of the biliary system, and the size, location, and number of hydatid cysts (Fig 51–18).

Although a posterolateral thoracotomy may be preferred if the cyst lies in a superior location or has undergone intrathoracic rupture, most hydatid cysts of the liver are approached from a midline abdominal incision. Involvement of both a superior, partially intrathoracic hydatid liver cyst and an inferior, abdominal cyst necessitates individual incisions and often separate timing of operations. In the majority of cases, however, an abdominal approach is useful, since it allows exploration of the peritoneum for concurrent hydatid implants as well as manual and sonographic evaluation of the entire liver for additional cysts. For patients with sus-

pected biliary involvement or obstruction, the abdominal approach is also helpful for proper exposure of the extrahepatic biliary system and intraoperative cholangiography. Once the cyst is managed operatively (see below), cholangiography is performed. If material is discovered within the common bile duct, the duct is explored and then decompressed with a transduodenal sphincteroplasty. A cholecystectomy concludes the procedure.

The hydatid cyst can be managed surgically by several methods. Once the cyst is exposed and isolated from the remainder of the operative field, partial or total cyst resection is performed. Partial resection, or conservative resection, consists of unroofing the hydatid cyst, removing its contents, including the laminated and germinal membranes, and leaving a portion of the pericyst behind (partial pericystectomy). If the cyst appears unilocular on a preoperative CT or sonogram, or intraoperative ultrasound, and the patient clinically has no signs of biliary involvement, an attempt at aspiration and sterilization is warranted before opening the cyst wall. Various methods of closed aspiration have been described, including the use of a freezing or suction cone, a plastic sheath sutured to the pericyst, or a laparoscopic trocar. Large suction devices are necessary as the cyst contents can be quite viscous. The cyst is aspirated and a scolicide is instilled into the cavity and allowed to remain for 5 to 10 minutes. This process then is repeated. Hypertonic saline (15%), chlorhexidine, 80% ethanol, 0.5% certrimide, 3% H_2O_2 and 0.5% silver nitrate solutions all

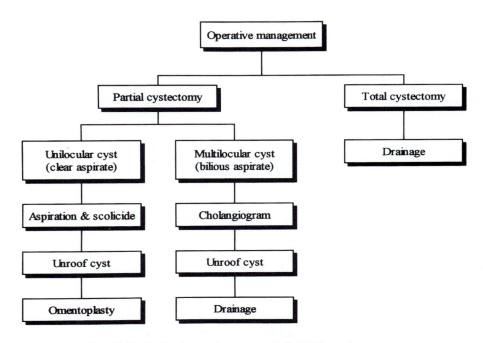

Figure 51–18. Algorithm for operative management of hydatid liver cysts.

have been used successfully as scolicides, killing 80% to 90% of organisms within the cyst. Formalin no longer is used for this purpose, since it may cause systemic acidosis or the development of sclerosing cholangitis if it enters the biliary system. Scolicides are incapable of sterilizing multilocular cysts and may cause inflammation and cholangitis if exposed to the biliary tree. Thus, if the hydatid cyst appears multilocular or the initial aspirate is bile-stained, no scolicide is used and the cyst is simply unroofed and cleared of its contents. Careful inspection of the pericyst may reveal small communications with bile ducts, which should be sutured closed. A final sterilization with a scolicide then is performed on all cysts before drainage or closure, and the edges of the remaining pericyst are oversewn to prevent leakage of bile.

The cavity resulting from a partial resection of a hydatid cyst can be managed in several ways. The pericystic cavity can be left open to the peritoneum, obliterated with omentum, externally drained, or reapproximated, a technique termed capitonnage. The use of open peritoneal communication should be limited to superficial, uncomplicated, unilocular hydatid cysts. Biliary fistulas develop frequently if this technique is used on multilocular cysts, and its employment for infected hydatid cysts is unwise. Capitonnage is associated with a decreased frequency of biliary fistulas, and is effective in cysts located deep within the liver. However, it is often difficult to perform in partially calcified pericysts with stiff walls. Experience with routine omentoplasty after conservative resection has been positive, and this procedure, coupled with external drainage of the resection site, also has proven efficacious in the management of secondarily infected hydatid liver cysts. External drains are indicated in cysts involving the biliary system and most infected cysts. However, the routine use of external drains after partial resection of uncomplicated hydatid liver cysts actually increases postoperative morbidity and prolongs the hospital stay.

There are several advantages to conservative surgical treatment of hydatid liver cysts. The procedure is faster and easier to perform than more complicated liver resections, as a plane usually exists between the pericyst and the laminated membrane. Blood loss is usually minimal during these procedures, since normal liver parenchyma is left intact. Conservative, or partial, resections are indicated for very large hydatid cysts, in which total resection would result in a major loss of normal liver tissue, and for hydatid cysts located deep within the substance of the liver. The major morbidity associated with conservative resections is the development of a postoperative biliary fistula. The mortality rate for these procedures is typically less than 2%.

Radical operative procedures, or total resection, of hydatid liver cysts consist of complete removal of the pericyst and the parasitic cyst contents. Examples include cystopericystectomy, wedge resections, and hepatic lobectomies. Because the cyst integrity is not breached with these procedures, aspiration and scolicidal agents are not necessary, and the risk of accidental contamination of the peritoneum is less than with conservative techniques. Radical resections often involve a substantial investment of time and considerable blood loss, since a clear plane of dissection is not found between the pericyst and normal hepatic parenchyma. Furthermore, a portion of normal liver tissue is invariably removed. Nevertheless, radical excisions in otherwise healthy patients are quite safe in experienced hands, with an operative mortality rate of less than 5%. Wedge resections and cystopericystectomies are useful for peripherally located, multiloculated hydatid cysts. Single or multiple hydatid cysts that occupy an entire hepatic lobe are best treated with a formal hepatic lobectomy.

Postoperative complications appear to be less frequent when complete excision of a hydatid cyst is performed. Biliary fistulas develop in 10% of these patients, compared to 25% of individuals treated with a more conservative operation. Cyst recurrence is also less frequent, with incidences of 2% and 16% being reported for hydatid cysts managed by total and partial resections, respectively.[56,57] For radial procedures, the necessity of external drainage of the excised cavity or liver depends on the extent of resection and the degree of hemostasis, but routine external drainage usually is performed in all but simple wedge resections.

Alveolar hydatid liver disease is managed by complete resection whenever possible, since the small size and thin wall of the cysts make aspiration and injection of scolicides impossible. Resections often involve a substantial portion of the liver parenchyma, gallbladder, and adherent omentum. If the cysts are successfully excised, the involved sites are irrigated with hypertonic saline solution and externally drained. Unfortunately, alveolar disease is much more aggressive and invasive than classic hydatid cysts, and many patients infected with *E multilocularis* have significant intrahepatic pathology that cannot be completely resected. The portal vein and common bile duct also may be completely encased by the parasitic process. Despite extensive debulking procedures, the outlook for these patients is quite grim.

COMPLICATIONS

Complications are seen in one-third of patients with hydatid liver cysts (Table 51–11). The most common complication is rupture of the cyst, which can occur internally or, less frequently, involve structures external to the hydatid cyst. Internal rupture may occur as a result of trauma or pressure necrosis from the growing cyst. In either case, the pericyst becomes separated from the laminated membrane, and a multiloculated cyst is

TABLE 51–11. COMPLICATIONS OF HYDATID LIVER CYSTS IN DECREASING ORDER OF FREQUENCY

Rupture
    Internal
    External
        Intrabiliary
        Intrathoracic
        Intraperitoneal
Secondary infection
Anaphylactic shock
Liver replacement

formed. Pressure necrosis of a neighboring bile duct may result in flow of bile into the cyst, resulting in an internal rupture, or flow of cyst contents into the biliary tree, an external rupture. When internal rupture from bile duct necrosis occurs, the hydatid cyst fluid may appear yellow and murky, similar to a pyogenic abscess. In such cases, however, a gram stain will not reveal microorganisms. Decompression of the cyst into the biliary system is the most common form of external rupture. When such decompression occurs, the patient, if previously symptomatic, often experiences a transient decrease in pain or dyspepsia as the cyst decompresses. Usually, however, the pain returns when cyst contents and fragments lead to obstructive jaundice, cholangitis, or secondary cyst infection. Intrathoracic rupture of a hydatid cyst occurs when a cyst reaching the posterior or superior liver capsule erodes through the diaphragm, a process heralded by the development of right shoulder pain. A local inflammatory effect within the pleural space allows the cyst to decompress within the lung parenchyma, and the patient may develop a hepatobronchial fistula and subsequent bronchobilia. Cysts localized to the anterior or inferior surface of the liver may rupture into the peritoneum. The resulting implantation and growth of hydatid organisms on and within the peritoneum and omentum is termed abdominal echinococcosis. Rarely, a cyst can grow large enough to replace the majority of the liver parenchyma and cause hepatic failure. Typically, however, the hydatid cyst will rupture before this complication develops.

Secondary infection of the cyst is relatively uncommon in hydatid disease and accounts for only 25% of all complications. Simple bacterial superinfections are decidedly rare. Instead, most secondary infections of hydatid cysts result from a communication between the cyst and the biliary system. Hyperbilirubinemia may develop in these patients as well, and the cyst fluid often appears bile-stained. Anaphylactic shock is the most acutely life-threatening complication of hydatid cyst disease, but fortunately the incidence of anaphylaxis is quite low. Sensitization to echinococcal parasites and their cysts develop when an internal rupture or small external leak results in various protein fragments accessing the bloodstream. Thus, the majority of patients with hypersensitivity responses to echinococcal antigens report a history of transient abdominal pain. Repeated exposure results in an IgE-mediated systemic allergic response, which is amenable to treatment with corticosteroids, antihistamines, and epinephrine. Complications of *E multilocularis* infection occur more frequently than with classic hydatid cyst disease and include severe cholestasis, portal hypertension, gastrointestinal hemorrhage, and dissemination of the disease to the lungs, brain, heart, and other organs.

PROGNOSIS

Liver replacement and subsequent death from *E granulosus* is usually slow, but unremittent, if the disease is left untreated. However, a small percentage of hydatid cysts do undergo spontaneous degeneration. With proper operative management of hydatid cysts, especially in centers experienced in liver surgery, survival rates for patients with hydatidosis approach 95%. The recurrence rate of hydatid liver cysts is typically less than 10% after a 5 year follow-up, with higher rates reported in those patients with ruptured or multiple cysts. Follow-up of all patients should consist of periodic hydatid serologies; serial ultrasound evaluations are also helpful. Cyst cavities should become homogenous and decrease in size within 6 months of operation, if complete sterilization was achieved. Unfortunately, the prognosis of alveolar hydatid disease remains poor despite rigorous medical and surgical management. The 5 year survival for these patients is approximately 50%, despite surgical therapy, with many patients dying from disseminated disease.

■ SUMMARY

Although uncommon in Western nations, infectious cystic masses within the liver may result from bacterial, amebic, or echinococcal organisms. Pyogenic and amebic processes result in true abscesses, while *E granulosum* infestation creates a hydatid cyst. A careful history and physical examination is helpful in determining the etiology of the mass, but the majority of signs, symptoms, and laboratory tests do not differentiate between the diseases. Thus, obtaining a specific diagnosis relies upon a combination of CT (or ultrasound, in selected cases) and serological testing for both amebic and echinococcal infection. The treatment of amebic liver abscesses is primarily by oral antibiotics, with surgery reserved for complications. Pyogenic abscesses require percutaneous or surgical drainage, whereas hydatid cysts are managed effectively with operative resection. The prognosis for amebic liver abscesses and classic hydatid liver cysts is excellent. However, significant mortality rates remain for individuals with pyogenic liver abscesses, owing to the coexisting pathological source of the infection as well as a patient population with a high frequency of chronic debilitation and malignancy.

REFERENCES

1. Ochsner A, DeBakey M, Murray S. Pyogenic abscess of the liver. *Am J Surg* 1938;40:292
2. Gyorffy EJ, Frey CF, et al. Pyogenic liver abscess. *Ann Surg* 1987;206:699
3. Miedema BW, Dineen P. The diagnosis and treatment of pyogenic liver abscesses. *Ann Surg* 1984;200:328
4. Schatten WE, Desprey JD, Holden WD. A bacteriologic study of portal-vein blood in man. *Arch Surg* 1955;71:404
5. Steele Jr. G. Cryoablation in hepatic surgery. *Semin Liver Dis* 1994;14:120
6. Cohen JL, Martin FM, et al. Liver abscess: the need for complete gastrointestinal evaluation. *Arch Surg* 1989;124:561
7. Minuk GY, Nicole LE, Sherman T. Cryptogenic abscess of the liver: evidence of underlying reticuloendothelial cell dysfunction. *Arch Surg* 1987;122:906
8. Pitt HA. Liver abscess. In: Zuidema GD, Turcotte JG (eds), *Shackelford's Surgery of the Alimentary Tract*, 3 ed Philadelphia, PA: WB Saunders; 1991:443
9. Grois N, Mostbeck G, et al. Hepatic and splenic abscesses—a common complication of intensive chemotherapy of acute myeloid leukemia (AML): a prospective study. *Ann Hematol* 1991;63:33
10. Moore-Gillon JC, Eykyn SF, Phillips I. Microbiology of liver abscesses. *Br Med J* 1981;283:819
11. Hague RA, Eastham EJ, et al. Resolution of hepatic abscess after interferon gamma in chronic granulomatous disease. *Arch Dis Child* 1993;69:443
12. Stain SC, Yellin AE, et al. Pyogenic liver abscess: modern treatment. *Arch Surg* 1991;126:991
13. Pitt HA, Zuidema GD. Factors influencing mortality in the treatment of pyogenic hepatic abscess. *Surg Gynecol Obstet* 1975;140:228
14. Rubinson HA, Isikoff MD, Hill MC. Diagnostic imaging of hepatic abscesses: a retrospective analysis. *AJR Am J Roentgenol* 1980;135:735
15. Mendez RJ, Schiebler ML, et al. Hepatic abscesses: MR imaging findings. *Radiology* 1994;190:431
17. Soriano V, Cobo J, et al. Espergillus hepatosplenic abscesses and chylous ascites: successful treatment with fluconazole. *Eur J Med* 1992;1:253
18. Attar B, Levendoglu H, Causay NS. CT-guided percutaneous aspiration and catheter drainage of pyogenic liver abscesses. *Am J Gastroenterol* 1986;81:550
19. Bertel CK, van Heerden JA, Sheedy PF. Treatment of pyogenic hepatic abscesses: Surgical vs percutaneous drainage. *Arch Surg* 1986;121:554
20. Northover JM, Jones BJM, et al. Difficulties in the diagnosis and management of pyogenic liver abscesses. *Br J Surg* 1982;69:48
21. McCorkell SJ, Niles NL. Pyogenic liver abscesses: Another look at medical management. *Lancet* 1985;1:803
22. Reynolds TB. Medical treatment of pyogenic liver abscesses. *Ann Intern Med* 1982;96:373
23. McFadzean AJ, Chang KP, Wong CC. Solitary pyogenic abscess of the liver treated with closed aspiration and antibiotics. *Br J Surg* 1953;41:141
24. Robert JH, Mirescu D, et al. Critical review of the treatment of pyogenic hepatic abscess. *Surg Gynecol Obstet* 1992;174:97
25. Lambiase RE, Deyoe L, et al. Percutaneous drainage of 335 consecutive abscesses: results of primary drainage with 1-year follow-up. *Radiology* 1992;184:167
26. Machi JM, Sigel B, et al. Ultrasonic examination during surgery for abdominal abscess. *World J Surg* 1983;7:409
27. Lee KT, Sheen PC, et al. Pyogenic liver abscess: multivariate analysis of risk factors. *World J Surg* 1991;15:372
28. Patterson M, Schoppe LE. The presentation of amoebiasis. *Med Clin North Am* 1982;66:689
29. Burrows RB. Prevalence of amebiasis in the United States and Canada. *Am J Trop Med* 1961;10:172
30. Guerrant RL. The global problem of amebiasis: current status, research needs and opportunities for progress. *Rev Infect Dis* 1986;8:218
31. Barnes PF, DeCock KM, et al. A comparison of amebic and pyogenic abscess of the liver. *Medicine* 1987;66:472
32. Conter RL, Pitt HA, et al. Differentiation of pyogenic from amebic hepatic abscesses. *Surg Gynecol Obstet* 1986;162:114
33. Boultbee JE, Simjee AE, et al. Experiences with grey scale ultrasonography in hepatic amoebiasis. *Clin Radiol* 1979;30:683
34. Ralls PW, Meyers HI, et al. Gray-scale ultrasonography of hepatic amebic abscesses. *Radiology* 1979;132:125
35. Fawcett HD, Lantieri RL, et al. Differentiating hepatic abscess from tumor: combined ^{111}In white blood cell and ^{99m}Tc liver scans. *AJR Am J Roentgenol* 1980;135:53
36. Powell SJ, Wilmot AJ, Elsdon-Dew R. Single and low dosage regimens of metronidazole in amoebic dysentery and amoebic liver abscess. *Ann Trop Med Parasitol* 1969;63:139
37. de la Rey NJ, Simjee AE, Patel A. Indications for aspiration of amoebic liver abscess. *S Afr Med J* 1989;75:373
38. Sheehy TW, Parmley LF, Jr., et al. Resolution time of an amebic liver abscess. *Gastroenterology* 1968;55:26
39. Van Allan RJ, Katz MD, et al. Uncomplicated amebic liver abscess: prospective evaluation of percutaneous therapeutic aspiration. *Radiology* 1992;183:827
40. Ken JG, von Sonneberg E, et al. Perforated amebic liver abscess: successful percutaneous treatment. *Radiology* 1989;170:195
41. Gibney EJ. Amoebic liver abscess. *Br J Surg* 1990;77:843
42. Rasaretnam R, Paul ATS, Yoganathan M. Pleural empyema due to ruptured amoebic liver abscess. *Br J Surg* 1974;61:713
43. Eggleston FC, Handra AK, Verghese M. Amebic peritonitis secondary to amebic liver abscess. *Surgery* 1982;91:46
44. Adams EB, MacLeod IN. Invasive amebiasis: amebic liver abscess and its complications. *Medicine* 1977;56:325

45. Ochsner A, DeBakey M: Diagnosis and treatment of amoebic abscess of the liver: a study based on 4,484 collected and personal cases. *Am J Dig Dis* 1935;2:47

46. Cohen HG, Reynolds TB. Comparison of metronidazole and chloroquine for the treatment of amoebic liver abscess. *Gastroenterology* 1975;69:35

47. Balasegaram M. Management of hepatic abscess. *Curr Probl Surg* 1981;18:282

48. Chuah SK, Chang-Chien CS, et al. The prognostic factors of severe amebic liver abscess: a retrospective study of 125 cases. *Am J Trop Med Hyg* 1992;46:398

49. McGreevy PB, Nelson GS. Larval cestode infections. In: Strickland GT (ed), *Hunter's Tropical Medicine*. Toronto, Canada: WB Saunders; 1984:771

50. Pitt HA, Korzelius J, Tompkins R. Management of hepatic echinococcosis in Southern California. *Am J Surg* 1986; 152:110

51. Ito A, Wang XG, Liu YH. Differential serodiagnosis of alveolar and cystic hydatid disease in the People's Republic of China. *Am J Trop Med Hyg* 1993;49:208

52. Shemesh E, Klein E, et al. Common bile duct obstruction caused by hydatid daughter cysts—management by endoscopic retrograde sphincterotomy. *Am J Gastroenterol* 1986; 81:280

53. Todorov T, Vutova K, et al. Chemotherapy of human cystic echinococcosis: comparative efficacy of mebendazole and albendazole. *Ann Trop Med Parasitol* 1992; 86:59

54. Acunas B, Rozanes I, et al. Purely cystic hydatid disease of the liver: treatment with percutaneous aspiration and injection of hypertonic saline. *Radiology* 1992;182:541

55. Simonetti G, Profili S, et al. Percutaneous treatment of hepatic cysts by aspiration and sclerotherapy. *Cardiovasc Intervent Radiol* 1993;16:81

56. Magistrelli P, Masetti R, et al. Surgical treatment of hydatid disease of the liver: a 20-year experience. *Arch Surg* 1991;126:518

57. Moreno Gonzalez E, Rico Selas P, et al. Results of surgical treatment of hepatic hydatidosis: current therapeutic modifications. *World J Surg* 1991;15:254

52

Cysts and Benign Tumors

Seymour I. Schwartz

Benign tumors of the liver are uncommon but have been reported with increasing frequency related, in part, to improvements in diagnostic technique and also to the widespread use of contraceptive medication. Edmondson documented the pathologic characteristics of these lesions and formulated the following classification.

1. Focal nodular hyperplasia
2. Adenoma
3. Adrenal rest tumor
4. Cystic mesenchymal hamartoma
5. Nonparasitic cysts
6. Cavernous hemangioma
7. Infantile hemangioendothelioma
8. Teratoma

The adrenal rest tumor and the teratoma are exceedingly rare; the remaining lesions are discussed individually because of unique characteristics.

■ NONPARASITIC CYSTS

Nonparasitic cysts of the liver may be single or multiple, diffuse or localized, unilocular or multilocular. The rarer varieties include blood and degenerative cysts, dermoid cysts, lymphatic cysts, and endothelial cysts (cystadenomas). The more common lesions are retention cysts, which are solitary simple cysts, or part of polycystic disease.

INCIDENCE

In 1856, Bristowe first reported a case of nonparasitic cystic disease of the liver and emphasized the association with polycystic renal disease. The same year, Michel recorded the first solitary, nonparasitic cyst. Hadad and associates reviewed almost 900 cases. An autopsy incidence of 0.15% to 0.5% has been reported.

Cystic disease of the liver has been reported at all ages. The disease most frequently makes its appearance during the fourth, fifth, and sixth decades. The average age of the patients with symptomatic, solitary cysts of the liver is 55 years. Polycystic disease occurs more frequently in the female patient, with a 2:1 ratio and solitary nonparasitic cysts occur four times more frequently in the female.

ETIOLOGY

Most investigators have regarded the condition as congenital, and it is postulated that aberrant ducts formed during embryonic development enlarge. Cyst formation is attributed to inflammatory hyperplasia of the ducts, or obstruction of the ducts with retention of fluid. Although some investigators believe that solitary cysts and polycystic liver disease are different manifestations of the same process, this opinion is not widespread.

SOLITARY NONPARASITIC CYSTS

These cysts usually are located on the anteroinferior surface of the right lobe of the liver. The cysts vary markedly in size from 1 to 15 cm. They may be more deeply placed; some have presented as pedunculated cysts. The external surface is smooth, glistening, and grayish-blue. The cyst wall is usually thin and opalescent or transparent and may be traversed by many dilated blood vessels. The cyst content is a clear, watery, or yellowish-brown material, but may appear bile stained. The cysts characteristically have a low internal pressure, in contrast to the high tension in parasitic cysts. The wall of the solitary cyst generally is composed of three layers: an inner layer of loose connective tissue that is rich in cellular elements, a circular dense middle layer, poor in cell nuclei, and an outer layer that contains segments of bile ducts and islands of liver cells, and a connective tissue framework that blends into the liver parenchyma. The inner lining may be cuboidal or columnar epithelium, at times ciliated, or there may be no distinct epithelial layer. Communication within the biliary tree may be expected in approximately one-fourth of solitary hepatic cysts.

POLYCYSTIC DISEASE

The affected portion of the liver is enlarged and deformed by numerous cysts of varying size on the surface of the organ (Fig 52–1). The cysts are surrounded by a capsule of fibrous tissue. On cut section, the appearance is that of a honeycomb with multiple cavities. The cysts contain a clear fluid, usually without bile. They commonly are distributed throughout the liver, but at times one lobe, more frequently the right, is preferentially involved. Hepatic function is seldom appreciably impaired, but polycystic livers have been implicated as a rare cause of portal hypertension. The lesion has been associated with atresia of the bile ducts, cholangitis, and hepatitis. Carcinoma, arising in the cyst wall, has been reported infrequently.

Microscopically, the epithelial lining of the cyst varies with the size and stage of development. In the larger cysts, the lining may have degenerated and is absent, or flattened. In medium-sized cysts, the lining is usually cuboidal, whereas columnar cells line the smaller cysts. The lining cells closely resemble those of normal bile ducts. Outside the epithelium, the wall is composed of a thin, collagenous tissue. Numerous nondilated bile ducts are seen in the surrounding tissue, and the islands of hepatic parenchyma between the cysts may be compressed, distorted, or normal.

Unlike the solitary, nonparasitic cyst, which is usually an isolated finding, polycystic disease is frequently associated with cystic involvement of other organs. The kidney is the most commonly involved, usually to a greater extent than the liver. In addition to the kidneys, cystic disease of the liver has been associated with cystic disease of the pancreas, spleen, ovary, and lungs.

CLINICAL MANIFESTATIONS

The great majority of patients with hepatic cysts are asymptomatic. Most cysts are incidental findings at operation or autopsy. When symptoms occur, they usually are related to the presence of an enlarging mass in the

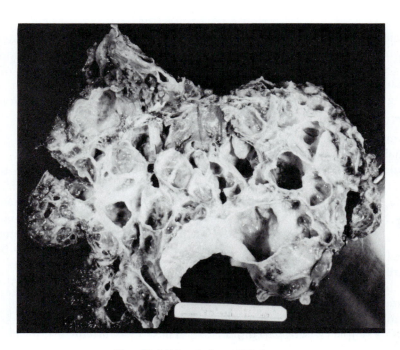

Figure 52–1. Polycystic disease of the liver.

upper abdomen, coupled with vague gastrointestinal complaints. The most common presentations of symptomatic cysts are abdominal mass (55%) with early satiety, hepatomegaly (40%), abdominal pain (33%), and jaundice (9%). Complications are rare and may account for symptoms. These include perforation, hemorrhage, and secondary infection. Torsion of a cyst on a pedicle may occur. Jaundice may develop secondary to compression of the common duct, and portal hypertension has been described with polycystic disease.

DIAGNOSTIC STUDIES

Studies of liver function are of little diagnostic aid. Serum bilirubin level and alkaline phosphatase are generally normal. With advanced polycystic disease of the kidneys, there are signs of impaired renal function, and excretory urograms are diagnostic. On plain x-ray examination, the diaphragm is frequently elevated and large cysts displace the colon down and to the left, in contrast to the anterior colonic displacement caused by renal masses. On lateral projection, the anterior location of the extrinsic pressure favors the diagnosis of a hepatic cyst. Isotopic scanning with technetium 99m (^{99m}Tc)- sulfur colloid may show areas of diminished uptake. Ultrasound examination offers a high yield, and the diagnosis is suggested if an anechoic area is defined. A computed tomography (CT) scan demonstrates a lower attenuation lesion (Figs 52–2 and 52–3). Ultrasonography may depict cysts as small as 2 cm in diameter. Arteriography, although usually unnecessary, will define an avascular mass.

DIFFERENTIAL DIAGNOSIS

Differentiation from primary tumors of the liver and from metastatic lesions is usually not a problem. Generally, differentiation from a hydatid cyst is not difficult; the latter diagnosis is suggested by eosinophilia, a positive Casoni test, and the deposition of calcium in the walls of the cyst. Calcareous deposits, however, have been noted in benign nonparasitic cysts.

TREATMENT

Solitary Cysts

With the exceptions of rupture, torsion, and intracystic hemorrhage, the operative treatment is elective and is based on the size and location of the cyst and the general status of the patient. Needle aspiration usually is associated with recurrence. Catheter drainage with or without injection of sclerosing solution usually is followed by recurrence. Wide unroofing of large cysts generally is effective and recurrence is rare. The inner wall should be inspected for a papillary tumor that would mandate excision. Excision of solitary cysts may be performed by developing a cleavage plane that leaves the outer wall adjacent to the liver parenchyma, but this is associated with more risk than the equally effective unroofing procedure. Resection or formal lobectomy may be required for large multiloculated cysts. Marsupialization is indicated only for infected cysts because it may be attended by prolonged drainage. Internal drainage into a Roux-en-Y loop may be used to drain a cyst that has a significant communication with the biliary channels, a very rare situation.

Polycystic Disease

Operation is indicated only for pain or symptoms caused by a mass effect. Resection of the dominant area of involvement can be facilitated by initial fenestration of larger cysts so that lines of resection can be defined. Formal lobectomy rarely can be performed. Unroofing of multiple cysts so that they drain into the peritoneal cavity usually results in recurrence of symptoms.

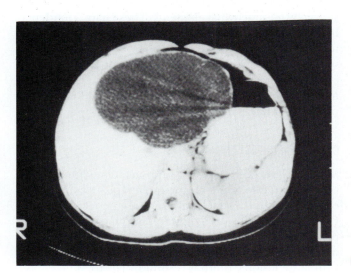

Figure 52–2. CT scan of a single cyst of the liver.

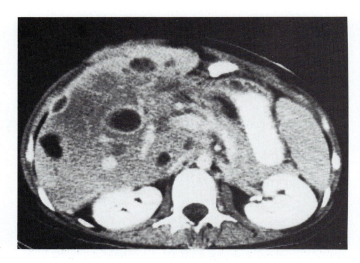

Figure 52–3. CT scan of a polycystic liver.

PROGNOSIS

Although the older literature reports mortality rates of approximately 20% for nonparasitic cysts treated by excision, limiting the cases to those reported subsequent to 1924, there were only 3 deaths in 122 patients subjected to operation.

Morbidity usually is related to the development of a persistent draining sinus in those patients subjected to marsupialization. Other complications include recurrence, extension of liver damage with hepatic failure and infection. The prognosis for the polycystic disease of the liver is essentially that of the accompanying polycystic renal disease. When the kidneys are involved insignificantly, the hepatic lesion is compatible with good health and long life. Hepatic failure, jaundice, esophageal varices, and ascites are extremely rare.

■ MESENCHYMAL HAMARTOMA

Mesenchymal hamartoma of the liver is a rare, benign tumor of childhood that was first reported by Maresh in 1903. This cystic hepatic tumor also has been termed "large solitary bile-cell fibroadenoma," "hamartoma," and "large, cavernous lymphangiomatoid lesion."

INCIDENCE

Approximately 50 cases of mesenchymal hamartoma have been reported. The lesion occurs much more frequently in infancy and childhood, but several cases have been reported in adults. The lesion usually was located in the right lobe (37 of 49 reported cases), rarely in the left lobe, and in three cases was present in both lobes. There was approximately equal distribution among females and males. The diagnosis was made during the first 2 years of life in the great majority of patients; in a few, the diagnosis was made during the first 3 months of life.

PATHOLOGY

The lesion usually appears as a single mass bulging from the liver on the inferior surface, and it is frequently pedunculated. One case was described as completely intralobar. The tumor is well-encapsulated and most frequently cystic. The contained fluid is usually watery, although on occasion it has a gelatinous, yellow color but does not contain bile. Histologically, according to Edmondson's criteria, the hamartomas are composed of tissues indigenous to the site. Mesenchymal harmatoma of the liver is characterized by an admixture of ductal structures in a copious, loose connective tissue stroma. The remnants of bile ducts and liver lobules are often associated with recognizable portal triads, all of which are overgrown by mesenchymal elements. These have a tendency to undergo cystic degeneration, and to accumulate fluid in quantities sufficient to create microscopic and macroscopic acellular spaces suggestive of lymphangiomatous channels but without an endothelial lining. Smaller cysts may have one layer of columnar or cuboidal lining cells, probably of bile duct origin (Fig 52–4).

CLINICAL MANIFESTATIONS

Most patients present with symptoms related to accelerated growth rate of the tumor and a rapid accumulation of fluid within the cyst. Symptoms are generally minor. Children present with a right upper quadrant mass that produces a bulge in the abdomen; the general physical condition, however, remains excellent. Occasionally, with large lesions, there is respiratory distress.

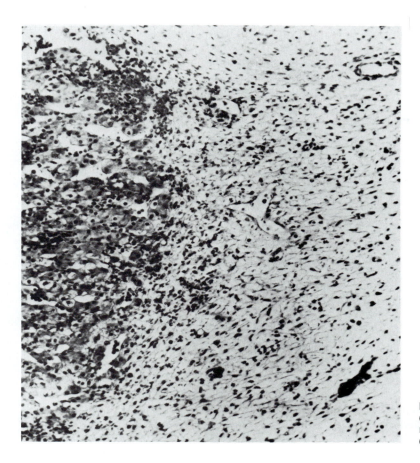

Figure 52–4. Section of the liver showing a large island of liver cells with clusters of smaller, darker staining hematopoietic cells on the left, and loose mesenchymal tissue on the right. (From Srouji MN, Chatten J, et al. Mesenchymal hamartoma of the liver in infants. Cancer 1978;42:2483)

DIAGNOSTIC STUDIES

^{99m}Tc-sulfur colloid scan defines a lack of uptake in the lesion and CT outlines the lesion. Angiography, useful in preoperative evaluation by delineating anatomic location, extent, and morphologic features, does not, however, define an abnormal vascularity. Exploration and biopsy are frequently necessary to define the diagnosis.

TREATMENT

The treatment is surgical excision, which depends on the location of the lesion. Pedunculated lesions are removed readily. If the tumor is well encapsulated, it may be enucleated. When the tumor is localized near the surface of the liver, a partial hepatectomy may be carried out. In rare instances, a formal lobectomy is required. Deeply located lesions should be left alone after histologic diagnosis has been established, since they do not grow rapidly or undergo malignant transformation. If the lesion is adherent to the inferior vena cava and involves both lobes of the liver, it may be treated by partial excision and marsupialization. Radiotherapy may effect some reduction in size of the lesion, owing to hyalinization of the mesenchymal components. Reduction in size should be followed by surgical excision.

■ HEMANGIOMAS

The most common benign tumor of the liver is the hemangioma, and the liver is the visceral organ most frequently affected by this lesion. Frerich is credited with the first description of hemangiomas of the liver in the medical literature, in 1861. Like other benign tumors, the majority are incidental findings, but lesions occasionally reach clinical significance in the adult. Symptoms include pain that is, at times, related to rapid expansion or intratumoral bleeding. In unusual circumstances, the hemangioma reaches a size that causes encroachment of adjacent viscera. Spontaneous hemorrhage rarely occurs; less than two dozen cases, mostly neonates, have been reported. In children, giant cavernous hemangiomas and infantile hemangioendotheliomas may produce cardiac failure, at times accompanied by a consumptive coagulopathy.

INCIDENCE

Autopsy series report an incidence of 0.4% to 7%. Ten percent of the lesions were multiple. In the adult, hepatic hemangiomas are found most frequently in patients in the third and fourth decades; the average age when the lesion is discovered is 44 years. Symptomatic hemangiomas in the adult occur in the female five times more frequently. In children, most cases present in the first month of life.

PATHOLOGY

Hemangiomas generally are classified into two types: capillary and cavernous. The lesions, as they appear in the liver, are almost always cavernous. They may be single or multiple and may be limited to the liver or involve other organs. They occasionally are associated with cysts of the liver and pancreas. An association also has been noted between focal nodular hyperplasia and hemangioma of the liver. The weight of the hemangioma of the liver varies from 1 gm to as much as 18 kg (40 lbs).

The lesions frequently are located immediately beneath Glisson's capsule, and the surface may be depressed, umbilicated, or, at times, elevated. On cut section, the hemangioma is purplish-red and spongelike in appearance; there are many cystic spaces filled with blood. The surrounding parenchyma is sharply demarcated, and there is an absence of communication between the tumor and the hepatic parenchyma. With increasing fibrosis, a condition termed "sclerosing hemangioma" may be produced.

Histologically, the tumor presents a typical appearance (Fig 52–5). It is composed of cystic spaces filled with blood and lined with epithelial cells separated by varying amounts of fibrous tissue. The hepatic plates between the blood spaces are absent or markedly compressed, but there is no distortion or compression of the adjacent hepatic parenchyma. Marked fibrosis may be present, contributing to the formation of a sclerosing hemangioma. Malignant degeneration does not occur, and the hemangioma must be distinguished from the hemangioendothelioma. The latter is represented by a widespread area of multicentric lesions, accompanied by vascular involvement of the skin and occurring in children with clinical manifestations in the first week of life.

The other lesion that must be distinguished from the hemangioma is peliosis hepatis, which consists of blood lakes surrounded by tissue without epithelial lining.

CLINICAL MANIFESTATIONS

Small hemangiomas are usually asymptomatic. Only patients in whom the lesion reaches a size > 4 cm develop symptoms. Larger lesions in adults usually present in one of three ways: as an asymptomatic abdominal mass, with pain or digestive symptoms related to encroachment of the tumor on the abdominal viscera, or as an intraperitoneal rupture. The presentations of giant hemangioma include obstructive jaundice, biliary colic, torsion of a pedunculated lesion, and gastric outlet obstruction. No conclusion can be made about the effect of pregnancy on cavernous hemangioma. Anecdotal re-

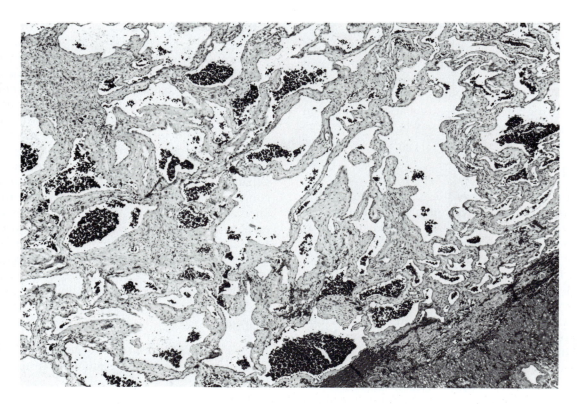

Figure 52–5. Hemangioma histology. Lesion is composed of cystic spaces filled with blood and lined with epithelial cells separated by varying amounts of fibrous tissue. (From Gutierrez OH, Schwartz SI: *Atlas of Hepatic Tumors and Focal Lesions.* New York, NY: McGraw-Hill; 1984:75)

ports chronicle rapid growth during pregnancy; others note no effect. On physical examination, if a mass is palpable, it is most commonly located in the epigastrium or the left upper quadrant. A bruit is heard only rarely. In patients with intraperitoneal hemorrhage, pain precedes shock by a day or more, thus suggesting subcapsular accumulation of blood. Rupture occurs in a greater proportion of children than adults. Rupture is not necessarily fatal. The potential for rupture per se is not an indication for excision.

Infants frequently present with an abdominal mass and a high-output frank congestive heart failure. A large liver, out of proportion to the degree of cardiac failure, an abdominal bruit, and cutaneous hemangiomas may be noted. The latter criteria are frequently absent.

DIAGNOSTIC STUDIES

Liver function tests are generally normal. In newborn infants with hepatic hemangiomas, thrombocytopenia is a rare complication, and it is probably the result of an increased mechanical destruction of platelets in the hemangioma. In a series of 38 cases reviewed by Linderkamp and associates, thrombocytopenia was present in six cases.

Routine x-ray examination may demonstrate a soft tissue mass, elevation of the diaphragm, and displacement of the stomach or colon. ^{99m}Tc-sulfur colloid scan may show single or multiple areas of decreased radioactivity. ^{99m}Tc-labeled red blood cells show pooling in the lesion. Although the echogenic pattern is variable, ultrasonography may be helpful in showing the extent of the lesion. A CT scan, when used with contrast material, will show differing degrees of pooling within the tumor. T2-weighted magnetic resonance imaging (MRI) provides tissue-specific characterizations of a hepatic hemangioma. Selective angiogram demonstrates the vascular character of the tumor, the tortuosity and enlargement of the feeding vessels, and the early venous drainage (Fig 52–6).

Percutaneous needle biopsy is hazardous because of the danger of hemorrhage.

TREATMENT

Surgical excision is the preferred treatment of clinically significant hemangiomas of the liver. The extent of resection is dependent upon the size and location of the lesion. Resection of the lesion, by enucleation or with a rim of normal tissue, is the treatment of choice for selected cavernous hemangiomas of the liver. Occasionally, large tumors present as pedunculated lesions that can be excised easily. Larger lesions are managed best by resection along anatomic planes. Few reports have documented reduction in the size of the lesion with radiation therapy. Hepatic arterial ligation has had no

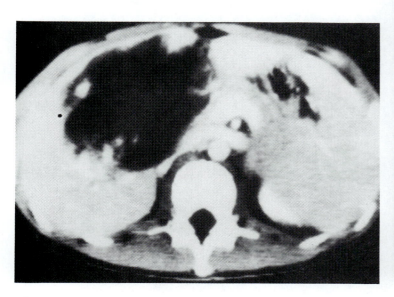

A

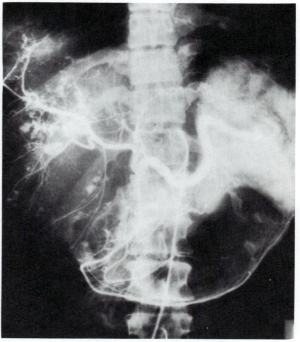

B

Figure 52–6. A. CT scan of a giant hemangioma. **B**. Angiogram showing the vascular character.

demonstrable effect. Control of bleeding from spontaneous hemorrhage of the cavernous hemangioma has been accomplished with packing and omental tamponade, but resection remains the treatment of choice.

The management of the newborn infant with hemangioma and consequent cardiac failure has proponents of both conservative and aggressive surgical management. Nguyen and associates successfully managed conservatively five children during the first year of life without steroids or radiotherapy. If complications were absent no active treatment was needed, since even large lesions are likely to resolve spontaneously. Goldberg and Fonkalsrud and Touloukian have used steroids successfully in extensive nonresectable tumors. Slovis and associates reported success with a regimen of digitalis and radiation therapy using approximately 350 rad in three treatments. In one patient, the size of the tumor regressed within 4 days. Another patient demonstrated dramatic decrease in liver size and cardiac failure within 3 days. De Lorimier was the first to report success for hepatic artery ligation as a means of reversing the cardiac failure; it seems the most appropriate method for cardiac failure due to diffuse hepatic hemangiomatosis. Linderkamp's review suggests that in infants with giant solitary hepatic hemangioma, excision of the tumor is the treatment of choice, since there was only 1 death among the 22 surgically treated patients with symptoms during the first year of life, whereas 15 of the conservatively treated patients died.

■ ADENOMA

INCIDENCE

The incidence has increased, as evidenced by the fact that Edmondson found only two hepatic cell adenomas in the review of 418 hepatic tumors in 50 000 autopsies over a 36 year period. Subsequent to the introduction of oral contraceptives, a marked increase in clinically manifest hepatic adenomas has been noted.

ETIOLOGY

Nissen and associates reporting on the role of oral contraceptive agents based on their registry data, indicate that all eight progesterones and both synthetic estrogens have been associated with the appearance of liver tumors. More than 60% of the patients were exposed to mestranol only, and 80% were exposed to a mestranol product. It is believed that inability to demethylate mestranol in the smooth endoplasmic reticulum of hepatocytes may allow massive accumulation of oncogenic metabolites.

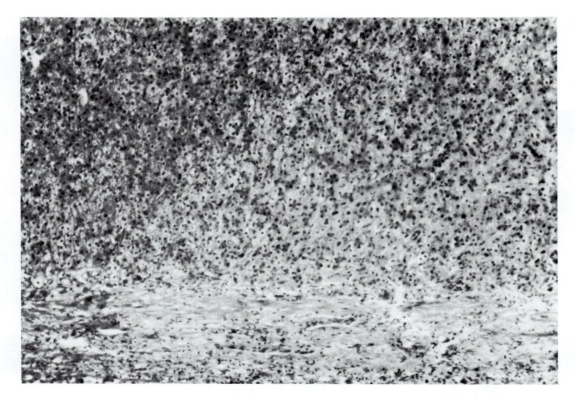

Figure 52–7. Hepatocellular adenoma. Peripheral section of an adenoma with a fibrous capsule component and a homogenous monotonous arrangement of hepatocyte cords without blood vessel or bile duct structures. (From Foster JH, Berman MM: *Solid Liver Tumors*. Philadelphia, PA: WB Saunders; 1977)

More than half the patients used the pill continuously for more than 5 years, and 85% of the women were exposed to contraceptive steroids for more than 4 years. The shortest duration of use was 6 months, by one patient, and the mean duration was 58.8 months. Peliosis hepatis, in other words, large blood spaces without endothelial linings, which is seen at the periphery of the tumor, has been noted in patients taking oral contraceptives and also in men on androgenic steroid therapy. Hepatic adenoma has been reported in a postmenopausal woman receiving hormonal replacement.

Liver cell adenomas that occur in women on oral contraceptive medication are more likely to undergo necrosis and to rupture than are adenomas occurring in patients who have not taken oral contraceptives. Occurrence of liver cell adenoma has been documented after cessation of oral contraceptives in some patients, but progression also has been reported. Transformation into hepatocellular carcinoma has been documented.

Adenomatosis, which is defined as more than ten adenomas, occurs with equal frequency in men and women.

PATHOLOGY

On gross examination, the lesions are soft, fleshy tumors with smooth surfaces that occasionally have large vessels coursing over the area. On cross-section, there are frequently areas of hemorrhage and necrosis. Microscopically, the hepatic adenomas are characterized by monotonous sheets of mature hepatocytes that are often smaller than normal and may contain glycogen (Fig 52–7). The lesion is devoid of bile ducts, portal triads, or central veins but may contain areas of dilated sinusoidal lakes or peliosis hepatis. Histologically, large

zones of necrotic ghost cells are noted in areas of hemorrhage. The lesions are separated from normal liver parenchyma by a connective tissue capsule.

CLINICAL MANIFESTATIONS

The lesions present in one of four ways: (1) as asymptomatic tumors noted incidentally during a CT scan, ultrasound, or at operation, (2) as a liver mass, (3) with pain in the upper abdomen, probably indicative of bleeding into the tumor and stretching of the liver capsule, and (4) with shock owing to rupture of the lesion and intraperitoneal hemorrhage. Recurrent pallor, diaphoresis, hypotension, and syncope have also been reported. About one-third of the reported patients have presented with intraperitoneal bleeding. The diagnosis should be considered particularly in a pregnant woman or a woman of childbearing age who has been on oral contraceptive medication and who presents with the triad of right upper quadrant or epigastric pain associated with shock and hemoperitoneum.

DIAGNOSTIC STUDIES

There are no currently available testing methods for identifying a patient at risk. In patients with established hepatic cell adenoma, the liver enzyme values are of limited usefulness. The α-fetoprotein is negative, as is the hepatitis B surface antigen determination. ^{99m}Tc-sulfur colloid liver scan will reveal a filling defect in about 85% of patients. Ultrasound generally defines a solid, filling defect with mixed echogenicity. CT scan and angiogram are particularly useful (Figs 52–8 and 52–9). The angiogram reveals a hypervascular lesion that may contain hypovascular regions related to tumor bleeding or ne-

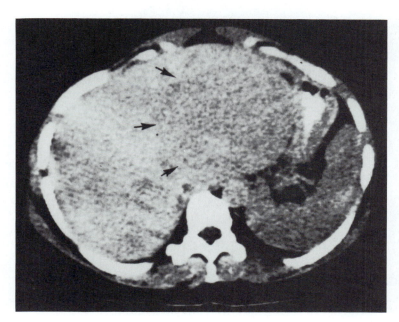

Figure 52–8. CT scan showing a solid, low-density mass occupying most of the left lobe of the liver (*arrows*). (From Gutierrez OH, Schwartz SI: *Atlas of Hepatic Tumors and Focal Lesions.* New York, NY: McGraw-Hill; 1984:83)

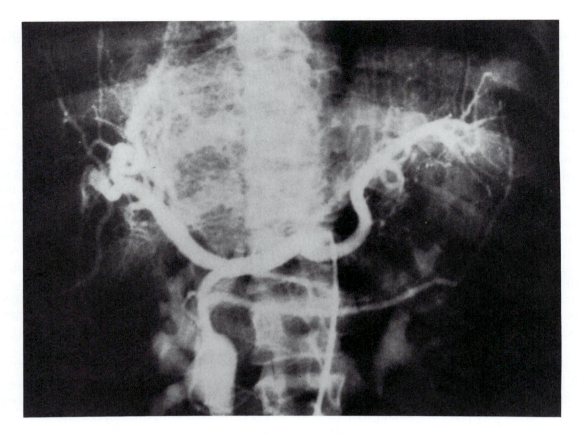

Figure 52–9. Angiogram showing a large hypervascular mass involving the entire left lobe of the liver. The tumor had a great number of tortuous, encased, and distorted vessels supplied by branches of the left hepatic artery. A vascular flush was apparent in the capillary phase. (From Gutierrez OH, Schwartz SI: *Atlas of Hepatic Tumors and Focal Lesions.* New York, NY: McGraw-Hill; 1984:84)

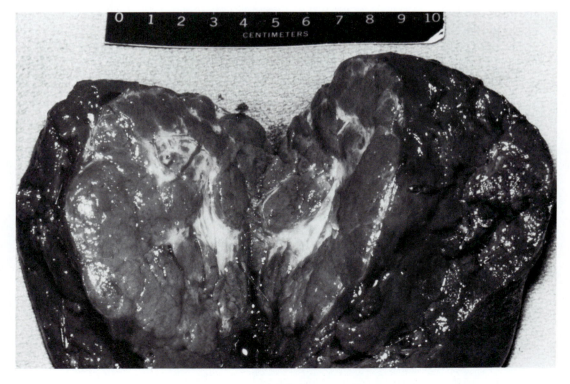

Figure 52–10. Cut section of FNH showing lesion with central stellate scar made of fibrous tissue.

crosis. There is frequently distortion and displacement of hepatic vessels, coupled with small tortuous abnormal vessels in the periphery of the lesion. Needle biopsy of the liver, previously thought to be contraindicated because of the danger of bleeding, is now advocated by some as a method for differentiating benign from malignant lesions, but the diagnostic yield is low.

TREATMENT

The management of small asymptomatic lesions is controversial. Regression, even disappearance, of radiographically defined lesions has been reported following cessation of contraceptive drugs. Lesions that do not regress should be removed. Because of the catastrophic consequences and the incidence of rupture during pregnancy, resection is advised for women who anticipate becoming pregnant. Prevention of hypoglycemia in patients with glycogen storage disease may lead to regression of tumor size.

Hepatic resection is indicated for large tumors or for painful lesions and intraparenchymal or intraperitoneal bleeding. Removal of only a small margin of normal liver is required but, in most instances, an anatomic segmentectomy or lobectomy is performed because of the location of the lesion. Recurrence following total resection has not been reported. Transplantation has been suggested for adenomatosis.

■ FOCAL NODULAR HYPERPLASIA

INCIDENCE

In the 1974 liver tumor survey, 63 cases met the criteria for focal nodular hyperplasia, contrasted with the 37 cases categorized as liver cell adenoma. Fifty-seven were female, and the majority of cases occurred between the ages of 20 and 50. Eight were seen in patients under the age of 10, the youngest, a 10 months of age male infant, and the oldest, a 70 years of age woman. Focal nodular hyperplasia was also more common in the Mayo Clinic experience, occurring almost twice as frequently as the hepatic cell adenoma. The mean age of the patients with focal nodular hyperplasia was much higher than that in patients with hepatic adenoma (41 versus 34 years).

ETIOLOGY

Since focal nodular hyperplasias (FNH) frequently occur in women who are not on oral contraceptive medication and also in males, many believe that the lesion is neither a neoplasm nor a hamartoma, but rather a reaction to injury. It has been suggested that FNH is a hyperplastic response of the parenchyma to a preexisting arterial spider-like malformation. When a reliable history is obtained, only 58% of women with focal nodular hyperplasia gave a history of oral contraceptive use, contrasted with almost 90% of women with hepatic cell adenoma.

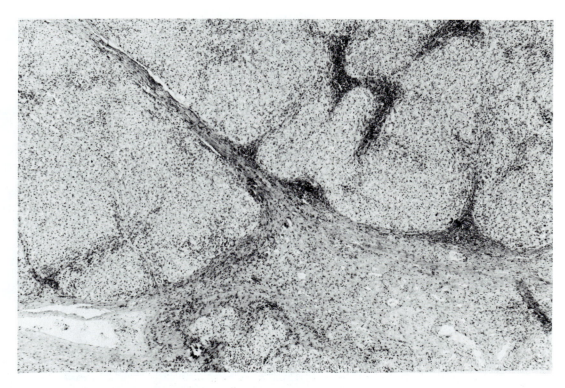

Figure 52–11. Microscopic section of FNH showing fibrous band containing bile ducts and surrounding hepatic tissue with nodular appearance. (From Gutierrez OH, Schwartz SI: *Atlas of Hepatic Tumors and Focal Lesions.* New York, NY: McGraw-Hill; 1984:99)

PATHOLOGY

The tumors are usually solitary and < 5 cm in diameter. They are frequently found near the free edge of the liver; they are grossly nodular, with surface scarring and blood vessels. On cut section they are tan in color and present with a classic central stellate fibrous scar (Fig 52–10). They may or may not have a capsule. The histologic appearance is characterized by fibrous bands that contain numerous bile ducts. The hepatocytes are arranged in cords and separated by sinusoids and the cells appear normal. The overall appearance resembles a regenerating nodule with the cirrhotic liver (Fig 52–11). The nuclei show no evidence of pyknosis or mitosis. Characteristically, there is absence of hemorrhage or necrosis.

CLINICAL MANIFESTATIONS

The overwhelming majority of cases of FNH have been discovered incidentally. A palpable mass or pain rarely occurs. Intraperitoneal hemorrhage has not been recorded in any of the large series. Two instances appear in the literature.

DIAGNOSTIC STUDIES

The liver function tests usually reveal no abnormalities. The serum markers for the hepatitis B virus and α-fetoprotein are negative. ^{99m}Tc-sulfur colloid scans could detect only half these lesions, and ultrasound and CT examinations also frequently fail to define the lesion, since the major bulk is isodense. The angiogram, however, may be diagnostic, demonstrating a hypervas-

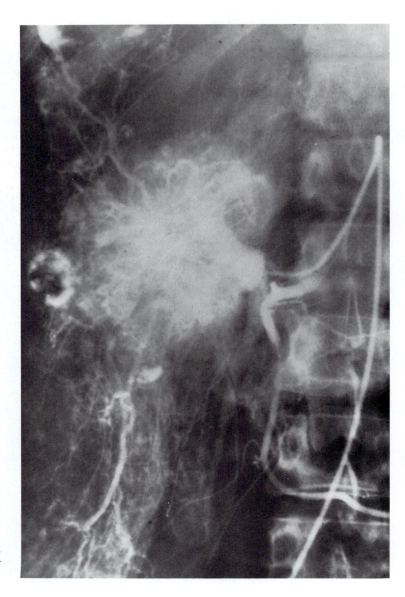

Figure 52–12. Angiogram demonstrating hypervascular tumor and characteristic stellate distribution of blood cells. Note hemangiomas in upper and lower portions of the right lobe.

cular tumor with large arteries and evidence of arteriovenous shunting in 85% of cases. There is a characteristic stellate distribution of the blood vessels (Fig 52–12). Needle biopsy is often nondiagnostic.

TREATMENT

Elective resection rarely is indicated. When FNH is found incidentally at laparotomy, a wedge biopsy should be performed. Smaller lesions may be removed, but the larger FNHs should be left. Oral contraceptive medication should be discontinued, and there is no suggestion that pregnancy should be discouraged in these patients because necrosis and rupture of these tumors during pregnancy rarely have been reported. The follow-up of patients subjected to resection has failed to reveal a single incidence of persistence, recurrence, or metastasis.

SELECTED READINGS

Alper A, Ariogul O, et al. Choledochoduodenostomy for intrabiliary rupture of hydatid cysts of liver. *Br J Surg* 1987; 74:243

Armitage NC, Blumgart LH. Partial resection and fenestration in the treatment of polycystic liver disease. *Br J Surg* 1984; 71:242

Brady MS, Coit DG. Focal nodular hyperplasia of liver. *Surg Gynecol Obstet* 1990;171:377

de Lorimier AA. Hepatic tumors of infancy and childhood. *Surg Clin North Am* 1977;57:443

DeMaioribus CA, Lally KP, et al. Mesenchymal hamartoma of the liver: a 35-year review. *Arch Surg* 1990;125:598

Edmondson HA. Tumors of the liver and intrahepatic bile ducts. In: *Atlas of Tumor Pathology.* Armed Forces Institute of Pathology, Section VII, Fascicle 25, 1958.

Edmondson HA, Reynolds TB, et al. Regression of liver cell adenomas associated with oral contraceptives. *Ann Intern Med* 1977;86:180

Edwards JD, Eckhauser FE, et al. Optimizing surgical management of symptomatic solitary hepatic cysts. *Am Surg* 1987;53:510

Fernandez M, Cacioppo JC, et al. Management of solitary nonparasitic liver cyst. *Am Surg* 1984;50:205

Goldberg SJ, Fonkalsrud E. Successful treatment of hepatic haemangioma with corticosteroids. *JAMA* 1969;208:2473

Hadad AR, Westbrook KC, et al. Symptomatic nonparasitic liver cysts. *Am J Surg* 1977;134:739

Ishak KG, Rabin L. Benign tumors of the liver. *Med Clin North Am* 1975;59:995

Kent DR, Nissen ED, et al. Maternal death resulting from rupture of a liver adenoma associated with oral contraceptives. *Obstet Gynecol* 1977;50:5

Kerlin P, Davis GL, et al. Hepatic adenoma and focal nodular hyperplasia: Clinical, pathologic, and radiologic features. *Gastroenterology* 1983;84:994

Koren E, Lazarovitch I, et al. Cystic hamartoma of the liver. *Int Surg* 1979;64:21

Leese T, Farges O, Bismuth H. Liver cell adenomas: a 12 year surgical experience from a specialist hepatobiliary unit. *Ann Surg* 1988;208:558

Linderkamp O, Hopner F, et al. Solitary hepatic hemangioma in the newborn infant complicated by cardiac failure, consumption coagulopathy, microangiopathic hemolytic anemia, and obstructive jaundice. *Eur J Pediatr* 1976;124:23

Litwin DE, Taylor BR, et al. Nonparasitic cysts of the liver: the case for conservative surgical management. *Ann Surg* 1987; 205:45

Lygidakis N. Diagnosis and treatment of intrabiliary rupture of hydatid cysts of the liver. *Arch Surg* 1983;118:1186

Moazam F, Rodgers BM, et al. Hepatic artery ligation for hepatic hemangiomatosis of infancy. *J Pediatr Surg* 1983;18:120

Nguyen L, Shandling B, et al. Hepatic hemangioma in childhood: medical management or surgical management. *J Pediatr Surg* 1982;17:576

Nissen ED, Kent DR, et al. Role of oral contraceptive agents in the pathogenesis of liver tumors. *Toxicol Environ Health* 1979;5:231

Rooks JB, Ory HW, et al. Epidemiology of hepatocellular adenoma: the role of oral contraceptive use. *JAMA* 1979;242: 644

Schwartz SI, Husser WC. Cavernous hemangioma of the liver: a single institution report of 16 resections. *Ann Surg* 1987; 205:456

Scott LD, Katz AR, et al. Oral contraceptives, pregnancy, and focal nodular hyperplasia of the liver. *JAMA* 1984;251:11

Shortell CK, Schwartz SI. Hepatic adenoma and focal nodular hyperplasia. *Surg Gynecol Obstet* 1991;173:426

Slovis TL, Berdan WE, et al. Hemangiomas of the liver in infants. *AJR Am J Roentgenol* 1975;123:791

Srouji MN, Chatten J, et al. Mesenchymal hamartoma of the liver in infants. *Cancer* 1978;42:2483

Stanley P, Geer GD, et al. Infantile hepatic hemangiomas: clinical features, radiologic investigations, and treatment of 20 patients. *Cancer* 1989;64:936

Wanless IR, Mawdsley C, Adams R. On the pathogenesis of focal nodular hyperplasia of the liver. *Hepatology* 1985;5:1194

Weinman MD, Chopra S. Tumors of the liver, other than primary hepatocellular carcinoma. *Gastroenterol Clin North Am* 1987;16:627

Williamson RCN, Ramus NI, et al. Congenital solitary cysts of the liver and spleen. *Br J Surg* 1978;65:871

53

Hepatocellular Carcinoma

Masatoshi Makuuchi ▪ *Seiji Kawasaki*

▪ EPIDEMIOLOGY

It is difficult to determine the incidence of hepatocellular carcinoma (HCC) accurately, since epidemiological data generally are based on vital statistics, the cancer registry, or autopsy; vital statistics and the cancer registry are based on diagnoses made by physicians, which often lack histological confirmation. Autopsy data are not very reliable, if the necropsy rate among patients who have died is low. Despite these limitations, epidemiological studies have shown clearly that HCC is one of the most common malignancies in the world, with a marked geographic variation.

The incidence of HCC is significantly higher in men than in women. The male/female ratio reportedly ranges up to 8:1 and tends to be higher in endemic than in nonendemic areas. The incidence rate tends to increase with age and to level off in old age. In endemic areas, HCC is seen frequently in individuals under 40 years of age, whereas it is extremely rare in low-risk populations. The main high-prevalence regions in the world are sub-Saharan Africa and Southeast Asia, and the tumor is less common in America, Europe, and Northern Africa. Age-standardized death rates owing to HCC, reported by the World Health Organization,[1–3] in selected countries are listed in Table 53–1. A relatively high variation in the incidence of HCC within a country also has been observed. This finding, and studies of migrating populations, both indicate that environmental factors rather than racial or genetic predisposition contribute much to hepatocarcinogenesis.

▪ PATHOPHYSIOLOGY

ETIOLOGY

It is estimated that more than 250 million people throughout the world are chronically infected with hepatitis B virus (HBV). A good geographic correlation between the incidence of HCC and the prevalence of HBsAg positivity has been demonstrated in some studies.[4] Several case-control studies[5,6] also have shown a significant incidence of HBsAg carriers among HCC patients in comparison with controls. The positivity rate of HBsAg patients ranged from 40% to 80% among HCC patients, compared with 5% to 10% among controls. Beasley and associates elegantly showed, in a controlled prospective study, that 70 cases of HCC developed among 3454 HBsAg carriers during a mean follow-up of 4.5 years, whereas only one case of HCC was observed during the same period in 19 253 noncarriers, giving a relative risk of 390 for an HBsAg carrier state.[7] All these studies have lent strong support to the etiological role of HBV in the development of HCC. A recent finding of a molecular biological study provides further strong evidence that HBV plays an important role in hepatocarcinogenesis. HBV-DNA can be integrated into the genomes of liver cell lines from HCC tissues in an experimental setting,[8] and integrated HBV-DNA actually has been found in malignant cells (and nonmalignant hepatocytes) obtained from HBsAg-positive HCC patients.[9]

Although HBV is a leading factor associated with the development of HCC in most of the high-prevalence re-

TABLE 53–1. AGE-ADJUSTED DEATH RATES FROM PRIMARY LIVER CANCER PER 100 000 POPULATION IN VARIOUS COUNTRIES[a]

Country	Male	Female
Hong Kong	29.1	7.8
Japan	22.8	7.3
Italy	11.8	5.2
France	9.0	1.8
Argentina	5.4	4.8
Sweden	4.4	2.8
Egypt	2.4	1.4
United States	2.1	0.9
Australia	2.0	0.9

[a]Death rates include primary and unspecified liver cancer.

gions throughout the world, this is not the case in some areas. In Japan, the number of patients who die from HCC has been increasing recently. However, this increase is not related to HBV infection but to non-A, non-B hepatitis, especially hepatitis C virus (HCV) infection. Currently, about 80% of cases of HCC in Japan are associated with chronic HCV infection. Similar results were documented by Bruix and associates in Spain, where the positivity rate for HCV antibody was 75% in patients with HCC.[10] Kiyosawa and associates reported that, in the case of HCV infection (anti-HCV-Ab-positive), the average intervals between blood transfusion (viral transmission) and diagnosis of chronic hepatitis, cirrhosis, and HCC were 10.0 ± 11.3 years, 21.2 ± 9.6 years, and 29.0 ± 13.2 years, respectively. Other Japanese researchers have reported similar results. In HBsAg-negative HCC patients, most of whom are anti-HCV-Ab-positive, the average age at which HCC is found is approximately 10 years older than in HBsAg-positive patients. Although HCV infection appears closely related to the development of HCC, its etiological role in hepatocarcinogenesis is probably different from that of HBV. HCV is a single-stranded RNA virus, so that integration of the viral genome into the human genome in hepatocytes does not occur as in the case of HBV. HCV also differs from HBV in other various aspects: (1) the possibility of vertical transmission (from mother to child) seems to be small, since the incidence of HCV infection is low in the younger generation, (2) it is not readily transmitted by sexual contact, (3) once transmitted to healthy adults, 50% to 60% of them develop chronic hepatitis, whereas in adult cases of HBV infection, the virus usually clears up after an episode of acute hepatitis.

The relationship between liver cirrhosis and HCC development is not clearly understood, since etiological agents such as HBV and HCV cause both cirrhosis and HCC, and it is uncertain whether the active regeneration process in the cirrhotic liver is closely related to hepatocarcinogenesis.

Alcohol is the most important factor responsible for liver cirrhosis in western countries, where the incidence of HCC is generally low. Although there is no evidence that alcohol itself is hepatocarcinogenic, there have been some case-control studies in which heavy drinkers have an increased risk of HCC. It has been reported that the majority of cases of alcoholic cirrhosis are micronodular, and that HCC develops in patients with alcoholic liver cirrhosis at an advanced stage (or at older age). By contrast, chronic viral hepatitis generally results in macronodular or mixed macro/micronodular cirrhosis, in which HCC tends to arise at an early stage.

It has been well-established that administration of aflatoxin, a mycotoxin produced by *Aspergillus flavus*, can cause liver tumors in certain animal species, and this agent has been considered to play an etiological role in HCC development in areas where foodstuffs are heavily contaminated by the toxin. Several studies have demonstrated that the amount of aflatoxin consumption is well correlated with HCC incidence.[12,13] Cocarcinogenic effects of aflatoxin with HBV also have been implicated, based on the finding that HCC tends to develop at a younger age in HBsAg-positive patients who live in highly contaminated areas.[14]

Alpha-1 antitrypsin deficiency and hemochromatosis also have been listed as conditions that increase the risk of HCC development.

NATURAL HISTORY

The natural course of patients with untreated hepatocellular carcinoma is generally dismal, although the survival period from the time of diagnosis varies somewhat according to the stage at which the diagnosis is made. Okuda and associates reported that the median survival of 229 patients with HCC who did not receive specific treatment was only 1.6 months.[15] If limited to the 33 patients in a favorable condition (tumor size <50% of the whole liver, no ascites, albumin level >3 g/dL, and bilirubin level <3 mg/dL), the median survival period was 8.3 months, in their series. Others have documented similar results for patients with advanced and symptomatic HCC, although some exceptional patients with advanced HCC have survived for a long time without any treatment.[16] The only report describing the natural history of minute HCC (<3 cm in diameter) gave survivals of 90.7%, 55%, and 12.8% at 1, 2, and 3 years, respectively, with an average of 20.7 ± 9.8 months.[17] The volume doubling time of a small HCC nodule is quite variable, ranging from 1.0 to 19.5 months (mean 6.5 ± 5.7 months) in one report[17] to 41 to 315 days in another.[18] Yoshino reported that the doubling time was short in patients with hepatitis B surface antigen (48 ± 8 days), compared with antigen-negative patients (140 ± 98 days).[18] Based on these reported values (the shortest doubling time was one month), it would take at least three months for a small round HCC nodule to double its diameter. Therefore, it is appropriate to perform follow-up examination, using ultrasound or CT for high-risk patients, every few months in order to detect small HCCs for which suitable treatment can be applied.

EARLY-STAGE HCC AND BORDERLINE LESIONS

Recent advances in imaging modalities and careful follow-up of high-risk patients have made it possible to detect small nodules in the liver frequently. Consequently, the number of liver resections for these small lesions has been increasing as surgical techniques become more refined. The resected specimens have been investigated by pathologists, who have thus accumulated considerable knowledge of early-stage HCC and so-called borderline or precancerous lesions.

The National Cancer Center group in Japan[19] defined "early HCC" as very well-differentiated tumor, corresponding to grade I of Edmondson and Steiner's classification,[20] without destruction of the underlying liver structure. Although Edmondson and Steiner classified cancer cell differentiation into four grades in 1954, few grade I tumors actually have been recognized until recently. The grade I early-stage HCC is usually <2 cm in diameter and demonstrates recognizable structural atypia with little cellular or nuclear atypia. An increase in the nuclear/cytoplasmic ratio compared with hepatocytes in the surrounding parenchyma, microacinar formation, increased basophilia or eosinophilia of the cytoplasm, and fatty change or clear cell change have been listed as histological diagnostic signs of early HCC.

Recently, adenomatous hyperplasia, which is recognized almost invariably as a sizeable nodule in a cirrhotic liver, has been implicated as a precancerous lesion on the basis of the following observations: (1) a high incidence of coexisting HCC and adenomatous hyperplasia was observed in an autopsy study,[21] (2) early-stage HCC has been detected within adenomatous hyperplasia, showing a nodule-in-nodule pattern, in some cases,[22] (3) in an HBsAg-positive patient with a minute lesion of early HCC within a nodule of adenomatous hyperplasia, DNA analysis indicated that both the HCC and surrounding adenomatous hyperplasia were derived from an identical clone,[23] (4) malignant transformation of nodules of biopsy-proven adenomatous hyperplasia has occurred during clinical follow-up.[24] A transitional state between early HCC and advanced HCC also has been recognized in some lesions where an area of advanced HCC (grade II or III tumor according to Edmondson and Steiner's classification) has existed within a nodule of early HCC. These findings suggest a multistep hepatocarcinogenesis sequence (liver cirrhosis to adenomatous hyperplasia to early HCC to advanced HCC) in humans,[25] although de novo occurrence of early or advanced HCC is another possible course. Some investigators have defined "atypical adenomatous hyperplasia" as a lesion intermediate between adenomatous hyperplasia and early HCC.[25,26] The nuclear/cytoplasmic ratio tends to increase in the following order: cirrhotic pseudolobule, adenomatous hyperplasia, atypical adenomatous hyperplasia, early HCC.

CLINICOPATHOLOGICAL FEATURES OF HCC

HCC has a strong tendency to invade the portal venous system. Once the tumor cells infiltrate the portal vein, they flow into the distal part of the liver and grow into daughter nodules. If these cells form a macroscopic tumor thrombus in the portal venous branch, the thrombus itself becomes a new source of cancer spread, as shown in Fig 53–1.[27] HCC also can invade hepatic vein tributaries and/or biliary ducts, although both occur less frequently than portal venous invasion. Extension of tumor thrombi in the hepatic vein into the inferior vena cava or even the right atrium is found in some cases.

Although cancer invasion into the biliary system rarely is encountered in a clinical setting, one autopsy study revealed that HCC growth into the hepatic duct and/or common bile duct was present in 6.1% of 439 cases.[28] Symptoms such as obstructive jaundice and hemobilia are clinical manifestations of this type of invasion.

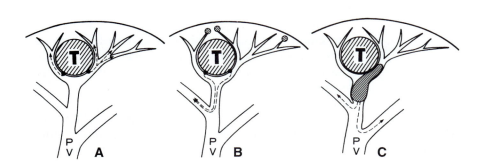

Figure 53–1. Intrahepatic extension and invasion of hepatocellular carcinoma. **A.** The tumor invades the portal venous branches, and tumor cells are carried to the distal part of the liver by the portal venous flow. **B.** These cells grow into microscopic tumor thrombi and then into daughter nodules. **C.** The tumor thrombus is, in turn, a source of wide tumor spread. T: tumor; PV: portal venous branch. (From Makuuchi M, Hasegawa H, et al. Ultrasonically guided subsegmentectomy. *Surg Gynecol Obstet* 1985;161:346)

The lung was found to be the most common site of extrahepatic metastases in an autopsy study,[29] followed by lymph nodes, intraperitoneal organs, the peritoneum, adrenal glands, bone, and brain.

■ DIAGNOSIS AND EVALUATION

SYMPTOMS

There is no distinctive symptom that indicates the presence of HCC. General malaise is the most common symptom, followed by anorexia, abdominal pain, abdominal fullness, and weight loss. However, these symptoms may be secondary to accompanying liver cirrhosis or chronic hepatitis. A large tumor sometimes can be palpated from the body surface. Ascites and edema also can occur as the first presenting symptoms, although again they merely may reflect exacerbation of underlying liver cirrhosis. Patients with a tumor thrombus in the main portal branch often suffer from diarrhea, ascites, and general malaise. Severe abdominal pain is associated with bleeding within the HCC nodule or tumor rupture into the peritoneal cavity. Tumor rupture leads to progressive anemia, shock, and abdominal fullness resulting from hemoperitoneum. Emergency abdominal angiography is indicated for the diagnosis and treatment of this condition. Jaundice can be observed in patients with HCC owing to either liver failure or tumor invasion of the biliary system. The latter frequently is associated with abdominal pain and hemobilia. In HCC patients with liver cirrhosis and portal hypertension, tumor invasion of the portal venous system may aggravate the portal hypertensive state and cause bleeding from esophagogastric varices or gastropathy. Extension of tumor growth through the hepatic vein into the inferior vena cava causes Budd-Chiari syndrome, characterized by ascites, edema of the lower extremities, dilated collateral veins in the abdominal wall, and hepatosplenomegaly. However, no radical treatment is indicated for the majority of patients presenting with the symptoms described above, since either the HCC itself or underlying liver cirrhosis is generally too advanced. Regular check-up of high-risk patients, including those with liver cirrhosis and/or chronic hepatitis, is important in order to detect small HCC, which is usually asymptomatic.

LABORATORY FINDINGS

Routine liver function tests do not disclose the presence of HCC; they can only detect underlying liver disease. Although both clinical signs and routine laboratory data can provide information on the degree of liver dysfunction to some extent, a more specific test, such as measurement of the indocyanine green retention rate, is useful for precise judgment in order to select the type of treatment for HCC patients with associated chronic liver disease.

Alpha-fetoprotein (AFP) and protein induced by absence of vitamin K or by antagonist II (PIVKA II)[30] have been accepted as specific tumor markers for HCC. In Japan, measurement of these tumor markers together with ultrasonography and CT scan are conducted as regular follow-up procedures in order to detect HCC in high-risk patients or to diagnose recurrence after hepatic resection. The reported incidence of an elevated serum AFP level (>200 ng/mL) in patients with HCC ranges from 65% to 75%,[31] while that of PIVKA-II is in the range 55% to 62%.[32,33] Measurements of AFP and PIVKA-II levels complement each other, and no significant correlation has been observed between the levels of the two markers. Ono and associates reported that 80.8% of HCC patients had elevated levels of one or both markers, suggesting the usefulness of simultaneous measurement of AFP and PIVKA-II for the diagnosis of HCC.[32]

RADIOLOGIC FINDINGS

Various imaging modalities, including ultrasonography, computed tomography (CT), magnetic resonance imaging (MRI), and angiography now are used in combination to make a correct diagnosis of HCC. Using these procedures, a HCC nodule should be differentiated from other nodular lesions, and its exact location should be investigated in relation to intrahepatic vascular and biliary structures.

Ultrasound

It is easy to differentiate HCC from metastatic liver tumor or hemangioma by ultrasound examination alone, if the tumor is a typical nodular-type HCC. A thin halo with lateral shadows and a mosaic pattern reflect the surrounding capsule and a nodule-in-nodule pattern with separating fibrous septa, respectively. Minimum ultrasound attenuation through a HCC nodule creates posterior echo enhancement on ultrasound images[34] (Fig 53–2). However, these characteristic ultrasound features of HCC may not necessarily be evident, especially when the tumor is at an early stage. Early-stage HCC appears as a homogeneously hyperechoic or hypoechoic mass on ultrasound, which is not easily differentiated from hemangioma, focal fatty change (hyperechoic), adenomatous hyperplasia (hyperechoic or hypoechoic), a large regenerative nodule, or an area without fatty infiltration in a steatotic liver (hypoechoic).

Ultrasonic detection of changes indicative of liver cirrhosis and portal hypertension, such as compensatory hypertrophy of the left lobe of the liver, splenomegaly, and dilated left gastric or paraumbilical veins, is useful

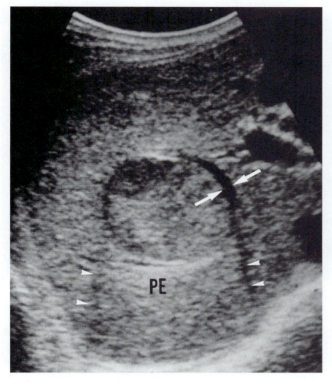

A

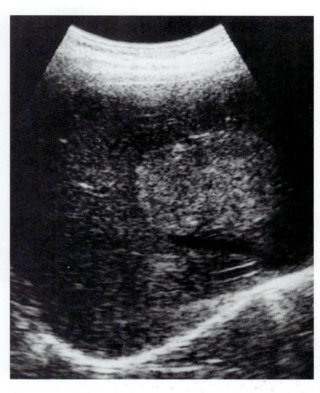

B

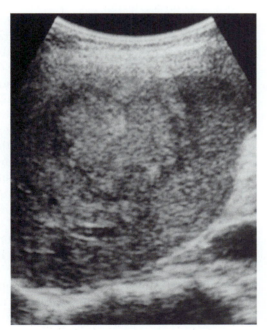

C

Figure 53–2. Differential diagnosis of HCC from cavernous hemangioma and metastatic liver tumor on ultrasound images. **A**. Nodular-type HCC. Characteristic features include a thin halo (*arrows*), lateral shadows (*arrow heads*), posterior echo enhancement (*PE*), and a mosaic-pattern appearance of the tumor. **B**. Cavernous hemangioma. This tumor appears as a hyperechoic lesion with a finely indented circular border. **C**. Metastatic liver tumor. The tumor shows a bosselated appearance with a wide, irregular hypoechoic rim.

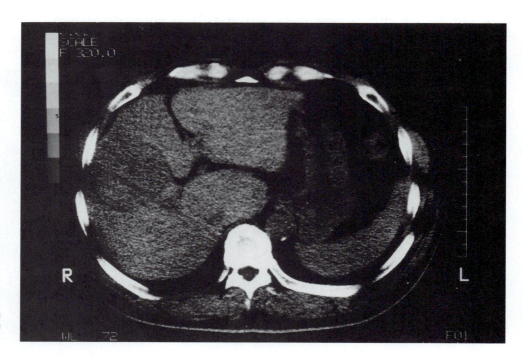

Figure 53–3. Plain CT image of HCC. A thin circular hypodense band corresponding to the fibrous capsule is evident.

for the differential diagnosis of HCC from lesions that usually develop in noncirrhotic liver. Tumor thrombi in the portal vein, hepatic vein, or inferior vena cava, which frequently are found by ultrasound examination, are highly suggestive of HCC and may change the indication for surgical treatment.

Unlike other diagnostic modalities, ultrasonic images can be obtained from various directions. This property allows accurate localization of the HCC nodule in relation to intrahepatic vascular structures, so that the type of liver resection can be selected preoperatively, although a final decision is made on the basis of intraoperative ultrasound investigation.[34]

Computed Tomography

CT scans with and without administration of contrast medium have been performed for the diagnosis of HCC. The fibrous capsule of HCC frequently is shown as a thin hypodense band surrounding the tumor on CT without contrast (Fig 53–3). In addition to these routine procedures, serial CT scans at the same slice level following bolus injection of contrast medium (dynamic CT) is very useful for differentiating HCC from other hepatic lesions. A typical HCC nodule is demonstrated as a hyperdense mass with an internal mosaic architecture in the early phase, and in the late phase as a hypodense lesion surrounded by an enhanced fibrous capsule (Fig 53–4). In contrast, cavernous hemangioma, which is the most common benign tumor with hypervascularity, shows prolonged enhancement on dynamic CT. However, these characteristic features are not evident in a small well-dif-

ferentiated HCC, since it is usually hypovascular and less frequently associated with a surrounding fibrous capsule. Other advanced methods of CT scanning have been developed and used for preoperative examination in order to diagnose HCC nodules precisely. These include CT scanning during injection of dye through the hepatic artery (arterial CT)[35] or during the portal venous phase following the injection of contrast medium into the superior mesenteric artery (portal CT)[36] (Fig 53–5). The latter method is sensitive for the detection of minute well-differentiated HCC, which is usually seen as a hypodense lesion since portal venous perfusion is decreased in the HCC nodule compared with the surrounding liver parenchyma. CT scanning 2 to 3 weeks after injection of iodized poppyseed oil through the hepatic artery (Lipiodol CT)[37] also has been advocated. This technique is especially useful for detecting small intrahepatic metastases of HCC (Fig 53–6).

Angiography

Angiography used to be the only accurate diagnostic imaging modality for the detection of HCC. However, its central role in the radiologic diagnosis of HCC gradually has been replaced by other imaging techniques. Angiography now is used in combination with CT as described above, or as a therapeutic approach in the form of transcatheter arterial chemoembolization for inoperable HCCs. A tortuous rich neovasculature is a typical feature of HCC in the arterial phase of hepatic angiography, and tumor staining is observed in the venous phase (Fig 53–7). Arterioportal venous shunting or portal perfusion

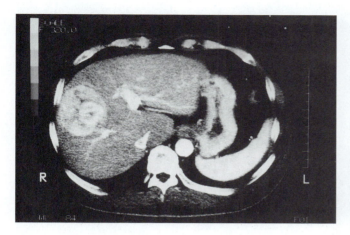

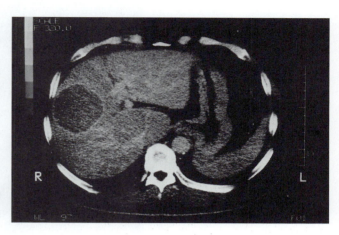

A

B

Figure 53–4. HCC on dynamic CT. **A.** Early phase. The tumor is seen as a hyperdense mass with a nodule-in-nodule appearance. **B.** Late phase. The tumor becomes hypodense, whereas the capsule is enhanced.

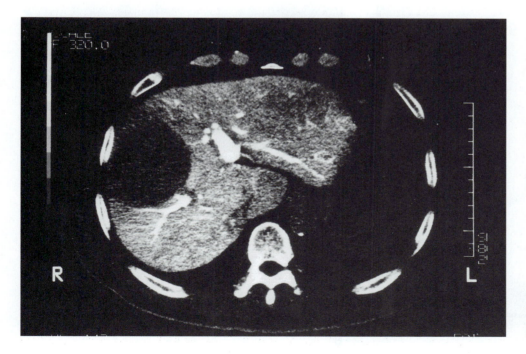

Figure 53–5. Portal CT (CT scanning during the portal venous phase after injection of contrast medium into the superior mesenteric artery). The tumor is totally hypodense since little portal blood flow feeds the HCC.

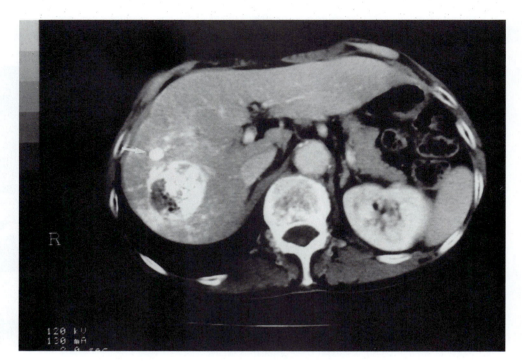

Figure 53–6. Lipiodol CT. A small lipiodol deposit indicating intrahepatic metastasis (*arrow*) is identified close to the main HCC nodule.

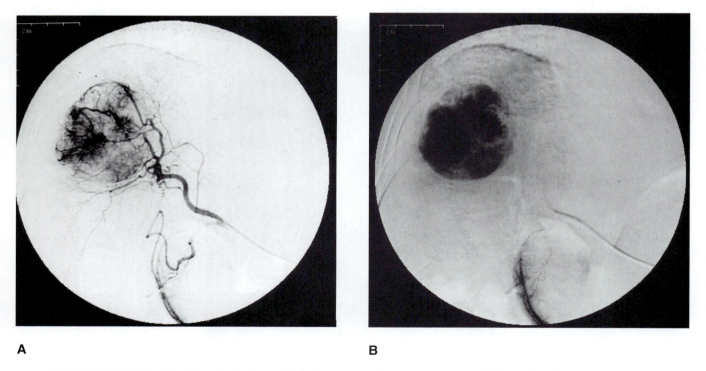

A

B

Figure 53–7. Hepatic arteriography. **A**. Arterial phase. Irregular tortuous arteries feeding the tumor are demonstrated. **B**. Tumor staining (a nodule-in-nodule appearance) is shown in the late phase.

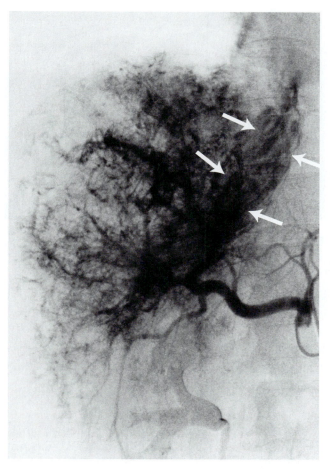

Figure 53–8. Advanced HCC occupying the right lobe. Fine arteries feeding a tumor thrombus in the hepatic vein (*white arrows*) are evident (thread and streaks sign).

defects corresponding to tumor thrombi in the portal vein are frequently seen on angiography for advanced-stage HCC. Several fine arteries feeding tumor thrombus in the portal and hepatic veins often are demonstrated as the "thread and streaks" sign (Fig 53–8).

Magnetic Resonance Imaging

Similar to other imaging techniques, MRI demonstrates characteristic features of HCC such as a thin fibrous capsule and mosaic pattern (Fig 53–9). The fibrous capsule can be seen clearly as a low-intensity ring on T1-weighted imaging. Fibrous septa within the tumor, which create a mosaic architecture, also are depicted as low-intensity bands. Tumor thrombi are revealed as high-intensity areas in the dilated portal vein, which appears hypointense. Whereas most tumors are shown as low-intensity areas on T1-weighted images, HCCs are demonstrated as high-intensity nodules in approximately half of all cases.[38] Adenomatous hyperplasia also shows characteristic high intensity on T1-weighted im-

ages and low intensity on T2-weighted images,[39] in contrast to MRI images of other kinds of tumors. MRI images with contrast enhancement using gadopentetate dimeglumine (Gd-DTPA) are of similar diagnostic usefulness to contrast or dynamic CT in the case of HCC.[40]

DIFFERENTIAL DIAGNOSIS

In patients with chronic hepatitis and/or liver cirrhosis who have been followed-up as high-risk patients, it is most likely that newly identified tumors in the liver are HCC or precancerous lesions. While metastatic tumors or cholangiocellular carcinoma are rare in these patients, cavernous hemagioma frequently is detected. Ultrasound findings such as a hyperechoic lesion with posterior echo enhancement and absence of a hypoechoic halo are highly suggestive of hemangioma. Multiplicity and an irregular shape are indirect findings indicative of hemangioma. A typical small hemangioma accompanied by a peripheral hyperechoic ring does not need further investigation, and follow-up should be conducted with ultrasound. Dynamic CT or MRI is indicated for atypical echogenic tumors >2 cm in diameter. Hemangioma is diagnosed on the basis of dense contrast enhancement from the tumor margin on dynamic CT,[41] and an extremely high signal in the T2-weighted image on MRI.[42] High values of AFP and PIVKA-II are other diagnostic clues for HCC, although there are some AFP-producing tumors other than HCC.

Differential diagnosis of HCC from other kinds of hypervascular tumor should be made cautiously in patients without chronic liver disease. Hypervascular tumors including lipoma, hemangiomyolipoma, focal nodular hyperplasia (FNH), liver cell adenoma (LCA), and cavernous hemangioma need to be differentiated from HCC, since most of these tumors do not require surgical treatment. Lipoma or hemangiomyolipoma is suggested when fat density is identified in the tumor on CT scan. A large artery entering the center of the tumor with a "spoked-wheel" appearance on arteriography is the typical sign of a large FNH. A central scar occasionally is demonstrated with ultrasound or CT. When colloid scintigraphy demonstrates uptake of 99Tc phytate, this is a definite sign of FNH, seen in 20% to 40% of cases. Kudo reported that ultrasound during angiography can demonstrate a small HCC as a tumor with a spoked-wheel appearance.[43] Fine arterial proliferation and faint staining for a very short period are seen in small LCA, but these findings also are evident in small HCC. In patients without chronic liver disease and in whom tumor markers for HCC are negative, fine-needle core biopsy is indicated in order to differentiate FNH and LCA from HCC. A diagnosis of FNH can be obtained when scar tissue and bile ductule proliferation are seen in the specimen. The characteristic histologi-

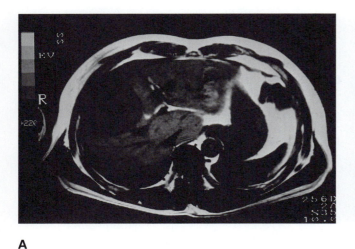

A

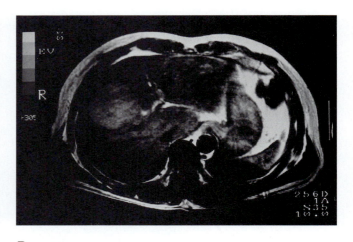

B

Figure 53–9. HCC on magnetic resonance imaging. **A.** T1-weighted image. **B.** T2-weighted image.

cal feature of LCA is proliferation of cytologically normal liver cells that are arranged in cord structures. Therefore, it is very difficult to differentiate LCA from borderline lesions and very well-differentiated HCC, even on histologic examination. All LCAs and FNH without definite findings on histology should be resected. It is difficult to differentiate between very small HCCs and borderline lesions ranging from 1.0 to 1.5 cm in diameter, even if fine-needle core biopsy is carried out. CT and angiography often fail to detect these small lesions. The best way of differentiating among these nodules is follow-up, since both very small HCCs and borderline lesions are very slow-growing. If a tumor is shown to grow 2 cm in diameter by ultrasound, CT scan and angiography are performed and the most appropriate treatment is selected. Prophylactic alcohol injection may be effective for borderline lesions.

A liver tumor with a target pattern and a bosselated surface on ultrasound is either a metastatic tumor or a cholangiocellular carcinoma. Surveillance of the gastrointestinal tract and pancreas is required in this setting.

■ TREATMENT

Current popular treatments for HCC are surgical resection, transcatheter arterial embolization, and percutaneous ethanol injection. Arterial ligation, arterial catheterization followed by chemotherapy through the catheter, arterial one-shot chemotherapy and systemic chemotherapy also are used, but are not as widely practiced as the former three modalities.

NONSURGICAL TREATMENTS

Transcatheter Arterial Embolization

Transcatheter arterial embolization (TAE) is used most commonly in patients with unresectable HCC. HCCs are generally hypervascular and fed almost exclusively by arterial blood, so that the tumor becomes necrotic, if its arterial blood supply is interrupted. TAE was performed first by Goldstein and associates,[44] and later was applied by Yamada and associates to patients with HCC.[45] TAE is highly effective for most HCCs, except early ones and those with faint staining.[46] TAE may not be indicated for patients whose total bilirubin level is >3 mg/dL, since it can produce severe liver dysfunction.[47] When the serum level of total bilirubin exceeds 2 mg/dL, the area to be embolized should be limited to one or two Couinaud segments. A tumor thrombus in the main portal trunk has been considered a contraindication for TAE. However, TAE is applicable, even in the presence of a tumor thrombus, if collateral circulation of the portal blood to the liver is demonstrated by arterial portography, or if one of the major portal venous branches is opacified. When one of the major portal venous branches is obstructed, the type of TAE should be selected according to the patient's liver functional status, in a manner similar to the indication for liver resection (Fig 53–10). It has been believed that dual blood supply to the liver (hepatic artery and portal vein) can prevent post-TAE damage to the liver. However, when the entire arterial blood supply is obstructed, the liver becomes necrotic in some patients. Furthermore, necrosis of the bile duct frequently is encountered.[48] These phenomena are experienced in liver transplantation when arterial thrombosis of the graft occurs. Necrosis of the non-

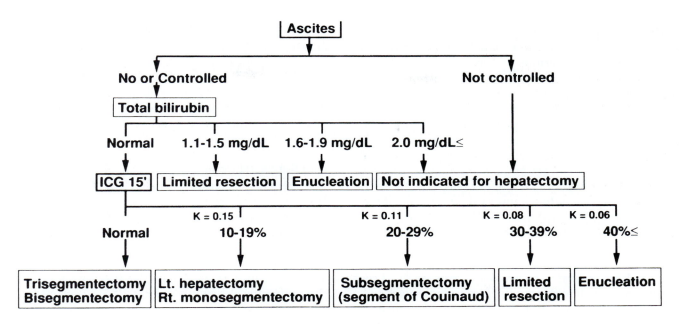

Figure 53–10. Decision tree for selection of operative procedures in patients with HCC and liver cirrhosis. (From Makuuchi M, Kosuge T, et al. Surgery for small liver cancers. *Sem Surg Oncol* 1993;9:298)

cancerous liver does not occur after TAE because there is portal blood flow and also a rich collateral blood supply to the liver through the bile duct and perivascular connective tissue.

In the current standard procedure of TAE, the femoral artery is punctured and a catheter is introduced into the common hepatic artery using the Seldinger technique. A thinner catheter then is advanced using the coaxial catheter system into the segmental or subsegmental hepatic arterial branches. Emulsion consisting of lipiodol, urografin, and anticancer drugs is administered, followed by injection of gelfoam cubes that are permeated by chemotherapeutic agents.[49,50] Injection of embolic material without any drug is performed only rarely, and some anticancer agents usually are coadministered. The most common complications associated with TAE are upper abdominal pain (59%) and fever (47%).[51] Ulceration of the stomach and duodenum, pancreatitis, and cholecystitis may occur when embolic materials flow into the arteries feeding these organs. Takayasu and associates reported that cholecystitis was observed in 53% of patients undergoing TAE, in their early series.[52] This complication can be prevented if the tip of the catheter is advanced beyond the site where the cystic artery branches off.

The response rate for TAE was reported to be 65%.[49] Necrosis of the main tumor was seen in 90% of patients. The rate of necrosis of HCC is highest in patients with tumors 2 to 3 cm in diameter,[53] whereas it is not effective for tumor thrombus, intracapsular infiltration, or

small intrahepatic metastasis.[50] The reported survival rates after TAE are approximately 40% to 60% at 1 year, 20% to 30% at 3 years, and 5% to 10% at 5 years. However, it can be quite variable, depending on the patient's condition. When tumor thrombi are present in the main portal vein, most patients die within 1 year after TAE. Okazaki and associates reported that 1 year survival rates for patients with and without tumor thrombi were 15% (n=163) and 69.1% (n=479), respectively.[47] In patients without tumor thrombi, a high serum albumin value, adjunctive hepatic resection, and a small (<2 cm) HCC appear to be significantly favorable prognostic factors after TAE.[53a]

Although preoperative TAE prior to hepatic resection used to be performed widely, it did not affect or even adversely affect the overall survival of the patient.[54] This finding may be explained by the fact that preoperative TAE makes it difficult to perform postoperative TAE for HCC recurrence after liver resection. Development of a collateral arterial blood supply to the liver, after TAE, is the major cause of tumor regrowth in the liver. Replaced hepatic arteries[55] and the right phrenic arteries often are embolized, but other anonymous small arteries and the gastroepiproic artery can enter the liver after all the major arteries have been obstructed.

Percutaneous Ethanol Injection Therapy

Absolute ethanol fixes all kinds of soft tissue. HCC is a soft and fragile tumor that can be permeated widely by injected alcohol. Percutaneous ethanol injection therapy (PEIT) for HCC was started by Shinagawa and associates, in 1985,[56] and now is used in patients with small HCC or borderline lesions.[57–59] Patients who have HCCs no more than 3 cm in diameter and no more than 3 nodules are considered to be good candidates for PEIT.[60] Under ultrasound guidance, a 22G needle is inserted into the tumor and 2 to 5 mL of absolute ethanol is injected according to the tumor size. When the tumor is large, injection proceeds from the deeper part of the tumor because bubbles of the alcohol disturb ultrasound monitoring. When the tumor is filled with alcohol bubbles and turns echogenic, injection of alcohol is stopped. This procedure is repeated several times on separate days. Contraindications are patient noncooperation and severe coagulation disorders. It is very important not to inject alcohol into vessels or ducts in order to avoid necrosis of the liver parenchyma or bile ducts, which may cause liver failure or jaundice. Koda and associates reported atrophy of the whole right lobe of the liver following PEIT.[61] Common complications of this procedure are fever and severe pain owing to leakage of alcohol into the abdominal cavity. Survivals at 1, 3, and 5 years after PEIT were documented to be higher than 90%, 60%, and 40%, respectively. Livraghi and associates recently reported that survival after PEIT reached 76% at 3 years in 207 patients with solitary HCCs <3 cm.[62] Our recent investigation, sponsored by the Ministry of Health and Welfare of Japan (directed by Shimamura) collected data on patients with HCC treated by surgical resection, TAE, or ethanol injection.[63] When the analysis was limited to patients whose tumor size and number were no more than 3 cm and three or less, respectively, the survival rates for the first 5 years were 94%, 87%, 78%, 66%, and 58% after hepatic resection (n=566), 75%, 68%, 42%, 22%, and 13% after TAE (n=84), and 98%, 94%, 87%, 61%, and 47% after ethanol injection (n=109), respectively (unpublished data). Thus, ethanol injection therapy seems to produce better survival than hepatic resection during the first few years, but thereafter, survival declines rapidly, showing the same tendency as for TAE. In addition, the background factors for the hepatic resection and PEIT groups differed in this study: 95% of patients who underwent surgery had HCC nodules >2 cm, whereas 65% of the PEIT group had tumors <2 cm in diameter. For HCC tumors no more than 2 cm in diameter, 82% of patients had well-differentiated HCC (early HCC) or a borderline lesion. In our experience, surgical resection for early HCC provides an excellent outcome, with a 5 year survival of 100%. Therefore, even for very small HCCs, surgical resection is the first choice of treatment and the indications for PEIT are limited, especially in institutions where there are experienced hepatic surgeons.

Using a similar technique, chemotherapeutic agents,[57] interleukin-2,[64] and OK-432[65] have been injected into the tumor. However, results were not as good as those of ethanol injection. Combination therapy using PEIT and TAE for HCCs >3 cm in diameter is now under investigation. Tanaka and associates documented that this combined therapy led to total necrosis of the HCC nodule in 83% of cases.[66]

Other Nonsurgical Treatments

Systemic chemotherapy, one-shot arterial injection of anticancer drugs, percutaneous catheterization into the hepatic artery, and radiation therapy have been carried out. Systemic chemotherapy was widely applied to patients with HCC after the introduction of doxorubicin. However, the drug dosage usually is limited owing to underlying liver disease, and the response rate after chemotherapy was found to be <10%, in recent studies.[67–70] If confined to patients who responded to treatment, the survival curve after systemic chemotherapy was similar to that of TAE. Since there are various effective therapeutic approaches for HCC patients, systemic chemotherapy is regarded as a last resort. Arterial chemotherapy has been performed either as a bolus injection during angiography or by infusing the chemotherapeutic agents through an infusion pump or port. It has been demonstrated that the drug concentration in the tumor is increased by its combined use with lipiodol, and that the lipiodol concentration in the tumor is related to the extent of tumor necrosis.[71,72] However, Kalayci and associates reported that the survival rate did not differ between patients given arterial injection of doxorubicin with lipiodol and those given intravenous administration of doxorubicin without lipiodol.[73] Mitoxantrone and cisplatin also have been used intraarterially, giving response rates of 25%[74] and 17%,[75] respectively. Arterial administration of cisplatin suspended in lipiodol has produced a response rate of 46%.[76] Recently, administration of fluorodeoxyuridine and mitomycin C from an implantable pump without lipiodol produced a 40% response rate.[77] Further study will be necessary to define whether coadministration of lipiodol and chemotherapeutic agents through the artery really enhances the anticancer effect.

Conventional radiation therapy rarely is indicated because it can produce significant damage to the noncancerous liver. A combination of radiation with other treatments, such as TAE, is worth attempting. Internal irradiation using iodine 131 (^{131}I)-labeled lipiodol was performed by Park and associates[78] and Kobayashi and associates[79] and was reported to be as effective as TAE.

Immunotherapy using lymphokine-activated killer cells,[80–82] tumor infiltrating lymphocytes,[83] and interferon[84] has been carried out. Monoclonal antibody against ferritin[85,86] and hyperthermia also have been tried. The effectiveness of these new therapies for HCC remains to be established.

The growth of HCC may be affected by hormones, and HCC has both androgen[87] and estrogen receptors.[88,89] While antiandrogen treatment does not seem to be effective, Farinati and associates reported that antiestrogen therapy, using tamoxifen, improved the survival time of patients with HCC.[90]

SURGICAL TREATMENTS

Indications for Hepatectomy

Liver Function Tests and Resectable Area of the Liver. Indications for hepatectomy are decided mainly by two factors, the spread of HCC and liver function. The Child-Pough classification has been applied widely for evaluating the liver functional reserve in patients with chronic liver disease. It is useful for deciding operative indications for portal hypertension. However, this classification does not indicate how much of the noncancerous liver can be removed together with the tumor in HCC patients with associated chronic liver disease. Various indicators have been advocated for this purpose, but no definite scheme has been established for predicting the safe limit of hepatectomy. Based on our own clinical experience, these authors have selected patients and decided the resection area using the criteria shown in Fig 53–10.[91,92] The primary selection criterion is the presence of ascites. If ascites is not easily controlled with diuretics, hepatectomy is not carried out. The second parameter is the serum total bilirubin level. Hepatic resection is not indicated when the total bilirubin level is persistently higher than 2 mg/dL. Limited resection and enucleation of the tumor can be performed safely in patients whose serum total bilirubin levels range from 1.1 to 1.4 mg/dL and from 1.5 to 1.9 mg/dL, respectively. If the total bilirubin level is normal, the indocyanine-green retention rate at 15 mins (ICG 15′) and its plasma disappearance rate (K-ICG) are used as parameters for selecting the type of hepatectomy. Major hepatic resection such as right hepatectomy and right or left trisegmentectomy can be tolerated if the ICG 15′ value is <10% (K-ICG >0.15). For patients with ICG 15′ within the range of 10% to 19%, one-third of the liver parenchyma can be resected. This resection corresponds to left hepatectomy, right anterior segmentectomy, or right posterior segmentectomy. Central bisegmentectomy also is included when the left medial segment is small. Segments 7 and 8 or segments 5 and 6 can be removed in combination. When the ICG 15′ value ranges from 20% to 29%, approximately one-sixth of the liver parenchyma can be resected. This resection roughly is equivalent to Couinaud's segments.

Limited resection[93] is indicated in patients whose ICG 15′ values are 30% to 39%. Enucleation of the tumor is applied in patients with an ICG 15′ value of >40%.

When the extension of HCC in the liver is limited to the resectable area defined according to the above criteria, hepatectomy is indicated even if multiple tumors are present. If tumor thrombus exists in the portal venous branch, all the portal areas distal to the tip of the tumor thrombus have to be removed. Therefore, right hepatectomy is indicated when the tumor thrombus buds into the right portal vein. The presence of tumor thrombus in the main portal vein precludes radical hepatic resection.

Preoperative Portal Venous Branch Embolization. When liver resections larger than or equal to Healey's segment are needed, volumetry of the segments and lobes is carried out by CT scan or MRI. If resection of the noncancerous liver exceeds 60% of the whole liver excluding the tumor, or if liver resection larger than the limit in Fig 53–1 is necessary for a HCC patient with liver dysfunction, portal venous branch embolization of the area to be resected is indicated, with the aim of inducing atrophy of the resection part and hypertrophy of the future remnant liver. This method was first introduced by our team in 1982 in patients with hilar bile duct carcinoma.[94] Since HCC grows faster than the bile duct carcinoma, and arterioportal shunting is common, TAE should be done before portal venous branch embolization. There are two routes of portal embolization, percutaneous portography and transileocolic portography technique.[95] The embolic materials used are gelfoam powder (2 gm), thrombin powder (5000 μ), meglumine sodium amidotrizoate (60% urografin, 40 mL) and gentamicin sulfate (40 mg). A 6-French (Fr) balloon catheter is inserted into the embolizing portal venous branch and the mixture of embolic materials is injected under fluoroscopic control until the blood flow becomes slow. Then the balloon is inflated and the embolic materials are added until all the portal venous branches to be embolized are filled with contrast material. A few minutes after injection of the embolus, the balloon is deflated. The balloon should be placed 1 or 2 cm away from the origin of the embolized portal venous branch to prevent the embolic material flowing back into the nonembolized part of the portal vein. Complications of portal embolization are rare. Fever, pain and elevation of liver enzymes levels are milder than those after TAE. One to six months later, hepatectomy is carried out. After hepatectomy, increment of the serum total bilirubin value, which is a sign of liver insufficiency, is usually not significant in patients who have undergone portal embolization.

Kinoshita and associates also have applied this method in order to enhance the effect of preoperative TAE on HCC.[96]

Varices and Hypersplenism. Esophageal varices and hypersplenism are common preoperative complications in patients with HCC. For treatment of esophageal varices before hepatic resection, sclerotherapy is indicated, since rupture of esophageal varices is life-threatening. Hassab's procedure (devascularization of the lower esophagus and upper stomach together with splenectomy) is selected for gastric varices. Since hypersplenism may raise the serum bilirubin level owing to overdestruction of red blood cells, it is difficult to evaluate the liver functional status precisely in terms of serum bilirubin in HCC patients with this complication. We carry out splenectomy for these patients, and judge the indications for hepatectomy 1 month later, according to Fig 53–1. Hassab's operation can be performed together with hepatectomy when the patient's ICC 15′ value is no more than 30%. If the tumor is located superficially and the liver mass to be resected is very small, hepatectomy together with Hassab's procedure is indicated for patients with an ICG 15′ of up to 40%.

Tumor Thrombus. Since tumor thrombus is one of the most common forms of tumor extension in HCC, a special effort should be made to detect its presence. In an autopsy study, tumor thrombi were demonstrated in the portal vein in 54% of HCC patients, in both the portal and hepatic veins in 28%, and in the hepatic vein only in 1.6%.[97] In our experience, 9.6% of 718 patients with HCC who underwent surgery had tumor thrombi. Patients with tumor thrombi in the portal vein generally have a poor prognosis. If a thrombus is located in the main portal vein or its bifurcation, the prognosis is dismal and hepatic resection usually is not indicated. Although some groups have attempted surgery for this type of tumor extension, the results have not been satisfactory.[98] On the other hand, tumor thrombus in the hepatic vein is potentially curable, especially when it is limited to within the liver. A small tumor thrombus budding into the inferior vena cava can be removed easily and the surgical outcome is not poor. Surgical intervention using cardiopulmonary bypass[99] has been reported for long extension of tumor thrombus into the right atrium, although this type of extension often is associated with lung embolism and/or lung metastasis.

Tumor thrombus in the bile duct is rare, and it has been seen in only 0.56% of our 718 patients with HCC. The first symptoms are obstructive jaundice and colicky pain. When a polypoid mass is identified in the bile duct on diagnostic imaging, this complication should be suspected. Small irregular masses detached from the major thrombus in the bile duct are frequently seen owing to the fragility and bleeding tendency of a HCC tumor thrombus. Tumor markers (AFP and PIVKA-II), serum markers of hepatitis virus, and tumors in the liver parenchyma need to be checked. When the bile ducts show significant dilation, percutaneous biliary drainage is indicated. A tumor thrombus in the bile duct generally responds well to TAE, unlike the case of thrombus in vessels. Hepatectomy should be considered after the patient has recovered from obstructive jaundice.

Rupture of HCC. Rupture of HCC has been seen in 3% of patients with resectable HCC, in our experience, and is an important issue in the treatment of HCC. TAE should be carried out for ruptured HCC if the serum total bilirubin value is no more than 3 mg/dL.[100] The liver function then is evaluated after the patient has recovered from shock status and post-TAE damage of the liver. Surgical indication is decided according to the criteria in Fig 53–1. Using this procedure (TAE + second-stage liver resection), long-term survival can be expected,[101] whereas almost all patients with ruptured HCC have been reported to die within 1 year after treatment by arterial ligation only[102,103] or TAE.[104]

When an angiographer is not available or if laparotomy has been done without suspecting a ruptured HCC, temporary packing or compression of the ruptured site should be done for hemostasis, and the arterial branch feeding the HCC is exposed at the hepatic hilus. A small sheathed needle is inserted into the hepatic arterial branch as far as possible, and intraoperative embolization is carried out. Complete hemostasis can be obtained by this procedure. Hepatectomy should be performed if resection of the tumor seems easy.

Operative Procedures

Perioperative Care. Liver resection should be avoided immediately after admission, in patients with chronic hepatitis and liver cirrhosis. A certain period of bedrest can improve the general condition of the patient and decrease the levels of transaminase.

Fresh frozen plasma (FFP) is transfused during hepatectomy. The amount of infusion usually is adjusted to exceed the amount of blood loss by 10% to 20%. Whole blood is not transfused unless the amount of bleeding exceeds 1,500 mL or unless the hematocrit value becomes <30%. Estimation of blood loss is not always reliable in patients with chronic liver disease, since a large amount of ascites and lymph fluid is included. Intraoperative infusion of sodium should be restricted, since FFP contains high sodium.

Just before starting division of the liver, 100 mg of hydrocortisone is administered in order to protect the liver from ischemia. A sufficient level of anesthesia and muscle relaxation is required in order to decrease the thoracic and right atrial pressures. The tidal volume of respiration is kept at a minimum level with the increase in respiratory rate. These forms of anesthetic management can help reduce the loss of blood during liver transection.[92] Blood inflow to the area of the liver scheduled for resection is occluded by Pringle's maneuver[105] or the selective vascular occlusion technique.[106] The presence of a left hepatic artery arising from the left gastric artery needs to be checked when the vascular occlusion technique is applied prior to liver transection. When the blood pressure is reduced as a result of bleeding from the hepatic vein or inferior vena cava, most anesthesiologists try to keep the depth of anesthesia shallow. However, this procedure may lead to air embolism, if the patient takes a deep spontaneous breath.

If the serum potassium level exceeds 4.0 mmol/L just after the operation, potassium-free solution is given. Acidosis owing to transfusion usually is not corrected because this turns alkalosis spontaneously after the operation and because the use of bicarbonate results in excessive sodium infusion. FFP is given at about 15 mL/kg/day until the total protein reaches 6.5 gm/dL. Chloride-rich amino acid solution is administered at 400 to 600 mL/day to prevent alkalosis resulting from citrate in the FFP. Electrolyte solution without sodium is infused at about 1 mL/kg/hr. The total amount of water, including FFP, is restricted to 40 to 45 mL/kg/day. Glucose is started at 0.1 gm/kg/hr and its administration is increased gradually by 0.05 gm/kg/hr until it reaches 0.25 gm/kg/hr. A sufficient amount of insulin is used to control the serum glucose level.

Once FFP administration has been discontinued, the amino acid solution is switched from a chloride-rich to an acid base–balanced one and a maintenance dose of sodium is added. Furosemide is given, if there is a water retention tendency. Potassium canrenoate is switched to spironolactone after the start of oral intake.

Intraoperative Ultrasonography.
After laparotomy has been accomplished, intraoperative ultrasonography (IOUS) is carried out to estimate the extent of HCC and the vascular architecture of the liver. Small tumors in a cirrhotic liver often are not recognizable from the liver surface.[107] Among 718 patients with HCC, 47% of them had at least one invisible and nonpalpable tumor nodule. In 371 patients with HCCs, no more than 5 cm in diameter and associated liver cirrhosis, this figure reached 66%. Therefore, precise liver resection is not possible without IOUS for these invisible and nonpalpable tumors. By IOUS, new nodules that are not detected preoperatively very often are found.[108] When a new minute lesion is demonstrated by IOUS and its histologic nature cannot be defined, thick-needle biopsy (14G, Tru-cut) is carried out and its histologic nature is confirmed by frozen section. Tumor thrombus was seen in 9.6% of HCC patients in our series. IOUS found 73% of the thrombi, whereas preoperative ultrasound and hepatic arteriography with arterial portography demonstrated only 26% and 19%, respectively. In our series,

hepatectomy was abandoned in 9 patients with HCC owing to extension of tumor thrombi, which were newly identified by IOUS.

IOUS is indispensable as a direct aid during dissection of the hepatic parenchyma, demonstrating the interrelationship between the tumor and vessels (Fig 53–11).[109] The portal vein, hepatic vein, and tumor are shown on a TV monitor two-dimensionally, and a three-dimensional effect can be achieved by moving the IOUS probe. Moreover, the transection line of the liver is visualized together with the tumor and vessels (Fig 53–12), so that the orientation of parenchymal division can be obtained.

Limited Resection and Enucleation.
In liver resection for patients with HCC and liver cirrhosis, preservation of the liver parenchyma is critical in order to prevent postoperative liver insufficiency. Even limited resection and enucleation are major surgical procedures for cirrhotic patients. Fifty-five percent of HCC patients in our series underwent limited liver resection or enucleation of the tumor. When the liver is cirrhotic and hard, a HCC nodule is softer than the liver parenchyma and therefore, not palpable during liver transection. Therefore, monitoring of the transection plane by IOUS is indispensable in limited resection and enucleation. If division of the liver parenchyma is carried out without the aid of IOUS, it is possible that the surgeon may fail to resect, or may cut into, the tumor. To avoid these events, IOUS guidance should be continued until the echogenic line of liver transection reaches the other side of the tumor (Fig 53–13).

When a tumor is attached to the major portal pedicle or hepatic veins and the patient has poor liver function, these veins have to be preserved, even though the capsule of the tumor is exposed. In HCC, the tumor usually grows expansively and does not infiltrate the adjacent vessels except in the case of tumor thrombus. Direct invasion to the connective tissue or venous wall is rare. Therefore, when an HCC nodule compresses the hepatic venous wall, it can be dissected from the venous wall except in cases of sclerosing or mixed-type HCC. This procedure is quite different from metastasectomy of colorectal cancer.

In limited resection, the amount of the noncancerous liver parenchyma to be resected, together with the tumor, varies according to the tumor location. The resection of a centrally located tumor requires much more sacrifice of the parenchyma than that of a superficially located one. Therefore, limited resection of a deep-seated tumor is more invasive for a patient with HCC, even though the resection itself is nonanatomical and nonradical, from the standpoint of the pathophysiologic nature of HCC (ie, spreading through the portal venous system) (Fig 53–1).

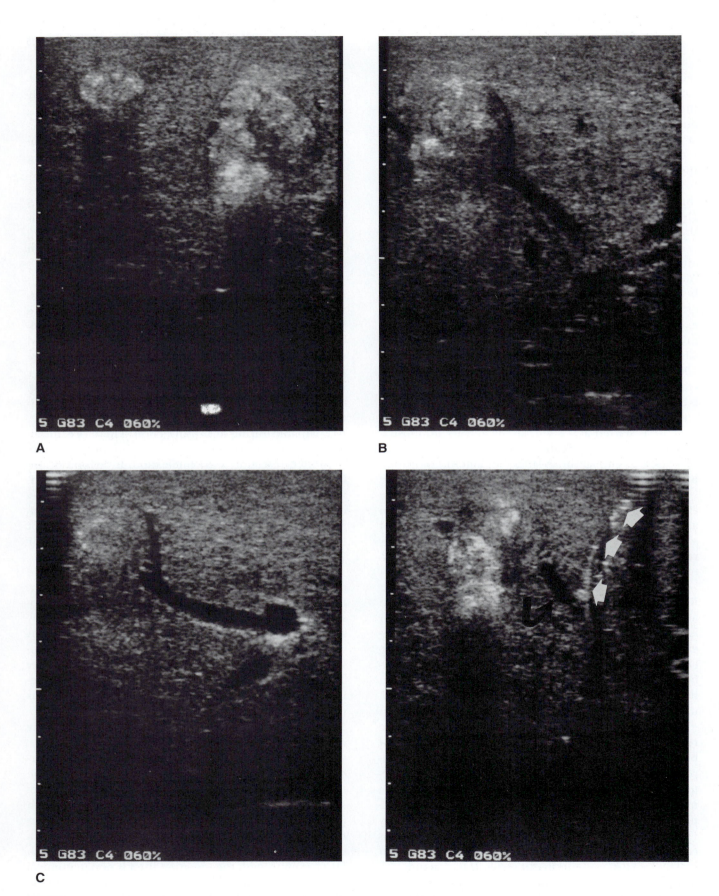

Figure 53–11. Intraoperative ultrasonography of the tumor and vessels. **A**. Two tumors in S8. Shadowing is owing to lipiodol accumulation in the tumor. **B**. Main tumor and draining middle hepatic vein. **C**. Portal venous branch feeding the tumor.

Figure 53–12. Extension of the transection plane (*arrow heads*) to the draining hepatic venous branch (*curved arrow*).

A

B

C

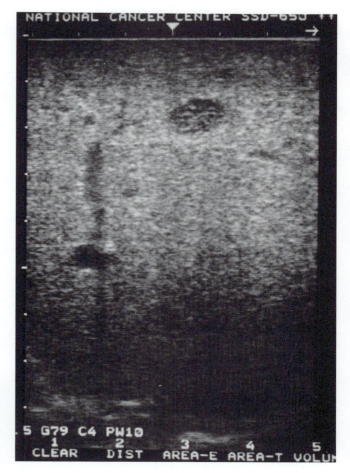

A

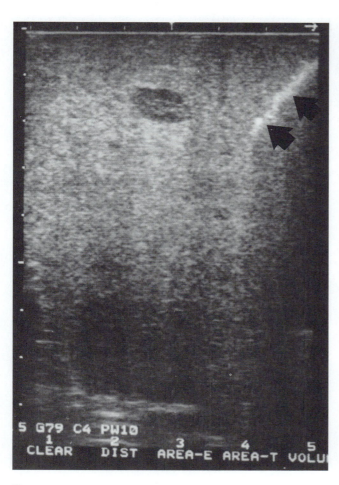

B

Figure 53–13. Small HCC and transection plane in the liver. **A**. Intraoperative ultrasonography demonstrates a hypoechoic nodule 1 cm in diameter in S8. **B**. The transected surfaces of the liver are put together in their natural position and the liver is scanned. The dividing line in the liver is visualized as an echogenic line (*arrows*). *Continued*

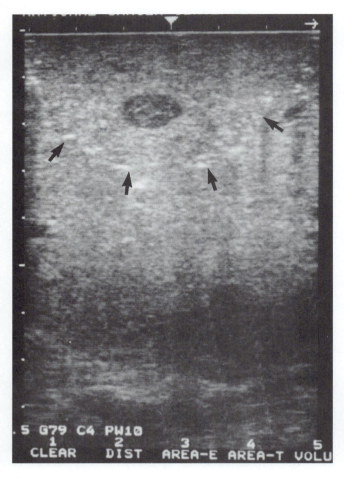

C

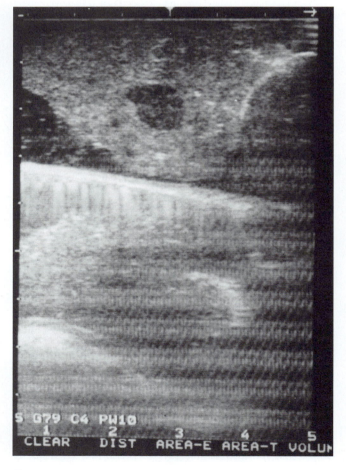

D

Figure 53–13, cont'd. C. Intraoperative ultrasonogram after more than half of the liver transection has been accomplished. Echogenic spot (*arrows*) indicates the transected surfaces of the liver. **D**. Intraoperative ultrasonogram of the resected specimen in a water bath. The surgical margin can easily be estimated. (From Makuuchi M, Kosuge T, et al. Recent technical advances in segmentectomy, subsegmentectomy, and limited resection in patients with small hepatocellular carcinoma and liver cirrhosis with special reference to intraoperative ultrasonography. In: *Early Detection and Treatment of Liver Cancer. Monograph on Cancer Research No. 38,* Tokyo, Japan: Japan Scientific Societies; 1991:179)

Subsegmentectomy and Segmentectomy. HCC cells infiltrate to the portal vein and spread via the portal blood flow, thereafter growing into intrahepatic metastases.[48] Other forms of metastasis are beyond the scope of surgical treatment. Therefore, anatomical resection, according to the architecture of the portal vein, has the potential to remove undetected cancerous foci that have scattered from the main tumor through the portal venous system. Such resection may ultimately improve the survival of patients with HCC. The segments of Couinaud in the left lobe (S2 to 4) can be identified by discoloration after ligating the portal venous and arterial branches in the umbilical fossa. The right anterior (S5+S8) and posterior segments (S6+S7) are similarly discolored by the same procedure in the right portal fissure. However, portal areas smaller than Couinaud's segment in the left lobe or Healey's segment in the right lobe cannot be identified by conventional hepatectomy procedures. For this purpose, systematic subsegmentectomy procedures (Fig 53–14), using IOUS, have been devised. Anatomical resection of an area of liver smaller than Healey's segment first was achieved by this surgical procedure.[48]

As an example of systematic subsegmentectomy, total resection of the right anterosuperior area (S8) is described briefly below.

An upper median incision is made, turning to the right lateral side about 5 cm above the umbilicus and entering the 9th intercostal space. The diaphragm is incised and the thoracic cavity is opened. The intercostal muscles are divided to the midpoint between the vertebra and the posterior axillary line (J shaped incision), and the xiphoid process is removed. The falciform ligament is divided and cholecystectomy is performed, preserving the full length of the cystic duct. The right and left portal veins, right hepatic artery, and the left and middle hepatic arteries, together with all the connective tissue to the left of the main portal vein, are taped. The anterior wall of the inferior vena cava, between the middle and right hepatic veins, is dissected from the liver until the index finger of the surgeon can be inserted between these vessels. The liver behind the right hepatic vein also is freed from the bare area to facilitate insertion of the index finger. Under ultrasound guidance, the dorsal portal venous branch of S8 is punctured and blue dye is injected after clamping the right hepatic artery (Fig 53–15). The stained area on the liver surface is marked by electrocautery. Puncture and staining of the ventral branch is carried out in the same manner. Figure 53–16 shows one example of staining of the portal area on the liver surface. If the portal area is not clearly stained, there are several possible explanations:

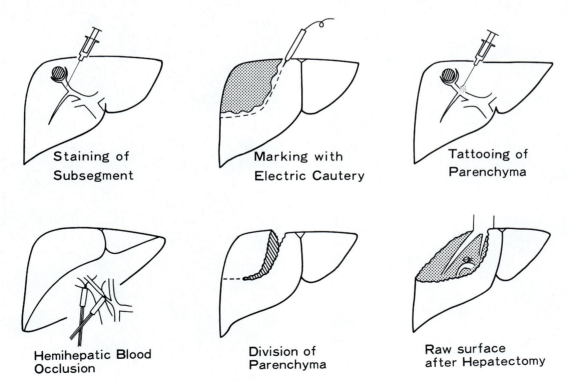

Staining of Subsegment

Marking with Electric Cautery

Tattooing of Parenchyma

Hemihepatic Blood Occlusion

Division of Parenchyma

Raw surface after Hepatectomy

Figure 53–14. Systematic subsegmentectomy procedure (From Makuuchi M, Hasegawa H, et al. Ultrasonically guided subsegmentectomy. *Surg Gynecol Obstet* 1985;161:346)

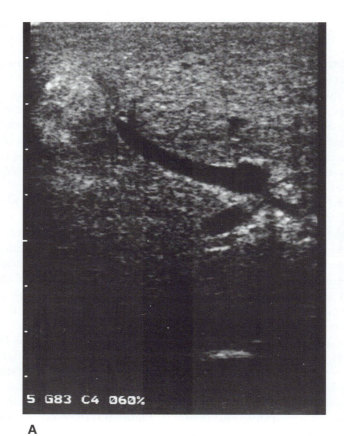

A

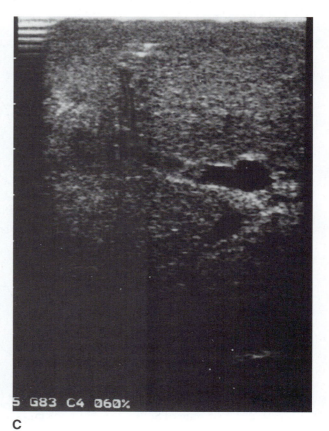

B   **C**

Figure 53–15. Ultrasound-guided puncture of the portal venous branch (same case as that in Fig 53–11). **A**. Portal venous branch feeding the tumor. **B**. Just after puncture of the portal venous branch. The tip of the needle is clearly evident in the portal vein. **C**. Injection of dye increases the echo level in the portal vein distal to the puncture site.

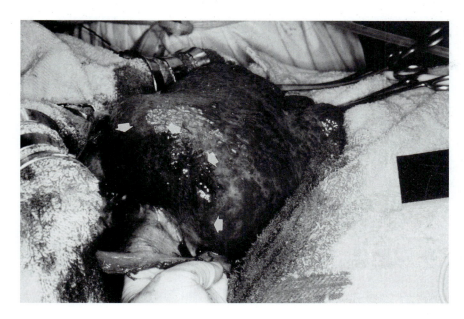

Figure 53–16. Surface of the liver after puncture of the portal venous branch and injection of blue dye. The dorsolateral area of S8 is clearly stained (*arrows*).

(1) puncture of the portal vein has failed, (2) injection of the dye has been too fast, causing regurgitation in the proximal portal vein, (3) arterioportal shunting may have occurred. The first eventuality can be avoided by practice in ultrasound-guided puncture techniques. The second can be prevented by puncturing the portal vein in a peripheral direction using a thin needle (22G), and by controlling the speed of dye injection using IOUS monitoring. The third possibility can be neglected if the hepatic arterial branch is properly occluded at the hepatic hilus.

After the blood supply to the left lobe has been occluded, division of the liver parenchyma is started 1 to 2 cm to the left of the Rex-Cantlie line. The parenchyma is crushed with a large Peans forceps and remaining vessels and connective tissue are ligated on the side of the remnant liver and clipped on the side for removal. When about two-thirds of the right side wall of the middle hepatic vein has been exposed on the raw surface, hemihepatic vascular occlusion is switched to the right lobe. Parenchymal division then proceeds along a line 1 cm caudal to the border between S8 and S5, and the portal branch feeding the ventral part of S5 is exposed. The bifurcation of the ventral branches of S5 and S8 is identified by IOUS, and the ventral portal pedicle of S8 is ligated and divided. Division of the liver then is continued along the cranial side of the anterior portal pedicle up to the dorsal branch of S8, which is located 1 to 2 cm dorsal to the ligation point of the ventral branch. The dorsal portal pedicle of S8 is fairly thick, and this is ligated and divided. The proximal one-third of the middle hepatic vein is fully exposed. Near the confluence with the inferior vena cava, there are a few thick tribu-

taries. If bleeding from these veins starts, the left index finger of the surgeon is inserted behind the middle hepatic vein, and the liver parenchyma in this region is lifted up gently. By this maneuver, bleeding can be controlled easily. At this point, the right wall of the middle hepatic vein is completely exposed as far as the inferior vena cava. Division of the liver parenchyma then is directed to the distal portion of the right hepatic vein under IOUS guidance. The anterior wall of the right hepatic vein is exposed from a caudal to cranial direction, dissecting, ligating, and dividing the small tributaries of the right hepatic vein. Similar to the middle hepatic vein, a few thick tributaries of the right hepatic vein always are encountered near the confluence with the vena cava. After the right hepatic vein has been freed from the liver parenchyma to be resected, there are no important vessels to be preserved. Thereafter, transection can proceed rapidly toward the premarked line on the liver between S8 and S7. The main right and middle hepatic veins are fully exposed on the raw surface of the liver after complete removal of S8. The stumps of the dorsal and ventral portal pedicles of S8, and the cranial part of the retrohepatic vena cava are also seen (Fig 53–17). If there is bleeding from the raw surface, it is controlled with sutures. The raw surface of the liver then is covered with a rubber sheet and gently compressed with gauzes for 15 minutes. After complete hemostasis, a bile leakage test, using a balloon catheter with a proximal-side hole, is carried out. The catheter is introduced from the remaining cystic duct to the distal common bile duct. The balloon is inflated and saline is injected. The site of saline leakage on the raw surface is sutured. Fibrin glue is spread on the raw surface, fol-

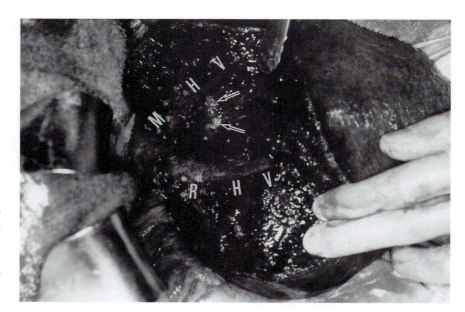

Figure 53–17. Raw surface of the liver after total resection of the anterosuperior area (S8). *Arrows* are the stumps of the dorsal and ventral portal pedicles of S8. MHV: middle hepatic vein; RHV: right hepatic vein. (From Makuuchi M. Segmentectomy and subsegmentectomy. In: Lygidakis NJ, Makuuchi M (eds), *Pitfalls and Complications in the Diagnosis and Management of Hepatobiliary and Pancreatic Diseases.* New York, NY: Georg Thieme Verlag; 1993:139)

lowed by further compression with the rubber sheet. The abdomen is closed and a drain is placed along the raw surface of the liver. Another drain is placed in the thoracic cavity. Subcutaneous tissue is tightly sutured so as not to create deadspace.

Other types of subsegmentectomy can be carried out in a similar manner. When the posterosuperior area (S7) is removed, the dorsal wall of the main right hepatic vein and the stump of the portal pedicle of S7 can be seen (Fig 53–18). The main hepatic veins are not exposed after resection of S5 or S6. If total resection of S5 is intended and there are several portal venous branches feeding it, the counterstaining technique is useful.[110] When the right distal tributaries of the middle hepatic vein draining S6 are thick, and S5 is totally removed, this hepatic venous branch should be preserved. The architecture of the portal pedicle of the area smaller than the Healey's segment of the right lobe is variable, and it is sometimes difficult to recognize the intersegmental plane between S5 and S8 or S6 and S7. However, any portal unit of the liver can be removed in an anatomical manner using the systematic subsegmentectomy procedure.[48] Subsegmentectomy accounts for 26% of all liver resections for HCC in our series. From a technical viewpoint, any two or three segments of Couinaud can be removed together or separately, such as resection of S3+S4[111] or S6+S8, and even hepatectomies preserving the inferior right hepatic vein (Fig 53–19) have been performed successfully.[112] Segmentectomy, such as right anterior[92] and posterior segmentectomies and their extension to the other adjacent segments, have been indicated in 12% of our cases. Right hepatectomy, extended right hepatectomy, and right

and left trisegmentectomies have been performed in only 6% of our patients with HCC because of impaired liver function.

Other Hepatectomy Procedures. In 1974, Fortner and associates introduced hepatic resection using in situ cold perfusion, although this technique was not popularized because of associated high mortality and morbidity.[113] However, since Picklmayr and associates reported their experience with in situ and ex situ hepatectomies, these operations have been carried out in major institutions throughout the world.[114] From our experience with more than 800 hepatectomies, a biopump was prepared in five cases, but hepatic resection was accomplished without its use in all cases. The growth pattern of HCC is not infiltrative but usually expansive, so that resection of the tumor combined with the hepatic venous wall or portal pedicle can be avoided. Except for tumor extension into the vena cava and right atrium, in situ or ex situ operations are not indicated for HCC. Even for HCC located in the caudate lobe and compressing the major vessels, complete removal of the caudate lobe is possible without sacrificing other parts of the liver parenchyma or vessels.[115] Partial autotransplantation of the liver is not necessary for HCC.[16]

We use Pringle's maneuver or the hemihepatic vascular occlusion technique during liver parenchymal dissection in order to reduce blood loss in patients with HCC. Huguet and associates proposed complete vascular isolation of the liver up to a period of 85 minutes for hepatic resections.[117] However, this technique cannot be applied for cirrhotic liver, since it may cause significant warm ischemic injury of the liver. As a result of the

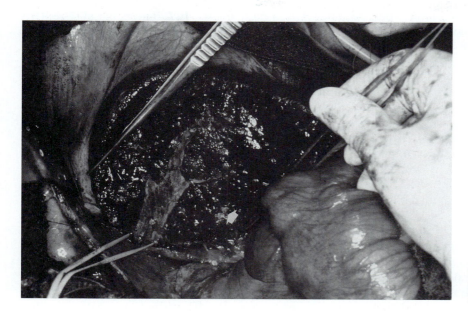

Figure 53–18. Raw surface of the liver after resection of the posterosuperior area (S7). *Arrow* indicates the stump of the portal pedicle of S7.

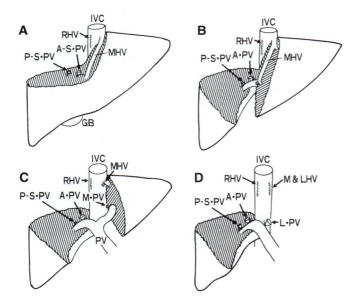

Figure 53–19. Four new hepatectomy procedures for resection of the right hepatic vein and preservation of the inferior right hepatic vein. (From Makuuchi M, Hasegawa H, et al. Four new hepatectomy procedures for resection of the right hepatic vein and preservation of the inferior right hepatic vein. *Surg Gynecol Obstet* 1987;164:68)

introduction of vascular occlusion techniques and non-transfusion protocol,[118] the average amount of blood loss in liver resection for HCC is now <1000 mL, and 70% to 75% of our patients do not receive blood transfusion. Lower blood loss and no transfusion improve operative mortality and long-term survival after hepatectomy.[119]

Results of Hepatectomy

Postoperative Complications. Immediately after surgery, it is necessary to pay attention to bleeding from the drain. If the amount of bleeding exceeds 100 mL/hr, reoperation should be done without hesitation. Hypovolemic shock has a detrimental effect on the cirrhotic liver and may result in liver insufficiency. If the serum total bilirubin level does not decrease by postoperative day 3, liver dysfunction is highly likely. If the level is >10 mg/dL within a week, in patients who have undergone hepatectomy, most are ultimately lost. No effective treatment exists for postoperative liver insufficiency except for liver transplantation. Ascites and pleural effusion are the most common complications. The intra-abdominal drain is removed if ascitic discharge continues for more than one week. The amount of protein lost in the ascitic discharge is calculated and substituted by FFP. When patients have fever, the intra-abdominal space close to the raw surface of the remnant liver needs to be investigated by ultrasound to determine whether there is fluid collection. Any abscess should be drained percutaneously under ultrasound guidance. Pleural effusion and a central venous catheter are common causes of fever. These are immediately removed and appropriate antibiotics are administered, if necessary. Postoperative hyperamylasemia often is encountered as a result of prolongation of Pringle's maneuver for liver resection.[120] Bile leakage has been seen in 8% of our patients. This leakage often follows drainage of an abscess at the site of liver resection. The drain should be left in place and irrigated until the leakage stops spontaneously. Since such leakage generally continues for a long time in cirrhotic patients, a bile leakage test should be performed routinely at the time of surgery.

Operative and hospital mortality after 1990 were 0.8% and 1.5%, respectively. Morbidity was 37%, including minor complications.

Survivals. Survival rates after hepatectomy in patients with HCC are listed in Table 53–1. Five year survival rates have reportedly ranged from 12% to 44%. If limited to recent reports, the rate has been higher than 25%. Survival of patients with HCCs ≤5 cm in diameter was better than that of patients with HCCs >5 cm. The rate reached 30% to 70% at 5 years, except for a report from Hong Kong.[121] Five year survival rates after hepa-

tectomy were 65% and 100% in patients with single minute HCCs ≤2 cm in diameter and those with single early HCCs, respectively. In our study, poor prognostic factors of HCC (≤5 cm) after hepatic resection were a large tumor size, multiple tumors (≥2), the presence of intrahepatic metastases, microscopic or macroscopic portal vein invasion, and capsular invasion.[92,122] These factors generally have been accepted as less favorable by other investigators. The degree of preoperative liver dysfunction and the type of liver resection are related to survival after liver resection. Several authors have claimed that associated liver cirrhosis is a significant prognostic factor.[123–125] Although general agreement has not been obtained with regard to positivity of the surgical margin,[121,126–128] this may be a less important prognostic factor in patients with HCC, which usually shows expansive growth. Survival rates of patients with small HCCs (<5 cm) have shown a dramatic improvement year by year. In our series, the five year survival rate was only 16.7% in patients who underwent hepatic resection before 1980. This figure improved to 32.2% between 1980 and 1984, and reached 50.4% after 1985. The improvement can be attributed mainly to refinement of surgical techniques and development of imaging modalities for accurate detection of tumor extension, such as tumor thrombus and intrahepatic metastases. Resection of HCC >10 cm always is challenging. The largest HCC specimen in our series weighed 5.5 kg. In this group of patients, the rate of combined liver cirrhosis was only 16%, whereas microscopic portal vein invasion and intrahepatic metastasis were observed in 95% and 79%, respectively. The survival curve for this group declined rapidly during the first three years after liver resection, but leveled off thereafter with a 5 year survival rate of 24%. It is necessary to perform surgical resection followed by multidisciplinary treatment in this group of patients because of the low incidence of associated liver cirrhosis.

Recurrence. The recurrence rate in HCC patients after hepatic resection is very high because a second or third primary lesion can develop in the remnant liver within a few years. Belghiti reported 100% recurrence at 5 years.[129] In our experience, the recurrence-free 5 year survival rate was 25% in patients who underwent curative resection.[122] Therefore, treatment for recurrent HCC is very important. The primary treatment of choice is repeated hepatic resection.[130–132] The results of repeated resections have shown good long-term survival rates without any significant increase in postoperative morbidity or mortality. Indications for repeated hepatectomy are evaluated in accordance with the same scheme as that for the first hepatectomy. Meticulous hemostasis is necessary in order to prevent significant blood loss during dissection of intraperitoneal adhesion resulting from the first opera-

TABLE 53–2. OVERALL SURVIVAL RATE AFTER HEPATIC RESECTION FOR HCC

First Author	Year	Cases resected	With cirrhosis (%)	Operative mortality (%)	Survival rate (%)				
					1 yr	2 yr	3 yr	4 yr	5 yr
Wu	1980	181	70	8.8	55.9	—	28.9	—	16.0
Okuda	1980	222	72	21.5	33.3	—	19.6	—	11.8
Tang	1981	153	—	12.5	56.3	—	31.5	—	23.6
Li	1982	114	—	11.4	58.6	—	32.7	—	20.5
Huang	1982	181	—	2.8	55.6	—	29.4	—	27.6
Lee	1982	165	85	20.0	35.0	24.4	20.0	—	19.0
Shen	1989	195	—	8.2	60.2	—	28.7	—	22.9
Lee	1985	109	—	—	84.0	72.0	52.0	28.0	—
Wu	1986	283	78	4.2	60.3	—	40.4	—	25.8
Nagasue	1986	118	85	7.6	—	59.3	—	29.7	—
Nagao	1987	94	75	19.0	73.0	—	42.0	—	25.0
Chen	1989	120	45.8	4.1	55.5	40.4	—	32.4	25.9
Choi	1990	174	65	15.5	45.5	—	21.0	—	15.0
Yamanaka	1990	295	80	—	76.0	—	44.0	—	31.0
LCSGJ[a]	1990	4354	82	—	67.1	—	39.6	—	28.5
Ringe	1991	131	17.6	12.2	67.5	54.4	42.3	38.8	35.8
Iwatsuki	1991	76	22.3	—	71.1	55.0	47.2	37.2	32.9
Kosuge	1993	480	63	2.1	86.6	—	62.7	—	44.1

[a]LCSGU: Liver Cancer Study Group of Japan

TABLE 53–3. SURVIVAL RATE AFTER RESECTION OF SMALL HCC

First Author	Year	Cases resected	With cirrhosis (%)	Operative mortality (%)	Survival rate (%)				
					1 yr	2 yr	3 yr	4 yr	5 yr
Kanematsu	1984								
standard		13	—	15.4	78.7	67.3	—	—	22.5
limited		37	—	10.8	79.9	60.3	—	—	32.6
Lee	1985	62	—	3.0	92.0		44.0	—	—
Hsu	1985	49	73	9.0	81.6	77.6	—	—	—
Li	1986	23	79	8.7	89.7	—	71.2	—	41.2
Wu	1986	65	78	4.2	83.1	—	73.9	—	64.0
Makuuchi	1989								
subseg[a]		87	—	0.8	85.5	78.3	60.7	49.0	45.4
limited		168	—	0.8	89.4	73.5	58.1	36.7	29.7
Tang	1989	132	89.6	2.3	—	—	—	—	67.9
Kawano	1989	57	72.0[b]	17.6[c]	86	75	60	40	35
Franco	1990	50	100	6.9	66.8	53.8	41.9	—	—
Lai	1991	36	84.6	7.7	59	—	28	—	11
Makuuchi	1993	349	73.5	1.7	90.2	79.2	66.2	50.8	43.7

[a]Hepatectomy procedures are divided into three categories: standard resection, limited resection and subsegmentectomy.
[b]Including large HCC.
[c]Hospital mortality from all HCCs.

tion. In our series of 24 second and 6 third hepatic resections, the mean amount of blood loss was not significantly different from that at the first hepatectomy. When hepatectomy is not indicated, TAE is the most popular treatment for patients with recurrent HCC. Survival after TAE for patients with tumor recurrence following hepatectomy was much better than for patients who underwent TAE for the primary HCC.[133] This was because cancerous nodules were detected at a less advanced stage owing to careful follow-up in patients with a previous history of liver resection, and because some of the collateral blood supply was obliterated by prior surgery, which may have enhanced the effects of TAE.

Surgical Treatments Other Than Hepatectomy

Arterial ligation or catheterization of the hepatic artery with implantation of a port has been carried out as an alternative surgical procedure for HCC. These procedures are indicated when HCC is found to be unexpectedly extended and judged to be unresectable after laparotomy. Simple arterial ligation is not significantly effective because a rich arterial blood supply through the collateral circulation can develop within a few days after ligation. However, Okamoto and associates reported that the effect of arterial ligation was the same as that of palliative liver resection, if an HCC nodule is fed by a single arterial branch.[134] Hepatic arterial ligation, together with portal venous infusion chemotherapy, can increase the response rate.[135] Arterial ligation also can facilitate the effect of postoperative TAE; the aberrant hepatic arteries and some branches of the common hepatic artery feeding extrahepatic organs are ligated, and cholecystectomy is performed. Division of the falciform, coronary, and triangular ligaments and dissection of the bare area are useful for preventing development of a collateral blood supply to the liver and the tumor.

Implantation of the port or pump can be performed in the same manner as that in the case of metastatic liver cancer. However, implantation rarely is indicated since TAE can be substituted for this procedure. If arterial chemotherapy is indicated and arterial ligation for postoperative TAE has been carried out during laparotomy, catheterization of the common hepatic artery can be performed using the Seldinger technique, at any time, without difficulty. Arterial catheterization is applied only for hypovascular types of HCC (mixed or sclerosing types) and for cholangiocellular carcinoma.

Wrapping of the tumor-bearing liver has been performed as an adjunct to TAE in order to prevent development of a collateral arterial blood supply.[136]

Palliative resection of the main HCC nodule may be indicated in patients with multiple HCCs if intrahepatic metastases are well controlled with TAE but an aberrant arterial blood supply to the main tumor develops.

Laser irradiation of the tumor using a specially designed probe for spherical dispersal of the radiation has been performed.[137] Cryosurgery for superficial tumor also has been reported.[138] Although these procedures are simply applied after laparotomy, there is some risk of injury to major vessels adjacent to the tumor.

Liver transplantation also has been carried out for HCC. However, its long-term outcome was not impressive[139] because of early recurrence in the transplanted liver and acceleration of tumor growth because of the immunosuppressive state of the patient.[140] Whereas patients with stage II disease showed better survival after transplantation compared with those after hepatic resection, poor outcome was observed after transplantation in patients with stage III or stage IV disease.[141]

Patients with unilobar HCC ≤5 cm in diameter and those with associated liver cirrhosis showed better survival after transplantation than those treated by hepatectomy.[142] Bismuth and associates have proposed the so-called 3-3 rule, which means that in patients with no more than 3 HCC nodules <3 cm in diameter, the survival after transplantation is higher than after hepatic resection.[143] Therefore, patients with small hepatoma and severe cirrhosis may be appropriate candidates for liver transplantation. However, patients with benign cholestatic diseases, hereditary metabolic diseases, or cryptogenic cirrhosis should be given first priority for transplantation ahead of patients with small HCCs and cirrhosis. Whether or not patients with small HCCs should be listed as candidates for transplantation depends mainly on organ availability. Recent results of perioperative chemotherapy may indicate improved survival after liver transplantation in HCC patients.[144]

REFERENCES

1. World Health Organization. Causes of death, by sex and age. In: *World Health Statistics Annual.* Geneva, Switzerland: WHO; 1991

2. World Health Organization. Causes of death, by sex and age. In: *World Health Statistics Annual.* Geneva, Switzerland: WHO; 1992

3. World Health Organization. Causes of death, by sex and age. In: *World Health Statistics Annual.* Geneva, Switzerland: WHO; 1993

4. Szmuness W. Hepatocellular carcinoma and the hepatitis B virus: evidence for a causal association. *Prog Med Virol* 1978;24:40

5. Lam KC, Yu MC, et al. Hepatitis B virus and cigarette smoking: risk factors for hepatocellular carcinoma in Hong Kong. *Cancer Res* 1982;42:5246

6. Yeh FS, Mo CC, et al. A serological case-control study of primary hepatocellular carcinoma in Guangxi, China. *Cancer Res* 1985;45:872

7. Beasley RP. Hepatitis B virus as the etiologic agent in hepatocellular carcinoma—epidemiologic considerations. *Hepatology* 1982;2:21S

8. Chakraborty PR, Ruiz-Opazo N, et al. Identification of integrated hepatitis B virus DNA and expression of viral RNA in an HBsAg-producing human hepatocellular carcinoma cell line. *Nature* 1980;286:531

9. Prince AM. Hepatitis B virus and hepatocellular carcinoma: molecular biology provides further evidence for an etiologic association. *Hepatology* 1981;1:73

10. Bruix J, Calvet X, et al. Prevalence of antibodies to hepatitis C virus in Spanish patients with hepatocellular carcinoma and hepatic cirrhosis. *Lancet* 1989;ii:1004

11. Kiyosawa K, Akahane A, et al. Hepatocellular carcinoma after non-A non-B posttransfusion hepatitis. *Am J Gastroenterol* 1984;79:777

12. Alper ME, Hutt MRS, et al. Association between aflatoxin content of food and hepatoma frequency in Uganda. *Cancer* 1971;28:253

13. Peers FG, Linsell CA. Dietary aflatoxin and liver cancer: a population-based study in Kenya. *Br J Cancer* 1973;27:473

14. Steiner PE. Cancer of the liver and cirrhosis in Trans-Saharan Africa and the United States of America. *Cancer* 1960;13:1085

15. Okuda K, Ohtsuki T, et al. Natural history of hepatocellular carcinoma and prognosis in relation to treatment: study of 850 patients. *Cancer* 1985;56:918

16. Davidson AR, Tomlinson S, et al. The variable course of primary hepatocellular carcinoma. *Br J Surg* 1974;61:349

17. Ebara M, Ohto M, et al. Natural history of minute hepatocellular carcinoma smaller than three centimeters complicating cirrhosis. *Gastroenterology* 1986;90:289

18. Yoshino M. Growth kinetics of hepatocellular carcinoma. *Jpn J Clin Oncol* 1983;13:45

19. Kanai T, Hirohashi S, et al. Pathology of small hepatocellular carcinoma: a proposal for a new gross classification. *Cancer* 1987;60:810

20. Edmondson HA, Steiner PE. Primary carcinoma of the liver: a study of 100 cases among 48 900 necropsies. *Cancer* 1954;7:462

21. Sasaki K. Adenomatous hyperplasia in liver cirrhosis: an approach from a microangiographical point of view. *Gann Monogr Cancer Res* 1980;25:127

22. Arakawa M, Kage M, et al. Emergence of malignant lesions within an adenomatous hyperplastic nodule in a cirrhotic liver. *Gastroenterology* 1986;91:198

23. Tsuda H, Hirohashi S, et al. Clonal origin of atypical adenomatous hyperplasia of the liver and clonal identity with hepatocellular carcinoma. *Gastroenterology* 1988;95:1664

24. Takayama T, Makuuchi M, et al. Malignant transformation of adenomatous hyperplasia to hepatocellular carcinoma. *Lancet* 1990;336:1150

25. Sakamoto M, Hirohasi S, et al. Early stages of multistep hepatocarcinogenesis: adenomatous hyperplasia and early hepatocellular carcinoma. *Hum Pathol* 1991;22:172

26. Nakanuma Y, Terada T, et al. Atypical adenomatous hyperplasia in liver cirrhosis: low grade hepatocellular carcinoma or borderline lesion? *Histopathology* 1990;17:27

27. Makuuchi M, Hasegawa H, et al. Ultrasonically guided subsegmentectomy. *Surg Gynecol Obstet* 1985;161:346

28. Kojiro M. Pathomorphology of advanced hepatocellular carcinoma. In: Tobe T, et al (eds), *Primary Liver Cancer in Japan*. Tokyo, Japan: Springer-Verlag; 1992:31

29. The Liver Cancer Study Group of Japan. Primary liver cancer in Japan. *Ann Surg* 1990;211:277

30. Liebman H, Furie BC, et al. Des-χ-carboxy (abnormal) prothrombin as a serum marker of primary hepatocellular carcinoma. *N Engl J Med* 1984;310:1427

31. Okuda K, Kasai Y, et al. Primary liver cancer in Japan. *Cancer* 1980;45:2663

32. Ono M, Ohta H, et al. Measurement of immunoreactive prothrombin, des-χ-carboxy prothrombin, and vitamin K in human liver tissues: overproduction of immunoreactive prothrombin in hepatocellular carcinoma. *Am J Gastroenterol* 1990;85:1149

33. Sakon M, Monden M, et al. Relationship between pathologic prognostic factors and abnormal levels of des-χ-carboxy prothrombin and α-fetoprotein in hepatocellular carcinoma. *Am J Surg* 1992;163:251

34. Makuuchi M, Hasegawa H, et al. Ultrasonic characteristics of the small hepatocellular carcinoma. In: Lerski RA, Morley P (eds), *Ultrasound '82*. Oxford, England: Pergamon; 1983:489

35. Prando A, Wallace S, et al. Computed tomographic arteriography of the liver. *Radiology* 1979;130:697

36. Matsui O, Kayoda M, et al. Dynamic sequential computed tomography during arterial portography in the detection of hepatic neoplasms. *Radiology* 1983;146:721

37. Ohishi H, Uchida H, et al. Hepatocellular carcinoma detected by iodized oil: use of anticancer agents. *Radiology* 1985;154:25

38. Inayoshi G, Nishimura H, et al. MR imaging of hepatocellular carcinoma (in Japanese). *Jpn J Mag Reson Med* 1989;9:216

39. Matsui O, Kadoya M, et al. Adenomatous hyperplastic nodules in the cirrhotic liver: differentiation from hepatocellular carcinoma with MR imaging. *Radiology* 1989;173:123

40. Yoshida H, Itai Y, et al. Small hepatocellular carcinoma and cavernous hemangioma: differentiation with dynamic FLASH MRI with Gd-DTPA. *Radiology* 1989;171:339

41. Itai Y, Frui S, et al. Computed tomography of the cavernous hemangioma of the liver. *Radiology* 1980;137:149

42. Ohtomo K, Itai Y, et al. Hepatocellular carcinoma and cavernous hemangioma: differentiation with MR imaging-efficacy of T2 values of 0.35 and 1.5T. *Radiology* 1988;168:621

43. Kudo M, Tomita S, et al. Hepatic focal nodular hyperplasia: specific findings at dynamic contrast-enhanced US with carbon dioxide microbubbles. *Radiology* 1991;179:333

44. Goldstein HM, Wallace S, et al. Transcatheter occlusion of abdominal tumors. *Radiology* 1976;120:539

45. Yamada Y, Sato M, et al. Hepatic artery embolization in 120 patients with unresectable hepatoma. *Radiology* 1983;148:397

46. Takayasa K, Wakao F, et al. Response of early-stage hepatocellular carcinoma and borderline lesions to therapeutic arterial embolization. *AJR Am J Roentgenol* 1993;160:301

47. Okazaki M, Higashihara H, et al. Transcatheter arterial embolization for inoperable hepatocellular carcinoma. *Jpn J Clin Radiol* 1991;36:592

48. Makuuchi M, Sukigara M, et al. Bile duct necrosis: com-

plication of transcatheter hepatic arterial embolization. *Radiology* 1985;156:331

49. Sasaki Y, Imaoka S, et al. A new approach to chemoembolization therapy for hepatoma using ethiodized oil, cisplatin and gelform sponge. *Cancer* 1987;60:1194

50. Nakamura H, Hashimoto T, et al. Transcatheter oil chemoembolization of hepatocellular carcinoma. *Radiology* 1989;170:783

51. Yamada R, Kishi K, et al. Transcatheter arterial embolization in unresectable hepatocellular carcinoma. *Cardiovasc Intervent Radiol* 1990;13:135

52. Takayasu K, Moriyama N, et al. Gallbladder infarction after hepatic artery embolization. *AJR Am J Roentgenol* 1985;144:135

53. Hasegawa H. Multidisciplinary treatment for hepatocellular carcinoma—hepatectomy after transcatheter arterial embolization. *Naika* 1983;52:555

53a. Shijo H, Okazaki M, et al. Hepartocellular carcinoma: a multivariant analysis of prognostic features in patients treated with hepatic arterial embolization. *Am J Gastroenterol* 1992;87:1154

54. Nagasue N, Galizia G, et al. Adverse effects of preoperative hepatic artery chemoembolization. *Surgery* 1989;106:81

55. Okazaki M, Higashihara H, et al. Chemoembolization for hepatocellular carcinoma via the inferior pancreaticoduodenal artery in patients with celiac artery stenosis. *Acta Radiol* 1993;34:20

56. Shinagawa T, Ukaji H, et al. Intratumoral injection of absolute ethanol under ultrasound imaging for treatment of small hepatocellular carcinoma—attempts in three cases. *Acta Hepatol Jpn* 1985;26:99

57. Livraghi T, Baietta E, et al. Fine-needle percutaneous intratumoral chemotherapy under ultrasound guidance: a feasibility study. *Tumori* 1986;72:81

58. Shiina S, Tagawa K, et al. Percutaneous ethanol injection therapy of hepatocellular carcinoma: Analysis of 77 patients. *AJR Am J Roentgenol* 1990;155:1221

59. Ohto M, Ebara M, et al. Ethanol injection. In: Okuda K, Tobe T, et al (eds), *Gann Monograph on Cancer Research No 38, Early Detection and Treatment of Liver Cancer.* Tokyo, Japan/London, England: Jpn Scientific Societies and Taylor & Francis; 1991:147

60. Shue JC, Sung JL, et al. Intratumor injection of absolute ethanol under ultrasound guidance for treatment of small hepatocellular carcinoma. *Hepatogastroenterology* 1987;34:255

61. Koda M, Okamoto K, et al. Hepatic vascular and bile duct injury after ethanol injection therapy for hepatocellular carcinoma. *Gastrointest Radiol* 1992;17:167

62. Livraghi T, Bolondi L, et al. Percutaneous ethanol injection in cirrhosis (a study on 207 patients). *Cancer* 1992;69:925

63. Ministry of Health and Welfare of Japan (directed by Shimamura).

64. Gandolfi L, Salmi L, et al. Intratumoral echoguided injection of interleukin-2 and lymphokine-activated killer cells in hepatocellular carcinoma. *Hepatogastroenterology* 1989;36:352

65. Huang G, Yang PM, et al. Intramural injection of OK-432

for the treatment of small hepatocellular carcinoma. *Hepatogastroenterology* 1990;37:439

66. Tanaka K, Nakamura S, et al. Hepatocellular carcinoma: treatment with percutaneous ethanol injection and transcatheter arterial embolization. *Radiology* 1992;185:457

67. Okazaki M, Yoshino M, et al. A controlled study of intravenous doxorubicin versus oral tegaful in patients with hepatocellular carcinoma. *J Jpn Soc Cancer Ther* 1985;20:556

68. Ravry MJR, Omura GA, et al. Phase II evaluation of cisplatin: a Southeastern Cancer Study Group trial. *Cancer Treat Rep* 1986;70:311

69. Davis RB, Van Echo DA, et al. Phase II trial of mitoxantrone in advanced primary liver cancer: a cancer and leukemia group B study. *Cancer Treat Rep* 1986;70:1125

70. Lai KH, Tsai YT, et al. Clinical trial of doxifluridine in the treatment of primary hepatocellular carcinoma. *Cancer Treat Rep* 1986;70:1339

71. Takayasu K, Shima Y, et al. Hepatocellular carcinoma treatment with intraarterial iodized oil with and without chemotherapeutic agents. *Radiology* 1987;162:345

72. Kanematsu T, Furuta T, et al. A 5 year experience of lipiodolization: selective regional chemotherapy for 200 patients with hepatocellular carcinoma. *Hepatology* 1989;10:98

73. Kalayci C, Johnson PI, et al. Intraarterial adriamycin and lipiodol for inoperable hepatocellular carcinoma: a comparison with intravenous administration. *J Hepatol* 1990;11:349

74. Shepherd FA, Evans WK, et al. Hepatic arterial infusion of mitoxantrone in the treatment of primary hepatocellular carcinoma. *J Clin Oncol* 1987;5:635

75. Falkson GF, Ryan LM, et al. A random phase II study of mitoxantrone and cisplatin in patients with hepatocellular carcinoma: a BCOG study. *Cancer* 1987;60:2141

76. Shibata J, Fujiyama S, et al. Hepatic arterial injection chemotherapy with cisplatin suspended in an oily lymphographic agent for hepatocellular carcinoma. *Cancer* 1989;64:1589

77. Atiq OT, Kemeny N, et al. Treatment of unresectable primary liver cancer with intraheptic fluorodeoxy uridine and mitomycin C through an implantable pump. *Cancer* 1992;69:920

78. Park CH, Suh JH, et al. Evaluation of intrahepatic I-131 ethiodol on a patient with hepatocellular carcinoma: therapeutic fesibility study. *Clin Nucl Med* 1986;11:514

79. Kobayashi H, Hidaka H, et al. Treatment of hepatocellular carcinoma by transarterial injection of anticancer agents in iodized oil suspension or of radioactive iodized oil suspension. *Acta Radiol Diag* 1986;27:139

80. Okuno N, Takagi H, et al. Treatment for unresectable hepatoma via selective hepatic arterial infusion of lymphokine-activated killer cells generated from autologous spleen. *Cancer* 1986;58:1001

81. Ichida T, Higuchi K, et al. Treatment of hepatocellular carcinoma utilizing lymphokine-activated killer cells and interleukin-2. *Cancer Chemother Pharmacol* 1989;23:545

82. Ohnishi S, Saibara T, et al. Adoptive immunotherapy with lymphokine-activated killer cells plus recombinant interleukin-2 in patients with unresectable hepatocellular carcinoma. *Hepatology* 1989;10:349

83. Takayama T, Makuuchi M, et al. Distribution and therapeutic effect of intraarterially transferred tumor-infiltrating lymphocytes in hepatic malignancies. *Cancer* 1991; 68:2391

84. Sachs E, Di Biscleglie AM, et al. Treatment of hepatocellular carcinoma with recombinant leucocyte interferon. *Br J Cancer* 1985;52:111

85. Order SE, Stillwagon GB, et al. Iodine 131 antiferritin: a new treatment modality in hepatoma: a Radiation Therapy Oncology Group study. *J Clin Oncol* 1985;3:1573

86. Tang ZY, Liu KD, et al. Radioimmunotherapy in the multimodality treatment of hepatocellular carcinoma with reference to second-look resection. *Cancer* 1990; 65:211

87. Nagasue N, Ito A, et al. Androgen receptors in hepatocellular carcinoma and surrounding parenchyma. *Gastroenterology* 1985;89:643

88. Nagasue N, Ito A, et al. Estrogen receptors in hepatocellular carcinoma. *Cancer* 1986;57:87

89. Ohnishi S, Murakami T, et al. Androgen and estrogen receptors in hepatocellular carcinoma and in the surrounding noncancerous liver tissue. *Hepatology* 1986; 6:440

90. Farinati F, Salvagnini M, et al. Unresectable hepatocellular carcinoma: a prospective controlled trial with tamoxifen. *J Hepatol* 1990;11:297

91. Makuuchi M, Hasegawa H, et al. Indication for hepatectomy in patients with hepatocellular carcinoma and cirrhosis (in Japanese). *Shindan to Chiryo* 1986;74:1225

92. Makuuchi M, Kosuge T, et al. Surgery for small liver cancers. *Semin Surg Oncol* 1993;9:293

93. Kanematsu T, Takenaka K, et al. Limited hepatic resection effective for selected cirrhotic patients with primary liver cancer. *Ann Surg* 1984;199:51

94. Makuuchi M, Takayasu K, et al. Preoperative transcatheter embolization of the portal venous branch for patients receiving extended lobectomy due to the bile duct carcinoma (in Japanese). *J Jpn Soc Clin Surg* 1984; 45:1558

95. Makuuchi M, Le Thai B, et al. Preoperative portal embolization to increase safety of major hepatectomy for hilar bile duct carcinoma: a preliminary report. *Surgery* 1990;107:521

96. Kinoshita H, Sakai K, et al. Preoperative portal vein embolization for hepatocellular carcinoma. *World J Surg* 1986;10:803

97. Kuwao S. Pathomorphological study on primary liver cancer (in Japanese). *Acta Hepatol Jpn* 1979;20:828

98. Yamaoka Y, Kumada AK, et al. Liver resection for hepatocellular carcinoma with direct removal of tumor thrombi in the main portal vein. *World J Surg* 1992; 16:1172

99. Fujisaki M, Kurihara E, et al. Hepatocellular carcinoma with tumor thrombus extending into the right atrium: report of a successful resection with the use of cardiopulmonary bypass. *Surgery* 1991;109:214

100. Okazaki M, Higashihara H, et al. Intraperitoneal hemorrhage from hepatocellular carcinoma: Emergency chemoembolization or embolization. *Radiology* 1991; 180:647

101. Chen MF, Jan YY, et al. Transcatheter hepatic arterial embolization followed by hepatic resection for the spontaneous rupture of hepatocellular carcinoma. *Cancer* 1986;58:332

102. Chearanai O, Plengvani JU, et al. Spontaneous rupture of primary hepatoma: report of 63 cases with particular reference to pathogenesis and rational treatment by hepatic artery ligation. *Cancer* 1983;51:1532

103. Lai ECS, Wu KM, et al. Spontaneous ruptured hepatocellular carcinoma: an appraisal of surgical treatment. *Ann Surg* 1989;210:24

104. Hsieh JS, Huang CJ, et al. Intraperitoneal hemorrhage due to spontaneous rupture of hepatocellular carcinoma: treatment of hepatic arterial embolization. *AJR Am J Roentgenol* 1987;149:715

105. Pringle JH. Notes on the arrest of hepatic hemorrhage due to trauma. *Ann Surg* 1908;48:541

106. Makuuchi M, Mori T, et al. Safety of hemihepatic vascular occlusion during resection of the liver. *Surg Gynecol Obstet* 1987;64:155

107. Makuuchi M, Hasegawa H, et al. Intraoperative ultrasonic examination for hepatectomy. *Jpn J Clin Oncol* 1981;11:367

108. Makuuchi M. Application of intraoperative ultrasonography to hepatectomy. In: Makuuchi M (ed), *Abdominal Intraoperative Ultrasonography*. New York, NY: Igaku-Shoin; 1987:89

109. Makuuchi M, Hasegawa H, et al. The use of operative ultrasound as an aid to liver resection in patients with hepatocellular carcinoma. *World J Surg* 1987;11:615

110. Takayama T, Makuuchi M, et al. A new method for mapping hepatic segment: counterstaining identification technique. *Surgery* 1991;109:226

111. Kawasaki S, Makuuchi M, et al. A new alternative hepatectomy method for resection of segments 3 and 4 of the liver. *Surg Gynecol Obstet* 1992;175:267

112. Makuuchi M, Hasegawa H, et al. Four new hepatectomy procedures for resection of the right hepatic vein and preservation of the inferior right hepatic vein. *Surg Gynecol Obstet* 1987;164:68

113. Fortner JG, Shiu MH, et al. Major hepatic resection using vascular isolation and hypothermic perfusion. *Ann Surg* 1974;180:644

114. Picklmayer R, Grosse H, et al. Technique and preliminary results of extracorporeal liver surgery (bench procedure) and of surgery on the in situ perfusion of the liver. *Br J Surg* 1990;77:21

115. Takayama T, Tanaka T, et al. High dorsal resection of the liver. *J Am Col Surg* 1994;179:72

116. Kumada K, Yamaoka Y, et al. Partial autotransplantation of the liver in hepatocellular carcinoma complicating cirrhosis. *Br J Surg* 1992;79:566

117. Huguet C, Addario-Chieco P, et al. Technique of hepatic vascular exclusion for extensive liver resection. *Am J Surg* 1992;163:602

118. Makuuchi M, Takayama T, et al. Restrictive versus liberal blood transfusion policy for hepatectomies in cirrhotic patients. *World J Surg* 1989;13:644

119. Yamamoto J, Kosuge T, et al. Perioperative blood transfusion promotes recurrence of hepatocellular carcinoma after hepatectomy. *Surgery* 1994;115:303

120. Miyagawa S, Makuuchi M, et al. Changes in serum amylase level following hepatic resection in chronic liver disease. *Arch Surg* (in press).

121. Lai ECS, Ng IOL, et al. Hepatic resection for small hepatocellular carcinoma: the Queen Mary Hospital experience. *World J Surg* 1991;15:654

122. Kosuge T, Makuuchi M, et al. Long-term results after resection of hepatocellular carcinoma: Experience of 480 cases. *Hepatogastroenterology* 1993;40:328

123. Kawano N, Ohmori Y, et al. Long-term prognosis of surgical patients with hepatocellular carcinoma. *Cancer Chemother Pharmacol* 1989;23(suppl):S129

124. Franco D, Capussotti L, et al. Resection of hepatocellular carcinomas results in 72 European patients with cirrhosis. *Gastroenterology* 1990;98:733

125. Sasaki Y, Imanaka S, et al. Influence of coexisting cirrhosis on long-term prognosis after surgery in patients with hepatocellular carcinoma. *Surgery* 1992;112:515

126. Yamanaka N, Okamato E, et al. Prognostic factors after hepatectomy for hepatocellular carcinomas: a univariate and multivariate analysis. *Cancer* 1990;65:1104

127. Shirabe K, Kanematsu T, et al. Factors linked to early recurrence of small hepatocellular carcinoma after partial hepatectomy: univariate and multivariate analysis. *Hepatology* 1991;14:802

128. Arii S, Tanaka J, et al. Predictive factors for intrahepatic recurrence of hepatocellular carcinoma after partial hepatectomy. *Cancer* 1992;69:913

129. Belghiti J, Panis Y, et al. Intrahepatic recurrence after resection of hepatocellular carcinoma complicating cirrhosis. *Ann Surg* 1991;214:114

130. Nagasue N, Yukaya H, et al. Second hepatic resection for recurrent hepatocellular carcinoma. *Br J Surg* 1986;73:434

131. Matsuda Y, Ito Y, et al. Rationale of surgical management for recurrent hepatocellular carcinoma. *Ann Surg* 1992;217:28

132. Kakazu T, Makuuchi M, et al. Repeat hepatic resection for recurrent hepatocellular carcinoma. *Hepatogastroenterology* 1993;40:337

133. Takayasu K, Wakao F, et al. Postresectional recurrence of hepatocellular carcinoma treated by arterial embolization: analysis of prognostic factors. *Hepatology* 1992;16:906

134. Okamoto E, Tanaka N, et al. Result of surgical treatment of primary hepatocellular carcinoma: some aspects to improve long-term survival. *World J Surg* 1984;8:360

135. Lai ECS, Choi TK, et al. Treatment of unresectable hepatocellular carcinoma: results of a randomized controlled trial. *World J Surg* 1986;10:501

136. Sasaki Y, Imaoka S, et al. Decollateralization with silicone rubber sheeting for advanced hepatocellular carcinoma: a preliminary report. *Surgery* 1990;108:840

137. Hashimoto D. Ultrasonically guided lasers and spheric laser. In: Rienann JF, Ell C (eds), *Lasers in Gastroenterology.* New York, NY: Thieme Verlag; 1989:134

138. Zhou XD, Tang ZY, et al. Clinical evaluation of criosurgery in the treatment of primary liver cancer, report of 60 cases. *Cancer* 1988;61:1889

139. Penn I. Hepatic transplantation for primary and metastatic carcinoma of the liver. *Surgery* 1991;110:726

140. Yokoyama I, Carr B, et al. Accelerated growth rates of recurrent hepatocellular carcinoma after liver transplantation. *Cancer* 1991;68:2095

141. Ringe B, Picklmayer R, et al. Surgical treatment of hepatocellular carcinoma: experience with liver resection and transplantation in 198 patients. *World J Surg* 1991;15:270

142. Iwatsuki S, Starzl TE, et al. Hepatic resection versus transplantation for hepatocellular carcinoma. *Ann Surg* 1991;214:221

143. Bismuth H, Chiche L, et al. Surgical treatment of hepatocellular carcinoma in cirrhosis: liver resection or transplantation? *Transplant Proc* 1993;25:1066

144. Carr BI, Starzl TE, et al. Aggressive treatment for advanced hepatocellular carcinoma (HCC): high response rates and prolonged survival. *Hepatology* 1991;14:103A

54

Hepatic Metastases

Peter W. Soballe ▪ *John M. Daly*

Surgical management of hepatic metastases has become increasingly important in the care of cancer patients. Although 25% to 50% of all patients dying of cancer are found to have hepatic metastases, advances in hepatic resection and regional anticancer therapies have produced measurable benefits in many of these cases. Thus, surgeons are increasingly called upon for reassessment and management of patients with hepatic metastases.

■ HISTORICAL BACKGROUND

Rokitansky, in 1855, first distinguished between primary and metastatic hepatic tumors. The first hepatic resections for metastatic diseases were reported by Garre, in 1888, and Keen, in 1899, and Wangensteen performed a total right lobectomy in 1949 for a metastasis from gastric cancer. In 1963, Woodington and Waugh first demonstrated that resection of hepatic colorectal metastases resulted in improved survival. Continuous hepatic artery infusion techniques were developed in 1959, and in 1972 an implantable pump was introduced for continuous hepatic infusion.

■ INCIDENCE

COLORECTAL

Nearly two-thirds of patients with colorectal cancer will develop hepatic involvement, and 80% to 90% of re-sections of hepatic metastases are for colorectal cancers. In these patients, synchronous hepatic metastases continue to be found in 15% to 25% of cases at the time of initial diagnosis, despite screening efforts designed to achieve earlier diagnosis of the primary tumor. An additional 40% to 50% of these patients will develop metachronous hepatic metastases after initial treatment of the primary tumor. About one-third of all patients with hepatic metastases will have their disease restricted to the liver and thus are amenable to resection. Based on an age-adjusted estimated annual incidence per 100,000 of 61 for men and 42 for women with an annual mortality of 40% of the incidence, this would represent about 5000 potentially resectable patients per year in the United States. About 1000 patients per year undergo hepatic resection, and one-fourth of these achieve long-term survival. There is room for major improvement in each of these statistics.

OTHER PRIMARIES

A variety of common primary sites often give rise to metastatic disease in the liver:

Colon	65%
Pancreas	63%
Breast	61%
Ovary	52%
Rectum	47%
Stomach	45%
Lung	36%
Kidney	27%

Hepatic metastases are also common in children with neuroblastoma and Wilms' tumor. In uncommon, hormonally active tumors such as carcinoid, they represent a special opportunity for symptom palliation. Careful selection of patients with hepatic metastases from Wilm's and carcinoid tumors will yield a subgroup of patients who will achieve a 40% long-term survival after resection. Selected patients with metastases from breast, stomach, kidney, adrenal, melanoma, and leiomyosarcoma primary sites will achieve 15% long-term survival after hepatic resection. Occasional patients with gynecologic tumors may benefit; symptomatic palliation of such hormonally active tumors as carcinoid, gastrinoma, and glucagonoma can be achieved.

■ PATHOGENESIS

The biologic steps involved in tumor progression are becoming more clearly characterized. In addition to loss of proliferative control, tumor cells must acquire imbalances in regulation of motility, adhesion, and stromal proteolysis in order to become competent for invasion and metastasis. The cell-surface protein encoded by the tumor suppressor gene DCC plays a prominent role in this process; its loss correlates with advanced invasiveness and metastasis in patients with colon and pancreatic carcinomas. Target tissues for metastases are determined by tumor adhesion to organ-specific endothelial and possibly parenchymal cell structures. Carcinoembryonic antigen (CEA) may be one of the molecules that contribute to this metastatic specificity. The genetic steps of progression are especially well-defined for colon carcinoma, and the clinical behavior of hepatic colorectal metastases seems to reflect underlying biologic determinants in these tumors. For example, survival following resection of solitary metastases is equivalent whether they are large or small, and is best when CEA levels are lowest, regardless of tumor size. Similarly, the finding of positive mesenteric nodes (Duke's C or N_1), or cytologic de-differentiation in the primary resection portends more aggressive hepatic metastases. The finding of extrahepatic metastases effectively eliminates any survival value of resection, even when the extrahepatic disease seems to be resectable.

Metastases reach the liver by four routes: (1) direct invasion (stomach, colon, bile ducts, and 50% to 72% of gallbladder tumors), (2) lymphatics (breast and lung via mediastinal nodes; also occurs with organs drained by the portal venous system), (3) hepatic artery (lung, melanoma), and (4) portal vein.

The portal vein is by far the most common route. Hepatic metastases are found in approximately half of the cases in which an organ drained by the portal vein is involved. Colorectal tumors lead the list as a consequence of their frequency and carcinoid syndrome is the most common small intestinal metastasis. Less commonly, genitourinary tumors invade portal vein tributaries and reach the liver.

Once established in the liver, however, metastases derive nearly the entire blood supply from the hepatic artery, and only the outer rim of rapidly growing cells continue to be supplied by the portal vein (Fig 54–1). Angiogenesis induced by proteolytic enzymes and

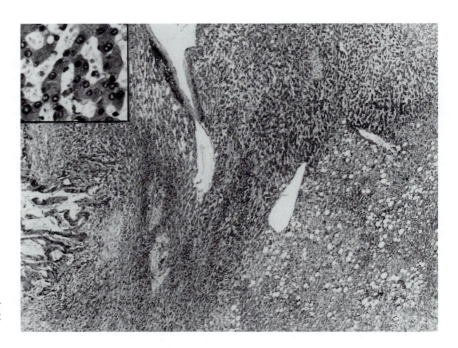

Figure 54–1. Metastatic adenocarcinoma of the colon to the liver (lower right) with an outer rim of infiltrated liver apparent. Insert demonstrates capillary neovascularization.

growth factors produced by tumor implants result in neovascularization that lacks smooth muscle, elastic tissue, and sympathetic innervation, and is insensitive to pharmacologic manipulations.

■ DIAGNOSIS

BEFORE TREATMENT FOR THE PRIMARY TUMOR

Extensive preoperative evaluation for metastatic disease is not warranted before operation for colorectal primaries, since surgical management of the primary tumor usually is required, regardless of synchronous metastases. However, careful palpation of the liver is mandatory at abdominal exploration. Intraoperative ultrasound (Fig 54–2) is a valuable adjunct to this exploration. The procedure is relatively simple, quick, and more sensitive than palpation or preoperative imaging. If a lesion is found, tissue should be obtained for pathologic confirmation.

AFTER TREATMENT FOR THE PRIMARY TUMOR

Two-thirds of all patients with liver metastases present with major symptoms referable to the liver, including pain, ascites, jaundice, anorexia, and weight loss. Patients with carcinoid syndrome present with flushing and profuse diarrhea. Hepatomegaly, often distinctly nodular, and tenderness are found commonly. But since symptomatic patients rarely respond significantly

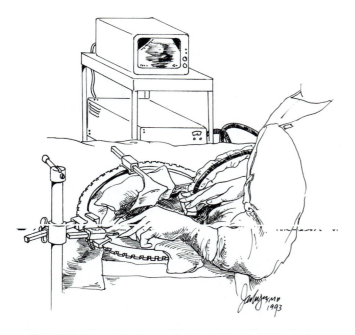

Figure 54–2. Intraoperative ultrasound is performed to evaluate the entire liver.

to any specific treatment, the challenge for physicians is to identify patients with asymptomatic hepatic metastases amenable to surgical resection.

The detection of metachronous hepatic metastases following resection of the primary tumor is only one goal of optimum management. In colorectal carcinoma, other potentially valuable goals include the detection of local (intestinal) recurrence and of the rare resectable pulmonary metastasis (2% incidence; 5 year survival, 15% to 35%).

When designing a specific diagnostic strategy for patients after resection of the primary tumor, it is important to remember that the early detection of asymptomatic but incurable disease generally serves no useful purpose, since palliative measures are not innocuous and may be equally effective when instituted at the onset of symptoms. Factors that may render any later hepatic metastasis incurable include co-existing medical conditions that will contraindicate major resection and any characteristics of the primary tumor that are predictive of a poor outcome for later metastases. Such prognostic characteristics of primary colorectal tumors include extreme de-differentiation and multiple positive mesenteric nodes. Conversely, factors that are predictive of a very low incidence of metastasis, such as low primary stage or grade, may not support the cost-effectiveness of extensive postoperative evaluations.

Plasma CEA levels will be elevated above normal in 89% to 95% of patients with colorectal hepatic metastases and will be the first positive test available in 67% of cases. However, early detection of hepatic metastases by plasma CEA levels may not significantly improve the survival rate following resection. While alkaline phosphatase levels can be useful, elevations are nonspecific, and liver enzyme levels, in general, are insufficiently reliable for routine evaluations.

Recommendations regarding methods of follow-up after resection of the primary tumor are potentially subject to rapid modification with the evolution of technology, such as tumor-specific antigens, which may be shown to increase diagnostic sensitivity and specificity. A reasonable follow-up regimen for colorectal carcinoma, which is based on current studies of cost effectiveness, is to perform history and physical examination and plasma CEA level every 3 months for 2 years after surgery. Endoscopy of the remaining colon should be done at 6 months and them biannually.

AFTER DISCOVERY OF HEPATIC METASTASES

Should routine evaluation reveal an abnormality in the liver, further studies are indicated. A modest elevation of the plasma CEA level should be repeated. Imaging with contrast-enhanced computer tomography (CT),

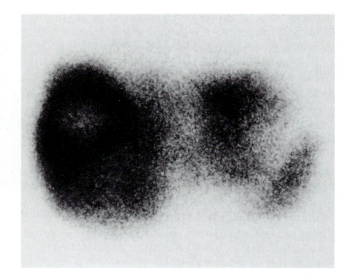

A

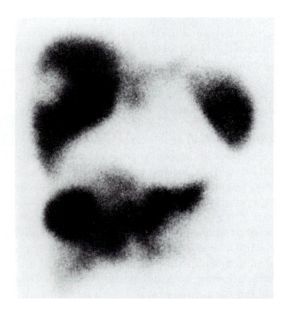

B

Figure 54–3. A. The radionuclide ^{99m}Tc-microaggregated arterial flow scan shows a hypervascular tumor "rim." **B**. The upper radionuclide done with ^{99m}Tc-sulphur colloid shows a "cold" area in the liver. The scan done with ^{99m}Tc-microaggregated albumin injected intra-arterially shows a "hot" spot due to tumor hypervascularity.

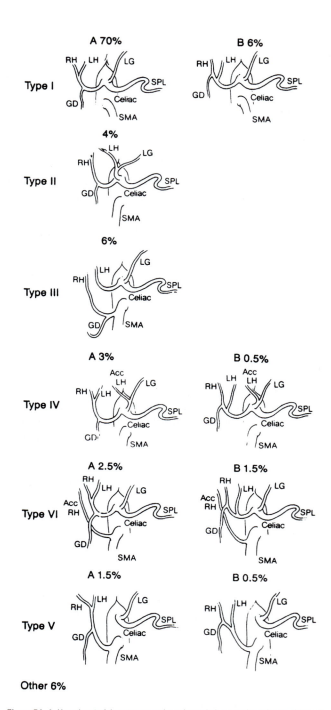

Figure 54–4. Hepatic arterial anatomy can be quite varied; approximately two-thirds of individuals have type I anatomy.

magnetic resonance imaging (MRI), or ultrasound should be used to establish the extent of hepatic and extrahepatic disease. Each of these tests has unique advantages and weaknesses; all are sensitive for hepatic metastases that are a minimum of 1 to 2 cm in diameter. CT portography is the most sensitive imaging tech-

nique; it requires arteriographic placement of a catheter into the superior mesenteric artery for contrast infusion. Radioimmunoscintigraphy with an indium-labeled anti-CEA antibody has detected hepatic metastases when conventional methods have failed, although widespread clinical usefulness of this promising approach has yet to be established. Hepatic scanning after injection of ^{99m}Tc-labeled microaggregated albumin into the hepatic artery defines the nutrient blood supply of tumor implants (Fig 54–3) and is predictive of tumor response to intraarterial chemotherapy. Although of little value in defining the extent of tumor, hepatic arteriography is often used preoperatively to define the hepatic arterial anatomy (Fig 54–4), especially if infusion pump implantation is contemplated. Pulmonary, intracranial, and bone metastases and metachronous colon cancer should be ruled out prior to hepatic resection. Finally, if surgery is to proceed, autologous blood should be secured if possible.

AT THE TIME OF HEPATIC RESECTION

Intraoperative ultrasound has proven extremely valuable as an adjunct to hepatic resection in defining the location of vital structures, the extent of resection required to obtain adequate margins, and the presence of additional unsuspected metastatic lesions. Further assistance is available with radioimmuno-guided surgery (RIGS), a new technique that changes the planned operative procedure in 50% of hepatic resections. An intraoperative (hand-held or laparoscopic) gamma detector is used to detect a radiolabeled antitumor antibody that has become localized to the tumor.

The goal of this extensive evaluation is to optimize decisions as to further therapy for the patient with hepatic metastases: curative resection, regional antitumor infusion, other surgical management, or nonsurgical systemic/palliative treatment.

■ RESECTION

Resection of hepatic metastases is the only potentially curative option available for this condition. Approximately 30% of patients survive beyond 5 years. Improvements in patients' outcomes will result from identification of those most likely to benefit from resection, application of optimal curative techniques for those selected, and minimization of operative morbidity and mortality.

INDICATIONS

Efforts to identify reliable prognostic factors to predict long-term outcome of patients undergoing hepatic resection continue to evolve, and the large number of patients that would be required to demonstrate probable survival differences make a randomized prospective trial improbable. Nonetheless, consideration of each of these factors is required prior to a decision to resect hepatic metastases (Table 54–1).

TABLE 54–1. FACTORS ADVERSELY CORRELATING WITH SURVIVAL IN PATIENTS WITH HEPATIC METASTASES

EXTENT OF METASTASES
  Presence of extrahepatic disease
  Unresectable with adequate margins
  Inadequate uninvolved liver to support life (50% to 60%)
  Numerous (>3) implants
  Markedly elevated plasma CEA level
  Elevated plasma alkaline phosphatase level
  Decreased serum albumin level
  Elevated serum bilirubin level
  Ascites
  Palpable hepatomegaly
  Weight loss (>5%), anorexia, hepatic pain/tenderness, fevers
  Blood transfusion required for resection

CHARACTERISTICS OF THE PRIMARY TUMOR
  Unresectable/bypassed tumor
  Extreme de-differentiation (high histologic grade)
  Extensive regional nodal metastases (Dukes C)
  Synchronous/short interval until metastases
  Elevated plasma CEA level preoperatively

CHARACTERISTICS OF THE PATIENT
  Cirrhosis
  Karnofsky performance scores <80%
  Other medical conditions making operative stress problematic

Extent of Hepatic Metastases

Evaluation of the extent of metastatic disease is the first consideration. A staging system has been developed (Table 54–2) in order to standardize descriptions of extent of hepatic metastases and facilitate comparison of results. There is a consensus that resectable tumor must be localized to the liver. Finding distant extrahepatic spread or positive portal lymph nodes generally contraindicates hepatic resection, despite occasional reports of success. Although up to two-thirds of the liver may be removed in noncirrhotic patients, resections for metastatic disease rarely require such extensive procedures. Removal of portions of contiguous structures, such as the diaphragm and abdominal wall, does not eliminate a successful outcome; in fact, the size of individual tumor implants has little bearing on prognosis. The total number of implants is an important factor; although satellites may be more favorable, a finding of more than three tumor implants reduces the likelihood of long-term success. Markedly elevated plasma CEA and alkaline phosphatase levels are negative considerations. Liver failure and ascites are usually indicators of end-stage disease and massive hepatic replacement. However, the presence of other symptoms, while a negative prognostic factor, does not sufficiently jeopardize the outcome to constitute a contraindication. Requirement for blood transfusion at the time of hepatic resec-

TABLE 54–2. INTERNATIONAL STAGING SYSTEM FOR HEPATIC METASTASES

Stage	% Hepatic Replacement	Extrahepatic	Symptoms	Code
0	resected	0	0	
I	<25	0	0	P1E0S0
II	25–75	0	0	P2E0S0
III	>75 or	+ or	+	P3 or... Any P with E1 or S1

Extent of hepatic and extrahepatic disease is determined by best imaging technique available in each institution. Symptoms must be attributable to hepatic metastases.

tion, although associated with the extent of the operation performed, may be an independent predictor of poor outcome.

Characteristics

Characteristics of the primary tumor also should be considered. Extreme de-differentiation and extensive regional nodal metastases are predictors of poor outcome after hepatic resection of metastases in most studies. Synchronous metastases or a very short interval between treatment of the primary and the discovery of metastases are negative factors in some studies, but do not contraindicate resection. The specific site of the colorectal primary does not correlate with outcome. Elevation of the plasma CEA level in colon cancer is associated with a poorer outcome in some series, but other tumor markers have not yet been demonstrated to distinguish, more reliably, biologically aggressive tumors.

Patient Characteristics

Characteristics of the patient are the final consideration. Advanced cirrhosis precludes a major hepatic resection owing to increased vascularity, lack of functional liver reserve, impaired regenerative capacity, and, perhaps, reduced systemic tumor defenses. For example, poor general health as reflected in low Karnofsky performance index scores is a significant negative factor. Other medical conditions must, of course, be sufficiently manageable to allow the stress of a major operation. Age and gender of the patient have no predictive values.

OPERATIVE CONSIDERATIONS

Techniques of hepatic resection are discussed in detail in Chapter 55. The most significant prognostic factor in the treatment of hepatic metastases is the ability to remove all apparent tumor with an adequate margin of liver tissue. Recurrence is virtually assured when mar-

gins of resection are positive for residual tumor. Malignant cells can be microscopically detected for a distance of only about 1 mm from the visible edge of an implant, and a margin of 1 cm has been demonstrated repeatedly to be optimal. Larger, anatomic resections do not offer a survival advantage compared with smaller wedge resections. Intraoperative design of the minimum safe operation required to achieve adequate margins around all metastatic disease thus is essential. This plan may be facilitated greatly by an intraoperative ultrasound study and RIGS. Glisson's capsule may be a natural barrier to tumor dissemination and it should be left intact. Adjacent soft tissues may be resected in continuity with the specimen in order to achieve this goal.

Minimization of blood loss is especially important in view of the possibly deleterious effect of transfusion on long-term outcome. Compression of the vessels in the porta hepatis (Pringle's maneuver) will reduce blood loss and may be safely maintained with a noncrushing clamp for up to 60 minutes at ambient temperature. Total vascular isolation of the liver should be considered for major resections. Autotransfusion should be achieved whenever possible, and intraoperative blood salvage and reinfusion is indicated; there is little risk of dissemination of viable malignant cells as long as the tumor is not entered and 1 cm margins are maintained.

Adequate exposure is a prerequisite to both operative planning and minimization of blood loss. Complete mobilization of the liver greatly facilitates this exposure, as does division of the appropriate portal vessels, if anatomic resection is anticipated. It is no longer routine to enter the right chest for hepatic resection, but extension through the chest wall and diaphragm should be considered whenever necessary to improve access to the hepatic veins and vena cava.

RESULTS OF RESECTION

Natural History

The natural history of hepatic metastases in colorectal carcinoma is better than for other common tumors metastasizing to the liver. However 5 year untreated survivors are nearly unprecedented. Median survival is usually <1 year (4 to 24 months), but median survival for the subgroup of untreated patients with less extensive disease, which would be amenable to resection, is about 20 months.

Survival after Resection

At five years, survival after resection is 25% to 30% overall, although it should be noted that all reported series represent selected patients. Median survival after resection is often no different from a comparable un-

TABLE 54–3. SURVIVAL AFTER RESECTION OF HEPATIC METASTASES

	Median Survival: Months		5 Yr Survival	
	Mean	*(Range)*	*Mean*	*(Range)*
OVERALL UNTREATED	11	(4–24)	0%	
CURATIVE RESECTIONS				
Solitary	20	(16–24)	36%	(0–90)
Multiple	15	(5–26)	26%	(0–50)
Synchronous	42	(n.a.)	27%	(0–38)
Metachronous	32	(24–40)	31%	(0–59)
			2 Yr Survival	
Small, Wedge	29	(24–45)	50%	(41–60)
Large, Anatomic	23	(11–34)	24%	(15–36)

treated subgroup, but 5 year survivals are clearly improved (Table 54–3). Studies of survival correlated with extent of resection represent heterogenous groups of highly selected patients, and differences are almost certainly the result of the extent of tumor replacement plus difficulty with securing clear margins. Disease-free intervals and median survivals for patients undergoing re-resection (one or two) of hepatic metastases are also better than those for untreated disease, although follow-ups are still too short to permit accurate estimates of long-term benefits in this subgroup.

Morbidity and Mortality

Morbidity and mortality figures continue to improve with advances in patient selection, technique, and perioperative support. Operative mortality is consistently reported at under 5%; significant morbidity is usually about 25% (3% to 62%).

Postoperative Follow-Up

Follow-up after hepatic resection should include frequent visits with intensive evaluation of any detected abnormality. Postoperative abdominal CT scan and plasma CEA level should be obtained to establish a baseline. Ten to twenty percent of these patients may develop a re-resectable recurrence. In order to minimize the extent of additional volume resected, early detection using plasma CEA levels is extremely important in the case of re-recurrence.

■ REGIONAL INFUSION

Direct infusion of antitumor agents into the hepatic artery has theoretical advantages for treatment of hepatic metastatic disease. The fact that metastases are supplied almost exclusively by the hepatic artery while the liver receives substantial alternate flow through the portal vein means that higher drug concentrations can be applied to the tumor while sparing toxicity to the liver. Since the antitumor agent passes first through the tumor neovasculature and capillary system, much will be extracted and higher doses can thus be administered without systemic toxicity. Since the tumor neovasculature is unable to respond to vasoactive drugs, relative tumor concentration of infused agents may be further boosted by pharmacologic manipulations.

Clear disadvantages to regional infusion also have emerged. Gastroduodenitis and ulceration, probably owing to infusion of the antitumor agent into the intestinal blood supply, are common (28%) but usually resolve with reduction in dose. Gastroduodenal complications may be avoided by meticulous ligation of the right gastric artery and collaterals, especially the supraduodenal artery near its origin from the gastroduodenal. However, rigorous dearterialization in the porta hepatis may contribute to a higher incidence of the other major complications of this procedure, biliary stricture, and sclerosing cholangitis. These complications require complete cessation of infusion therapy and can result in prolonged, severe side effects. The incidence of serious hepatobiliary toxicity (12%) may be reduced by alternating chemotherapeutic agents or by administering drugs in a circadian, rather than continuous, pattern.

The optimal antitumor protocol has yet to be established; indeed, the ultimate value of this procedure will depend on the development of more effective chemotherapeutic or biologic response-modifying agents. FUDR (floxuridine) is currently the most commonly infused agent for colorectal metastases. 5-fluoro-uracil (5-FU), a precursor to FUDR, also is used but achieves lower tumor concentrations. Leucovorin (folinic acid) may increase the effectiveness of FUDR but also increases its hepatobiliary toxicity.

INDICATIONS

The same principles that make hepatic infusion so attractive for hepatic metastases make it less effective for extrahepatic disease, where systemic therapy remains the only useful option. When preoperative imaging and intraoperative ultrasound and RIGS demonstrate unresectable synchronous or metachronous disease limited to the liver, infusion therapy may be considered. Patients who have failed systemic therapy for liver metastases but retain a good general performance standard also may benefit from this procedure. Finally, regional chemotherapy is theoretically very attractive in an adjuvant role following hepatic resection and may be significantly more effective than systemic therapy in this setting.

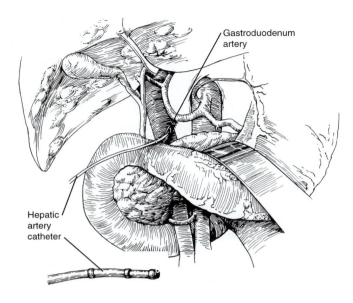

Figure 54–5. This schematic shows the catheter inserted into the gastroduodenal artery for hepatic infusion.

TECHNIQUE

Celiac and superior mesenteric arteriography define the highly variable anatomy of the hepatic arterial blood supply (Fig 54–4). Following this, the patient may be taken with the catheter in the common hepatic artery for angiographically enhanced CT (CT portography), a very sensitive determinant of the extent of disease. While a percutaneous catheter has been used for infusion therapy, risks of infection, inadequate catheter fixation, and nonexclusive hepatic infusion generally make this technique unwarranted.

An upper abdominal incision is used, and a careful exploration is done to confirm the absence of extrahepatic metastases. Extrahepatic disease probably negates any long-term benefit of regional infusion. Extent of liver replacement should be correlated with preoperative assessments and carefully documented to allow accurate later determinations of tumor response rates.

If present, the gallbladder is removed to prevent chemical cholecystitis. The hepatic arterial supply is exposed with dissection in the hepatoduodenal and hepatogastric ligaments medial to the common bile duct while the liver is retracted cephalad (Fig 54–5). Normally the catheter will be placed in the gastroduodenal artery, ligating it distally as well as ligating its posterior pancreaticoduodenal branch. Dissection is continued to the bifurcation of the proper hepatic artery into right and left hepatic arteries. All branches are ligated to prevent infusion of chemotherapy into the stomach and duodenum or into unsuspected branches to the com-

mon bile duct. Further dissection of the right and left hepatic arteries may reveal other important collateral branches. Injury to the common and left hepatic bile ducts must be avoided throughout this dissection. The catheter tip is fixed with ligatures to rest at the junction of gastroduodenal and proper hepatic arteries. Intraoperative fluorescein infusion will document adequate perfusion of the liver only. Postoperatively, technetium 99m (^{99m}Tc)-macroaggregated albumin infusion also will document exclusive perfusion, and the pattern of tumor uptake is predictive of response to infusion therapy.

Variable hepatic arterial supply may require alternate catheter placement. Celiac stenosis with retrograde flow through the gastroduodenal artery requires catheter insertion into the common hepatic artery with proximal ligation and with the tip at the junction of gastroduodenal and proper hepatic arteries. When there is <2 cms of proper hepatic artery prior to division into left and right hepatic, or if the left hepatic arises prior to the gastroduodenal, the catheter should be placed in the splenic artery with the tip at the junction of splenic artery and celiac trunk. If the left hepatic artery arises from the left gastric or directly from the celiac trunk, a second catheter in the left gastric artery is required. If the right hepatic artery arises from the superior mesenteric, a second catheter in the right hepatic artery is used.

A subcutaneous pocket is created through a separate incision, usually in the lower abdomen below the belt line. The gas-powered pump is implanted and the catheter tunneled through the abdominal wall, flushed with heparinized saline and placed into the appropriate artery.

RESULTS

Most patients presenting for regional infusion today are asymptomatic. Palliation, then, is not a satisfactory endpoint to measure the effectiveness of the procedure. Survival benefits have been difficult to document so far, although prospective studies are in progress. Median survivals usually are prolonged compared to historical controls (8 to 27 months), and objectively measured tumor responses of about 50% (35% to 75%) imply that substantial benefit may be shown for regional infusion. Widespread use of this procedure will require reduction of serious hepatobiliary morbidity and development of more effective antitumor regimens.

CURRENT INDICATIONS AND PROTOCOLS FOR THE IMPLANTABLE INFUSAID PUMP

Although there was initial widespread enthusiasm for the results from regional infusion for hepatic metastases from colorectal cancer, these results have been tempered by various reports that patient survival has not increased. Patients who are treated with implantable infusion pumps should be on a prospective study protocol. The current indications for the implantable pump are (1) patients who are operated on to undergo hepatic resection but who are found to have four or more metastases in the liver without evidence of disease outside of the liver, (2) those patients with disease limited to the liver who have received systemic chemotherapy, who have responded and then have lost the response to the systemic treatment and have a good performance status, and (3) potentially, those individuals who have both primary large bowel cancer and metastatic disease to the liver only and who undergo colon resection.

These current indications provide guidelines for the surgeon and/or institution to be prepared for full services to the patient with colorectal cancer. It is not uncommon to evaluate fully for metastatic colorectal cancer of the liver and discover at the time of surgery that the patient has a tumor confined to the liver, but in both lobes. If this is unanticipated, these patients are candidates for regional chemotherapy. However, it is helpful to know prior to surgery whether the patient has any aberrant anatomy of the hepatic arterial architecture. If regional chemotherapy is to be considered, prior hepatic arteriography should be performed.

For the second indication, patients usually receive systemic chemotherapy and have responded but have begun to fail in the liver again. Regional chemotherapy is only appropriate when there is disease confined to the liver. These patients should be fully informed and have a good performance status.

Those undergoing colon resection for their primary tumor at the same time that the metastatic disease is present in the liver can receive regional chemotherapy or alternatively, are candidates for systemic chemotherapy.

Current protocols using hepatic infusion pumps consist of multiple group trials comparing two forms of therapy after hepatic resection for colorectal metastatic disease. One form of therapy combines intrahepatic infusion and systemic chemotherapy, whereas the other form of therapy consists of no therapy. The infusion arm consists of intraarterial FUDR plus intravenous 5-FU. Another protocol consists of FUDR plus Leucovorin administered in the infusion pump compared with intravenous chemotherapy using 5-FU. Other protocols use a 6-week program in which the patient receives 1 week of intraarterial infusion consisting of FUDR followed by a 2 week rest and then three weekly injections of 5-FU with Leucovorin. All of these protocols currently are underway with endpoints looking at patient survival, tumor response, and complication rates of regional hepatic infusion.

■ OTHER SURGICAL TREATMENT

HEPATIC ARTERY LIGATION

Hepatic artery ligation has been used to reduce tumor blood supply and has been combined with portal infusion of chemotherapeutic agents with no apparent improvement over arterial infusion. However, transient hepatic artery occlusion with biodegradable starch microspheres (Fig 54–6), or chemotherapy-impregnated microcap-

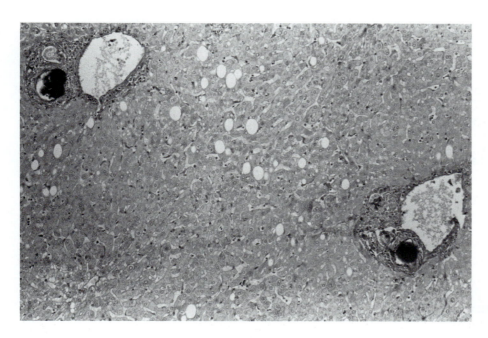

Figure 54–6. PAS stain of liver biopsy after hepatic artery infusion of biodegradable starch microspheres. Arterial occlusion is demonstrated.

TABLE 54–4. ARTERIAL VERSUS PORTAL INFUSION FOR HEPATIC COLORECTAL METASTASES

	Hepatic Artery	Portal Vein	Crossover: Vein to Artery
TUMOR RESPONSE			
Major (>50%)	40%	0	33%
Minor (25%–50%)	25%	0	...
PLASMA CEA LEVELS			
Reduced >50%	50%	25%	33%
TOXICITY			
Gastroduodenitis	25%	9%	33%
Increasing Serum Bilirubin	50%	9%	9%
DURATION OF RESPONSE	8 mo	...	8 mo

sules, has shown experimental and clinical promise and may prove to be a useful adjuvant to arterial infusion. Vasoconstrictive drugs may increase the ratio of tumor to parenchymal blood flow owing to the insensitivity of tumor neovascularity. Such manipulations may prove useful to increase the effectiveness of infusion chemotherapy.

PORTAL VEIN INFUSION

Portal vein infusion of hepatic metastases is of little benefit. Even intraportal infusion adjuvant to initial resection of high-risk primaries has not proven to be benefi-

cial. Although the rapidly growing outer rim of tumor implants may be supplied by the portal vein, direct comparison of arterial and portal infusions clearly establishes the superior effectiveness of hepatic artery infusion (Table 54–4).

HYPERTHERMIA

Hyperthermia applied by radiofrequency to unresectable metastases has produced a high level of tumor response in clinical trials, but any long-term benefits remain unproven.

CRYOTHERAPY

Cryotherapy, with the limits of freezing determined by intraoperative ultrasound, may be used to extend resectability or as treatment for unresectable metastases. Initial results have been encouraging, although long-term control of hepatic disease rarely has been achieved. Reported complications have been minimal.

LIVER TRANSPLANTATION

Liver transplantation, which could be an option when resection would not be tolerated owing to inadequate liver reserves, rarely is performed for metastatic disease because of the high risk of recurrence related to immunosuppression.

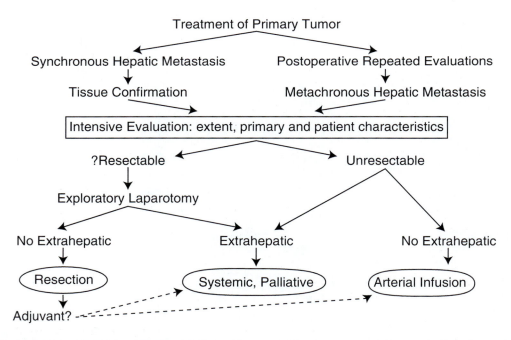

Figure 54–7. Decision tree for patients with hepatic metastases. Beginning with treatment of the primary tumor, optimal management depends on careful weighing of multiple factors and making the best individual treatment choice.

■ CONCLUSIONS

In recent years, the prognosis for some patients with hepatic metastases has improved greatly owing to advances in techniques of liver resection. Colorectal tumors are the most common hepatic metastases, and most liver resections are done for this condition. Nearly two-thirds of patients with this very common malignancy will develop hepatic metastases, but only 30% to 50% of these will be amenable to surgery. Mean 5 year survivals after resection for cure are 25% to 30% overall, and higher with careful case selection based on extent of metastases, characteristics of the primary tumor, and patient characteristics.

The biologic steps of tumor progression that lead to metastatic competence in colon cancer involve multiple genetic alterations; adhesive cell-surface molecules, such as DCC and CEA, are involved in this process and in organ-specific targeting. Hepatic metastases are supplied almost exclusively by the hepatic artery, but usually reach the liver via the portal vein. Once implanted, tumor implants induce neovascularity that is insensitive to vasoactive drugs.

Frequent clinical evaluations and plasma CEA levels should be part of postoperative monitoring for colorectal patients. When liver metastases are suspected, intensive diagnostic evaluation should be undertaken. CT portogram is the most accurate imaging technique overall, and operative ultrasound may be an extremely useful adjunct. Radioimmunoscintigraphy and radioimmunoguided surgery may become increasingly valuable with the development of better tumor antibodies. Preoperative angiography is an important diagnostic measure, and infusion scanning may well be incorporated with it.

Hepatic resection rarely should be undertaken in the presence of extrahepatic disease, and is contraindicated unless approximately 1-cm tumor-free margins can be safely obtained. Many other adverse prognostic signs must be considered, but none constitute absolute contraindications individually. Minimization of blood transfusions may be especially important during hepatic resection.

Patients who are not candidates for resection may benefit from regional infusion of antitumor agents via hepatic artery infusion. Arterial infusion also may be helpful as an adjuvant to resection. FUDR is currently the most frequently used drug. Demonstrated survival advantages are contingent upon development of optimal protocols and more effective agents. Other surgical options, such as hepatic artery ligation and occlusion, hyperthermia, cryosurgery, and liver transplantation, may prove useful, although their roles have not been clearly established.

The surgical management of patients with hepatic metastases involves sorting through a large number of variables and choosing an optimal course of action;

these decisions are summarized in Figure 54–7. Optimum selection of cases and technologic advances will continue to improve the outcome for patients with this previously hopeless condition.

SELECTED READINGS

Andrade SP, Bakhle YS, et al. Effects of tumour cells on angiogenesis and vasoconstrictor responses in sponge implants in mice. *Br J Cancer* 1992;66:821

Arnold MW, Schneebaum S, et al. Intraoperative detection of colorectal cancer with radioimmunoguided surgery and CC49, a second-generation monoclonal antibody. *Ann Surg* 1992;216:627

Aznavoorian S, Murphy AN, et al. Molecular aspects of tumor cell invasion and metastasis. *Cancer* 1993;71:1368

Ballantyne GH, Quin J. Surgical treatment of liver metastases in patients with colorectal cancer. *Cancer* 1993;71:4252

Blackshear PJ, Dorman FD, et al. The design and initial testing of an implantable infusion pump. *Surg Gynecol Obstet* 1972;134:51

Breedis C, Young G. The blood supply of neoplasms of the liver. *Am J Pathol* 1954;30:969

Cady B, Stone MD. The role of surgical resection of liver metastases in colorectal carcinoma. *Semin Oncol* 1991;18:399

Cho KR, Vogelstein B. Genetic alterations in the adenoma-carcinoma sequence. *Cancer* 1992;70:1727

Clarkson B, Young C, et al. Effects of continuous hepatic artery infusion of antimetabolites on primary and metastatic cancer of the liver. *Cancer* 1962;25:472

Daly JM. Hepatic arterial chemotherapy for colorectal liver metastases: a perspective. *Perspec Gen Surg* 1991;2:97

Daly JM, Butler J, et al. Predicting tumor response in patients with colorectal hepatic metastases. *Ann Surg* 1985;202:384

Daly JM, Kemeny N, et al. Long-term hepatic arterial infusion chemotherapy. *Arch Surg* 1984;119:936

Daly JM, Kemeny N, et al. Regional infusion for colorectal hepatic metastases: a randomized trial comparing the hepatic artery with the portal vein. *Arch Surg* 1987;122:1273

Didolkar MS, Elias EG, et al. Unresectable hepatic metastases from carcinoma of the colon and rectum. *Surg Gynecol Obstet* 1985;160:429

Doerr RJ, Abdel-Nabi H, et al. Detection of primary colorectal cancer with indium 111 monoclonal antibody B72.3. *Arch Surg* 1990;125:1601

Evans CW. Cell adhesion and metastasis. *Cell Biol Int Rep* 1992;16:1

Finan PJ, Marshall RJ, et al. Factors affecting survival in patients presenting with synchronous hepatic metastases from colorectal cancer: a clinical and computer analysis. *Br J Surg* 1985;72:373

Fortner JG, Silva JS, et al. Multivariate analysis of a personal series of 247 patients with liver metastases from colorectal cancer. *Ann Surg* 1984;199:317

Hohne MW, Halatsch ME, et al. Frequent loss of expression of the potential tumor suppressor gene DCC in ductal pancreatic adenocarcinoma. *Cancer Res* 1992;52:2616

Hostetter RB, Augustus LB, et al. Carcinoembryonic antigen

as a selective enhancer of colorectal cancer metastasis. *J Natl Cancer Inst* 1990;82:380

Hughes K, Scheele J, Sugarbaker PH. Surgery for colorectal cancer metastatic to the liver: optimizing the results of treatment. *Surg Clin North Am* 1989;69:339

Keen WW. Report of a case of resection of the liver for the removal of a neoplasm with a table of seventy-six cases of resection of the liver for hepatic tumors. *Ann Surg* 1899;30:267

Kelly CJ, Daly JM. Colorectal cancer: principles of postoperative follow-up. *Cancer* 1992;70:1397

Kemeny N, Cohen A, et al. Continuous intrahepatic infusion of floxuridine and leucovorin through an implantable pump for the treatment of hepatic metastases from colorectal carcinoma. *Cancer* 1990;65:2446

Kim JA, Triozzi PL, Martin E Jr. Radioimmunoguided surgery for colorectal cancer. *Oncology* 1993;7:55

Lorenz M, Hottenrott C, et al. Continuous regional treatment with fluoropyrimidines for metastases from colorectal carcinomas: influence of modulation with leucovorin. *Semin Oncol* 1992;19:163

Machi J, Isomoto H, et al. Intraoperative ultrasonography in screening for liver metastases from colorectal cancer: comparative accuracy with traditional procedures. *Surgery* 1987;101:678

Martin EW, Minton JP, Corey LC. CEA-directed second look surgery in the asymptomatic patient after primary resection of colorectal carcinoma. *Ann Surg* 1985;202:310

Mattsson J, Appelgren L, et al. Adrenergic innervation of tumor blood vessels. *Cancer Lett* 1977;3:347

Mavligit GM, Zukiwski AA, et al. Regional biologic therapy: hepatic arterial infusion of recombinant human tumor necrosis factor in patients with liver metastases. *Cancer* 1992;69:557

Metzger U, Mermillod B, et al. Intraportal chemotherapy in colorectal carcinoma as an adjuvant modality. *World J Surg* 1987;1:452

Mountain CF, Khalil KG, et al. The contribution of surgery to the management of carcinomatous pulmonary metastases. *Cancer* 1978;41:833

Nakamura S, Sakaguchi S, et al. Aggressive repeat liver resection for hepatic metastases of colorectal carcinoma. *Surg Today* 1992;22:260

Onik G, Rubinsky B, et al. Ultrasound-guided hepatic cryosurgery in the treatment of metastatic colon carcinoma: preliminary results. *Cancer* 1991;67:901

Patt YZ, McBride CM, et al. Adjuvant perioperative hepatic mitomycin C and floxuridine combined with surgical resection of metastatic colorectal cancer in the liver. *Cancer* 1987;59:867

Pihil E, Hughes ESR, McDermott FT. Lung recurrence after curative surgery for colorectal cancer. *Dis Colon Rectum* 1987;30:417

Ravikumar TS, Steele GJ, et al. Experimental and clinical observations on hepatic cryosurgery for colorectal metastases. *Cancer Res* 1991;51:6323

Ridge JA, Bading JR, et al. Perfusion of colorectal hepatic metastases: relative distribution of flow from the hepatic artery and portal vein. *Cancer* 1987;59:1547

Ridge JA, Daly JM. Treatment of colorectal hepatic metastases. *Surgery* 1985;161:597

Rifkin MD, Rosato FE, et al. Intraoperative ultrasound of the liver: an important adjunctive tool for decision making in the operating room. *Ann Surg* 1987;205:466

Roemeling R, Hrusheky WJM. Circadian patterning of continuous floxuridine infusion reduces toxicity and allows higher dose intensity in patients with widespread cancer. *J Clin Oncol* 1989;7:1710

Rosen CB, Nagorney DM, et al. Perioperative blood transfusion and determinants of survival after liver resection for metastatic colorectal carcinoma. *Ann Surg* 1992;216:493

Steeg PS. Invasion and metastasis. *Curr Opin Oncol* 1992;4:134

Sullivan RD, Miller E, Sikes MP. Antimetabolite-metabolite combination cancer chemotherapy: effects of intra-arterial methotrexate-intramuscular Citrovorum factor therapy in human cancer. *Cancer* 1959;12:1248

Sullivan RD, Norcross JW, Watkins E. Chemotherapy of metastatic liver cancer by prolonged hepatic artery infusion. *N Engl J Med* 1964;270:321

Trezona T, Butler JA, Vargas H. Angiotensin alteration of drug uptake in an experimental model of hepatic metastases. *J Surg Res* 1991;51:124

Vaillant JC, Balladur P, et al. Repeat liver resection for recurrent colorectal metastases. *Br J Surg* 1993;80:340

Wagman LD, Kemeny MM, et al. A prospective, randomized evaluation of the treatment of colorectal cancer metastatic to the liver. *J Clin Oncol* 1990;8:1885

Wolf RF, Goodnight JE, et al. Results of resection and proposed guidelines for patient selection in instances of noncolorectal hepatic metastases. *Surg Gynecol Obset* 1991;173:454

Woodington GF, Waugh JM. Results of resection of metastatic tumors of the liver. *Am J Surg* 1963;105:24

55

Hepatic Resection

Seymour I. Schwartz

The evolution of hepatic resection, from an imprecise removal of portions of the liver, frequently accompanied by extensive hemorrhage, to a controlled anatomic procedure with acceptable risk, represents a major advance in modern surgery. This accomplishment has been made possible by (1) an appreciation of the segmental distribution of blood vessels and bile ducts within the liver, (2) recognition of the functional reserve of the liver and the extreme potential for hepatic regeneration, (3) a better understanding of hepatic function and the metabolic needs of the liver, (4) improvements in surgical technique that have reduced the hazard of uncontrollable hemorrhage, and (5) data that have made a strong case for improved survival following resection of primary and metastatic malignancies of the liver.

■ HISTORICAL BACKGROUND

The first surgical removal of a portion of the liver was recorded in 1716 by Berta, who amputated the protruding portion of the liver in a patient with a self-inflicted knife wound. In 1870, Bruns resected a lacerated portion of the liver in a soldier wounded during the Franco-Prussian war. In 1886, Lius excised a solid tumor of the left lobe of the liver by cutting through a pedicled lesion; death owing to hemorrhage from the stump occurred 6 hours later. In 1888, Langenbuch successfully excised a pedicled tumor of the left lobe of the liver; the

patient had a long and difficult postoperative course but eventually recovered. Tiffany, in 1890, was the first American surgeon to report a case of hepatic resection for tumor. He excised a walnut-sized mass from the convex surface of the left lobe, using scissors and cauterization. In the United States, the first reported removal of a true neoplasm was accomplished by Keen who, in 1892, resected a cystic lesion from the edge of the right lobe of the liver. Keen resected an angioma in 1897 and a large primary carcinoma of the left lobe in 1899. Wendel has been credited with the first authentic case of near-total right lobectomy, performed in 1910 for a primary tumor; the patient survived 9 years. The right hepatic artery and the right hepatic duct were ligated at the hilus of the liver, but Wendel did not attempt ligation of the right portal vein in its extrahepatic position. In 1949, Wangensteen removed the entire right lobe of the liver for metastatic carcinoma of the stomach.

The modern era of anatomic hepatic lobectomy dates from the 1952 report of Lortat-Jacob and Robert, who used a thoracoabdominal approach and a technique designed to control hemorrhage by extrahepatic ligation of the contributing vessels. In 1953, Quattlebaum reported three cases of major hepatic resection, two by guillotine technique. The other represents the first recorded right hepatic lobectomy performed for primary hepatocellular carcinoma. In this patient, the technique of primary hilar ligation of the vessels and ducts was used.

Digitoclasia, or finger fracture, of the hepatic parenchyma has evolved during the last 30 years. In 1953, Quattlebaum, in his classic article, described breaking the liver with the handle of a knife and clamping the vessels within the plane of transection. In 1956, Fineberg and associates reported on right hepatic lobectomy for primary carcinoma of the liver; they carried out a quick parenchymal dissection with the finger on the back of the scalpel. In 1958, Tien Y. Lin and associates introduced a new technique in which the thumb and index finger are inserted into the liver tissue, after which the surgeon "fractures and crushes the tissue between the fingers, and when resistant vessels or ducts are encountered they are tied and divided." In 1963, Ton That Tung modified this technique by occluding the portal pedicle before finger fracture. More recently, Couinaud demonstrated a segmental anatomy of the liver leading to the use of anatomic segmentectomy.

■ INDICATIONS

The indications for hepatic resection include (1) parasitic and nonparasitic cysts, (2) granulomatous processes, (3) benign primary neoplasms, (4) malignant primary tumors, and (5) secondary tumors that involve the liver by direct extension or metastasis. The technique of planned anatomic resection generally is reserved for lesions that are large or located so that resection along an anatomic plane provides the opportunity for the most complete removal, coupled with the best control of vascular supply. Resection along anatomic planes with vascular control rarely is indicated for trauma, where the preferred approach is limited resectional debridement that permits removal of devitalized tissue and control of bleeding.

Advanced cirrhosis generally precludes a major hepatic resection, since intraoperative bleeding from collaterals and parenchymal vessels is increased significantly. The incidence of liver failure with resection is increased because of lack of reserve; hepatic regeneration is impaired, and reported cures for malignant tumors in cirrhotic patients are negligible.

■ SURGICAL ANATOMY

LIGAMENTOUS ATTACHMENTS

The peritoneal relationships of the liver relate to the embryologic development. Since the liver develops as a forward extension between two layers of ventral mesentery, a prehepatic and posthepatic portion of this original mesentery results. The ventral mesentery extends only to the umbilicus; the dorsal mesentery extends the entire length of the gut. The prehepatic portion of the ventral

mesentery persists in the adult as the falciform ligament (Fig 55–1). The liver is connected with the anterior abdominal wall and the diaphragm by the falciform ligament, the lower free border of which is termed the "ligamentum teres" and contains the obliterated left umbilical vein. The posthepatic portion of mesentery becomes the lesser omentum (gastrohepatic ligament) connecting the stomach with the liver. The lowermost portion of the lesser omentum extends beyond the stomach onto the duodenum. The lateral free portion of the lesser omentum is termed the "hepatoduodenal ligament."

The common pleuroperitoneal cavity is divided by the pleuroperitoneal membrane arising from the septum transversum and extending to the dorsal abdominal wall, becoming the diaphragm. This results in an anterior and posterior reflection of the serous lining of the abdominal cavity upon the liver. The reflection of the diaphragmatic peritoneum onto the parietal surface of the liver is termed the "anterior coronary ligament," present on both the right and left posterior coronary ligaments. The anterior and posterior coronary ligaments remain separate on the posterior surface of the liver; thus, the bare area of the liver maintains an extraperitoneal position. The anterior and posterior coronary ligaments on each side fuse laterally and become the right triangular ligament and the left triangular ligament, which is longer than its counterpart on the right side (Fig 55–2).

STRUCTURES WITHIN THE HEPATODUODENAL LIGAMENT

Bile Ducts

The relational anatomy of structures in the hepatoduodenal ligament is shown in Fig 55–3. The most lateral structure in the hepatoduodenal ligament is the extrahepatic bile duct system. The right and left hepatic ducts form the common hepatic duct in the porta hepatis, where the latter lies anteriorly in relation to other structures in this area. The common hepatic duct then descends a variable distance in the lateral portion of the hepatoduodenal ligament and is joined by the cystic duct coming in from the right side at a variable angle. These two ducts, the common hepatic on the left and the cystic on the right, and the liver above form the cystohepatic triangle of Calot, where the cystic and right hepatic arteries, as well as aberrant segmental right hepatic ducts and arteries, frequently are found.

The common hepatic duct averages about 4 cm in length but varies considerably, depending on the point of union with the cystic duct, which usually occurs 2.5 cm above the upper border of the duodenum. The common bile duct descends along the right margin of the hepatoduodenal ligament to the right of the hepatic artery and anterior to the portal vein. This supraduodenal portion continues beyond the first portion of the duodenum as a retroperitoneal portion.

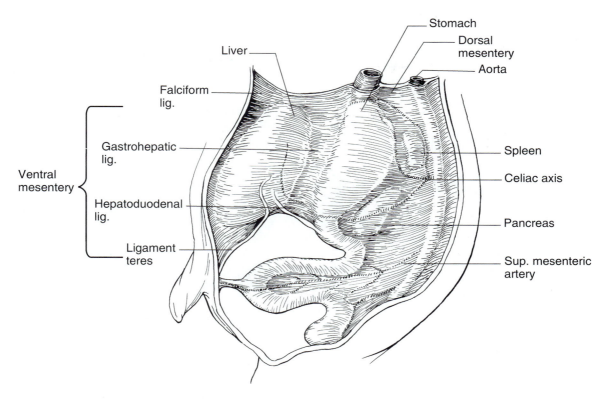

Figure 55–1. Embryonal stage showing relationship of the liver to the ventral mesentery. (Redrawn from Healey JE, Schwartz SI. Surgical diseases of the liver. In: Schwartz SI (ed), *Surgery of the Liver.* New York, NY: McGraw-Hill; 1964)

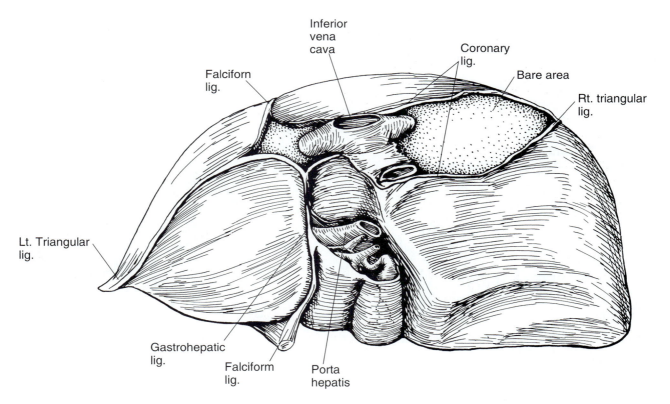

Figure 55–2. Peritoneal reflections. Rear view of the superior and visceral surfaces of the adult liver. (Redrawn from Healey JE, Schwartz SI. Surgical diseases of the liver. In: Schwartz SI (ed), *Surgery of the Liver.* New York, NY: McGraw-Hill; 1964. After Peter Ng)

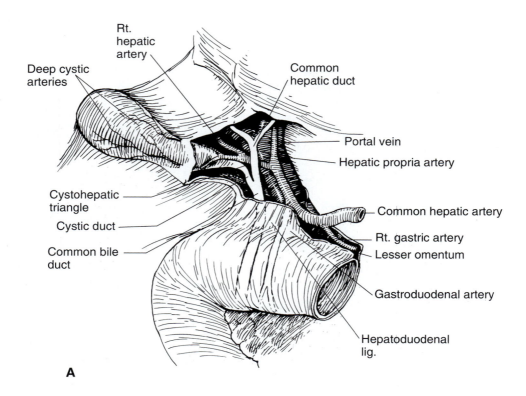

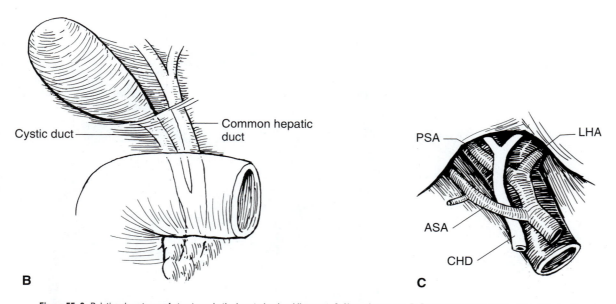

Figure 55–3. Relational anatomy of structures in the hepatoduodenal ligament. **A**. Normal anatomy. **B**. Frequent variation of the union of the cystic and common hepatic ducts (CHD). **C**. Rare variation, separate origin of the anterior (ASA) and posterior (PSA) segmental arteries; LHA: left hepatic artery. (Redrawn from Healey JE, Schwartz SI. Surgical diseases of the liver. In: Schwartz SI (ed), *Surgery of the Liver.* New York, NY: McGraw-Hill; 1964. After Peter Ng)

Hepatic Arteries

The common hepatic artery derives from the celiac artery and proceeds through the lesser omentum at the upper border of the first portion of the duodenum, where it gives rise to the right gastric artery and the gastroduodenal artery and continues as the hepatic propria, which ascends in the hepatoduodenal ligament to the left of the common bile duct and anterior to the portal vein. In its ascent, the hepatic propria bifurcates into a right and left branch; the bifurcation occurs at a variable point between the origin of the vessel and the porta hepatis. In the porta hepatis, the bifurcation is always to the left of the main lobar fissure and, as a consequence, the right hepatic artery is the longer of the two terminal branches. The preceding described origin of the common hepatic artery occurs in ≥90% of cases. The most frequent aberrant site of origin is directly from the superior mesenteric artery.

After its origin from the hepatic propria, the right hepatic artery courses to the right behind the common hepatic duct in 87% of cases. In 11% of cases, it passes in front of the duct; in 2% there is no true right hepatic artery, and there are separate branches of the anterior and posterior segmental arteries to the right lobe. The termination of the right hepatic artery is its division into an anterior and posterior segmental artery, which may occur within the hepatic parenchyma, extrahepatically in the porta hepatis to the right of the common hepatic duct, in the cystohepatic triangle, or, rarely, extrahepatically to the left of the common hepatic duct.

After originating from the hepatic propria in the region of the porta hepatis, the left hepatic artery courses obliquely upward to the left for only a short distance before it divides into its two terminal branches, the medial and lateral segmental arteries. The medial segmental artery arises from the undersurface of the left hepatic artery, descends into the portion of the liver known as the "quadrate lobe," and divides within the liver parenchyma into its superior and inferior branches. The lateral segmental artery ascends in the porta hepatis to gain a variable relationship with the lateral segmental bile duct and is located either on the superior or the inferior border of this duct.

A variety of abnormalities occur in the arterial circulation, and this is a major reason to mandate angiography in a patient who will undergo hepatic resection. In 17% of cases, the superior mesenteric artery is the site of origin of aberrant arteries to the right lobe of the liver. An aberrant right hepatic artery courses anteriorly and to the right of the portal vein in the hepatoduodenal ligament. The most frequent site of origin of an aberrant left hepatic artery is the left gastric artery (Fig 55–4).

Portal Venous System

The portal vein is formed behind the pancreas between the head and neck by a confluence of the splenic vein and the superior mesenteric vein and, in about 25% of cases, the inferior mesenteric vein. The portal vein passes from its origin behind the first portion of the duodenum and then enters the hepatoduodenal liga-

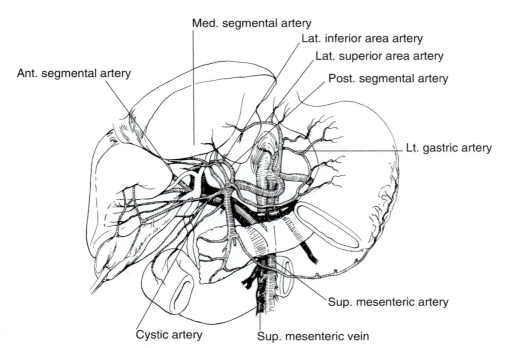

Figure 55–4. Findings in an adult cadaver in which five hepatic arteries were present, each supply a specific segment or subsegment of the liver. (Redrawn from Healey JE, Schwartz SI. Surgical diseases of the liver. In: Schwartz SI (ed), *Surgery of the Liver.* New York, NY: McGraw-Hill; 1964)

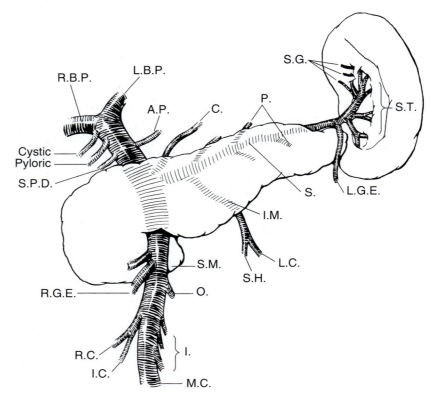

Figure 55–5. Anatomy of the extrahepatic portal venous system, anterior aspect. The termination of each vein is shown as it was encountered most frequently in the 92 dissections. The pancreas is represented by the shaded area. AP: accessory pancreatic vein; C: coronary vein; Cystic: cystic vein; I: intestinal veins; IC: ileocolic vein; IM: inferior mesenteric vein; IPD: inferior pancreaticoduodenal vein; L: liver; LBP: left branch of portal vein; LC: left colic vein; LGE: left gastroepiploic vein; MC: middle colic vein; O: omental vein; P: pancreatic veins; Pyloric: pyloric vein; RC: right colic vein; RGE: right gastroepiploic vein; RBP: right branch of portal vein; S: splenic vein; SG: short gastric vein; SH: superior hemorrhoidal vein; SM: superior mesenteric vein; SPD: superior pancreaticoduodenal vein; ST: splenic trunk. (Redrawn from Healey JE, Schwartz SI, Surgical diseases of the liver. In: Schwartz SI (ed), *Surgery of the Liver.* New York, NY: McGraw-Hill; 1964)

ment between the two layers of the lesser omentum in front of the foramen of Winslow. In the hepatoduodenal ligament, it ascends in an essentially straight line and resides posteriorly in relation to the hepatic artery and the bile ducts. In the porta hepatis, the portal vein divides into two branches: a short, wide right branch enters the right lobe, and a longer, narrower left branch passes transversely to the left of the porta hepatis and supplies the left lobe and the quadrate lobe. In the porta hepatis, the branches of the hepatic artery maintain their anterior relationship to the branches of the portal vein.

A variety of tributaries may enter the main portal vein; these include the coronary vein, the pyloric vein, the superior pancreaticoduodenal vein, an accessory pancreatic vein, and a cystic vein (Fig 55–5). The coronary vein (left gastric vein) passes from left to right in the lesser omentum along the lesser curvature of the stomach. It enters the portal vein, or the confluence of the splenic and mesenteric veins in about 75% of cases. It enters the portal vein itself in the hepatoduodenal ligament above the pancreas in about 25% of cases.

Hepatic Veins

The hepatic venous system begins as a central vein of a liver lobule. The central vein receives sinusoids from all sides and unites with the central vein of other lobules to

form the sublobular veins, which fuse to form collecting veins from various subsegments of the liver. The collecting veins gradually increase in size by joining other large intrahepatic collecting veins and finally coalesce to form the three major hepatic veins.

The three major veins are the right, left, and middle vein (Fig 55–6). The middle hepatic vein lies in the main lobar fissure, the left hepatic vein lies in the upper portion of the left segmental fissure, and the right hepatic vein is located in the right segmental fissure. As a consequence of their intersegmental positions, the hepatic veins drain adjacent segments. The left hepatic vein drains the entire lateral segment and the superior area of the medial segment. The right hepatic vein drains the entire posterior segment, as well as the superior area of the anterior segment. The inferior areas of the middle and anterior segments are drained by the middle hepatic vein. In the French nomenclature, segment is termed "sector," and "segment" represents a subdivision of a sector.

The middle and left hepatic veins, in 60% of cases, unite to form a single trunk before emptying into the inferior vena cava. The right hepatic vein usually drains directly into the vena cava. At the caval orifices, both the right and left veins vary in size from 0.8 to 2.0 cm in diameter.

In addition to the main branches, one or two constant branches from the caudate lobe, as well as incon-

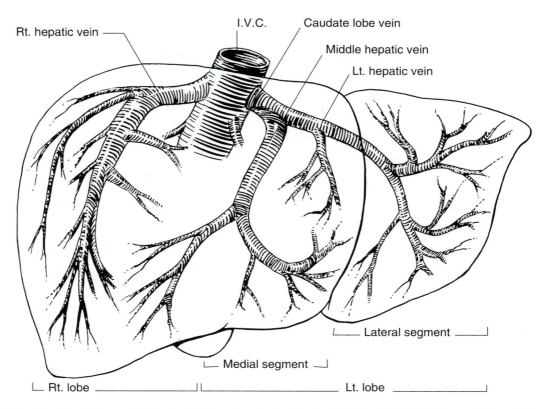

Figure 55–6. Prevailing pattern of drainage of hepatic veins in the human liver. (Redrawn from Healey JE, Schwartz SI. Surgical diseases of the liver. In: Schwartz SI (ed), *Surgery of the Liver.* New York, NY: McGraw-Hill; 1964)

stant branches from the posterior segment of the right lobe, may enter directly into the inferior vena cava caudad in relation to the entrance of the main hepatic veins. There are frequent variations in size and number of the hepatic veins entering the inferior vena cava.

LOBAR ANATOMY OF THE LIVER

An appreciation of the lobar, or the so-called functional anatomy of the liver was initiated by Cantlie in 1898, and was followed by the works of McIndoe and Counseller, Hjorstjo, Couinaud, and Goldsmith and Woodburne. This concept, which is applicable to hepatic resection, is based on a description of hepatic segmentation related to the distribution of the portal pedicles and the location of the hepatic veins.

The liver is divided into two lobes, or hemilivers, by the main portal fissure (scissura), which is also called Cantlie's line. The main portal fissure describes a 75° angle with a horizontal plane and extends from the anteroinferior gallbladder fossa posterosuperiorly to the left side of the inferior vena cava. The main portal fissure is a constant feature.

On each side of the main portal fissure, the organi-

zation of the right and left lobes of the liver is identical. Adjacent to the fissure there is a right or left paramedian sector. Lateral to each of these sectors there is a fissure, which is variable and without anatomic boundaries, separating the paramedian sector from the distal sector known as the right or left lateral sector (Figs 55–7 and 55–8).

The left lobe of the liver consists of the hepatic tissue to the left of the falciform ligament, plus the quadrate lobe and the caudate lobes of the old anatomic nomenclature. The right hepatic lobe consists of remaining hepatic tissue.

The right portal fissure divides the right lobe into an anteromedial and posterolateral sector. The right hepatic vein courses along this fissure. There is no external landmark to define this fissure. According to Couinaud, it extends from the anterior surface of the liver, midway between the right angle of the liver and the right side of the gallbladder, to the confluence between the inferior vena cava and the right hepatic vein posteriorly, describing an angle of 40° with the transverse plane (Fig 55–9).

The left portal fissure divides the left lobe into an anterior and posterior sector, and it is in this fissure that

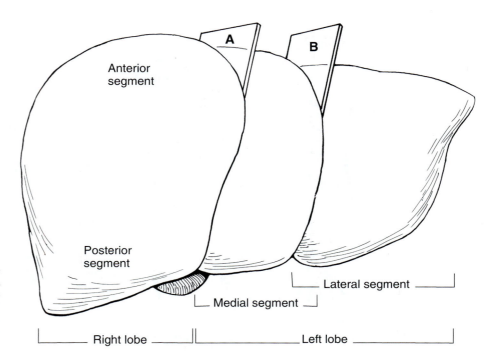

Figure 55–7. Lobar and segmental divisions of the liver. **A**. Lobar fissure. **B**. Left segmental fissure. A right segmental fissure divides the right lobe into its anterior and posterior segments. (Redrawn from Healey JE, Schwartz SI. Surgical diseases of the liver. In: Schwartz SI (ed), *Surgery of the Liver*. New York, NY: McGraw-Hill; 1964)

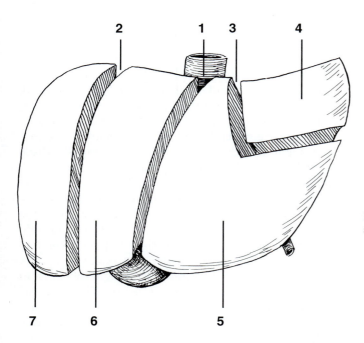

Figure 55–8. Symmetrical organization of the right liver. 1. Main portal fissure. 2. Right portal fissure. 3. Left portal fissure. 4. Left lateral segment. 5. Left paramedian sector. 6. Right paramedian sector. 7. Right lateral sector. Human liver is characterized by the atrophy of the left lateral sector. (Redrawn from Couinaud C. *Controlled Hepatectomies and Exposure of the Intrahepatic Bile Ducts*. Paris, France: C. Couinaud; 1981)

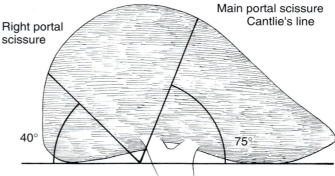

Figure 55–9. The obliquity of the middle and of the right portal scissurae. (Redrawn from Bismuth H. Surgical anatomy and anatomical surgery of the liver. *World J Surg* 1982;6:3)

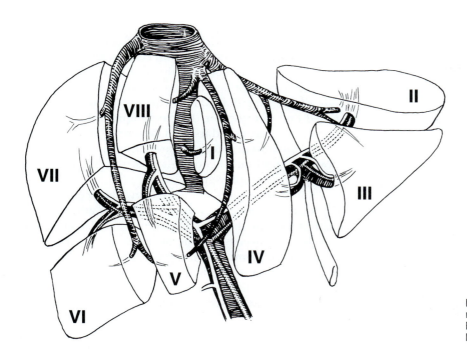

Figure 55–10. The functional division of the liver and the segments according to Couinaud's nomenclature. (Redrawn from Bismuth H: Surgical anatomy and anatomical surgery of the liver. *World J Surg* 1982;6:3)

the left hepatic vein courses. The left portal fissure is located posteriorly in relation to the ligamentum teres.

The liver is further divided into segments that, according to Couinaud, represent the smallest anatomic unit of the organ. In the right lobe, each of the two sectors is divided into two segments: the anteromedial sector is divided into segment V anteriorly and segment VIII posteriorly, while the posterolateral sector is divided into segment VI anteriorly and segment VII posteriorly. In the left lobe, the anterior sector is divided by the umbilical fissure into segment IV, the anterior part of which is the quadrate lobe, and segment III, which is the anterior part of the left lobe. The posterior sector is comprised of only one segment, segment II, which is the posterior part of the left lobe. The spigelian lobe, or segment I, is considered an autonomous segment, since it receives its vascularization independent of the portal division and the three main hepatic veins. It receives tributaries from both the right and left branches of the portal vein and hepatic artery, and its hepatic venous drainage is independent and may terminate directly into the inferior vena cava (Fig 55–10).

■ NOMENCLATURE OF HEPATIC RESECTION

Resection along the main portal fissure, separating the right and left lobes of the liver, is termed a right or left hepatic lobectomy (right and left hepatectomy, in French nomenclature). Resection of the entire right lobe and the medial segment (sector) of the left lobe,

the hepatic parenchyma to the right of the falciform ligament and ligamentum teres, is termed a right extended lobectomy (trisegmentectomy). Left lateral segmentectomy (lobectomy) consists of removal of segments II and III to the left of the falciform ligament and the ligamentum teres.

Unisegmentectomy refers to the removal of a single segment. Theoretically, each of the eight segments of the liver could be removed separately, but there is no practical value to removing segment II or III as a unisegmentectomy. Isolated segmentectomy I is also impractical, since access to the segment requires a preliminary removal of segments II and III. Segmentectomy IV usually refers to removal of the anterior and mobile part of that segment, located anterior to the liver hilus, corresponding to the quadrate lobe. Resection of segment VI alone, in other words, that portion of the liver anterior to the level of the hilus located to the right of the right lateral fissure, rarely is indicated. Segmentectomy VIII consists of resection of the superior part of the right paramedian segment. It is connected with the intrahepatic vena cava and with segment I, rendering isolated resection of this segment a difficult procedure.

Plurisegmentectomy, or removal of two or more segments at one time, may be performed. Removal of segments VI and VII is carried out along the right portal fissure and may be referred to as "right lateral sectorectomy." Bisegmentectomy IV and V finds its applicability in patients with carcinoma of the gallbladder extending into the liver. Bisegmentectomy V and VI rarely is performed. Removal of IV, V, and VI may be carried out as treatment for carcinoma of the gallbladder, since the cystic veins may enter in the portal branch of segment VI.

Removal of a small portion of the liver, either within a single segment or traversing segmental planes, constitutes a wedge resection.

■ PREOPERATIVE MANAGEMENT

An essential feature of the preoperative protocol is angiography of both the celiac and the superior mesenteric arteries to define the extent of hepatic involvement and thus the resectability, and also to demonstrate the vascular anatomy and segmental supply. A venous phase to determine involvement of the portal vein should be included. Computed tomography (CT) performed while radiopaque medium is infused directly into the hepatic artery provides the best definition of intrahepatic pathology.

The serum albumin, prothrombin time, activated partial thromboplastin time, and platelet count are all performed and, if abnormal, corrected. Cephalosporin is instituted on the day of operation. Significant blood loss should be anticipated, and an autotransfusion apparatus made available for use intraoperatively.

■ OPERATIVE TECHNIQUE

The more commonly performed major lobectomies and segmentectomies will be considered. Right hepatic lobectomy will be described in detail, and the description of left hepatic lobectomy will be omitted, since all of the principles detailed for right lobectomy apply. The descriptions of unisegmentectomies and plurisegmentectomies derive mainly from the experiences of Couinaud and of Bismuth.

GENERAL CONSIDERATIONS

The essential technical features that transcend all major hepatic resections include adequate mobilization of the portion of the liver to be removed, temporary or permanent control of the main vessels entering the liver, compression of blood vessels within the substance of the hepatic parenchyma, transection of the hepatic parenchyma, and efforts directed at the raw surface.

Mobilization of the lobes of the liver requires complete transection of the ligamentous attachments, including the appropriate triangular and coronary ligaments. Control of the main vessels entering the liver is accomplished permanently with ligature and transection or, temporarily, by occlusion using vascular tapes or vascular clamps. It now is known that the liver will tol-

erate inflow occlusion for 1 hour, even under normothermic conditions. Compression of the blood vessels within the hepatic parenchyma can be achieved using digital compression beyond the lines of resection or by the application of a compressive clamp placed on the side of the liver that will remain just beyond the proposed line of resection. The technique of Kouznetzoff and Pensky, proposed in 1896, described the introduction of hemostatic sutures parallel to the line of incision, using a blunt needle. At present, this technique usually is not employed.

Cautery dissection still is used in many centers, but digitoclasia (finger fracture) provides the advantage of disrupting only the hepatic parenchyma, isolating the vessels that traverse the line of resection to permit isolated ligation and transection. Ultrasonic dissection achieves the same effect. Persistent oozing from the raw surface of the liver may be controlled by the Argon beam coagulator, Gelfoam, oxidized cellulose, or micronized collagen. The raw surface may remain uncovered or may be covered by an omental graft. Control of minor oozing and reduction of the raw surface area can be accomplished by tying through-and-through absorbable sutures to coapt the anterior and posterior surfaces of Glisson's capsule.

RIGHT HEPATIC LOBECTOMY

A right subcostal incision is preferred, either with a left subcostal extension in a chevron fashion (Fig 55–11) or with an extension craniad over the xiphoid process. The

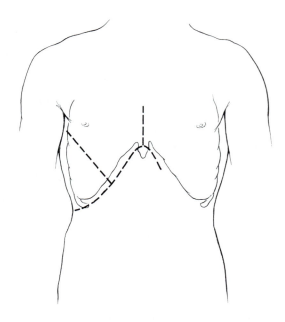

Figure 55–11. Choice of incisions for right hepatic lobectomy.

incision should be placed high enough to permit placement of an overhead retractor so that the sternum can be retracted toward the ceiling. The entire right rectus muscle is transected and the oblique muscles are split laterally almost to the tip of the right tenth rib. Transection of the medial portion of the left rectus muscle usually provides sufficient exposure. A vertical incision in the midline, extending from the xiphoid process to transect the transverse incision, facilitates exposure. A thoracic extension placed perpendicular to the right subcostal incision and extending through the seventh intercostal space rarely is used and is reserved for large lesions in the dome of the right lobe of the liver, with diaphragmatic involvement or encroachment on the suprahepatic inferior vena cava.

MOBILIZATION

Mobilization should be accomplished so that the right lobe can be delivered into the wound. The ligamentum teres is transected; a clamp can be left on the hepatic end to facilitate traction. The triangular ligament supporting the right lobe is divided, and the dissection is continued by transecting the anterior and posterior leaflets of the right coronary ligament to the inferior vena cava (Fig 55–2). This permits the entire right lobe of the liver to be mobilized toward the left. At times, complete mobilization is impaired by attachment of two or three small hepatic veins, and these may be ligated at the point where they enter the inferior vena cava. Following mobilization, laparotomy pads may be placed behind the right lobe of the liver to make the hilus more accessible.

HEPATODUODENAL DISSECTION

The cystic artery and duct are ligated and divided prior to dissection of the hepatoduodenal structures. It generally is easier to remove the gallbladder at this time, but it is sufficient to dissect the medial half of the gallbladder from the liver bed, since this will expose the interlobar fissure. The peritoneal reflection overlying the structures within the hepatoduodenal ligament is incised, and the right main hepatic artery is identified as the first step of the dissection, since it is the most anterior structure encountered. A vascular tape is placed around this vessel, and care is taken to ensure that the left main hepatic artery is protected. The right hepatic artery may be displaced and may arise from the superior mesenteric artery; this is readily defined by preoperative angiogram.

Dissection is continued craniad, and the right branch of the portal vein is identified in the posterior portion of the hepatoduodenal ligament. Exposure frequently is facilitated by rotating the mobilized right lobe of the liver anteriorly. A vascular tape then is passed around the right branch of the portal vein, taking care to protect the left main portal vein. The right main hepatic duct then is dissected free and a tape is passed around it. This maneuver represents the most craniad step in the dissection. The right hepatic artery, the right portal vein, and the right hepatic duct then may be doubly ligated in continuity and divided, or the vascular tapes may be snugged up to provide temporary occlusion (Fig 55–12).

After the structures in the porta hepatis have been ligated and divided or temporarily occluded, there are two potential approaches to the completion of hepatic lobectomy. The first involves securing the hepatic veins outside the liver as they drain into the inferior vena cava. In this circumstance the right lobe is rotated in a clockwise fashion, and the veins are isolated from below upward (Fig 55–13). The main right hepatic vein is large and managed by applying a Satinsky or Derra vascular clamp to the anterior aspect of the inferior vena cava so that it incorporates the right hepatic vein. A curved hemostat is applied to the hepatic side of the vein, and the hepatic vein then is transected and the caval side is sewn with continuous prolene suture. The operation is completed by incising the capsule of the liver and transecting the parenchyma, clamping, dividing, and ligating vessels and ducts as they traverse the interlobar plane.

The second approach, and the one that this author generally uses, involves transection of the hepatic parenchyma in the interlobar plane, beginning anteroinferiorly and progressing posterosuperiorly. A compressive liver clamp may be placed to the left of the lobar plane, but we rarely use it. Glisson's capsule is incised anteroinferiorly, and the parenchyma is transected by digital dissection, which disrupts the hepatic tissue but does not transect the vessels as they cross the interlobar fissure. These are doubly clamped and transected. The side of the vessel that will remain is ligated with silk, and the vessels on the specimen side are controlled with hemostatic clips. As the fingers divide the hepatic parenchyma in the anteroinferior portion of the liver, branches of the hepatic artery, portal vein, and duct are defined intrahepatically (Fig 55–14), doubly ligated, and transected.

The dissection continues posterosuperiorly to the region where the right main hepatic vein is encountered (Fig 55–15). The hepatic vein is isolated within the substance of the liver and doubly clamped with a vascular clamp applied on the caval side of the vein and a hemostat on the side to be removed. The vessel then is transected, and the caval side of the transected hepatic vein is closed with continuous vascular sutures.

This technique has the advantage of avoiding inadvertent ligation of a hepatic vein that serves as the efferent conduit from the remaining left lobe of the liver. It is also more rapid.

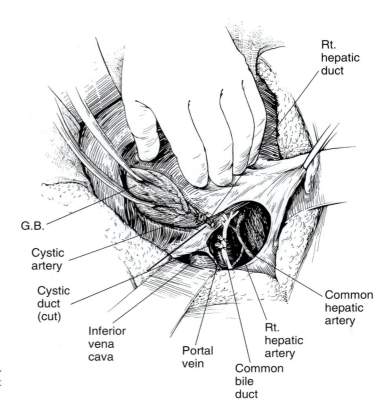

Figure 55–12. Hepatoduodenal dissection. (Redrawn from Schwartz SI. Liver resection. In: *Modern Technics in Surgery, Abdominal Surgery* 10:1. Mt. Kisco, NY: Futura; 1981)

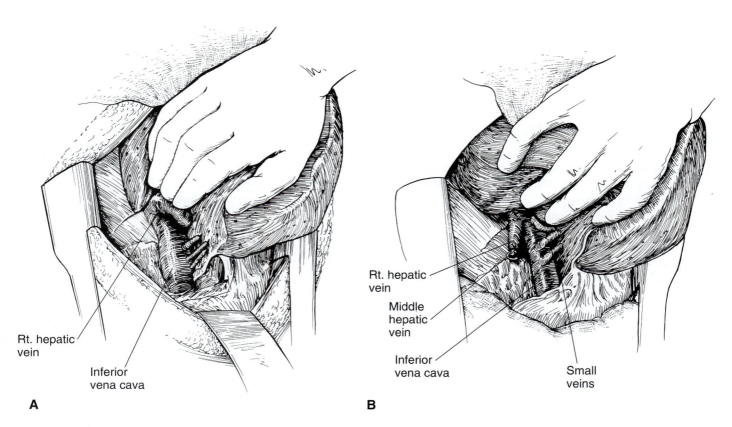

Figure 55–13. A and **B**. Retrohepatic dissection to achieve control of hepatic veins. (Redrawn from Schwartz SI. Liver resection. In: *Modern Technics in Surgery, Abdominal Surgery* 10:1. Mt. Kisco, NY: Futura; 1981)

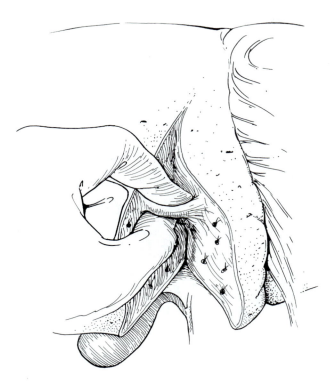

Figure 55–14. Finger fracture technique. Anteroinferior intraparenchymal dissection of portal structures.

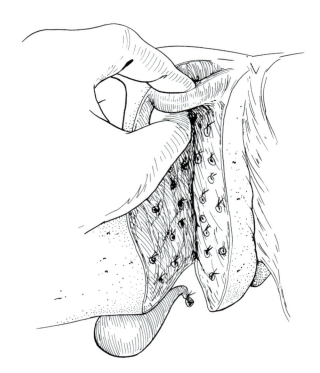

Figure 55–15. Finger fracture technique. Posterosuperior intraparenchymal dissection of the right hepatic vein.

Transection of the hepatic parenchyma in the interlobar plane may be performed with an ultrasonic scalpel, with a stream of saline irrigating the tip. At 80% to 90% of full power, the instrument is used in a probing motion, gradually deepening the incision from anterior to posterior. The parenchyma is transected, leaving skeletonized vessels that readily could be controlled by clamps or clips. When the larger vessels are approached posterosuperiorly, the power is reduced to about 70% to 80%, and the direction of the tip is changed so that it runs parallel to the vessels.

After transection of the parenchyma is complete, the specimen is removed. Following removal of the specimen, the vascular and ductal tapes can be released to determine that the bleeding and bile leak from the parenchymal surface are controlled completely. If arterial bleeding is encountered, the hepatic artery is ligated in the hepatoduodenal ligament. If portal bleeding is encountered, the portal vein is handled in a similar fashion. If there is evidence of bile leak, the hepatic duct can be ligated within the hepatoduodenal ligament. This usually is not required. The usual sequence that this author follows is the same as that endorsed by Bismuth (Fig 55–16).

The raw surface of the liver may be covered conveniently with pedicled omentum, but this is not neces-
sary. The anterior and posterior portions of the remaining Glisson's capsule can be approximated with interrupted catgut sutures to reduce the raw area and to provide a tamponade effect on the smaller vessels. Usually, two Jackson Pratt drains are placed in the subphrenic space that had been occupied by the resected specimen, brought out through one or two large stab wounds, and positioned in a suction bulb to provide a closed system of drainage. The common bile duct is not drained with a T tube

EXTENDED RIGHT HEPATIC LOBECTOMY (TRISEGMENTECTOMY)

The initial phases of the operation, including the incision, transection of the ligamentous attachments to the right lobe, and dissection of the hilus, proceed in the same fashion as described for right hepatic lobectomy. The right hepatic artery, right portal vein, and right hepatic duct are managed similarly.

Dissection in the region of the hilus continues, completing mobilization of the left branches of the portal structures (Fig 55–17). Two or three branches from the hepatic artery to the caudate lobe are ligated and several branches from the portal vein also are ligated in this region. This dissection is stopped short of the umbilical fissure. The right hepatic vein may be interrupted pos-

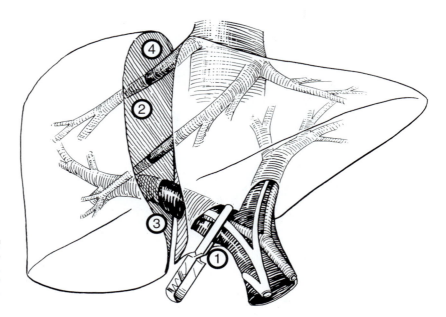

Figure 55–16. Sequence of events: 1. Temporary occlusion of structures in hepatoduodenal ligation. 2. Anterior parenchymal dissection. 3. Parenchymal dissection of portal structures. 4. Parenchymal dissection of the hepatic vein. (Redrawn from Bismuth H. Surgical anatomy and anatomical surgery of the liver. *World J Surg* 1982;6:3)

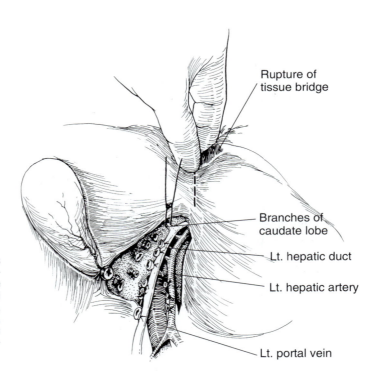

Rupture of tissue bridge

Branches of caudate lobe

Lt. hepatic duct

Lt. hepatic artery

Lt. portal vein

Figure 55–17. Nearly completed mobilization of the left branches of the portal triad. The tissue bridge is being broken down to permit access to the umbilical fissure. The final two branches before the main trunk reaches the umbilical fissure go to the left portion of the caudate lobe. These final branches, or at least the last one, should be preserved unless all of the caudate lobe is to be removed. Total caudate removal is not usually necessary. (Redrawn from Starzl T, Bell RH, et al: Hepatic trisegmentectomy and other liver resections. *Surg Gynecol Obstet* 1975;141:429. After J McC)

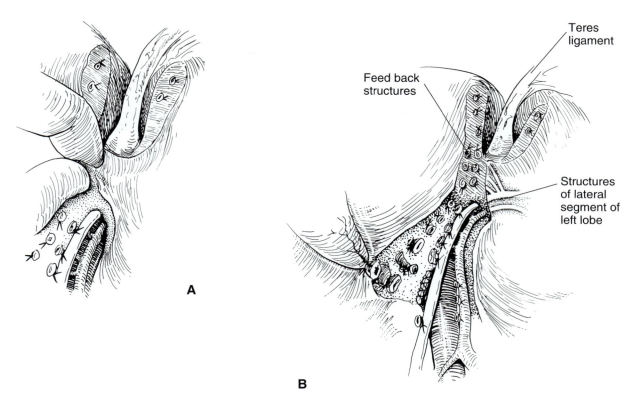

Figure 55–18. Structures feeding back from the umbilical fissure to the medial segment of the left lobe. **A**. These are encircled usually by blunt dissection within the liver substances just to the right of the falciform ligament and umbilical fissure without entering the fissure. Note that the hepatic tissue bridge concealing the umbilical fissure has been broken down. **B**. The three segments of the specimen now are devascularized. (Redrawn from Starzl T, Bell RH, et al: Hepatic trisegmentectomy and other liver resections. *Surg Gynecol Obstet* 1975;141:429. After J. McC)

teriorly at its junction with the inferior vena cava, or may be ligated within the parenchyma itself according to the two options described in the section on right hepatic lobectomy.

An incision is made just to the right of the falciform ligament and the parenchyma is crushed between fingers to permit access to the umbilical fissure. Vessels and ducts passing to the medial segment of the left lobe are divided, preserving the vessels and ducts to the lateral segment of the left lobe. If the right hepatic vein had not been ligated via the posterior approach, it can be managed at this time (Fig 55–18).

LEFT LATERAL SEGMENTECTOMY (LEFT LATERAL SECTORECTOMY—REMOVAL OF SEGMENTS II AND III)

This procedure can be performed through the same incision that is used for right lobectomy, or through an upper midline incision. The left lateral segment initially is mobilized by dividing its ligamentous attachments: the left triangular ligament, the left coronary ligaments, and the falciform ligament.

It then is possible to displace the portion to be resected downward and to expose the inferior surface of the porta hepatis. The segmental tributaries of the left branch of the portal vein, the left hepatic duct, and the left branch of the hepatic artery may be dissected within the hepatoduodenal ligament. These may be controlled by vascular tapes, but it may be simpler to temporarily occlude the entire contents of hepatoduodenal ligament with an atraumatic vascular clamp.

The plane for resection of the lateral segment of the left lobe is located 1 cm to the left of the falciform ligament. In this plane only the terminal branches supplying the lateral segment are encountered. There is no hazard of disturbing the ducts and vessels to the medial segment, since they reside in the umbilical fissure itself. After Glisson's capsule has been incised, the cleavage plane is established best by means of finger fracture to separate the liver parenchyma and to expose the larger ducts and vessels, which may be individually clamped and ligated, as they are encountered. The incision is continued posteriorly until the hepatic vein is demonstrated, doubly ligated, and transected. The entire procedure usually can be accomplished with sufficient facility so that preliminary vascular inflow occlusion may not be required.

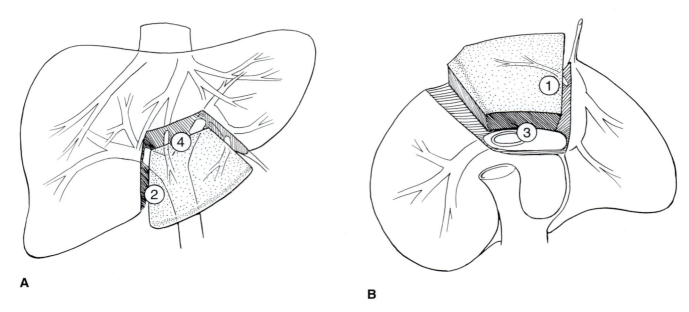

Figure 55–19. Anterior segmentectomy IV or resection of the quadrate lobe. The different steps of the technique: 1. Opening of the umbilical fissure. 2. Opening of the anterior part of the main scissura. 3. Ligation of the portal pedicles entering the posterior part of the quadrate lobe. 4. Transverse transection of the parenchyma. (Redrawn from Bismuth H, Houssin D, et al: Major and minor segmentectomies "Reglees" in liver surgery. *World J Surg* 1982;6:10)

UNISEGMENTECTOMY

Anterior Segmentectomy IV (Resection of the Quadrate Lobe)

This procedure was first performed by Caprio and has been used for gaining access to the upper portion of the biliary confluence.

The classic right upper quadrant chevron incision or a midline incision may be used. The anterior portion of the falciform ligament and the ligamentum teres are divided. Resection of the parenchyma begins by dividing the tissue between segments III and IV, by opening the umbilical fissure (Fig 55–19). The peritoneum at the inferior part of the ligamentum teres is divided, and several arterial and portal pedicles are dissected to the right of the ligamentum teres. The liver then is transected anteriorly along the main fissure, and this dissection is continued up to the hilus. The only vascular elements requiring ligation in this portion of the dissection are the left branches of the middle hepatic vein. Posteriorly, Glisson's capsule is incised in front of the peritoneum overlying the hilus, and arterial and portal branches of the quadrate lobe are ligated and divided. Finally, a transverse incision of Glisson's capsule is made anteriorly, joining the right and left lines of transection, and the specimen is removed.

Segmentectomy VI

Segmentectomy VI rarely is indicated but is performed with ease after the ligamentous attachments of the right lobe of the liver are divided to permit mobilization. The liver is transected along the right lateral fissure midway

between the gallbladder and the right edge of the liver. The transection is continued up to the level of the hilus, where the liver is transected tranversely toward its right lateral side. During dissection, the anterior part of the right hepatic vein and the portal pedicle of the segment are ligated (Fig 55–20).

Segmentectomy VIII

Segmentectomy VIII has been performed on occasion by Ton That Tung for chronic liver abscess situated superiorly in the liver. A right subcostal incision is made, and the falciform and right triangular and coronary ligaments are divided. Temporary hepatic inflow occlusion is effected. The right lateral and the main hepatic fissures are transected from the superior lip at the insertion of the right coronary ligament posteriorly, up to the level of the hilus anteriorly. These two lines of transection are joined by two transverse incisions along the insertion of the coronary ligament posteriorly and along the posterior part of the hilus anteriorly. During transection, hepatic veins of segment VIII are divided; attention must be directed to avoiding injury to the right and middle main hepatic veins (Fig 55–21).

PLURISEGMENTECTOMIES

Bisegmentectomy VI, V

This operation is indicated for carcinoma of the gallbladder. Through a subcostal incision the umbilical fissure is opened, and the parenchyma is split to the right of the falciform ligament. The right portal fissure then

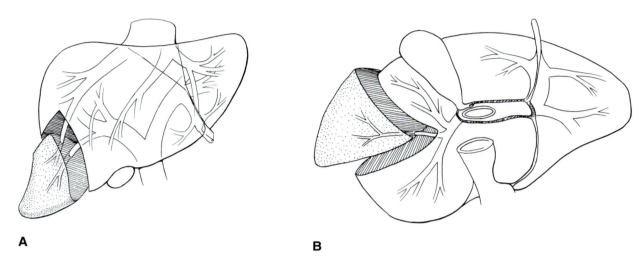

A   **B**

Figure 55–20. Segmentectomy VI. (Redrawn from Bismuth H, Houssin D, et al: Major and minor segmentectomies "Reglees" in liver surgery. *World J Surg* 1982;6:10)

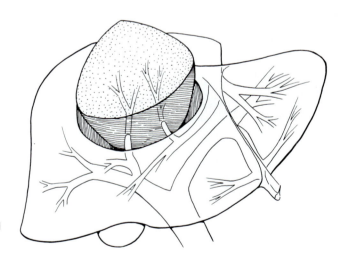

Figure 55–21. Segementectomy VIII. (Redrawn from Bismuth H, Houssin D, et al: Major and minor segmentectomies "Reglees" in liver surgery. *World J Surg* 1982;6:10)

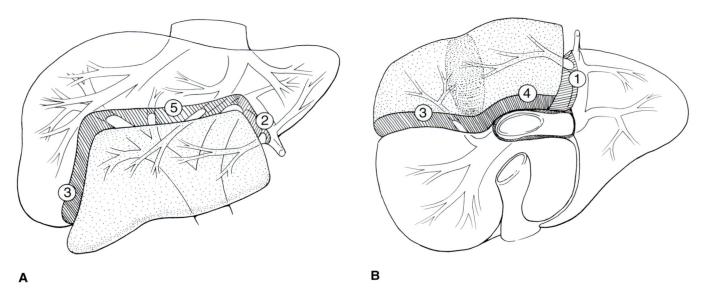

A

B

Figure 55–22. Bisegmentectomy IV and V. The different steps of the technique: 1. Opening of the umbilical fissure. 2. Splitting of the parenchyma to the right of the ligamentum teres. 3. Opening of the right portal scissura. 4. Ligation of the portal pedicles of the quadrate lobe and of the anterior portal pedicle of the right paramedian sector. (Redrawn from Bismuth H, Houssin D, et al. Major and minor segmentectomies "Reglees" in liver surgery. *World J Surg* 1982;6:10)

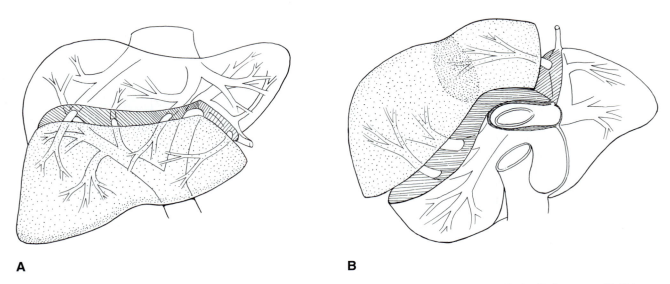

A

B

Figure 55–23. Trisegmentectomy IV, V, and VI. (Redrawn from Bismuth H, Houssin D, et al. Major and minor segmentectomies "Reglees" in liver surgery. *World J Surg* 1982;6:10)

is opened. The main step in the dissection is ligation of the portal pedicle of segments IV and V, avoiding damage to the main vascular supply to the right and left lobes of the liver. During transection of the hilus, the anterior branch of the large inferior and posterior right paramedian portal pedicle is ligated. The portal branch of the posterior part of the quadrate lobe then is ligated. The final step in the procedure is the posterior transection of the hepatic parenchyma joining the left and right incisions in front of the hilus. During this maneuver, the large middle hepatic vein is ligated and divided (Fig 55–22).

Trisegmentectomy IV, V, VI

The initial step is the same as that described for resection of segment IV, with division of the portal pedicles of the segment. The liver then is transected along the umbilical fissure, up to the level of the hilus. Anteriorly, Glisson's capsule is incised transversely to the right side of the liver, and the transection is continued deep to provide exposure of the divisions of the portal pedicles of segments V and VI. These are ligated and divided, as are branches of the right and middle hepatic veins (Fig 55–23).

Limited Resection

Intraoperative ultrasonographic guidance to remove the tumor and ≤1 cm of normal parenchyma can be performed in selected cirrhotic patients who have primary liver cancer. The presence of a capsule surrounding the tumor has been the most important factor correlating with recurrence.

■ POSTOPERATIVE MANAGEMENT

Gastric decompression usually is maintained for 1 to 2 days, after which oral intake is begun and rapidly advanced. Glucose infusions and albumin are given to maintain normal levels until the oral intake is adequate. Antibiotics generally are continued for 3 days. Following right lobectomy, hyperbilirubinemia and clinical jaundice are anticipated. These usually begin on day 2 or 3 and may continue for as long as 3 weeks. Hypoprothrombinemia also develops, but rarely reaches critical levels; if this becomes significant, it is readily corrected with fresh frozen plasma.

Continued bleeding in the immediate postoperative period generally is caused by ineffective mechanical hemostasis and not by a coagulopathy; thus, it usually requires early reexploration. Persistent leakage of bile or development of biliary fistula is extremely rare. The most common complication is a subphrenic abscess that usually becomes manifest on postoperative day 5. In the past, this required drainage through the lateral aspect of the major incision, but recently it has been managed successfully by ultrasonographically controlled placement of a pigtail catheter.

SELECTED READINGS

Bismuth H. Surgical anatomy and anatomical surgery of the liver. *World J Surg* 1982;6:3

Bismuth H, Houssin D, et al. Major and minor segmentectomies "Reglees" in liver surgery. *World J Surg* 1982;6:10

Bismuth H, Houssin D, et al. Liver resections in cirrhotic patients: a western experience. *World J Surg* 1986;10:311

Couinaud C. *Controlled Hepatectomies and Exposure of the Intrahepatic Bile Ducts.* Paris, France: C Couinaud; 1981

Franco D, Smadja C, et al. Segmentectomies in the management of liver tumors. *Arch Surg* 1988;123:519

Goldsmith NA, Woodburne RT. Surgical anatomy. In: Schwartz SI (ed), *Surgical Diseases of the Liver.* New York, NY: McGraw-Hill; 1964:1

Hodgson WJB, DelGuercio LRM. Preliminary experience in liver surgery using the ultrasonic scalpel. *Ann Surg* 1984; 95:320

Kinami Y, Takashima S, Miyazaki I. Hepatic resection for hepatocellular carcinoma associated with liver cirrhosis. *World J Surg* 1986;10:294

Makuuchi M, Hasegawa H, et al. The use of operative ultrasound as an aid to liver resection in patients with hepatocellular carcinoma. *World J Surg* 1987;11:615

Lin TY. A simplified technique for hepatic resection. *Ann Surg* 1974;180:225

Schwartz SI. Liver resection. In: *Modern Technics in Surgery, Abdominal Surgery* 10:1. Mt. Kisco, NY: Futura; 1981

Starzl T, Bell RH, et al. Hepatic trisegmentectomy and other liver resections. *Surg Gynecol Obstet* 1975;141:429

Tung TT. *Les Resection Majeures et Mineures du Foie.* Paris, France: Masson; 1979

56

Surgical Management of Ascites

Marshall J. Orloff ▪ *Mark S. Orloff*

The word *ascites* is derived from the Greek word *askos*, which means bag or sack. Ascites is the pathologic accumulation of fluid in the peritoneal cavity. As shown in Table 56–1, ascites occurs in a number of diseases but, in the United States, 80% or more of the cases are caused by cirrhosis of the liver.[1] Cirrhotic ascites has a poor prognosis. As shown in Fig 56–1, 50% of the patients succumb within two years.[2,3] The treatment of ascites depends on the cause. The therapy used in cirrhotic ascites is usually ineffective in ascites owing to peritoneal carcinomatosis, while tuberculous ascites responds only to specific antibacterial drug treatment.

A substantial majority of patients with cirrhosis and ascites respond satisfactorily to a medical regimen consisting of abstinence from alcohol, a nourishing diet, restriction of sodium intake, and one or more of a variety of diuretic and anti-aldosterone drugs. However, in a small but difficult group of patients, ascites is resistant to treatment with these measures. For these patients with *intractable* ascites, invasive procedures and surgical operations have been used.

The history of the surgical management of ascites is marked by a number of ingenious, but usually unsuccessful, operations. Included among these are various techniques designed to promote drainage of ascitic fluid, to create portasystemic communications, to reduce portal venous inflow, and to modify endocrine influences on fluid formation. In recent years, however, clarification of some of the hemodynamic abnormalities involved in the pathogenesis of ascites has provided a rational basis for surgical therapy that is effective.

▪ PATHOGENESIS OF CIRRHOTIC ASCITES

SINUSOIDAL HYPERTENSION

The pathogenesis of cirrhotic ascites is complex and involves a number of factors, some proven and others postulated. Included among these are increased hydrostatic pressure in the liver sinusoids, decreased serum protein osmotic pressure owing to hypoalbuminemia, renal sodium retention, activation of the sympathetic nervous system, and abnormal secretion of several hormones such as aldosterone, antidiuretic hormone, and atrial natriuretic peptide. The initiating and perpetuating abnormality, in many cases, appears to be sinusoidal hypertension resulting from hepatic venous outflow obstruction.

Almost one-fourth of the cardiac output is directed to the liver by way of the portal vein and hepatic artery, traverses the extensive network of liver sinusoids, is conducted out of the liver by the hepatic veins, and is returned to the heart by the inferior vena cava. The liver sinusoids make up the most permeable capillary bed in the body. They are lined by a single layer of endothelial cells that, in turn, are separated from the hepatocytes by a potential space called the space of Disse, where metabolic exchange takes place between the blood plasma and the hepatocytes. Because the sinusoidal endothelium is freely permeable to albumin, there is no oncotic gradient and hydrostatic pressure in the sinusoids controls the efflux of large quantities of fluid into the space of Disse. From the space of Disse, fluid is removed by the

TABLE 56–1. CAUSE OF ASCITES AND SURVIVAL RATES IN 1200 HOSPITALIZED PATIENTS IN THE UNITED STATES WHO UNDERWENT PARACENTESIS

Cause	% of 1200 Patients	Survival
Cirrhosis	81	50% at 2 yr
Alcoholic	65	—
Posthepatitic	10	—
Other	6	—
Cancer	10	Mean 20 wk
Heart Failure	3	50% at 2 yr
Tuberculosis	2	87%
Pancreatic Disease	1	82%
Dialysis	1	Mean 7 mo
Other	2	

(From Runyon BA. Care of patients with ascites. N Engl J Med 1994;330:337–342)

hepatic lymphatics and returned to the venous circulation via the thoracic duct.

Elevated hydrostatic pressure within the liver sinusoids may result from an increase in the pressure and rate of inflow or from interference with outflow of blood. Outflow obstruction is usually the cause of sinusoidal hypertension in patients with cirrhotic ascites. Histologic studies of cirrhotic livers obtained from patients with and without ascites have shown extensive obliterative fibrosis of the hepatic veins in the liver of patients with ascites; this fibrosis was particularly severe when the ascites was refractory to treatment.[4–7] Studies of corrosion casts of the hepatic vasculature revealed an absolute increase in the size of the portal venous and hepatic arterial inflow tracts and a concomitant absolute decrease in the size of the hepatic venous outflow tract in the liver obtained from patients with irreversible ascites.[4] Outflow occlusion combined with inflow dilation was not found in cirrhosis without ascites or with acute and reversible ascites. Volume studies of the hepatic vasculature were reported to have shown a striking diminution in hepatic venous outflow in patients with cirrhotic ascites.[8] In cinefluorographic studies, Britton, Brown and Shirey[9,10] demonstrated obliterative changes in the hepatic veins in all patients with cirrhotic ascites and observed a remarkably close correlation between the severity of the outflow block and the responsiveness of the ascites to medical therapy. These authors characterized cirrhotic ascites as being functionally similar to the Budd-Chiari syndrome.

Since the observation of Starling in 1894,[11] numerous studies have demonstrated a marked increase in the flow of lymph in the hepatic hilar lymphatics and thoracic duct in association with experimental ascites,[12–15] hepatic outflow obstruction,[11–18] and experimental cirrhosis.[19–25] A similar increase in lymph flow in the thoracic duct has been observed in human subjects with cirrhosis

[22,23] and the familiar enlargement of the lymphatics in the hilum of the cirrhotic liver has been documented by a histopathologic study.[24] Thoracic duct lymph flow rates as high as 20 L/day, which is 20 times the normal flow rate, have been observed in patients with cirrhosis and ascites. It has been suggested, on the basis of some indirect experiments, that altered sinusoidal permeability, resulting from the release of vasoactive substances by the damaged liver, may be responsible for the increased lymph production.[25,26] However, the bulk of evidence supports the proposal that the augmented formation of hepatic lymph is, in large part, a mechanical phenomenon resulting from obstruction of the outflow of blood from the liver sinusoid and the consequent spill-over of the plasma portion of the blood into the perisinusoidal spaces and lymphatics.[14,22,27] Ascites, in turn, is the result of the inability of the lymphatic system to accommodate the excessive formation of lymph, with resulting leakage of fluid into the peritoneal cavity from the over-burdened hepatic lymphatics.[6,14,18,22,27,28] Increased lymph flow in cirrhotic ascites is largely a reflection of elevated hydrostatic pressure in the liver (Fig 56–2).[29]

The contribution of lymph from the splanchnic bed to cirrhotic ascites is uncertain. In the presence of portal hypertension, splanchnic lymph formation undoubtedly is increased. However, the splanchnic capillary bed is much less permeable to fluid than the hepatic sinusoidal bed, and it is unlikely that the splanchnic lymphatics are a major site of ascites formation in most cases of cirrhosis. In experimental an-

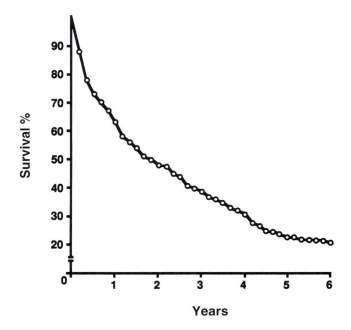

Figure 56–1. Survival in a series of 1155 patients with decompensated cirrhosis and ascites. (From D'Amico G, Morabito A, Pagliaro L, et al. Survival and prognostic indicators in compensated and decompensated cirrhosis. *Dig Dis Sci* 1986;31:468–475)

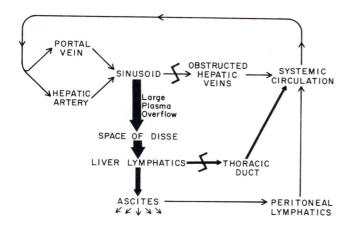

Figure 56–2. The chain of events in ascites formation. Hepatic venous outflow obstruction and the resultant sinusoidal hypertension play a primary role in causing transudation of ascitic fluid from the hepatic lymphatics. (From Orloff MJ. Pathogenesis and surgical treatment of intractable ascites associated with alcoholic cirrhosis. *Ann NY Acad Sci* 1966;3:213–236)

imals with cirrhosis, intestinal lymph flow increased only one-tenth as much as hepatic lymph flow, compared with controls.[30] Moreover, in portal venous hypertension in dogs, there was a reduction in intestinal blood flow that restricted, rather than favored, accumulation of intestinal interstitial fluid.

RENAL SODIUM RETENTION

There is marked retention of sodium by the kidneys in patients with cirrhotic ascites and, in fact, ascites does not occur in the absence of renal sodium retention. The question is whether retention of sodium is secondary to sinusoidal hypertension or is it a primary event. Normally, a decrease in effective circulating vascular volume is the stimulus to reabsorption of sodium at the proximal renal tubule. However, cirrhotic patients with established ascites have an increase in circulating blood volume,[31] and it is uncertain if initial hypovolemia is the primary stimulus for renal sodium retention.

There is increased sympathetic activity in patients with cirrhosis and ascites.[32,33] An increase in sympathetic tone is known to inhibit sodium excretion by the kidneys.[34] A number of studies suggest that increased sinusoidal pressure activates hepatic baroreceptors that produce renal sodium retention by neural and humoral mechanisms.[35–41]

PERITONEAL ABSORPTION OF ASCITES

Ascites is absorbed by the capillaries and lymphatics in the parietal and visceral peritoneum. The rates of fluid formation and absorption determine the amount of ascites that accumulates. The rate of ascites absorption is a reflection of the hydrostatic and oncotic pressures

on each side of the peritoneal capillary membrane, according to Starling's law. With diuretic therapy, a maximum of about 1L/day of ascites can be safely reabsorbed.[42,43] Increases in intraperitoneal pressure decrease the rate of ascites formation and increase the rate of reabsorption.[44–46] However, in cirrhotic patients with ascites, changes in intra-abdominal pressure are small and unlikely to influence the balance between ascites formation and absorption, except following large-volume paracentesis. Fibrosis and thickening of the peritoneum often occur in cirrhosis and may limit the resorption of ascites.[47] Nevertheless, peritoneal absorption of fluid is a secondary factor in the pathophysiology of ascites.

HYPOALBUMINEMIA

Oncotic pressure is determined largely by the concentration of albumin, the synthesis of which is markedly impaired in cirrhosis. Oncotic pressure in sinusoids of the cirrhotic liver would be decreased were it not for the fact that the hepatic sinusoids are freely permeable to albumin. Therefore, an oncotic gradient is not a significant determinant of fluid efflux into the space of Disse until liver disease becomes advanced and ascites is chronic. At that time, with progressive deposition of collagen, the sinusoidal endothelium loses its free permeability and comes to resemble intestinal capillaries, a change termed "capillarization" by Shaffner and Popper.[48] When this change occurs, efflux of fluid into the interstitium is governed by both hydrostatic and oncotic pressure gradients, resulting in ascites that is low in albumin.

HORMONAL INFLUENCES

Aldosterone

Substantial evidence indicates that humans with cirrhotic ascites secrete abnormally large quantities of aldosterone, and that the hyperaldosteronism plays an important role in the marked salt and water retention that characterizes this condition.[49–53] The cause and time of onset of the aldosterone hypersecretion are not known. Cirrhotic patients without ascites do not secrete excessive quantities of aldosterone,[50] which suggests that some mechanism peculiar to the ascites process is responsible. It has been proposed that a decrease in effective circulating blood volume is the initiating event that activates the renin-angiotensin system in the kidney to stimulate aldosterone secretion.[54] Alternatively, it has been suggested that early hyponatremia is the stimulus to renal release of renin. Evidence obtained in our laboratory indicates that increased intrahepatic pressure may be the underlying mechanism for aldosterone hypersecretion in cirrhotic ascites.

The effects of obstruction of the hepatic veins on aldosterone secretion were investigated in our laboratory in a series of experiments in conscious dogs.[56–58] Minimal hepatic outflow occlusion, insufficient to produce changes in vital signs, blood volume, or behavior, resulted in a prompt 4- to 50-fold increase in aldosterone secretion, suggesting the possibility that there was a sensitive baroreceptor mechanism in the liver that stimulated aldosterone secretion in response to an increase in intrahepatic pressure. The aldosterone response was abolished by bilateral nephrectomy, suggesting that the kidney and, presumably, the renin-angiotensin system, acted as a relay station in the efferent pathway between the liver and the adrenal cortex. Cross-circulation of blood from a nephrectomized donor dog undergoing gradual hepatic outflow occlusion to a normal recipient dog produced an immediate, marked, and highly significant increase in aldosterone secretion in the recipient, indicating that the aldosterone response to hepatic outflow occlusion was mediated by a potent humoral agent that arose in the liver. On the basis of these interesting experimental findings, it seems reasonable to postulate that the pressure within the liver is in some way involved in the regulation of aldosterone secretion. Furthermore, it seems plausible to speculate that intrahepatic hypertension plays a role in the hyperaldosteronism associated with cirrhotic ascites.

ANTIDIURETIC HORMONE

The role of antidiuretic hormone (ADH) in ascites formation, if any, is uncertain. Some evidence indicates that the decreased free-water clearance in cirrhotic ascites is owing to increased ADH secretion.[59,60] The stimulus to ADH secretion is believed to be a decrease in intravascular volume that sends a signal to the posterior pituitary via afferent volume receptors in the atria. It is doubtful that ADH plays an initiating role in ascites formation.

ATRIAL NATRIURETIC PEPTIDE

Atrial natriuretic peptide (ANP) is a group of peptides that have been isolated from the atria and have diuretic, natriuretic, and vasorelaxant properties. The role of ANP in cirrhotic ascites is doubtful. ANP levels have been found to be increased, normal, and decreased in various studies in patients with ascites owing to liver disease.[61–63]

OVERFLOW VERSUS UNDERFILL THEORIES

There are two theories regarding the initial pathophysiologic events leading to ascites formation.[64] According to the overflow theory, hepatic sinusoidal hypertension sends an as yet unidentified humoral signal to the kidney, causing abnormal reabsorption of sodium and water that precedes the appearance of ascites. The resul-

tant expansion of plasma volume, when combined with the high hydrostatic pressure in the liver sinusoids, leads to excessive efflux of sinusoidal fluid and ascites formation. Evidence for the overflow theory has come from a number of studies in animals and humans.[31–65]

The underfill theory proposes that hypovolemia is the initial event in ascites formation, not sodium retention. Hepatic outflow obstruction causes sinusoidal hypertension that leads to hypovolemia as a result of splanchnic pooling of blood and of excessive fluid loss from the sinusoids. Sodium retention by the kidney follows and is a result of the decreased intravascular volume. Support for the underfill theory has come from head-out water emersion studies in humans.[60]

It has been proposed that both the overflow and underfill mechanisms may be operative at different times in the evolution of ascites, with the overflow mechanism (renal sodium retention) occurring initially, and the underfill mechanism (hypovolemia) coming into play as intravascular fluid is lost into the peritoneal cavity.[64] Alternatively, Schrier and associates proposed another theory that combines the two hypotheses.[66] According to this theory, prior to the onset of ascites, decreased vascular resistance, peripheral arterial vasodilation, enlargement of the vascular compartment, and the consequent increase in cardiac output (the so-called hyperdynamic state) cause a decrease in effective blood volume (underfill) that, in turn, leads to renal sodium and water retention aimed at correcting the relative hypovolemia. Plasma volume expansion then ensues (overflow) and produces ascites.

It is important to recognize that regardless of which sequence of events in the evolution of ascites is correct, the underlying cause of cirrhotic ascites is a mechanical hemodynamic abnormality, namely, hypertension in the liver sinusoid owing to hepatic venous outflow obstruction.

■ DIAGNOSIS

HISTORY

Most patients with ascites have alcoholic liver disease, and the abdominal fluid collection often is the first sign of decompensation. Periods of abstinence from alcohol frequently are associated with disappearance of ascites so that patients experience wet-dry cycles of both alcohol consumption and ascites. On the other hand, patients with nonalcoholic cirrhosis usually develop ascites at an advanced stage of liver disease and the ascites tends to persist. Patients always should be questioned about causes of liver disease other than alcohol, such as intravenous drug use, blood transfusions, tattoos, acupuncture, and residence in or visits to a foreign country.

When ascites appears in a patient whose cirrhosis has been stable for a long time, the possibility of hepatocellular carcinoma should be considered.

Ascites in a patient with a history of cancer should raise the suspicion of malignancy-related ascites, particularly if the primary neoplasm involved the breast, colon, pancreas or ovary.[67] Such patients often have persistent abdominal pain, which is infrequent in cirrhotic ascites unless there is superimposed bacterial peritonitis or alcoholic hepatitis. Tuberculous peritonitis is characterized by ascites with fever and abdominal pain, in a recent immigrant from an endemic area. The picture can be confusing because many patients with tuberculosis also have cirrhosis. Cardiac ascites usually is associated with a history of cardiopulmonary disease and heart failure. Ascites in some alcoholics is the result of heart failure caused by alcoholic cardiomyopathy. Diabetic patients who develop edema and ascites should be suspected of having renal failure with cirrhotic ascites. Myxedema should be considered in patients with cold intolerance, lethargy, skin changes, and altered bowel mobility. Connective tissue diseases sometimes cause serositis with ascites.

PHYSICAL EXAMINATION

Ascites is estimated conventionally according to a semi-quantitative scale that ranges from 0 to 4+ as follows

0   No ascites
1+   Just detectable
2+   Easily detectable but of small volume
3+   Obvious but not tense
4+   Tense ascites

The diagnosis of ascites is suspected when there is abdominal fullness and bulging flanks. Percussion of the flanks with the patient supine demonstrates an air-fluid level that is higher than normal. Under such circumstances, shifting of the dullness with change in position usually is detected. Approximately 1.5 L of ascites is required to produce flank dullness and shifting dullness. Obesity and intestinal distension make detection of ascites difficult. Other signs of ascites include demonstration of a fluid wave and a puddle sign. The fluid wave sign is not very accurate and of limited value.[68] Demonstration of a puddle sign requires that the patient assume the hands-on-knees position, which is difficult or impossible for seriously ill patients to do. Sometimes it is necessary to perform paracentesis or abdominal ultrasound to determine whether or not ascites is present. Ultrasonography is particularly useful since as little as 100 mL of ascites can be detected.

Patients with ascites as a result of cirrhosis usually have other physical manifestations of chronic liver disease, such as muscle wasting, spider angiomata, palmar erythema, abdominal wall collateral veins, caput me-

dusa, breast hypertrophy in males, and lower extremity edema. Similarly, patients with cardiac ascites have signs of cardiac failure, nephrotic patients with ascites usually have anasarca, and patients with tuberculous peritonitis have abdominal tenderness and guarding or rigidity.

ABDOMINAL PARACENTESIS AND ASCITIC FLUID ANALYSIS

Abdominal paracentesis and ascitic fluid analysis are important diagnostic procedures that should be done in patients with new-onset ascites, those who are hospitalized with ascites, and ascitic patients whose condition deteriorates.[1,69–71] The incidence of complications, mainly hematomas of the abdominal wall, is ≤1%. Coagulopathy, which is present in most patients with cirrhosis, is not a contraindication to paracentesis, and preparation with transfusions of fresh-frozen plasma or platelets is not necessary.[69]

Table 56–2 shows the tests that are performed on the ascitic fluid. The cell count is done to immediately detect and initiate treatment of bacterial peritonitis; a neutrophil count of ≥250/mm³ indicates infection. Culture of the ascitic fluid by inoculation into blood-culture bottles at the bedside has been reported to have a sensitivity of about 85% in detecting infection.[72,73]

Determination of the serum-ascites albumin gradient by subtracting the albumin concentration in ascitic fluid from that in serum has a 97% correlation with the presence or absence of portal hypertension.[74,75] A gradient of ≥1.1 g/dL indicates the presence of portal hypertension, while a gradient of ≤1.1 g/dL indicates its absence. Table 56–3 shows how the serum-ascites albumin gradient can be used in the differential diagnosis of ascites.

Use of the total protein concentration to classify ascitic fluid as exudate (>2.5 g/dL) or transudate (<2.5 g/dL) has been shown to be considerably less helpful than the serum-ascites albumin gradient.[75] The same is true of the ratios of lactate dehydrogenase and total protein concentration in ascitic fluid to those in serum.[1] However, measurement of total protein concentration

TABLE 56–2. TESTS OF ASCITIC FLUID

Routine Tests	Optional Tests	Unusual Tests
Cell count	Glucose	Tuberculosis smear and culture
Albumin	Lactate dehydrogenase	Cytologic exam for cancer
Bacterial culture (in blood-culture bottles)	Amylase	
	Gram's stain	
Total protein		

(From Runyon BA. Care of patients with ascites. N Engl J Med 1994;330:337–342)

TABLE 56–3. DIFFERENTIAL DIAGNOSIS OF ASCITES ACCORDING TO THE SERUM-ASCITES ALBUMIN GRADIENT

HIGH GRADIENT ≥1.1 gm/dL	LOW GRADIENT <1.1 gm/dL
Cirrhosis	Peritoneal carcinomatosis
Alcoholic hepatitis	Peritoneal tuberculosis
Cardiac failure	Pancreatic ascites
Massive liver metastases	Biliary ascites
Fulminant hepatic failure	Nephrotic syndrome
Budd-Chiari syndrome	Serositis
Portal vein thrombosis	Bowel obstruction or infarction
Veno-occlusive disease	
Fatty liver of pregnancy	
Myxedema	
Mixed ascites	

(From Runyon BA. Care of patients with ascites. N Engl J Med 1994;330:337–342)

is helpful in detecting spontaneous bacterial peritonitis (<1.0 g/dL), and in differentiating spontaneous from secondary bacterial peritonitis (≥1.0 g/dL). The latter is a polymicrobial infection in which total protein concentration and lactate dehydrogenase in ascitic fluid are high, and glucose concentration is <50 mg/dL.[76]

Elevated amylase concentration in ascitic fluid indicates pancreatic ascites or gastrointestinal perforation.[77] Gram's staining of ascitic fluid is of little value in the diagnosis of spontaneous bacterial peritonitis, but may be helpful in detecting secondary peritonitis owing to gastrointestinal perforation.[73,76] When the cell count of ascitic fluid shows mainly lymphocytes and the serum-ascites albumin ratio is low, smears and cultures for tuberculosis and cytologic examination for malignant cells is indicated.[78]

■ COMPLICATIONS OF ASCITES

SPONTANEOUS BACTERIAL PERITONITIS

Spontaneous bacterial peritonitis (SBP) is the term used to describe bacterial infection of ascitic fluid without a detectable intra-abdominal source of infection. The prevalence of SBP in patients with cirrhotic ascites has been reported to be 10% to 27% at the time of hospital admission.[79,80] It is diagnosed by ascitic fluid analysis showing a neutrophil count ≥250/mm³ and a positive bacterial culture. One or the other of these findings, and preferably both, must be present to make the diagnosis. SBP is almost always monomicrobial, and enteric organisms are usually, but not always, the cause. When cultures show a polymicrobial infection, secondary bacterial peritonitis owing to perforation of the gastrointestinal tract should be suspected. The pathogenesis of SBP is uncertain, but it is presumed that the ascitic fluid is colonized by bacteria that have gotten into the systemic circulation as a result of the impaired reticuloendothelial function that occurs in advanced cirrhosis.

Once the diagnosis is suspected on the basis of an elevated ascitic fluid neutrophil count, antibiotic therapy should be started, even before bacterial culture results are available. The goals of antibiotic therapy are broad-spectrum coverage of common organisms causing SBP, adequate drug levels in ascitic fluid and avoidance of nephrotoxicity and superinfections.[81–85] Successful treatment is indicated by clinical improvement, a 50% or greater drop in the ascitic fluid neutrophil count, and sterile cultures. Use of a third generation cephalosporin, such as cefotaxime, is appropriate initial therapy that has been shown to be more effective and less toxic than ampicillin and an aminoglycoside. The antibiotic regimen can be changed when the sensitivities become known. Current practice is to treat the patient with intravenous antibiotics for 7 to 10 days.

The hospital mortality rate of SBP has been reported to be as high as 70%,[81] in large part owing to the advanced liver disease of the patients who get this complication. Recurrence of SBP after successful initial treatment has been reported to occur in more than half of the patients.[85]

TENSE ASCITES

When ascites distends the abdomen to the point that it becomes tense, breathing becomes difficult. In most cirrhotic patients, that point is reached when 10 L or more of fluid has accumulated, although in the occasional young patient who does not have muscle wasting, a smaller fluid volume produces a tense abdomen. Tense ascites must be relieved by therapeutic paracentesis. Contrary to old concepts based on anecdotal reports, tense ascites can be drained without untoward hemodynamic consequences.[86,87]

ABDOMINAL WALL HERNIAS

Patients with ascites commonly develop abdominal wall hernias, usually umbilical or incisional, sometimes inguinal. In one study, umbilical hernias were found in 17% of cirrhotic ascitic patients at the time of hospital admission; 14% were incarcerated, 35% developed skin ulceration, and 7% ruptured during follow-up of 4 years.[88] Rupture of an umbilical hernia has a mortality rate of 11% to 43%, often owing to bacterial peritonitis.[89] Abdominal wall hernias should be repaired surgically after the ascites is reabsorbed by medical treatment, since the recurrence rate is high in patients who are operated on in the presence of ascites.[90] Rupture of an umbilical hernia requires emergency surgical repair, even when substantial ascites is present.

PLEURAL EFFUSION

Patients with cirrhotic ascites commonly develop pleural effusions, usually on the right but sometimes bilateral, with the right greater than the left. The term hepatic hydrothorax is used when the effusion is large. Hepatic hydrothorax is the result of leakage of ascitic fluid into the pleural cavity through a small defect in the fibrous portion of the diaphragm.[91] Occasionally, a large pleural effusion is responsible for the presenting complaint of the patient, and the ascites initially is undetected.[92] Therapy is directed at treatment of the ascites with sodium restriction and diuretics. Therapeutic thoracentesis is used only to relieve significant difficulty in breathing. Continuous drainage of the pleural fluid by insertion of a chest tube is associated with serious problems owing to fluid and protein depletion, and should be avoided.[93] The chest tube is often difficult to remove.

BLOODY ASCITES

In the absence of liver disease and trauma, bloody ascites is usually due to cancer. Less than 5% of patients with cirrhotic ascites have bloody ascites, and usually it is an incidental finding.[94] The most common cause of bloody ascites is traumatic paracentesis in which the needle ruptures a venous collateral in the abdominal wall. Other causes of bloody ascites include spontaneous rupture of a portal-systemic collateral vein in the peritoneal cavity (often with hypovolemic shock), rupture of hepatocellular carcinoma, and traumatic rupture of the spleen or liver, sometimes from unnoticed trauma.

■ MEDICAL TREATMENT OF CIRRHOTIC ASCITES

SODIUM RESTRICTION

Restriction of dietary sodium intake is the mainstay of therapy of cirrhotic ascites. Sodium intake usually is restricted to 88 mEq/24 hrs (2 gm of salt/day), but if the ascites is refractory, it is necessary to reduce sodium intake to 44 mEq and even to 22 mEq/24 hrs. The importance of adherence to diet cannot be overemphasized. Treatment can be attempted in the outpatient clinic or office, but hospitalization greatly enhances therapy by assuring abstinence from alcohol, facilitating education of the patient and family in the limited sodium diet, and permitting close monitoring of body weight, abdominal girth, fluid intake and output, serum and urine electrolytes, renal function (serum concentrations of urea nitrogen and creatinine), and hepatic encephalopathy. Bedrest is not a necessary part of therapy, although it is widely used. Bedrest has not been shown to promote natriuresis,

and it has the disadvantage of furthering muscle wasting and predisposing to decubitus ulcers. A small percentage of patients develop diuresis with restriction of dietary sodium intake alone, but combining dietary therapy with use of diuretic drugs is much more effective. There is little justification for withholding diuretics.

WATER RESTRICTION

Patients with cirrhotic ascites have impaired excretion of water and regularly develop hyponatremia. Restriction of fluid intake of 1.5 L/day is routinely ordered in the therapy of ascites, but there is no solid data to support this convention. Severe hyponatremia (serum sodium <120 mEq/L) may produce neurologic manifestations and even permanent neurologic damage, and should be avoided.[95–97] Fluid restriction is not necessary in all patients with ascites but should be introduced if serum sodium falls below 130 mEq/L, and in patients who continue to gain weight despite stringent sodium restriction and use of diuretics.

DIURETIC THERAPY

Diuretic therapy should be started promptly in combination with dietary sodium restriction. The objective of diuretic therapy is to increase urinary sodium excretion and volume by blocking the sodium retaining mechanisms in the kidney. Table 56–4 shows the diuretics available for treatment of ascites and their renal sites of action. The two groups of drugs used most widely for ascites are agents that act on the distal tubule, particularly spironolactone, and diuretics that act on the loop of Henle, particularly furosemide.

Spironolactone inhibits sodium reabsorption in the distal tubules and collecting ducts by blocking the effects of aldosterone on tubular reabsorption of sodium. The onset of diuresis takes 10 to 14 days because of its long half-life, and it is a relatively weak diuretic; the maximal diuresis induced by spironolactone is only 2% of the filtered sodium load.[99] Spironolactone may cause hyperkalemia and a hyperchloremic acidosis, and sometimes causes painful gynecomastia. Amiloride is similar in its action to spironolactone, but it is more rapid acting and does not produce gynecomastia.[100]

Furosemide and other loop diuretics inhibit sodium transport in the thick ascending limb of the loop of Henle where 20% to 50% of the filtered sodium load is reabsorbed. Furosemide is a potent diuretic that can induce a natriuresis of up to 15% to 25% of the filtered load of sodium.[99] Furthermore, furosemide induces kaliuresis and causes hypokalemia and metabolic alkalosis. Thiazide diuretics, which act on the distal tubule, are about one-third as potent as furosemide and have similar side effects.[99]

TABLE 56–4. DIURETICS AND THEIR SITES OF ACTION IN THE KIDNEY

Filtration diuretics
  Aminophyline
  Glucocorticoids
Proximal tubular diuretics
  Mannitol
  Acetazolamide
Loop of Henle diuretics
  Furosemide
  Ethacrynic acid
  Bumetanide
  Piretanide
Distal tubular diuretics
  Potassium losing
    Thiazides
    Chlorthalidone
    Metolazone
  Potassium sparing
    Triamterene
    Spironolactone
    Amiloride
Collecting-ducts diuretics
  Lithium
  Demeclocycline

(From Linas SL, Anderson RJ, Miller PD et al. The rational use of diuretics in cirrhosis. In: Epstein M (ed), The Kidney in Liver Disease, 2nd ed. New York, NY: Elsevier North-Holland; 1983:555)

The combination of spironolactone and furosemide is the most effective regimen for obtaining prompt diuresis and avoiding potassium imbalance.[98,101–105] Typical starting doses are 100 mg of spironolactone and 40 mg of furosemide given by mouth once a day, in the morning, to facilitate compliance when out of the hospital and to minimize the necessity to awaken during the night to urinate. Use of divided doses is not supported by pharmacokinetic data.[99] Serial monitoring of body weight, fluid intake and output, and urinary sodium excretion helps to determine the optimal diuretic dose. The goal is a negative sodium and fluid balance with a weight loss of 0.5 kg/day. Weight loss in excess of 1.0 kg/day may precipitate renal insufficiency. If there is no decrease in body weight or an increase in urinary sodium excretion after 3 days, the daily doses are increased to 200 mg of spironolactone and 80 mg of furosemide and, ultimately, if necessary, to 400 mg and 160 mg, respectively. When combined with restriction of dietary sodium, treatment with spironolactone and furosemide is effective in >90% of cirrhotic patients, with no other treatment for ascites necessary.[89,99,101–105]

Ascites is considered intractable or refractory to medical treatment when satisfactory diuresis does not occur, or when the desirable weight loss (0.5 to 1.0 kg/day) is accompanied by azotemia, severe hyponatremia, or hepatic encephalopathy.

THERAPEUTIC PARACENTESIS

Substantial evidence indicates that therapeutic paracentesis, including large-volume (>5 L) paracentesis, is safe and appropriate treatment of ascites in the small minority of patients who are refractory to conventional medical therapy.[106–115] Use of plasma volume expansion following paracentesis by infusion of albumin or dextran is controversial. Investigators in Barcelona reported fewer abnormalities of electrolytes, creatinine, plasma renin, and aldosterone in patients who received albumin infusions after large-volume paracentesis for tense ascites than in those who did not.[111] Two other studies found little or no reduction in plasma volume after large-volume paracentesis in the absence of plasma volume expansion,[112,113] and another study found that albumin infusion in patients receiving repeated paracentesis had no influence on mortality rate or development of hepatorenal syndrome.[110] Recurrence of ascites following therapeutic paracentesis is frequent, and mortality rate after 1 year is 50% or greater.[107,111,115]

ASCITES REINFUSION

Ascitic fluid may be drained from the abdomen through a peritoneal dialysis catheter with the aid of a roller pump, concentrated by passage through a semipermeable membrane, and then reinfused into a peripheral vein.[116–121] Extracorporeal ultrafiltration and reinfusion of ascitic fluid conserves the proteins of the patients and probably is less expensive than albumin infusions. Two controlled trials comparing this form of therapy with paracentesis with albumin infusion showed similar effectiveness and mortality rate.[119–120] Fever and mild disturbances in coagulopathy have been observed in some patients, and may be alleviated by the recently described intraperitoneal reinfusion of the ascites concentrate.[121]

■ SURGICAL TREATMENT OF INTRACTABLE CIRRHOTIC ASCITES BY SIDE-TO-SIDE PORTACAVAL SHUNT

RATIONALE

The rationale for the use of portal-systemic shunts in the treatment of intractable cirrhotic ascites is directly related to the primary role of sinusoidal hypertension in the pathogenesis of ascites, and is based on the capacity of the shunt procedure to decompress the liver. The side-to-side portacaval shunt, and its equivalents, such as the mesocaval H-graft shunt and the central splenorenal shunt, accomplish sinusoidal decompression by shunting splanchnic blood away from the liver and by improving the outflow of hepatic blood via retrograde flow through the portal vein into the low-pressure vena cava. Numerous experimental and clinical studies have demonstrated, by use of contrast roentgenograms, dyes radioisotopes, and direct measurements of blood flow, that the valveless portal vein is capable of functioning as an outflow tract.[122–128] Moreover, pressure studies after side-to-side anastomosis in cirrhotic patients have shown that sinusoidal pressure is reduced markedly, often to normal levels, and that the objective hepatic decompression is accomplished.[129,130]

The end-to-side portacaval shunt accomplishes hepatic decompression by eliminating the contribution of portal venous blood to hepatic inflow and pressure. Documentation of this effect has been obtained by several studies that have shown a reduction in wedged hepatic vein pressure and hepatic blood flow in the majority of patients after end-to-side anastomoses.[6,131,132] However, end-to-side shunts generally have not reduced sinusoidal hypertension as much as side-to-side shunts, and in some patients high, sinusoidal pressures have persisted.[133–135] Moreover, the inability of the end-to-side shunt to improve the outflow of blood from the liver is a theoretic and, in some instances, an actual shortcoming of this procedure. While reduction of inflow often may overcome sinusoidal hypertension, in patients with severe outflow block or spontaneous reversal of portal flow, the end-to-side shunt actually may increase sinusoidal pressure by eliminating the possibility of retrograde flow in the portal vein.

The selective distal splenorenal shunt introduced by Warren and Zeppa does not decompress the hepatic sinusoids and is contraindicated in intractable cirrhotic ascites. In fact, ascites is a well-recognized complication of distal splenorenal shunt.

EXPERIMENTAL RESULTS

Experiments performed in our laboratory showed that side-to-side portacaval shunt was very effective in decompressing the liver and overcoming the effects of sinusoidal hypertension, while the end-to-side anastomosis was usually not effective. Construction of a side-to-side portacaval anastomosis at the same time that a cannula was inserted into the vena cava opposite the orifices of the hepatic veins consistently prevented ascites, while an end-to-side shunt failed to prevent ascites.[136] The side-to-side shunt usually cured ascites in dogs with well-established persistent ascites produced by ligation of the hepatic veins, while the end-to-side shunt usually had no effect on the accumulated fluid.[137] The marked hypersecretion of aldosterone associated with obstruction of the hepatic veins was prevented by side-to-side anastomosis but not by end-to-side shunt.[56,57] Finally, the greatly increased lymph flow in the thoracic duct in dogs with ascites produced by ligation of the hepatic veins was reduced almost to normal levels by the side-to-side shunt, while the end-to-side shunt had much less effect on lymph production.[12,13]

TABLE 56–5. PREOPERATIVE CLINICAL CHARACTERISTICS IN 32 PATIENTS WITH INTRACTABLE CIRRHOTIC ASCITES

Characteristic	% of Group
Age (yr)	
30–39	9
40–49	50
50–59	38
≥60	3
Male sex	75
Past history of bleeding varices	44
Cirrhosis proven by biopsy	100
Alcoholic	91
Posthepatitic	9
Jaundice	6
Portal-systemic encephalopathy-current or past history:	
None	81
Mild	13
Marked	6
Severe muscle wasting	100
Hyperdynamic state, cardiac output ≥6L/min	100
Total serum bilirubin ≤2.8 mg/dL	100
Serum albumin (g/dL)	
≤3.0	59
3.1–3.4	38
>3.4	3
BSP or ICG retention ≥18%/45 min (normal ≤6%/45 min)	100
Child-Pugh risk class[a]	
A	0
B	69
C	31

[a]Child-Pugh risk class was determined by the point scoring system proposed by Campbell and associates[140,141]

CLINICAL RESULTS

On the basis of our experimental observations, we began to use side-to-side portacaval shunt in the early 1960s to treat selected patients with truly intractable ascites owing to cirrhosis.[29,138,139] To date, we have operated on 32 selected patients, or approximately 1 patient per year. Their preoperative clinical characteristics are summarized in Table 56–5. The patients ranged in age from 36 to 60 years (mean age, 47.8 years), and 75% were men. Fourteen had a past history of bleeding from esophageal varices, but none had bled during the 6 months prior to operation. The primary indication for portacaval shunt in each case was intractable ascites. Based on the history, results of serologic tests for hepatitis, and microscopic findings in a liver biopsy obtained at operation, 91% of patients had alcoholic cirrhosis and 9% had posthepatitic cirrhosis. All of the patients had evidence of advanced cirrhosis that included, in addition to massive ascites, severe muscle wasting, a hyperdynamic cardiovascular state (cardiac output ≥6 L/min), marked retention of bromsulfalein or indocyanine-green dye, and a low serum albumin

TABLE 56–6. VOLUME OF ASCITES AND PORTAL PRESSURES IN 32 PATIENTS WHO UNDERWENT SIDE-TO-SIDE PORTACAVAL SHUNT FOR INTRACTABLE CIRRHOTIC ASCITES

	Mean	Range
Volume of ascites (L)	11.4	5.8–17.5
Preoperative corrected wedged hepatic vein pressure (mm saline)	294	230–364
Corrected free portal pressure at operation (mm saline)		
Preshunt	287	202–376
Postshunt	4	0–18

TABLE 56–7. METABOLIC DATA BEFORE AND AFTER SIDE-TO-SIDE PORTACAVAL SHUNT IN 32 PATIENTS WITH INTRACTABLE CIRRHOTIC ASCITES

	Preoperative		3 Weeks Postoperative	
	Mean	*Range*	*Mean*	*Range*
Months of medical therapy for ascites	13.5	5–22	—	—
Urine Na$^+$ (mEq/24hr)	1.3	0.4–2.7	43.0	32–53
Urine volume (mL/24hr)	531	158–823	2041	1562–2662
Serum Na$^+$ (mEq/L)	126	120–129	137	135–143
Serum K$^+$ (mEq/L)	3.5	3.1–4.1	4.6	4.0–5.2
Urine aldosterone (μg/24hr)[a] (n=10)	145	75–187	17	10–28

[a]Normal range is 2–26μg/24hr

concentration. However, only two patients had clinical jaundice, the serum total bilirubin concentration was ≤2.8 mg/dL in all patients and, although 19% of patients had a history of portal-systemic encephalopathy, it was recurrent and severe in only 2 patients. Child's risk classes determined by the quantitative point scoring system of Campbell and associates,[140,141] were C in 31% of patients, B in 69%, and A in none of the patients. Preoperatively, portal hypertension was demonstrated in all patients by hepatic vein catheterization. Wedged hepatic vein pressure, corrected by subtracting the inferior vena caval pressure, ranged from 230 to 364 mm saline and averaged 294 mm.

Prior to considering portacaval shunt, all patients received prolonged and intensive medical treatment for ascites during periods ranging from 5 to 22 months, consisting of abstinence from alcohol, a nutritious diet, rigorous dietary sodium restriction, spironolactone, a variety of potent diuretics and, in many instances, repeated therapeutic paracentesis. Operation was considered when the ascites failed to respond to medical therapy under ideal conditions during prolonged hospitalization. The criteria for intractable ascites were met in each patient.

The findings at operation are shown in Table 56–6. The volume of ascites ranged from 5.8 to 17.5 L and averaged 11.4 L. Corrected free portal pressure, obtained by subtracting the inferior vena caval pressure, ranged from 202 to 376 mm saline. In 21 patients (66%), the pressure on the hepatic side of a clamp occluding the portal vein (hepatic occluded portal pressure) was higher than the free portal pressure, suggesting the likelihood of spontaneous reversal of portal blood flow, and indicating the presence of severe hepatic outflow block. Side-to-side portacaval shunt reduced corrected free portal pressure from a mean of 287 mm saline to a mean of 4 mm saline, and in all patients to <20 mm saline.

Daily weight, girth, serum electrolytes, fluid balance, and sodium excretion were measured continuously while the patients were on a 44 mEq sodium diet for 10 to 28 days preoperatively and again 3 weeks postoperatively. In addition, 10 patients had daily measurements of urinary aldosterone excretion before and after operation. The results are summarized in Table 56–7. Preoperatively, all patients showed the characteristic pattern of sodium and fluid retention, with a low urine volume and sodium excretion, and a dilutional hyponatremia. No patient excreted more than 2.7 mEq/day of sodium. In addition, 27 (84%) of the 32 patients had hypokalemia, a common finding in cirrhosis. All 10 patients in whom urinary aldosterone excretion was measured had evidence of marked hyperaldosteronism, excreting 5 to 10 times the normal amount of aldosterone.

Side-to-side portacaval shunt produced marked diuresis and natriuresis in all 31 survivors. Within three weeks, sodium excretion reached normal levels. Urine volume increased markedly and negative fluid balance developed. Dilutional hyponatremia and hypokalemia disappeared. Urinary aldosterone excretion returned to the normal range, and intermittent determinations for 2 years showed that it remained normal.

Table 56–8 summarizes the long-term results of side-to-side portacaval shunt in the 32 patients with intractable cirrhotic ascites. All patients have been followed-up for more than 5 years or until death, if they died before 5 years. Ten year follow-up is 100% of the 25 patients who were operated on more than 10 years ago. There were two operative deaths; one in the operating room from bleeding; and one from hepatic failure on postoperative day 29. The remaining 30 patients (94%) were discharged from the hospital alive. Actual 5 year survival rate is 75%, and 10 year survival rate is 72%. There have been 8 late deaths between 2.5 and 11 years

TABLE 56–8. LONG-TERM RESULTS OF SIDE-TO-SIDE PORTACAVAL SHUNT IN 32 PATIENTS WITH INTRACTABLE CIRRHOTIC ASCITES

	% of Group
Length of follow-up	
>5 yr or until death (n=32)	100
>10 yr or until death (n=25)	100
Survival	
30 days and left hospital (n=32)	94
5 year (n=32)	75
10 year (n=25)	72
Ascites (n=31)	10*
Use of diuretics (n=31)	29#
Portal-systemic encephalopathy in 30 patients who left hospital alive	
Single episode	10
Recurrent episodes	7
Liver function 5 years postoperatively or at time of death (n=31)	
Improved	81
Same	6
Worse	13
Portacaval shunt patency	100

*Terminal ascites due to hepatoma in two patients, heart failure in one patient.
#Spironolactone was required for peripheral edema in nine patients, combined with furosemide in one patient.

postoperatively. Three of these deaths were from hepatic failure owing to continued alcoholism at 2.5, 3.5, and 4.2 years, respectively. Two deaths were from hepatoma at 2.5 and 4.5 years, respectively. One death each was from right heart failure due to pulmonary hypertension at 4.8 years, lung cancer at 9.5 years, and diabetic renal failure at 11 years, respectively.

All survivors were relieved of ascites. Three patients who were free of ascites for 2 to 4 years developed terminal ascites just prior to death from hepatoma (2 patients) and right heart failure (1 patient). All patients were continued on 88 mEq/day dietary sodium restriction as a precaution, but compliance was less than complete. Spironolactone was required intermittently in 9 patients for treatment of peripheral edema, not ascites, and one of these patients also received a brief course of furosemide.

During follow-up, the 4-test index described by Conn and associates was used to detect portal-systemic encephalopathy at each clinic visit.[142–144] Three (10%) patients had a single episode of encephalopathy, and two (7%) patients, both consumers of alcohol, had recurrent encephalopathy requiring dietary protein reduction. We attribute the low incidence of encephalopathy to our rigorous, lifelong follow-up program in which there is continuing emphasis on abstinence from alcohol and limitation of protein intake to 60 gm/day.

In the 31 survivors, liver function 5 years postopera-

tively or at the time of death improved in 81%, was unchanged in 6%, and was worse in 13%. Child's risk class improved in the vast majority of patients. Most patients experienced striking improvements in nutrition in the form of sizeable gains in both lean tissue mass and body fat. The portacaval anastomosis was shown to be patent and functioning effectively in every patient by Doppler duplex ultrasonography or angiographic studies performed every 1 to 2 years. No patient bled from esophagogastric varices or any other cause related to portal hypertension during long-term follow-up.

Fig 56–3 shows photographs of a 42-year-old male patient before and 6 weeks after side-to-side portacaval shunt. He had massive ascites, hepatomegaly, and the usual stigmata of alcoholic cirrhosis, but had never had jaundice, encephalopathy, or gastrointestinal bleeding. He was in Child's class B. He was treated during two hospital admissions and weekly outpatient clinic visits during a period of 5 months, with stringent dietary sodium restriction, spironolactone, four potent diuretics, and therapeutic paracentesis. The ascites responded initially to treatment, but then became intractable. He abstained from alcohol throughout the period of medical therapy. Fig 56–4 shows the results of a 2 month–long metabolic balance study performed in this patient. Preoperatively, he excreted a mean 151 μg/day of aldosterone, a 10-fold increase above normal, and was unable to excrete more than 2 mEq/day of sodium. Following side-to-side portacaval shunt, he had a marked diuresis and natriuresis, and urine aldosterone excretion returned to normal within 4 weeks. The large reductions in body weight and girth associated with operative removal of 16 L of ascites were sustained. Three months after operation, he resumed work as a merchant seaman, and when last seen 13 years postoperatively, he was regularly employed. He remained free of ascites, edema, encephalopathy and gastrointestinal bleeding. His sodium restriction was casual, and he did not require diuretics at any time during follow-up.

Side-to-side portacaval shunt is very effective treatment of cirrhotic ascites. However, it only should be used in carefully selected patients who have been proven to have intractable ascites during a period of intensive medical therapy and study in the hospital, and who have some chance of prolonged survival. The usual effectiveness of medical therapy combined with careful selection of patients who have failed medical treatment in the hospital are the reasons why we have performed side-to-side portacaval shunt in only one patient per year. It is inappropriate to use portacaval shunt to relieve ascites in patients whose liver disease is so far advanced that they will die of hepatic failure whether or not their ascites is abolished.

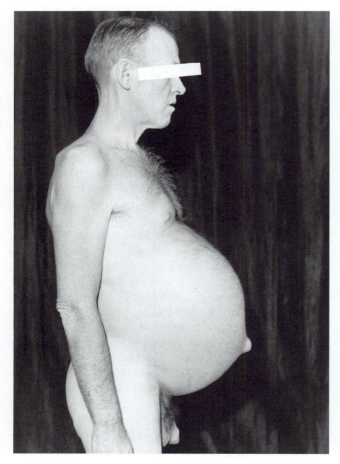

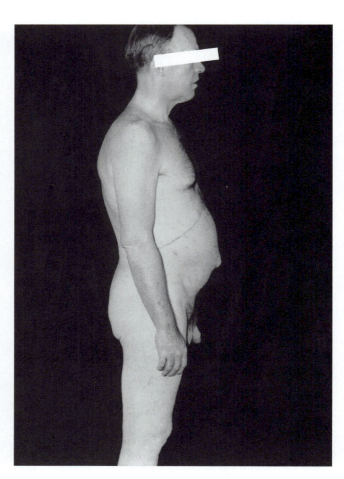

A

B

Figure 56–3. Photographs of a patient with cirrhosis and intractable ascites taken before and 6 weeks after side-to-side portacaval shunt. **A**. Preoperatively, when ascites was massive. **B**. Six weeks after side-to-side portacaval shunt. (From Orloff MJ. Effect of side-to-side portacaval shunt on intractable ascites, sodium excretion, and aldosterone metabolism in man. *Am J Surg* 1966;112:287–298)

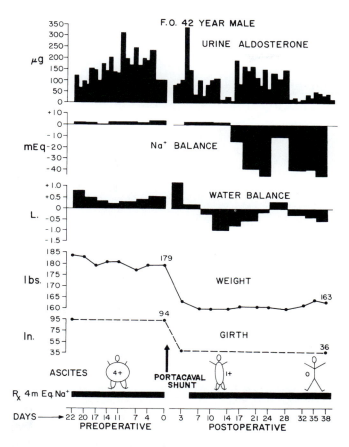

Figure 56–4. Results of a metabolic balance study of the patient shown in Fig 56–3, conducted before and after treatment of intractable ascites by side-to-side portacaval shunt. (From Orloff MJ. Effect of side-to-side portacaval shunt on intractable ascites, sodium excretion, and aldosterone metabolism in man. *Am J Surg* 1966;112:287–298)

SURGICAL TECHNIQUE

During the past 36 years, the authors and their associates have performed side-to-side portacaval shunt for portal hypertension in more than 1500 patients, with a resultant long-term shunt patency rate of 99.7%. From our experience, we have concluded that, with proper technique, a satisfactory side-to-side anastomosis can be performed in almost every patient who has a patent portal vein. The technique used by the authors is illustrated in Figs 56–5 through 56–14.[145,146] Important technical features of the operation are

1. The position of the patient on the operating table is crucial and can make the difference between an easy and difficult operation.
2. A long right subcostal incision is associated with fewer postoperative complications than a thoracoabdominal incision and is used routinely.
3. Use of electrocautery throughout the operation substantially reduces operating time and blood loss.

4. Bleeding from the many portasystemic collateral vessels is managed best by pressure with gauze sponge packs. Most of the bleeding stops as soon as the portacaval anastomosis is completed and the portal hypertension is relieved. Attempts to control each of the bleeding collateral with ligatures and sutures prolongs the operation and increases blood loss. The objective is to decompress the portal system as rapidly as possible.
5. Circumferential mobilization of the inferior vena cava (IVC) between the entrance of the renal veins and its disappearance behind the liver is essential for the side-to-side anastomosis and is neither hazardous nor difficult to perform. Apposition of the two vessels is greatly facilitated by elevation of the IVC toward the portal vein.
6. Mobilization of a long segment of portal vein, which includes division of the tough fibrofatty tissue that binds the portal vein to the pancreas and sometimes includes division of a bit of the head of the pancreas, is essential for the side-to-side anastomosis.
7. Resection of an enlarged caudate lobe of the liver to facilitate apposition of the two vessels is rarely necessary and may be hazardous.
8. Pressures in the IVC and portal vein should always be measured after completion of the portacaval shunt. A pressure gradient of >50 mm saline is unacceptable and requires revision of the anastomosis.

Fig 56–5 shows the position of the patient on the operating table, viewed from the right side of the patient. The patient is positioned with the right side elevated at an angle of 30° to the table, and the table is "broken" at the level of the costal margin and at the knees so as to widen the space between the right costal margin and the right iliac crest.

Fig 56–6 shows the position viewed from the left side of the patient, and the incision. A long right subcostal incision extending from the xiphoid to well into the flank is made 2 fingerbreadths below the costal margin. The skin is incised superficially with the scalpel, and the other layers with the electrocautery, which greatly reduces blood loss and shortens operating time. The right rectus abdominis, external oblique, and transversus abdominis muscles are completely divided and the medial 3 to 4 cm of the latissiums dorsi muscle often is incised. The peritoneum often contains many collateral blood vessels and is incised with electrocautery to obtain immediate haemostatis.

Fig 56–7 shows the exposure of the operative field. The viscera are retracted by three Deaver retractors positioned at right angles to each other. The inferior re-

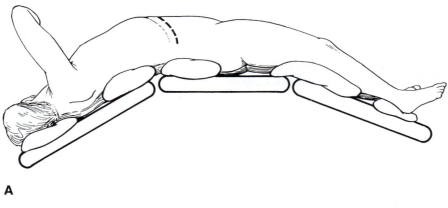

A

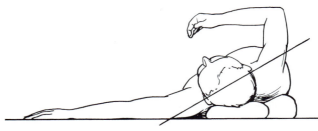

B

Figure 56–5. Position of the patient for side-to-side portacaval shunt. (Redrawn from Orloff MJ: Budd-Chiari syndrome and veno-occlusive disease. In: Blumgart LH (ed). *Surgery of the Liver and Biliary Tract.* London, England: Chruchill-Livingston; 1988:1425–1453)

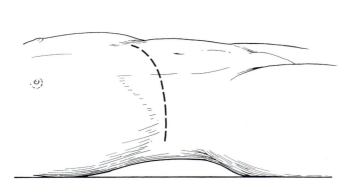

Figure 56–6. Long right subcostal incision used for side-to-side portacaval shunt. (Redrawn from Orloff MJ: Budd-Chiari syndrome and veno-occlusive disease. In: Blumgart LH (ed). *Surgery of the Liver and Biliary Tract.* London, England: Churchill-Livingston; 1988:1425–1453)

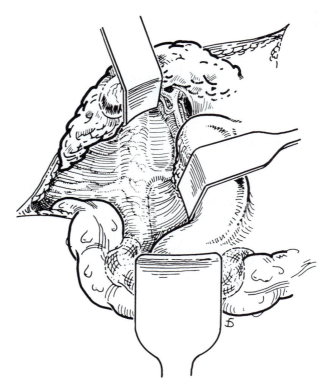

Figure 56–7. Exposure of the operative field for side-to-side portacaval shunt. (From Orloff MJ. Budd-Chiari syndrome and veno-occlusive disease. In: Blumgart LH (ed). *Surgery of the Liver and Biliary Tract.* London, England: Churchill-Livingston; 1988: 1425–1453)

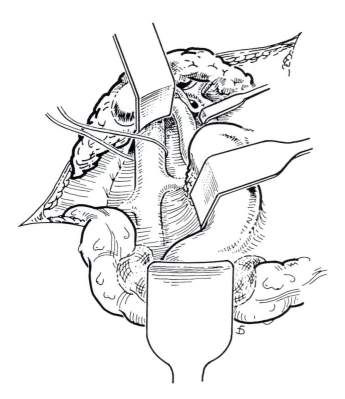

Figure 56–8. Circumferential isolation of the IVC between the renal veins and the liver in preparation for side-to-side portacaval anastomosis. (From Orloff MJ. Budd-Chiari syndrome and veno-occlusive disease. In: Blumgart LH (ed). *Surgery of the Liver and Biliary Tract.* London, England: Churchill-Livingston; 1988:1425–1453)

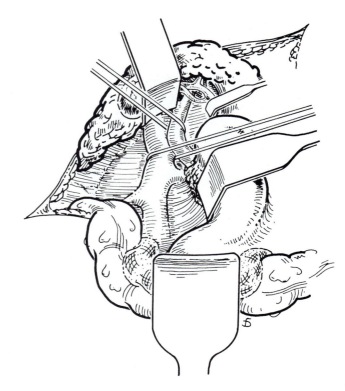

Figure 56–9. Exposure of the portal vein in preparation for side-to-side portacaval anastomosis. (From Orloff MJ. Budd-Chiari syndrome and veno-occlusive disease. In: Blumgart LH (ed). *Surgery of the Liver and Biliary Tract.* London, England: Churchill-Livingston; 1988:1425–1453)

tractor retracts the hepatic flexure of the colon toward the feet, the medial retractor displaces the duodenum medially, and the superior retractor retracts the liver and gallbladder toward the head. Alternatively, a self-retaining retractor may be used to accomplish the same exposure. The posterior peritoneum overlying the IVC is incised with electrocautery by an extended Kocher maneuver just lateral to the descending duodenum, and the retractors are repositioned to retract the head of the pancreas medially, and the right kidney caudally.

Fig 56–8 shows the isolation of the IVC. The anterior surface of the IVC is cleared of fibroareolar tissue, and the IVC is isolated around its entire circumference from the entrance of the right and left renal veins, below, to the point where it disappears behind the liver, above. The IVC is encircled with an umbilical tape. To accomplish the isolation, several tributaries must be ligated in continuity with fine silk ligatures and then divided. These tributaries often include the right adrenal vein, one or two pairs of lumbar veins that enter on the posterior surface, and the caudal pair of small hepatic veins that enter on the anterior surface of the IVC directly from the liver. When the IVC has been mobilized completely, it can be lifted up toward the portal vein. Failure

to isolate the IVC circumferentially is one major reason for the erroneous claim that the side-to-side portacaval shunt often cannot be performed because the portal vein and IVC are too widely separated.

Fig 56–9 shows the exposure of the portal vein. The superior retractor is repositioned medially so that it retracts the liver at the point of entrance of the portal triad. The portal vein is located in the posterolateral aspect of the portal triad and is approached from behind. The fibrofatty tissue on the posterolateral aspect of the portal triad, which contains nerves, lymphatics, and lymph nodes, is divided by blunt and sharp dissection. This technique is a safe maneuver because there are no portal venous tributaries on this aspect of the portal triad. As soon as the surface of the portal vein is exposed, a vein retractor is inserted to retract the common bile duct medially. The portal vein is mobilized circumferentially at its midportion and is encircled with an umbilical tape. It then is isolated up to its bifurcation in the liver hilum. Several tributaries on the medial aspect are ligated in continuity with fine silk and divided.

Fig 56–10 shows the mobilization of the portal vein behind the pancreas. Using the umbilical tape to pull the portal vein out of its bed, the portal vein is cleared

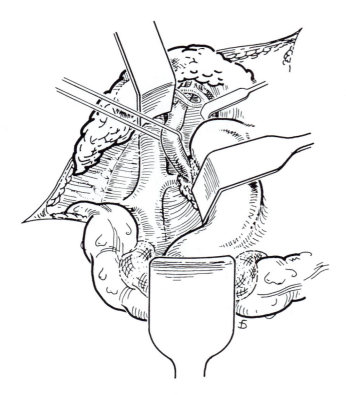

Figure 56–10. Mobilization of a long length of portal vein, including the segment behind the pancreas, in preparation for side-to-side portacaval anastomosis. (From Orloff MJ: Budd-Chiari syndrome and veno-occlusive disease. In: Blumgart LH (ed). *Surgery of the Liver and Biliary Tract*. London, England: Churchill-Livingston; 1988:1425–1453)

to the point where it disappears behind the pancreas. The tough fibrofatty tissue that binds the portal vein to the pancreas must be divided. Several tributaries that enter the medial aspect of the portal vein and one tributary that enters the posterolateral aspect are divided. It is usually not necessary to divide the splenic vein. Wide mobilization of the portal vein is essential for performance of a side-to-side portacaval anastomosis. Failure to mobilize the portal vein behind the pancreas is a second major reason for difficulty in accomplishing the side-to-side shunt. In some patients, it is necessary to divide a bit of the head of the pancreas between right-angled clamps to obtain adequate mobilization of the portal vein. Bleeding from the edges of the divided pancreas is controlled with suture ligatures. Division of a small amount of the pancreas is a very helpful maneuver and we have never observed postoperative complications, such as pancreatitis, from its performance.

Fig 56–11 shows measurement of pressures in the IVC and portal vein before performance of the portacaval anastomosis. Fig 56–12 through 56–14 show the performance of the side-to-side portacaval anastomosis. After it is determined that the IVC and portal vein can be brought together without excessive tension, a Satin-

sky clamp is placed obliquely across a 5-cm segment of the anteromedial wall of the IVC in a direction that is parallel to the course of the overlying portal vein, and the IVC is elevated toward the portal vein. A 5-cm segment of the portal vein is isolated between two angled vascular clamps, and the portal vein is depressed toward the IVC, bringing the two vessels into apposition (Fig 56–12A). A 2.5-cm long strip of the IVC and a 2.5-cm long strip of the portal vein are excised with scissors (Fig 56–12B). It is important to excise a longitudinal segment of the wall of each vessel rather than simply to make an incision in each vessel. A retraction suture of 5/0 vascular suture material is placed in the lateral wall of the IVC opening and is weighted by attachment to a hemostat to keep the IVC orifice open. The clamps on the portal vein are momentarily released to flush out any clots. The openings in both vessels then are irrigated with saline. The anastomosis is started with posterior continuous over-and-over suture of 5/0 vascular suture material (Fig 56–12C). The posterior continuous suture is tied at each end of the anastomosis. The anterior row of sutures consists of an everting continuous horizontal mattress stitch of 5/0 vascular material started at each end of the anastomosis (Fig 56–13). The suture started at the inferior end of the anastomosis is discontinued after 3 or 4 throws and is deliberately left loose so that the interior surface of the vessels can be visualized as the anastomosis is completed. In this way, inadvertent inclusion of the posterior wall in the anterior row of sutures is avoided. The suture started at the superior end of the anastomosis is inserted with continuous tension until it meets the inferior suture, at which point the inferior suture is drawn tight and the two sutures are tied to each other. Before drawing the inferior suture tight, the clamps on the portal vein are released momentarily to flush out any clots, and the anastomosis is thoroughly irrigated with saline.

Fig 56–14 shows the completed anastomosis. Upon completion of the anastomosis, a single interrupted-tension suture is placed just beyond each end of the anastomosis to take tension off the anastomotic suture line. The clamp on the IVC is removed first, the clamp on the hepatic side of the portal vein is removed next, and finally, the clamp on the intestinal side of the portal vein is removed. Bleeding from the anastomosis infrequently occurs; it can be controlled by one or two well-placed interrupted sutures of 5/0 vascular suture material.

Pressures in the portal vein and IVC must be measured after the anastomosis is completed. Usually the postshunt pressures in the portal vein and IVC are similar. A pressure gradient >50 mm saline between the two vessels indicates that there is an obstruction in the anastomosis, even when no obstruction can be palpated. In such circumstances, the anastomosis should be opened to remove any clots and, if necessary, the en-

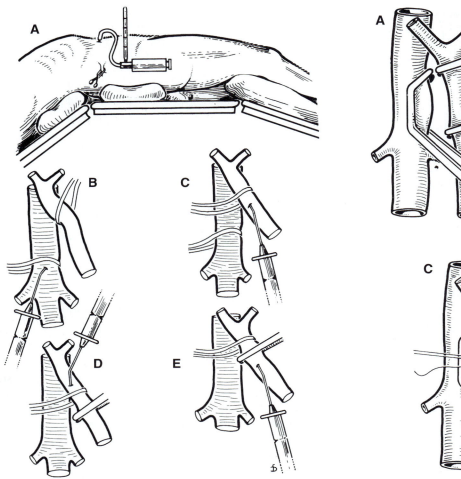

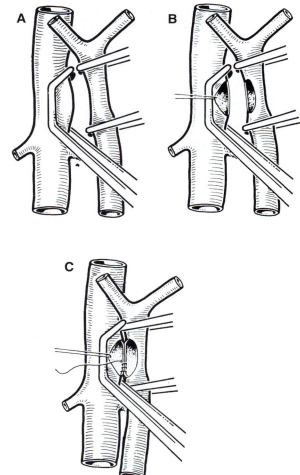

Figure 56–11. Measurement of pressures in the IVC and portal vein with a saline (spinal) manometer by direct needle puncture before performance of the portacaval anastomosis. All portal pressures are corrected by subtracting the IVC pressure from the portal pressure. Pressures in the IVC and portal vein are measured again after completion of the shunt. **A**. For all pressure measurements, the bottom of the manometer is positioned at the level of the IVC, which is marked on the skin surface of the body with a towel clip. **B**. IVC pressure (IVCP). **C**. Free portal pressure (FPP). **D**. Hepatic occluded portal pressure (HOPP), obtained on the hepatic side of a clamp occluding the portal vein. **E**. Splanchnic occluded portal pressure (SOPP), obtained on the intestinal side of a clamp occluding the portal vein. (From Orloff MJ. Budd-Chiari syndrome and veno-occlusive disease. In: Blumgart LH (ed). *Surgery of the Liver and Biliary Tract*. London, England: Churchill-Livingston; 1988:1425–1453)

Figure 56–12. Side-to-side portacaval anastomosis. **A**. Placement of clamps on IVC and portal vein. **B**. Strips of IVC and portal vein 2.5-cm long have been excised. **C**. Placement of posterior row of continuous 5/0 vascular suture from inside lumina of IVC and portal vein. (From Orloff MJ. Budd-Chiari syndrome and veno-occlusive disease. In: Blumgart LH (ed). *Surgery of the Liver and Biliary Tract*. London, England: Churchill-Livingston; 1988:1425–1453)

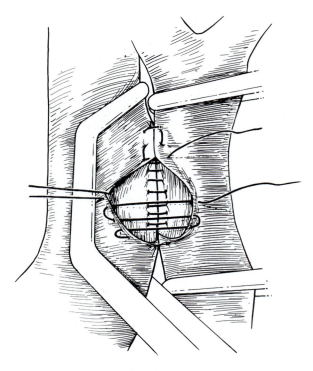

Figure 56–13. Side-to-side portacaval anastomosis. Placement of anterior row of two continuous everting sutures of 5/0 vascular material. (Redrawn from Orloff MJ. Budd-Chiari syndrome and veno-occlusive disease. In: Blumgart LH (ed). *Surgery of the Liver and Biliary Tract.* London, England: Churchill-Livingston; 1988:1425–1453)

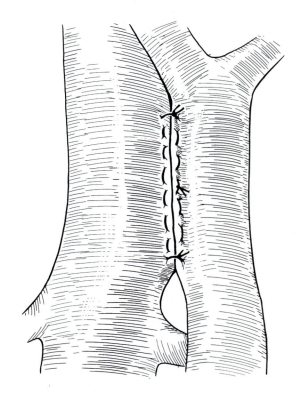

Figure 56–14. Completed side-to-side portacaval anastomosis. (Redrawn from Orloff MJ. Budd-Chiari syndrome and veno-occlusive disease. In: Blumgart LH (ed). *Surgery of the Liver and Biliary Tract.* London, England: Churchill-Livingston; 1988:1425–1453)

tire anastomosis should be taken down and done again. It is essential that there be no more than a 50-mm saline gradient between the portal vein and IVC to achieve permanently adequate portal decompression and avoid ultimate thrombosis of the shunt.

■ OTHER THERAPEUTIC MEASURES FOR INTRACTABLE CIRRHOTIC ASCITES

PERITONEOVENOUS SHUNT

LeVeen and associates described a pressure-activated one-way valve for use in a previously described device that shunted ascitic fluid from the high-pressure peritoneal cavity to the low-pressure superior vena cava.[147] The LeVeen shunt contains a diaphragm-type of valve attached to silicone struts. The struts act like springs, keeping the valve closed. One limb of the shunt lies free in the peritoneal cavity. The efferent limb is inserted through the internal jugular vein into the superior vena cava so that its venous opening lies near the entrance to the right atrium. Flow in the shunt is maintained if there is a 30- to 50-mm saline pressure gradient between the valve and its venous end, as occurs with inspiration. The valve closes when the gradient falls below 30 mm, preventing blood from flowing back into the tubing. Several other shunts that include a pumping mechanism for manually clearing the tubing and increasing flow, such as the Denver shunt and the Minnesota shunt, have been introduced.[148–150]

Insertion of a peritoneovenous shunt (PVS) is followed by increases in cardiac output, plasma volume, glomerular filtration rate, renal plasma flow, and creatinine clearance; decreases in plasma or serum levels of catecholamines, renin, and aldosterone; and natriuresis and diuresis.[151–155] Diuretics and sodium restriction are usually necessary to initiate and maintain natriuresis after insertion of the shunt, but the responsiveness of the patient to diuretics is enhanced.

In the 1980s, PVS was widely used for the treatment of ascites, often in patients who did not have intractable ascites. However, enthusiasm for this modality diminished considerably with reports of a high incidence of complications, substantial mortality, frequent shunt malfunctions, and recurrence of ascites in many patients.[148–173] Table 56–9 lists the complications of PVS. Evidence of disseminated intravascular coagulation (DIC) has been observed, in three-fourths of patients, in blood tests showing prolonged prothrombin

TABLE 56–9. COMPLICATIONS OF PERITONEOVENOUS SHUNT

Early	Late
Shunt occlusion or malfunction	Shunt occlusion or malfunction
Disseminated intravascular coagulation	Sepsis and bacterial peritonitis
Sepsis and bacterial peritonitis	Abdominal abscess
Congestive heart failure and pulmonary edema due to fluid overload	Central venous thrombosis
Bleeding varices	Pulmonary emboli
Air embolism	Abdominal wall infection
Allergic fever	Bleed varices
Ascites leakage	Adhesive intestinal obstruction

and partial thromboplastin times, decreased fibrinogen and platelet count, and increased fibrin split products.[157–161] About one-third of patients have been reported to develop bleeding following shunt placement.[159–161] It has been suggested that DIC is caused by an activator in ascitic fluid, and that DIC might be prevented by removal of ascitic fluid and replacement with saline at the time of shunt insertion. Bacterial peritonitis and/or sepsis, often due to *Staphylococcus aureas,* has been reported in ≤25% of patients, and is a very serious complication, with a mortality rate as high as 83%.[156,161,163,164] Treatment consists of prompt removal of the PVS and administration of intravenous antibiotics. Thrombosis of the jugular vein and superior vena cava has been observed in ≤30% of patients, causing recurrence of ascites, the superior vena cava syndrome, and pulmonary emboli that may be fatal.[149,161–163,170,171] Variceal hemorrhage as the result of an increase in portal pressure from rapid expansion of the plasma volume is an ever present risk following insertion of PVS.[161] At least 50% of patients have one or more of these complications.[161,163,165,170] Most shunts have been reported to develop occlusion in <1 year.[1,150,161,170]

Substantial evidence indicates that the ultimate failure rate of PVS is high.[104,115,148,149,166,170,173] Ascites has been reported to recur within one year, in >50% of patients whose ascites was relieved initially. Moreover, prospective randomized trials have shown no influence of PVS on survival or hepatic function, compared with medical therapy.[104,115,173] The 1-year mortality rate has exceeded 50%. In hepatorenal syndrome, PVS has had no effect on the outcome.[167] Many authorities have concluded that PVS is rarely indicated in cirrhotic ascites.

Technique of PVS

The operation is performed under local anesthesia (Fig 56–15). With the neck of the patient extended, an incision is made on the right side, 1 cm above the medial third of the clavicle at the insertion of the sternocleido-

mastoid muscle. The clavicular and sternal heads of the sternocleidomastoid muscle are retracted in opposite directions, exposing the internal jugular vein, which then is encircled with tapes.

A 6-cm abdominal incision then is made 6 cm below the right costal margin in the anterior axillary line. The oblique muscles are divided in the direction of their fibers and two purse-string sutures are placed in the transversus abdominus muscle and peritoneum, demarcating a circle 2 cm in diameter. An incision is made in the center of the circle and a Poole suction device is inserted into the peritoneal cavity to remove as much ascitic fluid as possible. The Poole suction device then is replaced with the peritoneal tube of the PVS, which is directed toward the pelvis. The one-way valve is placed in the extraperitoneal pocket, and the purse-string sutures are tied tightly around the nipple on the extraperitoneal surface of the valve. If the Denver shunt is used, a second 2 cm transverse incision is made over the costal margin for placement of the valve box subcutaneously, immediately above this incision.

Local anesthesia is instilled in the proposed subcutaneous tunnel, and the tunnel is bluntly fashioned just beneath the skin from the abdominal incision up to the neck incision. The venous tube of the PVS then is passed through the tunnel and out the cervical incision. A small venotomy is made in the right internal jugular vein, and the venous tube is inserted and passed down into the superior vena cava for a distance of about 9 to 11 cm. The venotomy is closed with interrupted 4-0 vascular sutures. The internal jugular vein is not ligated. A chest x-ray is obtained to ensure that the tip of the catheter is at the lower end of the superior vena cava. The wounds are closed without drainage.

Postoperatively, the patient is placed on a diet restricted to 44 mEq sodium/day, and diuretic therapy with furosemide and spironolactone is continued. Antibiotics are given for 4 days. The bed is kept flat, the abdomen is wrapped with a velcro abdominal binder, and the patient is encouraged to perform inspiratory exercises.

TRANSJUGULAR INTRAHEPATIC PORTAL-SYSTEMIC SHUNT (TIPS)

The most recent therapy to be proposed for the treatment of portal hypertension and its complications is percutaneous transjugular intrahepatic portal-systemic shunt, or TIPS. This procedure was introduced in 1969 but became clinically feasible only recently, as a result of the introduction of expandable metallic stents (Palmaz stent and Wallstent) that maintain patency of the shunt.[174] TIPS is a type of side-to-side portacaval shunt and theoretically, should have the same hemodynamic effects as a surgical side-to-side portacaval shunt. The

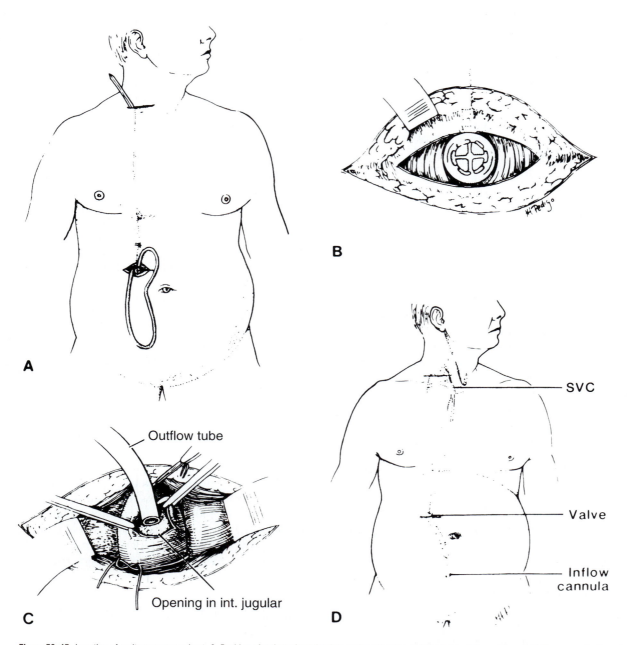

Figure 56–15. Insertion of peritoneovenous shunt. **A**. Position of catheter insertion into peritoneal cavity and cervical incision and tunnel. **B**. One-way valve is positioned superficial to posterior rectus sheath. **C**. Insertion of outflow tube into interior jugular vein. **D**. Position of venous and peritoneal cannulae. (From Greenlee HB, Stanley MM. Peritoneovenous shunt for ascites. In: Schwartz SI (ed). Abdominal Surgery. Installment IV, Vol. 16 of Modern Technics in Surgery. Mount Kisco, NY: Futura; 1982:9–14)

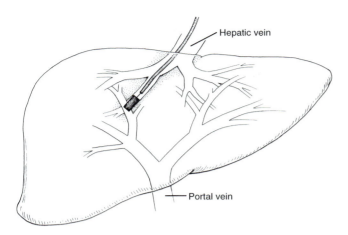

Hepatic vein

Portal vein

Figure 56–16. Diagram of a TIPS stent connecting a hepatic vein and the right portal vein. (Redrawn from Conn HO. Transjugular intrahepatic porta-systemic shunts: the state of the art. *Hepatology* 1993;17:148–158)

technique involves percutaneous passage of a catheter through the internal jugular vein, down the superior vena cava, through the heart, down the suprahepatic inferior vena cava, and into a hepatic vein in the liver, under fluoroscopic control. A needle then is passed through the catheter and an intrahepatic branch of the portal vein is punctured. The needle is replaced by a balloon catheter across the parenchymal tract, and the balloon is inflated with contrast medium to a diameter of 10 mm. An expandable metallic stent is introduced into the dilated parenchymal tract, and expanded to a diameter of 8 to 12 mm. Fig 56–16 is a diagram of a TIPS.

TIPS has been used mainly for elective treatment, and, to a lesser extent, emergency treatment of bleeding esophagogastric varices. In patients with variceal hemorrhage who also happened to have ascites, TIPS has provided relief of the ascites in short-term observations.[175,176] Data on the efficacy of TIPS in controlling intractable ascites is lacking. Anecdotal reports involving a small number of patients have been published in abstact form, describing some short-term success, some hepatic insufficiency, and some deaths.[177–183] In our institution, seven patients have undergone TIPS for cirrhotic ascites and four have developed occlusion of the shunt with recurrent ascites after short-term improvement.

There are two major potential problems with TIPS, shunt occlusion and portal-systemic encephalopathy.[174–176,183,184] The incidence of stenosis and occlusion of the shunt in relatively short-term follow-up has ranged from 33% to >50%. Although it has been possible to re-open many shunts by balloon dilation and to insert a second TIPS, the likelihood of long-term patency of a foreign body stent that is holding open a parenchymal tract in the venous system does not appear high. A major cause of stenosis and occlusion appears to be pseudointimal hypertrophy or hyperplasia that develops as the parenchymal tract heals.

There has been a high incidence of portal-systemic encephalopathy following TIPS. In our institution, the incidence has exceeded 50%. It has been suggested that the high incidence is owing to the lack of an organized program of follow-up treatment of the underlying liver disease in most reported series of TIPS.

Unfortunately, there have been no long-term prospective clinical trials of the use of TIPS in the treatment of portal hypertension. It is clear that the efficacy of TIPS can only be determined by such trials.

ORTHOTOPIC LIVER TRANSPLANTATION

In recent years, orthotopic liver transplantation (OLT) has been used with increasing frequency for the treatment of alcoholic cirrhosis in selected patients. One year survival rates after OLT in alcoholic cirrhotic patients have been 66% to 90%, which are comparable to those obtained in adult patients undergoing OLT for other hepatic disease.[185–190] In short-term follow-up, <20% of the transplanted patients have resumed alcohol consumption. On the basis of these promising results, it has been suggested that OLT be used regularly for patients in Child-Pugh class C who have developed complications, in the absence of any contraindications.[191] Data in support of this suggestion are lacking.

There has been no reported experience with the use of OLT specifically for treatment of intractable cirrhotic ascites. However, OLT must be considered a therapeutic option when other forms of therapy have failed and the patient meets the eligibility criteria for transplantation.

REFERENCES

1. Runyon BA. Care of patients with ascites. *N Engl J Med* 1994;330:337–342
2. Ginès P, Quintero E, Arroyo V, et al. Compensated cirrhosis: natural history and prognostic factors. *Hepatology* 1987;7:122–128
3. D'Amico G, Morabito A, Pagliaro L, et al. Survival and prognostic indicators in compensated and decompensated cirrhosis. *Dig Dis Sci* 1986;31:468–475
4. Madden JL, Lore JM Jr, Gerold FP, et al. The pathogenesis of ascites and a consideration of its treatment. *Surg Gynecol Obstet* 1954;99:385–391
5. Walker RM. The pathology and treatment of portal hypertension. *Lancet* 1952;ii:729–733
6. Gray HL. Clinical and experimental investigation of the circulation of the liver. *Ann R Coll Surg* 1951;8:354–365
7. Theron P, Allan JC. Ascites. A clinical and experimental study. *Acta Med Scand* 1955;152:145–154

8. Welch CS, Welch HJ, Carter JH. The treatment of ascites by side-to-side portacaval shunt. *Ann Surg* 1959;150:428–444

9. Britton RC, Shirey EK. Cineportography and dynamics of portal flow following shunt procedures. *Arch Surg* 1962;84:25–33

10. Britton RC, Brown CH, Shirey EK. Intrahepatic veno-occlusive disease in cirrhosis with chronic ascites: diagnosis by hepatic phlebography and results of surgical treatment. *Ann Surg* 1963;158:370–382

11. Starling EH. The influence of mechanical factors on lymph production. *J Physiol* 1894;16:224–267

12. Orloff MJ, Goodhead B, Windsor CWO, et al. Effect of portacaval shunts on lymph flow in the thoracic duct: experiments in normal dogs and dogs with cirrhosis and ascites. *Am J Surg* 1967;114:213–221

13. DeBenedetti MJ, Wright PW, Orloff MJ. Dynamics of hepatic lymph and blood flow in experimental liver disease and ascites. *Surg Forum* 1964;15:110–111

14. Bolton C, Barnard WG. The pathological occurrence of the liver in experimental venous stagnation. *J Pathol Bacteriol* 1931;34:701–709

15. Adams JT, Schwartz SI. Dynamics of blood, lymph, and ascitic fluid interchange. *Surg Forum* 1964;15:110–111

16. Brauer RW, Holloway RJ, Leong GF. Changes in liver function and structure due to experimental passive congestion under controlled hepatic vein pressures. *Am J Physiol* 1959;197:681–692

17. Morris B. The exchange of protein between the plasma and the liver and intestinal lymph. *Q J Exp Physiol* 1956;41:326–340

18. Van der Heyde MN, O'Keefe D, Welch CS. Thoracic duct lymph flow with variations in hepatic hemodynamics. *Surgery* 1964;56:1121–1128

19. Cain JC, Grindlay, JH, Bollman JL, et al. Lymph from liver and thoracic duct: An experimental study. *Surg Gynecol Obstet* 1947;85:559–562

20. Nix JT, Flock EV, Bollman JL. Influence of cirrhosis on the proteins of cisternal lymph. *Am J Physiol* 1951;164:117–118

21. Nix JT, Mann FC, Bollman JL, et al. Alterations of protein constituents of lymph by specific injury to the liver. *Am J Physiol* 1951;164:119–122

22. Dumont AE, Mulholland JH. Alterations in thoracic duct lymph flow in hepatic cirrhosis. *Ann Surg* 1962;156:668–677

23. Leger L, Premont M, Devissaguet P. Le drainage du canal thoracique dans les cirrhoses ascitiques. Etude du debit lymphatique. *Presse Med* 1962;70:1643–1646

24. Baggenstoss AH, Cain JC. The hepatic hilar lymphatics in man. Their relation to ascites. *N Engl J Med* 1957;256:531–535

25. Schwartz SI, Adesola AO. Influence of vasoactive agents on ascites. *Surgery* 1965;58:215–224

26. Zeppa R, Womack NA. Humoral control of hepatic lymph flow. *Surgery* 1963;54:37–44

27. Hyatt RE, Lawrence GH, Smith JR. Observations on the origin of ascites from experimental hepatic congestion. *J Lab Clin Med* 1955;45:274–280

28. Courtice FC: Ascites. The role of the lymphatics in the accumulation of ascitic fluid. *Med J Aust* 1959;2:945–951

29. Orloff MJ. Pathogenesis and surgical treatment of intractable ascites associated with alcoholic cirrhosis. *Ann NY Acad Sci* 1966;3:213–236

30. Barrowman JA, Granger DN. Effects of experimental cirrhosis on splanchnic microvascular fluid and solute exchange in the rat. *Gastroenterology* 1984;87:165–172

31. Lieberman FL, Denison EK, Reynolds TB. The relationship of plasma volume, portal hypertension, ascites, and renal sodium retention in cirrhosis: the overflow theory of ascites formation. *Ann NY Acad Sci* 1970;70:202–206

32. Keller U, Gerber PPG, Buhler FR, et al. Role of the splanchnic bed in extracting circulating adrenaline and noradrenaline in normal subjects and in patients with cirrhosis of the liver. *Clin Sci* 1984;67:45–49

33. Arroyo V, Planas R, Gaya J, et al. Symphatetic nervous activity, renin-angiotensin system, and renal excretion of prostaglandin E_2 in cirrhosis: relationship to functional renal failure and sodium and water excretion. *Eur J Clin Invest* 1983;13:271–278

34. DiBona GF, Swain LL. Renal nerves in renal adaptation to dietary sodium restriction. *Am J Physiol* 1983;245:F322–F328

35. Azer M, Gannon R, Kaloyanides GJ. Effect of renal denervation on the antinatriuresis of caval constriction. *Am J Physiol* 1972;222:611–616

36. Echtenkamp SF, Davis JO, DeForrest JM, et al. Effects of indomethacin, renal denervation, and propranolol on plasma renin activity in conscious dogs with chronic thoracic caval constriction. *Circ Res* 1981;49:492–500

37. Sweet WD, Freeman RH, Davis JO, et al. Ganglionic blockade in conscious dogs with chronic caval constriction. *Am J Physiol* 1985;249:H1038–H1044

38. Levy M, Wexler MJ. Sodium excretion in dogs with low-grade caval constriction: role of hepatic nerves. *Am J Physiol* 1987;253:F672–F678

39. Levy M. Sodium retention and ascites formation in dogs with experimental portal cirrhosis. *Am J Physiol* 1977;233:F572–F585

40. Levy M, Wexler MJ. Renal sodium retention and ascites formation in dogs with experimental cirrhosis but without portal hypertension or increased splanchnic vascular capacity. *J Lab Clin Med* 1978;91:520–536

41. Unikowsky R, Wexler MJ, Levy M. Dogs with experimental cirrhosis of the liver but without intrahepatic hypertension do not retain sodium or form ascites. *J Clin Invest* 1983;72:1594–1604

42. Shear LS, Ching S, Gabuzda GJ. Compartmentalization of ascites and edema in patients with hepatic cirrhosis. *N Engl J Med* 1970;282:1391–1395

43. Pockros P, Reynolds TB. Rapid diuresis in patients with ascites from chronic liver disease: the importance of peripheral edema. *Gastroenterology* 1986;90:1827–1833

44. Zink J, Greenway CV. Control of ascites absorption in anesthetized cats: effects of intraperitoneal pressure, protein, and furosemide diuresis. *Gastroenterology* 1977;73:1119–1124

45. Zink J, Greenway CV. Intraperitoneal pressure in forma-

tion and reabsorption of ascites in cats. *Am J Physiol* 1977;233:H185–H190

46. Buhac I, Flesh L, Kishore R. Intraabdominal pressure and resorption of ascites in decompensated liver cirrhosis. *J Lab Clin Med* 1984;104:264–270

47. Buhac I, Jarmolych J. Histology of the intestinal peritoneum in patients with cirrhosis of the liver and ascites. *Dig Dis Sci* 1978;23:417–422

48. Schaffner F, Popper H. Capillarization of hepatic sinusoids in man. *Gastroenterology* 1963;44:239–242

49. Axelrad BJ, Cates JE, Johnson BB, et al. Aldosterone in urine of normal man and of patients with oedema: its increased recovery after hydrolysis with acid and B-glucuronidase. *BMJ* 1955;1:196–199

50. Wolff HP, Koczorek KhR, Buchborn E. Aldosterone and antidiuretic hormone (Adiuretin) in liver disease. *Acta Endocrinol* 1958;27:45–58

51. Wolff HP, Bette L, Blaise H, et al. Role of aldosterone in edema formation. *Ann NY Acad Sci* 1966;139:285–294

52. Chart JJ, Shipley ES. The mechanism of sodium retention in cirrhosis of the liver. *Clin Invest* 1953;32:560 (Abstract)

53. Luetscher JA, Johnson BB. Observations on the sodium retaining corticoid (aldosterone) in the urine of children and adults in relation to sodium balance and edema. *Clin Invest* 1954;33:1441–1446

54. Bernardi M, Trevisian Santini C, DePalma R, et al. Aldosterone related blood volume expansion in cirrhosis before and during the early phase of ascites formation. *Gut* 1983;24:761–766

55. Epstein FH: Underfilling versus overflow in hepatic ascites. *N Engl J Med* 1982;307:1577–1578

56. Orloff MJ, Ross TH, Baddeley RM, et al. Experimental ascites VI: the effects of hepatic venous outflow obstruction and ascites on aldosterone secretion. *Surgery* 1964;56:83–98

57. Orloff MJ, Baddeley RM, Ross TH, et al. Regulations of aldosterone secretion by a humoral mediator. *Surg Forum* 1964;15:74–76

58. Orloff MJ, Lipman CA, Noel SM, et al. Hepatic regulation of aldosterone secretion by a humoral mediator. *Surgery* 1965;58:225–247

59. Bichet D, Szatalowicz V, Chaimovitz C, et al. Role of vasopressin in abnormal water excretion in cirrhotic patients. *Ann Intern Med* 1982;96:413–417

60. Epstein M. Renal effects of head out water immersion in man: implications for an understanding of volume homeostasis. *Physiol Rev* 1978;58:529–581

61. Ginès P, Jiménez W, Arroyo V, et al. Atrial natriuretic factor in cirrhosis with ascites: plasma levels, cardiac release, and splanchnic extraction. *Hepatology* 1988;8:636–642

62. Salerno F, Badalamenti S, Incerti P. Renal response to atrial natriuretic peptide in patients with advanced liver cirrhosis. *Hepatology* 1988;8:21–26

63. Morgan TR, Imada T, Hollister S, et al. Plasma human atrial natriuretic factor in cirrhosis and ascites with and without functional renal failure. *Gastroenterology* 1988;95:1641–1647

64. Levy M: Pathophysiology of ascites formation. In: Esptein

M (ed), *The Kidney in Liver Disease*. 3rd ed. Baltimore, MD: William & Wilkins; 1988:209–237

65. Levy M. Sodium retention and ascites formation in dogs with expermental portal cirrhosis. *Am J Physiol* 1977;233:572–585

66. Schrier RW, Arroya V, Bernardi M, et al. Peripheral arterial vasodilatation hypothesis: a proposal for the initiation of renal sodium and water retention in cirrhosis. *Hepatology* 1988;8:1151–1157

67. Runyon BA, Hoefs JC, Morgan TR. Ascitic fluid analysis in malignancy-related ascites. *Hepatology* 1988;8:1104–1109

68. Cattau EL Jr., Benjamin SB, Knuff TE. The accuracy of the physical exam in the diagnosis of suspected ascites. *JAMA* 1982;247:1164–1166

69. Runyon BA. Paracentesis of ascitic fluid: a safe procedure. *Arch Intern Med* 1986;146:2259–2261

70. McVay PA, Toy PT. Lack of increased bleeding after paracentesis and thoracentesis in patients with mild coagulation abnormalities. *Transfusion* 1991;31:164–171

71. Pinzello G, Simonetti RG, Craxi A, et al. Spontaneous bacterial peritonitis: a prospective investigation in predominantly nonalcoholic cirrhotic patients. *Hepatology* 1983;3:545–549

72. Runyon BA, Antillon MR, Akriviadis EA, et al. Bedside inoculation of blood culture bottles with ascitic fluid is superior to delayed inoculation in the detection of spontaneous bacterial peritonitis. *J Clin Microbiol* 1990;28Z:2811–2812

73. Runyon BA, Canawati HN, Akriviadis EA. Optimization of ascitic fluid culture technique. *Gastroenterology* 1988;95:1351–1355

74. Hoefs JC. Serum protein concentration and portal pressure determine the ascitic fluid protein concentration in patients with chronic liver disease. *J Lab Clin Med* 1983;102:260–273

75. Runyon BA, Montano AA, Akriviadis EA, et al. The serum-ascites albumin gradient is superior to the exudate-transudate concept in the differential diagnosis of ascites. *Ann Intern Med* 1992;117:215–220

76. Akriviadis EA, Runyon BA. Utility of an algorithm in differentiating spontaneous from secondary bacterial peritonitis. *Gastroenterology* 1990;98:127–133

77. Runyon BA. Amylase levels in ascitic fluid. *J Clin Gastroenterol* 1987;9:172–174

78. Runyon BA, Hoefs JC, Morgan TR. Ascitic fluid analysis in malignancy-related ascites. *Hepatology* 1988;8:1104–1909

79. Pinzello G, Simonetti RG, Craxì A, et al. Spontaneous bacterial peritonitis: a prospective investigation in predominantly non-alcoholic cirrhotic patients. *Hepatology* 1983;3:545–549

80. Runyon BA. Low-protein-concentration ascitic fluid is predisposed to spontaneous bacterial peritonitis. *Gastroenterology* 1986;91:1343–1346

81. Hoefs JC, Canawati HN, Sapico FL, et al. Spontaneous bacterial peritonitis. *Hepatology* 1982;2:399–407

82. Gerding DN, Hall WH, Schierl EA. Antibiotic concentrations in ascitic fluid of patients with ascites and bacterial peritonitis. *Ann Intern Med* 1977;86:708–713

83. Ariza J, Gudiol F, Dolz C, et al. Evaluation of aztreonam in

the treatment of spontaneous bacterial peritonitis in patients with cirrhosis. *Hepatology* 1986;6:906–910

84. Felisart J, Rimola A, Arroyo V, et al. Cefotaxime is more effective than is ampicillin-tobramycin in cirrhotics with severe infections. *Hepatology* 1985;5:457–462

85. Titó L, Rimola A, Ginès P, et al. Recurrence of spontaneous bacterial peritonitis in cirrhosis: Frequency and predictive factors. *Hepatology* 1988;8:27–31

86. Reynolds TB. Therapeutic paracentesis: have we come full circle? *Gastroenterology* 1987;93:386–388

87. Titó L, Ginès P, Arroyo V, et al. Total paracentesis associated with intravenous albumin management of patients with cirrhosis and ascites. *Gastroenterology* 1990;98:146–151

88. Belghiti J, Rueff B, Fekete F. Umbilical hernia in cirrhotic patients with ascites. *Gastroenterology* 1983;84:1363 (Abstract)

89. Lemmer JH, Strodel WE, Knol JA. Management of spontaneous umbilical hernia disruption in the cirrhotic patient. *Ann Surg* 1983;198:30–34

90. Runyon BA, Juler GL. Natural history of umbilical hernia in patients with and without ascites. *Am J Gastroenterol* 1985;80:38–39

91. Lieberman FL, Hidemaura R, Peters RL, et al. Pathogenesis and treatment of hydrothorax complicating cirrhosis with ascites. *Ann Intern Med* 1965;64:341–351

92. Rubinstein D, McInnes IA, Dudley FJ. Hepatic hydrothorax in the abscence of clinical ascites: diagnosis and management. *Gastroenterology* 1985;88:188–191

93. Runyon BA, Greenblatt M, Ming RHC: Hepatic hydrothorax is a relative contraindication to chest tube insertion. *Am J Gastroenterol* 1986;81:566–567

94. DeSitter L, Rector WG. The significance of bloody ascites in patients with cirrhosis. *Am J Gastroenterol* 1984;79:136–138

95. Arieff AI: Hyponatremia associated with permanent brain damage. *Adv Intern Med* 1987;32:325–344

96. Henry ML, Laureno R, Illowsky BP, et al. Therapy of hyponatremia. *N Engl J Med* 1986;315:1351–1355

97. Ayus JC, Krothapalli RK, Arieff AI. Treatment of symtomatic hyponatremia and its relation to brain damage. *N Engl J Med* 1987;317:1190–1195

98. Linas SL, Anderson RJ, Miller PD, et al. The rational use of diuretics in cirrhosis. In: Esptein M (ed), *The Kidney in Liver Disease*, 2nd ed. New York, NY: Elsevier North-Holland; 1983:555–568

99. Sungaila I, Bartle WR, Walker SE, et al. Spironolactone pharmacokinetics and pharmacodynamics in patients with cirrhotic ascites. *Gastroenterology* 1992;102:1680–1685

100. Yamada S, Reynolds TB. Amiloride (MK-870), a new antikaluretic diuretic: comparison to other antikaluretic diuretics in patients with liver disease and ascites. *Gastroenterology* 1970;59:833–841

101. Fogal MR, Sawheny VK, Neal EA, et al. Diuresis in the ascitic patient: a randomized controlled trial of three regimens. *J Clin Gastroenterol* 1981;3(suppl 1):73–80

102. Perez-Ayuso RM, Arroyo V, Planas R, et al. Randomized comparative study of efficacy of furosemide versus spironolactone in nonazotemic cirrhosis with ascites: relationship between the diuretic response and the activity of the renin-aldosterone system. *Gastroenterology* 1983;84:961–968

103. Stanley MM, Ochi S, Lee KK, et al. Perotoneovenous shunting as compared with medical treatment in patients with alcoholic cirrhosis and massive ascites. *N Engl J Med* 1989;321:1632–1638

105. Gatta A, Angeli P, Caregaro L, et al. A pathophysiological interpretation of unresponsiveness to spironolactone in a stepped-care approach to the diuretic treatment of ascites in non-azotemic cirrhotic patients. *Hepatology* 1991;1:231–236

106. Reynolds TB. Renaissance of paracentesis in the treatment of ascites. *Adv Int Med* 1990;35:365–374

107. Ginès P, Arroyo V, Quintero E, et al. Comparison of paracentesis and diuretics in the treatment of cirrhotics with tense ascites: results of a randomized study. *Gastroenterology* 1987;93:234–241

108. Ascione A, Burroughs AK. Paracentesis for ascites in cirrhotic patients. *Gastroenterol Int* 1990;3:120–123

109. Titó L, Ginès P, Arroyo V, et al. Total paracentesis associated with intravenous albumin management of patients with cirrhosis and ascites. *Gastroenterology* 1990;98:146–151

110. Antillon MR, Runyon BA. Postparacentesis plasma expansion prevents asymptomatic laboratory abnormalities, but does it have any impact on morbidity or mortality? *Gastroenterology* 1991;101:1455–1457

111. Ginès P, Titó L, Arroyo V, et al. Randomized comparative study of therapeutic paracentesis with and without intravenous albumin in cirrhosis. *Gastroenterology* 1988;94:1439–1502

112. Kao HW, Rakov NE, Savage E, et al. The effect of large volume paracentesis on plasma volume—a cause of hypovolemia? *Hepatology* 1985;5:403–407

113. Pinto PC, Amerian J, Reynolds TB: Large-volume paracentesis in nonedematous patients with tense ascites: its effect on intravascular volume. *Hepatology* 1988;8:207–210

114. Planas R, Ginès P, Arroyo V, et al. Dextran-70 versus albumin as plasma expanders in cirrhotic patients with tense ascites treated with total paracentesis: results of a randomized study. *Gastroenterology* 1990;99:1736–1744

115. Ginès P, Arroyo V, Vargas V, et al. Paracentesis with intravenous infusion of albumin as compared with peritoneovenous shunting in cirrhosis with refractory ascites. *N Engl J Med* 1991;325:829–835

116. Parbhoo SP, Ajdukiewicz A, Sherlock S. Treatment of ascites by continuous ultrafiltration and reinfusion of protein concentrate. *Lancet* 1974;i:949–952

117. Wilkinson SP, Henderson J, Davidson AR, et al. Ascites reinfusion using the rhodiasit apparatus—clinical experience and coagulation abnormalities. *Postgrad Med J* 1975;51:583–587

118. Lai KN, Leung JWC, Vallance-Owen J. Dialytic ultrafiltration by hemofilter in treatment of patients with refractory ascites and renal insufficiency. *Am J Gastroenterol* 1987;82:665–668

119. Smart HL, Triger DR. A randomized prospective trial comparing daily paracentesis and intravenous albumin

with recirculation in diuretic refractory ascites. *J Hepatol* 1990;10:191–197

120. Bruno S, Borzio M, Romagnoni M, et al. Comparison of spontaneous ascites filtration and reinfusion with total paracentesis with intravenous albumin infusion in cirrhotic patients with tense ascites. *BMJ* 1992;304: 1655–1658

121. Cadranel JF, Gargot D, Grippon P, et al. Spontaneous dialytic ultrafiltration with intraperitoneal reinfusion of the concentrate versus large paracentesis in cirrhotic patients with intractable ascites: a randomized study. *Int J Artif Organs* 1992;15:432–435

122. Child CG III, McDonough EF, DesRochers GC. Reversal of hepatic venous circulation in dogs. *Ann Surg* 1959; 150:445–454

123. David C, Bollman JL, Grindlay JH, et al. An experimental study of the effectiveness of the portal vein as a hepatic outflow tract. *Surg Gynecol Obstet* 1963;117:67–70

124. Long RTL, Lombardo CR, Morrow AG. The demonstration and quantification of reverse flow in the proximal portal vein following side-to-side portacaval anastomosis. *Surgery* 1960;47:125–131

125. Murray JF, Mulder DG. The effects of retrograde portal venous flow following side-to-side portacaval anastomosis: a comparison with end-to-side shunts. *J Clin Invest* 1961;40:1413–1420

126. Herrick FC. An experimental study into the cause of the increased portal pressure in portal cirrhosis. *J Exper Med* 1907;9:93–104

127. Longmire WP Jr, Mulder DG, Mahoney PS, et al. Side-to-side portacaval anastomosis for portal hypertension. *Ann Surg* 1958;147:881–894

128. Mulder DG, Murray JF. An evaluation of the side-to-side portacaval shunt. *Surg Forum* 1960;11:278–279

129. Warren WD, Muller WH Jr. A clarification of some hemodynamic changes in cirrhosis and their surgical significance. *Ann Surg* 1959;150:413–427

130. Reynolds TB, Mikkelsen WP, Redeker AG, et al. The effect of a side-to-side portacaval shunt on hepatic hemodynamics in cirrhosis. *J Clin Invest* 1962;41:1242–1248

131. Gliedman ML, Sellers RD, Burkle JS, et al. Cirrhosis with ascites: hemodynamic observations. *Ann Surg* 1962;155: 147–152

132. Eckman CA. Portal hypertension. Diagnosis and surgical treatment. *Acta Chir Scand* 1957;113:328–329

133. Taylor WJ, Meyers JD. Occlusive hepatic venous catheterization in the study of the normal liver, cirrhosis of the liver, and noncirrhotic portal hypertension. *Circulation* 1956;13:368–380

134. Gliedman ML, Sellers RD, Grant RN, et al. Observations on the effect of portacaval anastomosis upon the hemodynamics of the liver. *Surg Gynecol Obstet* 1959;108: 223–229

135. Krook H. Circulatory studies in liver cirrhosis. *Acta Med Scand* 1956;156:1–160

136. Orloff MJ, Snyder GB. Experimental ascites. II. The effects of portacaval shunts on ascites produced with an internal vena cava cannula. *Surgery* 1961;50:220–230

137. Orloff MJ, Spitz BR, Wall MH, et al. Experimental ascites. IV. comparison of the effects of end-to-side and side-to-

side portacaval shunts on intractable ascites. *Surgery* 1964;56:784–799

138. Orloff MJ. Effect of side-to-side portacaval shunt on intractable ascites, sodium excretion, and aldosterone metabolism in man. *Am J Surg* 1966;112:287–298

139. Orloff MJ. Surgical treatment of intractable cirrhotic ascites. In: Longmire WP Jr (ed), *Portal Hypertension.* Chicago, IL: Year Book Medical; 1966:28–51

140. Campbell DP, Parker DE, Anagnostopoulos CE. Survival prediction in portacaval shunt: a computerized statistical analysis. *Am J Surg* 1973;126:748–751

141. Orloff MJ, Orloff MS, Rambotti M, et al. Is portal-systemic shunt worthwhile in Child's class C cirrhosis? Long-term results of emergency shunt in 94 patients with bleeding varices. *Ann Surg* 1993;216:256–268

142. Conn HO, Leevy CM, Vlahcevic ZR, et al. Comparison of lactulose and neomycin in the treatment of chronic portal-systemic encephalopathy. a double-blind controlled trial. *Gastroenterology* 1977;72:573–583

143. Conn HO, Lieberthal MM. *The Hepatic Coma Syndromes and Lactulose.* Baltimore, MD: Williams & Wilkins; 1978

144. Pappas SC, Jones EA. Methods for assessing hepatic encephalopathy. *Semin Liver Dis* 1983;3:298–307

145. Orloff MJ. Portal hypertension: Portacaval anastomosis. In: Dudley H, Pories W, Carter D (eds), *Rob and Smith's Operative Surgery, Alimentary Tract and Abdominal Wall,* 4th ed. Condon, England: Butterworth's; 1983: 546–569

146. Orloff MJ, Orloff MS. Bleeding oesophageal and gastric varices: shunts. In: Jamieson GG, Debas HT (eds), *Rob and Smith's Operative Surgery.* 5th ed. London, England: Chapman & Hall; 1994:493–515

147. LeVeen HH, Christoudias G, Ip M, et al. Peritoneovenous shunting for ascites. *Ann Surg* 1974;180:580–591

148. Epstein M. Role of peritoneovenous shunt in the management of ascites and hepatorenal syndrome. In: Epstein M (ed), *The Kidney in Liver Disease,* 2nd ed. New York, NY: Elsevier Biomedical; 1983:583–600

149. Moscovitz M. The peritoneovenous shunt: expectations and reality. *Am J Gastroenterol* 1990;85:917–929

150. Fulenwider JT, Galambos JD, Smith RB III, et al. Denver peritoneovenous shunts for intractable ascites of cirrhosis. *Arch Surg* 1986;121:351–355

151. Epstein M. Peritoneovenous shunt in the management of ascites and the hepatorenal syndrome. *Gastroenterology* 1982;82:790–799

152. Schroeder ET, Anderson GH. Effects of the peritoneovenous shunt on the renin-angiotensin system and renal function in cirrhosis. In: Epstein M (ed), *The Kidney in Liver Disease,* New York, NY: Elsevier Biomedical: 1983: 569–582

153. Blendis LM, Greig PD, Langer B, et al. Renal and hemodynamic effect of the peritoneovenous shunt for intractable hepatic ascites. *Gastroenterology* 1979;77: 250–257

154. Blendis LM, Sole MJ, Campbell P, et al. The effect of peritoneovenous shunting on catecholamine metabolism in patients with hepatic ascites. *Hepatology* 1987;7: 143–148

155. Greig PD, Blendis LM, Langer B, et al. Renal and hemo-

dynamic effect of the peritoneovenous shunt. II. long-term effects. *Gastroenterology* 1981;80:119–125

156. Norfray JF, Henry HM, Givens JD, et al. Abdominal complications from peritoneal shunts. *Gastroenterology* 1979; 77:337–340

157. Schwartz ML, Swaim WR, Vogel SB. Coagulopathy following peritoneovenous shunting. *Surgery* 1979;85:671–676

158. Harmon DC, Demirjian Z, Ellman L, et al. Disseminated intravascular coagulation with the peritoneovenous shunt. *Ann Intern Med* 1979;90:774–776

159. Tawes RL Jr, Sydorak GR, Kennedy PA, et al. Coagulopathy associated with peritoneovenous shunting. *Am J Surg* 1981;142:51–55

160. Ragni MW, Lewis JH, Spero JA. Ascites-induced LeVeen shunt coagulopathy. *Ann Surg* 1983;198:91–95

161. Fulenwider JT, Smith RB III, Redd SC, et al. Peritoneovenous shunts: lessons learned from an eight-year experience with 70 patients. *Arch Surg* 1984;119:1133–1137

162. Foley WJ, Elliott JP Jr., Smith RF, et al. Central venous thrombosis and embolism associated with peritoneovenous shunts. *Arch Surg* 1984;119:713–720

163. Greig PD, Langer B, Blendis LM, et al. Complications after peritoneovenous shunting for ascites. *Am J Surg* 1980;139:125–131

164. Wormser GP, Hubbard RC. Peritonitis in cirrhotic patients with LeVeen shunts. *Am J Med* 1981;71:358–362

165. LeVeen HH, Wapnick S, Grosberg S, et al. Further experience with peritoneovenous shunts for ascites. *Ann Surg* 1976;184:574–581

166. Lossing A, Greig PD, Blendis L, et al. The LeVeen shunt: a nine-year experience. *Hepatology* 1984;4:1092 (Abstract)

167. Linas SL, Schaefer JW, Moore EE, et al. Peritoneovenous shunt in the management of hepatorenal syndrome. *Kidney Intr* 1986;30:736–740

168. LeVeen HH, Piccone VA, Hutto RB. Management of ascites with hydrothorax. *Am J Surg* 1984;148:210–213

169. Greenlee HB, Stanley MM, Reinhardt GF. Intractable ascites treated with peritoneovenous shunts (LeVeen). *Arch Surg* 1981;116:518–524

170. Bernhoft RA, Pellegrini CA, Way LW. Peritoneovenous shunt for refractory ascites. *Arch Surg* 1982;117:631–635

171. LeVeen HH, Vujic I, d'Ovidio NG, et al. Peritoneovenous shunt occlusion. *Ann Surg* 1984;200:212–223

172. Bories P, Garcia-Compean D, et al. The treatment of refractory ascites by the LeVeen shunt: a multi-centre controlled trial (57 patients). *J Hepatol* 1986;3:212–218

173. Greenlee HB, Stanley MM. Peritoneovenous shunt for ascites. In: Schwartz SI (ed), *Abdominal Surgery. Installment IV. Modern Technics in Surgery* vol. 16 Mount Kisco NY: Futura; 1982:9–14

174. Conn HO. Transjugular intrahepatic portal-systemic shunts: the state of the art. *Hepatology* 1993;17:148–158

175. Rossle M, Haag K, Ochs A, et al. The transjugular intrahepatic portosystemic stent-shunt procedure for variceal bleeding. *N Engl J Med* 1994;330:165–171

176. LaBerge JM, Ring EJ, Gordon RL, et al. Creation of transjugular intrahepatic portosystemic shunts with the Wall-

stent endoprosthesis: results in 100 patients. *Radiology* 1993;187:413–420

177. Grange JD, Boudghene F, Dussaule JC, et al. Transjugular intrahepatic portosystemic shunts (TIPS) in cirrhotic patients with refractory ascites: clinical efficacy and acute effects on aldosterone and atrial natriuretic factor. *Gastroenterology* 1993;104:A909 (Abstract)

178. Garcia-Villarreal L, Zozaya JM, Quiroga J, et al. Transjugular intrahepatic portosystemic shunt (TIPS) for intractable ascites—preliminary results. *J Hepatology* 1992; 16(suppl):S36 (Abstract)

179. Ochs A, Sellinger M, Haag K, et al. Transjugular intrahepatic portosystemic stent-shunt (TIPS) for treatment of refractory ascites and hepato-renal syndrome: results of a pilot study. *Gastroenterology* 1992;102:A863 (Abstract)

180. Sanyal AJ, Freedman AM, Luketic VA, et al. Transjugular intrahepatic portosystemic shunt (TIPS) and pathophysiology of portal hypertension (PH): endoscopic, radiologic and biochemical correlations. *Am J Gastroenterol* 1992;87:1305 (Abstract)

181. Somberg KA, Lake JR, Tomlanovich SJ, et al. Transjugular intrahepatic portosystemic shunt for refractory ascites: assessment of clinical and humoral response and renal function. *Gastroenterology* 1993;104:A998 (Abstract)

182. Strauss RM, Martin LG, Kaufman SL, et al. Role of transjugular intrahepatic portosystemic shunt (TIPS) in the primary management of refractory cirrhotic hydrothorax. *Hepatology* 1992;16:85A (Abstract)

183. Lind CD, Malisch TW, Chong WK, et al: Incidence of shunt occlusion or stenosis with transjugular intrahepatic portosystemic shunts (TIPS). *Gastroenterology* 1993; 104(suppl):A941 (Abstract)

184. Freedman AM, Sanyal AJ, Tesnado J, et al. Complications of transjugular intrahepatic portosystemic shunt: a comprehensive review. *Radiographics* 1993;13:1185–1210

185. Starzl TE, Van Thiel DH, Tzakis A, et al. Orthotopic liver transplantation for alcoholic cirrhosis. *JAMA* 1988; 260:2542–2544

186. Kumar S, Stauber RE, Gavaler JS, et al. Orthotopic liver transplantation for alcoholic liver disease. *Hepatology* 1990;11:159–164

187. Lucy MR. Liver transplantation for the alcoholic patient. *Gastroenterol Clin North Am* 1993;22:243–256

188. Bird GLA, O'Grady JG, Harvey FA, et al. Liver transplantation in patients with alcoholic cirrhosis: Selection criteria and rates of survival and relapse. *BMJ* 1990; 301:15–17

189. Lucy MR, Merion RM, Henley KS, et al. Selection for and outcome of liver transplantation in alcoholic liver disease. *Gastroenterology* 1992;102:1736–1741

190. Bonet H, Maney R, Kramer D, et al. Liver transplantation for alcoholic liver disease: survival of patients transplanted with alcoholic hepatitis plus cirrhosis as compared with those with cirrhosis alone. *Alcohol Clin Exp Res* 1993;17:1102–1106

191. Bismuth H, Adam R, Mathur S, et al. Options for elective treatment of portal hypertension in cirrhotic patients in the transplantation era. *Am J Surg* 1990;160:105–110

57

Portal Hypertension

J. Michael Henderson

Normal portal pressure is 7 to 8 mm Hg. Portal hypertension is present when portal venous pressure exceeds 10 mm Hg. In clinical practice, portal pressure usually is measured indirectly as the hepatic venous pressure gradient (HVPG), which is the wedged hepatic minus free hepatic vein pressure. The presence of esophageal varices at endoscopy or the finding of varices on abdominal imaging studies indicate portal hypertension.

■ HISTORY

Portal hypertension usually presents with one or more of the following symptoms: hepatosplenomegaly, variceal bleeding, ascites, or portal systemic encephalopathy. Whatever the signs and symptoms at presentation, the suspicion of portal hypertension demands full investigation. In the United States, the etiology is most commonly cirrhosis, but other etiologies, such as a prehaptic portal or splenic vein thrombosis, or other intraparenchymal liver diseases, such as schistosomiasis or granulomatous liver disease, should be excluded. Identification and full definition of these other causes is important since long-term prognosis is more dependent on the underlying disease than on the presenting complication. A full evaluation should not only characterize the presenting symptom, be it variceal bleeding, ascites, or encephalopathy, but also must characterize thoroughly the underlying disease. Knowledge of the cause of portal hypertension, of the ongoing activity of any liver disease, and of the likely natural history of the underlying disease are the most important determinants of outcome.

The medical literature is replete with writings about portal hypertension. Recognized by the Greeks and highlighted by Shakespeare, no therapy was available to treat portal hypertension until the last century. Eck demonstrated the practicality of decompressing portal hypertension in 1880, and since that time controversies have raged over when and how this should be done. The benefits of decompressing portal hypertension, balanced against the risk of liver failure caused by diverting portal flow, are the major factors that contribute to this management controversy. In the past 20 years a better understanding of the pathophysiology of portal hypertension, combined with more sophisticated evaluation of liver diseases and improved methods for their management, have led to broader therapy options. We now know that portal hypertension can be reduced pharmacologically, that esophageal varices often can be obliterated endoscopically, that most ascites can be controlled with diuretics, that selective decompression of gastroesophageal varices can be achieved while maintaining portal flow to the cirrhotic liver and finally, that the diseased cirrhotic liver can be removed and replaced by a normal liver with transplantation. The challenge in the 1990s is to develop optimal treatment strategies utilizing all of the above therapeutic approaches, and selecting the right patient for the right therapy.

Liver transplantation has changed the face of hepatology in the last decade, in that there is now a viable treatment for end-stage liver disease. Transplantation has changed how patients with liver disease and portal hypertension are evaluated. The question always should be asked of the patient who presents with one of the complications of portal hypertension: are they now or in the future a candidate for transplant? The answer to this question may alter the whole treatment strategy. However, not every patient who presents with one of the complications of portal hypertension does have end-stage liver disease, or is a candidate for liver transplant. In such patients, it is important to fully evaluate their disease and develop an appropriate treatment strategy for both their presenting symptoms and for their overall management.

■ PATHOPHYSIOLOGY

High portal venous pressure is only one of the hemodynamic changes in these patients. Increased resistance to portal flow, splanchnic hyperemia, and portal systemic shunting also are found in the portal circulation. In addition, systemic hemodynamic changes accompany portal hypertension with increased cardiac output, low total systemic vascular resistance, and relative systemic arterial hypotension. Finally, patients with portal hypertension have increased plasma volume.

Precise mechanisms have not been clarified, but experimental models have defined the sequence of changes.[1,2] Increased resistance to portal flow is the primary factor in raising portal pressure. Development of portal systemic collaterals then occurs, with plasma volume expansion preceding the development of the hyperdynamic systemic circulation. Splanchnic vasodilation, in part owing to local vasodilatory humoral responses and in part, to the hyperdynamic systemic circulation, contributes to maintenance and exacerbation of portal hypertension.

■ RISKS OF VARICEAL BLEEDING AND TIME POINTS OF THERAPY

- 30% of patients with cirrhosis develop portal hypertension.
- 30% of patients with cirrhosis will bleed from their varices in the 2 years following the finding of varices.
- 70% of patients who have bled from varices will rebleed within 18 to 24 months.
- Mortality of acute variceal bleeding is between 20% and 50%.
- Prophylactic therapy for variceal bleeding refers to treatment initiated before the first bleed.

- Therapy for acute variceal bleeding is management, given at the time of the acute bleeding episode.
- Therapeutic management for variceal bleeding is prevention of rebleeding after stabilization from the acute bleed.

■ MANAGEMENT ALGORITHM

Fig 57–1 outlines a management algorithm for variceal bleeding, and will form the basis for further discussion. Alternatives do exist at some of the steps indicated and will be presented within the text in subsequent sections. Centers managing patients with variceal bleeding should develop an algorithm such as this, with defined management methods for prophylaxis, management of acute variceal bleeding, and management methods to prevent recurrent bleeding.

■ EVALUATION OF PATIENTS WITH PORTAL HYPERTENSION

Evaluation must define the extent, size, and risk factors of the varices; the degree of portal hypertension and the portal venous anatomy; the underlying cause of the portal hypertension; and the etiology, activity, and prognosis of underlying liver disease.

UPPER GASTROINTESTINAL ENDOSCOPY

Upper gastrointestinal endoscopy is used to assess varices. Risk factors for bleeding have been defined by Beppu, Paquet, and the North Italian Endoscopic Club.[3–5] Size of varices, the overall extent, tortuosity, and the red color signs are risk factors defined as the major endoscopic predictors of bleeding. An elective endoscopy in a hemodynamically stable patient with an adequate central blood volume should be part of the assessment. This endoscopy should classify varices for the above factors, but also should assess the gastric mucosa for evidence of portal hypertensive gastropathy, and exclude other upper gastrointestinal bleeding pathology. Inspection of the lesser curve, antrum, pylorus, and duodenum should exclude peptic ulcer disease. Inspection of the body and fundus should look for cobblestoning and congestion of portal hypertensive gastropathy. Gastric varices may appear either as the continuation of esophageal varices across the gastroesophageal junction, or as individual gastric fundal varices that look like a bunch of grapes. Video endoscopy has improved the accuracy with which varies can be evaluated and allows review by the whole managing team.

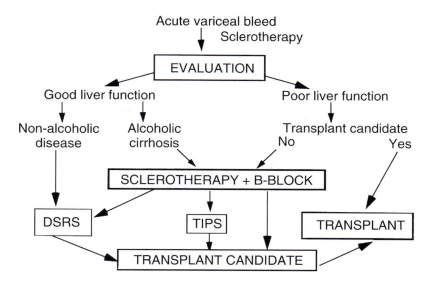

Figure 57–1. Algorithm for the management of variceal bleeding.

ANGIOGRAPHY

This technique remains the gold standard for assessment of portal venous anatomy and measurement of portal venous pressure.[6] Other imaging modalities such as ultrasound combined with Doppler, computed tomography scan (CT) or magnetic resonance imaging (MRI) may play a role in screening of patients with portal hypertension. The components of arteriography that fully assess a patient with portal hypertension and, therefore, should be included are HVPG, superior mesenteric and splenic artery injections followed through their venous phase, and assessment of left renal vein and vena caval anatomy. In some patients, more invasive studies such as splenoportography or transhepatic portography may be indicated.

HVPG is measured from the wedged or occluded hepatic venous pressure minus the free hepatic venous pressure.[7] This measurement is done in one of the major hepatic veins with a balloon catheter inserted from a peripheral vein though the vena cava. Normal hepatic venous pressure gradient will be 6 to 8 mm Hg. In most patients with cirrhosis and portal hypertension, a level >12mm Hg is indicative of portal hypertension. Selective superior mesenteric arterial injection, when followed through to the venous phase, allows visualization of the superior mesenteric vein, the portal vein, and any significant collateral filling of the coronary vein or retrograde filling of the inferior mesenteric vein. In addition to demonstrating the patency of these major veins, it also provides some semiquantitative information as to portal venous flow patterns and quantity. Selective splenic arterial injec-

tion allows visualization of the splenic vein and collaterals arising from it on venous phase injection. Splenoportography is reserved for those patients in whom venous phase arterial studies do not adequately demonstrate the venous anatomy.

Catheterization and injection of the left renal vein shows the anatomy of this vein and the inferior vena cava. Up to 20% of the population have some anomaly of the left renal vein, which is usually not a contraindication to distal splenorenal shunt (DSRS). However, such anomalies should be defined preoperatively.

Doppler ultrasound is a useful screening method for demonstrating the portal vein and directional flow. Depending on body habitus and bowel gas pattern, it may also be possible to demonstrate the splenic and superior mesenteric veins and their flows. However, this technology does not allow demonstration of the major collateral pathways or pressure assessment. As such, it is probably inadequate if surgical intervention is being considered, but may be sufficient for screening those patients in whom surgery is not being considered.

ETIOLOGY

The etiology of portal hypertension must be defined. The many etiologies are shown in Fig 57–2. While most patients in the United States and Europe have cirrhosis as the underlying cause, it is important to look for those other causes that have a better prognosis. Presinusoidal causes of portal hypertension usually are associated with normal hepatocellular function, so that if bleeding is

Causes and Site of Block for Portal Hypertension

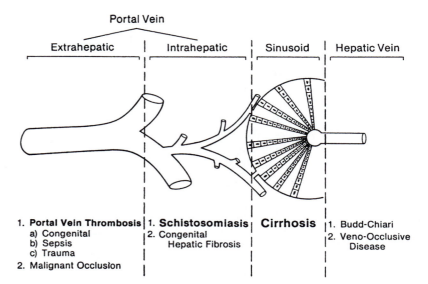

Figure 57–2. Sites for obstruction in portal hypertension. In the United States and Europe, most patients have a sinusoidal block secondary to cirrhosis. Other causes must be considered.

adequately controlled, survival is excellent. Portal vein thrombosis requires angiography for diagnosis, and the patient also should have a liver biopsy to document a normal liver. When this is the case, there is usually excellent portal perfusion through collaterals to the normal pressure sinusoids, the so-called cavernous transformation. Similarly, schistosomiasis, when occurring without associated hepatitis, usually is associated with normal liver function and carries an excellent prognosis, if bleeding is controlled. When the etiology is cirrhosis, the focus of evaluation is on the liver disease, since this is the most important determinant of outcome.

LIVER EVALUATION

Evaluation of the liver is based on clinical findings and laboratory studies.[8,9] Jaundice, ascites, encephalopathy, and malnutrition clearly define a patient with end-stage liver disease. However, many patients who present with variceal bleeding do not show these obvious clinical symptoms, and the status of their liver has to be defined by other means. Standard laboratory tests help to assess liver disease in different ways. Serum bilirubin, albumin, and prothrombin time give an overall picture of severity and some indication of synthetic function. Disease activity can be partially assessed from aminotransferases, gamma glutamyl-transpeptidase, and alkaline phosphatase. Etiology may be defined by serology specific for viral hepatitis or other liver disease markers, such as antimitochon-

drial antibody, α_1 antitrypsin, or ceruloplasmin. These markers should be measured in any patient with cirrhosis. Alpha-fetoprotein should be measured as a screening test for hepatoma. Quantitative liver function testing with studies such as indocyaine green clearance, galactose elimination capacity, and MEG-X formation are advocated by some.

Liver morphology is also important in evaluation. An ultrasound should be performed to make certain there are no focal lesions. If there are suspicions of hepatoma, by ultrasound or an elevated alpha-fetoprotein, a contrast-enhanced CT scan should be performed. Further assessment of morphology may require a liver biopsy either to assess the overall activity and status of cirrhosis or, in the case of focal lesions, a specific biopsy of that abnormal area.

TIMING

Timing of evaluation is important. Once a patient has been stabilized from their acute variceal bleeding, they then should have full evaluation during the next few days. The etiology of portal hypertension must be defined accurately, and for patients with cirrhosis, a decision made whether they have good or poor liver function (see algorithm, Fig 57–1). An assessment of the expected natural history of the liver disease should be made, if possible. However, a commitment to follow the patient and re-evaluate their liver status over the next few months may be required.

■ THERAPIES

PHARMACOTHERAPY

In the patient with acute variceal bleeding, portal hypertension can be reduced by intravenous infusion of vasopressin or somatostatin. These two drugs can lessen severity of bleeding, often stop the bleeding, but have not been shown to alter survival. Vasopressin acts by splanchnic vasoconstriction, but has the side effect of significant systemic vasoconstriction. The normal dose is an infusion of 0.1 to 0.4 U/min, which should have a concomitant infusion of nitroglycerin titrated to maintain a systolic blood pressure of 100 mm Hg. The starting dose of nitroglycerin is 40 μg/min and needs to be titrated to the above blood pressure. More recently, somatostatin, or its long-acting analog, Octreotide, have been shown to be equally efficacious to Pitressin.[10] In controlled studies, Octreotide infused at 50 μg/hr has been shown to control acute variceal bleeding as effectively as sclerotherapy.[11]

Pharmacologic therapy for long-term reduction of portal hypertension has received considerable attention in the last decade.[12] Noncardioselective beta blockade with Inderal or Nadolol has been widely applied with many randomized controlled trials evaluating efficacy. Initially studied for prevention of rebleeding, it was shown that hepatic venous pressure gradient (HVPG) and rebleeding are significantly reduced. However, improvement in long-term survival has had variable outcomes, in randomized studies.

Overall, these studies show a rebleeding rate between 30% and 40% at 2 yr follow-up.[13] In some patients, beta blockade may be appropriate therapy; however, the high risk of rebleeding must be kept in mind. Many other pharmacologic agents have been looked at for reduction of portal hypertension. Long-acting nitrates, serotonin antagonists, α_2 agonists, and calcium channel blockers all have been studied.[12] At the present time, there are no clear guidelines as to which combination therapy may prove most efficacious, and application has been limited by side effects. This remains an area of intensive clinical investigation.

Pharmacologic therapy for reducing portal hypertension has established a place in prophylaxis of the initial variceal bleed, and Inderal and Nadolol have been shown to significantly reduce the risk of the initial bleed in portal hypertension, with an overall significant improvement in survival.[14] Current recommendations are to use noncardioselective beta blockers once varices are identified.

ENDOSCOPIC SCLEROTHERAPY

Endoscopic sclerotherapy aims to either obliterate varices by intravariceal injection of a thrombotic sclerosing solution, or to create fibrosis in the mucosa overlying varices by paravariceal injection. Initially introduced in a limited way with the rigid esophagoscope, sclerotherapy now is performed through a fiberoptic flexible scope and is applied widely. Many agents have been used to produce sclerosis, but none has been shown clearly to be superior to the others. Whether varices should be injected intravariceal or paravariceal has likewise not been defined clearly. Both injection locations appear to work. Studies on the frequency of injection indicate that more frequent sessions over the first 4 to 6 weeks will achieve earlier obliteration and better control of bleeding.[15] However, the frequency of injection may be limited by the presence of mucosal ulceration. Variceal banding is gaining popularity and offers a good alternative to sclerotherapy.

Endoscopic sclerotherapy has a clearly defined role in management of acute variceal bleeding and is currently the treatment of choice. Its role in preventing rebleeding is less clear. A course of four to six sessions of endoscopic sclerotherapy can obliterate varices in some patients and prevent rebleeding. However, in randomized controlled trials in which sclerotherapy has been one form of treatment, rebleeding has been between 48% to 60% in studies conducted for at least four years of follow-up.[16] Controlled studies comparing sclerotherapy to long-term propranolol have shown an identical rebleeding and mortality rate in both treatment methods. Sclerotherapy appears to lessen the risk of early rebleeding, and buys time for full evaluation. This added timeframe may provide the window to define the etiology and the anticipated course of the underlying liver disease. As such, sclerotherapy plays a very important role in overall management. However, it probably should be considered as a temporizing measure with alternative treatment strategies planned for patients in whom varices cannot be obliterated or in whom rebleeding occurs.

DECOMPRESSIVE SHUNTS

Decompression of gastroesophageal varices with various shunting procedures has been demonstrated to be the most efficacious way of stopping bleeding. The reason that these have not been widely applied is the effect of such shunt surgery on liver function. Total portal diversion compromises the liver, will precipitate encephalopathy, and accelerate hepatic failure in patients with cirrhosis. However, not all shunts are alike, and it is important to look at the effects of different types of shunts both for controlling bleeding and for their effect on portal perfusion and liver function. In broad terms, shunts fall into the following categories: (1) total portal systemic shunts that divert all portal flow away from the liver,[17–19] (2) partial portal decompression in which a shunt of a sufficiently small caliber reduces portal pressure, but only diverts part of portal venous flow,[20,21] and

(3) selective variceal decompression that only decompresses the gastroesophageal and splenic segment, but allows continuing maintenance of portal hypertension and portal perfusion of the cirrhotic liver.[22,23]

The field has become more complicated in the last few years with the advent of a radiologic approach to variceal decompression by transjugular intrahepatic portal systemic shunt (TIPS). TIPS is a variation of a side-to-side portal systemic shunt[21] and will be discussed in that section.

Total Portal Systemic Shunts

Pathophysiologically there are two types of total portal systemic shunts, the end-to-side portocaval shunt and the various types of side-to-side shunts. The end-to-side portocaval shunt illustrated in Fig 57–3 divides the portal vein at its bifurcation and turns the mesenteric end of the portal vein down to anastomosis with the side of the inferior vena cava. This procedure totally decompresses the splanchnic and gastroesophageal venous beds and controls variceal bleeding. However, the obstructed sinusoids maintain their high pressure and thus, the operation does not alleviate ascites.

Side-to-side total portal systemic shunts may be created by any anastomosis between the portal vein or one of its major tributaries and inferior vena cava or one of its major tributaries. To be a total shunt, the anastomosis must be ≥10 mm in diameter. Side-to-side portacaval, mesocaval, mesorenal, or central splenorenal shunt all fall into this category (Fig 57–4).

Pathophysiologically, this differ from the end-to-side portacaval shunt in that the portal vein acts as an out-

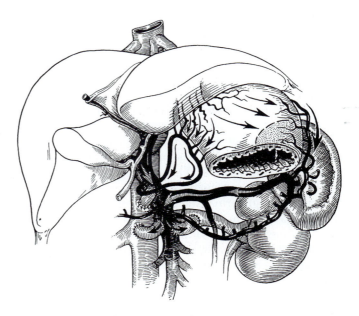

Figure 57–4. Side-to-side portal systemic shunts. Portacaval, mesocaval, and mesorenal shunts are shown. The portal vein acts as an outflow from obstructed sinusoids, decompressing the liver as well as varices and the splanchnic circulation.

flow tract from the obstructed sinusoids. These shunts not only decompress varices, but also decompress the obstructed sinusoids and will alleviate ascites.

Transjugular intrahepatic portosystemic shunt (TIPS) is a type of side-to-side portal systemic shunt. This radiologically inserted shunt creates an anastomosis between the portal vein and one of the major hepatic veins within the liver (Fig 57–5). When dilated to a diameter of 10 mm or greater, this is a totally diverting portal systemic shunt with the same advantages and disadvantages as those that are created surgically.

The indications for total portal systemic shunt in the 1990s are few. Side-to-side shunts may be indicated for acute Budd-Chiari Syndrome to decompress the congested liver. A side-to-side shunt may be indicated in a patient with continued massive bleeding who will exsanguinate if decompression is not provided. However, it must be recognized that this is a temporizing measure that will be accompanied by accelerated liver failure. As such, it may be considered as a bridge to liver transplantation. Are there some patients with massive variceal bleeding who still have adequate hepatocellular reserve to tolerate total portal diversion? These may be the 20% of patients who, historically, have been shown to tolerate total portal systemic shunts.[17,19] No clear data have been able to prospectively define which patients fall into this group, but if they could be identified, there might be a role for this type of decompression.

In the 1990s, if a total portal systemic shunt is performed, it is probably important to avoid the liver hilus,

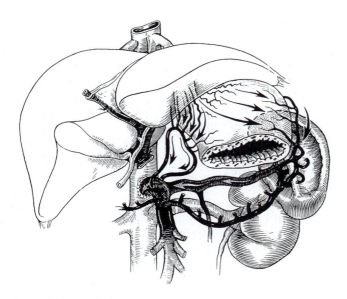

Figure 57–3. End-to-side portacaval shunt. This shunt decompresses varices and the splanchnic circulation. Sinusoidal pressure remains high in the cirrhotic liver.

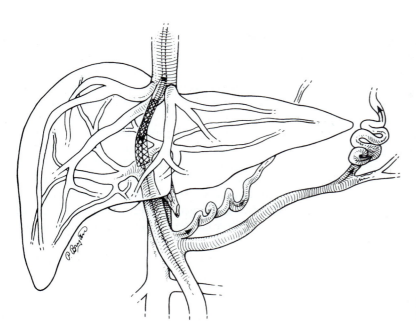

Figure 57–5. TIPS. This side-to-side shunt has variable hemodynamic effect depending on its diameter.

since the potential for subsequent liver transplantation must be considered. Avoiding the hilus will simplify liver transplantation. At the present time, TIPS is probably the procedure of choice for such side-to-side decompression. However, if TIPS is not possible, or concerns with patency dictate an operative approach, side-to-side portocaval or mesocaval shunts may be considered.

Portacaval Shunt. The patient is positioned with the right side elevated and a long, right subcostal incision is made. Adequate retraction of the liver upwards, and of the transverse colon and hepatic flexure downwards, expose the hepatoduodenal ligament. This ligament is incised along its right lateral margin, behind the common bile duct, to allow exposure of the portal vein on its right side. Exposure is facilitated further by a Kocher maneuver of the duodenum, which also will facilitate the subsequent visualization of the inferior vena cava. With the bile duct retracted to the left, the portal vein is freed approximately 2 to 3 cm upward to its bifurcation. Ideally, the portal vein is freed circumferentially for full control, but an alternative is simply to free sufficient vein to side clamp it. The vena cava then is exposed in the retroperitoneum, below the liver and behind the duodenum. The distance between the portal vein and the vena cava is dictated by the size of the caudate lobe of the liver. The vena cava must be cleared for a distance adequate to allow for safe side clamping. The anatomosis may be fashioned either with a direct portal vein to vena caval side-to-side anatomosis, or using a 2 to 3 cm long interposition graft, usually 14 to 16 gauge Goretex. This shunt is of a large caliber, anastomosing large and robust vessels and is performed easily. While exposure of the vessels may be somewhat difficult with bleeding, once the shunt is opened it is dramatic how rapidly the bleeding stops with relief of the portal hypertension.

Mesocaval Shunt. A mesocaval shunt achieves the same hemodynamic outcome as the side-to-side portacaval shunt, but is done at a more remote distance from the hepatic hilus. With the patient in a supine position, a transverse supraumbilical abdominal incision is made. The transverse colon is held superiorly and the retroperitoneum incised along the base of the transverse mesocolon. The superior mesenteric vein is identified readily, with the middle colic vein used to aid identification. The middle colic vein usually should be divided close to the superior mesenteric vein. The superior mesenteric vein then is traced up behind the pancreas to its junction with the splenic vein. Sufficient length (2 to 3 cm) should be circumferentially isolated for subsequent anastomosis. The inferior vena cava is identified by mobilizing the junction of the second and third portion of the duodenum superiorly. The more the duodenum is mobilized, the shorter the length of the graft for a mesocaval shunt. Sufficient vena cava must be isolated for side clamping and subsequent anastomosis. The graft usually is made with a 12 to 14 reinforced Goretex that is initially anastomosed to the inferior vena cava. With that anastomosis complete, the graft is brought up with as short a distance as possible to the right lateral side of the superior mesenteric vein. As a totally diverting portal systemic shunt, bleeding in the operative field usually ceases dramatically once this shunt is opened.

Postoperative Management. Postoperative management for these side-to-side total portal systemic shunts requires some attention to details. Patients are usually managed in the ICU for 24 to 72 hours depending on their pre-operative condition. Hemodynamics are stabilized in those patients who may have required significant volume resuscitation prior to operation. Blood, blood products, or fluid volume are used as indicated. Antibiotics should be continued while intravenous lines are present in patients with a prosthetic graft. Liquid diet is started with return of bowel function and advanced over the next few days. Protein restriction to 60 gm is advisable in patients with total portal diversion. Ascites is not usually a major problem, since side-to-side shunts alleviate all portal hypertension. Continued monitoring of the liver status is critical at this time, since some patients may show acute decompensation of their liver with total portal diversion. A rising bilirubin, increasing prothrombin time and clinical signs of overt encephalopathy, even to coma, will indicate such a course. Should this situation arise, the only possible salvage procedure is liver transplantation.

Partial Portal Decompression

When a side-to-side portal systemic shunt is reduced to 8 mm in diameter, portal pressure will be decompressed to approximately 12 mm Hg, some of the portal flow will be partially diverted through the shunt, and maintenance of some portal flow to the liver will be achieved in 80% of patients.[24] Current studies suggest that this type of shunt controls bleeding and has a lower risk of hepatic failure and encephalopathy. This partial decompression may be achieved with a small bore surgical shunt or with a TIPS of 8-mm diameter.

Small Bore Portacaval Shunt. This technique has been championed by Sarfeh and associates.[20] The technique for placing this shunt is very similar to that previously described for a side-to-side portacaval shunt. A 3 to 4 cm long, ringed 8-mm Goretex graft with beveled ends is anastomosed between the portal vein close to its bifurcation and the inferior vena cava. Pressure injecting the graft with heparin prior to insertion to fill its interstices reduces the risk of thrombosis. Careful follow-up study with documentation of graft patency prior to hospital discharge in a week to 10 days is an important component of postoperative care.

TIPS. This technique is currently the popular alternative for partial portal decompression.[25] Insufficient randomized studies or prolonged follow-up are available to clearly define its role. Procedurally, TIPS is placed via the right internal jugular vein. The right hepatic vein is catheterized and a needle punctured through the hepatic parenchyma to enter the main right portal vein.

A balloon is placed over a guidewire to dilate this parenchymal tract and finally, a metallic stent is placed in the dilated tract. Attention to detail in stent placement is important. Stents must bridge all the parenchyma between the portal and hepatic veins, but not protrude significantly into either of the veins. Portography before and after stent placement should document both flow patterns to the liver and varices, as well as measuring pressure. The portal to hepatic pressure gradient should be reduced to ≤12 mm Hg. Many different stents have been used over the last several years to create these shunts. Currently, the Wallstent, a self-expanding stent, is the most widely used. However, an adequately dilated tract must be created prior to its deployment. The risks for this procedure are similar to the risks for any portal systemic shunt, with bleeding, infection, and precipitation of liver failure as the main risks. In addition, there have been reports of rupture of the liver from perforation of the capsule, of hemobilia, of arterioportal fistulas, and of intravascular embolization of misplaced stents. The management during and after the procedure should parallel care of the operative patient. As with other minimally invasive surgical procedures, hospital stay can be shortened. However, the immediate fluid management, antibiotic coverage, and liver monitoring guidelines should be followed strictly. The major problem with TIPS at this time is stenosis or occlusion of the shunts in the first 6 months.[26,27] Follow-up protocols, usually based on Doppler ultrasound, should be in place so that evidence of stenosis or occlusion can be acted upon promptly, with shunt catheterization and redilation, if possible.

Selective Variceal Decompression

The distal splenorenal shunt (DSRS) provides selective decompression of gastroesophageal varices.[25] This shunt leaves the spleen in situ and anastomoses the splenic vein to the left renal vein. At the same time, portal hypertension is maintained in the splanchnic/hepatic axis to keep portal flow to the cirrhotic liver (Fig 57–6). The alternative approach to selective variceal decompression is coronary caval shunt;[23] however, this technique has not received the widespread acceptance of DSRS. DSRS is the most widely used operative shunt for management of variceal bleeding. With improved selection of patients, the results are much better than previously obtained.[29]

Variceal bleeding is controlled in 90% of patients managed by DSRS, a rate equivalent to total shunts. The goal of maintaining portal perfusion can be achieved in > 90% of patients with nonalcoholic cirrhosis, but is less well achieved in patients with alcoholic liver disease.[30] In alcoholic patients, portal perfusion is better maintained when the splenic vein is entirely dissected out of the pancreas.[31]

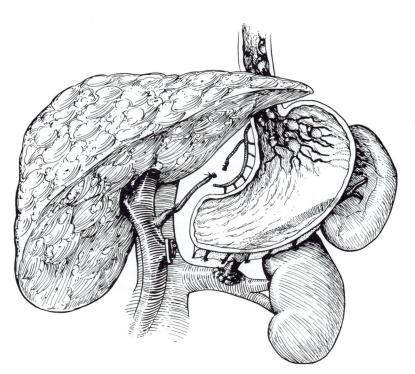

Figure 57–6. Distal splenorenal shunt. Varices are decompressed transplenic to the left renal vein. Portal hypertension is maintained in the splanchnic bed to keep prograde portal flow to the liver.

Distal Splenorenal Shunt. Distal splenorenal shunt is done with the patient in a supine position on the table, slightly hyperextended to open the gap between the costal margin and pelvis. A long left subcostal incision is made with extension across the right rectus. The lesser sac is opened by taking down the gastrocolic omentum from the pylorus to the short gastric vessels. Further exposure and compartmentalization of the left upper quadrant is achieved by taking down the splenic flexure of the colon. This method opens the plane to the posterior surface of the pancreas and also prevents development of collaterals along the mesocolon from the high-pressure portal vein to the low-pressure (shunted) splenic vein. With the stomach retracted superiorly, the pancreas then is mobilized fully along its inferior margin from the mesenteric vessels to the splenic hilus. The splenic vein is identified on the posterior surface of the pancreas and dissected free of the pancreas along a sufficient length to allow it to come down to the left renal vein without kinking. Initial safe dissection is along the posterior margin of the splenic vein, which should be freed entirely. The small perforating vessels from the pancreas into the splenic vein require meticulous dissection for their isolation and ligation on the vein side, and clip on the pancreas side. The vein is ligated flush with the superior mesenteric vein at the junction with the portal vein. A single ligature with a large clip placed behind it has proved to be the most satisfactory way of

dealing with this stump. The left renal vein is identified in the retroperitoneum and must be mobilized fully. This mobilization is achieved by identifying and ligating the left adrenal vein, usually leaving the gonadal vessel intact. The renal vein then can be brought up in a side clamp and the end of the splenic vein brought down for an end-to-side anastomosis. To complete the operation, the left gastric vein should be identified at its origin on the portal vein behind the pancreas and, in addition, ligated above the pancreas as it approaches the gastroesophageal junction. Thus, the components of this operation are the splenorenal anastomosis and adequate portal/splenic disconnection.

Postoperative management requires attention to details. The initial 24 hours usually are spent in the intensive care unit, with further hospitalization requiring 7 to 10 days. Meticulous fluid management is important because, with maintenance of portal hypertension, the risk of postoperative ascites is significant. These patients should not receive excess perioperative or postoperative intravenous fluids. Free sodium should be restricted as much as possible. Additionally, division of lymphatics around the left renal vein creates the risk of a chylous ascites. A diet with 2 gm sodium, 30 gm fat restriction is initiated for the initial 1 to 2 months. Patients usually require Aldactone in a dose sufficient to block sodium reabsorption over this time period. Prior to hospital discharge, shunt catheterization is performed to measure the pressured gradient and document shunt patency. A patent distal splenorenal shunt has excellent long-term patency. Early thrombosis usually is due to a technical problem and should be addressed with reoperation.

DEVASCULARIZATION PROCEDURES

This group of operations approaches the problem of variceal bleeding by interruption of inflow to varices. The components for these procedures are usually splenectomy, gastric devascularization, esophageal devascularization and occasionally, esophageal transection (Fig 57–7). The efficacy of these procedures appears to be related to the aggressiveness with which devascularization is undertaken. Popularized in Japan by Sugiura,[32] and in Egypt by Hassab,[33] good results have been achieved with extensive and aggressive devascularization for control of bleeding. More recent application in Mexico by Orozco and colleagues likewise has achieved good results in selected patients.[34] Poorer results have been obtained in Europe and North America, which, in part, may be related to poorer risk patients or to less aggressive devascularization. The advantage of devascularization procedures is that they do not reduce portal hypertension and thus, portal perfusion of the cirrhotic liver is maintained. The disadvantage is the relentless recollateralization of varices across the stomach and up the esophagus, with the risk of rebleeding.

The operative approach for devascularization operations may be entirely transabdominal, or a combined transabdominal and transthoracic approach. The advantage of the transthoracic approach is that more extensive esophageal devascularization can be performed. However, this must be weighted against the disadvantage of a thoracotomy. In the transabdominal approach, a splenectomy initially is performed, followed by extensive devascularization of the greater curve of the stomach. Care and attention also must be paid to the esophageal devascularization. Anatomic studies of the gastroesophageal junction have clearly defined the large paraesophageal collaterals with perforating veins that penetrate all layers of the esophageal wall to lie in the submucosa for approximately 2 cm at the gastroesophageal junction.[35,36] This segment is the site for >90% of variceal bleeding. In performing esophageal devascularization, it is important that all of the perforating veins be identified and totally cleared along this segment. In practical terms, this means circumferential clearing of approximately 7 cm of esophagus above the gastroesophageal junction. The vagus nerves should be identified and preserved, with devascularization continued down along the lesser curve of the stomach, in a manner similar to dissection for a proximal gastric vagotomy. By completing this dissection, the main inflow from the left gastric vein is totally interrupted. The role of esophageal transection to complete this operation is advocated by some, but not considered necessary by others. Many of these patients have received extensive sclerotherapy, which leaves considerable thickening in the distal esophagus. Transection is more difficult in such patients, and provided devascularization is sufficiently extensive, is probably not required. The extensive dissections involved in this operation leave many raw surfaces that are not decompressed. Hemostasis can be tedious in these procedures.

Postoperative management focuses on meticulous fluid and electrolyte management of the patient with cirrhosis. This management is important to minimize ascites. These patients have maintained portal hypertension, a positive factor in maintaining prograde portal flow, but a negative factor in the risk for ascites formation. Minimizing sodium intake, both intravenously and in the diet, will reduce the risk of ascites. Many of these patients will require diuretic therapy, at least in the initial postoperative period. Return of normal gastric emptying can be slow in these patients and initial recommendations are for a full liquid diet during the first two to four weeks. This diet can be advanced cautiously depending on how the patient tolerates it.

For longer term follow-up, this author recommends repeat endoscopy between 3 to 6 months to document the degree of obliteration of varices. The trend, in the course of time, is for recurrence of varices that, if seen, may warrant therapy with a pharmacologic agent.

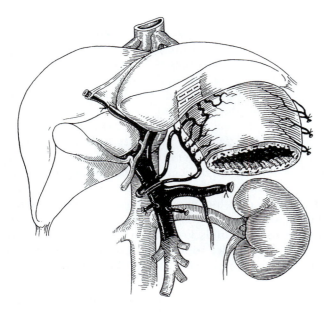

Figure 57–7. Gastroesophageal devascularization for variceal bleeding. Splenectomy, gastric and esophageal devascularization, and esophageal transection are the components of these operations.

LIVER TRANSPLANT

The final surgical approach to portal hypertension and variceal bleeding is liver transplantation.[37] However, the indication for transplant is end-stage liver disease, not variceal bleeding. The decision to proceed to transplantation should be based on full evaluation following stabilization of the initial bleed. Frequently, the exact nature of the liver disease, its severity or its activity is not clear at this time. Continued management of the patient with sclerotherapy during the next month or two may provide an opportunity to better assess these variables. In borderline patients, stabilization from the bleed may allow a better definition as to whether these patients will improve to Child-Pugh class A or whether they have more advanced disease (Child-Pugh class C). Quantitative liver function testing can help make this definition.[29] The Child-Pugh class C patient with variceal bleeding may require liver transplantation.

The benefit of liver transplantation in the patient with variceal bleeding and end-stage disease is that it not only decompresses the varices and controls bleeding but also restores functional hepatic mass. The disadvantage is that liver transplantation requires long-term immunosuppression with its associated morbidity. However, survival rate achieved in this patient subset are significantly better than the outcome historically achieved with other forms of therapy.

Details of the transplant procedure and perioperative management are provided in Chapter 58.

■ MANAGEMENT STRATEGIES

PROPHYLAXIS

Reduction of the risk of initial variceal bleed can be achieved with pharmacologic therapy.[14] Randomized controlled trials do not support a role for either prophylactic endoscopic schlerotherapy or prophylactic operative intervention.[38]

Noncardiac selective beta blockade with propranolol will reduce the risk of initial variceal bleed to approximately 15% to 20% 2 years following diagnosis of varices. Data from prospective randomized studies of endoscopic sclerotherapy have shown results varying from highly favorable to detrimental.[38] A new round of studies trying to define patients at higher risk of initial bleed may define a role for prophylactic sclerotherapy in such a subpopulation. However, there are insufficient data to advocate prophylactic sclerotherapy at this time. Surgical intervention for prophylaxis was tested in the 1970s with total portal systemic shunts. Those studies showed an increased mortality rate in patients undergoing shunt surgery.[39] However, there have been significant surgical advances since that time, and a single

multicenter study out of Japan has showed significant improval in patients undergoing nonportal decompressive surgery for control of their variceal bleeding in a prophylactic setting.[40] However, this single study does not justify the widespread application of prophylactic surgery in patients with varices.

ACUTE VARICEAL BLEEDING

Management of patients with acute variceal bleeding may require several treatment modalities. If the patient is massively bleeding, pharmacologic therapy may slow or even stop the acute bleed. Historically, pitressin has the established role. However, more recent studies show that somatostatin is equally efficacious, with fewer side effects. Early endoscopy, both for diagnosis and for acute sclerotherapy, is the mainstay of treatment. Sclerotherapy is conducted at the time of initial endoscopy, and a direct intravariceal injection with obliteration of the varix is probably most efficacious. In the occasional patient in whom the bleeding cannot be controlled with sclerotherapy, balloon tamponade with a Sengstaken-Blackmore tube may be required. It is this author's belief that this is necessary in <5% of patients. If tamponade is required, the tube should not be left down for more than 12 to 24 hours. Furthermore, it should be used only as a temporizing measure while other treatments are implemented. When bleeding cannot be controlled or there is recurrent bleeding on a daily basis, emergent surgery with decompression or TIPS may be required.

EVALUATION

Once the patient is stabilized from an acute variceal bleed, a full evaluation should be undertaken as outlined in the text. This is the step that is frequently forgotten. With this evaluation, the patient's disease is defined, and a long-term treatment strategy developed for each individual patient. Plans are based on a knowledge of the severity of the bleeding, the risk of further bleeding, the underlying liver disease, and the expected natural history of that disease.

PREVENTION OF RECURRENT BLEEDING

Decisions for the prevention of recurrent bleeding are based on whether the patient has good underlying hepatic function or is approaching end-stage liver disease. In patients with advanced liver disease, a full evaluation for consideration of liver transplant should be done. The decision as to how to manage the variceal bleeding in these patients depends on the outcome of transplant evaluation. If the patient is an acceptable candidate for transplantation, a temporizing method may be required to control bleeding during the waiting period. Endoscopic sclerotherapy or an intrahepatic shunt are the best options. High-risk or recurrent variceal bleeding may accelerate the patient's course towards transplantation and increase their priority ranking on the waiting list.

Patients with adequately maintained liver function may be managed in other ways. Equally, patients who are not candidates for liver transplantation must be managed with alternative therapies. The choice of optimal therapy is based on several variables: the available local expertise, the expected natural history of the underlying liver disease, the activity or inactivity of the liver disease, and patient preference. If varices can be obliterated easily with endoscopic sclerotherapy, this may be primary therapy. However, it must be kept in mind that the risk of a significant rebleeding is high and a more definitive management method may be appropriate. If the patient has stable liver disease with good hepatocellular reserve, the emphasis must be on control of bleeding. A distal splenorenal shunt will control bleeding and will not accelerate the course of the underlying liver disease.

When there are uncertainties as to the severity of the underlying liver disease and its likely rate of progression, temporizing measures may again be appropriate. These measures are achieved best with endoscopic sclerotherapy with or without a noncardioselective beta blocker. The managing physician has an obligation to follow these patients closely and make sure that the bleeding is controlled, that the liver disease is stabilized, and that, if there is persistence of high-risk varices or recurrence of bleeding, other appropriate steps are implemented. To allow a good-risk patient with good hepatocellular reserve to keep rebleeding and rapidly progress to becoming a poor-risk patient who can only be managed by transplantation is not acceptable.

Therefore, it is apparent, in the 1990s, that there are many treatment options open to the management of variceal bleeding and portal hypertension. There is no single therapy that is ideal for all patients. A clear understanding of the etiology of the problem, the risks associated for that particular patient, and the available treatment options will provide the best management.

■ OTHER TYPES OF PORTAL HYPERTENSION

PORTAL VEIN THROMBOSIS

This less common cause of portal hypertension and variceal bleeding is important to identify because the normal liver of such patients dictates a good prognosis. It should always be considered in a patient with variceal bleeding and excellent liver function. While findings on Doppler/ultrasound, CT or MRI scan can be suggestive of portal vein thrombosis, it requires angiography to confirm the diagnosis. Typically, the patient has cavernous

transformation, which are large collaterals that have collateralized from the high-pressure splanchnic bed to the low-pressure liver sinusoids. These collaterals can mimic the portal vein on some imaging studies and require angiography for full definition. They do, however, assure good continued portal perfusion of the liver. Liver biopsy is important to confirm normal liver histology.

Control of bleeding is the important issue in management since these patients do not die of progressive liver disease. While these patients can do well with scherotherapy, they have a rebleeding rate of approximately 30%.[41] Distal splenorenal shunt is technically feasible in about 80% of these patients, and has better control of bleeding.[42] Finally, it is important to complete a full hematologic evaluation on these patients, particularly when no etiologic factors can be defined. Hypercoagulable states and myeloproliferative disorders can be identified in many of these patients and need to be managed simultaneously with treatment of bleeding.

LEFT-SIDED (SINISTRAL) PORTAL HYPERTENSION

Left-sided (sinistral) portal hypertension occurs with isolated splenic vein thrombosis in patients with normal liver function.[43] Etiology is most commonly secondary to pancreatitis or pancreatic carcinoma. However, rarer causes, such as trauma or hematologic disorders, also can lead to this complication. These patients are important to identify since they are the only group whose variceal bleeding is cured by splenectomy. The diagnosis should be considered in patients with large gastric varices and a history of any of the above predisposing factors. Angiography usually is required for definitive diagnosis, which not only confirms splenic vein thrombosis, but, for this entity, also shows a patent portal vein and normal HVPG.

BUDD-CHIARI SYNDROME

Budd-Chiari Syndrome (BCS) is relatively uncommon.[44] This is a diagnosis that is often missed, but must always be considered in a patient with unexplained ascites. Early diagnosis leads to better outcome. The syndrome brings together all causes of hepatic venous outflow obstruction that result in sinusoidal congestion, centrilobular necrosis, hepatocellular death, lobular collapse, and ultimately, fibrosis. There is a spectrum of presentations depending on the acuteness and completeness of the hepatic venous obstruction. At one end of the spectrum, minor obstruction of a single hepatic vein will lead to damage of a single lobe, will not affect total hepatic function, and often will not be noted clinically. At the other end of the spectrum, complete obstruction of all lobes may lead to fulminant liver failure. Many patients lie somewhere in the middle of the spectrum; the syndrome frequently presents with a confusing and insidious course.

Pathophysiology and Etiology

The syndrome results from hepatic vein occlusion usually secondary to thrombosis in a major hepatic vein. Consequently, the sinusoids initially become congested. With increasing pressure, there is centrilobular necrosis that leads ultimately to hepatocyte death, collapse, and fibrosis.

The most common causes of Budd-Chiari Syndrome are chronic myeloproliferative disorders.[45] The increasing sophistication with which these can be elucidated has led to an increased recognition of their role in BCS. Such a disorder now can be defined in >50% of patients. The most common disorder is polycythemia rubra vera, but any stem-cell proliferation may lead to a hypercoagulable state. Other etiologies include paroxysmal nocturnal hemoglobinuria, other hypercoagulable problems such as protein C, protein S or antithrombin 3 deficiency, oral contraceptives, and pregnancy.

Finally, there is a group of mechanical etiologies for BCS. These include membranous webs of major hepatic veins or the vena cava, which are more common in the Far East and Africa, and extrinsic hepatic vein occlusion by liver tumors.

Clinical Course

Patients with Budd-Chiari Syndrome typically present with an insidious course. Ascites and hepatomegaly, with some right upper quadrant abdominal pain, are the most constant features. Laboratory studies often show minimal change, thus diverting attention away from the liver. The diagnosis is frequently overlooked.

Unexplained ascites should always raise the suspicion of BCS and lead to ultrasound of the hepatic vein and possible liver biopsy. Sudden occlusion of all veins can present with a more dramatic picture with massive and tense ascites, severe right upper quadrant pain, and marked elevation of serum transaminases. Diagnosis in such patients is relatively easy, but this is not the most common presentation. The key in determining the clinical course is the degree of outflow obstruction. When obstruction is severe and there is ongoing hepatocyte necrosis, the continuing liver injury becomes irreversible once there is lobular collapse. A diagnosis made before the lobules collapse will allow the sinusoids to be decompressed, with recoverable liver function.

Evaluation

The three key elements in evaluation are (1) hepatic vein imaging, (2) liver biopsy, and (3) hematologic evaluation.[46] Other adjunctive investigations may help in establishing the diagnosis, but these steps must be completed.

A Doppler ultrasound of the hepatic veins can be used as a screening test. If the main hepatic veins are visualized with phasic flow, this precludes a diagnosis of Budd-Chiari syndrome. Other imaging modalities, such as CT and MRI scan, may have some use in screening but do not provide definitive information. Hepatic venography is indicated if the screening tests fail to confirm patent hepatic veins, or the index of suspicion is high. The typical finding at hepatic venography is a "spider's web." Impaction of a catheter into a hepatic vein with injection of contrast fails to fill normal vein but rather fills multiple collaterals attempting to decompress the sinusoids. At the time of hepatic venography, the angiography also should study the intrahepatic inferior vena cava. Pressure should be measured in the right atrium, the intrahepatic vena cava, and the infrahepatic vena cava. Assessment of the degree of obstruction of the cava by the swollen liver of BCS is important in planning any sinusoidal decompression.

Percutaneous liver biopsy is essential. The sicker the patient, the more important the biopsy. If necessary, tense ascites should be drained and any coagulopathy corrected. Separate biopsies should be taken of the right and left lobes, since there is frequently a different degree of injury if outflow obstruction is different for the two lobes. The essential features to be looked for on biopsy are the degree of sinusoidal congestion, the presence of centrilobular necrosis, the presence of lobular collapse and the development of fibrosis.

Hematologic evaluation requires the involvement of a hematologist with an interest in myeloproliferative disorders. The findings can be deceptive in these patients, particularly if they have already developed splenomegaly.

Management

Nonsurgical management is justified only if there is no evidence of ongoing cell necrosis on multiple biopsies. It is reasonable to observe such patients and simply manage the ascites with diuretics. However, this scenario is unusual and repeat biopsies should be performed in 3 to 6 months. If there is a hypercoagulable state, anticoagulation should be considered. Occasionally, thrombolytic agents, such as streptokinase, may be indicated. When there is a major thrombus to be lysed, usually there is also severe ongoing hepatocellular necrosis. It is important to document that any therapy used stops ongoing hepatocyte necrosis.

Occasionally, balloon dilation of membranous webs in the hepatic vein or vena cava may be appropriate. In the United States this procedure is unusual, but it should be considered in the Far East where webs are more common.

Surgical management is frequently indicated for BCS.[46,47] The two main surgical options are a decompressive shunt or liver transplantation. In a liver that is acutely damaged and in which there is no lobular collapse, a side-to-side portacaval shunt or one of its variants, that allows the portal vein to serve as an outflow

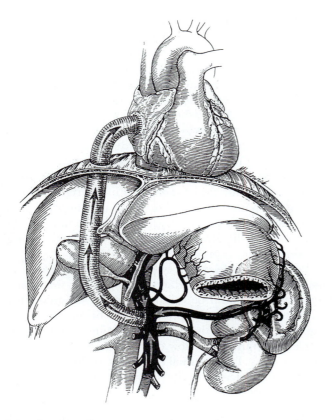

Figure 57–8. Mesoatrial shunt. The side-to-side portosystemic shunt may be needed to decompress the liver in Budd-Chiari Syndrome when the inferior vena cava is obstructed.

tract from the obstructed sinusoids is indicated. When the liver is severely damaged with collapse and fibrosis, the only remedy is transplantation.

The decision-making steps in using a decompressive shunt are (1) documentation of ongoing necrosis, (2) demonstration of intact lobular architecture, and (3) definition of the status of the intrahepatic inferior vena cava. When the vena cava is open, and the first two conditions are present, an infrahepatic side-to-side shunt should be used. If there is thrombosis or severe compression of the intrahepatic inferior cava, a mesocaval shunt is indicated (Fig 57–8). Prior to undertaking either of these shunts, it is important to complete the hematologic work-up. Failure to diagnose a hypercoagulable state will lead to thrombosis of the shunt. Concurrent management of that hematologic disorder is essential to maintain patency.

Long-term follow-up of patients appropriately selected for side-to-side shunts has been good. Serial biopsies have shown that the ongoing necrosis is halted and that usually only minimal, centrilobular fibrosis persists. Hepatocellular function has been well-maintained, and at follow-up 5 to 8 years later, encephalopathy has not

been a problem. The 10 to 20 year outcome for such patients has not been documented yet.[46]

Liver transplantation is indicated when there is severe liver damage.[46–48] Biopsy is again the main clue as to the degree of fibrosis. Further indications for transplantation may come from severe distortion seen on other imaging modalities, and significant hepatocellular dysfunction, as indicated by prolonged prothrombin time low serum albumin. In this author's own experience, quantitative function tests also have contributed to this differentiation.

REFERENCES

1. Mahl TC, Groszmann RJ. Pathophysiology of portal hypertension and variceal bleeding. *Surg Clin North Am* 1990; 70:251–266

2. Bosch J, Pizcueta P, Fen F, et al. Pathophysiology of portal hypertension. *Gastroenterol Clin North Am* 1992;21:1–14

3. Beppu K, Inokuchi K, Kayanagi N, et al. Prediction of variceal hemorrhage by esophageal endoscopy. *Gastrointest Endosc* 1981;27:213–218

4. Paquet KJ. Prophylactic endoscopic sclerosing treatment of the esophageal wall in varices—a prospective controlled trial. *Endoscopy* 1982;27:213–218

5. de Franchis R, and the North Italian Endoscopic Club. Prediction of the first variceal hemorrhage in patients with cirrhosis of the liver and esophageal varices. *N Engl J Med* 1988;319:983

6. Nordlinger BM, Nordlinger DF, Fulenwider JT, et al. Angiography in portal hypertension: clinical significance in surgery. *Am J Surg* 1980;139:132

7. Groszmann RJ, Glickman M, Blei AT, et al. Wedge and free hepatic venous pressure measured with a balloon catheter. *Gastroenterology* 1979;76:254–258

8. Galambos JT. Evaluation of patients with portal hypertension. *Am J Surg* 1990;160:14–18

9. Reichen J. Liver function and pharmacological considerations in pathogenesis and treatment of portal hypertension. *Hepatology* 1990;11:1066–1076

10. Jenkins SA, Baxter JN, Corbett WA, et al. A prospective randomized controlled trial comparing somatostatin and vasopressin in controlling acute variceal hemorrhage. *Brit Med J* 1985;290:270–278

11. Sung JJY, Chung SCS, Lai C-W, et al. Octreotide infusion or emergency sclerotherapy for variceal hemorrhage. *Lancet* 1993;342:637–641

12. Lebrec D: Current status and future goals of the pharmacologic reduction of portal hypertension. *Am J Surg* 1990; 160:19–23

13. Rodriguez-Perez F, Groszmann RJ. Pharmacologic treatment of portal hypertension. *Gastroenterology Clin North Am* 1992;21:15–40

14. McCormick PA, Burroughs AK. Prophylaxis for variceal hemorrhage. *Gastrointest Endosc Clin North Am* 1992;2: 167–182

15. Westaby D, Melia WM, MacDougall BRD, et al. Injection

sclerotherapy for oesophageal varices: a prospective randomized trial of different treatment schedules. *Gut* 1984; 25:129

16. Westaby D, Williams R. Status of sclerotherapy for variceal bleeding in 1990. *Am J Surg* 1990;160:32–37

17. Orloff MJ, Bell RH. Long-term survival after emergency portacaval shunting for bleeding varices in patients with alcoholic cirrhosis. *Am J Surg* 1986;151:176–183

18. Drapanas T. Interposition mesocaval shunt for treatment of portal hypertension. *Ann Surg* 1972;176:435

19. Reynolds TB, Donovan AJ, Mikkelsen WP, et al. Results of a 12-year randomized trial of portacaval shunt in patients with alcoholic liver disease and bleeding varices. *Gastroenterology* 1981;80:1005–1011

20. Rypins EB, Sarfeh IJ. Small-diameter portacaval H-graft for variceal hemorrhage. *Surg Clin North Am* 1990;70: 395–404

21. Richter GM, Noeldge G, Palmaz JC, et al. Transjugular intrahepatic portacaval stent shunt: preliminary clinical results. *Radiology* 1990;174:1027–1030

22. Warren WD, Zeppa R, Foman JS. Selective transplenic decompression of gastroesophageal varices by distal splenorenal shunt. *Ann Surg* 1967;166:437

23. Inokuchi K. A selective portocaval shunt. *Lancet* 1968;2:51

24. Sarfeh IJ, Rypins EB, Mason GR. A systemic appraisal of portacaval H-graft diameters: clinical and hemodynamic perspectives. *Ann Surg* 1986;204:356–363

25. Conn HO. Transjugular intrahepatic portalsystemic shunts: the state of the art. *Hepatology* 1993;17:148–158

26. Lind CD, Malish TW, Chang WK, et al. Incidence of shunt occlusion or stenosis with transjugular intrahepatic portosystemic shunts. *Gastroenterology* 1993;104:A941

27. Benner K, Sahagun G, Meyer RA, et al. Shunt patency after transjugular intrahepatic portosystemic shunt. *Gastroenterology* 1993;104:A876

28. WD Warren. Memorial Issue. *Am J Surg* 1990;160:1–138

29. Henderson JM, Gilmore GT, Hooks MA, et al. Selective shunt in the management of variceal bleeding in the era of liver transplantation. *Ann Surg* 1992;216:248–255

30. Henderson JM, Gong-Liang J, Galloway J, et al. Portaprival collaterals following distal splenorenal shunt: incidence, magnitude, and associated portal perfusion changes. *J Hepatol* 1985;1:649–661

31. Henderson JM, Warren WD, Millikan WJ, et al. Distal splenorenal shunt with splenopancreatic disconnection: a four year assessment. *Ann Surg* 1989;210:332–341

32. Sugiura M, Futagawa S. Esophageal transection with paraesophagogastric devascularization (the Sugiura procedure) in the treatment of esophageal varices. *World J Surg* 1984;8:673–682

33. Hassab MA. Nonshunt operations in portal hypertension without cirrhosis. *Surg Gynec Obstet* 1967;131:648–654

34. Orozco H, Mercado MA, Takahashi T, et al. Elective treatment of bleeding varices with the Sugiura operation over 10 years. *Am J Surg* 1992;163:585–589

35. Kitano S, Terblanche J, Kahn D, et al. Venous anatomy of the lower esophagus in portal hypertension: practical implications. *Br J Surg* 1986;73:525–531

36. Spence RAJ. The venous anatomy of the lower esophagus in normal subjects and in patients with varices: an image analysis study. *Br J Surg* 1984;71:739–744

37. Starzl TE, Demetris AJ, Van Thiel DH. Medical progress: liver transplantation. *N Engl J Med* 1989;321:1014–1022, 1092–1099

38. McCormick PA, Burroughs AK. Prophylaxis for variceal hemorrhage. *Gastrointest Endosc Clin North Am* 1992;2: 167–182

39. Conn HO, Lindenmuth WW, May CJ, et al. Prophylactic portacaval anastomosis. a tale of two studies. *Medicine* 1972;51:27–40

40. Inokuchi K, and Cooperative Study Group of Portal Hypertension in Japan. Improved survival after prophylactic portal nondecompressive surgery for esophageal varices: a randomized controlled trial. *Hepatology* 1990; 02:1–6

41. Kahn D, Krige JE, Terblanche J, et al. A 15 year experience of injection sclerotherapy in adult patients with extrahepatic portal venous obstruction. *Ann Surg* 1994; 219:34–39

42. Warren WD, Henderson JM, Millikan WJ, et al. Management of variceal bleeding in patients with noncirrhotic portal vein thrombosis. *Ann Surg* 1988;207:623–634

43. Moosa AR, Godd MA. Isolated splenic vein thrombosis. *World J Surg* 1985;9:384–390

44. Shill M, Henderson JM, Tavill AS. The Budd-Chiari Syndrome Revisited. *Gastroenterologist* 1994;2:27–38

45. Valla D, Casadevall N, Lacombe C, et al. Primary myeloproliferative disorders and hepatic vein thrombosis: a prospective study of erythroid colony formation in vitro in 20 patients with Budd-Chiari syndrome. *Ann Int Med* 1985;103:329–334

46. Henderson JM, Warren D, Millikan WJ, et al. Surgical options, hematologic evaluation and pathologic changes in Budd-Chiari syndrome. *Am J Surg* 1990;159:41–50

47. Klein AS, Stizmann JV, Coleman J, et al. Current management of Budd-Chiari syndrome. *Ann Surg* 1990;212: 144–149

48. Shaked A, Goldstein RM, Klintmalm GB. Portosystemic shunt versus orthotopic liver transplantation for the Budd-Chiari syndrome. *Surg Gynecol Obstet* 1992;174:453–459

58

Liver Transplantation

Douglas G. Farmer ▪ *J. Michael Millis* ▪ *Ronald W. Busuttil*

In the last 40 years, liver transplantation has evolved from an experimental procedure confined to the laboratory to a clinically therapeutic intervention that is applied worldwide to virtually all forms of end-stage liver disease. In 1992 alone, 4810 liver transplants were performed in 157 transplant centers.[1] This rapid expansion of clinical liver transplantation is founded largely in the pioneering work of Dr. Thomas E. Starzl.[2,3]

▪ HISTORY

The first attempted liver transplant was heterotopically positioned and reported in 1955 by Welch, using a canine model;[4] while the first attempted orthotopic liver transplant was described in 1956 by Cannon in a canine model.[5] Shortly thereafter, experimental success was realized by Goodrich and Welch (heterotopic model),[6] Moore and associates in Boston (orthotopic model)[7] and Starzl and associates in Chicago (orthotopic model).[8] This early experimental work provided the basis for the first human trials that followed.

In 1963, Starzl described orthotopic transplantation in three patients with end-stage liver disease secondary to biliary atresia, Laennec's cirrhosis combined with hepatocellular carcinoma, and bile duct carcinoma.[9] Immunosuppression was achieved with various combinations of thymectomy, splenectomy, azathioprine, prednisone, actinomycin C, and azaserine. Although no patient survived more than 8 days, the technical feasibility of the procedure was established. Five other transplants were attempted in the early 1960s in Colorado, Los Angeles, Boston, and Paris with no patient surviving beyond 23 days.[10–12] Table 58–1 outlines the first seven of these patients.

The first human orthotopic transplants with extended survival took place at the University of Colorado between July 1967 and March 1968.[13] Seven patients with hepatocellular carcinoma (n=2) or biliary atresia (n=5) between the ages of 13 months and 16 years underwent the procedure. Immunosuppression was maintained with azathioprine, prednisone, and antilymphocyte globulin. Although four patients died within 6 months, three were reported alive from 33 to 269 days after transplantation. One patient in particular represented the first long-term human survivor after liver transplantation. This 19-month-old female with hepatocellular carcinoma received a liver graft from an 18 month–old donor with microencephaly. She survived >1 year before succumbing to recurrent tumor.

Encouraged by these early successes, two centers, the University of Colorado in the United States and King's College, Cambridge in England, led continued efforts. In 1976 and 1977, these centers separately published the first major series describing a total of 153 orthotopic liver transplants in adults and children.[14,15] Azathioprine, prednisone, and antilymphocyte globulin were used for immunosuppression in the majority of recipients. Together, 33 patients lived ≥1 year, with the longest survival >6 years.

TABLE 58–1. THE FIRST TRIALS OF ORTHOTOPIC LIVER TRANSPLANTATIONS

No.	Location (ref.)	Age (yr)	Disease	Survival (days)	Main cause of death
1	Denver (1)	3	Extrahepatic biliary atresia	0	Hemorrhage
2	Denver (1)	48	Hepatocellular cancer, cirrhosis	22	Pulmonary emboli, sepsis
3	Denver (1)	68	Duct cell carcinoma	7.5	Sepsis, pulmonary emboli, gastrointestinal bleeding
4	Denver (2)	52	Hepatocellular cancer, cirrhosis	6.5	Pulmonary emboli, ? hepatic failure, pulmonary edema
5	Boston (3)	58	Metastatic colon carcinoma	11	Pneumonitis, liver abscesses, hepatic failure
6	Denver (2)	29	Hepatocellular cancer, cirrhosis	23	Sepsis, bile peritonitis, hepatic failure
7	Paris (4)	75	Metastatic colon carcinoma	0	Hemorrhage

The first seven attempted human orthotopic liver transplants along with the diagnosis and outcome are shown. The single attempted transplant at UCLA is not shown in the table. Technical failure and sepsis limited the survival to less than 23 days.
(From Starzl TE, Iwatsuki S, Van Thiel DH, et al. Evolution of Liver Transplantation. *Hepatology* 1982;2:614–636)

Following these two reports, worldwide enthusiasm increased and a number of transplant centers began to organize liver transplant units. Broader application was facilitated by the discovery[16] and application[17,18] of cyclosporine A to liver transplantation, resulting in improved patient and graft survival (Fig 58–1).[19] Endorsement of liver transplantation for treatment of many primary hepatic diseases by a National Institutes of Health consensus conference in 1983,[20] led to a rapid expansion of transplant centers and activity. Improvements in graft preservation (Fig 58–2)[21–23] and operative technique[12,24] solidified the role of liver transplantation for patients with end-stage liver disease.

PATIENT SELECTION

The list of hepatic diseases treated by transplantation has dramatically expanded since the first human trials. In general, liver transplantation represents the definitive treatment for all forms of end-stage liver disease. Careful patient selection for both donors and recipients is essential for successful transplantation. Table 58–2 represents an abbreviated list of indications for liver transplantation, and Table 58–3 includes contraindications to the procedure.

DONOR SELECTION

The concept of the ideal solid organ donor has undergone gradual evolution since the initiation of brain death legislation in the 1960s.[25] Without question, the ideal donor is a young, previously healthy, brain-dead, heart-beating victim of an accident. In reality, organ shortages coupled with expansion of the recipient indications for liver transplantation has led to liberalization of the classic donor criteria. As recent as the late 1980s, the classic criteria included strict age, pressor, hemodynamic, and hospitalization limitations (Table 58–4).[26] In fact, some centers advocated criteria which precluded the acceptance of as many as 80% of potential

donors.[27] However, owing to the pattern of organ supply and demand, less strict criteria are used now by some centers for donor acceptance and most so called "marginal" donors are only rejected after operative evaluation.[28] Still, several areas of controversy exist regarding donor selection.

Age continues to be one such controversy. At our institution, the mean donor age has increased from 23.7 ± 6.5 years between 1984 and 1987 to 35.4 ± 13.6 years (*P*<.05) between 1991 and 1992, with the oldest donor being 71 years.[26] During the same interval, an increased incidence of primary graft nonfunction was not seen and 78% of grafts from older donors were functioning at 1 year. Similarly, Teperman and associates compared the recipient outcome after transplantation of grafts from older donors (>50 years of age) with that of grafts from younger donors (<50 years of age). There was a 100% recipient survival rate in the older donor group as compared with 91% in the younger group. These studies support the use of suitable older donors, but contrasting data has been reported by other groups.[30]

At the opposite extreme of age, premature and anencephalic infants remain controversial sources of donor organs. The central issues are illustrated by Peabody and associates who examined the outcome of twelve anencephalic infants considered for organ donation.[31] Six were treated with early resuscitation and intensive care monitoring before clinical instability commenced while the others were treated with resuscitation and intensive care monitoring only after evidence of clinical instability. In the early resuscitation group, the majority (5/6) had organs suitable for donation but clinical brain death criteria were never met. In the late group, the majority were found to have organs not considered suitable for donation. Clearly, the ethical and legal issues associated with the use of these infants as well as premature infants functionally preclude organ donation. The applicability of current legal brain death criteria to anencephalic donors is suspect.[32,33] This prob-

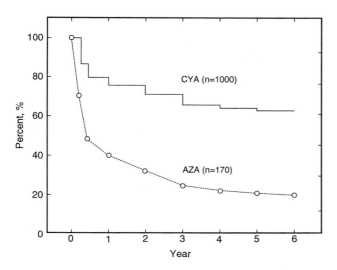

Figure 58–1. Actuarial percent patient survival is graphically demonstrated. Superior survival in 1000 patients treated with cyclosporine A–based immunotherapy over 170 patients receiving azathioprine-based immunotherapy is shown. (Redrawn from Iwatsuki S, Starzl TE, Todo S, et al. Experience in 1000 liver transplants under cyclosporine-steroid therapy: a survival report. *Transplant Proc* 1988;20:498–504)

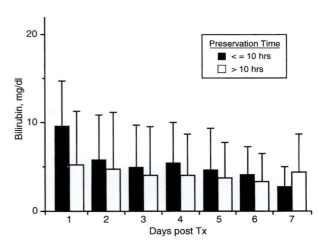

Figure 58–2. The effectiveness of the University of Wisconsin solution for liver preservation is demonstrated by the mean serum total bilirubin after liver transplantation in 8 patients with liver grafts preserved less than 10 hours (mean 8.0 hours, black bar) as compared with 9 patients with grafts preserved more than 10 hours (mean 12.7 hours, white bar). There were no episodes of primary graft nonfunction and no significant differences in total bilirubin during the first postoperative week. These results represented improved preservation over conventional Euro-Collins solution.[23] (From Kalayoglu M, Sollinger HW, Stratta RJ, et al. Extended preservation of the liver for clinical transplantation. *Lancet* 1988;March 19:617–619)

TABLE 58–2. RECIPIENT INDICATIONS FOR LIVER TRANSPLANTATION

Cirrhosis
    Viral - Hepatitis B, C, delta, CMV
    Alcoholic
    Autoimmune
    Cryptogenic
Biliary
    Sclerosing cholangitis
    Primary biliary cirrhosis
    Secondary biliary cirrhosis
    Biliary atresia (extrahepatic and intrahepatic)
    Byler disease (familial cholestasis)
    Alagile's syndrome
Metabolic
    α_1-antitrypsin deficiency
    Wilson's disease
    Hemochromatosis
    Protoporphyria
    Type IV hyperlipidemia
    Tyrosinemia
    Galactosemia
    Glycogen storage diseases (type I and IV)
    Congenital hepatic fibrosis
Vascular
    Budd-Chiari Syndrome
Malignancy
    Primary hepatocellular carcinoma
    Hepatoblastoma
    Neuroendocrine tumors
Fulminant

TABLE 58–3. RECIPIENT CONTRAINDICATIONS TO LTX

Absolute	Relative
Advanced cardiopulmonary disease	Active infection
Active substance abuse	Active hepatitis B infection
HIV infection	Metastatic hepatic malignancy
Extrahepatic malignancy	
Patient noncompliance	

TABLE 58–4. DONOR EXCLUSION CRITERIA GROUP 1

Age >45
Dopamine >10 mcg/kg/min
Cardiac arrest >15 min
Hospitalization >3 days
Transaminases >3 × normal
Malignancy
Systemic infection
HIV, HTL VIII, HbsAg+
Suspicious history or history of alcohol
"Bad-looking" liver

Criteria for donor exclusion in the first 100 liver transplants performed at UCLA from February 1, 1984 to November 1, 1987. Strict limitations on donor age, hemodynamic instability, length of hospitalization, liver function, malignancy and infection were routinely applied.
(From Busuttil RW, Shaked A, Millis JM, et al. One thousand liver transplants: the lessons learned. *Ann Surg* 1994;219:490–499)

TABLE 58–5. DONOR ASSESSMENT AND EARLY GRAFT FUNCTION ARE POORLY CORRELATED

Early Function	Donor Rating		Total
	Good	Poor	
Good	95	26	121
Fair	49	16	65
Poor	24	9	33
Total	168 (10)	51 (5)	219

Parentheses: number of grafts that never functioned.

lem, combined with technical considerations in these small donors, make organ donation in anencephalic and premature infants unlikely. It should be noted however, that the use of neonatal donors has been successfully reported.[34]

The utility of standard liver function tests for donor selection also remains controversial. Traditional policy has been to reject donors with elevated serum bilirubin, aspartate aminotransferase, alanine aminotransferase, and alkaline phosphatase. However, several studies have failed to support this practice (Table 58–5).[35–37] Clearly, further research is needed to develop alternate methods of quantitative liver function testing and to determine their usefulness in predicting donor outcome.[38–40] Until that time, donor selection decisions should not be based solely on nonquantitative liver function testing.

In our opinion, serious consideration should be given to all donors, regardless of age, who are without abdominal/hepatic trauma, history of liver disease, extracranial malignancy, human immunodeficiency virus infection, hepatitis B infection, or systemic infections. Operative evaluation of donors traditionally considered "marginal" is strongly recommended. Rejection of grafts with histologic evidence of significant necrosis, hepatitis, cirrhosis or macrosteatosis (>40 percent)[41] is recommended with all other potential grafts utilized for transplantation.

RECIPIENT SELECTION

Recipient selection remains one of the most important considerations for successful outcomes. An evaluation committee consisting of surgeons, hepatologists, cardiologists, pulmonologists, nephrologists, neurologists, gastroenterologists, infectious disease specialists, pediatricians, psychiatrists, anesthesiologists, transplant coordinators, and social workers commonly is employed at most centers and strongly recommended.[42] Acceptance for candidacy requires that a patient have irreversible end-stage liver disease associated with evidence of portal hypertension, hepatic encephalopathy, hyperbilirubinemia, and poor hepatic synthetic function. Increas-

ingly, indications for candidacy are broadening into quality of life issues.[43] These are patients considered and accepted for candidacy who manifest evidence of end-stage liver disease mainly through limitations of lifestyle such as intractable ascites, encephalopathy, pruritis, and fatigue. With improvements in the results of liver transplantation, these issues are now accepted as legitimate indications for liver replacement.

Strict contraindications continue to persist. Extrahepatic malignancy, advanced disease of other organ systems, patient noncompliance, human immunodeficiency virus infection or ongoing substance abuse are considered absolute contraindications (Table 58–3). Other relative contraindications are changing but include active systemic infection, infection with the hepatitis B virus, and anatomic abnormalities.

In the face of these broad selection criteria, the recipient indications have expanded dramatically. The most common indications in early series included biliary atresia, hepatocellular carcinoma, Laennec's cirrhosis, and cryptogenic cirrhosis.[14,15,44] Today, a broad list of primary hepatic diseases are common indications for liver transplantation (Table 58–2).

Age limitations for potential recipients have undergone significant re-evaluation. An upper limit of 55 years of age was arbitrarily established in most early series, probably based upon a theoretical ability of the younger age groups to tolerate major surgical intervention.[10,42,44] With technical refinements, consideration of the older recipient is now commonplace. Data from the University of Pittsburgh has demonstrated that outcome in patients more than 60 years of age is nearly identical to that for young patients.[45] At the University of California-Los Angeles (UCLA), 90% of recipients older than age 60 were alive at one year. Similar results have been seen at other institutions (Fig 58–3).[46,47] Together, the data indicate the successful outcome in older recipients and confirm the requirement for selection on a case by case basis. A similar evolution has occurred for the opposite extreme of age, although the very young age group remains controversial.[48,49]

Meticulous screening of potential candidates is essential to ensure excellent outcome. Several groups have attempted to identify recipient variables predictive of outcome after liver transplantation. Shaw and associates retrospectively evaluated 118 patients undergoing liver transplantation using a scoring system based upon several preoperative variables.[50] Patient scores then were used to categorize the potential 6-month survival where high-risk patients had a survival of 22% compared with 74% for low-risk patients. Operative blood loss, pretransplant hepatic coma, malnutrition, serum bilirubin, prothrombin time, and date of transplantation had a significant correlation with 6 month mortal-

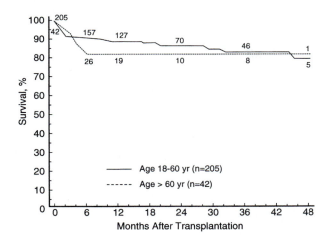

Figure 58–3. Patient outcome based on actuarial percent survival rate is demonstrated graphically. Survival at all time intervals for patients over the age of 60 did not significantly differ from those less than 60. (Redrawn from Keeffe EB, Esquivel CO. Controversies in patient selection for liver transplantation. *West J Med* 1993;159:586–593

ity rates. Shaw and associates found the same scoring system to accurately distinguish low- and high-risk patients.[51]

Similarly, a retrospective evaluation of pretransplant variables in 229 recipients[52] identified the Child-Pugh C classification, the presence of encephalopathy, intensive care requirement, and renal dysfunction as preoperative variables significantly associated with postoperative mortality.

At present, these systems have limited applicability and should not be utilized solely for patient selection purposes. These variables may help identify high-risk patients undergoing liver transplantation.

■ OPERATIVE TECHNIQUE

DONOR HEPATECTOMY

Techniques for harvesting abdominal organs from brain-dead, heart-beating donors have been previously described.[53–55] This discussion will be limited to procurement of the hepatic graft alone and interested readers are referred to other texts for more information on multiple organ procurement.[56]

The majority of liver grafts are obtained as part of a multi-organ procurement. Careful coordination and communication between surgical teams is mandatory for the optimal use of these scarce resources. Supine positioning and standard skin preparation from the neck to the pubis provide optimal exposure. A midline incision is made from the suprasternal notch to the pubis.

The round and falciform ligaments are divided. This approach ensures optimal access to the abdominal and thoracic organs and obviates the need for further subcostal incisions.

Visual and manual inspection of the liver as well as other intra-abdominal viscera is mandatory. The procedure should be abandoned only in instances of significant hepatic trauma, cirrhosis, or an extremely poor-appearing hepatic graft. Marginal grafts should be harvested with decisions on later engraftment made based upon a combination of donor quality, liver function testing, and graft histopathology, as well as the condition of the recipient.

The Traditional Technique

After adequate exposure is obtained, delineation of the vascular anatomy is initiated. First, inspection of the gastrohepatic ligament to identify and preserve a replaced left hepatic artery is accomplished (Fig 58–4).[57] Palpation of the hepatic hilum is undertaken next to identify a common hepatic artery as well as a replaced right hepatic artery. Division of the common bile duct and flushing of the gallbladder is performed. Control of the distal aorta then is obtained, followed by isolation and control of the inferior mesenteric vein.

After ligation of both the right gastric artery and the gastroduodenal artery, the main hepatic artery is dissected back to the aorta. The splenic and left gastric arteries should be ligated during this maneuver, except in the presence of arterial aberrancy.

Control of the portal circulation is addressed. Access to the portal vein is obtained superior to the pancreas and the coronary vein is ligated. The portal vein is freed back to the confluence of the superior mesenteric and splenic veins. Here, portal canulation later may be accomplished or the inferior mesenteric vein may be utilized.

After this dissection is completed, the infradiaphragmatic aorta is usually cross-clamped and instillation of preservation solution into the aortic and portal venous circulation is accomplished. The graft then is removed.

This technique is usually more time consuming than those subsequently described. However, most of the anatomic dissection occurs in vivo prior to the onset of ischemia.

The UCLA Technique

The gastrohepatic ligament is inspected to determine if a replaced left hepatic artery is present. When present, this artery must be spared. The right colon, and the second, third, and fourth portions of the duodenum are mobilized. The superior aspects of both renal veins are identified. The inferior mesenteric vein is cannulated and chilled plasmalyte solution is slowly instilled into the portal circulation. The aorta is encircled just above

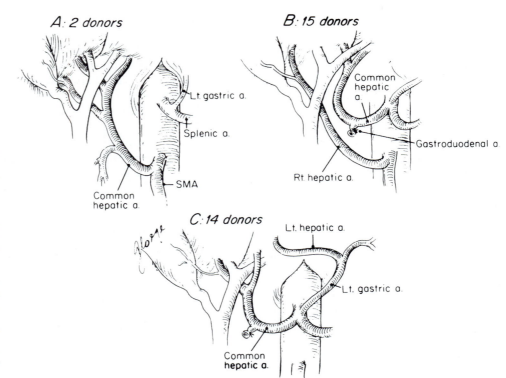

Figure 58–4. Frequently encountered hepatic arterial anomalies are depicted schematically. In this series, 77% of donors had type 1 or normal hepatic arterial anatomy (not pictured). Origination of the entire common hepatic artery off the superior mesenteric artery (type 5) is shown in **A** and occurred in two of 172 donors (1.2%). A replaced right hepatic artery (type 3) originating off the superior mesenteric artery is shown in **B** and was found in 15 of 172 donors (8.7%). A replaced left hepatic artery (type 2) originating off the left gastric artery was seen in 14 of 172 donors (8.1%). Other anomalies encountered include a simultaneous replaced left and right hepatic artery (type 4, 4.1%) and a common hepatic artery arising directly off the aorta (type 6, 0.5%). (Redrawn from Brems JJ, Millis JM, Hiatt JR, et al. Hepatic artery reconstruction during liver transplantation. *Transplantation* 1989;47:403–406)

the bifurcation and the inferior mesenteric artery is ligated. The common bile duct is divided and saline is instilled into the biliary tree via an incision into the gallbladder. Finally, the supraceliac aorta is encircled.

The donor then is heparinized and a large-bore cannula is placed into the distal aorta and connected to the University of Wisconsin (UW) solution. With all teams present and in coordination, the right atrium is incised, the supraceliac aorta is clamped, and the aortic and portal cannulas are allowed to flow freely with UW preservation solution. Ice is placed on all the organs to be harvested (Fig 58–5).[58]

After 2 to 3 L of chilled UW solution are infused, the hepatic artery then is dissected. This dissection is initiated by identifying and dividing the gastroduodenal artery. The hepatic artery is followed down and the splenic artery is divided similarly. Once the dissection has proceeded to the level of the aorta, its anterior surface is dissected and the aorta is divided at the level of the diaphragm. The pancreas is next divided and the portal vein is identified. The superior mesenteric vein and the splenic vein are divided and reflected towards the liver. The base of the mesentery is inspected to identify the superior mesenteric artery. The superior mesenteric artery is dissected from the retropancreatic portion of the aorta to determine if a replaced right hepatic artery exists (Fig 58–4). The infrahepatic vena cava is then divided just above the renal veins. All vascular

structures now have been divided and the liver is freed of any remaining ligamentous attachments. We have reported that 23% of donors will have aberrant arterial anatomy; maintenance of these vessels is critical for successful liver transplantation.[57]

After bilateral donor nephrectomy, the iliac arteries and veins are removed in case arterial or venous grafts are necessary.[59] The liver then is transported back to the recipient hospital and cleanly dissected on the bench. This bench work consists of trimming the suprahepatic cuff and tying the origins of the phrenic vessels. The infrahepatic cuff also is checked for the adrenal vein. The portal vein is freed to its bifurcation. The hepatic artery is dissected to the level of the gastroduodenal artery and any vascular reconstruction is performed involving conduits or cuffs. After completion of this process, the graft is now ready for recipient implantation.

This technique closely resembles the rapid flush technique first introduced at the University of Pittsburgh.[60] Both techniques are particularly useful in the hemodynamically unstable patient.[60]

Few studies exist to compare the traditional and rapid flush techniques. Miller and associates retrospectively compared 157 rapid flush grafts with 280 traditional-technique grafts based on donor and recipient parameters, and primary nonfunction.[61] No significant difference was noted between either donor or recipient group, except for a slightly longer ischemic time when

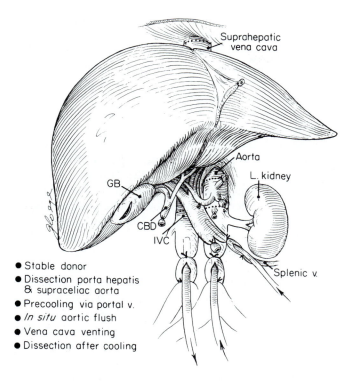

- Stable donor
- Dissection porta hepatis & supraceliac aorta
- Precooling via portal v.
- *In situ* aortic flush
- Vena cava venting
- Dissection after cooling

Figure 58–5. A schematic representation of the donor liver prepared for harvesting. The gallbladder (GB) is shown after incision and drainage and the common bile duct (CBD) is ligated. The suprahepatic and infrahepatic inferior vena cava, celiac trunk, aorta, and portal venous system have been dissected. In this drawing, cannulas have been inserted into the infrarenal aorta and splenic vein for infusion of preservation solution and cooling. A cannula has been placed in the infrahepatic inferior vena cava for venting. (Redrawn from Busuttil RW, Colonna JO II, Hiatt JR, et al. The first 100 liver transplants at UCLA. *Ann Surg* 1987;206:387–402)

using the traditional technique. Grafts harvested by the rapid flush technique demonstrated significantly lower peak aspartate aminotransferase and alanine aminotransferase levels postoperatively, although nonsignificant differences in the prothrombin time and primary graft failure rate were noted. These results establish the rapid flush technique as a safe, reliable procedure capable of producing graft outcomes comparable to those of the conventional technique. However, the rapid flush technique requires complete and expert mastery of the anatomy and should not be performed until the surgeon is fully trained in the traditional method of liver harvesting.

RECIPIENT HEPATECTOMY

In many instances, dissection and removal of the recipient liver is the most demanding part of liver transplantation. Previous abdominal operations, severe hepatic disease, coagulopathy and portal hypertension create technically demanding conditions. However, careful dissection with or without the routine use of venove-

nous bypass allows successful hepatectomy in the face of surgically difficult situations.

Optimal recipient exposure is accomplished using a bilateral subcostal incision with an upper midline extension. The falciform ligament is taken down and dissection is begun in the porta hepatis. The use of venovenous bypass (see below) influences the timing and steps of the hepatectomy. The hepatic artery is ligated first in an attempt to diminish potential bleeding from the hepatic surface. Further hilar dissection allows transection of the bile duct as close to the liver as possible. The portal vein then is isolated and circumferential control is obtained. At this point, patients may be placed on venovenous bypass by cannulating the portal vein as described below. In our opinion, the development of venovenous bypass has facilitated the recipient hepatectomy and subsequent graft implantation. Many centers, including our own, use venovenous bypass almost exclusively in adults.[26]

Passive venous bypass for liver transplantation was first developed in early experimental models.[7,8] Primarily because of the requirement for recipient systemic anticoagulation, its use was not applied to human liver transplantation until almost 20 years later. Persistently significant operative mortality rates without the use of venovenous bypass renewed interest in its use in the early 1980s. Collaboration between cardiothoracic and transplant surgeons led to the development of pump-driven venovenous bypass without heparin.[62–64] The safety of venovenous bypass was demonstrated shortly thereafter.[65]

The application of venovenous bypass to the recipient operation changes the operative approach. Systemic bypass usually is accomplished via the femoral and axillary veins. Splanchnic decompression is accomplished through the portal vein (Fig 58–6). The initial approach to the porta hepatis is undertaken to cannulate and distally ligate the portal vein with subsequent dissection accomplished as described above. Alternatively, bypass can be instituted after complete dissection of the recipient liver and cross-clamping of the venous circulation demonstrates hemodynamic instability. However, in the authors' opinion, one of the major benefits of bypass is to have both the splanchnic and systemic venous systems decompressed during the retrohepatic dissection.

With the portal vein cannulated on bypass, the infrahepatic dissection and circumferential control of the inferior vena cava is obtained easily. The hepatic triangular ligaments are taken down and the suprahepatic inferior vena cava identified. Circumferential control is obtained, ensuring adequate length for construction of a venous cuff. After cross-clamping the suprahepatic and infrahepatic inferior vena cava, these vessels are transected and the diseased liver removed.

Proponents of venovenous bypass cite data that

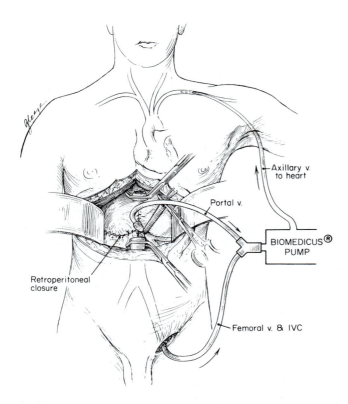

Figure 58–6. The technique of venovenous bypass is represented schematically. Note the femoral and portal veins are cannulated and drained into an external pump. Reinfusion into the systemic circulation is accomplished through the axillary vein. Using this technique, decompression of the splanchnic circulation and restoration of venous drainage from the lower body alleviates hemodynamic instability produced by cross-clamping the inferior vena cava. (Redrawn from Busuttil RW, Colonna JO II, Hiatt JR, et al. The first 100 liver transplants at UCLA. *Ann Surg* 1987;206:387–402)

demonstrate the maintenance of near-normal physiology during the anhepatic phase, a lower requirement for intraoperative blood transfusion, improved postoperative renal function, and a better 30 day mortality rate.[65,66] In contrast, other studies have demonstrated no improvement in patient survival after 180 days, similar renal function and intraoperative transfusion requirements in patients transplanted without the use of venovenous bypass as compared with those using bypass.[67] Overall, most centers prefer the use of venovenous bypass, primarily because of the hemodynamic stability it affords during the anhepatic phase.

An alternative exists that eliminates the need for venovenous bypass. The piggyback technique, introduced at the University of Pittsburgh, allows anastomosis of the suprahepatic inferior vena cava with total diversion of systemic venous return.[68]

RECIPIENT IMPLANTATION

The techniques of graft implantation originally were developed in animal models[7,8] and subsequently ap-

plied to humans.[12,24] The current techniques have been described previously.[55,58]

After removal of the recipient liver, the donor graft is situated in the orthotopic position. The order of the vascular anastomoses usually proceeds with suprahepatic inferior vena cava, infrahepatic inferior vena cava, portal vein, and hepatic artery (Fig 58–7). For reconstructing the suprahepatic and infrahepatic inferior vena cava anastomoses, use of adequate venous cuffs, especially in the suprahepatic location, is crucial (Fig 58–8).[69]

The suturing technique for the suprahepatic and infrahepatic vena caval anastomoses involves the use of a 4-0 polypropolene monofilament. The posterior layer is sewn in a continuous manner from the inside, creating an everting intima-to-intima approximation (Fig 58–9).[9,70] The anterior layer is sutured externally using either an interrupted or continuous technique.

In all vascular anastomoses, particularly in children and young adults, incorporation of a growth factor is essential for prevention of later anastomotic strictures. The technique involves the use of a continuous anterior and posterior polypropylene monofilament anastomosis in which the rows are tied loosely together to allow for anastomotic expansion (Fig 58–10).[71] In experienced hands, the growth factor has minimal bleeding problems and prevents future anastomotic stricture.

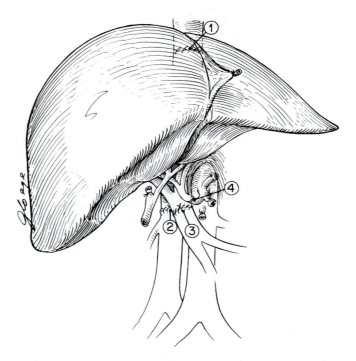

Figure 58–7. The order of vascular anastomoses during graft implantation is demonstrated. (1) Suprahepatic to suprahepatic inferior vena cava, (2) infrahepatic to infrahepatic inferior vena cava, (3) portal to portal vein, and (4) hepatic artery to artery. See text for further details. (Redrawn from Busuttil RW, Colonna JO II, Hiatt JR, et al. The first 100 liver transplants at UCLA. *Ann Surg* 1987;206:387–402)

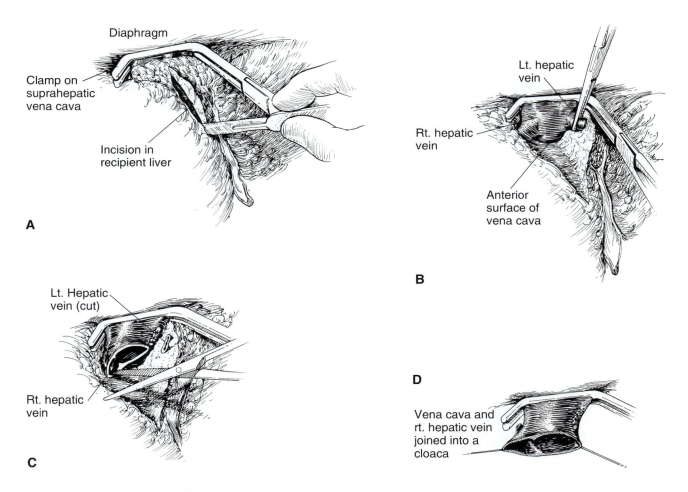

Figure 58–8. The creation of sufficient suprahepatic inferior vena cava cuff is paramount to successful revascularization. Chronic disease states and hepatic inflammation can produce a shortened infradiaphragmatic suprahepatic inferior vena cava segment. One method to rectify this situation is schematically represented here. **A** and **B.** Adequate suprahepatic inferior vena cava length may be obtained by the intraparenchymal dissection of the hepatic veins and suprahepatic inferior vena cava. **C.** Oversewing one hepatic vein (the left in this case). **D.** Creation of a common cloaca between the opposite hepatic vein and the inferior vena cava creates an adequate cuff for anastomosis. (Redrawn from Starzl TE, Koep LJ, Weil R III, Halgrimson CG. Development of a suprahepatic recipient vena cava cuff for liver transplantation. *Surg Gynecol Obstet* 1979;149:76–77

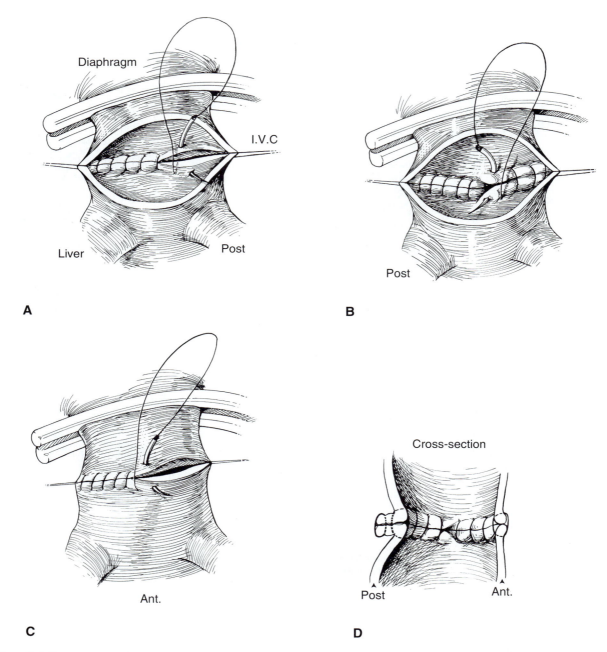

Figure 58–9. The technique for inferior vena cava reconstruction is shown diagramatically. From left to right, the anastomosis of the inferior vena cava is completed from the inside on the posterior layer (step 1 and 2) and from exterior on the anterior layer (step 3). The everting technique resulting from intima to intima approximation is shown in cross-section. (From Starzl TE, Marchioro TL, Von Kaulla KN, et al. Homotransplantation of the liver in humans. *Surg Gynecol Obstet* 1963;117:659–676)

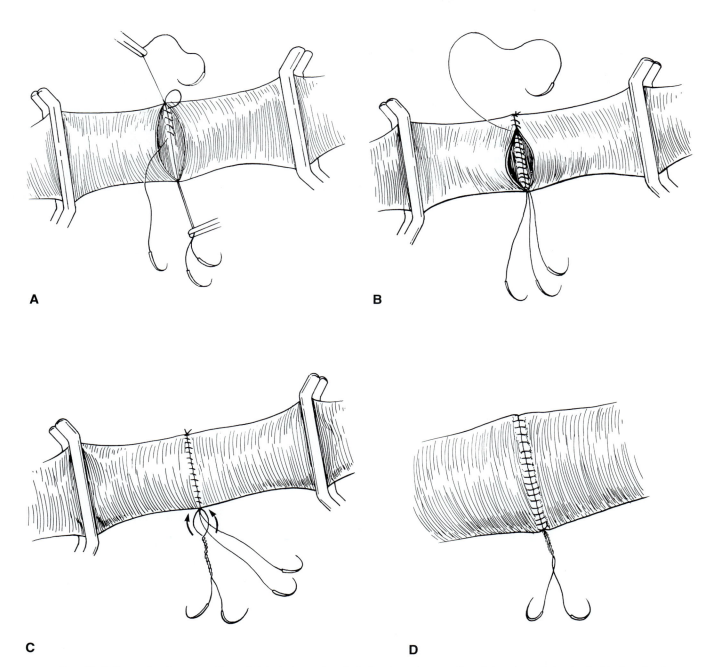

A

B

C

D

Figure 58–10. The creation of an anasomotic growth factor is shown schematically. **A.** polypropylene monofilament stay sutures are placed on the lateral margins of the vessels. The anterior and posterior layers are completed in a continuous fashion. **B.** The free ends are tied in an air knot which is approximately one-third the vessel circumference. Upon release of the clamps, the slack is reincorporated into the anastomosis leaving a bulging suture line. (Redrawn from Starzl TE, Iwatsuki S, Shaw Jr BW. A growth factor in fine vascular anastomoses. *Surg Gynecol Obstet* 1984;159:164–165)

Alternatively, absorbable monofilament suture can be used to prevent anastomotic strictures. The University of Chicago recently reported their experience using polyglyconate for all venous anastomoses.[72] No venous complications related to the suture material were reported, leading the group to advocate the use of absorbable monofilaments for vascular anastomoses during liver transplantation.

Alterations in the standard implantation techniques are employed when anomalies in the inferior vena cava exist. Although infrequent (<4% of patients),[73–75] these anomalies include interrupted inferior vena cava between the renal veins and diaphragm, and noncommunicating retrohepatic inferior vena cava. To efficiently handle such anomalies without compromising graft function, simple oversewing of the donor infrahepatic inferior vena cava is recommended. Alternate methods using allograft or bioartificial conduits have been described but are time consuming and offer no real advantages.

The third anastomosis, restoring portal continuity, is accomplished using standard techniques as described above for the inferior vena cava. Fine (6-0 to 7-0) polypropylene suture is employed and a growth factor included as needed. Since the transplanted liver has few collaterals and relies heavily on portal venous flow for viability, inadequate inflow or technical mistakes can be disastrous.

Further increasing the complexity of this anastomosis is the frequently encountered presence of portal venous pathology. Central shunts in the form of end-to-side or side-to-side portocaval shunts require dismantling during graft implantation. Techniques for shunt dismantling have been described (Fig 58–11) and are usually initiated after the completion of the suprahepatic inferior vena cava anastomosis.[76] The easiest shunt to dismantle is the mesocaval H graft which requires simple ligation. The end-to-side and side-to-side portocaval shunts are more difficult to dismantle and are associated with higher intraoperative blood loss, increased incidence of primary nonfunction and longer hospitalization.[76,77] Distal shunts (splenorenal) usually do not require takedown after implantation.[78]

Once considered a contraindication to liver transplantation,[79] the presence of portal vein thrombosis now does not preclude graft implantation. This conclusion was first realized at the University of Pittsburgh where two patients with portal vein thrombosis were successfully engrafted using iliac vein graft from the confluence of the superior mesenteric vein (SMV) and splenic vein.[80] Subsequently, publications from the same[74,81] as well as other centers[77,82] have confirmed the technical feasibility of transplantation in the face of portal vein thrombosis. Operative techniques applied to the thrombosed vein include thrombectomy of the native vessel, retrograde dissection to the splenomesenteric junction and the use of venous conduits. Most series report few venous complications,[74,80,82,83] while others have noted increased incidences of primary non-

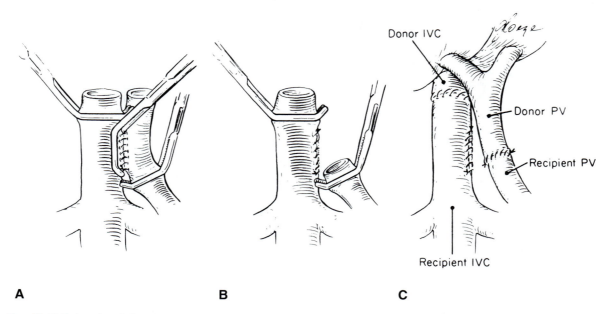

A   **B**   **C**

Figure 58–11. During orthotopic liver transplantation, the presence of proximal portocaval shunts increases the complexity of the procedure. A technique for dismantling end to side portacaval shunts is shown schematically. **A.** After completion of the suprahepatic inferior vena cava anastomosis, a vascular clamp is applied to occlude inflow from the portal vein and distal inferior vena cava. **B.** The shunt is dismantled. **C.** The vessels repaired. (Redrawn from Brems JJ, Hiatt JR, Klein AS, et al. Effect of prior portasystemic shunt on subsequent liver transplantation. *Ann Surg* 1989;209:51–56)

function, prolonged hospital stay, and higher 90 day mortality rates.[77] Despite this controversy, successful engraftment has been achieved in patients with portal vein thrombosis.

Flushing of the graft prior to revascularization is essential for removal of the preservation solution and trapped air within the graft. The initial flush, occurring prior to completion of the infrahepatic inferior vena cava anastomosis, is accomplished through a cannula present in the portal vein using cold lactated Ringer's solution. A second flush may take place after completion of the portal anastomosis using splanchnic blood vented out the infrahepatic inferior vena cava anastomosis. We recommend inclusion of the second flush only if there is a special concern of hemodynamic instability secondary to hyperkalemia at the conclusion of reperfusion. Restoration of blood flow to the hepatic graft is initiated after the completion of the portal anastomosis and prior to commencing arterial anastomosis.

The principles of hepatic arterialization during graft implantation include ensuring pulsatile inflow through a large caliber vessel over a short length. Arterial inflow is crucial to postoperative graft function, primarily because the transplanted liver lacks collateral flow and is extremely sensitive to ischemia. Furthermore, the blood supply of the bile duct is derived exclusively from the hepatic artery.

The anastomotic technique involves the use of a fine (6-0 to 7-0) polypropylene monofilament to create an end-to-end anastomosis. The vessel is sewn from the outside and rotated to achieve the most precise anastomosis. A continuous or interrupted suturing technique can be used. Application of the branch-patch technique is strongly urged to reduce postoperative arterial complications (Fig 58–12).[84]

Aberrant hepatic arterial anatomy is seen in 45% of patients at autopsy[85] and 33% of organ donors (Fig 58–6).[55,57,58] Preservation of accessory arteries is essential for complete arterialization. For type 3 anatomy (replaced right hepatic artery), back-table, ex vivo reconstruction of the arterial supply to create a single inflow vessel can simplify the recipient operation (Fig 58–13). Type 2 (replaced left hepatic artery) anatomy requires no further manipulation other than preservation of the left gastric artery during procurement. Likewise, type 5 (common hepatic artery originating off the superior mesenteric artery) and type 6 (common hepatic artery originating off the aorta) anatomy require only careful identification and preservation during organ procurement and implantation. Type 4 anatomy (right hepatic

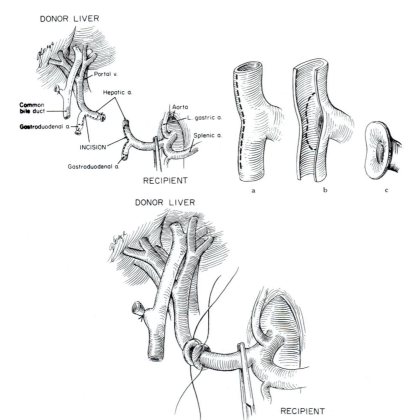

Figure 58–12. The branch patch technique for hepatic arterialization is shown schematically. **A.** An arterial bifurcation is chosen for application of this technique as shown, where the hepatic-gastroduodenal artery bifurcation is utilized. **B.** Creation of a patch from both branches is shown. **C.** Anastomosis of donor and recipient arteries follows. (Redrawn from Quinones-Baldrich WJ, Memsic L, Ramming K, et al.)

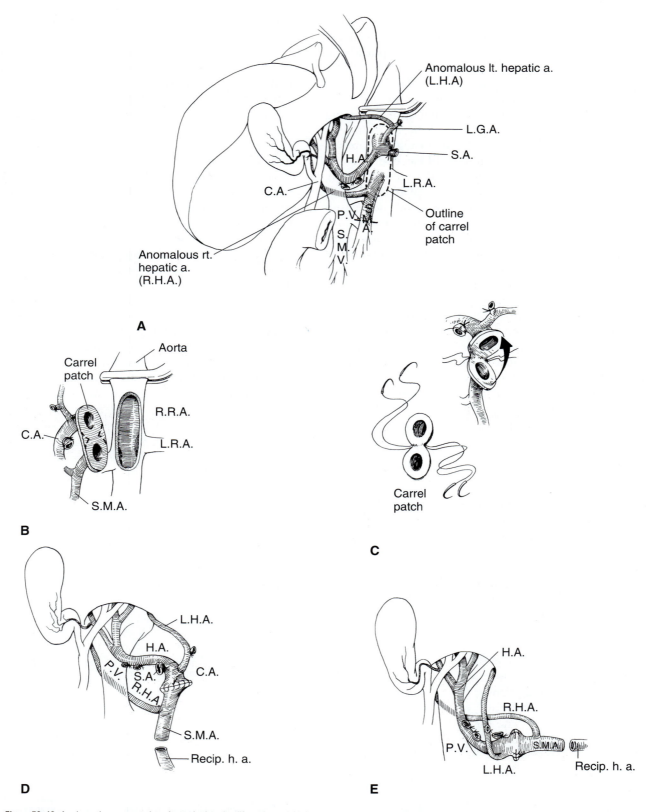

Figure 58–13. A schematic representation of a method to simplify graft arterial inflow in type 4 (shown here), 3, or 2 hepatic arterial anatomy. **A.** The native anatomy demonstrates an anomalous or replaced right hepatic artery off the superior mesenteric artery as well as a replaced left hepatic artery off the left gastric artery. **B.** Procurement involves a carrel patch of the aorta that includes the celiac trunk and superior mesenteric artery. **C** and **D.** The end-to-end anastomosis of the celiac trunk and superior mesenteric artery to create a single inflow vessel is demonstrated. **E.** The proper vascular orientation is shown. (Redrawn from Gordon RD, Shaw BW Jr, Iwatsuki S, et al. A simplified technique for revascularization of homografts of the liver with a variant right hepatic artery from the superior mesenteric artery. *Surg Gynecol Obstet* 1985;160:475–476)

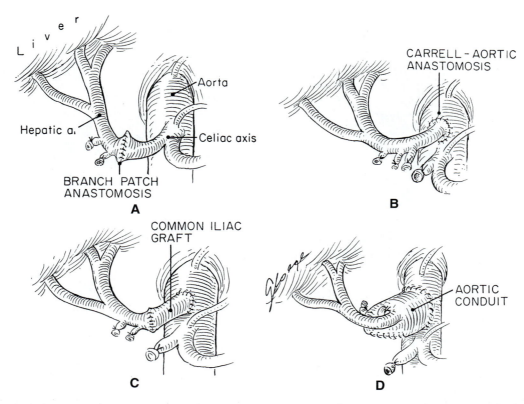

Figure 58–14. Alternatives for arterial inflow are represented schematically. **A.** A standard hepatic to hepatic arterial anastomosis using the branch patch technique is demonstrated. **B.** Arterial inflow is obtained from the supraceliac aorta using a Carrel patch of the donor hepatic artery or celiac trunk. In **C.** a donor iliac artery interposition graft is shown. **D.** A donor aortic conduit is represented. (Redrawn from Shaked A, Takiff H, Busuttil RW. The use of the supraceliac aorta for hepatic arterial revascularization in transplantation of the liver. *Surg Gynecol Obstet* 1991;173:198–202)

artery originating off the superior mesenteric artery combined with the left hepatic artery originating off the left gastric artery) is encountered less frequently and is reconstructed in a similar manner to a replaced right hepatic artery alone.[57]

When adequate arterial inflow cannot be obtained through the recipient native hepatic artery, the use of arterial conduits is indicated. Inflow originating from both the infrarenal and supraceliac aorta has been described. Advocates for an infrarenal approach report no difference in arterial complications (compared with standard arterial inflow through the native vessels) and feel that the infrarenal aorta provides technically simpler access.[87,88] Those in favor of supraceliac inflow (including the authors), cite the use of a shorter conduit distance, lower incidence of hepatic artery thrombosis and avoidance of retropancreatic dissection as proof of superiority.[89,90] In either case, the anastomotic techniques are similar, with only the path of the graft tunnel differing (Fig 58–14).[89] In both, utilization of donor arterial conduits is preferred.

Completion of vascular anastomoses is followed by the establishment of biliary continuity. The most common methods used are choledochocholedochostomy (bile duct to bile duct) and choledochojejunostomy (bile duct to jejunum). Factors influencing the method used include the size of the donor and recipient common bile duct and the presence of preexisting biliary pathology. In general, choledochojejunostomy is utilized in pediatric recipients, recipients (both pediatric and adult) with preexisting biliary pathology, including sclerosing cholangitis and malignancy. Choledochocholedochostomy can be utilized safely in all other recipients. The technical aspects of the biliary anastomosis involve ensuring a tension-free anastomosis, the use of fine absorbable monofilament suture and anastomotic stents (Fig 58–15).[58]

Alternatives have been described. A technique utilizing the gallbladder as a conduit has been largely abandoned.[24] More recently, techniques successfully employing side-to-side choledochocholedochostomy[91] and end-to-end choledochocholedochostomy without T tube stenting[92] have been reported.

AUXILIARY TRANSPLANTATION

Heterotopic positioning of the liver graft during transplantation was first described in the early experimental animal studies by Welch and associates.[4,6] The graft was placed in the right lower abdomen and vascular conti-

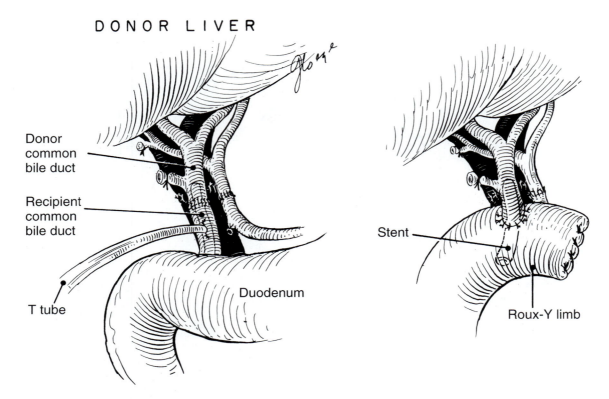

Figure 58–15. Methods of biliary reconstruction are demonstrated schematically. A choledochocholedochostomy over a T tube stent is shown on the left. A choledochoenterostomy over an internal stent is demonstrated on the right. See text for indications. (Redrawn from Busuttil RW, Colonna JO II, Hiatt JR, et al. The first 100 liver transplants at UCLA. *Ann Surg* 1987;206:387–402)

nuity was achieved by anastomosing the donor suprahepatic inferior vena cava to the recipient infrahepatic inferior vena cava, the donor celiac axis to the abdominal aorta, and the donor portal vein to the recipient distal inferior vena cava. The donor infrahepatic inferior vena cava was ligated and the recipient liver was left in its native position. The authors reported success, defined as survival more than 5 days and bile production for at least one day, in 21 to 49 heterotopic transplants. However, heterotopic positioning soon was found to be associated with graft atrophy, which limited the utility of the procedure.

In an elegant series of experiments, Starzl and his associates addressed the problem of liver atrophy and, in the process, identified hepatotrophic substances in the splanchnic blood. In their first publication,[93] auxiliary liver transplantation was performed in dogs with total portal venous blood or splanchnic venous (from SMV only) diverted to the graft. Atrophy was noted only in the livers that did not receive portal venous flow. Inflow via the SMV alone failed to prevent this process. In a follow-up study, the same group surgically produced either partial portacaval transposition or partial splanchnic flow diversion into separate hepatic lobes of dogs.[94] Lobes that received either portal blood flow or inflow

from the pancreatic, gastroduodenal, and splenic circulation demonstrated hypertrophy. Hepatic lobes receiving either systemic or splanchnic (SMV alone) venous inflow demonstrated marked atrophy. This hepatotrophic effect of the portal blood was further investigated in a third publication from the same group.[95] Total portacaval shunts were created in dogs with one lobe of the liver perfused via a portal venous cannula using either insulin, glucagon, or a combination of both. Insulin produced a strong hepatotrophic response, while glucagon demonstrated either no effect or a negative effect. As a result of these works, the importance of portal venous blood, and specifically insulin, on hepatic viability was elucidated and auxiliary liver transplantation was reinstituted as a viable clinical option.

The clinical application of auxiliary transplantation has been limited. Initially, nine human attempts in the 1960s using this technique failed, resulting in death within 34 days.[96] Clinical successes were reported in 1973 by Fortner and associates.[97] Grafts were placed in the right paravertebral region with arterial inflow via the infrarenal aorta, portal venous inflow via the SMV, and venous outflow through the infrahepatic inferior vena cava. The suprahepatic inferior vena cava was ligated (Fig 58–16). One patient was reported alive while

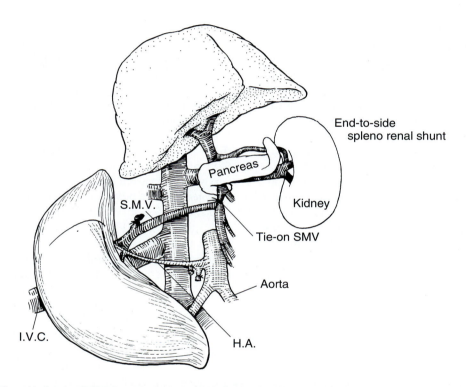

Figure 58–16. The positioning of an auxiliary liver transplant is shown schematically. The native, disease liver is left in the orthotopic position. The transplanted graft is placed in the right paracolic gutter. Arterial and portal venous inflow is obtained from the infrarenal aorta and the superior mesenteric vein, respectively. Venous outflow is into the infrarenal inferior vena cava via the donor infrahepatic inferior vena cava. Note the donor suprahepatic inferior vena cava is oversewn. (Redrawn from Fortner JG, Kinne DW, Shiu MH, et al. Clinical liver heterotropic (auxiliary) transplantation. *Surgery* 1973;74:739–751)

the other two died 37 and 240 days after transplantation, respectively, from nontechnical causes. The authors acknowledged the technical feasibility of the procedure. Other centers have subsequently reported attempted heterotopic transplantation.[98–102] Terpstra and associates[98] reported six patients who underwent heterotopic transplantation for end-stage liver disease secondary to hepatitis B, primary sclerosing cholangitis and α-1-antitrypsin deficiency. No increased perioperative morbidity was noted and all patients were reported alive with functioning grafts with a mean follow-up of 14 months.

Despite these efforts, auxiliary liver transplantation in humans has been slow to gain acceptance. The reasons are multifactorial but mainly related to the tremendous success of orthotopic liver transplantation. The technique of auxiliary liver transplantation persists and remains an option for patients with end-stage liver disease. Proponents tout its potential advantages, including decreased morbidity associated with removal of the native liver, diminished patient mortality related to graft failure (the native graft remains in place), and fewer donor size restrictions.[98] In addition, auxiliary liver transplantation is advocated as a "bridge" in patients with potentially reversible fulminant hepatic failure.[103] However, opponents cite overall poor clinical outcome, the continued presence of the diseased native liver, and the success of orthotopic grafting as reasons for limited application of auxiliary transplantation.[103] Regardless, auxiliary transplantation holds a prominent historical position related to the development of the technical and physiological aspects of liver transplantation and still has limited clinical application in very select transplant candidates.

REDUCED-SIZE, SPLIT, AND LIVING-RELATED TRANSPLANTATION

Shortages in donor organs, particularly in the pediatric population, has led to innovative techniques designed to expand the donor pool. Reduced-size liver transplants, in which a hepatic lobe is transplanted into a smaller donor, was first introduced successfully in 1981.[104] Shortly thereafter, the concept of split liver transplantation, in which two recipients receive a hepatic lobe from the same donor, was introduced.[105] The techniques of both split- and reduced-sized liver grafting are derived from anatomical description of hepatic segments (Fig 58–17).[101,106]

The successful application of these techniques is demonstrated in a University of Chicago study in which 61 procedures (26 reduced, 30 split, and 5 living-related liver transplants) were performed.[101] Biliary atresia was the most common indication for transplantation, and 62% of patients were <2 years of age. Overall patient survival rates varied by the type of graft used. Split-graft recipients had a 67% survival rate, reduced-graft recipients had a 78% survival rate, and living-related graft recipients had a 100% survival rate. These rates did not differ markedly from recipients of whole grafts. Furthermore, although split liver grafts were associated with the highest complication rate, the overall rate

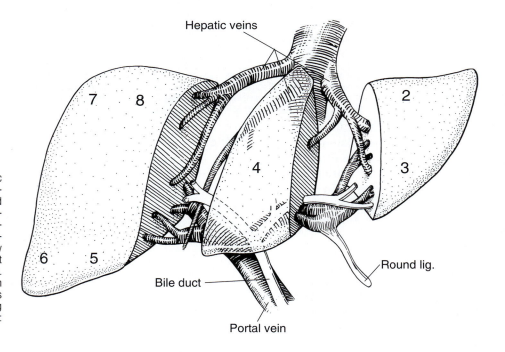

Figure 58–17. A schematic representation of hepatic segmental anatomy is shown. The principles of hepatic resection, split-grafting and reduced-sized grafting are based upon a thorough knowledge of hepatic segmental anatomy. The division of the 8 segments is based upon portal venous branching and hepatic venous drainage. The relation of the biliary ducts and the hepatic artery (not shown) also must be taken into account when splitting liver segments. (Redrawn from Broelsch CE, Emond JC, Whitington PF, et al. Application of reduced-size liver transplants as split grafts, auxiliary orthotopic grafts, and living related segmental transplants. *Ann Surg* 1990;212: 368–377)

again did not differ from recipients of full-size grafts. The results led the authors to recommend the application of these techniques as a viable method of increasing the donor pool, especially for pediatric recipients. Similar results and conclusions have been reported by other groups.[106]

■ IMMUNOSUPPRESSION

GENERAL

A detailed discussion of all immunosuppressive options is beyond the scope of this chapter. The success of clinical liver transplantation has, however, been directly related to the development of newer immunosuppressive agents. The art of administering immunosuppressive regimens lies in the ability to achieve a delicate balance between rejection and infection, thus maximizing patient survival and minimizing morbidity.

AZATHIOPRINE

Azathioprine (Imuran) and its metabolite 6-mercaptopurine interfere with DNA synthesis through their ability to impair purine biosynthesis.[108] The earliest experimental and human trials involved the use of either no immunosuppression or various combinations of azathioprine, prednisone, actinomycin C, azaserine, antithymocyte globulin along with thymectomy or splenectomy.[9] The use of azathioprine as a primary immunosuppressant was clinically introduced in the early 1960s[9] with the most successful regimen being a double or triple drug combination based upon azathioprine and prednisone with or without antilymphocyte globulin. Actual patient survival at 1 year was 10% to 19% in adults and 36% in children.[15,86] Azathioprine is no longer used as a primary immunosuppressant but instead is incorporated into combination drug therapy.

CYCLOSPORINE

Perhaps no other immunosuppressive agent has radically impacted transplantation as much as the introduction of cyclosporine (Sandimmune) in 1976.[16] Cyclosporine A is a peptide isolated from the fungus *Tolypocladium inflatum Gams*. Its immunosuppressive properties are exerted on T lymphocytes through inhibition of cell activation and proliferation.[109] By 1978, the first clinical trials using cyclosporine A as a primary immunosuppressant were published in patients undergoing renal allotransplantation.[17]

In 1979, the application of cyclosporine A to clinical liver transplantation produced revolutionary results.[17] Large series from the University of Pittsburgh,[19] UCLA,[58] and in Europe[110] demonstrated 1 and 2 year survival rates as high as 74% and 73% respectively. These results were three times higher than those seen previously using noncyclosporine A–based immunosuppression (Fig 58–1). Later series reported further progress with 1 year patient survival rates of 88% mostly owing to improved intensive care monitoring, expanded experience, improved operative techniques, and advances in antimicrobial treatment.[26]

OKT3

OKT3 (Orthoclone) was first developed in 1979 using hybridoma technology.[111] It is a murine monoclonal IgG_{2A} antibody specific for the CD3 complex found on all circulating T lymphocytes.[112] The binding of OKT3 to this molecule interferes with the process of antigen recognition and signal transduction that is normally accomplished via the T-cell receptor and adjacent CD3 complex.[112] To this end, OKT3 has tremendous immunosuppressive potential.

In 1981, OKT3 was first introduced into clinical transplantation through trials in renal transplant recipients by Cosimi and associates.[113] Its prophylactic use as a primary agent was reported in several studies from UCLA.[114,115] In a randomized study, OKT3 combined with low-dose steroids (n=46) was compared with cyclosporine A, azathioprine, and steroids (n=39) as primary immunosuppression regimens. With a mean follow-up of nearly 2 years, no differences in the regimens were seen when comparing the number of rejection episodes in the first month, long-term renal function, infectious episodes, graft- or patient-survival. A significant difference in the number of rejection episodes during the first 14 postoperative days favoring the OKT3 group was noted in an earlier study.[114] In contrast, Fung and associates, in a review of prophylactic OKT3 use,[116] found improved short- and long-term renal function while also reporting no differences in long-term patient or graft outcome. As a result, the prophylactic use of OKT3, particularly in patients with preoperative renal dysfunction, is frequently employed.

FK-506

The isolation and introduction of FK-506 from the fungus *Streptomyces tsukubaensis* was reported in 1986.[117] It is a potent immunosuppressant of the macrolide antibiotic family which exerts its effects primarily by inhibiting activation and proliferation of T lymphocytes.[118] The first clinical trials utilizing this agent were reported by Starzl and associates for liver, kidney and pancreas transplantation.[119]

The first trial comparing this agent with cyclosporine A for liver transplantation was completed in 1991.[120] Eighty-one patients were enrolled in the study with no statistically significant difference noted in patient (93%

for FK-506 vs 81% for cyclosporine A) or graft (90% for FK-506 vs 70% for cyclosporine A) survival rates at 1 year. Significant differences favoring FK-506 were seen in the mean time to first rejection (21.5 days vs 9.9 days, $P<.005$), the rejection-free rate at 1 month (18% vs 61%, $P<.001$), and the mean number of steroid boluses per patient required in the first 90 days (0.50 vs 0.99, $P<.01$). Fewer FK-506 patients required OKT3, while 29 of 40 cyclosporine A–treated patients were converted to FK-506 mainly owing to rejection.

More recently, a study involving 12 transplant centers and 529 patients comparing the two agents was published.[121] Two hundred and sixty-three patients were randomized to the FK-506 limb and 266 to the cyclosporine A limb. No significant difference were seen between agents with regard to 1 year patient survival and graft survival. Significant differences favoring the FK-506 group were noted in the number of patients with biopsy-proven rejection, requiring OKT3 for rejection, and with refractory rejection. Adverse reactions, seen frequently in both groups, were significantly more frequent in the FK-506 group and included gastrointestinal symptoms, neurologic effects, renal effects, electrolyte abnormalities, and anemia.

These results, in addition to the lower steroid requirement and lower incidence of hypertension with FK-506, confirm the effectiveness of FK-506 as a primary immunosuppressant in patients undergoing liver transplantation. At present, it can be concluded that FK-506 provides a consistent alternative to cyclosporine A for primary immunosuppression in liver transplantation. Furthermore, FK-506 provides another option for rescue therapy in refractory rejection.

■ TECHNICAL COMPLICATIONS

GENERAL

Technical complications were formerly the leading cause of failure following liver transplantation. Advances in surgical techniques have reduced the incidence and impact of these complications. Presently, primary nonfunction, hepatic artery thrombosis, portal vein thrombosis, biliary problems, infection, and rejection represent the most common postoperative complications.

PRIMARY NONFUNCTION

Strictly speaking, primary nonfunction can be defined as poor initial graft function after transplantation not attributable to technical problems. Clinically, characteristic poor graft function manifested by inadequate bile production, coagulopathy, markedly elevated transaminases, encephalopathy, and acidosis are the hallmark findings in the early postoperative period. Graft recovery is unlikely and patient mortality is as high as 80% unless retransplantation is undertaken.[122]

The etiology of primary nonfunction is unknown. Investigation has focused on the role of preservation injury and prolonged ischemia.[122] Animal models have demonstrated that the hepatic sinusoidal endothelium is more sensitive to ischemia than hepatocytes and may contribute to the development of primary nonfunction.[123] In one study, research attempting to identify donor variables associated with this development has been conflicting, with donor age, length of hospitalization, and temperature implicated.[124] Others have found donor criteria to be unreliable and unpredictable in regards to graft outcome.[37] One variable, graft steatosis, is a reliable predictor of primary nonfunction,[41] leading most surgeons to reject donor livers with >40% macrosteatosis.[26]

Regardless, primary nonfunction occurs in 4% to 20% of grafts after liver transplantation.[26,110,122] Early recognition and urgent retransplantation is imperative for patient survival. Nonsurgical therapies have not proven efficacious to date. Potential medical treatments include the use of intravenous prostaglandin E_1,[122] but randomized control trials are needed to determine their effectiveness.

HEPATIC ARTERY THROMBOSIS

Hepatic artery thrombosis is a potentially devastating early postoperative technical complication. Liver grafts, having been subjected to ischemia and lacking collateral circulation, are particularly sensitive to the loss of hepatic arterial perfusion. Acutely, hepatic artery thrombosis typically presents as a sudden elevation of transaminases, prolongation of the prothrombin time, encephalopathy, and hemodynamic instability, although as many as 20% to 30% may be asymptomatic.[2] Diagnosis is confirmed using angiography or duplex ultrasonography. False-negative results have been reported using the latter technique.[125]

The incidence of hepatic artery thrombosis is 3% to 5% in adult and 10% to 20% in pediatric recipients.[57,126,127] Risk factors associated with its development include a small-diameter vessel, long inflow length, technically difficult anastomosis, and uncontrolled rejection. Preexisting donor arterial anomalies have been shown in several studies not to increase the incidence.[126]

The treatment of hepatic artery thrombosis is related to the chronicity of the problem as well as the resulting liver function. For acute, early hepatic artery thrombosis in which hepatic function is significantly impaired, therapy typically involves prompt identification and retransplantation. Increasingly, hepatic artery reconstruction and thrombectomy have been successfully applied to grafts after acute hepatic artery thrombosis. Rethrombosis, however, remains a problem.[128,129] Regardless, the mortality remains as high as 58%.[126] Hepatic artery thrombosis without significant liver dysfunction, regardless of the chronicity, can be managed expectantly, at least for the short-term. However, in the majority of patients, biliary strictures will result in cholangitis, with the need for ultimate regrafting.

PORTAL VEIN THROMBOSIS

Postoperative portal vein thrombosis is infrequently seen after liver transplantation. The incidence is reported to occur in less than 3% of recipients.[74] Preoperative portal vein thrombosis, the presence of portosystemic shunts, and the use of vein grafts/conduits have been identified as risk factor predisposing to postoperative thrombosis.[74,77] Patients may present with a clinical picture of acute liver failure or esophageal varices. Alternatively, symptoms may be absent, as seen in a study from the University of Pittsburgh in which 43% of patients had good liver function despite the presence of portal vein thrombosis.[74]

The diagnosis is usually confirmed using venous duplex sonography or angiography.[130] Treatment depends largely on hepatic function and can include thrombectomy, anastomotic revision, portosystemic shunts, retransplantation, or observation. The prognosis varies, with long-term survivors reported using all modalities.[74,77]

BILIARY COMPLICATIONS

Biliary reconstruction was once described as the "Achilles heel" of the recipient procedure.[10] Complications occur in as many as 34% of these patients after liver transplantation.[58,131] Most commonly, these complications include anastomotic leaks, anastomotic strictures, or intrahepatic strictures.[132] A higher frequency of biliary complications has been seen in recipients of ABO-incompatible grafts.[133] The association between hepatic artery thrombosis and biliary complications is well documented.[134] In a study by Colonna and associates, 9 of 25 patients with anastomotic or intrahepatic postoperative biliary strictures were found to have hepatic artery thrombosis.[135] This association is explained by the fact that the blood supply to the common bile duct is exclusively derived from the hepatic artery. Furthermore, this relation mandates that hepatic artery thrombosis be investigated in all liver transplantation patients with biliary complications.

As mentioned previously, two methods of biliary reconstruction, choledochocholedochostomy and choledochojejunostomy, are most commonly employed. Choledochojejunostomy can carry a higher complica-

tion rate than choledochocholedochostomy.[131,135] The major reason for this difference relates to the use of choledochojejunostomy in pediatric recipients, recipients with small ducts, previous underlying duct pathology, or difficult anastomosis.

Methods of handling biliary complications are evolving and are dependent on recipient liver function and condition.[135] Conservative management has been applied successfully to patients with stable liver function and no systemic compromise. Surgical intervention is reserved for patients with biliary sepsis, intra-abdominal sepsis or impaired liver function. Surgical options include anastomotic revision or conversion to choledochojejunostomy. Less invasive methods such as CT-guided drainage of bile collections, transhepatic stenting and drainage and endoscopic retrograde pancreaticography have been employed with increasing success.[131,136] A systematic approach to management is strongly recommended (Fig 58–18).[135] Using a multimodality management approach, patient and graft survival has achieved 76% and 64%, respectively, in some series.[135] Clearly, continued efforts to improve techniques are needed.

INFECTION

Infection remains one of the most serious and frequent complications in patients undergoing liver transplantation. Up to 83% of all recipients experience a significant postoperative infectious episode.[137,138] Many of the early (within 6 months) postoperative deaths are directly attributable to infectious complications.[137] Bacterial infections are most common, followed by viral and then fungal infections.[137,138] The most frequent organisms isolated within each category are gram-negative bacteria, cytomegalovirus (CMV) and *Candida*, respectively. The onset is usually within the first two postoperative months,[139] contributing significantly to postoperative morbidity and mortality.

Early identification is crucial for successful treatment, particularly in transplant recipients in whom the presence of immunosuppression significantly impairs the ability to resist rapid progression and dissemination of invading micro-organisms. Most transplant centers rely heavily on routine surveillance cultures and aggressive work-up of constitutional symptoms for detection. Analysis of factors contributing to infectious susceptibility have revealed that surgical factors are the most important.[137] Specifically, prolonged operating time, multiple abdominal operations, biliary complications and hepatic artery thrombosis demonstrate the strongest association.

The use of antimicrobial prophylaxis is now routine because of the frequency and gravity of postoperative infections in the transplant population. Administration of prophylactic antibiotics protects against postoperative in-

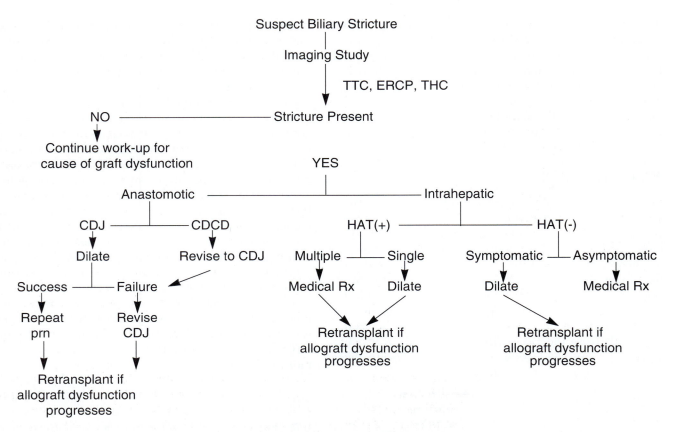

Figure 58–18. A suggested algorithm for the management of biliary strictures after liver transplantation. Abbreviations used include T tube cholangiogram (TTC), Endoscopic retrograde cholangiopancreatography (ERCP), transhepatic cholangiogram (THC), hepatic artery thrombosis (hepatic artery thrombosis), choledochojejunostomy (CDJ), choledochocholedochostomy (CDCD). (Redrawn from Colonna JO II, Shaked A, Gomes AS, et al. Biliary strictures complicating liver transplantation: incidence, pathogenesis, management, and outcome. *Ann Surg* 1992;216:344–350)

fections by specific microorganisms.[137] Antimicrobial agents targeted against a broad-spectrum of bacterial agents are mandatory during the first 48 hours after transplantation. Prophylactic administration of trimethoprim-sulfamethoxazole (Bactrim) is effective in reducing the incidence of posttransplant *Pneumocystis carinii*.[139,140] The prophylactic administration of both acyclovir (Zovirax) and ganciclovir (Cytovene) reduces the postoperative incidence of CMV infection in transplant recipients.[141,142] Caution should be exercized with prophylactic antibiotic administration resulting from the association between prolonged antibiotic use and fungal infection.[143] In high-risk cases requiring prolonged antibiotic administration, prophylactic amphotericin should be considered.

When infection is present, treatment should be based upon suspected etiology. Early, broad-spectrum antimicrobial therapy should be initiated after pertinent cultures have been obtained. Aggressive search for site of origin should be undertaken using radiography, sonography, and computerized tomography (CT). Percutaneous or surgical drainage of fluid collections or

abscesses should be emergently performed. Despite an aggressive approach, infectious-related mortality after liver transplantation is as high as 14%.[138] Minimization of immunosuppression and advances in antimicrobial agents should help reduce this rate.

REJECTION

General

Rejection presents a diagnostic and therapeutic dilemma after liver transplantation. Almost all recipients experience at least one rejection episode, most of which are classified as mild or moderate.[58,144] Severe rejection, although occurring less frequently, historically has negatively impacted survival. In a study from UCLA, 21 (25%) of 83 patients experienced a rejection episode that was refractory to steroid therapy.[58] Thirteen of these patients had a complete response and 8 had a partial response to therapy with OKT3. In this latter group, two patients (25% of patients with refractory rejection) required retransplantation with a survival rate of 57%. This data represent the potential morbidity and mortality associated with severe rejection, although newer therapeutic options now have been introduced as discussed below.

Prompt identification and treatment of rejection is essential for effective reversal. Although acute allograft rejection is the most common cause of early postoperative graft dysfunction,[145] other causes, such as primary nonfunction, hepatic artery thrombosis, cholestasis, infectious hepatitis, drug toxicity, and sepsis must be ruled out. Evaluation of all suspected rejection episodes should consider cultures of body fluids, broad-spectrum antibiotics, hepatic duplex sonography, HIDA scanning, cholangiogram, and percutaneous liver biopsy.

Acute Rejection

Diagnostic confirmation of rejection is achieved using a combination of clinical, laboratory, and histopathologic criteria. Acute liver rejection presents with classic constitutional symptoms and physical signs such as fever, anorexia, malaise, decreased bile output, and a change in bile color. Laboratory evaluation reveals variable degrees of elevation in serum transaminases, cholestasis, and impaired hepatic synthetic function. Definitive diagnosis can be difficult without tissue confirmation.

Percutaneous liver biopsy is a safe, effective means to assist with definitive diagnosis of posttransplant graft dysfunction. Large series from the University of Pittsburgh and UCLA have demonstrated that liver biopsy specimens in the setting of postoperative graft dysfunction confirm the presence of rejection in up to half of the specimens.[145,146] Other causes of graft dysfunction are seen in up to 51%, although as many as 15% were nondiagnostic. Biopsy complication rates were <1%, in experienced hands.[145]

Several histologic patterns have been described in acute allograft rejection.[145–147] These include portal inflammation with bile duct injury, hepatocyte ballooning, hepatocyte necrosis (either focal or confluent), or a mixed histologic picture containing elements of more than one of the aforementioned predominant patterns. The presence of cholestasis is a common but nonspecific finding in acute hepatic allograft rejection.

An algorithmic approach to management of suspected acute rejection is recommended. An intravenous bolus of methylprednisolone (20 mg/kg) for 2 days is employed. Prompt, complete clinical response requires no further treatment. Failure to normalize liver function tests requires an intravenous methylprednisolone recycle for 5 days, starting with 30 mg/kg and tapering to 0.3 mg/kg. Responders require no further treatment, while nonresponders mandate additional intervention, including consideration of repeat biopsy.

For steroid-resistant rejection, the effectiveness of OKT3 has been demonstrated in several studies.[148–150] Colonna and associates reported 25 patients with steroid-resistant rejection treated with a 10 to 14 day course of OKT3 using a dose of 2.5 to 5.0 mg/day.[148] Ninety-six percent of patients had either complete or partial response to therapy, with 80% of grafts salvaged and 88% of patients saved. Adverse reactions included constitutional symptoms (≤72%), viral infections (20%), and recurrent rejection responsive to steroids (40%). Serum antibodies against the murine component of OKT3 have been detected in nearly all patients undergoing therapy.[149] Their presence does not preclude successful repeat therapy[150] although the dosage required may be higher.

Retransplantation is the last option available to treat refractory rejection. It is reserved primarily for patients with irreversible hepatic failure secondary to uncontrolled acute rejection. While occuring infrequently, acute rejection is reported the cause of death in ≤20% of patients.[10] Survival after retransplantation for rejection is diminished. Shaw and associates report a 1 year survival rate of 42% after retransplantation[152] while Brems and colleagues[144] report a 33% survival rate for the same situation. Clearly, patient salvage is possible but alternative means of controlling acute rejection are needed.

Chronic Rejection

Chronic rejection (along with the vanishing bile duct syndrome) is characterized by the progressive deterioration in liver function primarily manifested as cholestasis.[10] The histopathologic picture is one of progressive thickening of the intima of hepatic artery branches by fat-laden macrophages, rapid disappearance of the interlobular bile ducts, dense mononuclear portal infiltrate, centrolobular cholestasis, and deposition of reticulin bands.[10,12] The process is not readily reversed by changes in immunosuppression. Retransplantation represents the only treatment option at this time.

Antibody-Mediated Rejection

Once thought not to exist in hepatic transplantation,[12] antibody-mediated or "hyperacute" rejection is now a recognized entity. Particularly with ABO-incompatible grafts, antibody-mediated rejection in the early postoperative period has been described.[153,154] Its presence has also been reported after ABO-identical liver transplantation.[155] Strict defining criteria includes the absence of other causes of early graft failure, characteristic histopathologic findings, presensitized recipient state and demonstration of donor-specific antibodies.[153] Potentially, hyperacute rejection may represent a larger proportion of early graft loss previously attributed to primary nonfunction.[154] Retransplantation represents the only treatment for antibody-mediated rejection.

The question of donor cross-matching remains an issue. Early human and experimental liver transplantation suggested that the liver is less susceptible than other organs to immunological-mediated injury.[3,14] Furthermore, successful liver transplantation across ABO barriers,[10] in the presence of preformed antibodies,[156] and in the absence of human leukocyte antigen (HLA) matching[157] questions the need for donor typing.

However, evidence is accumulating to challenge these dictums. In a study from the University of Pittsburgh, a higher acute graft failure rate (46% vs 11%, *P*<.02) was seen in recipients of ABO-incompatible grafts as compared with ABO-compatible grafts.[153] A graft-versus-host-like reaction manifested by hemolysis resulting from iso-hemagglutinins derived from the graft has been described.[158,159] Under FK-506 immunosuppression, a lower 6 month actuarial graft survival has been demonstrated (49% vs 92%) in patients with a >50% positive and panel reactive antibodies as compared with those without presensitization.[160] Furthermore, a recent study from the University of Wisconsin involving 236 patients demonstrated a significant correlation between HLA matching of class I molecules and graft survival.[161] Together, these studies raise questions related to the need for standard tissue typing in liver transplantation. However, until further data is available, current practices using ABO matching only should be continued.

■ OUTCOME

GENERAL

Overall, recipient outcome after liver transplantation has improved dramatically over the past two decades (Fig 58–19). The reasons behind this improvement are multifactorial.

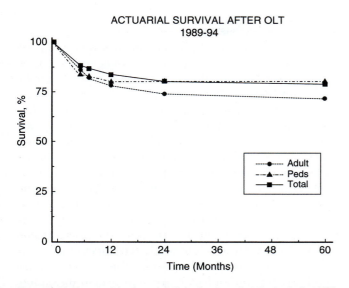

ACTUARIAL SURVIVAL AFTER OLT 1989-94

Figure 58–19. The actuarial patient survival after liver transplantation for the first 1000 liver transplants performed at UCLA is shown. Adults, pediatric and overall rates are included.

BILIARY ATRESIA

Although early portoenterostomy can be curative in some infants with biliary atresia, the majority of patients continue to manifest liver failure requiring transplantation. Biliary atresia remains the most common indication for pediatric liver transplantation at most centers, including our own.[162] Although earlier reports indicated otherwise,[163] the results after liver transplantation for biliary atresia in more recent studies demonstrate 1 and 3 year survival rates of 78% and 75%, respectively.[164–166] Improved outcome is realized with early referral for liver transplantation, fewer pretransplant abdominal surgical procedures, and flexible utilization of reduced-, split- or living-related grafts.

PRIMARY BILIARY CIRRHOSIS AND PRIMARY SCLEROSING CHOLANGITIS

Primary biliary cirrhosis and primary sclerosing cholangitis are common causes of cholestatic end-stage liver disease. Both diseases are characterized by a variable natural history, thereby making the timing of liver transplantation crucial. Several mathematical models based upon patient variables have been developed in an effort to predict the optimal timing for liver transplantation in these patients.[167–169] Inevitably, timing is based upon clinical condition and rate of deterioration of liver function.

Outcome after liver transplantation for primary sclerosing cholangitis was recently analyzed by Abu-Elmagd and associates.[170] Two hundred sixteen patients underwent transplantation and were compared with a control group of 392 patients whose outcome was predicted by the Mayo Clinic mathematical model. With a mean follow-up of 34 ± 25 months, the actual survival at 1 and 5 years was 86% and 73%, respectively. The survival rate represents a significantly improved outcome when compared with the control group (Fig 58–20). Other centers also have reported excellent outcomes in these patients.[171] Similar results were reported by Markus and associates for primary biliary cirrhosis (Fig 58–21).[172] Together, these studies provide evidence supporting the efficacy of appropriately timed liver replacement in patients with primary sclerosing cholangitis and primary biliary cirrhosis.

ALCOHOLIC CIRRHOSIS

Transplantation for alcoholic/Laennec's cirrhosis, although one of the earliest indications for liver transplantation, has been slow to gain acceptance. Ethical considerations and high potential recidivism rates have been responsible for this trend. In 1988, Starzl and associates reported 41 patients with alcoholic cirrhosis.[173] Survival after liver transplantation in these recipients

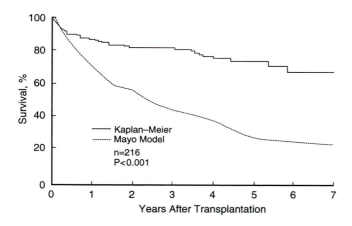

Figure 58–20. The actual survival after liver transplantation in patients with primary sclerosing cholangitis as compared to a cohort of patients predicted by the Mayo model. Statistically significant survival was seen at all time points. Borrowed with permission from *Surg Gynecol Obstet* (1993);335–344

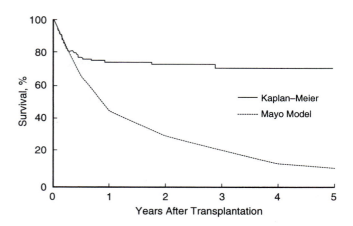

Figure 58–21. The actual survival of 161 patients with primary biliary cirrhosis is shown compared to a control cohort of 312 patients whose survival was predicted using the Mayo model. The differences in survival reached significance after the first three post-transplant months. (Redrawn from Markus BH, Dickson ER, Grambsch PM, et al. Efficacy of liver transplantation in patients with primary biliary cirrhosis. *N Engl J Med* 1989;320:1709–1713)

did not significantly differ from that of patients with other types of cirrhosis, and a low recidivism rate (5.7%) was reported. Subsequent studies have confirmed the excellent survival statistics, albeit with slightly higher recidivism rates (<20%) (Fig 58–22).[43,46,174]

Transplantation for alcoholic cirrhosis has steadily increased. At UCLA, 1% of all candidates between 1984 and 1986 suffered from alcoholic cirrhosis, compared with 20% between 1991 and 1992.[26] Strict criteria should be employed in the patient selection process. At UCLA, that criteria includes participation and completion of a substance abuse rehabilitation program, proven abstinence for at least 6 months prior to transplantation, preoperative psychological assessment, and the presence of strong support groups. Only after these criteria have been met should consideration for transplantation be undertaken.

HEPATITIS B VIRUS

Transplantation for hepatitis B virus-associated liver disease remains controversial. Although those with hepatitis B virus-induced fulminant liver failure or chronic hepatitis B virus cirrhosis associated with delta infection may have lower recurrence rates (<30%), patients with chronic hepatitis B virus-induced cirrhosis suffer from high reinfection rates and reduced survival.[175–178] Jurim and associates reported 45 patients with chronic hepatitis B virus cirrhosis undergoing liver transplantation.[179] Overall, Asians fared significantly worse than non-Asians, with recurrent hepatitis B virus infection rates as high as 72% and mortality owing to reinfection as high as 87% (Table 58–6). This poor outcome is

probably a result of circulating or extrahepatic hepatitis B virus reinfection of the transplanted graft. Patients with active pretransplant hepatitis B virus replication, as demonstrated by hepatitis Be antigen or hepatitis B virus DNA in the serum, have higher recurrence rates than do patients without active viral replication, with associated delta infection or those with fulminant hepatitis B virus liver failure.[177] The facilitating role of immunosuppression remains controversial.[179]

The poor outlook recently has been improved with the use of antiviral prophylaxis. First introduced at King's College, Cambridge in 1978,[180] the use of passive anti-hepatitis B surface antigen prophylaxis has shown promise. Samuel and associates have used a protocol of long-term anti-hepatitis B surface antigen immunoprophylaxis in patients undergoing liver transplantation for all forms of hepatitis B virus.[181] The actuarial recurrence rates at 1 and 2 years were 17% and 29%, respectively. Again, patients with fulminant hepatitis B virus or hepatitis B virus with delta infection fared better than those with chronic hepatitis B virus cirrhosis. Those with evidence of active viral replication pretransplant demonstrated the worse outcome, with 2 year actuarial recurrence rates of 96%. Other methods of prophylaxis, such as anti-hepatitis B surface antigen vaccination, recombinant interferon-α, or Vidarabine, have been attempted with limited results.[179] As a result, our policy in patients with liver disease secondary to hepatitis B virus is to transplant only using immunoprophylaxis with polyclonal anti-hepatitis B surface antigen, which is administered long-term. Patients are serially monitored and the serum anti-hepatitis B immunoglobulin is maintained greater than 100 IU/mL.

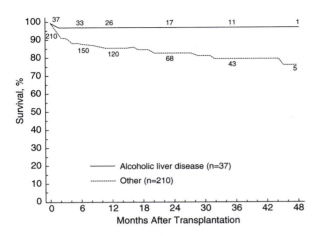

Figure 58–22. The actuarial percent survival of patients undergoing liver transplantation for alcoholic cirrhosis as compared to those undergoing transplantation for other indications is shown. Superior survival is demonstrated at all time intervals. (Redrawn from Keeffe EB, Esquivel CO. Controversies in patient selection for liver transplantation. *West J Med* 1993;159:586–593)

HEPATITIS C VIRUS

Hepatitis C virus (HCV), first identified in 1989, accounts for the majority of cases of non-A, non-B hepatitis in the United States and produces a high rate of chronic liver disease after infection.[182] Hepatitis C virus is most often acquired through blood transfusion or intravenous drug use, although up to 50% of patients have no identifiable risk factor.[182]

Patients undergoing liver transplantation for HCV-induced chronic liver disease almost uniformly manifest evidence of recurrent infection. In a study by Shiffman and associates, 25 patients with cirrhosis secondary to hepatitis C virus were followed for an average of 22 ± 1.9 months after liver transplantation.[183] Five patients died from causes unrelated to hepatitis C virus infection and four underwent retransplantation unrelated to hepatitis. Recurrent hepatitis C infection was documented in all patients with at least 6 months follow-up, although most cases were reported to be mild or subclinical. An 88% 1 year survival rate was reported. The results led the authors to support the use of liver transplantation in patients with end-stage liver disease secondary to hepatitis C virus.

Other important considerations prudent to hepatitis C virus and liver transplantation include the potential peritransplant acquisition of the virus from blood transfusion or organ donors.[182] As a result, further evaluation of hepatitis C virus and liver transplantation is ongoing. Until more data are available, continued application of liver transplantation to appropriate candidates with hepatitis C virus is appropriate.

HEPATOCELLULAR CARCINOMA

Transplantation for primary hepatic malignancies has changed significantly over the last decade. Today, the major malignancy for which liver transplantation is indicated is hepatocellular carcinoma. Large series from the University of Pittsburgh,[184] King's College, Cambridge[185] and UCLA,[186] report overall survival rates as high as 64% at 1 year and 45% at 5 years. The controversy lies in the significant recurrence rates (as high as 65%) seen after transplantation. By examining subgroups of patients with hepatocellular carcinoma, patients with a more favorable prognosis can be identified.

Few would argue that transplantation for hepatocellular carcinoma with extrahepatic spread is not indicated and that transplantation for incidental hepatocellular carcinoma (stage I disease by the American Joint Committee on Cancer staging) is associated with excellent survival. The controversy involves patients with lesions confined to the liver of a more advanced stage. This issue was closely examined in a recent review from UCLA[187] that concluded that patients with lesions confined to the liver but unresectable by conventional techniques can benefit from liver transplantation. Furthermore, patients with significant liver dysfunction in the setting of hepatocellular carcinoma are treated best by transplantation due to the higher mortality associated with hepatic resection in patients with cirrhosis.[185] Factors associated with lower recurrence rates and improved survival are smaller tumors (<5 cm), the fibrolammellar histological variant, well-differentiated subtypes, multifocality with three or fewer nodules, and a lack of vascular invasion.[187] Multimodality therapy combining surgery and adjuvant chemotherapy,[187,188] or transarterial chemoembolization,[187] appears to offer an improved outlook over transplantation alone. As a result, most centers continue to perform transplants in patients with hepatocellular carcinoma but use careful screening to determine those who will most benefit from the procedure.

TABLE 58–6. RESULTS OF OLT FOR ASIANS AND NON-ASIANS

	Asians	Non-Asians
Total no. of patients	16	29
Early mortality	5/16 (31%)	1/29 (3%) $P<0.05$
Recurrent HBV infection	8/11 (72%)	9/28 (32%) $P<0.05$
Mortality due to recurrent HBV infection	7/8 (87%)	2/9 (22%) $P<0.05$

The results of liver transplantation in patients with chronic HBV cirrhosis is demonstrated according to race. Asians fared significantly worse than other groups with significantly higher early mortality, recurrent HBV infection and late mortality rates.
(From Shiffman ML, Contos MJ, Luketic VA, et al. Biochemical and histological evaluation of recurrent hepatitis C following orthotopic liver transplantation. Transplantation. 1994;57:526–532)

TABLE 58–7. LIVER TRANSPLANTATION PROCEDURE CHARGES[a]

Item	Charge ($)
Laboratory	52,304
Organ procurement	26,456
Intensive care unit room and board	20,240
Semiprivate room and board	19,113
Operating room, recovery room, anesthesia	17,394
Pharmacy and intravenous solutions	14,305
Radiology	8395
Blood processing	8341
Respiratory therapy	6346
Medical and surgical supplies	3193
CT	2374
Other ancillary procedures (including but not limited to EEG, EKG, physical therapy, and diet instruction)	1809
Average professional fees for surgeons, anesthesiologists, and radiologists	36,000
Total	216,000

[a]Estimates are based on an average hospital stay of 46 days: 13 in intensive care and 33 in a semiprivate room.
Data from Children's Hospital of Pittsburgh, based on liver transplants done in fiscal year 1986–87; Presbyterian-University Hospital.

■ FULMINANT HEPATIC FAILURE

In some centers, up to 15 percent of patients undergo LTx for fulminant hepatic failure.[165] The most common etiology of fulminant liver failure is viral hepatitis secondary to non-A, non-B hepatitis, HBV, and hepatitis A virus.[1,2] Traditionally, these patients have experienced a poorer outcome due to their premorbid condition. However, the outlook is improving.

Ascher and associates from the University of California, San Francisco reported 35 patients who underwent LTx for fulminant hepatic failure.[192] A 92 percent 1- and 2-year actuarial patient survival rate and an 83 percent graft survival was achieved. No patient with non-A, non-B, non-C hepatitis developed a recurrence. Twenty-nine percent of patients with fulminant hepatitis secondary to HBV developed a recurrence within 2 years of transplantation. The authors attributed these exceptional results to a systematic approach to pretransplant management, early listing for organ donors and careful patient selection.

In general, donor organ availability has been a significantly limiting factor in patient survival from fulminant hepatic failure. Improvements may be forthcoming with the development of bioartificial livers[3], the innovative use of donor livers,[4,101] the exploration into xenotransplantation,[193] auxiliary transplantation and the utilization of prolonged anhepatic phase.[194,195]

■ RETRANSPLANTATION

Irreversible graft failure after LTx is fatal unless retransplantation is undertaken. The incidence of re-transplantation varies by transplant center and indication for LTx with most centers reporting rates less than 27%.[196] The highest retransplantation rates are seen in patients with primary sclerosing cholangitis.[196] The most common indications for retransplantation in adults include PNF, HAT and chronic rejection[197] while HAT is the leading indication in children.[197]

Historically, the outcome after retransplantation has differed markedly from that after primary transplantation.[155] Recent data from several centers has demonstrated a more optimistic outlook. At UCLA, the first 100 patients undergoing LTx between 1984 and 1986 were compared to the last 200 patients between 1991 and 1992[26]. The 1-year survival rate after retransplantation improved during that interval from 54% to 74%, respectively. Further analysis has shown a significant difference in outcome when patients undergoing "elective" retransplantation are compared to those undergoing "emergent" retransplantation. Survival rates for the former are more similar to that of primary, elective transplantation, as demonstrated in studies from the University of Wisconsin[197] and Baylor University.[196] Still, the most common cause of death in patients undergoing retransplantation remains sepsis and multiorgan system failure.[155] Attempts to identify clinical criteria which may favorably influence clinical outcome after retransplantation have been limited.[197]

This data present an ethical delimma that continues to be source of debate. Are the limited resources of organs and money best applied to those in need of primary LTx or those in need of retransplantation? Furthermore, should recipients be limited in the number of grafts they receive? These questions obviously have no easy solution. One can conclude from the current state of affairs that retransplantation is a practical option in select patients and that the timing of retransplantation is critical to patient outcome.

■ FINANCIAL CONSIDERATIONS

Financial considerations promise to play an ever increasing role in health care allocation in general, and in transplantation, specifically. As this country enters a health care revolution, policy-makers, insurors, hospital administrators, and physicians will continue to reevaluate the allocation medical procedures which carry a significant financial impact. Organ transplantation is one such procedure.

Liver transplantation is the most expensive single surgical procedure. The average cost of LTx for the acute phase is close to 200 000 although considerable variation has been reported in numerous studies.[198] The actual breakdown of this cost (Table 58–6) reveals a significant proportion allocated towards laboratory, organ procurement, and professional fees.[198] Factors related to increased cost include race, multiple transplantations, pre-transplant recipient status, teaching hospitals, and more active programs.[198] Furthermore, ongoing outpatient follow-up, rehospitalizations and medication cost certainly increase this figure by an estimated $20,556.[198]

Reimbursement for the procedure is primarily from third-party payors. Prior to endorsement by the National Institutes of Health concensus conference in 1983,[20] few third party payors covered LTx. Currently, it is estimated that over 80% of private and public insurance carriers cover the procedure.[198] In 1988, nearly 70% of all liver transplants were paid for by private insurance.[198] However, third party reimbursement does not necessarily equate with hospital procedural cost leading to a potential money-losing discrepancy for hospitals.

Already, efforts are underway at many centers to reduce the expense of LTx. Early patient referral as well as advances in intensive care monitoring, operative techniques, antimicrobial prophylaxis, and immuno-suppression promise to improve patient outcome and decrease patient hospital stay. Continued progress in this regard can help solidify the use of the procedure on future potential recipients.

■ CONCLUSION

Since the initial trials in the late 1950's, the results after LTx have continued to improve. Today, the procedure is performed daily in many centers worldwide. Survival rates have climbed to as high as 88 percent at 1-year and operative mortality rates have dropped to as low as zero percent.[26] The reasons behind this improvement are multiple and include:

1) Advances in the donor hepatectomy and graft preservation techniques have afforded extended preservation times and improved early recipient survival. Expansion of the donor pool has been created through the evaluation and use of older donors, suitable "marginal" donors, and living-related donors as well as through the application of innovative graft splitting techniques. Still, no reliable assay of donor variables as yet exists to predict postoperative graft function.

2) Prudent recipient selection has provided LTx for those best able to tolerate the procedure and for those with hepatic diseases are most amendable to transplantation. Simultaneously, a trend toward earlier evaluation and transplantation of patients with ESLD has led to improved operative outcomes. Critical evaluation of those recipients with controversial indications such as HBV and hepatic malignancy should continue.

3) The widespread use of venovenous bypass has in-

creased patient tolerance of the procedure, decreased the intraoperative blood loss, and improved the technical difficulty of the procedure. Further improvements in surgical technique involving vascular anastomoses and biliary reconstruction have led to decreased operative times and postoperative complications. Furthermore, technical advances have allowed successful transplantation in patients with inadequate arterial inflow or PVT.

4) Early identification and aggressive treatment of postoperative complications such as PNF, HAT, PVT and biliary problems has led improved patient survival.

5) Advances in immunosuppression and antimicrobial prophylaxis have reduced the incidence and impact of postoperative rejection and infection. Newer forms of immunotherapy such as FK-506 and RS-61443 have provided alternative methods of treatment for refractory rejection diminishing the requirement for retransplantation.

Overall, the future of LTx remains promising. Potential future obstacles include organ shortages, expanding recipient pool and financial constraints. Current research efforts in the fields of immunomodulation, rejection and molecular biology may favorably impact the prognosis after LTx. Further effort directed toward improving patient survival and expanding the donor pool is needed.

REFERENCES

1. *Clinical Transplants 1992.* Los Angeles, CA: UCLA Tissue Typing Laboratory; 1992:656
2. Starzl TE, Demetris AJ, Van Thiel D. *Liver transplantation* Part 1. *N Engl J Med* 1989;321:1014–1022
3. Starzl TE, Demetris AJ, Van Thiel D. Liver transplantation Part 2. *N Engl J Med* 1989;321:1092–1099
4. Welch CS. A note on transplantation of the whole liver in dogs. *Transplant Bull* 1955;2:54–55
5. Cannon JA. Letter. *Transplant Bull* 1956;3:7
6. Goodrich EO Jr, Welch HF, Nelson JA, et al. Homotransplantation of the canine liver. *Surgery* 1956;39:244–251
7. Moore FD, Wheeler HB, Demissianos HV, et al. Experimental whole-organ transplantation of the liver and of the spleen. *Ann Surg* 1960;152:374–387
8. Starzl TE, Kaupp HA Jr, Brock DR, et al. Reconstructive problems in canine liver homotransplantation with special reference to the postoperative role of hepatic venous flow. *Surg Gynecol Obstet* 1960;111:733
9. Starzl TE, Marchioro TL, Von Kaulla KN, et al. Homotransplantation of the liver in humans. *Surg Gynecol Obstet* 1963;117:659–676
10. Busuttil RW, Goldstein LL, Danovitch GM, et al. Liver transplantation today. *Ann Intern Med* 1986;104:377–389
11. Fonkalsrud EW, Stevens GH, Joseph WL, et al. Orthotopic

liver allotransplantation using an internal vascular shunt. *Surg Gynecol Obstet* 1968;127:1051–1057

12. Starzl TE, Iwatsuki S, Van Thiel DH, et al. Evolution of liver transplantation. *Hepatology* 1982;2:614–636

13. Starzl TE, Groth CG, Brettschneider L, et al. Orthotopic homotransplantation of the human liver. *Ann Surg* 1968; 168:392–415

14. Starzl TE, Porter KA, Putnam CW, et al. Orthotopic liver transplantation in ninety-three patients. *Surg Gynecol Obstet* 1976;142:487–505

15. Calne RY, William R. Orthotopic liver transplantation: the first 60 patients. *Br Med J* 1977;1:471–476

16. Borel JF, Feurer C, Magnee C, Stahelin H. Effects of the new antilymphocytic peptide cyclosporin A in animals. *Immunology* 1977;32:1017–1025

17. Calne RY, Rolles K, White DJG, et al. Cyclosporin A initially as the only immunosuppressant in 34 recipients of cadaveric organs: 32 kidneys, 2 pancreases, and 2 livers. *Lancet* 1979; November 17:1033–1036

18. Calne RY, Rolles K, White DJG, et al. Cyclosporin-A in clinical organ grafting. *Transplant Proc* 1981;13:349–358

19. Iwatsuki S, Starzl TE, Todo S. Experience in 1000 liver transplants under cyclosporine-steroid therapy: a survival report. *Transplant Proc* 1988;20:498–504

20. National Institutes of Health Concensus Developmental Conference Statement: Liver Transplantation—June 20–23, 1983. *Hepatology* 1984;4:107s–110s

21. Jamieson NV, Sundberg R, Lindell S, et al. Preservation of the canine liver for 24–48 hours using simple cold storage with UW solution. *Transplantation* 1988;46:517–522

22. Kalayoglu M, Sollinger HW, Stratta RJ, et al. Extended preservation of the liver for clinical transplantation. *Lancet* 1988; March 19:617–619

23. Olthoff KM, Millis JM, Imagawa DK, et al. Comparison of UW solution and Euro-Collins solutions for cold preservation of human liver grafts. *Transplantation* 1990;49:284–290

24. Calne RY, Williams R. Liver transplantation. *Curr Prob Surg* 1979;16:3–44

25. Beecher HK. A definition of irreversible coma: report of the Ad Hoc Committee of the Harvard Medical School to examine the definition of brain death. *JAMA* 1968;205: 337–340

26. Busuttil RW, Shaked A, Millis JM, et al. One thousand liver transplants: the lessons learned. *Ann Surg* 1994;219: 490–499

27. Mora NP, Turrion VS, Pardo F, et al. Relevance of donor liver selection and graft viability in a liver transplantation program. *Transplant Proc* 1988;20:978–979

28. Mor E, Klintmalm GB, Gonwa TA, et al. The use of marginal donors for liver transplantation: a retrospective study of 365 liver donors. *Transplantation* 1992;53:383–386

29. Teperman L, Podesta L, Mieles L, Starzl TE. The successful use of older donors for liver transplantation. *JAMA* 1989;262:2837

30. Ploeg RJ, D'Alessandro AM, Knechtle SJ, et al. Risk factors for primary dysfunction after liver transplantation—a multivariate analysis. *Transplantation* 1993;55:807–813

31. Peabody JL, Emery JR, Ashwal S. Experience with anencephalic infants as prospective organ donors. *N Engl J Med* 1989;321:344–350

32. Brink LW, Ballew A. Care of the pediatric organ donor. *AJDC* 1992;146:1045–1050

33. Diaz JH. The anencephalic organ donor: a challenge to existing moral and statutory laws. *Crit Care Med* 1993;21: 1781–1786

34. Yokoyama I, Tzakis AG, Imventarza O, et al. Pediatric liver transplantation from neonatal donors. *Transpl Int* 1992;5: 205–208

35. Avolio AW, Agnes S, Magalini SC, et al. Importance of donor blood chemistry data (aspartate aminotransferase, serum sodium) in predicting liver transplant outcome. *Transplant Proc* 1991;23:2451–2452

36. Pruim J, Hesselink EJ, de Vos R, et al. The validity of clinical parameters for the selection of liver donors. *Transplant Proc* 1988;20:973

37. Makowka L, Gordon RD, Todo S, et al. Analysis of donor criteria for the prediction of outcome in clinical liver transplantation. *Transplant Proc* 1987;19:2378–2382

38. Schroeder TJ, Pesce AJ, Ryckman FC, et al. Selection criteria for liver transplant donors. *J Clin Lab Anal* 1991;5: 275–277

39. Burdelski M, Oellerich M, Lamesch P, et al. Evaluation of quantitative liver function tests in liver donors. *Transplant Proc* 1987;19:3838–3839

40. Shimada M, Yanaga K, Higashi H, et al. Pretransplant assessment of human liver grafts by plama lecithin:cholesterol acyltransferase (LCAT) activity in multiple organ donors. *Transpl Int* 1992;5:27–30

41. Todo S, Demetris AJ, Makowka L, et al. Primary nonfunction of hepatic allografts with preexisting fatty infiltration. *Transplantation* 1989;47:903–905

42. Busuttil RW, Memsic LDF, Quinones-Baldrich W, et al. Liver transplantation at UCLA: program development, organization, initiation, and early results. *Am J Surg* 1986;152:75–80

43. Lake JR. Changing indications for liver transplantation. *Gastroenterol Clin North Am* 1993;22:213–229

44. Van Der Putten ABMM, Bijleveld CMA, Slooff MJH, et al. Selection criteria and decisions in 375 patients with liver disease, considered for liver transplantation during 1977–1985. *Liver* 1987;7:84–90

45. Stieber AC, Gordon RD, Todo S, et al. Liver transplantation in patients over sixty years of age. *Transplantation* 1991;51:271–273

46. Keeffe EB, Esquivel CO. Controversies in patient selection for liver transplantation. *West J Med* 1993;159:586–593

47. Castaldo P, Langnas AN, Stratta RJ, et al. Liver transplantation in patients over 60 years of age. *Gastroenterology* 1991;100:a727

48. Belani KG, Batra YK, Naasz M, et al. Infants are a higher intraoperative risk group for orthotopic liver transplantation. *Transplant Proc* 1994;26:196–197

49. Beath S, Brook G, Kelly D, et al. Improving outcome of liver transplantation in babies less than 1 year. *Transplant Proc* 1994;26:180–182

50. Shaw BW Jr, Wood RP, Gordon RD, et al. Influence of selected patient variables and operative blood loss on six-month survival following liver transplantation. *Semin Liver Dis* 1985;5:385–393

51. Shaw BW Jr. Exclusion criteria for liver transplant recipients. *Transplant Proc* 1989;21:3484–3486

52. Baliga P, Merion RM, Turcotte JG, et al. Preoperative risk factor assessment in liver transplantation. *Surgery* 1992; 112:704–711

53. Hiatt JR, Quinones-Baldrich WJ, Ramming KP, Busuttil RW. Orthotopic transplantation. *Surg Rounds* 1986;9:17–27

54. Starzl TE, Hakala TR, Shaw BW Jr, et al. A flexible procedure for multiple cadaveric organ procurement. *Surg Gynecol Obstet* 1984;158:223–230

55. Starzl TE, Iwatsuki S, Esquivel CO, et al. Refinements in the surgical technique of liver transplantation. *Semin Liver Dis* 1985;5:349–356

56. Merkel FK, Jonasson O, Bergan JJ. Procurement of cadaveric donor organs: evisceration technique. *Transplant Proc* 1972;4:585–589

57. Brems JJ, Millis JM, Hiatt JR, et al. Hepatic artery reconstruction during liver transplantation. *Transplantation* 1989;47:403–406

58. Busuttil RW, Colonna JO II, Hiatt JR et al. The first 100 liver transplants at UCLA. *Ann Surg* 1987;206:387–402

59. Starzl TE, Halgrimson CG, Koep LJ, et al. Vascular homografts from cadaveric organ donors. *Surg Gynecol Obstet* 1979;149:737

60. Starzl TE, Miller C, Broznick B, Makowka L. An improved technique for multiple-organ harvesting. *Surg Gynecol Obstet* 1987;165:343–348

61. Miller C, Mazzaferro V, Makowka L, et al. Rapid flush technique for donor hepatectomy: safety and efficacy of an improved method of liver recovery for transplantation. *Transplant Proc* 1988;20:948–950

62. Cutropia JC, Coratolo F, Spinetta A, et al. Transplante hepatico ortotopico experimental. *Revista Exspanola de las Enfermedades del Aparato Digestivo* 1972;38:553–570

63. Denmark SW, Shaw BW Jr, Starzl TE, Griffith BP. Venovenous bypass without systemic anticoagulation in canine and human liver transplantation. *Surg Forum* 1983; 34:380–382

64. Griffith BP, Shaw BW Jr, Hardesty RL, et al. Venovenous bypass without systemic anticoagulation for transplantation of the human liver. *Surg Gynecol Obstet* 1985;160: 270–272

65. Shaw BW Jr, Martin DJ, Marquez JM, et al. Venous bypass in clinical liver transplantation. *Ann Surg* 1984;200: 524–534

66. Shaw BW Jr, Martin DJ, Marquez JM, et al. Advantages of venous bypass during orthotopic transplantation of the liver. *Semin Liver Dis* 1985;5:344–348

67. Wall WJ, Grant DR, Duff JH, et al. Liver transplantation without venovenous bypass. *Transplantation* 1987;43: 56–61

68. Tzakis A, Todo S, Starzl TE. Orthotopic liver transplantation with preservation of the inferior vena cava. *Ann Surg* 1989;210:649–652

69. Starzl TE, Koep LJ, Weil R III, Halgrimson CG. Development of a suprahepatic recipient vena cava cuff for liver transplantation. *Surg Gynecol Obstet* 1979;149:76–77

70. Starzl TE, Groth CG, Brettschneider L. An everting technique for intraluminal vascular suturing. *Surg Gynecol Obstet* 1968;127:125

71. Starzl TE, Iwatsuki S, Shaw BW Jr. A growth factor in fine vascular anastomoses. *Surg Gynecol Obstet* 1984;159:164–165

72. Contis JC, Heffron TG, Whitington PF, Emond JC. Use of absorbable suture material in vascular anastomoses in pediatric liver transplantation. *Transplant Proc* 1993;25: 1878–1880

73. Boillot O, Sarfati PO, Bringier J, et al. Orthotopic liver transplantation and pathology of the inferior vena cava. *Transplant Proc* 1990;22:1567–1568

74. Lerut J, Tzakis AG, Bron K, et al. Complications of venous reconstruction in human orthotopic liver transplantation. *Ann Surg* 1987;205:404–414

75. Farmer DG, Shaked A, Olthoff KM, et al. Evaluation, operative management and outcome after liver transplantation in children with biliary atresia and situs inversus. *Ann Surg* 1994;222:47–50

76. Brems JJ, Hiatt JR, Klein AS, et al. Effect of prior portasystemic shunt on subsequent liver transplantation. *Ann Surg* 1989;209:51–56

77. Shaked A, Busuttil RW. Liver transplantation in patients with portal vein thrombosis and central portacaval shunts. *Ann Surg* 1991;214:696–702

78. Esquivel CO, Klintmalm G, Iwatsuki S, et al. Liver transplantation in patients with patent splenorenal shunts. *Surgery* 1987;101:430–432

79. Van Thiel DH, Schade RR, Starzl TE, et al. Liver transplantation in adults. *Hepatology* 1982;2:637–640

80. Shaw BW Jr, Iwatsuki S, Bron K, Starzl TE. Portal vein grafts in hepatic transplantation. *Surg Gynecol Obstet* 1985; 161:67–68

81. Tzakis A, Todo S, Stieber A, Starzl TE. Venous jump grafts for liver transplantation in patients with portal vein thrombosis. *Transplantation* 1989;48:530–531

82. Burdick JF, Pitt HA, Colombani PM, et al. Superior mesenteric vein inflow for liver transplantation when the portal vein is occluded. *Surgery* 1990;107:342–345

83. Kirsch JP, Howard TK, Klintmalm GB, et al. Problematic vascular reconstruction in liver transplantation part II, portovenous conduits. *Surgery* 1980;107:544–548

84. Quinones-Baldrich WJ, Memsic L, Ramming K, et al. Branch patch for arterialization of hepatic grafts. *Surg Gynecol Obstet* 1986;162:489–490

85. Michels NA. Newer anatomy of the liver and its variant blood supply and collateral circulation. *Am J Surg* 1966; 112:337–347

86. Gordon RD, Shaw BW Jr, Iwatsuki S, et al. A simplified technique for revascularization of homografts of the liver with a variant right hepatic artery from the superior mesenteric artery. *Surg Gynecol Obstet* 1985;160: 475–476

87. Shaw BW Jr, Iwatsuki S, Starzl TE. Alternate methods of arterialization of the hepatic graft. *Surg Gynecol Obstet* 1984;159:491–493

88. Goldstein RM, Secrest CL, Klintmalm GB, Husberg BS. Problematic vascular reconstruction in liver transplantation, part I, arterial. *Surgery* 1990;107:540–543

89. Shaked A, Takiff H, Busuttil RW. The use of the supraceliac aorta for hepatic arterial revascularization in transplantation of the liver. *Surg Gynecol Obstet* 1991;173: 198–202

90. Stewart MT, Millikan WJ Jr, Henderson JM, et al. Proximal abdominal graft for arterialization during hepatic transplantation. *Surg Gynecol Obstet* 1989;169:261–262

91. Neuhaus P, Blumhardt G, Bechstein WO, et al. Technique

and results of biliary reconstruction using side-to-side choledochocholedochostomy in 300 orthotopic liver transplants. *Ann Surg* 1994;219:426–434

92. Rolles K, Dawson K, Novell R, et al. Biliary anastomosis after liver transplantation does not benefit from T tube splintage. *Transplantation* 1994;57:402–404

93. Marchioro TL, Porter KA, Dickinson TC, et al. Physiologic requirements for auxiliary liver homotransplantation. *Surg Gynecol Obstet* 1965;121:17–31

94. Starzl TE, Francavilla A, Halgrimson CG, et al. The origin, hormonal nature, and action of hepatotrophic substances in portal venous blood. *Surg Gynecol Obstet* 1973;137:179–199

95. Starzl TE, Watanabe K, Porter KA, Putnam CW. Effects of insulin, glucagon, and insulin/glucagon infusions on liver morphology and cell division after complete portacaval shunt in dogs. *Lancet* 1976;1:821–825

96. Starzl TE, Groth C, Makowka L. *Clio Chirurgica: Liver Transplantation.* Austin, Tx:Silvergirl, Inc, 1988:286–288

97. Fortner JG, Kinne DW, Shiu MH, et al. Clinical liver heterotopic (auxiliary) transplantation. *Surgery* 1973;74:739–751

98. Terpstra OT, Schalm SW, Weimar W, et al. Auxiliary partial liver transplantation for end-stage chronic liver disease. *N Engl J Med* 1988;319:1507–1511

99. Bismuth H, Houssin D. Partial resection of liver grafts for orthotopic or heterotopic liver transplantation. *Transplant Proc* 1985;17:279–283

100. Armenti V, Radomski J, Carabasi RA, et al. Heterotopic liver transplantation for fulminant hepatic failure—a bridge to recovery. *Transplantation* 1990;50:524–526

101. Broelsch CE, Emond JC, Whitington PF, et al. Application of reduced-size liver transplants as split grafts, auxiliary orthotopic grafts, and living related segmental transplants. *Ann Surg* 1990;212:368–377

102. Gubernatis G, Pichlmayr R, Kemnitz J, Gratz K. Auxiliary partial orthotopic liver transplantation (APOLT) for fulminant hepatic failure: first successful case report. *World J Surg* 1991;15:660–666

103. Shaked A, Busuttil RW. Auxiliary liver transplantation: a negative viewpoint. *Hepatology* 1990;12:173–175

104. Bismuth H, Houssin D. Reduced-sized orthotopic liver graft in hepatic transplantation in children. *Surgery* 1984;95:367–370

105. Emond JC, Whitington PF, Thistlethwaite JR, et al. Transplantation of two patients with one liver: analysis of a preliminary experience with 'split-liver' grafting. *Ann Surg* 1990;212:14–22

106. Goldsmith NA, Woodburne RT. The surgical anatomy pertaining to liver resection. *Surg Gynecol Obstet* 1957;195:310–318

107. de Ville de Goyet J, Hausleithner V, Reding R, et al. Impact of innovative techniques on the waiting list and results in pediatric liver transplantation. *Transplantation* 1993;56:1130–1136

108. Flye MW. Immunosuppressive therapy. In: Flye MW (ed), *Principles of Organ Transplantation,* Philadelphia, PA: WB Saunders Company; 1989:155–175

109. Kahan BD. Cyclosporine. *N Engl J Med* 1989;321:1725–1737

110. Bismuth H, Castaing D, Ericzon BG, et al. Hepatic transplantation in Europe: first report of the European liver transplant registry. *Lancet* 1987;2:674–676

111. Kung PC, Goldstein G, Reinherz EL, Schlossman SF. Monoclonal antibodies defining distinctive human T cell surface antigens. *Science* 1979;206:347–349

112. Goldstein G. An overview of orthoclone OKT3. *Transplant Proc* 1986;18:927–930

113. Cosmi AB, Burton RC, Colvin RB, et al. Treatment of acute renal allograft rejection with OKT3 monoclonal antibody. *Transplantation* 1981;32:535–539

114. Millis JM, McDiarmid SV, Hiatt JR, et al. Randomized prospective trial of OKT3 for early prophylaxis of rejection after liver transplantation. *Transplantation* 1989;47:82–88

115. McDiarmid SV, Busuttil RW, Levy P, et al. The long-term outcome of OKT3 compared with cyclosporine prophylaxis after liver transplantation. *Transplantation* 1991;52:91–97

116. Fung JJ, Starzl TE. Prophylactic use of OKT3 in liver transplantation: a review. *Dig Dis Sci* 1991;36:1427–1430

117. Kino T, Hatanaka H, Miyata S, et al. A novel immunosuppressant isolated from a *Streptomyces,* II immunosuppressive effect of FK-506 in vitro. *J Antibiotics* 1987;XL:1256–1265

118. Kay JE, Moore AL, Doe SEA, et al. The mechanism of action of FK-506. *Transplant Proc* 1990;22:96–99

119. Starzl TE, Todo S, Fung J, et al. FK-506 for liver, kidney, and pancreas transplantation. *Lancet* 1989;ii:1000–1004

120. Fung J, Abu-Elmagd K, Jain A, et al. A randomized trial of primary liver transplantation under immunosuppression with FK-506 vs cyclosporine. *Transplant Proc* 1991;23:2977–2983

121. Busuttil RW, McDiarmid SV, Klintmalm GBG. Comparison of FK-506 and cyclosporine for immunosuppression in liver transplantation. *N Engl J Med* in press.

122. Greig PD, Woolf GM, Abecassis M, et al. Treatment of primary liver graft nonfunction with prostaglandin E_1 results in increased graft and patient survival. *Transplant Proc* 1989;21:2385–2388

123. Otto G, Wolff H, David H. Preservation damage in liver transplantation: electron-microscopic findings. *Transplant Proc* 1984;16:1247–1248

124. Pruim J, van Woerden WF, Knol E. Donor data in liver grafts with primary nonfunction—a preliminary analysis by the European Liver Registry. *Transplant Proc* 1989;21:2383–2384

125. McDiarmid SV, Hall TR, Grant EG, et al. Failure of duplex sonography to diagnose hepatic artery thrombosis in a high-risk group of pediatric liver transplant recipients. *J Pediatr Surg* 1991;26:710–713

126. Todo S, Makowka L, Tzakis AG, et al. Hepatic artery in liver transplantation. *Transplant Proc* 1987;19:2406–2411

127. Shaked A, McDiarmid SV, Harrison RE, et al. Hepatic artery thrombosis resulting in gas gangrene of the transplanted liver. *Surgery* 1992;111:462–465

128. Klintmalm GB, Olson LM, Nery JR, et al. Treatment of hepatic artery thrombosis after liver transplantation with immediate vascular reconstruction: a report of three cases. *Transplant Proc* 1988;20:610–612

129. Yanaga K, Lebeau G, Marsh JW, et al. Hepatic artery re-

construction for hepatic artery thrombosis after orthotopic liver transplantation. *Arch Surg* 1990;125:628–631

130. Tessler FN, Gehring BJ, Gomes AS, et al. Diagnosis of portal vein thrombosis: value of color doppler imaging. *Am J Roentgenol* 1991;157:293–296

131. Donovan J. Nonsurgical management of biliary tract disease after liver transplantation. *Gastroenterol Clin North Am* 1993;22:317–336

132. Greif F, Bronsther OL, Van Thiel DH, et al. The incidence, timing and management of biliary tract complications after orthotopic liver transplantation. *Ann Surg* 1994;219:40–45

133. Sanchez-Urdazpal L, Batts KP, Gores GJ, et al. Increased bile duct complications in liver transplantation across the ABO barrier. *Ann Surg* 1993;218:152–158

134. Zajko AB, Campbell WL, Logsdon GA, et al. Biliary complications in liver allografts after hepatic artery occlusion: a 6-1/2 year study. *Transplant Proc* 1988;20(suppl 1):607–609

135. Colonna JO II, Shaked A, Gomes AS, et al. Biliary strictures complicating liver transplantation: incidence, pathogenesis, management, and outcome. *Ann Surg* 1992;216:344–350

136. Sherman S, Shaked A, Cryer HM, et al. Endoscopic management of biliary fistulas complicating liver transplantation and other hepatobiliary operations. *Ann Surg* 1993;218:167–175

137. Markin RS, Stratta RJ, Woods GL. Infection after liver transplantation. *Am J Surg Pathol* 1990;14(suppl 1):64–78

138. Colonna JO II, Winston DJ, Brill JE. Infectious complications in liver transplantation. *Arch Surg* 1988;123:360–364

139. Paya CV, Hermans PE, Washington JA II, et al. Incidence, distribution, and outcome of episodes of infection in 100 orthotopic liver transplantations. *Mayo Clin Proc* 1989;64:555–564

140. Brayman KL, Stephanian E, Matas AJ, et al. Analysis of infectious complications occurring after solid-organ transplantation. *Arch Surg* 1992;127:38–48

141. Balfour HH Jr, Stapleton JT, Simmons RL, Fryd DS. A randomized, placebo-controlled trial of oral acyclovir for the prevention of cytomegalovirus disease in recipients of renal allografts. *N Engl J Med* 1989;320:1381–1387

142. Winston DJ, Ho WG, Bartoni K, et al. Ganciclovir prophylaxis of cytomegalovirus infection and disease in allogeneic bone marrow transplant recipients. *Ann Intern Med* 1993;118:179–184

143. Kusne S, Dummer JS, Singh N. Infections after liver transplantation: an analysis of 101 consecutive cases. *Medicine* 1988;67:132–143

144. Brems JJ, Hiatt JR, Colonna JO II, et al. Variables influencing the outcome following orthotopic liver transplantation. *Arch Surg* 1987;122:1109–1111

145. Colonna JO II, Brems JJ, Goldstein LL, et al. The importance of percutaneous liver biopsy in the management of the liver transplant recipient. *Transplant Proc* 1988;20(suppl 1):682–684

146. Demetris AJ, Lasky S, Van Thiel DH, et al. Pathology of hepatic transplantation: a review of 62 adult allograft recipients immunosuppressed with a cyclosporine/steroid regimen. *Am J Pathol* 1985;118:151–161

147. Ray RA, Lewin KJ, Colonna JO, et al. The role of liver biopsy in evaluating acute allograft dysfunction following liver transplantation: a clinical histologic correlation of 34 liver transplants. *Hum Pathol* 1988;19:835–848

148. Colonna JO II, Goldstein LI, Brems JJ, et al. A prospective study on the use of monoclonal anti-T3-Cell antibody (OKT3) to treat steroid-resistant liver transplant rejection. *Arch Surg* 1987;122:1120–1123

149. Cosmi AB, Cho SI, Delmonico FL, et al. A randomized clinical trial comparing OKT3 and steroids for treatment of hepatic allograft rejection. *Transplantation* 1987;43:91–95

150. Starzl TE, Fung JJ. Orthoclone OKT3 in treatment of allografts rejected under cyclosporine-steroid therapy. *Transplant Proc* 1986;18:937–941

151. Woodle ES, Thistlethwaite JR Jr, Emond JC, et al. OKT3 therapy for hepatic allograft rejection: differential response in adults and children. *Transplantation* 1991;51:1207–1212

152. Shaw BW Jr, Gordon RD, Iwatsuki S, Starzl TE. Retransplantation of the liver. *Semin Liver Dis* 1985;5:394–401

153. Demetris AJ, Jaffe R, Tzakis A, et al. Antibody-mediated rejection of human orthotopic liver allografts: a study of liver transplantation across ABO blood group barriers. *Am J Pathol* 1988;132:489–502

154. Imagawa DK, Noguchi K, Iwaki Y, Busuttil RW. Hyperacute rejection following ABO-compatible orthotopic liver transplantation—a case report. *Transplantation* 1992;54:1114–1117

155. Bird G, Friend P, Donaldson P, et al. Hyperacute rejection in liver transplantation: a case report. *Transplant Proc* 1989;21:3742–3744

156. Iwatsuki S, Iwaki Y, Kano T, et al. Successful liver transplantation from crossmatch-positive donors. *Transplant Proc* 1981;13:286–288

157. Markus BH, Duquesnoy RJ, Gordon RD, et al. Histocompatibility and liver transplant outcome: does HLA exert a dualistic effect? *Transplantation* 1988;46:372–377

158. Ramsey G, Nusbacher J, Starzl TE, Lindsay GD. Isohemagglutinins of graft origin after ABO-unmatched liver transplantation. *N Engl J Med* 1984;311:1167–1170

159. Triulzi DJ, Shirey RS, Ness PM, Klein AS. Immunohematologic complications of ABO-unmatched liver transplants. *Transfusion* 1992;32:829–833

160. Takaya S, Bronsther O, Iwaki Y, et al. The adverse impact on liver transplantation of using positive cytotoxic crossmatch donors. *Transplantation* 1992;53:400–406

161. Knechtle SJ, Kalayoglu M, D'Alessandro AM, et al. Histocompatibility and liver transplantation. *Surgery* 1993;114:667–672

162. Imagawa DK, Strange SM, Shaked A, et al. Liver transplantation at UCLA: report of clinical activities. In: Terasaki P (ed), *Clinical Transplants 1991*, Los Angeles, CA: UCLA Tissue Typing Laboratory; 1991:127–134

163. Iwatsuki S, Shaw BW Jr, Starzl TE. Liver transplantation for biliary atresia. *World J Surg* 1984;8:51–56

164. Lynch SV, Akiyama T, Ong TH, et al. Transplantation in children with biliary atresia. *Transplant Proc* 1992;24:186–188

165. Millis JM, Brems JJ, Hiatt JR, et al. Orthotopic liver trans-

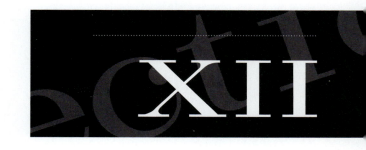

GALLBLADDER AND BILE DUCT

59

Choledochal Cysts

Pamela A. Lipsett ▪ *Charles J. Yeo*

A choledochal cyst is defined as an isolated or combined congenital dilation of the extrahepatic or intrahepatic biliary tree. The disease is much more common in Asians and in females. In children, the classic findings include a right upper quadrant abdominal mass, jaundice, and abdominal pain. In adults, the diagnosis is often confused with benign biliary tract or pancreatic disease. Complications of choledochal cyst disease include cholangitis, jaundice, pancreatis, portal hypertension, and cholangiocarcinoma. Cyst excision, rather than cyst bypass, is the treatment of choice.

▪ HISTORICAL PERSPECTIVE

In 1723, Vater and Ezler described the anatomic details of a choledochal cyst,[1] but Douglas is credited with the first clinical description of a case of a choledochal cyst.[2] Douglas' patient was a 17 year-old female with a 3 year history of intermittent abdominal pain, fever, and jaundice, who was found to have a choledochal cyst at postmortem examination. The cyst occupied the entire right side of her abdomen and contained a half-gallon of yellow, thin, foul-smelling fluid. The hepatic ducts were dilated but the gallbladder and cystic duct were not. The patient was treated with "hot fermentations and purgatives. Blisters were of some service." Douglas proposed repeated trocar aspirations of the cyst in future cases.[2] The first excision of a choledochal cyst was reported by McWhorter.[3] This patient was an adult

woman who had been treated unsuccessfully for her symptoms with cholecystostomy, although she was found to have no gallstones. Fourteen years later, she was treated with cyst excision, cholecystectomy, and hepaticoduodenostomy. She had relief of her symptoms for the subsequent 13 years of follow-up, until her death from unrelated causes.

Alonso-Lej and associates reviewed the literature in 1959 and proposed an early classification system for choledochal cysts that is still used by some surgeons today.[4] Todani and his associates modified the Alonso-Lej classification in 1977, to account for the combination of intra- and extrahepatic cystic dilation.[5]

There are several excellent reviews[4–8] and published experiences[9–11] on choledochal cyst disease that we recommend to the reader.

▪ INCIDENCE/EPIDEMIOLOGY

Once considered a rare congenital lesion of children, choledochal cysts have been reported in over 3300 patients, with many recent reports including adult patients. More than two-thirds of all reported cases have originated in Asia, where the hospital admission rate for choledochal cyst disease is as high as 1 per 1000 admissions. In Western countries, the incidence of choledochal cyst disease is between 1 in 100 000 and 1 in 150 000 live births. In Madrid, Spain, between January 1983 and December 1986, only 9 children had surgery for choledochal cyst disease out of 27 107 children undergoing an operation.[12] In most series, the female/male ratio varies between 3:1 and 4:1, and in most of the older series, the disease was most often recognized in children less than 10 years of age. However, many recent reports have emphasized that this disease also is seen in adults. In the adult population, choledochal cyst disease is probably under-recognized and under-reported.

■ ANATOMY/PATHOLOGY

Cystic dilation of the biliary tree can occur in the extrahepatic or intrahepatic biliary tree or in both. The most common type of choledochal cyst is confined to the extrahepatic biliary tree, commencing just below the bifurcation of the right and left hepatic ducts and extending into or near the pancreatic parenchyma. Typically, the cystic duct enters the choledochal cyst and the gallbladder is of normal size. Histologically, two major types of choledochal cysts are seen: (1) in the *glandular* type, the normal cuboidal epithelium is seen, but there are glandular cavities in the mucosal layer associated with a chronic inflammatory cell infiltrate, (2) in the *fibrotic* type, the bile duct is thickened, with well-developed collagen fibers and a paucity of inflammation (Figs 59–1 and 59–2). A close relationship has been described between the fibrotic type and the cystic dilation of the bile duct seen most often in young children and is associated with a palpable mass.[13]

In most uncomplicated cases of choledochal cyst disease, there are no significant abnormalities of liver his-

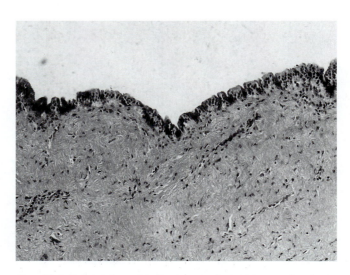

Figure 59–2. Choledochal cyst of the fibrotic type, stained with hematoxylin and eosin (×10). Note the thickened bile duct wall with well-developed collagen and the paucity of inflammation.

tology. However, in some cases, mild inflammatory changes may be seen in the portal tracts with a minor degree of periportal fibrosis. In Caroli's disease (isolated intrahepatic biliary dilation) the intrahepatic cyst can be associated with congenital hepatic fibrosis, with extensive fibrosis extending from the portal triads outward into the periphery of the hepatic lobules.[14] When this degree of hepatic fibrosis is present, patients are at risk for the development of cirrhosis and portal hypertension.

In 1959, Alonso-Lej and associates proposed the first widely used classification system of choledochal cysts.[4] This classification did not account for isolated intrahepatic disease and Todani and associates proposed the following classification scheme[5] (Fig 59–3) which has gained widespread acceptance:

- Type I: Dilation of the extrahepatic biliary tree: Ia-cystic, Ib-focal, or Ic-fusiform
- Type II: Saccular diverticulum of extrahepatic bile duct
- Type III: Biliary tree dilation within the duodenum; choledochocele
- Type IVa: Dilation of the intrahepatic and extrahepatic biliary tree
- Type IVb: Multiple extrahepatic cysts
- Type V: Dilation confined to the intrahepatic ducts (Caroli's disease).

Type I cysts are seen in 40% to 60% of cases. Of the three subtypes of Type I cysts, the cystic and fusiform varieties are the most common, with the cystic variety being five times more common than the fusiform. Type IVa disease, combined intrahepatic and extrahepatic

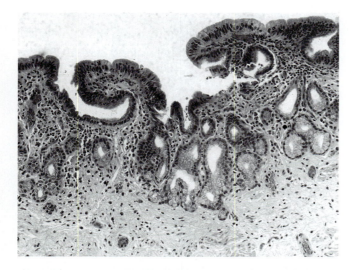

Figure 59–1. Section of a choledochal cyst with glandular features stained with hematoxylin and eosin (×10). In the glandular type, the normal cuboidal epithelium is seen and glandular cavities are seen associated with chronic inflammatory cells.

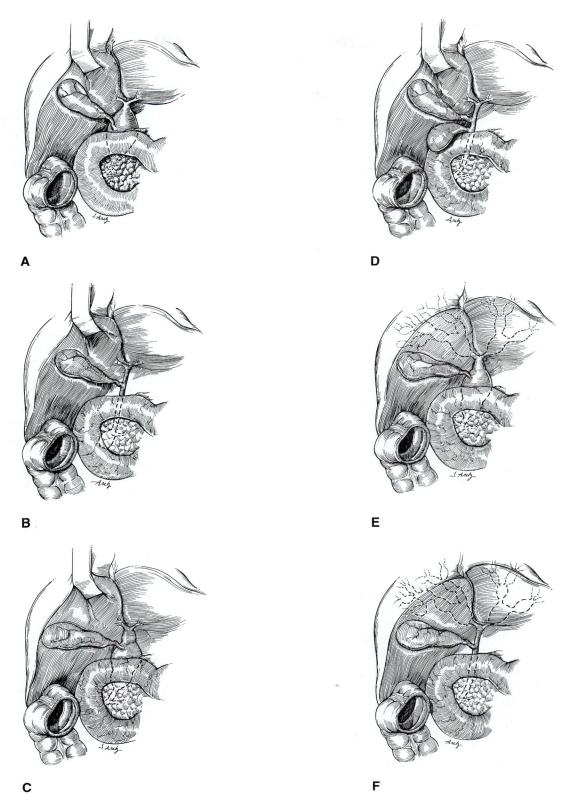

A

B

C

D

E

F

Figure 59–3. Illustrations of the Todani[5] classification of choledochal cysts **A.** Type Ia, **B.** Type II, **C.** Type III, **D.** Type IVa, **E.** Type IVb, and **F.** Type V.

TABLE 59–1. REVIEW OF RECENT SERIES OF CHOLEDOCHAL CYSTS

	Johns Hopkins n=42	Northwestern[11] n=21	Hannover[9] n=13	Kyushu[10] n=46
Mean age (yrs)	23	3	47	24
Sex (F:M)	36:6	17:4	10:3	41:5
Cyst type[5]				
I	21 (50)	14-IA (67)	7 (54)	26 (57)
II	1 (2)	7-IB (33)	1 (8)	0 (0)
III	2 (5)	1 (0)	2 (5)	
IVa	14 (33)	2 (15)	17 (37)	
IVb	3 (7)	1 (8)	1 (2)	
V	1 (2)	1 (8)	0 (0)	

Numbers in parentheses denote percentages.

biliary dilation, is present in 20% to 40% of patients, while isolated intrahepatic dilation (Type V) is rarely seen.[5,9,10,15]

Our recent series of 42 patients with choledochal cyst disease treated at The Johns Hopkins Hospital included 21 (50%) patients with type I cysts, one type II patient, two type III patients, 14 (33%) type IVa patients, 3 type IVb patients and one type V patient.[16] Other recent series are listed in Table 59–1.

■ ETIOLOGY

The pathogenesis of choledochal cysts remains controversial. Three theories of choledochal cyst formation include: (1) the anomalous pancreatic duct–biliary junction theory; (2) the abnormal canalization of the bile duct theory; and (3) the theory concerning abnormalities of autonomic innervation of the extrahepatic biliary tree. Babbitt proposed that an abnormal relationship between the pancreatic duct and the common bile duct could result in reflux of pancreatic juice into the common duct, with subsequent exposure of the bile duct to the higher pressure than normally occurs in the pancreatic duct.[17] In 19 patients, he found that a small common bile duct entered the pancreatic duct at a right angle, 2.0 to 3.5 cm away from the ampulla. Iwai and associates noted this abnormal pancreatic–biliary junction in 25 of 26 patients, and furthered the analysis of choledochal cyst disease by describing a correlation between cyst type and the type of abnormal choledochopancreatic duct junction.[18] If a small bile duct joined a prominent pancreatic duct, then patients had a cystic choledochal cyst. Alternatively, if the pancreatic duct appeared to join a prominent common bile duct, then a fusiform choledochal cyst was seen. In both settings, high concentrations of pancreatic amylase were found in the biliary tree and manometry confirmed a pressure gradient favoring reflux of pancreatic exocrine secretions into the biliary tree.

The embryologic development of the pancreatic and common bile duct is complete by 8 weeks of gestation.[19] An abnormal choledochopancreatic duct junction could form if the pancreatic duct and common bile duct develop abnormally, failing to descend into the duodenum under normal sphincteric muscle control. Under these conditions, the length of the common channel between the pancreatic and bile duct is abnormally long, and amylase-rich pancreatic secretions could then reflux into the biliary tree.[20] Although this choledochopancreatic duct junction abnormality is seen in most patients with choledochal cyst disease, it is also seen in patients without cystic dilation. Thus, the role of this anomalous pancreatic–biliary duct junction in the causation of choledochal cyst disease remains unclear.

A second theory of choledochal cyst development concerns abnormal canalization of the bile duct during embryogenesis, with distal obstruction. The distal obstruction is theorized to cause increased proximal pressure that leads to further weakening of the common duct wall. In experimental models, ligation of the common duct and the subsequent development of cystic dilation varies with the age of the animal at the time of ligation. In both neonatal rats and lambs, ligation of the common duct results in dilation similar to a type I choledochal cyst. However, in adult rats and lambs, ligation of the common duct results in diffuse extrahepatic and intrahepatic ductal dilation, without formation of a choledochal cyst.[21,22]

The third theory of choledochal cyst pathogenesis involves abnormalities of autonomic innervation of the extrahepatic biliary tree. Autonomic dysfunction has been demonstrated in a choledochal cyst, with a reduction in the number of postganglionic cholinergic cells in the narrow distal portion of the cyst when compared with the dilated portion.[23] The number of ganglion cells in the distal narrow portion of the cyst wall was only 14% to 41% of that in the dilated portion of the cyst. Additionally, cholecystokinin has been demonstrated to produce smaller contractions in the muscle of the narrow part of the cyst when compared with the dilated cystic muscle. Further, nicotine and γ-aminobutyric acid, two known prokinetic agents, produced no contractions, indicating intrinsic dysfunction of the postganglionic neurons. Thus, numerous factors including an anomalous choledochopancreatic duct junction, abnormal bile duct canalization, and autonomic neural abnormalities all may be important in choledochal cyst formation.

■ CLINICAL PRESENTATION AND DIFFERENTIAL DIAGNOSIS

Traditionally, choledochal cysts have been diagnosed in early infancy. In our series from The Johns Hopkins Hospital, the diagnosis was established in utero in two patients.[16] In most reported series, over one-half of the patients have been diagnosed before 10 years of age. However, we and others have recognized an increased number of adults who have been diagnosed with choledochal cyst disease. In our series, 31 of 42 patients presented in adulthood with a choledochal cyst, with the oldest patient being 62 years of age at presentation.

The classic triad of jaundice, right upper quadrant mass, and abdominal pain is present in a minority of patients (5% to 30%). Most children (40% to 80%) have two of these three findings at diagnosis. Nausea and vomiting are present in about one-third of patients. Adults are likely to present with pancreatitis (related to biliary calculi or sludge), a symptom mimicking biliary colic or acute cholecystitis. Jaundice is present in one-third of all adult patients, and some adults may have cholangitis as their initial presenting symptom.

In the group of 42 patients reviewed at The Johns Hopkins Hospital during the last 16 years, 11 children and 31 adults with choledochal cysts were identified. Eight of the 11 children were diagnosed and treated prior to 4 years of age, while the 31 adults were identified and treated at a median age of 30 years (range 17 to 62 years of age). Children and adults presented with different signs and symptoms (Table 59–2). A palpable abdominal mass was significantly more common in children, while abdominal pain, pancreatitis, or history of cholecystectomy for biliary symptoms were more common in adults. Only one child and no adults had the classic triad of abdominal pain, right upper quadrant mass, and jaundice. However, two of these three findings were present in eight (73%) of 11 children, but only seven (23%) of 31 adults.

■ DIAGNOSTIC STUDIES

The diagnosis of a choledochal cyst is established easily once considered. However, in the absence of the classic triad of symptoms and signs, the diagnosis often is not considered, particularly in adults. Several diagnostic studies are now available to define the presence and anatomy of a choledochal cyst. Thus, the diagnosis should virtually always be established preoperatively.

Although numerous nonspecific investigations may suggest an abnormality of the biliary tree, ultrasonography, computerized tomography (CT) and cholangiography are the most useful studies to establish the diagnosis of a choledochal cyst and to classify the cyst type. Table 59–3 lists the common investigations that are often obtained during the evaluation of this disease.

Plain abdominal radiographs may demonstrate a right upper quadrant mass effect, radiopaque calculi within the cyst, or a calcified cyst, but these findings are rare. Likewise, a barium upper gastrointestinal study may confirm displacement of the duodenum by a mass effect, or may show esophageal varices, if cirrhosis or portal vein thrombosis with resultant portal hypertension is present. Neither of these investigations are sufficiently sensitive or specific for the accurate diagnosis of a choledochal cyst.

Oral or intravenous cholangiography previously was performed in the evaluation of patients with suspected choledochal cyst. Such studies have now been abandoned, in favor of either endoscopic or percutaneous cholangiography (Figs 59–4 and 59–5). Endoscopic retrograde cholangiopancreatography (ERCP) has the advantage of defining the lower ductal anatomy (Figs 59–6 and 59–7), and specifically, the presence of an anomalous choledochopancreatic duct junction (ACDPDJ). However, with large extrahepatic cysts, the volume of contrast necessary to fill the cyst and define the intrahepatic anatomy is large, and full visualization of the extrahepatic

TABLE 59–2. SYMPTOMS AND SIGNS OF 42 PATIENTS PRESENTING WITH A CHOLEDOCHAL CYST

	Children (n=11)	Adults (n=31)
Abdominal mass	9 (82)	4 (13)[a]
Abdominal pain	4 (36)	27 (87)[a]
Jaundice	7 (64)	13 (42)
Fever	2 (18)	8 (26)
Nausea/Vomiting	2 (18)	9 (29)
Pancreatitis	0 (0)	7 (23)[b]
Prior cholecystectomy	0 (0)	16 (52)[b]

Numbers in parentheses denote percentages.
*$P \leqslant .01$ vs. children, by chi-square; #$P=.06$ vs children, by chi-square.

TABLE 59–3. COMMON INVESTIGATIONS UTILIZED IN THE DIAGNOSIS OF CHOLEDOCHAL CYST DISEASE

INVESTIGATION
Plain abdominal radiograph
Barium upper gastrointestinal series
Ultrasound
CT scan
Radionuclide imaging studies
ERCP
Percutaneous transhepatic cholangiography

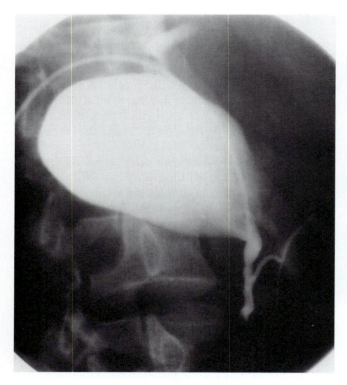

Figure 59–4. Percutaneous transhepatic cholangiogram via the right ductal system. A large type I choledochal cyst is seen. In this view, the gallbladder is not seen, but an anomalous choledochopancreatic duct junction is seen.

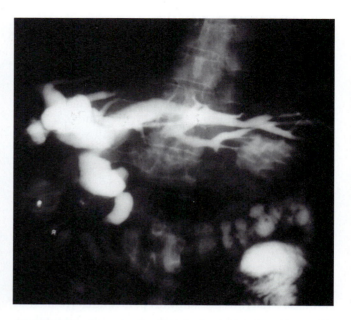

Figure 59–5. Percutaneous transhepatic cholangiogram of a patient with a type IVa choledochal cyst. Note both extrahepatic and intrahepatic sacculations of the biliary tree.

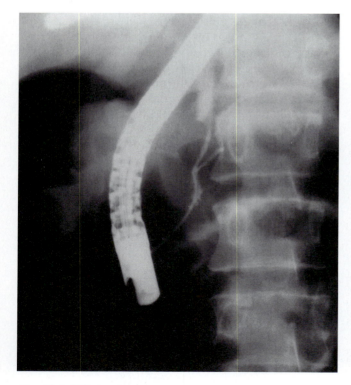

Figure 59–6. ERCP of a patient with an anomalous choledochopancreatic duct junction. This patient had a type I choledochal cyst not seen on this view.

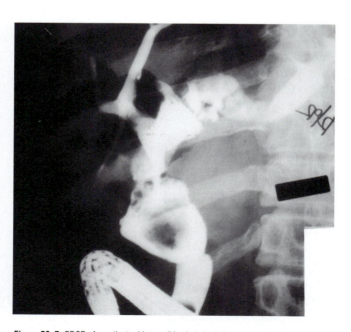

Figure 59–7. ERCP of a patient with type IVa choledochal cyst disease. The intraluminal filling defects seen are extrahepatic and intrahepatic stones.

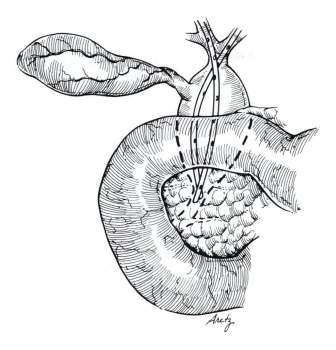

Figure 59–8. Illustration of the extrahepatic dilation of a type IVa choledochal cyst. Bilateral transhepatic stents have been placed preoperatively and the stents have been left above the anomalous choledochopancreatic duct junction.

and intrahepatic biliary tree can be problematic. Percutaneous cholangiography and preoperative placement of percutaneous transhepatic stents can be particularly helpful in cases with associated intrahepatic disease (types IV and V), or when an extrahepatic cyst approaches close to the bifurcation of the common hepatic duct. Complications of both endoscopic and trans-hepatic cholangiography include cholangitis, bacteremia, and pancreatitis. The development of pancreatitis is almost certainly related to the ACDPDJ, where the long common channel increases the risk of pancreatic duct hypertension or obstruction. In order to lessen the risk of catheter-induced pancreatitis, preoperatively placed transhepatic stents should be left within the choledochal cyst and are not advanced through the long common channel into the duodenum (Fig 59–8).

Ultrasonography can diagnose a choledochal cyst.[8,24,25] High resolution real-time scanning is accurate in determining the size, contour, and location of choledochal cysts. In the Johns Hopkins series, two of 11 children had the antenatal diagnosis of choledochal cyst established by ultrasonography. Although ultrasonography done at our institution was always diagnostic, 16 of 32 of our adult patients had been treated by cholecystectomy alone for biliary tract disease, primarily based on sonograms performed at outside institutions. At the time of cholecystectomy, choledochal cysts then were recognized at laparotomy or laparoscopy, but left untreated. Thus, ultrasonography may be misleading, if the diagnosis of choledochal cyst disease is unsuspected or not considered.

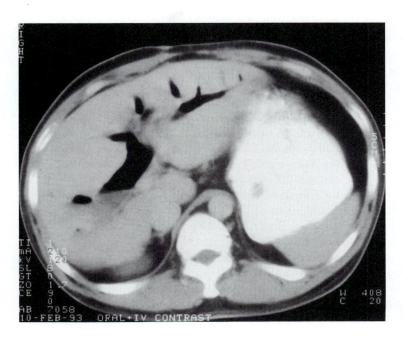

Figure 59–9. CT scan of the patient in Fig 59–7 with a type IVa choledochal cyst. In the right ductal system, debris is seen layered posteriorly.

Radionuclide hepatobiliary scanning has been championed by some as the investigation of choice in determining the presence of choledochal cyst disease. Images obtained early after radionuclide administration often demonstrate a filling defect in the liver, while later images may show contrast accumulation in the choledochal cyst. In deeply jaundiced patients, the radionuclide may be retained within the liver for up to 24 hours. Although hepatobiliary scans have been found to be helpful in the diagnosis of choledochal cyst,[26] in our series, such scans suggested the diagnosis in less than one-half of the patients in whom they were performed, and always prompted another confirmatory investigation. Thus, radionuclide scanning does not appear to be necessary or cost-effective in the evaluation of a patient with symptoms and signs of a choledochal cyst.

CT can delineate the size, location, and extent of intrahepatic and extrahepatic biliary dilation in patients with a choledochal cyst. This evaluation may be particularly useful in the adult patient in whom another etiology for biliary obstruction may be present, such as a pancreatic or periampullary mass. Most patients with a choledochal cyst have significant extrahepatic dilation alone. If intrahepatic dilation is present, typically it involves the central portions of the liver without peripheral involvement (Fig 59–9). On the other hand, patients with extrahepatic biliary obstruction secondary to acquired conditions, such as stones or neoplasms, most often have intrahepatic biliary dilation that extends beyond the central portion and toward the periphery of the liver.

Choledochal cysts are most easily diagnosed by ultrasonography or CT scan. Cyst type and associated biliary anatomy are delineated by endoscopic or percutaneous cholangiography. In children, if preoperative cholangiography is not available, operative cholangiography can be performed easily through the cystic duct or the common hepatic duct. In these instances, one must avoid overfilling of the cyst, obscuring either proximal intrahepatic anatomy or distal filling of an ACDPDJ.

■ COMPLICATIONS AND NATURAL HISTORY

Many complications of choledochal cyst disease have been reported. Jaundice, recurrent cholangitis, pancreatitis, gallstones, cholecystitis and carcinoma of the gallbladder and biliary tree are the most common complications of biliary cystic dilation. Additional rare complications include cirrhosis with portal hypertension, portal vein thrombosis with resultant portal hypertension, and in rare cases, cyst rupture, either spontaneously or in association with pregnancy.[27,28] No association between cyst rupture and the size of the cyst has been identified. Hepatic fibrosis and cirrhosis may not

be a complication of choledochal cyst disease alone but may represent an associated finding in some neonates with a choledochal cyst. This form of disease may require hepatic transplantation, being irreversible even after extrahepatic cyst excision. Milder forms of biliary cirrhosis have regressed after definitive biliary surgery cyst drainage, with hepatic recovery to yield normal histology.[29]

Adults often present with nausea, vomiting, and abdominal pain typical of pancreatitis. Hyperamylasemia may be present. Although many of these patients will have acute pancreatitis, hyperamylasemia also may result from reflux of pancreatic juice into the choledochal cyst, with subsequent absorption into the systemic circulation.[30] Further support for this thesis is provided in a report demonstrating an elevated amylase level in 12 children with a type I choledochal cyst, without evidence of pancreatic injury or pancreatitis.[31]

The presence of stones within the gallbladder and choledochal cyst has not been commonly reported. However, an 8% incidence of gallstones in 1433 cases of choledochal cyst in Japan have been reported.[8] In the Johns Hopkins series, 16 of 31 adults previously had undergone cholecystectomy for acute biliary tract symptoms. Histologically, the resected gallbladder always had evidence of inflammation. Furthermore, 12 of 16 patients had gallstones, and one patient had gallbladder carcinoma. Three of forty-two patients had stones within the choledochal cyst at the time of resection of their choledochal cyst, and these same three patients have had intrahepatic stones form in sacculations within the intrahepatic biliary tree after extrahepatic biliary excision, without anastomotic strictures.

Cancers of the biliary tree, gallbladder, pancreas, liver and duodenum have been associated with choledochal cyst disease. This association was first recognized by Irwin and Morison in 1944.[32] In a review of 48 cases of choledochal cyst-related cancer, it was estimated that the incidence of malignant change was approximately 3% of all cases.[23] Most commonly, the carcinoma has been found to be a cholangiocarcinoma involving the extrahepatic biliary tree, thus stressing the importance of excision of the biliary cyst. Several reviews of malignant change associated with choledochal cysts have been reported.[34–37] Patients with choledochal cyst–associated cholangiocarcinoma are diagnosed typically in the fourth decade of life, 30 years prior to the mean age of diagnosis of patients with cholangiocarcinoma without choledochal cyst. The higher incidence and young age of presentation at diagnosis of malignant change within the gallbladder and biliary tree is believed to be related to the ACDPDJ and resulting reflux of pancreatic enzymes into the biliary tree. Changes in bile acids, ranging from cholate to the secondary unconjugated bile acids, deoxycholate and lithocholate, were reported in one patient with choledochal cyst.[38] This class of bile acids has demonstrated carcinogenic potential in the Ames assay, using the TA100 strain of *Salmonella typhimurium* in a model of mammalian mutagenicity. Furthermore, the detection of mutations with the *K-ras* gene, which is associated with many human tumor cell types, has been identified in a patient with biliary papillomatosis and a choledochal cyst.[39] Although no definite malignant change was found in this patient, the presence of this *K-ras* mutation suggests a high probability of progression to malignancy. Thus, the secondary bile acids that can form from bacterial overgrowth in choledochal cysts may serve as promotor carcinogens in patients genetically susceptible to cancer.

■ SURGICAL MANAGEMENT

In recent years, choledochal cyst excision, with reconstruction via a biliary-enteric Roux-en-Y anastomosis, has become the treatment of choice for most types of choledochal cyst. Exceptions to this standard practice involve treatment of intraduodenal type III choledochal cysts (choledochocele), and isolated type V intrahepatic disease (Caroli's disease).

Enteric drainage of choledochal cyst disease was once considered appropriate therapy. Such drainage via choledochocystojejunostomy is no longer considered the treatment of choice in patients with choledochal cyst disease for two reasons. First, although construction of a Roux-en-Y loop and dependent drainage of the cyst is technically straightforward, the site of anastomosis on the cyst wall often involves abnormal mucosa, with inflammation and fibrosis. A 68% incidence of anastomotic strictures with associated cholangitis and stone disease when cyst walls were used as sites of biliary-enteric anastomosis has been reported.[40] Second, the risk of a malignancy developing in a retained dilated ductal structure is believed to be unacceptably high, although accurate data on such malignant transformation are not available. In our recent series, a woman 23 years of age was re-explored 7 years after choledochal cyst drainage/bypass, and was found to have widespread metastatic cholangiocarcinoma. One additional patient had cyst excision 8 years after drainage/ bypass, with histologic findings of metaplasia and dysplasia found in the resected cyst specimen.

Choledochocele (type III cysts) have been effectively treated with transduodenal sphincteroplasty or sphincterotomy.[5,41-43]

External drainage of choledochal cysts is not recommended. If severe cholangitis is present, decompression of the cyst can be accomplished by percutaneous or endoscopic routes. Occasionally, choledochal cysts may be drained externally when the diagnosis is not considered, or when the surgeon is not comfortable with the technique of cyst excision and biliary-enteric reconstruction. In such circumstances, subsequent definitive therapy to include cyst excision and biliary reconstruction is indicated.

For the majority of biliary tract cysts, radical excision and biliary reconstruction is the treatment of choice. For patients with type III cysts (choledochocele), transduodenal sphincteroplasty or endoscopic sphincterotomy may be considered appropriate therapy (see Chapter 62). For patients with type V cysts (Caroli's disease) (see Chapter 52).

PREOPERATIVE PREPARATION

Patients are routinely prepared for elective surgery. Patients with jaundice or cholangitis should be assessed carefully for normal blood coagulation parameters. In some patients, the operative procedure may be performed as a same-day admission. Mechanical and antibiotic bowel preparation are not necessary. Prophylactic antibiotics should be administered immediately prior to the skin incision and continued postoperatively for 24 hours. In many patients, the use of preoperatively placed percutaneous transhepatic drainage catheters may assist in the operative dissection and reconstruction.[44] Prophylaxis against deep venous thrombosis should be instituted. Blood should be cross-matched, although usually it is not required. Preoperative radiographic studies should be displayed in the operating room. Intraoperative cholangiography and choledochoscopy should be available.

OPERATIVE TECHNIQUE

Although a high transverse incision often is used in children, in adults, either an upper midline or a generous right subcostal incision provides adequate exposure. Mechanical retractors can facilitate visualization. A general inspection of the abdomen is performed, specifically assessing for portal hypertension, character of the liver, size of the spleen, and status of the pancreas. The size and location of the choledochal cyst and gallbladder are noted (Fig 59–10) and compared with the preoperative radiographic studies.

Initially, the gallbladder and cystic duct are mobilized, taking care to identify the right hepatic artery, which may be anomalous or adherent to the cyst wall. Once the gallbladder is dissected out of the gallbladder fossa, the anterior wall of the cyst is identified in the porta (Fig 59–11). This plane usually is found without difficulty. Inflammation rarely is problematic. The dissection should proceed in a caudal fashion until the entire retroduodenal portion of the cyst is freed, extending to the entry point of the common bile duct into the posterior aspect of the pancreatic parenchyma. After

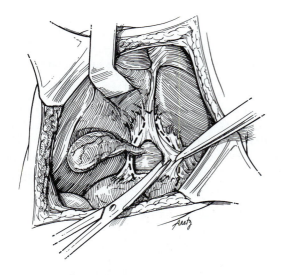

Figure 59–10. Radical excision of a choledochal cyst.

freeing both sides of the cyst, the posterior aspect of the cyst is identified and dissected, and a vessel loop is passed behind the cyst. The anterior wall of the cyst is opened, the preoperatively placed transhepatic catheters are extracted and the posterior wall of the cyst is divided (Fig 59–12). Care must be taken to avoid injury to the pancreatic duct at this point. If cholangiography and pancreatic duct anatomy are not known preoperatively, cholangiography should be performed before division of the extrahepatic biliary tree. In most cases, the common bile duct is divided distally at or near an intrapancreatic location, when the cyst diameter has narrowed to near normal caliber. After transection, the distal common bile duct is oversewn carefully, avoiding injury to the anomalously high junction of the pancreatic duct with the bile duct. Once the choledochal cyst has been divided distally, the anterior, lateral, and posterior aspects of the cyst are dissected from this transection point proximally, and the cyst is dissected free from the portal vein and hepatic artery. Dissection will typically proceed proximally until a normal caliber common hepatic duct is found (Figs 59–13 through 59–15). In most cases, the bifurcation is uninvolved with cystic dilation, and an anastomosis between the common hepatic duct and a Roux-en-Y limb of jejunum can be performed. However, if the cystic dilation involves the bifurcation of the common hepatic duct, then bifurcation resection can be performed. In such cases, preoperative placement of transhepatic catheters into both the right and left hepatic ductal systems may facilitate intraoperative dissection and postoperative anastomotic decompression and allow for postoperative cholangiography (Fig 59–16). If preoperative cholangiographic assessment of the intrahepatic biliary tree has not been possi-

ble, either intraoperative choledochoscopy or cholangiography can be performed.

Reconstruction of the biliary tree is accomplished using a 60-cm retrocolic Roux-en-Y loop of jejunum. An end-to-end hepaticojejunostomy is created, using a single layer of absorbable sutures (4-0 Vicryl or Dexon) (Fig 59–17). A transanastomotic, transhepatic stent is left in place, if it had been placed preoperatively (Fig 59–18). Anastomotic stenting is used routinely by some groups, and rarely by others. In children, stenting is rarely utilized.

Modifications of Operative Technique

Lilly suggested that, in cases of severe pericystic inflammation, the posterior aspect of the cyst wall can be left intact, so as not to injure the portal vein and hepatic artery during efforts at cyst excision.[45] To accomplish this technique, the cyst is opened transversely between stay sutures. The anterior, lateral, and medial walls of the cyst are completely excised, but the posterior wall is divided into a thick inner and thin outer layer. The inner layer is removed by blunt dissection, and the outer layer is left adherent to the portal vessels. Such a procedure rarely is indicated. Additionally, the risk of subsequent malignant degeneration of the retained posterior outer layer of the choledochal cyst is unknown.

In cases of cystic dilation of the entire common hepatic duct and its bifurcation, the left and right hepatic ducts may be independently anastomosed to the Roux-en-Y limb, or they may be amenable to ductoplasty with

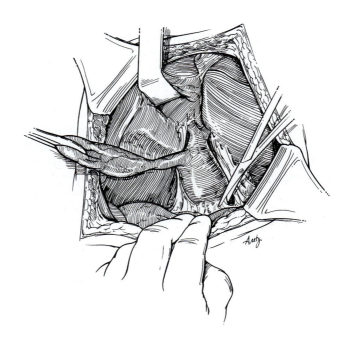

Figure 59–11. Exposure of the cyst and gallbladder.

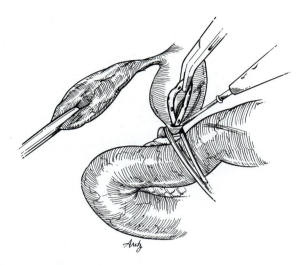

Figure 59–12. Cholecystectomy and anterior dissection of the distal choledochal cyst.

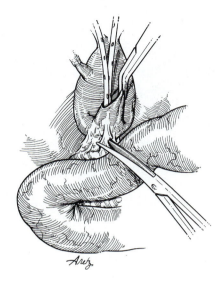

Figure 59–13. Distal extent of the cyst identified, encircled, and opened.

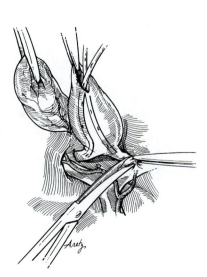

Figure 59–14. Posterior dissection proceeds caudad to cephalad.

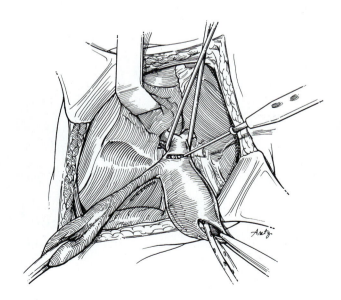

Figure 59–15. Dissection proceeds until normal hepatic duct is identified.

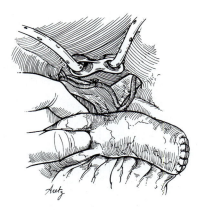

Figure 59–16. Cyst is transected and removed at normal duct.

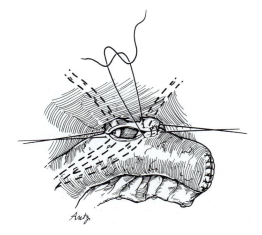

Figure 59–17. Excision is complete; reconstruction proceeds with Roux-en-Y hepaticojejunostomy. If the bifurcation is involved, right and left duct hepaticojejunostomies can be performed.

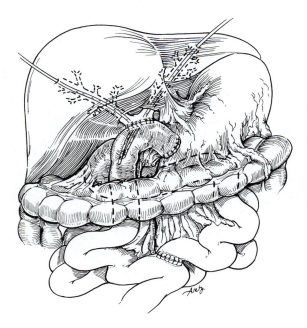

Figure 59–18. One-layer hepaticojejunostomy at the hepatic bifurcation; completed Roux-en-Y hepaticojejunostomy.

lateral incisions, thereby creating a single common opening allowing for a wide anastomosis.

Reconstruction with a valved jejunal anastomosis has been suggested[11] and is touted as being more physiologic. As described above, the choledochal cyst is excised in its entirety. Biliary reconstruction is established via an isolated jejunal limb. A segment of jejunum on a narrow pedicle is brought through the right mesocolon and the cephalad end is closed. An intussusception valve 1.5 to 2 cm in length is created with nonabsorbable sutures in this jejunal conduit. The common hepatic duct is anastomosed end-to-side to the antimesenteric border of the conduit, proximal to the valve. The distal end of the jejunal conduit is sutured to the second portion of the duodenum. Jejunal continuity is re-established with an end-to-end anastomosis. This operation is designed to allow physiologic drainage of bile into the duodenum without reflux or stasis. To date, reconstruction in this manner has been performed on only a limited number of children. Problems with this method of reconstruction include failure of the intussusception valve (with either obstruction to bile flow or reflux of enteric contents), leakage at the site of jejunoduodenostomy, or ischemia of the short-segment jejunal conduit from compromise of its mesentery.

COMPLICATIONS OF SURGICAL MANAGEMENT

In experienced hands, postoperative complications following choledochal cyst excision and biliary reconstruction are relatively uncommon. Typically, the postoperative length of hospital stay is 7 to 10 days. A leak at the biliary-enteric anastomosis can occur and usually is recognized easily by the presence of bile in an operatively placed drain and confirmed by cholangiography. Most patients will heal such a small anastomotic biliary leak with additional external biliary drainage. If transhepatic biliary stents are used, hemobilia can occur postoperatively. Most commonly, stent-associated hemobilia is self-limited. Occasionally, large-volume hemobilia caused by an iatrogenic hepatic artery–bile duct fistula will require angiographic embolotherapy.

In addition to biliary complications, pancreatic duct complications with subsequent pancreatitis can develop if the distal dissection of the choledochal cyst has been too extensive or if sutures have been placed that occlude pancreatic ductal flow. Careful preoperative or perioperative identification of the common duct–pancreatic duct junction will avoid such pancreatic duct injuries.

The long-term development of a biliary stricture was commonly reported when cyst-bypass procedures were performed. The incidence of anastomotic stricture following cyst excision and Roux-en-Y hepaticojejunostomy should be quite low (≤15%) at long-term follow-up. Patients with type IVA disease, in whom the bifurcation has been resected, may benefit from long-term stenting, since it is in this small group of patients in whom postcyst excision, intrahepatic stone disease has been problematic.

REFERENCES

1. Vater A, Ezler CS. Dissertatio de scirrhis viserum occasione sections viri typanite defunte. *Wittenburgae, 4 Pamphlers* 1723;881:22
2. Douglas AH. Case of dilation of common bile duct. *Monthly J Med Sci (London)* 1852;14:97–101
3. McWhorter GL. Congenital cystic dilation of the common bile duct. *Ann Surg* 1924;8:604–626
4. Alonso-Lej F, Rever WB Jr, et al. Congenital choledochal cysts, with a report of 2, and an analysis of 94 cases. *Surg Gynecol Obstet* 1959;108:1–30
5. Todani T, Watanabe Y, et al. Congenital bile duct cysts: classification, operative procedures, and review of thirty-seven cases including cancer arising from choledochal cyst. *Am J Surg* 1977;134:263–269
6. Longmire WP Jr, Manidiola SA, et al. Congenital cystic disease of the liver and biliary system. *Ann Surg* 1971; 174:711–724
7. Flanigan DP. Biliary cysts. *Ann Surg* 1975;182:635–643
8. Yamaguchi M. Congenital choledochal cysts: analysis of 1,433 patients in the Japanese literature. *Am J Surg* 1980; 140:653–657
9. Schmid C, Meyer HJ, et al. Cystic enlargement of extrahepatic bile ducts. *Surgery* 1993;114:65–70
10. Chijiiwa K, Koga A. Surgical management and long term followup of patients with choledochal cysts. *Am J Surg* 1993;165:238–242
11. Coséntino CM, Luck SR, et al. Choledochal duct cyst: resection with physiologic resection. *Surgery* 1992;112: 740–748
12. Gonzalez EM, Garcia IG, et al. Choledochal cyst resection and reconstruction by biliary-jejuno-duodenal diversion. *World J Surg* 1989;13:233–237
13. Okada A, Nakamura T, et al. Congenital dilation of the bile duct in 100 instances and its relationship with anomalous junction. *Surg Gynecol Obstet* 1990;171:291–298
14. Caroli J, Soupalt R, et al. La digitation polykstique congenitale des voico biliares intraheptiques; essai de classification. *Sem Hop Paris,* 1958;34:488–495
15. Deziel D, Rossi RL, et al. Management of bile duct cysts in adults. *Arch Surg* 1986;121:410–415
16. Lipsett PA, Pitt HA, et al. Choledochal cyst disease: a changing pattern of presentation. *Ann Surg* 1994;220: 644–652.
17. Babbitt DP. Congenital choledochal cysts. New etiological concepts on anomalous relationships of the common bile duct and pancreatic bulb. *Ann Radiol* 1969;12:231–240
18. Iwai N, Yanagihara J, et al. Congenital choledochal dilation with emphasis on pathophysiology of the biliary tract. *Ann Surg* 1992;215:27–30
19. Wong KC, Lister J. Human fetal development of the he-

pato-pancreatic duct junction—a possible explanation of congenital dilation of the biliary tract. *J Pediatr Surg* 1981; 16:139–145

20. Tanaka M, Ikeda S, et al. The presence of a positive pressure gradient from pancreatic duct to choledochal cyst demonstrated by duodenoscopic microtransducer manometry: clue to pancreaticobiliary reflux. *Endoscopy* 1982; 14:45

21. Ohkawa H, Sawaguchi S, et al. Experimental analysis of the ill effect of anomalous pancreaticobiliary ductal union. *J. Pediatr Surg* 1982;17:7

22. Spitz L. Experimental production of cystic dilation of the common bile duct in lambs. *J. Pediatr Surg* 1977;12:39

23. Kusunoki M, Saitoh N, et al. Choledochal cysts oligioganglionosis in the narrow portion of the choledochus. *Arch Surg* 1988;123:984–986

24. Dewbury KC, Aluwihare M, et al. Prenatal ultrasound demonstration of a choledochal cyst. *Br J Radiol* 1980; 53:906

25. Young W, Blane C, et al. Congenital biliary dilation: a spectrum of disease detailed by ultrasound. *Br J Radiol* 1990;63:333–336

26. Componovo E, Buck JL, et al. Scintigraphic features of choledochal cyst. *J Nucl Med* 1989;30:622–628

27. Chesterman JT. Choledochous cyst complicating pregnancy and the puerperium. *J Obstet Gynaecol Br Emp* 1944; 51:512

28. Yamashiro Y, Sato M, et al. Spontaneous perforation of a choledochal cyst. *Eur J Pediatr* 1982;138:193

29. Yeong ML, Nicholson GI, et al. Regression of biliary cirrhosis following choledochal cyst drainage. *Gastroenterology* 1982;82:332

30. Stringel G, Filler RM. Fictitious pancreatitis in choledochal cyst. *J Pediatr Surg* 1982;17:359

31. Tan KC, Howard ER. Choledochal cyst: a 14-year surgical experience with 36 patients. *Br J Surg* 1988;75: 892–895

32. Irwin ST, Morison JE. Congenital cyst of the common bile-duct containing stones and undergoing cancerous change. *Br J Surg* 1944;32:319

33. Kagawa Y, Kashihara S, et al. Carcinoma arising in a congenitally dilated biliary tract: report of a case and review of the literature. *Gastroenterology* 1978;74:1286–1294

34. Ackerholm P, Benediktsdottir K, et al. Cholangiocarcinoma in a patient with biliary cysts. *Acta Chir Scan* 1981; 147:605

35. Bedikian AY, Valdivieso M, et al. Cancer of the extrahepatic bile ducts. *Med Pediatr Oncol* 1980;8:53

36. Todani T, Watanabe Y, et al. Congenital choledochal cyst with intrahepatic involvement. *Arch Surg* 1984;119: 1038–1043

37. Rossi RL, Silverman ML, et al. Carcinomas arising in cystic conditions of the bile ducts: a clinical pathologic study. *Ann Surg* 1987;205:377–386

38. Reveille RM, Van Stiegmann G, et al. Increased secondary bile acids in a choledochal cyst: possible role in biliary metaplasia and carcinoma. *Gastroenterology* 1990;99: 525–527

39. Ohta H, Yamaguchi Y, et al. Biliary papillomatosis with the point mutation of *K-ras* gene arising in congenital choledochal cyst. *Gastroenterology* 1993;105:1209–1212

40. Rattner DW, Schapiro RH, et al. Abnormalities of the pancreatic and biliary ducts in adult patients with choledochal cysts. *Arch Surg* 1983;118:1068–1073

41. Klotz D, Cohn BD, et al. Choledochal cysts: diagnosis and therapeutic problems. *J Pediatr Surg* 1973;8:271

42. Venu RP, Geenen JE, et al. Role of endoscopic retrograde cholangiopancreatography in the diagnosis and treatment of choledochocele. *Gastroenterology* 1984;87: 1144–1149

43. Shemesh E, Czerniak A, et al. The role of endoscopic retrograde cholangiopancreatography in the diagnosis and treatment of adult choledochal cyst. *Surg Gynecol Obstet* 1988;167:423–426

44. Yeo CJ, Cameron JL. Transhepatic biliary stents in high benign and malignant biliary tract obstructions. In: Nyhus LM, Baker RJ (eds), *Mastery of Surgery*, 2nd ed. Boston, MA: Little Brown; 1992:967

45. Lilly JR. Total excision of choledochal cysts. *Surg Gynecol Obst* 1979;146:254–256

SELECTED READING

Gatrad AR, Gatrad AH. The association of choledochus cyst with congenital hepatic fibrosis. *Br J Clin Pract* 1979; 33:182

Joseph VT. Surgical techniques and long term results in the treatment of choledochal cyst. *J Ped Surg* 1990;25: 782–787

Kato T, Hebiguchi T, et al. Action of pancreatic juice on the bile duct: pathogenesis of congenital choledochal cyst. *J Pediatr Surg* 1981;16:146

Komi N, Tamura T, et al. Nationwide survey of cases of choledochal cysts: analysis of coexistent anomalies, complications and surgical treatment in 645 cases. *Surg Gastroenterol* 1984; 3:69–73

Lake DNW, Smith PM, et al. Congenital hepatic fibrosis and choledochus cyst. *Br Med J* 1977;186:549

Lopez RR, Pinson CW, et al. Variation in management based on type of choledochal cyst. *Am J Surg* 1991;161: 612–615

Martin LW, Rowe GA. Portal hypertension secondary to choledochal cyst. *Ann Surg* 1979;190:638

Mata Y, Susaki F, et al. Surgical treatment of congenital biliary dilation associated with pancreaticobiliary malfunction. *Surg Gynecol Obstet* 1993;176:581–587

Mercadier M, Chigot JP, et al. Caroli's disease. *World J Surg* 1984;8:22–29

O'Neil JA, Templeton JM Jr, et al. A recent experience with choledochal cyst. *Ann Surg* 1987;205:533–540

Oguchi Y, Okada, et al. Histopathologic studies of congenital dilation of the bile duct as related to an anomalous junction of the pancreaticobiliary ductal system: clinical and experimental studies. *Surgery* 1988;103:168–171

Sarris GE, Tsang D. Choledochocele: case report, literature review and a proposed classification. *Surgery* 1989;105: 408–414

Todani T, Watanabe Y, et al. Cylindrical dilation of the chole-dochus: A special type of congenital bile duct dilation. *Surgery* 1985;98:964–968

Todani T, Watanabe Y, et al. Carcinoma related to chole-dochal cysts with internal drainage operation. *Surg Gynecol Obstet* 1987;164:61–64

Todani T, Watanabe Y, et al. Reoperation for congenital choledochal cyst. *Ann Surg* 1988;207:142–147

Todani T, Tabuchi K, et al. Carcinoma arising in the wall of congenital bile duct cysts. *Cancer* 1979;44:1134–1141

Trout HH, Longmire WP Jr. Long term followup study of pa-tients with congenital cystic dilation of the common bile duct. *Am J Surg* 1971;121:68–86

Vanderpool D, Lane BW, et al. Choledochal cysts. *Surg Gynecol Obstet* 1988;167:447–451

Voyles CR, Smadja C, et al. Carcinoma in choledochal cysts: age-related incidence. *Arch Surg* 1983;118:986–988

60

Cholelithiasis and Cholecystectomy

Joseph Karam ■ *Joel J. Roslyn*

■ HISTORY

Archaeological excavations demonstrating the presence of gallstones in young Egyptian women have confirmed that cholelithiasis has plagued mankind for over 2000 years.[1] During the last several centuries, numerous innovative and creative techniques have been introduced in an effort to manage patients with symptomatic gallstone disease. During the Middle Ages, alchemists frequently recommended to patients suffering from biliary colic the ingestion of waters rich in magnesium sulfate. While they appreciated that this empiric treatment was effective in minimizing such painful episodes, these early clinician/scientists probably did not understand the pathophysiological basis for their therapy. Today, we recognize that magnesium sulfate is a potent stimulus for gallbladder contraction, and may have helped evacuate the gallbladder of small stones. Nonetheless, the treatment for symptomatic gallstone disease remained relatively primitive and ineffective until the late 1800s. As surgical techniques began to evolve, John Bobbs, an Indiana surgeon, and others attempted to perform cholecystolithotomy, removing the stone from the gallbladder and leaving the organ in situ. While this proved to be effective in ameliorating acute symptoms, physicians were disappointed by the recurrence of symptoms in many of these patients. In 1882, Karl Langenbuch, a noted German surgeon, performed the first successful cholecystectomy.[2] This event marked the beginning of the successful management of a disease that continues to be a national and international health disorder. During the last 100 years, open cholecystectomy has remained the gold standard for the definitive management of patients with symptomatic cholelithiasis.

Despite the efficacy and safety of cholecystectomy, physicians have long pursued and investigated other less invasive options. The earliest attempts at medical dissolution for cholesterol gallstones were reported in the mid 1920s. These early pioneering studies ultimately paved the way for the development of bile acid dissolution therapy. Although two agents for oral dissolution are now commercially available, their utility has been limited by stone recurrence, side effects and toxicity, cost, and by the availability of other, more effective treatment modalities. The development of a potent cholesterol solvent, methyl turt-butyl ether, provided the opportunity for the introduction of a form of gallstone dissolution in which a catheter is placed percutaneously in the gallbladder and the agent is directly instilled. This technique, while theoretically attractive, has found limited utility because of its invasive nature, as well as problems with gallstone recurrence. The management of patients with gallstone disease has been revolutionized during the last seven years with the introduction and evolution of laparoscopic cholecystectomy. This technique is rapidly emerging as the gold standard for the treatment of patients with symptomatic gallstone disease, and is now available throughout most parts of the world. This technique has a number of advantages as compared to conventional therapy, including improved patient compliance and satisfaction, and reduced cost.

Its primary advantage over nonoperative modalities for the treatment of gallstone disease is that the gallbladder is completely removed with a laparoscopic cholecystectomy, and the recurrence rate is therefore essentially zero. Proper training in laparoscopic techniques, patient selection, and careful follow-up are essential in assessing the proper role of this technique in the treatment of patients with gallstone disease. As our ability to safely remove the gallbladder and access the bile duct laparoscopically improves, surgeons are being confronted by a new set of challenges and need to re-evaluate traditional algorithms for decision-making. Patient selection criteria for open versus laparoscopic cholecystectomy, the role of preoperative endoscopic retrograde cholangiopancreaticography (ERCP) in evaluating patients with presumed common bile duct stones, and indications for laparoscopic choledochotomy, are but a few of the questions that are being addressed and defined. One can only anticipate that well-designed outcome analyses will help clarify and define the most appropriate and cost-effective treatment for gallstone disease, particularly insofar as it affects such a significant percentage of the population in many countries throughout the world.

■ CLASSIFICATION OF GALLSTONES

The schema for classifying gallstone disease may be based on stone composition, location, and etiology. Worldwide, pigment stones (brown or black) account for the majority of calculi. These stones are endemic in parts of Asia. Cholesterol or mixed cholesterol and pigment stones are the most common type of stones found in the United States, and account for approximately 70% of all stones in the United States and most Western nations.

Biliary calculi may be found either in the gallbladder, extrahepatic biliary tract, or within the intrahepatic ductal system. Although most Western patients with cholelithiasis have stones exclusively in the gallbladder, up to 15% of patients will have, in addition, common bile duct stones. Primary common bile duct stones forming exclusively in the intrahepatic or extrahepatic bile ducts is unusual, and accounts for probably <5% of all ductal stone disease. Most stones found in the common bile duct are actually gallbladder stones that pass into the common bile duct, either through the cystic duct or, occasionally, through a biliary fistula. Intrahepatic stone disease is a well-recognized clinical entity that occurs predominantly in parts of Asia and probably results from a sequence of events initiated by chronic biliary infection, leading to stricture formation, stasis, and the biochemical deconjugation of bilirubin resulting in the precipitation of calcium bilirubinate.

■ PATHOGENESIS OF CHOLESTEROL GALLSTONES

The pathogenesis of gallstones is certainly multifactorial and, although there are certain elements common to both cholesterol and pigment stone disease, there are significant etiologic differences between these two clinical entities. A clearer understanding of the pathogenesis of gallstone disease has provided a rational basis for the development of nonoperative modalities designed to dissolve or prevent gallstone formation. Many years ago, the prevailing opinion suggested that the formation of cholesterol calculi was the result of specific alterations in hepatic metabolism and that the gallbladder was "an innocent bystander." More recent studies suggest that neither the liver nor the gallbladder alone has an exclusive etiologic role in the formation of calculi. Moreover, it appears that cholesterol calculi form as the result of a dynamic interaction between the liver and the gallbladder, wherein factors present within cholesterol-saturated bile induce a series of alterations in gallbladder function that promote nucleation and stone growth.[3] The solubilization of cholesterol is critical to the formation of cholesterol gallstones, and understanding the factors that regulate this process has provided new insights into gallstone disease. It is helpful to arbitrarily view gallstone formation as occurring in three stages: cholesterol saturation, nucleation, and stone growth (Fig 60–1).

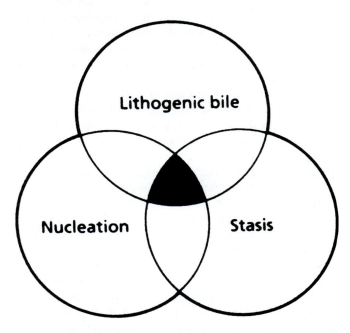

Figure 60–1. Three elements necessary for gallstone formation. The shaded area represents the interaction of all three. (From Abedin MZ, Roslyn JJ. Gallstone pathogenesis. In: Darzi A, et al (ed), *Techniques in the Management of Gallstones.* Oxford, England: Blackwell Scientific; 1995

CHOLESTEROL SATURATION

Cholesterol is virtually insoluble in bile, and is dependent on some other mechanism for its solubilization. For many years, it was thought that the key to maintaining cholesterol in solution was the formation of mixed bile acid-lecithin-cholesterol micelles. Bile acids are amphipathic compounds, with one end being hydrophilic and polar, while the other end is hydrophobic and nonpolar. Although bile acids exist as individual ionized molecules when in dilute solutions, these molecules undergo a physical transformation when present in a sufficient concentration, and form micelles. These cylindrical aggregates are oriented such that the hydrophobic end is oriented inward, and the polar, hydrophilic end points outward. Incorporation of lecithin into the micelle allows water to penetrate the structure, causing swelling. This process increases the ability of the micelle to transport greater amounts of cholesterol. Any alteration in the relative molar concentration of bile acids, lecithin, and cholesterol, will disturb the homeostasis and presumably lead to cholesterol precipitation. The critical nature of this relationship was described in 1968 by Admirand and Small in their now classic paper.[4] More recent information indicates that perhaps no more than 30% of biliary cholesterol is transported in micelles. Several independent investigators have demonstrated that much of the biliary cholesterol normally present in bile actually exists in a vesicular form.[5,6] These vesicles are made up of lipid bilayers similar to those found in cell membranes, and are capable of solubilizing greater quantities of cholesterol. The relative amounts of cholesterol transported in vesicles or micelles is related to the degree of bile saturation, and alteration of this delicate equilibrium would appear to be a key determinant of crystal precipitation, and ultimately stone formation. Regardless of the mode of cholesterol transport, failure to solubilize all cholesterol present, either as a result of excessive quantity or alteration of the vehicle, is considered to be a critical step in the formation of gallstones. Theoretically, an increase in cholesterol concentration relative to bile acids and lecithin can occur as a result of altered secretion of any of these three biliary lipids. It is generally accepted that the cholesterol content of bile exceeds the solubilizing capacity in patients with cholesterol gallstones. Cholesterol supersaturated bile can occur secondary to secretion of hepatic bile with either increased amounts of cholesterol or decreased amounts of bile acids or lecithin. The former situation has been established as a cause of lithogenic bile in most patients. Healthy patients, without cholesterol gallstones, have bile that is nearly saturated with cholesterol and exhibit the secretion of cholelithogenic bile during periods of fasting or starvation. This finding suggests that factors other than cholesterol saturation of bile may play an important etiologic role in the formation of cholesterol gallstones.

NUCLEATION

Nucleation refers to the process by which cholesterol monohydrate crystals form and agglomerate to become macroscopic stones. The realization that healthy humans without gallstones may secrete cholesterol-saturated bile and form crystals during various times of the day, suggest that there must be specific factors present or absent in bile that promote or retard the process of nucleation. Evidence has emerged that suggests that aggregation of cholesterol-phospholipid vesicles is critical to nucleation and formation of cholesterol crystals. Nucleation occurs more rapidly in the gallbladder bile of patients with cholesterol gallstones as compared to individuals with saturated bile, but without stones. Data are conflicting regarding the presence of antinucleating factors in bile of patients who fail to form gallstones versus the presence of pronucleating factors in gallstone patients.[7–9] Several specific heat labile glycoproteins in the bile of gallstone patients have been identified as potential pronucleating factors. It has been proposed that specific proteins within cholesterol-saturated bile induce vesicular aggregation and ultimately, promote stone growth. Nucleation time of gallbladder and hepatic bile correlates with nucleation time of vesicles, as opposed to micelles. Similar relationships between nucleation time and total protein, as well as vesicular cholesterol concentration, have been noted.

Diet-induced cholesterol gallstone formation in animal models is characterized by increased gallbladder mucin secretion. This mucous gel can serve as a nucleating agent and as a matrix on which crystals can agglomerate and cluster. Human gallbladder mucin has been shown to accelerate nucleation of cholesterol in artificial bile.[10] Separation of vesicular and micellar fractions of cholesterol indicate that nucleation of cholesterol crystals is accelerated significantly in the presence of bovine gallbladder mucin only in cholesterol-containing vesicles and not in mixed micelles. The physicochemical behavior of gallbladder mucin and bile is influenced by both mucin and electrolyte concentrations at the epithelial surface of the gallbladder, activities that have been shown to be altered in experimentally induced cholesterol gallstone formation. These data suggest that mucin may be a pronucleating factor. Moreover, administration of pharmacologic doses of aspirin to an animal model significantly inhibits mucous secretion, and simultaneously reduces the incidence of diet-induced gallstones. The relationship between mucin secretion and vesicle formation and stability suggests that a clear understanding of the factors responsible for vesicle formation may help elucidate and further clarify the mechanism by which nucleation and gallstone formation occurs. Nucleation occurs from the metastable phase as opposed to the more stable micellar phase. Efforts are underway to understand the physiologic balance between nucleation-inhibiting and pronucleating factors, and the manner in which this balance may be disturbed during cholesterol gallstone formation.

Stasis of bile within the gallbladder has been identified in a number of clinical settings associated with an increased incidence of cholelithiasis.[11–13] Moreover, experimental studies have demonstrated specific motor defects, including decreased gallbladder motility and emptying, and increased cystic duct resistance in diet-induced models of cholesterol gallstones.[14–17] Theoretically, a stagnant pool of bile within the gallbladder may result in a decrease in the amount of bile salts available for cholesterol solubilization, and therefore predispose to saturation and crystal formation. Although data has been conflicting, recent evidence suggests that the formation of cholesterol gallstones in humans is indeed associated with alterations in gallbladder motor activity.[18,19] Stasis of bile within the gallbladder is thought to provide an ideal milieu for the precipitation of specific factors present in gallbladder bile. The relationship between gallbladder stasis and the concentration of nucleating or antinucleating factors in gallbladder bile continues to be investigated. Other factors presumed to be important to the nucleation process include increased concentrations of biliary calcium, alterations in gallbladder prostaglandin metabolism, and alterations in gallbladder absorptive and secretory function.

STONE GROWTH

The growth of cholesterol gallstones has been traditionally viewed as a natural consequence of cholesterol precipitation and agglomeration. Whether, in fact, stone formation is an inevitable consequence of agglomeration of cholesterol crystals remains unclear. The exact cascade of events by which stone growth occurs has not been well studied.

■ PATHOGENESIS OF PIGMENT STONES

Although the pathogenesis of cholesterol gallstones has been the subject of considerable investigation, there has been limited effort to study the mechanisms by which pigment gallstones form. A number of factors may explain this phenomenon, including the relative infrequency with which pigment gallstones are found in the United States, lack of a suitable animal model, and the heterogenous nature of pigment gallstones. Despite the diverse settings in which pigment gallstones are known

to occur, the final common pathway in the pathogenesis of the various types of pigment calculi is altered solubilization of unconjugated bilirubin with precipitation of calcium bilirubinate and insoluble salts. Pigment stones are classified as either brown or black stones. Brown stones have a characteristic appearance and consistency, and are typically found in Asia. These stones are similar in composition to primary common bile duct stones, and presumably occur as a result of infection.[20,21] Free, unconjugated bilirubin produced by bacterial deconjugation combines with calcium and bile to produce a calcium bilirubinate matrix. This structure appears to be the predominant component of most pigment gallstones. Bacteria are found within the calcium bilirubinate–protein matrix of brown pigment stones, but are conspicuously absent from either black pigment or cholesterol gallstones. The release of beta glucuronidase by gram-negative bacteria has long been thought to be the critical factor in the formation of brown pigment gallstones. This enzyme results in the enzymatic hydrolysis of bilirubin glucuronide into free bilirubin and glucuronic acid. The free, unconjugated bilirubin, which is insoluble in water, combines with calcium in the bile to produce a calcium bilirubinate matrix. The finding that endogenously synthesized beta glucuronidase is secreted in human bile suggests another possible factor in the pathogenesis of brown pigment gallstones.

Epidemiologic studies have failed to define any relationship between formation of black pigment stones and infected bile. These stones typically are found in patients with hemolytic disorders or cirrhosis. The absence of bacteria from most patients with black pigment stones suggest that other factors may be operational. A high incidence of pigment gallstones in patients with hemolytic disorders probably results from excessive loads of bilirubin being presented to the liver for excretion. Two possible explanations for the high incidence of pigment gallstones in cirrhotics include hypersplenism leading to increased hemolysis, and impaired hepatic conjugation of bilirubin. It has been proposed that unconjugated bilirubin may be secreted directly into hepatic bile, where, in the presence of increased amounts of cholesterol, the bilirubin moiety is driven out of the micelle and is available for precipitation with calcium. The presumed role of calcium in the pathogenesis of pigment gallstone formation has been substantiated by the finding that bile is supersaturated with calcium bilirubinate. In a manner similar to cholesterol solubilization, mixed micelles are thought to be an important factor in regulating calcium binding. Increased concentrations of biliary calcium in animals and humans with pigment gallstones have been correlated with specific change in bile acid composition. It has been proposed that changes in the relative concentrations of individual bile acids associated with gallstone formation may alter phospho-lipid—bile acid micelles, resulting in a reduction of biliary calcium solubility and promotion of nucleation. This entire process may be facilitated by stasis of bile within the gallbladder.

■ DEMOGRAPHIC AND EPIDEMIOLOGIC CONSIDERATIONS

INCIDENCE

The incidence of biliary calculus disease varies widely throughout the world. Approximately 10% of the population in the United States has documented cholelithiasis. In addition to the 25 million people with known gallstone disease, another 800 000 new cases are diagnosed each year in the United States. A decade ago, it was generally viewed that over 90% of gallstone patients in the United States had cholesterol stones. More recent studies would suggest that there is a trend towards an increasing incidence of pigment gallstones. This probably reflects the changing ethnic composition of the United States population. The incidence of gallstone disease in Asia is considerable, and constitutes a problem of enormous magnitude. As stated previously, most patients in the Far East with cholelithiasis have pigment stones. The incidence of cholesterol gallstones is increasing in Asia for reasons that may be related to environmental and dietary considerations. The incidence of gallstones in Africa is quite low, and this has been attributed to genetic and/or dietary factors.

AGE

Epidemiologic studies have clearly demonstrated a linear relationship between increasing age and the prevalence of cholelithiasis.[22] Although gallstones are rarely seen in the pediatric population, children with hemolytic disorders, ileal disorders, and/or short gut syndrome maintained on long-term parenteral nutrition are predisposed to the formation of pigment stones. A number of factors have been proposed as possible explanations for the increased incidence of gallstone disease noted in the elderly population. The proportion of cholesterol present in bile and the cholesterol saturation index are significantly increased in elderly women compared with younger subjects. A change in the ratio of androgen and estrogen that is physiologic in elderly males has been associated with specific alterations in biliary lipid metabolism and gallbladder motility, and may contribute to the increased incidence of gallstones that has been observed in elderly men. Ultrasonographic studies indicate that gallbladder sensitivity to cholecystokinin (CCK), the primary hormonal stimulus for gall-bladder contraction, decreases with aging. Although serum concentrations of pancreatic polypeptide increase with aging, its etiologic relationship with gallbladder motor activity and stone formation remains unclear. Further studies are needed to clarify the effects of these and other endogenous peptides on gallbladder contractility and absorptive function in the geriatric population.

GENDER AND HORMONES

For centuries, physicians and the lay public have been aware that gallstone disease is found much more commonly in women than in men. Moreover, the association between the number of pregnancies and the incidence of gallstone disease also has been well recognized. Biliary tract symptoms frequently are found in women in the second and third trimesters of pregnancy, and the development of acute cholecystitis postpartum is a well-established clinical entity. The propensity to form gallstones in women is almost certainly owing to hormonal-mediated changes in gallbladder motor function and biliary lipid metabolism. Gallbladder motility is altered during pregnancy as manifested by decreased gallbladder emptying and a concomitant increase in absolute and residual gallbladder volume after contraction. These effects are due to progesterone and result in incomplete gallbladder emptying and biliary stasis. Estrogen-induced alterations in cholesterol metabolism have been well documented in premenopausal women, as well as women receiving exogenous estrogen administration. Experimental studies suggest that estrogen decreases activity of the hepatic enzyme responsible for the conversion of cholesterol to bile acids, resulting in a decrease in bile acid synthesis and secretion, and an associated increase in cholesterol saturation of bile. The effects of decreased gallbladder emptying and increased cholesterol saturation of bile create an ideal environment for the formation of cholesterol gallstones.

OBESITY AND RAPID WEIGHT LOSS

Obesity has long been recognized as a risk factor for the formation of cholesterol gallstones. Epidemiologic evidence suggests there is a twofold to threefold increase in the incidence of cholelithiasis among morbidly obese patients, compared with age-matched normal weight individuals. Over 50% of women 45 to 55 years of age who are classified as morbidly obese have a history of cholelithiasis and gallbladder disease. Moreover, morbidly obese patients are more resistant to drug therapy to dissolve gallstones than are normal weight individuals. Metabolic studies indicate that obese patients secrete hepatic bile that has an increased concentration of cholesterol relative to the other biliary lipids. Presumably, it is this propensity to secrete cholelithogenic bile that predisposes to the formation of cholesterol gallstones in this patient population. Clinical evidence suggests that 25% to 30% of patients undergoing bariatric surgery as primary therapy for morbid obesity have had a prior cholecystectomy. An additional 10% to 15% of these patients will be noted to have gallstones preoperatively, if routine ultrasonography is performed. It has been of some interest that rapid weight loss in previously morbidly obese patients has been associated with secretion of cholesterol-saturated bile and an increased incidence of gallstones. Although the mechanism for this phenomenon remains unclear, a major factor is probably sequestration of bile acids and the concomitant reduction in bile acid pool.

DIABETES

Clinical experience has long suggested that patients with diabetes mellitus have an increased risk of developing gallstones, as compared to nondiabetics. A rational explanation for this finding is derived from the observations that diabetic patients have bile that is usually supersaturated with cholesterol, a reduced bile acid pool, and impaired gallbladder motor activity. Furthermore, there is some evidence to suggest that treatment of diabetics with insulin actually exacerbates the predisposition to gallstone formation by increasing the degree of cholesterol saturation of bile.

The clinical significance of this presumed etiological relationship between diabetes and gallstone formation has been the subject of some debate and controversy during recent years.[23,24] Traditional teaching suggests that diabetics with gallstones were more likely to develop acute cholecystitis and be at greater risk for postoperative septic complications. This dogma led to the recommendation that diabetics with even asymptomatic stones were candidates for prophylactic cholecystectomy. More recent data indicate that the incidence of gallbladder perforation, wound infection, and overall morbidity and mortality was not significantly different between the diabetic and nondiabetics undergoing cholecystectomy. Although these and other studies have suggested that diabetes itself is not a significant risk factor for severe biliary tract disease nor postoperative complications following cholecystectomy, the exact relationship between diabetes and postoperative morbidity and mortality remains poorly defined.

CIRRHOSIS

The exact frequency with which cholelithiasis occurs in patients with alcohol-induced cirrhosis remains unclear. Nonetheless, autopsy studies do indicate that the incidence of gallstone disease is increased significantly in patients with alcoholic cirrhosis, compared to the general population. Interestingly enough, these stones would appear to be primarily pigment stones. Recent experimental data suggest that alcohol consumption in an animal model may actually be protective regarding the development of cholesterol gallstone disease. Biliary lipid studies indicate that bile from patients with cirrhosis has a greater cholesterol solubilizing capacity than bile from normal subjects. Specific alterations in bile acid metabolism have been proposed as critical to the pathogenesis of cirrhosis-induced pigment gallstones.

It has been well documented that, regardless of the type of gallstones present, cholecystectomy, when performed in cirrhotic patients, is associated with significant morbidity and mortality.[25,26] Most of the difficulties associated with operation in these patients relate to propensity to bleeding and difficulty in controlling hemorrhage. Several factors are responsible for this, including portal hypertension, thrombocytopenia secondary to hypersplenism, and coagulopathy owing to impaired hepatic synthetic function. Recognition that the perioperative morbidity may approach 40% to 50% in this selected group of patients has led to the recommendation that indications for open or laparoscopic cholecystectomy in a cirrhotic patient should be more restrictive than in normal, healthy individuals. Operation should be undertaken only in those patients who are truly symptomatic or who require operative intervention because of an acute complication from their biliary tract disease. Many surgeons have advocated performing a partial cholecystectomy in cirrhotic patients, leaving the posterior wall of the gallbladder attached to the hepatic bed, so as to minimize the propensity for bleeding.

VAGOTOMY

In years gone by, there was great interest in defining the possible etiologic relationship between truncal vagotomy and an increased risk of cholesterol gallstone formation. Although early clinical studies suggested that truncal vagotomy was associated with a twofold increase in the incidence of gallstones, other studies failed to confirm this hypothesis. While ultrasonographic studies suggest that truncal vagotomy is associated with a dilated gallbladder, numerous experimental studies have been unable to demonstrate any increased incidence of gallstone formation following bilateral truncal vagotomy.

TOTAL PARENTERAL NUTRITION AND GALLSTONE FORMATION

In the 1970s, the development and introduction of total parenteral nutrition (TPN) as a means of providing nutritional support for critically ill patients who are unable to consume oral nutrition revolutionized the practice of medicine and surgery. While we now believe that the enteral administration of calories may have significant advantages over the parenteral route, the contribution that TPN has made to the management of surgical diseases should not be minimized. In addition to potential catheter and other technically related complications, the administration of long-term TPN also has been associated with a variety of metabolic complications and a purported increased risk of gallstone formation. Early anecdotal reports suggested that the long-term administration of TPN predisposed to both acalculous and calculus cholecystitis. A number of large clinical studies subsequently have confirmed the etiologic relationship between TPN and gallstone formation in both children and adults.[27,28] Ultrasonographic studies have helped identify the scientific basis for gallstone formation in this subset of population, and have focused our attention on the relationship between altered gallbladder motor activity, decreased stimulation for gallbladder contraction, and the formation of sludge and ultimately, biliary lithiasis. Preliminary studies suggest that most de novo stones in this setting are composed primarily of calcium bilirubinate.

The clinical importance of TPN-induced gallbladder disease is underscored by the observation that asymptomatic and symptomatic gallstone disease forms in approximately 45% of patients (both children and adults) who are maintained on long-term TPN. Many of these patients have underlying gastrointestinal disorders, or have recently undergone other abdominal operations. This clinical setting often makes the diagnosis of biliary tract disease difficult. One report has indicated that 40% of patients with TPN-induced gallbladder disease require emergent cholecystectomy, and that severe acute cholecystitis was present in more than 50% of these patients.[29] Furthermore, these authors suggest that the perioperative morbidity and mortality in this subset of patients is significantly greater as compared to other patients undergoing cholecystectomy for symptomatic gallstone disease. These observations have led some authors to conclude that prophylactic cholecystectomy should be considered in patients who are committed to a long-term course of TPN and who are undergoing exploratory laparotomy for other indications. In addition, experimental and clinical studies have indicated a beneficial role for pharmacologic prophylaxis with periodic stimulation of gallbladder contraction in the reduction and prevention of TPN-induced gallbladder disease.

■ CLINICAL PRESENTATION

NATURAL HISTORY

It is impossible to view gallstone disease as a single, homogeneous entity. The spectrum of clinical syndromes associated with biliary stone disease is as varied as the etiologies and risk factors that have been associated with the formation of gallstones. The large number of patients in the United States and throughout the world who harbor gallstones has made it essential that we develop a rational approach to the management of patients with this disorder. Understanding the natural history of asymptomatic and symptomatic gallstones, therefore, becomes essential both from a medical and economic perspective. It generally is believed that, at least in the United States, up to 50% of all patients with gallstones are asymptomatic. The remaining patients may have intermittent episodes of recurring biliary colic, or present with acute cholecystitis, symptoms secondary to choledocholithiasis or gallstone pancreatitis. Recently completed prospective longitudinal studies have attempted to trace the natural history of asymptomatic gallstone disease in several well-defined patient populations.[30,31] Although both of these studies would suggest that only a small percentage of patients with asymptomatic gallstone disease develop serious complications within a finite period of time, questions continue to linger about how best to identify patients at risk for developing complications from their stone disease. Death from uncomplicated gallstone disease is uncommon, and <1% of all patients requiring hospitalization for management of the initial manifestation of gallstone disease will have a fatal outcome. Nonetheless, there are numerous questions that continue to exist regarding the ideal management of patients with asymptomatic gallstone disease. The importance of resolving this issue is underscored by the recognition of the large number of patients harboring asymptomatic gallstones.

The inability to precisely define what constitutes an asymptomatic patient and moreover, how to identify such patients, has made resolution of this issue difficult. It is apparent that a significant number of patients with cholelithiasis do not have postprandial pain, but instead are plagued by dyspepsia, vague epigastric discomfort, or even mildly increased flatulence as the primary manifestation of their biliary stone disease. Gallstone patients who complain of nonspecific dyspeptic symptoms without biliary colic are less likely to have a satisfactory outcome following cholecystectomy. However, the fact that up to 70% of such patients will derive significant benefit from surgical removal of the gallbladder suggests that nonspecific symptomatology may be attributable to biliary calculi. Should these patients be considered as asymptomatic when one discusses the optimal treatment for patients with asymptomatic stones? This author believes not, and would propose that one should apply the strictest of criteria to patients when considering the optimal management for asymptomatic stone disease. At this point in time, it is truly impossible to accurately define the natural history of patients with asymptomatic cholelithiasis and moreover, it is extremely difficult to select a priori, those patients who would benefit from prophylactic cholecystectomy. The economic consequences of performing routine prophylactic cholecystectomy on all patients with asymptomatic gallstones would be staggering. Nonetheless, early cholecystectomy should be considered in any patient with asymptomatic gallstones who is particularly concerned about developing complications from biliary tract disease or in patients who have major risk factors and on whom operation is not contraindicated because of poor medical condition. In addition, it is perfectly acceptable to perform cholecystectomy in patients who are asymptomatic and are undergoing laparotomy for other reasons. Medical dissolution with oral agents as a primary therapeutic modality for cholelithiasis has been disappointing, and therefore this modality cannot be recommended for the management of patients with asymptomatic gallstone disease. Similar thoughts would apply to contact dissolution with MTBE, as well as biliary lithotripsy. The role of laparoscopic cholecystectomy in the management of patients with asymptomatic gallstone disease is beginning to emerge as a controversial issue. Most authors believe that the same criteria that have been established for open cholecystectomy and asymptomatic stone disease should be applied for this new technology as well.

RISK OF GALLBLADDER CARCINOMA

The development of gallbladder carcinoma has long been recognized as a potential complication of patients with gallstone disease.[32] In particular, this complication would appear to develop in patients with longstanding single large stones. Seventy to ninety percent of all patients with gallbladder cancer have gallstones, and about 0.4% of all patients with gallstones will ultimately develop carcinoma of the gallbladder. The risk of carcinoma of the gallbladder is particularly high in patients with single stones >3 cm in diameter. Although there is an increased risk of cancer formation in patients with such stones, the potential risk is so low that prophylactic cholecystectomy cannot be recommended in this group of patients. Calcification of the gallbladder wall, or so-called porcelain gallbladder, has been associated with a 25% to 60% incidence of carcinoma.[33] In this small subgroup of patients, cholecystectomy probably is warranted to prevent the formation of cancer, even in patients who are completely asymptomatic.

BILIARY COLIC AND CHRONIC CHOLECYSTITIS

The term "colic" is commonly used to describe the pain associated with gallbladder disease. Unfortunately, this is somewhat of a misnomer, since the pain is actually constant in most patients, as opposed to the usual intermittent, crescendo-type pain normally associated with ureteral stones or small bowel obstruction. The symptoms that comprise biliary colic result from the impaction of a gallstone in the cystic duct or in the infundibulum of the gallbladder. Obstruction of the outlet causes contraction of the gallbladder against resistance, with failure of the gallbladder to empty. Classically, the onset of pain is within 30 to 60 minutes after consumption of a meal, and usually lasts for several hours. Although the inciting meal is classically described as fatty, any meal can stimulate gallbladder contraction and therefore, biliary colic. In most cases, the pain associated with biliary colic is self-limiting. It is intense, escalates rapidly, and generally is of a steady quality before it dissipates. Nausea and vomiting often accompany the abdominal pain and represent constitutional manifestations of visceral obstruction. The frequency with which attacks of biliary colic occur is unpredictable and is neither linked to the size nor the number of stones present within the gallbladder. For reasons that are unclear, once patients begin to have attacks of biliary colic, these episodes tend to occur with increasing frequency and intensity. There is no concrete evidence that avoidance of specific foods will, in fact, alter the natural history of this disease.

The pain of biliary colic is typically located in the right upper quadrant, or midepigastrium. Pain will frequently radiate laterally around the back to the inferior medial aspect of the right scapula. Based on the dermatomal distribution, pain also may be referred to the right shoulder. Patients experiencing biliary colic will not manifest any evidence of peritonitis on clinical examination. They may, however, demonstrate some right upper quadrant tenderness on palpation. The remainder of the physical examination is frequently unremarkable. Laboratory tests are often not helpful in diagnosing biliary colic. The diagnosis is suggested by clinical presentation, and is confirmed by documenting the presence of gallstones.

ACUTE CHOLECYSTITIS

Acute inflammation of the gallbladder is the most common complication of gallstone disease. This clinical entity is similar in many regards to biliary colic in terms of etiology and pathophysiology. The initiating factor is impaction of a stone either in the cystic duct or in the infundibulum of the gallbladder. The onset and character of pain associated with acute cholecystitis is often indistinguishable from that which is observed initially in patients with biliary colic. The pain of acute cholecystitis may be more intense and, unlike biliary colic, persists for several days. The exact frequency with which acute cholecystitis occurs is unclear. It is a frequent indication for exploration for intra-abdominal emergencies, particularly in middle-aged women and in the elderly. It has previously been estimated that 15% to 20% of the 500 000 to 700 000 cholecystectomies performed annually in this country are done for acute cholecystitis. In recent years, there is evidence to suggest that this trend actually may be changing, and that the frequency with which acute cholecystitis occurs is increasing.[34,35] This trend is somewhat disturbing, and probably relates to changes in health care economics and access to health care.[36] As stated above, acute inflammation of the gallbladder is associated with cystic duct obstruction. The mechanism by which cholecystitis develops, however, remains unclear. The combination of cystic duct occlusion and altered biliary lipid composition appears to initiate the cascade of events which culminate in the mucosal release of inflammatory agents from the gallbladder. There is both direct and indirect evidence that prostaglandins may be important mediators of the inflammatory process. A number of experimental studies suggest that alterations in prostanoid metabolism occur during gallstone formation. In clinical studies, indomethacin, a prostaglandin synthetase inhibitor, has been shown to be effective in the management of pain secondary to acute cholecystitis. Further studies are needed to define more clearly the role of prostaglandins and other cellular mediators in the inflammatory response. Although bacteria are cultured in approximately 50% of patients with acute cholecystitis, these organisms generally are thought to play a secondary role in the pathogenesis of cholecystitis. The gross changes that occur with acute cholecystitis have been well described, and include edema, hypervascularity, venous engorgement, and gallbladder distension. At the time of laparotomy, the acutely inflamed gallbladder often is surrounded by omentum or is adherent to the duodenum and contiguous structures. Depending on the evolution of the disease process, there may be gross evidence of ischemia, particularly in the least vascularized portion of the gallbladder, the fundus.

In the early stages of acute cholecystitis, the character of the pain may be indistinguishable from biliary colic. However, unlike biliary colic, in which the pain lasts for minutes to hours, the pain of acute cholecystitis tends to be progressive. With time and the progression of the inflammatory process, the gallbladder becomes even more distended, and may ultimately result in inflammation of the contiguous parietal peritoneum. At this point in time, the patient typically complains of well-localized right upper quadrant pain. Many of these patients will experience anorexia, nausea, and vomiting, and may manifest a low-grade fever. As a result of associated peritoneal irritation, the patient is often reluctant to move, and is most comfortable lying relatively still and calm. Palpation of the abdomen frequently elicits localized tenderness in the right upper quadrant, which is associated with guarding and rebound tender-

ness. The classic physical finding of acute cholecystitis is a positive Murphy's sign, which refers to inspiratory arrest during deep palpation in the right upper quadrant. There is clearly a wide variation in the spectrum of complaints and physical findings in patients with acute cholecystitis. While most patients with uncomplicated acute cholecystitis will have right upper quadrant pain, fever, and evidence of leukocytosis, the diagnosis also may be suggested by the persistance of right upper quadrant pain in excess of 4 to 6 hours, without any other associated findings. A mass is found in only 20% of patients with acute cholecystitis and typically is secondary to adherent omentum overlying the inflamed gallbladder. Most patients with uncomplicated acute cholecystitis will have a leukocytosis in the range of 12 000 to 15 000. Values much above 20 000 should suggest the possibility of gangrenous cholecystitis, perforation, cholangitis, or some other more serious complication of biliary tract stone disease. The differential diagnosis of acute cholecystitis includes other common causes of acute abdominal pain, including acute appendicitis, perforated ulcer, pancreatitis, pyelonephritis, right lower lobe pneumonitis, myocardial infarction, and cholangitis.

Although bacteria do not play a primary role in the pathogenesis of acute cholecystitis, septic complications continue to be a source of significant morbidity after cholecystectomy when the indication for operation is acute cholecystitis. In normal, healthy subjects without gallstones, the incidence of positive bile cultures is essentially zero. The incidence of positive bile cultures in patients with chronic cholecystitis who undergo elective operation for biliary colic, is probably ≤20%. In contrast, bacteria can be cultured from the bile of 50% to 70% of patients with acute cholecystitis. Bacteria typically isolated are of enteric origin, with the most common species being *Escherichia coli*. Other bacteria which may be present include *Enterobacter* or *Klebsiella*. *Enterococcus* is emerging as an important biliary pathogen, particularly in the elderly or patients with complications of cholecystitis such as empyema, gangrene, or perforation. The presence of bacteria in the bile of patients with acute cholecystitis is a source of significant morbidity and mortality, and is a predictor of the organism that would be isolated from a wound infection or intra-abdominal abscess following cholecystectomy. A number of studies have tried to identify risk factors that would be predictive of septic complications. These risk factors include patients >70 years of age, indication for operation being acute cholecystitis, history of obstructive jaundice, and the presence of common duct stones. These factors form a rational basis for prophylactic antibiotics in patients undergoing cholecystectomy. The goal of antimicrobial therapy should be the establishment of adequate serum and tissue levels of antibiotic rather than achieving specific biliary concentrations of drug. Appropriate antibiotic regimens should therefore provide coverage against gram-negative aerobes. If septic complications develop postoperatively, the choice of antibiotics should be based on operative cultures as well as on cultures from the wound or intra-abdominal fluid collections.

CHRONIC CHOLECYSTITIS

Chronic cholecystitis is a term that adds little to our understanding of the clinical manifestations of gallstone disease. In patients who have had recurring bouts of biliary colic, or longstanding gallstones, it is not unusual to find that there is evidence of fibrosis and round-cell infiltration with some thickening of the gallbladder wall. In those patients, the mucosa is intact in this setting. Although patients with recurring biliary colic are thought histologically to have chronic cholecystitis, there is a subset of patients who despite having chronic inflammation of the gallbladder, do not have recurring pain. Some of these patients will indeed complain of dyspepsia, as manifested by excessive belching or flatus, postprandial abdominal bloating, fullness or discomfort, fatty food intolerance, epigastric burning, and nausea or vomiting. In the absence of other demonstrable gastrointenstinal disorders, these symptoms may be attributed to chronic cholecystitis.

■ DIAGNOSIS

OVERVIEW

The presence of gallstone disease is suggested by the appropriate clinical setting. The suspicion that an individual patient has symptoms referable to biliary tract stone disease is an indication for further diagnostic studies. To date, there are no serum or other laboratory tests that are absolutely specific for the presence of gallstones. As has already been mentioned, laboratory evaluation of patients with biliary colic generally is unrevealing. In the setting of acute cholecystitis, most patients will manifest a leukocytosis and may have a mild elevation of their transaminases and alkaline phosphatase. Significant hyperbilirubinemia is often indicative of biliary obstruction, and either common duct stones or neoplastic processes should be considered in this setting. Most clinicians rely on one of a number of imaging studies to confirm the diagnosis of cholelithiasis or cholecystitis.

ABDOMINAL RADIOGRAPHY

Supine and upright abdominal radiographs are of limited value in identifying gallstones. Visualization of gallstones on plain abdominal radiographs is possible only in that 20% of patients whose stones are grossly calcified. Nonetheless, gallstones are so common that they

are the most frequent cause of discrete right upper quadrant calcifications. Gallstones in this area may be confused with renal calculi, contrast material or calculi in diverticuli of the hepatic flexure of the colon, vascular calcifications, or other problems such as granulomas or hepatic cysts. The small number of calcified gallstones that will be seen on plain films are indicative of the fact that the majority of stones in the United States are cholesterol based and contain little calcium. Despite the overall limited utility of plain abdominal films in the diagnosis of gallstone disease, such radiographic examinations may be very helpful in eliminating other causes of acute abdominal pain.

ORAL CHOLECYSTOGRAPHY

In 1924, Graham and Cole introduced the concept of oral cholecystography (OCG) (Fig 60–2).[37] For many years, this test was considered the mainstay and gold standard for the diagnosis of gallstone disease. The technique, introduced more than 70 years ago, was based on two physiologic principles: halogenated dyes are excreted into bile, and the gallbladder is capable of concentrating bile eight- to ten-fold. In a normally functioning gallbladder, dye is concentrated as a result of the absorptive function of the gallbladder, and it will appear opacified. The presence of gallstones is suggested

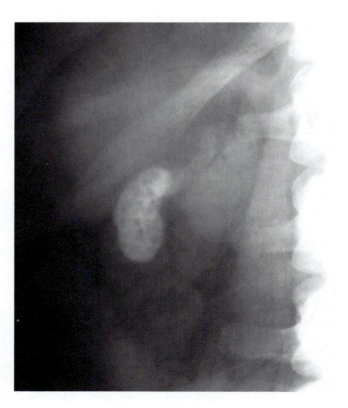

Figure 60–2. Oral cholecystogram

by the appearance of filling defects in an otherwise opacified gallbladder, or by nonvisualization. The latter is indicative of reduced absorption, which is consistent with chronic cholecystitis. The accuracy of oral cholecystography is reported to be between 95% to 99%. Such figures probably are inaccurate, and represent an underestimation of false negative studies. False-positive cholecystograms are quite rare. However, it is unclear how frequently patients are thought to have a normal OCG but, in fact, have gallstones (false-negative). One of the major criteria for establishing OCG evidence of gallstone disease has been nonopacification of the gallbladder after two successive doses of oral contrast medium. This has traditionally been thought to be indicative of gallstone disease in >90% of patients. However, it is now clear that there are a number of other factors that may account for nonopacification, including failure to ingest the contrast agent, failure of the agent to reach the small bowel, hepatic parenchymal disease or biliary obstruction, prolonged fasting, pancreatitis, hyperalimentation, and prior cholecystectomy. All of these factors, plus overall patient compliance, have been quite limiting in the efficacy and utility of oral cholecystography. Since 1976, it has been estimated that the number of oral cholecystograms performed has decreased by more than 80%. This trend has largely been due to the introduction and development of abdominal ultrasonography. Oral cholecystography is, however, more accurate than sonography in terms of quantification of number of stones and their size.

ABDOMINAL ULTRASONOGRAPHY

Cholecystosonography was introduced in the mid 1970s. This technology has evolved during the last 20 years, and has emerged as the preferred test for the evaluation of patients with suspected cholelithiasis or cholecystitis.[38,39] Initial studies of cholecystosonography suggested that the sensitivity for cholelithiasis was between 65% and 85%. More recent data suggests a sensitivity of 95% to 99%, with a very low false-positive and false negative rate. The performance of abdominal ultrasonography has been greatly enhanced by the development of real-time imaging. This technology has replaced static scanning. This newer technology provides better visualization and is able to allow the experienced scanner to more readily distinguish stones from other sources of shadow (Fig 60–3). In general, ultrasonography has distinct advantages over conventional oral cholecystography. These include absence of radiation exposure, independence of patient compliance, and the lack of a requirement for an intact digestive and hepatic system. A number of ultrasonographic criteria have been developed to allow for the identification of gallbladder stones or sludge. Limitations with sonography include the difficulty in actually measuring large stones and in quantifying more than three to five stones. Although abdominal ultrasonography is most useful in identifying gallstones, it also may facilitate the diagnosis of acute cholecystitis.[40] This diagnosis is suggested by the size and shape of the gallbladder, gallbladder wall thickness, and the presence of pericholecystic fluid collections. A sonographic Murphy's sign has been described, in which the technician probes the point of maximal tenderness and correlates this with the location of the gallbladder. Several studies have suggested that this sign has an 85% accuracy rate in diagnosing acute cholecystitis. Nonetheless, it should be recognized that ultrasonography is most beneficial in identifying the presence or absence of gallstones, and not whether or not a patient has

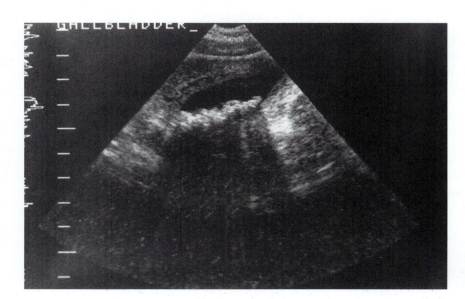

Figure 60–3. Gallbladder ultrasound showing multiple small echogenic foci (stones) in the dependent portion of the gallbladder. Note the acoustic shadows behind the stones.

acute cholecystitis. In addition to identifying stones within the gallbladder or bile duct, abdominal ultrasonography provides important ancillary information regarding the anatomy of bile ducts, pancreas, and other structures in the upper abdomen.

COMPUTED TOMOGRAPHY

Computed tomography (CT) scans are not a first-line test for the diagnosis of cholelithiasis.[41] Obvious gallstones frequently are missed by routine CT, although they may be seen as incidental findings, if they are densely calcified. In addition to failing to demonstrate calculi that might be seen more easily by ultrasonography or oral cholecystography, CT has the additional disadvantage, compared to cholecystosonography, of relying on ionizing radiation for images. Utilizing x-rays striking a series of sensitive detectors, images are created by computers, based on different sections and individual levels, and the entire body can be visualized. Although this test is not particularly sensitive for identifying gallstones, it does provide important information regarding the nature, extent, and location of biliary dilatation and masses in and around the biliary tract and pancreas. In general, this test provides more useful information than ultrasonography when the concern is extrahepatic obstruction owing to causes other than choledocholithiasis. Limiting factors for CT scanning include patient exposure to ionizing radiation and cost.

MAGNETIC RESONANCE IMAGING

Magnetic resonance imaging (MRI) provides images that may appear similar to CT. The images, however, result from the different magnetic properties of tissues, and rely on the use of a contrast material, gadolinium. This material, which is administered intravenously, affects the magnetic properties of tissues. Gallstones, when sufficiently large, may be visualized with MRI as low-intensity filling defects within the gallbladder bile. The majority of gallstones, however, produce no signal whatsoever with this modality. Therefore, its role in the evaluation of patients with cholelithiasis remains unclear at this time.

HEPATOBILIARY SCINTIGRAPHY

In the late 1970s, the introduction of technetium 99m (^{99m}TC)-labeled iminodiacetic acid (IDA) agents facilitated the development of radionuclide imaging as a diagnostic modality for suspected acute cholecystitis. This family of radionuclides provides direct imaging of the gallbladder and biliary tract. These agents, administered intravenously, are cleared from the blood by hepatocytes and excreted in an unconjugated form directly into the biliary ductal system. Currently, two commercially available IDA agents are in common use: disofenin and mebrofenin. These agents are superior to those that we used in earlier years, and make possible the evaluation of patients despite elevated bilirubin levels. In addition, these isotopes have a relatively short half-life and this provides for improved visualization with less radiation exposure for the patient. This test provides information on the patency of the bile ducts and cystic duct (Fig 60–4). Recognition that cystic duct obstruction is present represents the hallmark of the diagnosis of acute cholecystitis.[42] Cystic duct obstruction, and by implication acute cholecystitis, is diagnosed when there is normal imaging of the liver and common bile duct with prompt visualization of the duodenum but absence of label within the gallbladder. Failure to visualize the gallbladder after 60 minutes is diagnostic of cystic duct obstruction, and highly suggestive of acute cholecystitis. Delayed visualization of the cystic duct and gallbladder after four hours, even in patients with al-

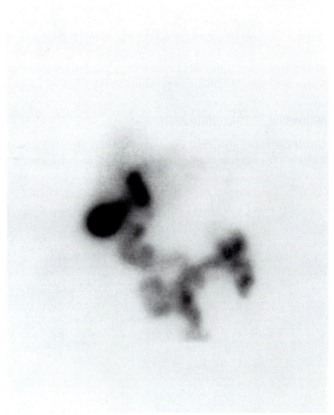

A

Figure 60–4. HIDA scan. **A.** shows a normal scan with visualization of the gallbladder (*arrow*). *Continued*

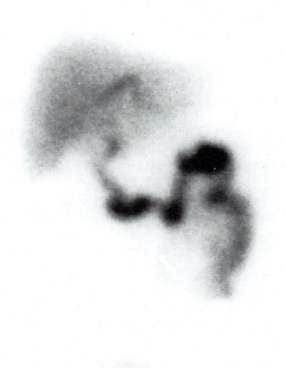

B

Figure 60–4. cont'd. B. Demonstrates radionucleotide in the common bile duct and small intestine; however the gallbladder does not fill, consistent with acute cholecystitis.

tered hepatocellular function, is also highly suggestive of cholecystitis. False-positives include patients maintained on long-term total parenteral nutrition, or in the midst of a prolonged fast. Caution should be exercised in over-interpreting a scan in which imaging of the liver is obtained without evidence of radionuclide in any portion of the extrahepatic biliary system. Although these findings occasionally may be observed in patients with complete extrahepatic obstruction secondary to either stones or tumor, this scenario is more frequently indicative of diffuse hepatic parenchymal disease. Most large series suggest that biliary scintigraphy has a diagnostic accuracy for acute cholecystitis of 98%. Although this test is extremely sensitive in diagnosing acute cholecystitis, it is often superfluous in the clinical evaluation of patients suspected of having this diagnosis. Biliary scintigraphy does not demonstrate the presence of gallstones. Often, the diagnosis of acute cholecystitis is made based on clinical criteria and the ultrasonographic demonstration of the presence of stones.

■ MEDICAL THERAPY FOR GALLSTONE DISEASE

The nonoperative therapy for the management of gallstones has long fascinated physicians. During this century, dissolution of existing gallstones with pharmacologic agents was a dream that has been realized recently. In the 1920s, the recognition that excess biliary cholesterol was critical to the formation of cholesterol gallstones paved the way for a series of studies that attempted to identify agents that could reduce bile lithogenicity and dissolve cholesterol gallstones. The earliest agents tested were selected because of their ability to expand the bile acid pool, but these were largely ineffective. Years of intense investigation culminated in the identification and subsequent commercial release of chenodeoxycholic acid (CDCA). This agent desaturates bile and dissolves cholesterol gallstones by a mechanism that is independent of simple expansion of the bile salt pool. CDCA is a specific inhibitor of HMG-CoA reductase, the rate-limiting enzyme for cholesterol biosynthesis. Data from the National Cooperative Gallstone

Study, which included more than 900 patients, helped establish the rate and frequency of stone dissolution with CDCA.[43] Patients meeting criteria for selection were randomly assigned to receive high-dose CDCA, low-dose CDCA, or placebo. The rate of complete stone disappearance was only 13.5% in the high-dose CDCA group and another 28% experienced partial dissolution. In addition to this disappointingly low rate, initial enthusiasm for CDCA was tempered by the realization that many patients experienced diarrhea and a few developed reversible hepatic toxicity. Patient selection is absolutely critical for success with CDCA. Factors for success relate to gallbladder function, stone size, and stone composition. Ideal candidates are young, thin females who have tiny (<5mm) radiolucent, floating stones. Ninety percent of such selected patients will undergo total dissolution, but will require 6 to 12 months of intense therapy. Unfortunately, <5% of patients with gallstones meet these criteria. In addition, most patients will require a lifetime of maintenance therapy to prevent recurrence of stones. Actuarial life table analysis indicates that the risk of gallstone recurrence in patients who have undergone dissolution of gallstones with oral bile acid therapy is 12.5% after 1 year, 50% by 5 years, and 61% by 11 years. Cost analyses studies have suggested that bile acid therapy is not cost effective, as compared to cholecystectomy for younger patients, but may in fact be appropriate from a fiscal and economic perspective in patients more than 65 years of age.

Ursodeoxycholic acid (UCDA) is now commercially available. Similar to CDCA, UCDA, when taken orally, can dissolve cholesterol gallstones in selected patients. Neither CDCA nor UDCA has any efficacy for patients with pigment stones. These two bile acids are similar in structure, differing only in the orientation of a hydroxyl group. Nonetheless, this singular difference alters the solubility and detergent action and makes UDCA less injurious to biological membranes. It therefore does not cause nearly as much secretory diarrhea as CDCA and does not appear to be hepatotoxic. Initial data suggested that UDCA was, in fact, a better, safer, and more effective drug for gallstone dissolution than CDCA.[44] UDCA facilitates conversion of hepatic cholesterol to bile acid and, in addition, reduces cholesterol absorption in the intestine. There is also some preliminary evidence that suggests that UDCA may have a primary effect on cholesterol nucleation. A number of large studies would suggest that the administration of UDCA results in approximately a 40% rate of complete gallstone dissolution. The criteria for patient selection in predicting success with UDCA are identical to that which has been discussed above for CDCA. Unfortunately, a similarly small number of patients are candidates for this type of therapy, based on selection criteria. The disappointingly low rate of complete dissolution with CDCA and UDCA, coupled with the recurrence rate and need for maintenance therapy, have severely limited the indications and use of these drugs in clinical medicine. The ultimate role of oral bile dissolution therapy remains to be more clearly defined. To date, medical dissolution of gallstones has only been accomplished for cholesterol gallstones. Limited information is available regarding the dissolution of noncholesterol, calcium bilirubinate stones. A series of in vitro investigations, however, suggest that pigment gallstone material can be solubilized by a solvent system that contains a mucolytic agent, a chelating agent, and a strong detergent. Such drugs require further identification and study.

DIRECT CONTACT DISSOLUTION

The development and refinement of percutaneous transhepatic cholangiography and catheter placement has facilitated a technique for gallstone dissolution based on instillation of solvents directly into the gallbladder. Pioneered by Thistle and his colleagues at the Mayo Clinic in the late 1980s,[45] percutaneous transhepatic cholecystolitholysis (direct contact dissolution) has been utilized in only a small number of centers. The procedure involves the percutaneous placement of a pigtail catheter through the liver and directly into the gallbladder, with rapid alternating infusion and aspiration of a specific agent that dissolves cholesterol. Gallbladder puncture and intubation can be accomplished using local anesthesia with fluoroscopic or ultrasonographic guidance. Methyl tert-butyl ether (MTBE) is an aliphatic ether that is liquid at body temperature and rapidly dissolves cholesterol. This agent is potentially explosive, and can be toxic when allowed to enter the bile duct and/or duodenum. MTBE has been used in only a small number of patients. Patient selection is critical, and current criteria include high-risk patients with symptomatic stones or who refuse operation, and who have a patent cystic duct, as demonstrated by oral cholecystography or biliary scintigraphy. This procedure is invasive and associated with potential side effects and risks, including hemorrhage, catheter displacement, transient abdominal pain, nausea, emesis, duodenitis, and sedation. Stones have been documented to reoccur in approximately 10% of patients who have been followed for 36 months. The use of contact dissolution with MTBE should probably be limited to a few specific centers with specific interest and expertise in this area. Other percutaneous mechanical techniques, including rotary contact lithotripsy, are being investigated, but remain experimental at this time.

EXTRACORPOREAL SHOCK WAVE LITHOTRIPSY

In 1980, the management of patients with nephroureterolithiasis was revolutionized by the introduction and subsequent development of extracorporeal shock wave lithotripsy (ESWL). The basis for this technology is the observation that shock waves can exert a destructive effect on solids without damaging (passing harmlessly) tissues with the same acoustic impedance as water. Currently available mechanisms of shock wave generation include (1) electromagnetic, (2) spark gap, and (3) piezoelectric. The efficacy of each modality is variable and is influenced by the nature of the interface between the shock wave generated, time, and stone characteristics. This technology is used widely in the management of close to 1 million patients with kidney stones, and has largely replaced open surgical procedures for the management of this disorder.

The success of ESWL for genitourinary (GU) stones led to a number of trials examining the role of this technology for patients with biliary tract stones. Although the inherent anatomic and physiologic differences between the GU and biliary tracts prompted early concern about the efficacy and potential side effects of biliary lithotripsy, considerable experience has been gained with ESWL. Potential advantages of biliary lithotripsy include shortened hospitalization, avoidance of surgical intervention and associated complications, and high rate of acceptance by patients. Preliminary studies performed in Germany suggested stone-free rates of up to 90% could be realized by the combination of ESWL and litholytic therapy with CDCA or UDCA.[46] Unfortunately, more recent prospective studies performed in the United States and other countries have been disappointing. Data from the Dornier National Biliary Lithotripsy study indicated that only 22% of patients treated with ESWL and litholytic therapy were stone free at 6 months. A number of selection criteria have been proposed based on the collective experience with ESWL: history of biliary tract pain, one to three radiolucent gallbladder stones with diameters <30 mm, and a functioning gallbladder, as demonstrated by oral cholecystography. Patients who should be excluded specifically from consideration for ESWL therapy include patients with more than three stones, very large or calcified stones, a nonfunctioning gallbladder, or presence of acute cholecystitis, cholangitis, jaundice, or pancreatitis. Applying present criteria, the suitability for ESWL has been assessed in 100 consecutive patients who underwent cholecystectomy at a university center.[47] The results from this study suggest that <20% of patients in the United States undergoing cholecystectomy would be eligible for ESWL. This figure is similar to that reported in the European literature. Cost-effectiveness analyses also have been disappointing and raised our concern about the value of ESWL as a first line of therapy for gallstone patients.[48,49]

The major problem with ESWL for gallstones continues to be the high rate of stone recurrence.[50] As with other nonoperative therapies that leave the gallbladder in situ, patients undergoing ESWL can expect a recurrence rate of 10% per year for the first 5 years. What remains unclear, however, is what percentage of patients who develop recurrent stones ultimately develop symptoms requiring additional therapy? Nonetheless, this observation, coupled with limitations based on selection criteria, and the development of laparoscopic techniques have caused a re-evaluation of its role in the treatment strategy of gallstone patients.

■ OPERATIVE MANAGEMENT OF CHOLELITHIASIS

Historically, initial efforts to surgically manage gallstone disease focused on cholecystolithotomy (removal of stones with the gallbladder remaining intact). The realization and demonstration, in 1882, that the gallbladder could be removed safely heralded the era of modern day surgical management of gallstone disease. For the last 100 years, this operation has been the mainstay of therapy for this disease. During the 1970s and 1980s, it was estimated that each year between 500 000 and 700 000 patients in the United States underwent cholecystectomy. The introduction of laparoscopic cholecystectomy in 1988 has revolutionized our approach to patients with symptomatic gallstone disease. There are still numerous challenges and unanswered questions that remain regarding issues related to the application of laparoscopic techniques to this very common clinical disorder.

OPEN CHOLECYSTECTOMY

Indications

Experience with open cholecystectomy is vast and spans generations of surgeons. This operation has been performed in virtually every country throughout the world. Traditionally, open cholecystectomy has been the gold standard for all patients with symptomatic gallstone disease, regardless of whether the indication for intervention was recurring biliary colic, acute cholecystitis or one of the complications of biliary stone disease. Although laparoscopic techniques have largely supplanted traditional methods of performing open cholecystectomy for most patients with chronic, uncomplicated cholecystitis and cholelithiasis, the open approach continues to be a safe and effective therapy for the treatment of complicated gallstone disease. The most common indication for surgical removal of the gallbladder is recurrent biliary colic. There are no established criteria for how many episodes are tolerated before cholecystectomy should be recommended, and this decision generally is dictated by both the symptoms of the patient and the experience of the physician. In most situations throughout the world, laparoscopic cholecystectomy is the procedure of choice for patients with recurring biliary colic. There are a number of clinical situations that, when present, make the laparoscopic approach more difficult and should prompt consideration of the open approach. Morbid obesity, cirrhosis, portal hypertension, severe obstructive lung disease, previous surgery, and pregnancy are all factors for which laparoscopic cholecystectomy may be difficult and associated with increased risk. Although there have been anecdotal reports of successful laparoscopic cholecystectomy in pregnant women,[51] there continues to be concern over the effects of prolonged carbon dioxide pneumoperitoneum on the fetus and the technical challenges presented by the gravid uterus.[52]

Early experience suggested that acute cholecystitis was a relative contraindication to performing laparoscopic cholecystectomy. A number of recent reports indicate that laparoscopic cholecystectomy indeed can be done safely for patients with acute inflammation of the gallbladder, but should be performed in this setting only by experienced laparoscopic surgeons.[53–55] One should not hesitate to convert to an open cholecystectomy if significant adhesions or inflammation are identified during laparoscopy. In addition, open cholecystectomy should be considered the procedure of choice in patients with severe cholecystitis, empyema of the gallbladder, acute cholangitis, gallbladder perforation, cholecystenteric fistulae, or a suspected gallbladder neoplasm.

The optimal management of the gallbladder in patients with choledocholithiasis is evolving. While open cholecystectomy, choledocholithotomy with common bile duct exploration have been viewed as the standard of care, a number of minimally invasive techniques have been recently described that have prompted re-evaluation of this teaching. The magnitude of the problem is underscored by the realization that 10% to 15% of patients with cholelithiasis will be proven to have common bile duct stones. There is increasing evidence to suggest that ideal management from both a quality and economic perspective includes preoperative ERCP with papillotomy, followed by laparoscopic cholecystectomy.[56,57] Unfortunately, many patients are not candidates for this approach since their stones are discovered at the time of cholecystectomy. Although laparoscopic techniques for stone removal are now available, most surgeons are not proficient in these procedures. Conversion to open cholecystectomy should be considered by most surgeons when confronted with common bile duct stones identified during a laparoscopic procedure.

A number of technical and anatomic considerations may preclude laparoscopic cholecystectomy or make its performance unwise. Control of hemorrhage and difficulty in identifying ductal and vascular anatomy are important considerations in deciding the most appropriate way of removing the gallbladder. It is ultimately the responsibility of the surgeon to assess which procedure should be performed. Surgeons must be comfortable in their ability to safely perform the procedure laparoscopically; significant concerns based on laparoscopic findings should prompt conversion to open cholecystectomy. Despite the advent of minimally invasive technology, open cholecystectomy continues to be a perfectly acceptable method for removal of the gallbladder under any circumstances and should certainly be considered if proper facilities for performance of laparoscopic surgery are not available or if the surgeon is not adequately trained in this technology.

Operative Technique

The technical aspects of performing an open cholecystectomy have not changed significantly since Langenbuch's description of this procedure more than 100 years ago. Although this operation can be performed safely through a midline, paramedian, or right subcostal incision, most surgeons prefer the right subcostal incision. Appropriate retractors should be inserted to optimize visualization of the hepatoduodenal ligament and its structures, gallbladder, and the triangle of Calot. Meticulous dissection and positive identification of the cystic duct, its junction with the common bile duct, and the cystic artery are absolutely mandatory and significantly reduce the likelihood of bile duct injury (Fig 60–5). Most experienced surgeons prefer to identify these important structures before beginning dissection of the gallbladder from the hepatic bed. When a large distended gallbladder is encountered, removal can be facilitated by trocar decompression of the gallbladder. Acute inflammation or chronic scarring may preclude this approach and in most cases, the gallbladder can be removed safely by dissecting the fundus initially, and the ductal and vascular structures subsequently, after the organ has been separated from the liver. Careful ligation of the cystic duct is essential in preventing not only a biliary leak, but also in reducing the possibility of bile duct injury and stricture. Ligation of the cystic duct in close proximity to its junction with the common bile duct has long been considered an essential component of open cholecystectomy. Recent experience with laparoscopic cholecystectomy suggests that the size of the cystic duct stump is not a critical factor and probably does not significantly contribute to postcholecystectomy syndrome, a poorly defined clinical entity characterized by pain following gallbladder removal. The cystic artery should be dissected carefully free as it passes from left to right within the triangle of Calot (space between cystic duct and hepatic duct). This vessel should be doubly ligated and divided. This will reduce bleeding associated with division of the peritoneum investing the

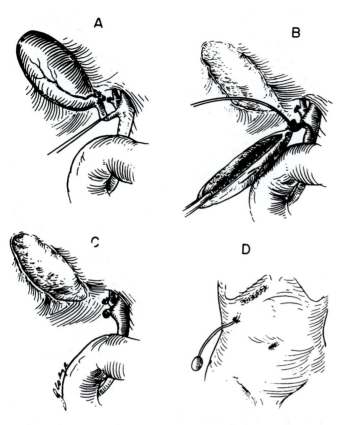

Figure 60–5. Technique of open cholecystectomy. **A.** Gallbladder in situ with the cystic duct isolated and the cystic artery ligated and divided. **B.** The gallbladder has been taken down from liver bed and a catheter placed in the cystic duct for an intraoperative cholangiogram. **C.** Gallbladder completely removed with the cystic duct stump and proximal stump of the cystic artery remaining. **D.** The abdomen is closed with a closed-suction drain placed through a separate stab incision.

gallbladder and separation of areolar tissue between the gallbladder and the liver. At this juncture, intraoperative cholangiography can be performed at the discretion of the surgeon. For many years, traditional teaching indicated that routine cholangiography was essential. More recent data suggest that selective cholangiography is appropriate with indications of a history of jaundice or biliary pancreatitis, abnormal liver function tests suggestive of extrahepatic obstruction, a dilated common bile duct, or palpable stones. Throughout the procedure, care should be exercised to minimize spillage of bile into the peritoneal cavity. Drains are not mandatory and are indicated only if the surgeon is concerned about identifying or controlling a possible bile leak.

Morbidity and Mortality

Despite the frequency with which open cholecystectomy has been performed, our knowledge of current practice patterns and outcome data has been limited. Early studies focused on large numbers of patients, but

were flawed because they were either longitudinal studies extending for a long period of time or represented data from a single institution. In a series of over 10 000 patients undergoing open cholecystectomy during a 40 year period at a single university center, the average mortality exceeded 1%.[58] Given the enormity of the changes that occurred in perioperative management during this period, the relevance of this data to current clinical practice is suspect. In a report of 1035 consecutive patients undergoing open cholecystectomy by a small group of practitioners during a 5 year period, the reported mortality was 0.5%.[59] All of these 5 deaths occurred in elderly patients undergoing emergent operation for complications of gallstone disease. More recently, a population-based study examined the outcome of all open cholecystectomies performed in a 12 month period in two states in the United States.[60] In this series of 42 474 patients, representing approximately 8% of all cholecystectomies performed annually in the United States, the overall mortality rate was 0.17% (Table 60–1). The morbidity rate of 14.7% includes all reported complications, including minor problems such as electrolyte imbalances, atelectasis, urinary retention, and other assorted difficulties that often occur following any surgical procedure. Perhaps the most significant complication that can arise during open or laparoscopic cholecystectomy is bile duct injury. Numerous reports in the literature, including this large population-based study indicate that the risk of bile duct injury during open cholecystectomy is between 0.1% and 0.2%. Similar morbidity and mortality data has been reported by other large series.[61] These data confirm that open cholecystectomy continues to be a very safe operation that can be performed with near zero mortality. In elective situations, open cholecystectomy is being performed in most hospitals throughout the world on patients who are admitted the day of surgery, with an overall stay of 2 to 4 days.[62,63]

TABLE 60–1. IMPACT OF DISEASE STATUS ON OUTCOME

| | Disease Status | | |
	Chronic	Acute	Complicated
Number	27,892	13.246	1336
Percent of group	65.7	31.2	3.1
Morbidity rate (%)	11.9	19.4*	25.2[a]
Number of deaths	29	34	8
Mortality rate (%)	0.10	0.26*	0.60*
Length of stay (days)	4.8	6.6*	8.6*
Charges ($)	5881	9043*	12,510*

[a]p <0.0001 vs. chronic cholecystitis

LAPAROSCOPIC CHOLECYSTECTOMY

Indications

In 1988, anecdotal reports suggested that the gallbladder could be removed laparoscopically, without the need for laparotomy. Published series began to appear shortly thereafter.[64,65] During the last several years, this minimally invasive procedure has emerged world-wide as the preferred treatment for patients with uncomplicated cholelithiasis and cholecystitis.[66–70] Theoretical benefits of this approach include reduced hospitalization and associated costs, decreased pain, avoidance of a large incision with improved cosmetic outcome, and reduced postoperative recovery with quicker return to work. The indications for laparoscopic cholecystectomy (LC) are analogous to open cholecystectomy and include the presence of symptomatic gallstones. Occasionally, asymptomatic patients or individuals with atypical symptoms or complaints suggestive of biliary dyskinesia should be considered for gallbladder removal, which can be accomplished either laparoscopically or with the open technique. As experience with this technology has increased, recommendations regarding contraindications for laparoscopic cholecystectomy have evolved. Absolute contraindications include inability to perform LC because of inadequate training or equipment, patient factors contributing to status as a poor candidate for general anesthesia, uncorrectable coagulopathy, peritonitis, or suspected gallbladder carcinoma.

Judgment should be exercised when considering LC in patients with acute cholecystitis. Laparoscopic removal of an acutely inflamed gallbladder is made more challenging by the inability to exert adequate traction on a friable, edematous gallbladder and by the distortion of ductal and vascular anatomy. This procedure should only be undertaken by experienced laparoscopists. Surgeons should be cognizant of specific principles that may apply to performance of safe LC in the setting of acute cholecystitis. This procedure is made more difficult by the inability to exert adequate traction on a friable, edematous gallbladder wall and by distorted ductal and vascular anatomy. This has raised the concern about bile duct injury and the safety and wisdom of performing LC in this clinical setting. LC should be considered for patients with typical signs and symptoms of acute cholecystitis only if the surgeon is experienced in laparoscopic surgery. Several authors have shown that laparoscopic cholecystectomy can be performed safely with minimal morbidity in patients with acute cholecystitis. Patient selection is key and the operator should have a low threshold for conversion to laparotomy. The reported conversion rate in patients with uncomplicated stone disease is 3% to 7%. For patients with acute cholecystitis, several studies suggest the conversion rate from laparoscopy to open procedure

TABLE 60–2. REASONS TO CONSIDER OPEN CHOLECYSTECTOMY

Severe cholecystitis
Empyema of the gallbladder
Emphysematous cholecystitis
Cholangitis
Gallbladder perforation
Cholecystoenteric fistula
Gallbladder neoplasm
Severe obstructive pulmonary disease
Morbid obesity
Cirrhosis
Portal hypertension
Previous upper abdominal surgery
Pregnancy

From: Roslyn JJ, Binns GS, Hughes EF, et al. Open cholecystectomy: a contemporary analysis of 42,474 patients. *Ann Surg* 1993; 218:129.

exceeds 20%. Moreover, the decision to convert to laparotomy should be made prior to a complication. When these principles are followed, the incidence of common bile duct injury is similar to patients undergoing elective cholecystectomy (Table 60–2).

Role of Intraoperative Cholangiography

Common bile duct stones are found in approximately 8% to 12% of all patients who undergo cholecystectomy for symptomatic gallstone disease. Intraoperative cholangiography (IOC) continues to be an effective way of identifying common bile duct stones at the time of surgery. This can be accomplished, in most cases, by the placement of a small catheter through the cystic duct with installation of 10 to 20 mL of dye. After many years of discussion, consensus seems to have been reached amongst surgeons that IOC should be performed selectively in patients undergoing open cholecystectomy (OC). More recently, considerable discussion has focused on the role of IOC in the performance of LC.[71–73] Initial recommendations included routine IOC so as to identify ductular anatomy and hopefully reduce the incidence of common bile duct injury. With greater experience, many authors have begun to recommend selective cholangiography for LC. IOC is technically more challenging than with OC and may be associated with a greater incidence of false-positives than is OC. When anatomical structures are not clearly distinguishable during LC, IOC is mandated in order to avoid serious injury to vital structures. Surgeons performing LC should be well versed with the technique of IOC so that it can be utilized when appropriate.

Role of ERCP

Stones are present in 10% to 15% of patients undergoing cholecystectomy. Patients in whom common bile duct stones are identified at the time of open cholecystectomy have traditionally been managed by common bile duct exploration and choledocholithotomy. In recent years, the preoperative identification of patients at risk for having common bile duct stones (history of jaundice or abnormal liver function tests (LFTs) frequently resulted in ERCP and sphincterotomy with stone removal as possible therapeutic options. Although ERCP clearly has been shown to be of enormous benefit in patients with retained common bile duct stones, its role as a preoperative diagnostic and potentially therapeutic examination remains unsettled.[74] In part, because the laparoscopic techniques for common bile duct stone extraction are not practiced universally and continue to evolve, there has been renewed interest in the preoperative identification of patients who may be harboring ductal stones. A number of studies suggest that preoperative ERCP should be considered prior to laparoscopic cholecystectomy in patients believed at risk for common bile duct stones. Lingering concerns remain, however, regarding the number of negative endoscopic evaluations that will be performed. Most authors recommend performing laparoscopic cholecystectomy the day following ERCP and common bile duct stone removal. This issue will be discussed more fully in a subsequent chapter.

Morbidity and Mortality

Since the introduction of laparoscopic cholecystectomy in 1988, this operation has emerged as the preferred treatment for patients with symptomatic gallstone disease. Several large series have been published that underscore the safety of this procedure when performed by appropriately trained surgeons and for properly selected patients.[75,76] In patients undergoing elective operation, the conversion rate to open laparotomy is between 2% and 9%. This figure rises to 25% to 35% in patients with acute cholecystitis. Major complications occur in 1% to 5% of patients. The incidence of common bile duct injury is difficult to ascertain, although most authors suggest that this complication occurs in up to 0.7% of patients. A number of studies indicate that there is a learning curve associated with this technology and that careful judgment should be exercised until sufficient experience has been obtained. The mortality for laparoscopic removal of the gallbladder is comparable to data reported for the open approach and is dependent on age and the presence of comorbid diagnoses such as cardiac, cerebrovascular, and/or pulmonary disease. In 1992, the National Institute of Health sponsored a consensus conference focusing on the treatment of gallstone disease.[77] This group concluded that laparoscopic cholecystectomy was the treatment of choice for many patients and had distinct advantages over open laparotomy, including decreased pain and disability, reduced cost, and more rapid return to normal activity. However, they pointed out that outcome was influenced directly by the level of training, experi-

ence, skill, and judgment of the surgeon. They recommended that future efforts should focus on the refinement of laparoscopic techniques to optimize outcome and cost effectiveness.

■ ACALCULOUS CHOLECYSTITIS

Acalculous cholecystitis is an unusual, but potentially lethal complication of gallbladder disease.[78] Although the etiology of this disorder is, by definition, not related to gallstone disease, it is appropriate to discuss its pathophysiology and clinical presentation in the context of this chapter. The precise cause and pathogenesis of this disorder has yet to be determined. The estimated incidence of acute acalculous cholecystitis is about 3% of all surgical biliary tract cases treated in most large centers. Acalculous cholecystitis has been reported in critically ill patients in the intensive care unit (ICU) setting (particularly in patients with multisystem organ failure), following severe trauma or burn, and as a postoperative complication after virtually any major procedure. Most postoperative patients who develop this problem have undergone a major abdominal or thoracic procedure 2 to 14 days prior to the onset of symptoms. The clinical setting in which acalculous disease occurs has provided important insights into its possible pathogenesis. Stasis of bile within the gallbladder has long been considered an important factor in the development of this disorder. Biliary stasis can occur as a result of ampullary spasm secondary to administration of narcotics, decreased gallbladder emptying during periods of prolonged fasting, or cystic duct occlusion secondary to edema. Moreover, altered viscosity of bile as a result of dehydration and multiple transfusions with an associated increase in pigment load has also been implicated as an important factor. The combination of biliary stasis and increased bile viscosity may lead to altered concentration of specific biliary lipids and other luminal factors that may predispose to irritation and inflammation of the gallbladder mucosa. A cascade of events is initiated with release of specific biochemical mediators of the inflammatory response. The role of ischemia is speculative in this process, but, because the cystic artery is an end artery, the gallbladder has little collateral circulation and may predispose to organ ischemia. While these hypotheses are attractive, they remain to be confirmed.

The diagnosis of acalculous cholecystitis poses a considerable challenge to the clinician, especially when it occurs in ICU patients. These patients typically have multiple medical and surgical problems and, as a result, the diagnosis may be delayed. Biliary scintigraphy is often not helpful in this situation because the false-positive rate is quite high owing to the fasting state. Early ultrasonography and a high index of suspicion based on the clinical setting are the keys to diagnosis. Several studies suggest that the associated morbidity and mortality of acalculous cholecystitis, when it occurs in ICU patients, is between 40% and 60%. The liberal use of ultrasonography (portable units are available in most hospitals and can be brought to the bedside) and a high index of clinical suspicion may facilitate early diagnosis and operative treatment, thereby reducing mortality associated with this disease. Surgical management is warranted in all patients with acute acalculous cholecystitis. Cholecystectomy may be contraindicated because of the unstable overall condition of the patient. Under these circumstances, a cholecystostomy should be considered. This procedure often can be accomplished using local anesthesia, with minimal compromise of the patient's overall status. Recent experience with percutaneous cholecystotomy using radiologic guidance confirms the safety and utility of this potentially life-saving measure. While this procedure allows for decompression and drainage of infected gallbladder bile, it obviously will not be curative for those patients with gangrenous changes of the gallbladder. Percutaneous cholecystotomy should be viewed as a temporizing measure in a critically ill patient.

■ COMPLICATIONS OF ACUTE CHOLECYSTITIS

GALLBLADDER PERFORATION

Perforation of the gallbladder is a not uncommon complication of gallstone disease, being present in approximately 3% of all patients undergoing cholecystectomy. It is helpful to consider this complication as being manifested in one of three ways: acute, free perforation with bile peritonitis; subacute perforation with abscess; and chronic perforation with fistula formation.[79] Acute, free perforation of the gallbladder is a relatively rare event, occurring in <1% of all patients with acute cholecystitis and accounting for approximately 10% of patients with gallbladder perforation. The presentation is often dramatic and mimics an acute abdomen with obvious signs of peritonitis. This complication has been documented to occur more frequently in elderly patients with other signs of peripheral vascular disease, and in patients who are immunocompromised secondary to organ transplantation, neoplasm, or immunosuppressive therapy for any malady. The treatment is early cholecystectomy. Subacute perforation with abscess is the most common variant of gallbladder perforation and is believed to result from chronic gallstone disease with pressure necrosis from a stone, resulting in perforation into a contiguous structure. If the inflammatory process is walled off by the omentum, a pericholecystic abscess may result. Management includes drainage of the abscess and chol-

ecystectomy. This procedure can be performed at the same time or may be staged, depending on the size of the collection and specific patient circumstances. Perforation into an adjacent organ will result in a biliary-enteric fistula. Most commonly, the fistula forms between the gallbladder and the duodenum (cholecystoduodenal fistula). Other organs that are less frequently involved in this type of process include colon, stomach, small bowel, or skin. Many of these patients are relatively asymptomatic and the fistula is only discovered when, for example, a large stone becomes impacted in the intestine and causes small bowel obstruction. Patients with so-called gallstone ileus present with symptoms, signs, and radiographic findings suggestive of mechanical small bowel obstruction. Clues to the diagnosis include the presence of gallstones in the gallbladder and air in the biliary tract that can be identified on plain abdominal radiographs. The site of the obstruction is usually the terminal ileum, just proximal to the ileocecal valve. This corresponds to the segment of the intestine with the smallest diameter. Treatment priority should focus on relief of the obstruction. This usually can be accomplished by "milking" the stone retrograde, and then extracting it after a controlled enterotomy. In most cases, the gallbladder disease is not acute, and a decision to deal primarily with the gallbladder and biliary fistula should be determined by the condition of the patient. Deferring the biliary procedure to another time often may be the most appropriate course of action.

EMPHYSEMATOUS CHOLECYSTITIS

Emphysematous cholecystitis refers to an unusual variant of cholecystitis, which is characterized by severe infection and the presence of gas generated by gas-producing enteric bacteria. This disorder is typically seen in elderly patients, although diabetics account for approximately 25% of cases. Clostridial species are the most prevalent bacteria isolated from patients with emphysematous cholecystitis. Other bacteria that may be present include *Escherichia coli, Klebsiella,* and streptococci. Whether there are additional factors that predispose to this complication remains unclear. The clinical presentation mimics acute cholecystitis, although the patients are often more toxic. The treatment is surgical removal of the gallbladder.

REFERENCES

1. Shehadi WH. The biliary system through the ages. *Int Surg* 1979;64:63
2. Beal JM. Historical perspective of gallstone disease. *Surg Gynecol Obstet* 1984;158:181
3. LaMorte WW, Schoetz DJ Jr, Birkett DH, Williams LF Jr. The role of the gallbladder in the pathogenesis of cholesterol gallstones. *Gastroenterology* 1979;77:580

4. Admirand WH, Small DM. The physiochemical basis of cholesterol gallstone formation. *J Clin Invest* 1968;47:1043

5. Halpern Z, Dudley MA, Kibe A, et al. Rapid vesicle formation and aggregation in abnormal human biles. *Gastroenterology* 1986;90:875

6. Holzbach RT. Current concepts of cholesterol transport and crystal formation in human bile. *Hepatology* 1990;12:26S

7. Harvey PRC, Somjen, Gilat T, et al. Vesicular cholesterol in bile: relationship to protein concentration and nucleation time. *Biochem Biophys Acta* 1988;958:10

8. Burnstein MJ, Ilson RG, Petrunka CN, et al. Evidence for a potent nucleating factor in the gallbladder bile of patients with cholesterol gallstones. *Gastroenterology* 1983;85:801

9. Holzbach RT, Kibe A, Theil E, et al. Biliary proteins: unique inhibitors of cholesterol crystal nucleation in human gallbladder bile. *J Clin Invest* 1984;73:35

10. Levy PF, Smith BF, LaMont JT. Human gallbladder mucin accelerates nucleation of cholesterol in artificial bile. *Gastroenterology* 1984;87:270

11. Braverman DZ, Johnson ML, Kern F Jr. Effect of pregnancy and contraceptive steroids on gallbladder function. *N Engl J Med* 1980;302:362

12. Holzbach RT. Gallbladder stasis: consequence of long-term parenteral hyperalimentation and risk factor for cholelithiasis. *Gastroenterology* 1983;84:1055

13. Tompkins RK, Kraft AR, Zimmerman E, et al. Clinical and biochemical evidence of increased gallstone formation after complete vagotomy. *Surgery* 1972;71:196

14. Roslyn J, DenBesten L, Pitt H, Kuchenbecker S, Polarek JW. Effects of cholecystokinin on gallbladder stasis and cholesterol gallstone formation. *J Surg Res* 1981;30:22

15. Pitt HA, Roslyn JJ, Kuchenbecker S, DenBesten L. The role of increased cystic duct resistance in the pathogenesis of cholesterol cholelithiasis. *J Surg Res* 1981;30:508

16. Doty JE, Pitt HA, Kuchenbecker SL, DenBesten L. Impaired gallbladder emptying before gallstone formation in the prairie dog. *Gastroenterology* 1983;85:168

17. Friedhandler TM, Davison JS, Shaffer EA. Defective gallbladder contractility in the ground squirrel and prairie dog during the early stages of cholesterol gallstone formation. *Gastroenterology* 1983;85:830

18. Pomeranz IS, Shaffer EA. Abnormal gallbladder emptying in a subgroup of patients with gallstones. *Gastroenterology* 1985;88:787

19. Jazrawi RP, Pazzi P, Petroni ML, et al. Postprandial gallbladder motor function: refilling and turnover of bile in health and in cholelithiasis. *Gastroenterology* 1995;109:582

20. Maki T. Pathogenesis of calcium bilirubinate gallstones: role of E. coli, B-glucuronidase and coagulation of inorganic ions, polyelectrolytes, and agitation. *Ann Surg* 1966;164:90

21. Stewart L, Smith AL, et al. Pigmented gallstones form as a composite of bacterial microcolonies and pigment solids. *Ann Surg* 1987;206:242

22. Kahng KU, Roslyn JJ. Surgical issues for the elderly patient with hepatobiliary disease. *Surg Clin North Am* 1994;74:345

23. Ikard RW. Gallstones, cholecystitis and diabetes. *Surg Gynecol Obstet* 1990;171:528

24. Aucott JN, Cooper GS, Bloom AD, Aron DC. Management of gallstones in diabetic patients. *Arch Intern Med* 1993;153:1053

25. Doberneck RC, Sterling WA Jr, Allison DC. Morbidity and mortality after operation in nonbleeding cirrhotic patients. *Am J Surg* 1983;146:306

26. Aranha GV, Kruss D, Greenlee HB. Therapeutic options for biliary tract disease in advanced cirrhosis. *Am J Surg* 1988;155:374

27. Roslyn JJ, Pitt HA, Mann LL, Ament ME, DenBesten L. Gallbladder disease in patients on long-term parenteral nutrition. *Gastroenterology* 1983;84:148

28. Roslyn JJ, Brequist WE, Pitt HA, et al. Increased risk of gallstones in children on total parenteral nutrition. *Pediatrics* 1983;91:784

29. Roslyn JJ, Pitt HA, Mann LL, Fonkalsrud EW, DenBesten L. Parenteral nutrition-induced gallbladder disease: a reason for early cholecystectomy. *Am J Surg* 1984;148:58

30. Gracie WA, Ransohoff DF. The natural history of gallstones; the innocent gallstone is not a myth. *N Engl J Med* 1982;307:798

31. McSherry CK, Festenberg H, et al. The natural history of diagnosed gallstone disease in symptomatic and asymptomatic patients. *Ann Surg* 1985;202:59

32. Diehl AK. Gallstone size and the risk of gallbladder cancer. *JAMA* 1983;250:2323

33. Ashur H, Siegal B, Oland Y, et al. Calcified gallbladder (porcelain gallbladder). *Arch Surg* 1978;113:594

34. Diettrich NA, Cacioppo JC, Davis RP. The vanishing elective cholecystectomy: trends and their consequences. *Arch Surg* 1988;123:810

35. Reiss R, Nudelman I, Gutman C, Deutsch AA. Changing trends in surgery for acute cholecystitis. *World J Surg* 1991;14:567

36. Saunders-Kirkwood KD, Aizen B, Thompson JE Jr. Cholecystectomy. The impact of social change. *Ann Surg* 1992;215:318

37. Graham EA, Cole WH. Roentgenologic examination of the gallbladder: preliminary report of a new method utilizing intravenous injection of tetrabromophthalein. *JAMA* 1924;82:613

38. Cooperberg PL, Burhenne HJ. Real-time ultrasonography. Diagnostic technique of choice in calculous gallbladder disease. *N Engl J Med* 1980;302:1277

39. Krook PM, Allen FH, Bush WH, et al. Comparison of real-time cholecystosonography and oral cholecystography. *Radiology* 1980;135:145

40. Ralls PW, Colletti PM, Lapin SA, et al. Real-time sonography in suspected acute cholecystitis: prospective evaluation of primary and secondary signs. *Radiology* 1985;155:767

41. Marzio LM, Innocenti P, Genovesi N, et al. Role of oral cholecystography, real-time ultrasound, and CT in evaluation of gallstones and gallbladder function. *Gastrointest Radiol* 1992;17:257

42. Suarez CA, Block F, et al. The role of HIDA/PIPIDA scanning in diagnosing cystic duct obstruction. *Ann Surg* 1980;191:131

43. Schoenfield LT, Lachin JM, The Steering Committee, The National Cooperative Gallstone Study Group. Chen-

odiol (chenodeoxycholic acid) for dissolution of gall-stones; the National Cooperative Gallstone Study: a controlled trial of efficacy and safety. *Ann Intern Med* 1981; 95:257

44. Roda E, Bazzoli F, et al. Ursodeoxycholic acid vs. chenodeoxycholic acid as cholesterol gallstone dissolving agents: a comparative study. *Hepatology* 1982;2:804

45. Thistle JL, May GR, Bender CE, et al. Dissolution of cholesterol gallbladder stones by methyl ter-butyl ether administered by percutaneous transhepatic catheter. *N Engl J Med* 1989;320:633

46. Sackman M, Delius M, Sauerbruch T, et al. Shock-wave lithotripsy of gallbladder gallstones. *N Engl J Med* 1988; 318:393

47. Magnuson TH, Lillemoe KD, Pitt HA. How many Americans will be eligible for biliary lithotripsy? *Arch Surg* 1990; 124:1185

48. Bass EB, Steinberg HP, Pitt HA, et al. Cost-effectiveness of extracorporeal shock-wave lithotripsy versus cholecystectomy for symptomatic gallstones. *Gastroenterology* 1991; 101:189

49. Nealon WH, Urrutia F, Fleming D, Thompson JC. The economic burden of gallstone lithotripsy: will cost determine its fate? *Ann Surg* 1991;213:645

50. Sackmann M, Ipposch E, Sauerbruch T, et al. Early gallstone recurrence rate after successful shock-wave therapy. *Gastroenterology* 1990;98:392

51. Soper NJ, Hunter JG, Petrie RH. Laparoscopic cholecystectomy during pregnancy. *Surg Endosc* 1992;112:856

52. Haglund U, Norlen K, Rasmussen I, Flowers JL. Complications related to pneumoperitoneum. In: Bailey RW, Flowers JF (eds), Complications of Laparoscopic Surgery, St. Louis, MO: Quality Medical; 1995:26–57

53. Rattner DW, Ferguson C, Warshaw AL. Factors associated with successful laparoscopic cholecystectomy for acute cholecystitis. *Ann Surg* 1993;217:233

54. Zucker KA, Flowers JL, Bailey RW, et al. Laparoscopic management of acute cholecystitis. *Am J Surg* 1993; 165:508

55. Singer JA, McKeen RV. Laparoscopic cholecystectomy for acute or gangrenous cholecystitis. *Ann Surg* 1994;56:402

56. Brodish RJ, Fink AS. ERCP, cholangiography, and laparoscopic cholecystectomy. *Surg Endosc* 1993;7:3

57. Graham SM, Flowers JL, Scott TR, et al. Laparoscopic cholecystectomy and common bile duct stones. The utility of planned perioperative endoscopic retrograde cholangiography and sphincterotomy: experience with 63 patients. *Ann Surg* 1993;218:61

58. Glenn F. Trends in surgical treatment of calculous disease of the biliary tract. *Surg Gynecol Obstet* 1975;140:877

59. Ganey JB, Johnson PA Jr, Prillaman PE, McSwain GR. Cholecystectomy: clinical experience with a large series. *Am J Surg* 1986;151:352

60. Roslyn JJ, Binns GS, Hughes EX, et al. Open cholecystectomy: a contemporary analysis of 42 474 patients. *Ann Surg* 1993;218:129

61. Morgenstern L, Wong L, Berci G. Twelve hundred open cholecystectomies before the laparoscopic era: a standard for comparison. *Arch Surg* 1992;127:400

62. Moss G. Discharge within 24 hours of elective cholecystectomy: the first 100 patients. *Arch Surg* 1986;121:1159

63. Hall RC. Short hospital stay: two hospital days for cholecystectomy. *Am J Surg* 1987;154:510

64. Dubois F, Icard P, Berthelot G, et al. Coeliscopic cholecystectomy: preliminary report of 36 cases. *Ann Surg* 1990; 211:609

65. Southern Surgeons Club. A prospective analysis of 1,518 laparoscopic cholecystectomies. *N Engl J Med* 1991;324: 1073

66. Schirmer BD, Edge SB, Dix J, et al. Laparoscopic cholecystectomy: treatment of choice for symptomatic cholelithiasis. *Ann Surg* 1991;213:665

67. Gadacz TR. U.S. experience with laparoscopic cholecystectomy. *Am J Surg* 1993;165:450

68. Barkun JS, Barkun AN, Meakins JL. Laparoscopic versus open cholecystectomy: the Canadien experience. *Am J Surg* 1993;165:455

69. Kimura T, Kimura K, Katshuhiko S, et al. Laparoscopic cholecystectomy: the Japanese experience. *Surg Laparosc Endosc* 1993;3:194

70. Perissat J. Laparoscopic cholecystectomy: the European experience. *Am J Surg* 1993;165:444

71. Sackier JM, Berci G, Phillips E, Carroll B, Shapiro S, Paz-Partlow M. The role of cholangiography in laparoscopic cholecystectomy. *Arch Surg* 1991;126:1021

72. Soper NJ, Dunnegan DL. Routine versus selective intraoperative cholangiography during laparoscopic cholecystectomy. *World J Surg* 1992;16:1133

73. Traverso LW, Hauptmann EM, Lynge DC. Routine intraoperative cholangiography and its contribution to the selective cholangiographer. *Am J Surg* 1994;167:464

74. Stiegmann GV, Goff JS, Mansour A, Pearlman N, Reveille RM, Norton L. Precholecystectomy endoscopic cholangiography and stone removal is not superior to cholecystectomy, cholangiography, and common duct exploration. *Am J Surg* 1992;163:227

75. Steiner CA, Bass EB, Talamini MA, Pitt HA, Steinberg EP. Surgical rates and operative mortality for open and laparoscopic cholecystectomy in Maryland. *N Engl J Med* 1994;330:403

76. Deziel DJ, Millican KW, Economou SJ, Doolas A, Ko ST, Airan MC. Complications of laparoscopic cholecystectomy; a national survey of 4292 hospitals and an analysis of 77 604 cases. *Am J Surg* 1993;165:9

77. NIH Consensus Development Panel on Gallstones and Laparoscopic cholecystectomy. Gallstones and Laparoscopic Cholecystectomy. *JAMA* 1993;269:1018

78. Babb RR. Acute acalculous cholecystitis: a review. *J Clin Gastroenterol* 1992;15:238

79. Roslyn JJ, Thompson JE Jr, Darvin H, DenBesten L. Risk factors for gallbladder perforation. *Am J Gastroenterol* 1987;82:636

61

Choledocholithiasis and Cholangitis

Ronald K. Tompkins

Common bile duct stones are the most common cause of obstructive jaundice and cholangitis. In many patients, the stones also may be associated with pancreatitis. Thus, it is important to know about the pathophysiology of choledocholithiasis, as well as the diagnostic and therapeutic maneuvers that are most useful for managing patients with this disorder.

■ CLASSIFICATION OF COMMON DUCT STONES

Biliary stones, in general, may be classified as predominantly cholesterol or predominantly pigment in composition. Over 95% of gallstones fall into one of these two groups with the majority being composed of cholesterol. The remaining 5% or so of gallstones are calcium stones. The pathogenesis of these various types of stones has been well described in the literature[1,2] and is beyond the scope of this chapter.

PRIMARY COMMON DUCT STONES

There can be no doubt that stones do form per primam in the common bile duct. These stones are called primary stones to distinguish them from those stones originating in the gallbladder and are, thus, secondary stones. Almost all primary common duct stones are of the pigment type. There have been a few recent reports, however, of primary common duct and intrahepatic stones composed of cholesterol.[3,4]

Two types of pigment stones have been identified; black and brown. Both types have calcium bilirubinate as their principal compound. Brown pigment stones occur primarily in the common bile duct and are closely associated with bacteria.[5] Black pigment stones are found chiefly in the gallbladder. Scanning electron microscopic studies have shown bacteria, or their residual spaces, in brown pigment stones but not in black pigment stones.[6,7] Furthermore, in one study, bile cultures were positive in all patients with brown pigment stones but were positive in only 13% and 14% of patients with cholesterol and black pigment stones, respectively.[7]

The surgical significance of primary common duct stones is that they are the product of two conditions that the surgeon must correct in treating the disease. These two conditions are bile duct stasis, and infection. Disturbance in the flow of bile as well as the introduction of infected material into the biliary tract may be associated with previous operations that disturb the usual motility dynamics of the sphincter, such as sphincterotomy or sphincteroplasty, and biliary-enteric anastomoses. Patients with cystic diseases of the biliary tract usually have stasis as a major component of their condition. Stasis also occurs with conditions that obstruct the flow of bile into the duodenum, such as sphincter fibrosis, chronic pancreatitis, and periampullary (periVaterian) duodenal diverticula.[8]

Bacterial infection of the biliary system occurs in approximately two-thirds of patients with common bile duct stones.[9] In most cases, it is thought that the infection is secondary to either the stones themselves, many of which have come from the gallbladder, or to the obstruction caused by the stones. In the case of primary stones, which occur much less frequently than secondary stones, the role of bacteria is thought to be primary in their formation.

SECONDARY (RETAINED) COMMON DUCT STONES

Secondary common duct stones are those that have migrated into the biliary system from the gallbladder. As is the case with primary stones, they may be found in the intrahepatic as well as the extrahepatic bile ducts, or in both areas. Approximately 11% of patients with gallbladder stones will have associated common duct stones at the time of operation. This incidence may climb to 18% in older patients who have had gallstones for a longer period of time. Between 5% and 7% of common duct stones found at operation may be unsuspected by preoperative evaluation and are discovered by cystic duct cholangiography during the cholecystectomy.[10]

Retained common duct stones are those that present themselves at some point in time following cholecystectomy, with or without concomitant bile duct exploration, and which have the characteristics of secondary rather than primary stones. Some authors have suggested an arbitrary time period following cholecystectomy as a defining criterion for retained stones versus primary stones. However, such time periods are really not helpful and the visual (or occasionally, chemical) analysis of the stone, in most situations, should be used as the criterion to diagnose retained versus primary stones.

■ DIAGNOSIS AND EVALUATION

In the last decade, many refinements have been made to technologies in radiology, endoscopy and clinical laboratory testing that have improved the diagnosis and evaluation of patients with choledocholithiasis and cholangitis. In some respects, the available tests are so numerous that care must be exercised to avoid overutilizing them. A careful old-fashioned but time-honored history and physical examination will point the clinician in the proper direction, in most cases.

SIGNS AND SYMPTOMS

Patients with symptomatic common duct stones usually present with abdominal pain that may be constant but, more commonly, is intermittent. The pain usually presents as a deep visceral, midepigastric pain and often is associated with nausea and/or vomiting.[11] In those patients with associated cholangitis, fever also will be present. Depending upon the severity of the disease, the patient may complain of itching, jaundice, acholic stools, and dark urine. In approximately 20% of patients, back pain may be a prominent symptom and raises the possibility of associated pancreatitis. More complete discussions of jaundice and pancreatitis will be found in Section II and Section XIII, respectively.

On physical examination, the clinician searches for vital signs of fever, tachycardia, hypotension and malnutrition or weight loss. Jaundice may be evident in the sclerae, under the tongue or in the skin. Excoriations of the extremities and/or trunk may point to pruritus as an early sign of biliary obstruction.

In many cases, the abdominal examination of primary or retained common duct stones may be unremarkable, especially after subsidence of an attack. During episodes of pain, the patient may exhibit tenderness over the liver with or without voluntary guarding in the upper abdomen. In patients who have concomitant gallstones in the gallbladder, there may be a tender gallbladder as well. Patients with cholangitis associated with common duct stones very often will have tenderness to examination in the upper abdomen that is more pronounced than in patients without cholangitis. If the patient exhibits severe abdominal signs on examination, with rebound tenderness or rigidity, the clinician must think of disease processes other than choledocholithiasis and cholangitis as explanations for these findings.

LABORATORY FINDINGS

In most patients with common duct stones, the serum alkaline phosphatase will be elevated along with the serum gamma glutamyl transpeptidase (GGTP). These tests are among the most sensitive laboratory indicators of biliary obstruction and may be elevated even when the total bilirubin is in the normal range. Patients with fully developed obstruction will show elevations of the alkaline phosphatase, GGTP, and bilirubin. Often the alanine aminotransferase (ALT or SGPT) and aspartate aminotransferase (AST or SGOT) levels are mildly elevated with longer standing obstruction. The latter two tests are more markedly elevated in patients who have associated cholangitis, as is the white blood cell count.

RADIOLOGIC FINDINGS

Abdominal ultrasound is the preferred first radiologic examination in most patients in whom biliary tract obstruction is suspected. The presence of associated gallbladder stones can be confirmed in >98% of patients with gallstones and the dilation of the intrahepatic biliary system can be identified in most. If intestinal gas is not excessive, the extrahepatic biliary system also may be visualized and stones demonstrated. Diagnostic ultrasound, especially the real-time mode, has been the single most valuable screening test in the jaundiced patient in recent years (Fig 61–1). In some instances, real-time ultrasound has shown the passage of common duct

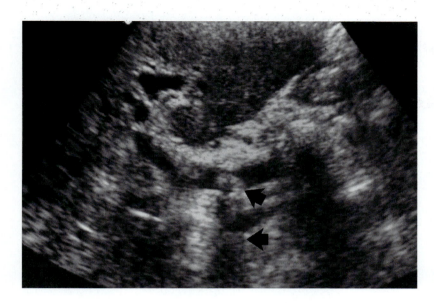

Figure 61–1. Ultrasound study demonstrating common duct stones. The shadowing produced by the stones is indicated by the *arrows*.

stones into the duodenum during the examination. More complete discussions of this and other radiologic procedures is to be found in Section I.

When biliary dilation has been demonstrated by ultrasound, the clinician must consider the next radiologic procedure to be done. In most cases in our experience, this should be a *cholangiogram.*

Cholangiograms may be obtained by many different techniques. In almost no case of obstructive jaundice will an intravenous cholangiogram (IVC) be of value. For this reason, IVC seldom has been used in recent years, even with refinements in tomographic techniques.

The preferred types of cholangiograms in most medical centers today are the percutaneous transhepatic cholangiograms (PTC) done by the radiologists, in most centers, and the endoscopic retrograde cholangiogram (ERC) done by surgical or medical endoscopists. The decision as to which procedure is chosen depends on several factors. First, one should use the procedure that is most readily available in the medical environment where the patient presents. If both techniques are equally available, then the decision may be made on the basis of the previous ultrasound findings. For example, if the ultrasound has shown dilated intrahepatic ducts, but the extrahepatic system is not dilated or has not been visualized, a PTC will offer a chance to visualize the upper tract and to demonstrate the site and nature of the obstruction (Fig 61–2). In addition, this route offers opportunities for interventional procedures, such as decompressive stenting and biopsies (see Section I).

In the situation where the ultrasound has demonstrated both intrahepatic and extrahepatic biliary dilation, the clinician may be better off choosing an ERC to demonstrate the pathology (Fig 61–3). This approach offers capabilities additional to the cholangiogram itself. By the endoscopic approach, it is possible to examine the stomach, duodenum, and especially the ampulla of Vater for other causes of biliary obstruction. The endoscopic route also allows stenting and decompression of the biliary system, which may be important in the emergency management of patients with cholangitis associated with common duct stones. In certain patients with primary or retained common duct stones, endoscopic methods may be the sole treatment for this condition.

Plain abdominal films are of very limited value in the diagnosis of choledocholithiasis with or without cholangitis, since <15% of stones are radiopaque.

Computed tomography (CT) usually is not of additional help in the diagnosis or management of patients with choledocholithiasis, with or without cholangitis. It has a lower diagnostic yield in these conditions and offers no therapeutic additional advantages and is also very expensive. The use of CT is therefore to be discouraged as an initial test in the evaluation of the jaundiced patient. It should probably be reserved for use in those patients in whom ultrasound and PTC or ERC have not yielded clear diagnoses or in whom some other hepatic or pancreatic lesions are suspected.

Magnetic resonance imaging (MRI) has not demonstrated any superiority in the diagnosis of choledocholithiasis to those tests mentioned above. As with CT, MRI is expensive and should not be used as an initial diagnostic test.

Endoscopic ultrasound has recently been evaluated in patients with obstructive jaundice. This test, performed by endoscopic placement of an ultrasound probe in the duodenum, is capable of detecting lesions in the pancreas, distal bile duct and ampulla that may be causing

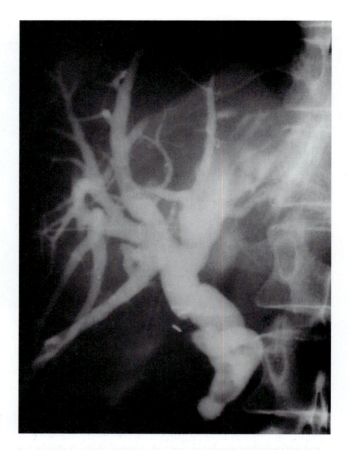

Figure 61–2. Transhepatic cholangiogram demonstrating stones in a postcholecystectomy patient. The stones were primary, owing to a fibrotic stricture at the distal end of the bile duct.

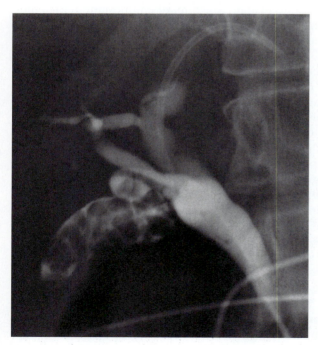

A

Figure 61–3. Endoscopic studies in a patient with cholelithiasis, choledocholithiasis, and cholangitis. **A.** Nasobiliary tube inserted to decompress the biliary system. Multiple stones in gallbladder are visible. **B.** Endoscopic removal of CBD stones was done. Patient subsequently underwent elective laparoscopic cholecystectomy.

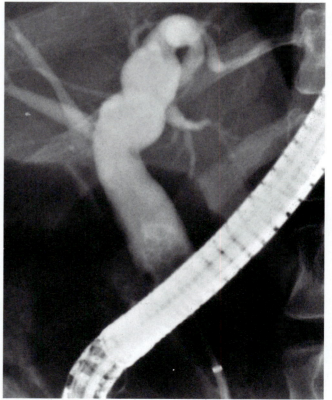

B

the obstruction. It has the current drawbacks of not being readily available, requiring expensive hardware, and being greatly operator dependent. Further studies are required to assess the proper place of this new technique in the diagnosis of biliary tract obstruction.

Operative cholangiography is a diagnostic test of great value in the discovery of common duct stones. While preoperative testing has improved greatly during the past decade, the fact remains that about 5% to 7% of common duct stones are unsuspected at the time of operation and are discovered only by operative cystic duct cholangiography. The techniques of properly performing cystic duct cholangiography have been well described in a photographic essay.[12] The accuracy of intraoperative cholangiography has been enhanced greatly by improvements in imaging offered by newer portable C-arm fluoroscopic equipment with image enhancement.[13]

Surgeons continue to quarrel about whether cystic duct cholangiograms should be done routinely at every cholecystectomy or whether they should be performed only in those patients whose preoperative tests place them in a group at high risk of having common bile duct (CBD) stones (selective cholangiography).

Proponents of routine cholangiography cite the 5% to 7% of patients who have stones found at operation and who had no preoperative indicators that the stones were present.[14] Routine cystic duct cholangiography is felt to reduce bile duct injury rates by identifying ductal anomalies in approximately 14% of patients.[15] Proponents also cite the benefits in efficiency of doing cholangiography routinely because of familiarity with the procedure by all operating room personnel and the improved success rates because of better education of operating room personnel and resident surgeons. Also, a study of cost-benefits has concluded that the overall cost of doing routine cholangiography is lower than doing selective cholangiography.[16]

Opponents of routine cholangiography argue that many of the unsuspected stones found on routine cholangiography will pass spontaneously and, hence, are clinically insignificant. They show data that retained stone rates in series of selective cholangiography are as low as those in series with routine cholangiography. Unfortunately, the end points in these studies are clinical follow-ups that are incomplete or too short, or both. There is a need for a more objective follow-up of patients in both groups, routine and selective, to answer the question definitively. In the meantime, each group will continue to pursue its practices based on the data each has chosen to highlight.

Laparoscopic cholecystectomy has added to the cholangiogram controversy in two distinct ways. With the recognition of increased numbers of bile duct injuries associated with laparoscopic cholecystectomy, proposals have been made that intraoperative cholangiograms are mandatory to identify ductal anomalies on the one hand, and to help the surgeon know exactly where the dissection is taking place, on the other hand.[17] The data to support the role of routine cholangiography in laparoscopic cholecystectomy in preventing or reducing bile duct injury is incomplete and controlled studies have not been done.

The second way in which laparoscopic cholecystectomy has increased the cholangiogram controversy is in the recommendation that endoscopic retrograde cholangiopancreatography (ERCP) be used preoperatively to identify and treat patients with common duct stones. This recommendation carries with it a number of serious considerations. First, it assumes that patients can be clearly identified preoperatively to be at risk for harboring common duct stones. Second, the performance of ERCP carries with it a distinct, well-documented mortality and morbidity risk that is added to the risk of the laparoscopic procedure subsequently performed. Third, it assumes that a negative ERCP done a few days before the laparoscopic cholecystectomy will remain negative until the cholecystectomy; it does not allow for the possibility that gallstones may migrate into the CBD in the period between ERCP and cholecystectomy or even *during* cholecystectomy.

In a recent prospective nonrandomized study reported from the Brigham and Women's Hospital in Boston, 514 patients were screened before laparoscopic cholecystectomy by history, physical exam, abdominal ultrasound and liver chemistries.[18] Based on the results of these tests, the patients were classified as: unlikely, likely, or indeterminate to have common duct stones. Four hundred forty-one (86%) of the 514 patients were classified as unlikely to have CBD stones and they had no cholangiograms done. Three of these patients had symptomatic retained stones in the postoperative period; the incidence of asymptomatic retained stones could not be determined since no cholangiograms were done. All 25 patients (5% of total) who were classified as likely to have CBD stones underwent preoperative ERCP. Only six patients (24% of likely group) had CBD stones identified and removed. No retained stones had been identified in this group at the time of report. Twelve additional patients (2% of total) had had ERCP by referring physicians at various time intervals prior to cholecystectomy. One of these patients who had a negative ERCP 6 weeks before underwent laparoscopic cholecystectomy without cholangiogram and had a symptomatic retained stone at 7 days after cholecystectomy and required another ERCP with sphincterotomy.

Of the 36 patients (7% of total) who were classified as having an intermediate likelihood of CBD stones, 30 (83%) had cholangiography successfully completed. One patient (3%) in this group had a CBD stone. No retained stones were identified in the follow-up period in the remainder of the patients.

This study purported to evaluate and disprove the necessity of routine cholangiography during laparoscopic cholecystectomy. However, it did not prospectively study the utility of cholangiography in the unlikely group (86% of the patients) in whom previous studies have demonstrated a 5% to 7% incidence of unsuspected stones. Furthermore, the length of follow-up was not stated, nor was the completeness of follow-up to search for retained stones detailed. Experience has shown that many patients who have recurrent symptoms following cholecystectomy do not return to their original surgeon for care, especially in large metropolitan areas. Therefore, the message in this study must be viewed in terms of the inherent bias in not doing cholangiography on a large percentage of the patients. As far as ERCP is concerned, when it was done in the group judged most likely to have CBD stones, it was negative in 76%. The risk of ERCP is considerably higher than the negligible risk of intraoperative cholangiogram and its cost is also considerably greater. Further discussions of this subject are to be found in recent publications.[19–21]

DIFFERENTIAL DIAGNOSIS

The differential diagnoses to be considered are all of those that produce jaundice, elevated liver enzymes, fever, and upper abdominal pain. During the evaluation process, it should be attempted, first of all, to separate hepatocellular diseases (medical jaundice) from obstructive diseases (surgical jaundice). Findings which are initially helpful in this distinction are acholic stools, an elevated alkaline phosphatase and/or GGTP with relatively normal aminotransferases and dilated bile ducts on ultrasound, all of which suggest a surgical jaundice versus a medical cause.

When this initial distinction has been made, more refined testing may be performed to more precisely delineate the etiology. For example, in patients with presumed medical jaundice, distinctions will be made between drug-induced jaundice versus viral etiologies such as hepatitis. In patients demonstrating a surgical type of jaundice, distinctions must be made between benign and malignant causes of jaundice and treatment directed appropriately.

■ TREATMENT

The management of choledocholithiasis with or without cholangitis depends upon many variables, including patient condition, skill of interventional radiologists and endoscopists, location of treatment and experience of the surgeon. The following discussion will attempt to

place these options in perspective. The details of operative techniques of laparoscopic cholecystectomy, choledochoduodenostomy, and common bile duct exploration and drainage will be covered in other chapters.

COMMON DUCT STONES ASSOCIATED WITH GALLBLADDER STONES

The majority of patients with common duct stones will present for treatment of these stones in conjunction with treatment of their cholelithiasis. The majority of these patients will be treated electively, as opposed to urgently, for their combined stone diseases. In many of the patients with common duct stones, the presence of stones will be suspected preoperatively and the procedure will be planned appropriately.

It is now agreed that laparoscopic cholecystectomy is the procedure of choice for most patients with symptomatic gallstones.[22]

Suspected common duct stones prior to planned laparoscopic cholecystectomy may be managed in different ways. If the surgeon and team are experienced in laparoscopic techniques of CBD stone removal, the patient may be taken to the operating suite with this procedure in mind. An intraoperative cholangiogram should be done to confirm the presence of CBD stones and their position. Transcystic common duct stone removal via choledochoscope or choledochotomy by laparoscopic means have been utilized by experienced surgeons to clear the common duct of stones.[23–25]

In the procedure of transcystic common bile duct stone removal, the cystic duct size is a limiting factor to stone removal. Smaller cystic ducts may be dilated carefully with balloons to accommodate the instruments needed to remove the CBD stones. However, large stones (>1 cm) usually are not removable by this approach. Similarly, stones situated in the upper ductal system (common hepatic duct or intrahepatic ducts) are very difficult to remove by this method since cephalad angulation of the instruments is very difficult to perform. In these situations, choledochotomy via laparoscopic approach has been done by experienced surgeons. This approach allows complete access to the biliary system but requires additional operating time and special skill in suturing laparoscopically to close the choledochotomy. Reported success rates have been between 95% to 100% in the hands of skilled operators.[23,24]

If the surgical team is not experienced with laparoscopic methods of common duct stone removal, they may elect to refer the patient with suspected CBD stones to an endoscopist for a preoperative ERCP. If the ERCP is positive for stones, the endoscopist may perform a sphincterotomy and stone extraction. This procedure has a reported success rate of >90% in removing CBD

TABLE 61–1. ENDOSCOPIC SPHINCTEROTOMY IN PATIENTS WITH GALLBLADDERS IN SITU

AUTHOR	NO. PATIENTS	CBD STONES CLEARED (%)	MORTALITY (%)	MORBIDITY (%)	FOLLOW-UP MOS.	LATE DEATHS (%)	SUBSEQUENT GB REMOVAL (%)	REMAINING WITH SYMPTOMS (%)
Hansell[27]	121	95	6	4	12–72 (Median 24)	2	18	6
Lamont[28]	75	96	0	4	Mean 30.4	26	26	2
Hill[29]	218	89	1	8	Mean 38	26	11	NA
Kullman[30]	148	88	4	16	1–97 (Mean 42)	42	11	NA

stones, but has an overall mortality rate of about 1% and a complication rate of 6% to 10%, in experienced centers.[19,26] This morbidity and mortality risk must be added to that of the subsequent laparoscopic cholecystectomy that the patient will undergo to remove the gallbladder. If one accepts a mortality risk of 0.3% and a complication rate of 5% for the laparoscopic cholecystectomy, the total mortality risk for a patient treated by the two procedures would be 1.3% and the morbidity risk, 11% to 15%.

These figures assume that the patient is under 70 years of age and is not acutely ill. In such patients, the risk of open cholecystectomy with common duct exploration would be similar or less. This option would be well worth considering by surgical teams experienced in biliary tract surgery. The opportunity to complete the treatment in one procedure is still an attractive one for many patients, even though it means a longer hospitalization and recovery period.

For elderly, poor-risk patients with gallstones and CBD stones, some have recommended ERCP and sphincterotomy as the sole treatment, leaving the gallbladder and its stones in situ. Several studies have reported the success rates of removal of CBD stones as being between 88% to 96%.[27–30] Mortality rates ranged from 0% to 6%. Subsequent cholecystectomies were required in 11% to 26% of patients in follow-ups averaging up to 42 months after the endoscopic procedure (Table 61–1). Given these figures, one could recommend sphincterotomy alone for those patients with life expectancies of <2 years.

A study from the University of Southern California group compared results of preoperative endoscopic sphincterotomy plus surgery with those of surgery alone, in a prospective randomized fashion.[31] Fifty-two patients with gallbladder stones and choledocholithiasis were evaluated. In the patients having preoperative endoscopic sphincterotomy plus surgery, only 65% were free of stones, whereas 88% were free of stones after surgery alone (P<.05). The authors concluded that preoperative endoscopic sphincterotomy could not be recommended as a technique for clearance of CBD stones on the basis of efficacy, morbidity rate, or cost.

Unsuspected common duct stones found at the time of cholecystectomy may prove to be a bigger problem for the surgical team. As previously discussed, in a program of routine cystic duct cholangiography during cholecystectomy, approximately 5% to 7% of patients will be found to have unsuspected stones in the CBD.[10,14]

If the surgical team is performing cholecystectomy by the laparoscopic route, and the cholangiogram reveals unsuspected stones, they must decide whether they have the expertise to explore the CBD laparoscopically. If not, they then must decide whether to convert the operation to an open procedure and remove the common duct stones or to complete the cholecystectomy and refer the patient postoperatively for ERCP and attempted stone removal.

Conversion to an open procedure must never be considered either a failure of the surgical team or a complication. It is prudent to explain preoperatively to all patients that their laparoscopic procedure may have to be converted to a standard open procedure, based upon unforeseen factors, including discovery of unsuspected CBD stones. Most surgeons regard such conversions as a demonstration of good surgical judgment. The surgeon owes the patient every effort to correct the biliary pathology in one procedure, under one anesthetic, if possible.

Referral for a postoperative ERCP attempt to remove the CBD stone, in lieu of doing an open operation, must be done on the basis of individual considerations, including patient demands. It should be recognized that patients with large CBD stones or prior gastric surgery may be unsatisfactory patients for ERCP. Also, the surgeon must consider the additive morbidity and mortality risks of the ERCP and spincterotomy, in addition to the likelihood of success in removing the stones as well as the additional cost. It is felt that most surgeons inexperienced in laparoscopic bile duct surgery, but experienced in open biliary surgery, will make the decision to convert such a patient to an open procedure if the condition of the patient permits.

COMMON DUCT STONES PRESENTING AFTER CHOLECYSTECTOMY

The majority of such stones are found to be retained rather than primary or recurrent. Previous discussion has indicated methods for differentiating between these two types of CBD stones.

Common duct stones in the immediate postoperative period are found most often by postoperative T tube cholangiogram in those patients who had concomitant cholecystectomy and common duct exploration (Fig 61–4). These stones are clearly retained and are more likely to occur in those patients who had numerous common duct stones removed at the original operation.

Preventive measures for such retained stones at the original procedure are the uses of both operative cholangioscopy and completion T tube cholangiogram on the table, prior to closing the abdominal incision. Combined use of these two modalities has been demonstrated to reduce the postoperative retained stone rate significantly and even to zero in many institutions.[32–35]

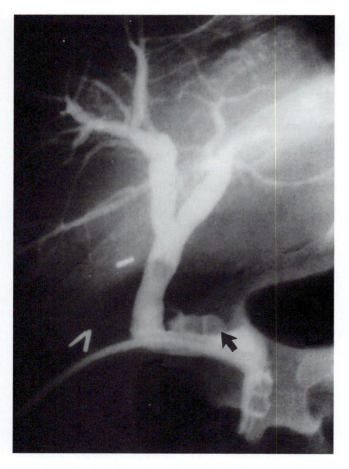

Figure 61–4. T tube cholangiogram demonstrates retained CBD stones in a postoperative patient. Note distal migration of T tube in the duct and the cystic duct stones (*arrow*).

In most patients who have retained CBD stones discovered postoperatively, T tube drains are in place and should be left in for access to the biliary tree and the retained stones. The most frequently chosen method of treatment in these patients is to allow the T tube tract to mature for approximately 4 weeks and then to refer the patient for interventional radiologic removal of stones. If a 14-Fr tube or larger has not been placed at operation, the radiologists may need to perform a series of dilations of the tract over several days prior to removing the stone(s). The success rate of complete stone removal by the radiologic method has been reported to be as high as 98%.[36]

Some reports of chemical dissolution of common bile duct stones have suggested that monooctanoin might be useful. It is instilled via the T tube and its limiting factors have been that the patient must have cholesterol stones, be monitored for pressure in the biliary tree to prevent cholangitis, and be in a hospital setting for many days while being infused. A review of 48 patients undergoing monooctanoin infusion showed that only 35 patients completed a full course of treatment. Of these 35, only nine (26%) had clearance of their stones at the end of treatment. Subsequent clearance by ERCP was obtained in eight additional patients, for a total clearance rate of 49%. Patients with stones >2 cm in diameter were not able to be cleared.[37]

In an attempt to dissolve both cholesterol and calcium pigment stones, German investigators have studied compounds containing both monooctanoin and ethylene-diamine-tetra-acetic acid (EDTA).[38] These authors reported 75% complete dissolution rates after infusion periods of 2 to 15 days.

As an alternative to radiologic extraction of stones, surgeons at Boston University treated a large number of patients by using fiberoptic choledochoscopy via the T tube tract.[39] Of 126 patients treated, extraction was successful in 94% of patients, including patients with multiple stones and hepatic duct stones. Some patients required electrohydraulic lithotripsy or laser fragmentation of the stones in order to remove them. No serious complications or deaths occurred in this group of patients. Because of its high success rate and avoidance of radiation exposure, this method was recommended for treatment of retained CBD stones when a T tube is in place.

It can be appreciated that, because of the many alternatives to reoperation in patients with retained stones in the CBD and a T tube in place, the need to treat such patients surgically should occur in only 2% to 5% of all cases.

Common duct stones found at a time much later from the original operation may be either retained or primary. Since a T tube usually is not present beyond a few weeks in most of these patients, the previously described methods of extraction or dissolution do not pertain.

Although attempts at dissolution of common duct stones via endoscopically placed nasobiliary tubes have been described, the poor patient acceptance and low results have made this a procedure of last resort, if used at all.[37,38]

Most of the patients in this category will be referred initially to an endoscopist for an attempt at endoscopic papillotomy and retrieval of stones.[40,41] Success rates of between 85% and 95% have been reported. It seems best suited for the elderly, poor surgical risk patient. The complication rate for endoscopic sphincterotomy ranges from 6.5% to 8.7% and the mortality rate ranges from 0% to 1.3%.[40] Long-term follow-up studies have shown that restenosis and/or recurrent stones occurred in 7% of patients, usually within 2 years.[42] In a prospective study of the complications of endoscopic sphincterotomy in 423 patients, Sherman and associates demonstrated an overall complication rate of 6.9% (10.8% in an Oddi dysfunction group versus 4.3% in a stone, tumor, and miscellaneous group) and a 30 day mortality rate of 1.7%.[43] This is one of the few studies to provide 30 day figures that can be compared with standard surgical mortality reporting.

In patients in whom endoscopic sphincterotomy and stone extraction has been unsuccessful, the use of extracorporeal shock-wave lithotripsy (ESWL) has proven beneficial. A multi-institutional study of 42 patients treated at 11 institutions showed that stone fragmentation could be obtained in 95% of patients.[44] However, 50% of the patients required adjunctive procedures to clear the bile duct stones, including endoscopic extraction, biliary lavage, and stenting. Only two patients required operation to clear the bile duct stones. In most of the patients in this study, previous attempts to clear the bile ducts by endoscopic or chemical means had failed.

In a study from Germany of ESWL, 29 patients of a group of 220 had failed endoscopic removal of CBD stones.[45] ESWL achieved fragmentation in 80% of these 29 patients and complete stone clearance was achieved in these 80%. Surgical removal of stones was required in 4 patients. No deaths occurred and complications were said to be mild.

Some researchers have utilized the transhepatic route in attempting to remove common duct stones. Using a modified Dormia basket inserted through a percutaneous transhepatic catheter, a Boston group reported successful clearance of CBD stones in 93% of 50 patients treated.[46] All of these patients either had contraindications to surgery or had undergone unsuccessful endoscopic attempts at removal. Twenty-nine patients in this group required either monooctanoin or methyl tert-butyl ether infusions to reduce stone size or remove residual debris. The authors reported a 13% morbidity and a 4% mortality rate.

The percutaneous transhepatic route has also been used as a method of passing a cholangioscope to visualize and remove the biliary stones. In a report of 50 patients treated, the success rate in stone removal was 78%.[47] Sixty percent of the patients had intrahepatic bile duct stones only; 24% had common bile duct stones only; and 16% had stones in both intrahepatic and common bile ducts. Overall, 221 procedures were required in the 50 patients and complications included pain intolerance (14%), minor bleeding (14%), and massive bleeding (10%).

Many investigative reports on innovative techniques are available. These include endoscopic introduction of electrohydraulic lithotripters by use of "mother-daughter" endoscopic techniques,[48] endoscopic introduction of intracorporeal shock-wave lithotripters into the bile duct,[49] percutaneous transhepatic insertion of electrohydraulic lithotripters,[50] and insertion of laser lithotripters via T tube tracts.[51] While these technologic advances are interesting, they remain to be proven effective and economical.

It is likely that patients who fail endoscopic removal with or without ESWL, will be strongly considered for open removal of their CBD stones, at least at the time of this writing.

INTRAHEPATIC STONES

There is a clear ethnic predilection for intrahepatic stones in patients from Asian countries (5% to 15%) as compared with natives of the United States (0.5%) (Fig 61–5). In the latter group, the disease presents as (1) associated intrahepatic stones with extrahepatic duct stones, (2) associated with ductal cystic dilations (Caroli's disease) or (3) occurring in segments of ducts dilated behind strictures of traumatic, neoplastic, or idiopathic origin. Intrahepatic stones are found more often in the left hepatic duct. This location may make certain nonoperative approaches, such as percutaneous cholangioscopy and stone removal, more difficult since many radiologists find left hepatic duct punctures technically more difficult.

Intrahepatic stones associated with extrahepatic duct stones are the most common presentation and are most often removed during cholecystectomy and common duct exploration. The techniques for these procedures will be described in chapter 12.

Intrahepatic stones associated with cystic disease of the intrahepatic ducts (Caroli's disease) are very often diagnosed by the occurrence of cholangitis and/or abscess. Surgeons also must be aware that these stones, in the setting of Caroli's disease, may coexist with cholangiocarcinoma.[52]

Nonoperative attempts at removal of stones from Caroli's patients are minimally successful owing to the

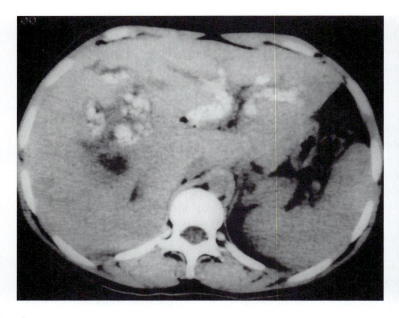

A

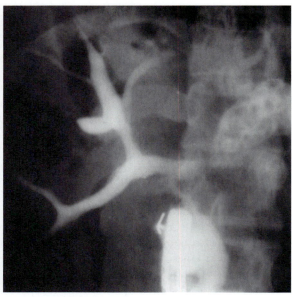

B

Figure 61–5. A. CT scan demonstrating intrahepatic stones in an Asian patient. **B.** Endoscopic removal of the intrahepatic stones in the left duct was accomplished via Roux-Y hepaticocutaneous-jejunostomy.

anatomic abnormalities that convert the intrahepatic biliary system into a "chain of lakes." The strictures that occur also make primary attempts at nonoperative stone removal likely to fail.

The operative approach to Caroli's patients should be to perform cholecystectomy and common duct exploration. The intrahepatic stones should be removed with the aid of the choledochoscope and strictures should be dilated as much as possible to aid in stone removal. Biopsies of strictured areas should be performed because of the high incidence of associated malignancy in these patients.

If stone removal can be completed at operation, the surgeon may elect to close the common bile duct over a large T tube (14-Fr or greater diameter sidearm) and to follow the patient with postoperative cholangiograms. Some have suggested that the patient be given ursodeoxycholic acid orally for a period of a few months in order to promote a choleresis and to prevent stone recurrence. To our knowledge there is no controlled trial that demonstrates this to be effective.

The T tube may be removed 3 to 6 weeks later if postoperative cholangiograms show the ducts to be clear. However, patients with Caroli's disease deserve careful long-term follow-up for recurrent stones, development of biliary cirrhosis, abscesses of liver, and/or malignancy.

If the surgeon encounters an abscess in one of the cystic dilations, then consideration must be given to hepatic resection to remove the affected portion of the biliary system (see Section XI).

Not unusually, the surgeon is unable to clear all of the stones from the bile ducts at operation. In this situation, it should not be assumed that biliary-enteric drainage by choledochoduodenostomy or choledochojejunostomy, or even sphincteroplasty, will allow the stones to pass in the postoperative period. A decision must be made at the time of the initial operation as to the best long-term management of the unremovable stones. If the stones are located in one area of the liver, strong consideration for hepatic resection must be given. If the stones are more diffuse, the surgeon should consider a high hepaticojejunostomy using a Roux-Y limb with the blind end implanted in the abdominal wall for future easy access to the biliary tract (see below) (Fig 61–6).[53]

Intrahepatic stones associated with strictures of the biliary system occur in approximately 25% of patients with intrahepatic stones of all causes. The strictures may be primary in the course of the disease, such as those owing to bile duct injuries, where the stones occur in the dilated static system behind the stricture. In other cases, the stones may lead to inflammation and scarring of the bile ducts and thus further complicate the disease. As in the patients with Caroli's disease, biopsies of the strictured areas are important to rule out occult malignancy.

In all the important principles, the management of intrahepatic stones in this setting is essentially the same as for those in the clinical setting of Caroli's disease.

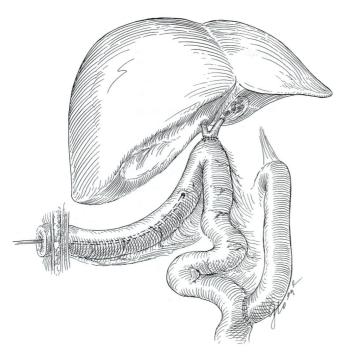

Figure 61–6. Diagram of Roux-Y hepaticojejunostomy with cutaneous stoma. Illustrated is the use of a flexible choledochoscope to remove intrahepatic stones in the left ductal system.

The group from the Queen Mary Hospital in Hong Kong have recently reviewed their series of 162 patients treated for intrahepatic stones between January 1984 and July 1991.[54] In 41 of these patients, a decision was made to perform a Roux-Y hepaticojejunostomy with the blind proximal end of the jejunal limb brought to the abdominal wall either as a stoma or anchored to the subcutaneous fascia or peritoneum, for possible future opening.

The indications used to perform this procedure were either recurrent stones or strictures in a patient who previously had been operated on or had a high likelihood of recurrent stones or strictures after the first laparotomy.

While the majority of the biliary-enteric connections were made at the common hepatic duct, technical difficulties made it necessary to perform some anastomoses to the bifurcation or parts of the left ductal system. The stoma itself was placed on either the right or left side of the abdomen, generally on the contralateral side to the most severely involved liver lobe, in order to allow easier access to the involved ductal system.

Postoperative choledochoscopy was used via the stoma in two-thirds of the patients, beginning at about the second week postoperatively. From one to fifteen choledochoscopies per patient were required to clear the residual stones. Ninety-three percent of the pa-

tients had their stones completely removed by choledochoscopy, which in some cases also required electrohydraulic lithotripsy and balloon dilation of strictures. The stomas subsequently were closed, under local anesthesia, at a median of 2 months after operation. Twenty-nine percent of the patients developed recurrent symptoms at a median time of 27 months postoperatively, with reestablishment of the stoma and repeat flexible choledochoscopy required.

This series from one of the leading biliary surgery groups treating intrahepatic stones serves as a benchmark for the management of these stones and also provides important technical advice for the biliary surgeon who may require repeated postoperative access to the biliary tract.

■ CHOLANGITIS

The classic presentation of patients with cholangitis was described as fever, jaundice and abdominal pain by Charcot.[55] In fact, a third to one-half of patients with acute cholangitis will not present with the complete triad. Reynolds and Dargan added the presenting symptoms of shock and mental obtundation to the triad to describe a group of patients with severe forms of the disease.[56]

INITIAL MANAGEMENT

Patients presenting with signs suggestive of cholangitis deserve urgent hospitalization and treatment. The initial management is directed to replacement of fluids and general resuscitation along with antibiotics. Current treatment often consists of empiric administration of a broad-spectrum penicillin (mezlocillin or piperacillin) until cultures and sensitivities are available.[57] Multiple organisms are recovered from bile cultures (mostly aerobic bacteria) and approximately 25% of blood cultures also will grow the same organisms.[58]

Following initial treatment, the patient must be observed frequently for signs of worsening condition. Experience has shown that about 17% of patients will require emergency biliary surgery in the first 24 hours; of the remainder, two-thirds will require definitive treatment in the first 72 hours.[58]

BILIARY DECOMPRESSION

The *sine qua non* of treatment of acute cholangitis is to relieve pressure in the obstructed biliary system. In most centers, this is attempted first by endoscopic means. Early endoscopy allows not only diagnosis by cholangiography and direct visualization of the ampulla but also permits attempts at biliary decompression.

Endoscopic attempts at biliary decompression in this setting consist of sphincterotomy and endoscopic removal of stones, as previously described. In a prospective, randomized study of 82 patients, 41 were assigned to surgical decompression and 41 were randomized to endoscopic drainage followed by definitive treatment.[59] Complications related to treatment occurred in 34% of the endoscopic group and 66% of the surgical group and the time for temperature and blood pressure normalization was similar in the two groups. The hospital mortality was 10% for the endoscopic group and 32% for the surgical group ($P<.03$).

If the stones cannot be removed, a nasobiliary catheter or stent should be inserted to decompress the biliary tract. One review of 127 patients so treated found that placement of these tubes was successful in 98%.[60] Clearance of stones was ultimately achieved in 43% by endoscopic means and in 21% by surgical treatment. Poor-risk patients, who were followed for a mean of 15.9 months, without stone clearance, and who required stent changes for cholangitis were successfully managed. Thirty day mortality was 3%. In another report of similar management of 104 patients, no pancreatitis occurred, but 17% of patients became jaundiced and 3% developed cholangitis.[61] All were controlled by antibiotics and stent changes and only 2% of patients required biliary surgery.

Transhepatic percutaneous biliary decompression also has been proven to be effective in the urgent treatment of cholangitis.[62] However, with the readily available expertise in endoscopic management in most institutions, radiologic decompression has not been as frequently utilized. Newer instrumentation has been described previously that is available for stone removal by the percutaneous route; however, the chief use of the transhepatic route is for emergency biliary decompression in situations where endoscopic early management is not available.

Surgical biliary decompression is indicated in those severely ill patients who cannot be managed by endoscopic or percutaneous means. In such patients, emergency operation consists of common duct exploration and T tube drainage. If the condition of the patient permits, attempts to remove CBD stones are made along with cholecystectomy. The use of the choledochoscope has greatly improved the stone clearance rate in these patients and has not been associated with increased complication rates.[63,64]

In patients too ill to tolerate a long procedure, choledochotomy and T tube insertion, leaving stones in place for later treatment, may result in salvage of an otherwise hopeless situation.

In those patients who have been stabilized by medical treatment alone, or who have had endoscopic or percutaneous decompression, definitive surgical treatment should be electively undertaken. This treatment consists, at a minimum, of removal of the diseased gallbladder, choledochotomy with exploration of the duct and preferably, endoscopic verification of complete stone clearance. T tube drainage generally is recommended so that a completion cholangiogram can be performed before abdominal wound closure and also to provide access to the biliary tract in the postoperative period.

Some studies have reported prospectively randomizing patients to primary closure of the choledochotomy versus T tube drainage.[65,66] The results of these studies have indicated that primary closure is as effective as drainage in most patients fitting within specific inclusion criteria. Patients with emergency conditions such as cholangitis are generally not included in such studies.

Laparoscopic surgery for the emergency management of the patient with acute cholangitis has not yet attained the level of efficacy of the open operation. Reasons for this are undoubtedly related to the longer operative time for laparoscopic procedures and the relative inexperience of surgeons in exploring the common bile duct via the laparoscopic route. In acutely ill patients, these factors make laparoscopic treatment less satisfactory than open operation.

In the patient who is stabilized on medical management and is to have elective surgical removal of CBD stones with or without cholecystectomy, the laparoscopic approach should be considered more seriously, since it is an elective situation.

SURGICAL PROCEDURES FOR BILIARY DECOMPRESSION

The surgeon performing open operation for the correction of common bile duct obstruction has several choices to make. First, can the stone(s) in the CBD be removed? Previous discussion has focused on newer techniques for stone fragmentation and removal. The decision often is made to open the duodenum and perform sphincterotomy to attempt removal of difficult, impacted stones. This increases the magnitude of the operation as well as the risk of morbidity and mortality. In a review of their experience with thirty-two patients with impacted distal bile duct stones, Thompson and Bennion were able to remove all stones in a retrograde fashion without need for spincter ablation.[67] Acute cholangitis was present in 22% of their patients. There was no mortality; two patients had mild pancreatitis and one patient had a retained intrahepatic stone.

In another report of 100 consecutive CBD explorations, Pappas and associates needed to open the duodenum for extraction of difficult stones in only two patients.[68] There was a 5.3% incidence of retained stones in this series; no mortality occurred; major complications occurred in 7.4% of the patients.

Thus, it appears that the need for a surgeon to perform duodenotomy to extract difficult stones should be infrequent. An exception may be in the unusual patient who has a small common bile duct with stones. Cameron and associates have reported on transduodenal common duct exploration after spincteroplasty in 28 patients.[69] They chose this method because of the risk of producing ductal injury or late stricture if the usual choledochotomy and exploration were used. No mortality occurred; one patient had postoperative pancreatitis with jaundice and cholangitis; the overall morbidity was 29%.

A second choice to be made by the surgeon is whether to perform a biliary enteric anastomosis at the time of removal of CBD stones. Generally, indications for such a procedure have been an older patient with a dilated ductal system and multiple stones. These indications were promulgated before the refinements of endoscopic stone removal, but are still considered by surgeons today.

If a decision is made to perform such an operation, the surgeon must choose which of the available procedures should be done. For many years, the favored method of biliary enteric anastomosis in this department has been the Roux-Y choledochojejunostomy or hepaticojejunostomy. Reasons for this have been a generally lower incidence of cholangitis and reflux of undigestible intestinal contents into the biliary tree. A drawback of the Roux-Y procedure had been an increased incidence of postoperative peptic ulcer disease.[70] However, with the routine use of preoperative and postoperative histamine-receptor antagonists, this complication has been avoided in our later experience. Long-term follow-up of such patients shows a high degree of success. One study has reported a 98% good result in patients followed a median of 8 years.[71]

Many surgeons have utilized the choledochoduodenostomy as their procedure of choice for biliary-enteric anastomosis in the patient with CBD stones. They favor this procedure because of the usually easy anastomosis of the distal duct to the adjacent duodenum. Drawbacks to this procedure have been a higher incidence of cholangitis when the anastomosis has narrowed or is initially too small.

The risk of leakage of the duodenal suture line is also present. Another drawback has been the development of the "sump syndrome" in patients with a side-to-side choledochoduodenostomy.[72] The cause of this is the accumulation of stones, undigestible food matter, or both in the segment of the distal bile duct which then obstructs the anastomotic opening and causes cholangitis and pain. This complication also is favored by a small anastomotic opening. Surgical clearance and conversion to an end-to-side choledochoenterostomy may be required to correct the situation, although some patients have been successfully treated by endoscopic sphincterotomy and removal of debris and stones by this route.

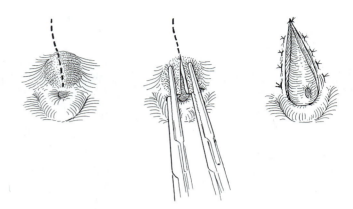

Figure 61–7. Diagram of surgical sphincteroplasty for removal of impacted stone and drainage of bile duct. The incision is made in the 11 o'clock position.

Long-term follow-up studies of patients with choledochoduodenostomies has shown a very high rate of success when the anastomosis has been 15 mm or greater in diameter.[73]

Surgical sphincteroplasty alone may be all that is required to provide good drainage to the biliary tree (Fig 61–7). In patients in whom the duct is dilated down to the terminal few millimeters, this procedure may offer lasting relief without the fear of "sump syndrome" or the need to perform an anastomosis. A drawback of this procedure is the necessity to open the duodenum and the small but real risk of duodenal leakage postoperatively. This risk is increased in patients with pancreatitis or those who develop pancreatitis postoperatively. The technical details of these procedures will be presented in other chapters in this section.

Much of the success of treatment of patients with choledocholithiasis, with or without associated cholangitis, depends on close consultation and collaboration between the surgeon, radiologist, and endoscopist. In this area, as in all areas of surgery, the experience and judgment of the surgeon is an important factor. No computer or machine has yet been developed that comes close to matching the abilities of the brain and hands of the surgeon.

REFERENCES

1. Diliberto JP, Marks JW, Schoenfield LJ. Classification and pathogenesis of gallstones. In: Braasch JW, Tompkins RK (eds), *Surgical Disease of the Biliary Tract and Pancreas.* Chicago, IL: Mosby Year-Book, 1994 (in press)
2. Saunders KD, Cates JA, Roslyn JJ: Pathogenesis of gallstones. In: Pitt HA (ed), *The Surgical Clinics of North America: Biliary Tract Surgery.* Philadelphia, PA: WB Saunders; 1990:1197–1216

3. Schillio Y, Amouyal G, Gayet B, et al. Primary intrahepatic cholesterol stones: report of one case and treatment with ursodeoxycholic acid. *Dig Dis Sci* 1992;37:1460–1463

4. Strichartz S, Abedin MZ, Ippoliti AF, et al. Intrahepatic cholesterol gallstones: a rationale for oral dissolution therapy. *Gastroenterology* 1991;100:228–232

5. Vitetta L, Sali A, Little P, et al. Primary "brown pigment" bile duct stones. *HPB Surg* 1991;4:209–220

6. Smith AL, Stewart L, Fine R, et al. Gallstone disease. The clinical manifestations of infectious stones. *Arch Surg* 1989;124:629–633

7. Kaufman HS, Magnuson TH, Lillemoe KD, et al. The role of bacteria in gallbladder and common duct stone formation. *Ann Surg* 1989;209:584–591

8. Hall RI, Ingoldby CJ, Denyer ME. Periampullary diverticula predispose to primary rather than secondary stones in the common bile duct. *Endoscopy* 1990;22:127–128

9. Chetlin SH, Elliott DW. Biliary bacteremia. *Arch Surg* 1971;102:303–307

10. Kakos GS, Tompkins RK, Turnipseed W, et al. Operative cholangiography during routine cholecystectomy: a review of 3012 cases. *Arch Surg* 1972;104:484–488

11. Zollinger RM. Significance of pain and vomiting in cholelithiasis. *JAMA* 1935;105:1647–1652

12. Jolly PC, Walker JH. Operative cholangiography in biliary tract surgery. *Hospital Practice,* February, 1972

13. Berci G, Shore JM, Hamlin JA, et al. Operative fluoroscopy and cholangiography: the use of modern radiologic techniques during surgery. *Am J Surg* 1977;135:32–35

14. Shively EH, Wieman TJ, Adams AL, et al. Operative cholangiography. *Am J Surg* 1990;159:380–384

15. Berci G, Hamlin JA. Biliary ductal anomalies. In: Berci G, Hamlin JA (eds), *Operative Biliary Radiology.* Baltimore, MD: Williams & Wilkins; 1981:109–141

16. Barnes BA, Barnes AB. Evaluation of surgical therapy by cost-benefit analysis. *Surgery* 1977;82:21–28

17. Phillips EH, Berci G, Carroll B, et al. The importance of intraoperative cholangiography during laparoscopic cholecystectomy. *Am Surg* 1990;56:792–795

18. Clair DG, Carr-Locke DL, Becker JM, et al. Routine cholangiography is not warranted during laparoscopic cholecystectomy. *Arch Surg* 1993;128:551–555

19. Fink AS. To ERCP or not to ERCP: that is the question. [Editorial]. *Surg Endosc* 1993;7:375–76

20. Surick B, Washington M, Ghazi A. Endoscopic retrograde cholangiopancreatography in conjunction with laparoscopic cholecystectomy. *Surg Endosc* 1993;7:388–392

21. Fink AS. Current dilemmas in management of common duct stones. *Surg Endosc* 1993;7:285–291

22. Kalser SC, Bray EA, Burton BT, et al. National Institutes of Health Consensus Development Conference Statement on gallstones and laparoscopic cholecystectomy. *Am J Surg* 1993;165:390–398

23. Hunter JG. Laparoscopic transcystic common bile duct exploration. *Am J Surg* 1992;163:53–56

24. Carroll BJ, Phillips EH, Daykhovsky L, et al. Laparoscopic choledochoscopy: an effective approach to the common duct. *J Laparoendosc Surg* 1992;2:15–21

25. Phillips EH, Carroll BJ, Pearlstein AR, et al. Laparoscopic choledochoscopy and extraction of common bile duct stones. *World J Surg* 1993;17:22–28

26. Cotton PB. Endoscopic retrograde cholangiopancreatography and laparoscopic cholecystectomy. *Am J Surg* 1993;165:474–478

27. Hansell DT, Millar MA, Murray WR, et al. Endoscopic sphincterotomy for bile duct stones in patients with intact gallbladders. *Br J Surg* 1989;76:856–858

28. Lamont DD, Passi RB. Fate of the gallbladder with cholelithiasis after endoscopic sphincterotomy for choledocholithiasis. *Can J Surg* 1989;32:15–18

29. Hill J, Martin DF, Tweedle DE. Risks of leaving the gallbladder in situ after endoscopic sphincterotomy for bile duct stones. *Br J Surg* 1991;78:554–557

30. Kullman E, Borch K, Dahlin LG, et al. Long-term follow-up of patients with gallbladder in situ after endoscopic sphincterotomy for choledocholithiasis. *Eur J Surg* 1991;157:131–135

31. Stain SC, Cohen H, Tsuishoysha M, et al. Choledocholithiasis: endoscopic sphincterotomy or common bile duct exploration. *Ann Surg* 1991;213:627–633

32. Nora PF, Berci G, Dorazio RA, et al. Operative choledochoscopy: results of a prospective study in several institutions. *Am J Surg* 1977;133:105–110

33. Berci G. Intraoperative and postoperative biliary endoscopy (choledochoscopy). *Endoscopy* 1989;21:330–332

34. Nagorney DM, Lohmuller JL. Choledochoscopy. A cost-minimization analysis. *Ann Surg* 1990;211:354–359

35. Takada T, Yasuda H, Uchiyama K, et al. Choledochoscopy during biliary surgery for reducing the risk of overlooked stones. *Surg Endosc* 1991;5:192–195

36. Braghetto I, Csendes A, de la Cuadra R, et al. Treatment of residual common bile duct stones after cholecystectomy. *Hepatogastroenterology* 1989;36:123–127

37. Stock SE, Carlson GL, Lavelle MI, et al. Treatment of common bile duct stones using monooctanoin. *Br J Surg* 1992;79:653–654

38. Klueppelberg U, Baumgaertel H, Schusdziarra V, et al. Dissolution of bile duct stones by a hydrophilized glyceromonooctanoin-bile-acid-EDTA emulsion. *Klin Wochenschr* 1991;69:76–82

39. Hieken TJ, Birkett DH. Postoperative T tube tract choledochoscopy. *Am J Surg* 1992;163:28–30

40. Sivak MV Jr. Endoscopic management of bile duct stones. *Am J Surg* 1989;158:228–240

41. Gordon RL, Shapiro HA. Nonoperative management of bile duct stones. In: Pitt HA (ed), *Surgical Clinics of North America.* Philadelphia, PA: WB Saunders; 1990;70:1313–1328

42. Kullman E, Borch K, Liedberg G. Long-term follow-up after endoscopic management of retained and recurrent common duct stones. *Acta Chir Scand* 1989;155:395–399

43. Sherman S, Ruffolo TA, Hawes RH, et al. Complications of endoscopic sphincterotomy: a prospective series with emphasis on the increased risk associated with sphincter of Oddi dysfunction and nondilated bile ducts. *Gastroenterology* 1991;101:1068–1075

44. Bland KI, Jones RS, Maher BW, et al. Extracorporeal shock-wave lithotripsy of bile duct calculi: an interim re-

port of the Dornier United States. Bile Duct Lithotripsy Prospective Study. *Ann Surg* 1989;209:743–753

45. Harz C, Henkel TO, Kohrmann KU. Extracorporeal shock-wave lithotripsy and endoscopy: Combined therapy for problematic bile duct stones. *Surg Endosc* 1991;5: 196–199

46. Stokes KR, Falchuk KR, Clouse ME. Biliary duct stones: update on 54 cases after percutaneous transhepatic removal. *Radiology* 1989;170:999–1001

47. Jeng KS, Chiang HJ, Shih SC. Limitations of percutaneous transhepatic cholangioscopy in the removal of complicated biliary calculi. *World J Surg* 1989;13:603–610

48. Hixson LJ, Fennerty MB, Jaffee PE, et al. Peroral cholangioscopy with intracorporeal electrohydraulic lithotripsy for choledocholithiasis. *Am J Gastroenterol* 1992;87: 296–299

49. Riemann JF, Kohler B, Weber J, et al. Intraductal shockwave lithotripsy in complicated common bile duct stones. *Clin Investig* 1992;70:148–151

50. Bonnell DH, Ligoury CE, Cornud FE, et al. Common bile duct and intrahepatic stones: results of transhepatic electrohydraulic lithotripsy in 50 patients. *Radiology* 1991;180: 345–348

51. Josephs LG, Birkett DH. Laser lithotripsy for the management of retained stones. *Arch Surg* 1992;127:603–604

52. Dayton MT, Longmire, WP Jr, Tompkins RK. Caroli's disease: a premalignant condition. *Am J Surg* 1983;145:41

53. Fang K, Chou TC. Subcutaneous blind loop—a new type of hepaticocholedochojejunostomy for bilateral intrahepatic calculi. *Chin Med J* 1977;3:413–418

54. Fan ST, Mok F, Zheng SS, et al. Appraisal of hepaticocutaneous jejunostomy in the management of hepatolithiasis. *Am J Surg* 1993;165:332–335

55. Charcot JM. *Leçons sur les Maladies du Foie, des Voies Biliares et des Reins.* Paris, France: Faculté de Médicin de Paris, Bourneville et Sevestre, 1877

56. Reynolds BM, Dargan EL. Acute obstructive cholangitis: a distinct clinical syndrome. *Ann Surg* 1959;150:299

57. Sawyer RG, Hanks JB. Antibiotic selection in biliary tract surgery. In: Cameron JL (ed), *Current Surgical Therapy.* Chicago, IL: BC Decker-Mosby Year-Book; 1992:389–394

58. Thompson JE Jr, Tompkins RK, Longmire WP Jr. Factors in management of acute cholangitis. *Ann Surg* 1982;195: 137–145

59. Lai EC, Mok FP, Tan ES, et al. Endoscopic biliary drainage for severe acute cholangitis. *N Engl J Med* 1992;326: 1582–1586

60. Cairns SR, Dias L, Cotton PB, et al. Additional endoscopic procedures instead of urgent surgery for retained common bile duct stones. *Gut* 1989;30:535–540

61. Nordback I. Management of unextractable bile duct stones by endoscopic stenting. *Ann Chir Gynaecol* 1989;78: 290–292

62. Nahrwold DL. Acute cholangitis. *Surgery* 1992;112: 487–488

63. Dayton MT, Conter R, Tompkins RK. The incidence of complications with operative choledochoscopy. *Am J Surg* 1984;147:139–142

64. Lau WY, Chu KW, Yuen WK, et al. Operative choledochoscopy in patients with acute cholangitis: a prospective randomized study. *Br J Surg* 1991;78:1226–1229

65. De Roover D, Vanderveken M, Gerard Y. Choledochotomy: Primary closure versus T tube: a prospective trial. *Acta Chir Belg* 1989;89:320–324

66. Sheen-Chen SM, Chou FF. Choledochotomy for biliary lithiasis: is routine T tube drainage necessary? A prospective controlled trial. *Acta Chir Scand* 1990;156:387–390

67. Thompson JE Jr, Bennion RS. The surgical management of impacted common bile duct stones without sphincter ablation. *Arch Surg* 1989;124:1216–1219

68. Pappas TN, Slimane TB, Brooks DC. 100 consecutive common duct explorations without mortality. *Ann Surg* 1990;211:260–262

69. Rotych RE, Sitzmann JV, Lillemoe KD, et al. Transduodenal exploration of the common bile duct in patients with non-dilated ducts. *Surg Gynecol Obstet* 1991;173:49–53

70. McArthur MS, Longmire WP Jr. Peptic ulcer disease after choledochojejunostomy. *Am J Surg* 1971;122:155–159

71. Gouma DJ, Konsten J, Soeters PB, et al. Long-term follow-up after choledochojejunostomy for bile duct stones with complex clearance of the bile duct. *Br J Surg* 1989;76: 451–453

72. Miros M, Kerlin P, Strong R, et al. Post-choledochoenterostomy 'sump syndrome.' *Aust NZ J Surg* 1990;60: 109–112

73. Escudero-Fabre A, Escallon A Jr, Sack J, et al. Choledochoduodenostomy: analysis of 71 cases followed for 5 to 15 years. *Ann Surg* 1991;213:635–642

62

Disorders of the Duodenal Ampullae

David W. Rattner ▪ *Andrew L. Warshaw*

▪ DISORDERS OF THE DUODENAL AMPULLAE

Clinical entities discussed in this chapter involve the orifice of the termini of the bile duct and the pancreatic ducts, either in producing a disease or in preventing its spontaneous resolution. Included are benign ampullary tumors, stenosis and dyskinesia of the sphincter of Oddi, stenosis of the orifice of the duct of Wirsung, and stenosis of the accessory papilla associated with pancreas divisum. Patients with these disorders have pain, pancreatitis, jaundice, or cholangitis, and malignancy must be excluded. Treatment of these conditions, in each instance, must consider elimination or bypass of the terminal sphincter mechanism.

▪ TOOLS FOR DIAGNOSIS

BLOOD TESTS

The most sensitive blood test indicating biliary obstruction is determination of the serum alkaline phosphatase level. It is often elevated, whereas the bilirubin remains at normal levels. The levels of serum transaminase (alanine and aspartate aminotransferases; SGPT, SGOT) commonly rise modestly (up to 200 units, although they can reach levels of 1000 to 2000 units), which can cause diagnostic confusion by suggesting hepatitis. The serum amylase level remains the simplest and most useful index of acute pancreatitis. It is elevated in 70% to 95% of cases, the usual exceptions being those that come to medical attention late after the amylase level has already returned to normal, and flares of acute inflammation in chronic pancreatitis, in which the gland is thought to have insufficient remaining secretory capacity. There are many causes of hyperamylasemia, other than pancreatitis, that must be kept in mind for differential diagnosis (Table 62–1). Measurement of other pancreatic enzymes in the serum, including lipase, and determination of the amylase-creatinine clearance ratio have not contributed to diagnosis.

PANCREATIC FUNCTION TESTS

Ampullary stenosis, with the exception of iatrogenic injuries, is virtually never complete enough to cause clinical malabsorption. Pancreatic function (fecal fat measurement, pancreaolauryl test) is usually normal.

RADIOGRAPHIC TESTS

Dilation of the biliary and pancreatic ducts can be demonstrated by ultrasonography and computed tomography (CT), but stones can be detected in the common duct in only 10% to 20% of cases, when present. Changes in diameter of a few millimeters of the bile duct, and as little as 1 mm of the pancreatic duct, are detectable. Real definition of the ducts, as well as the precise location and configuration of a blockage, requires opacification with contrast material (eg, as used in transhepatic cholangiography (THC) and endoscopic retrograde cholangiopancreatography (ERCP). ERCP (Fig 62–1) has the advantage of showing both systems, al-

TABLE 62–1. NONPANCREATIC CAUSES OF HYPERAMYLASEMIA

Renal disease	Acute and chronic renal failure
Salivary gland disease	Mumps, parotitis, sialadenitis, maxillofacial surgery and other trauma
Liver disease	Cirrhosis, fulminant hepatitis, trauma
Gastrointestinal tract disorders	Common bile duct stones, acute cholecystitis, penetrating peptic ulcer, intestinal obstruction, afferent loop syndrome, acute appendicitis, Crohn's disease, ruptured aortic aneurysm, aortic dissection, mesenteric infarction, postoperative metabolic dysfunction
Diabetic ketoacidosis	
Pulmonary disorders	Pneumonia, pulmonary infarction
Neoplastic disease	Lung (primary and metastatic), prostate, parotid, colon, ovary, and breast carcinoma
Gynecologic disorders	Ruptured ectopic pregnancy, ruptured graafian follicle, ovarian cysts, salpingitis, endometritis
Intracranial trauma	Cerebral trauma
Macroamylasemia	
"Normal" hyperamylasemia	

lowing visualization and biopsy of the ampulla, and providing at least an estimate of the ampullary orifice size. In competent hands, the papilla can be cannulated in >90% of cases. This success rate has led some to state that inability to cannulate the papilla is an indicator of stenosis. However, this statement generally has not correlated with surgical findings and can be attributed more frequently to technical features of the procedure or the unique anatomy of the patient. When a retrograde cholangiogram is obtained, the presence of a dilated common bile duct (>12 mm) in the absence of structural causes of common duct dilation is a reliable indicator of ampullary disease. Delayed emptying of contrast material from the common bile duct (>45 mins) also may indicate an element of ampullary obstruction (Fig 62–2). The absence of these findings does not exclude ampullary disease. In patients with suspected ampullary stenosis without evidence of biliary disease, information derived from pancreatograms may be useful in predicting the response to sphincteroplasty. Incomplete filling of the pancreatic duct, cyst formation, or changes compatible with chronic pancreatitis often predict sphincteroplasty failure.

Biliary excretion scans also have been used to detect delayed emptying and may be abnormal in extreme cases. Shaffer used DISIDA to measure tracer uptake and clearance by the liver and biliary excretion. Patients with manometrically documented sphincter of Oddi dysfunction had prolonged times to peak excretion of the tracer. Endoscopic sphincterotomy shortened the time to peak excretion, although it did not return to normal values. This test is based on the premise that sphincter of Oddi dysfunction is defined best in terms of bile flow. With cholescintigraphy, delayed emptying can be detected and, therefore, this test may be a suitable screen for assessing persistent pain after cholecystectomy and the results of ampullary surgery.

EVOCATIVE TESTS

Evocative tests are intended to bring out a subtle abnormality that is not apparent on routine testing. In the morphine-prostigmine test championed by Nardi, prostigmine (1 mg intramurally) is given to increase pancreatic secretion, while morphine (10 mg intramurally) is given to induce sphincter spasm. A positive test result is defined as the reproduction of the patient's pain concomitant with a three-fold rise of the serum amylase or lipase level. Several prospective studies have not found this test to be useful.

The ultrasound-secretin test is based on an interesting new concept and is under continuing evaluation. Secretin (1 U/kg) is given intravenously to induce pancreatic hypersecretion while the size of the pancreatic duct is monitored with ultrasonography. The normal response is a transient (up to 3 minutes) dilation followed by a return to baseline values. In the presence of outflow tract stenosis or dysfunction, the pancreatic duct has been observed to remain dilated for up to 30 minutes or longer (Fig 62–3), unless the gland is fibrotic and unable to respond. The sensitivity of the test has been estimated at 70% (Fig 62–4). Consistent changes in the bile duct have not been noted.

MANOMETRY

It has been widely accepted by biliary surgeons, but never verified, that the inability to pass a 3-mm Bakês dilator or 10-Fr rubber catheter through the ampulla during common duct exploration is indicative of ampullary stenosis. Whether one ought to proceed with sphincteroplasty solely on the basis of this finding is controversial. Intraoperative flow manometry can be used to measure the perfusion pressure in the common bile duct, the flow rate into the duodenum, and the opening pressure of the sphincter. These techniques depend on the assumption that obstruction at the ampullary level will cause an elevation of intrabiliary pressure or a reduction of flow through the sphincter. White found that the combination of abnormal resting pressure, decreased flow rate, and a dilated common duct was 99.1% accurate in detecting ampullary obstruction and that manometry detected abnormalities not appreciated on operative cholangiograms. Others have cast doubt on the utility of this technique, and few surgeons seem to use it. With the advent of preoperative endoscopic manometry, we see little use for intraoperative flow manometry.

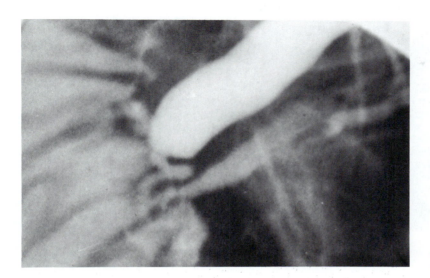

Figure 62–1. Detail of ERCP showing the bile duct and pancreatic duct entering the duodenum.

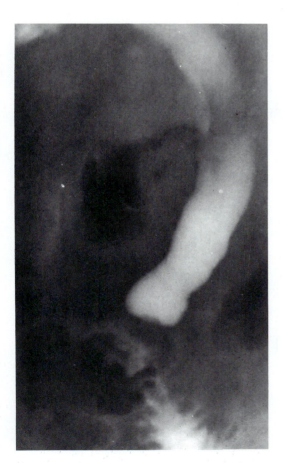

Figure 62–2. Endoscopic retrograde cholangiogram showing retention of contrast in the bile duct, which has not emptied 15 minutes after filling with contrast and removal of the catheter.

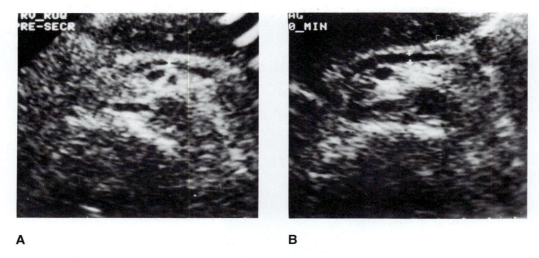

Figure 62–3. Ultrasound examination of the pancreas. The pancreatic duct in the body is indicated with markers before and 30 minutes after secretion. The prolonged 30 minute dilation is distinctly abnormal and probably indicates ampullary obstruction.

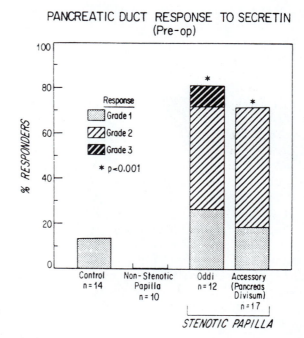

Figure 62–4. Pancreatic duct response to preoperative secretin-ultrasound testing in 24 patients without ampullary stenosis and 2 patients with major and minor papilla stenosis.

Endoscopic Transampullary Manometry

The systems used for transampullary manometry consist either of triple lumen catheters with continuous fluid perfusion (open system), or a pressure-sensitive micro-transducer catheter (closed system). The closed systems measure pressure in the common bile duct or pancreatic duct, whereas the open triple-lumen system also records intrasphincteric pressure. It is important to remember that most reports of common duct manometry are based on patients who have had a prior cholecystectomy. If the gallbladder is present it acts as a low-pressure reservoir for the biliary system and may decrease elevations in common duct pressure induced by morphine.

Measurement of the sphincter pressures and contraction rhythms can be accomplished by introduction of transducers via an endoscope. The normal pressure within the sphincter of Oddi may reach 30 mm Hg with regular anterograde contraction waves. Abnormally high pressures and a variety of arrhythmias (eg, "tachyoddia" or retrograde contractions) have been described. Elevated basal pressure, owing either to spasm or fibrosis, is the only manometric abnormality that has been associated with symptomatic relief following sphincterotomy. In a study of patients with suspected sphincter of Oddi dysfunction, Toouli and associates defined four types of manometric sphincter abnormalities. Most patients in this series were females between 30 and 60 years of age. If a patient had abnormal liver function tests and/or a dilated common bile duct, manometric abnormalities of the sphincter of Oddi invariably were found. The most common abnormality was excessively frequent retrograde propagation of phasic contractions. This abnormality is felt to prevent emptying from the ampulla of Vater and has been noted by other authors to be associated with common duct stones. Nearly as common was a high frequency of sphincter of Oddi phasic contractions, so-called tachyoddia. The symptoms of these patients often correlated with bursts of phasic contractions. These contractions also have been shown to obstruct flow into the ampulla by shortening the diastolic interval, whereby filling of the intra-ampullary segment of the common bile duct ceases. Nearly one-third of the study group demonstrated a paradoxical response to intravenous cholecystokinin (CCK), manifested by increased frequency of phasic contractions, by absence of change in the frequency of phasic contractions, or by an increase in basal pressure. These manometric changes occurred while the patients experienced pain. It is possible that these abnormalities represents a disordered control mechanism of the sphincter of Oddi such that bile flow is retarded after eating, with consequent common bile duct dilation and pain. Finally, as in most other series, there was a subgroup of patients with an abnormally elevated basal sphincter of Oddi pressure owing either to fibrosis or spasm. Unresponsiveness of the basal sphincter of Oddi pressure to CCK suggests the presence of a fixed structural stenosis. The implications for therapy of tachyoddia and retrograde contractions have not been established. Finally, transampullary manometry has been associated with a high incidence of postprocedure pancreatitis, particularly in patients being evaluated for causes of recurrent acute pancreatitis. In our practice, therefore, we have not found the benefits of manometry worth its risks of serious complications.

■ AMPULLARY OBSTRUCTION, STENOSIS, AND DYSFUNCTION

The term *ampullary stenosis* is used in this discussion to include both fixed ampullary stenosis and motility disorders. Fixed ampullary stenosis most commonly is the result of inflammation and fibrosis. This situation usually develops in association with cholelithiasis and is postulated to be caused by chronic inflammation from repeated passage of small stones or sludge. Iatrogenic injury to the ampulla during common bile duct exploration also can produce fibrosis. Small ampullary tumors can create ampullary obstruction, either in a continuous fashion or by a "ball-valve" mechanism, with resultant right upper quadrant pain, jaundice, or recurrent pancreatitis. Such tumors include adenomas, villous adenomas, small adenocarcinomas, and a spectrum of neuroendocrine tumors. Motility disorders include muscular hyperplasia, dysfunction, or dyskinesia without a fixed fibrotic stricture. Patients without a demonstrable fixed obstruction or proximal dilation of the ducts are the most troublesome to treat. In the absence of any objective lesion, it is easier, and possibly safer, to be skeptical rather than overtreating a pain syndrome that is erroneously attributed to ampullary stenosis.

MANIFESTATIONS

The presenting symptoms and signs of ampullary stenosis may be those of obstructive jaundice, cholangitis, pancreatitis, or pain. Pain is most often in the right upper quadrant of the abdomen, but also may be in the epigastrium and may radiate around the right side or straight through to the back. It is usually intermittent, but can be food-induced or constant.

Jaundice or cholangitis rarely occurs as a primary presentation (Fig 62–5). A dilated bile duct with or without an increased serum alkaline phosphatase level is more common. Ampullary stenosis, in combination with stasis, also may lead to formation of primary common duct stones.

Pancreatitis that is ascribed to ampullary stenosis is usually mild and recurrent. The symptom of recurrent pain, without accompanying signs of pancreatic inflam-

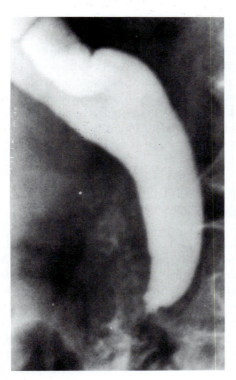

Figure 62–5. Biliary obstruction owing to fibrotic ampullary stenosis in a patient who presented with acute cholangitis.

mation or hyperamylasemia, is considered part of this syndrome (Nardi, Moody, Warshaw). Progression to chronic pancreatitis rarely occurs. The obstruction may involve either the dorsal segment (duct of Santorini, accessory or minor papilla), the ventral segment (duct of Wirsung, major papilla, or papilla of Vater) or both, depending on ductal anatomy (Fig 62–6).

VENTRAL/MAJOR AMPULLARY STENOSIS

Ventral/major ampullary stenosis (Fig 62–7) has had its proponents and detractors for many years. The number of patients with unequivocal fibrosis of the duct orifice is small. It is unknown whether the fibrosis is congenital or acquired; the lesion responding to sphincterotomy has been described in children, but most cases are seen in adults. Some cases are attributed to the traumatic passage of gallstones. For the last 40 years, surgeons have treated ventral ampullary stenosis by transduodenal sphincterotomy with varying success. Symptomatic improvement has been reported in no more than 70% of patients. Failures are due in part to the inclusion of patients in whom the diagnosis was either unproved or incorrect. Some writers have contended that the sphincterotomy is too short for ablation of the entire sphincter mechanism to include the

duodenal wall component (sphincter of Boyden) (Figs 62–8 and 62–9). Others have emphasized the pathogenic role of the septum between the end of the duct of Wirsung and the terminal segment of the bile duct, and advocated the routine addition of septotomy-sphincterotomy of the pancreatic duct orifice in addition to the choledochal sphincter (Fig 62–10). Recently, the claim has been made that a "misplaced pancreatic duct orifice," opening among the muscular fibers of the sphincter of Oddi, is an important cause of recurrent obstructive pancreatitis.

Endoscopists have now entered into competition to treat stenosis or spasm of the sphincter of Oddi. Electrosurgical papillotomy has been used widely. The relative safety of the procedure has been established, but its efficacy remains debatable. In addition to the difficulty of accurately identifying candidates for treatment when the objective indices are sparse or lacking, endoscopic papillotomy has two disadvantages: (1) it may be impossible to cannulate the papilla when it is genuinely stenotic, and (2) the usual papillotomy divides only the choledochal portion of the sphincter. Extending the procedure by cutting the septal segment of the duct of Wirsung greatly increases the risk of pancreatitis, which is sometimes severe. Conversely, if the pancreatic duct orifice is not opened, the significant point of stenosis may elude treatment. At the Massachusetts General Hospital, we have seen several patients who continue to have recurrent pancreatitis after endoscopic papillotomy but who seem to have benefited from subsequent surgical septotomy.

Safe attempts at relief of obstruction of the orifice of the pancreatic duct have been made with balloon dilation of the sphincter and placement of endoprosthetic stents. The benefits accruing from balloon dilation are short-lived and the incidence of postdilation pancreatitis is high. Therefore, this approach has been abandoned by most centers. However, enthusiasm for stenting the pancreatic duct orifice persists, championed by Geenen. In our view, a brief trial of stenting of the pancreatic duct may provide useful diagnostic information. Patients who are free of pain or who have relief of recurrent pancreatitis are likely to derive long-term benefit from surgical sphincteroplasty. If the stent remains in place for more than 2 months, granulation tissue forms in the pancreatic duct caused by the mechanical irritation of the stent, leading to fibrosis. When this occurs, the strictures are too proximal in the pancreatic duct to be opened via a transampullary sphincteroplasty. Thus, we can endorse stenting as a diagnostic maneuver in patients without clear-cut objective parameters of ampullary stenosis, but condemn its use for long-term therapy. From what we have seen thus far, we are skeptical that stenting will be either as safe or as effective as surgical sphincteroplasty.

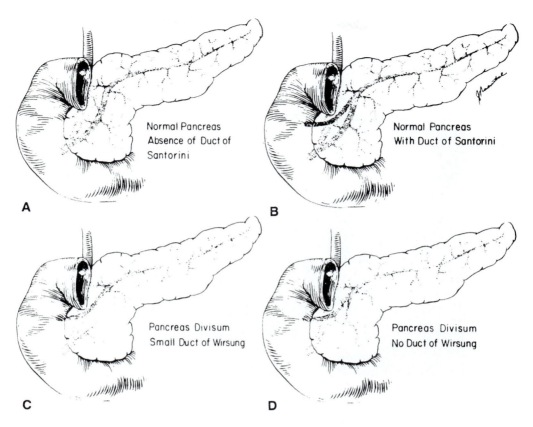

Figure 62–6. Variations of ventral (Wirsung) and dorsal (Santorini) duct anatomy. Small, functionally inadequate intercommunication is also common (10% to 20%). We use the term "dominant dorsal duct" for the latter, as well as C and D.

DORSAL DUCT OBSTRUCTION

Dorsal duct obstruction may occur in patients with pancreas divisum (Fig 62–11). The latter term originally described a failure of fusion of the duct system of the primitive embryologic dorsal and ventral pancreatic anlage (Fig 62–6). In this entity, the dorsal duct cannot empty through the ampulla of Vater but must drain through the accessory or minor papilla. The concept since has been expanded to include other variants of dorsal duct dominance requiring the major fraction of pancreatic secretions to egress from the accessory papilla (Fig 62–12). A dominant dorsal pancreatic duct occurs in at least 9% of the population, as shown by both autopsy analyses and endoscopic pancreatography. The association of pancreas divisum and recurrent pancreatitis or pancreatic pain has been both upheld and disputed. Because the pancreas rarely is resected in this condition, histologic evidence is scarce. However, two reports have documented convincing chronic obstructive changes confined to the dorsal duct distribution in a few selected patients.

Cotton, summarizing the consensus of an international workshop held in London in 1984, indicated that pancreas divisum is probably a genuine factor in a syndrome of obstructive pancreatitis in some patients. Stenosis of the accessory papilla superimposed on pancreas divisum, rather than pancreas divisum alone, appears to be the critical combination. In addition, the term "pancreas divisum" is misleading because it does not include the other variants of dominant dorsal duct. Distinguishing patients with genuine accessory papillary stenosis from those with clinically insignificant pancreas divisum is difficult, and is the greatest cause of differing conclusions concerning the association of the dominant dorsal duct with pancreatitis and the efficacy of accessory papilla sphincteroplasty. ERCP can readily establish the presence of a dominant dorsal duct, but endoscopic calibration of the papillary orifice size has not been successful. Recently, endoscopic measurements of dorsal duct pressure and sphincter function have suggested that hypertension of the sphincter and dorsal duct pressures may be a genuine phenomenon. Prolonged dorsal duct dilation after secretin administration has, in our ex-

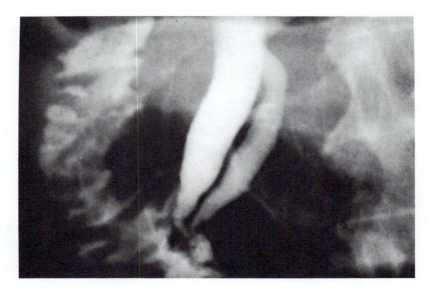

A

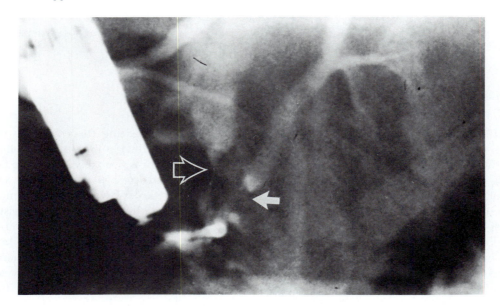

B

Figure 62–7. Two examples of ampullary stenosis. **A.** Dilated bile and pancreatic ducts in a man with recurrent discrete attacks of acute pancreatitis. **B.** Narrowed ampullary segments of the bile duct (*open arrow*) and pancreatic duct (*closed arrow*) in a woman with persistent pain, normal serum amylase, and a positive secretin-ultrasound test. Both were cured by transduodenal sphincteroplasty and transampullary septectomy.

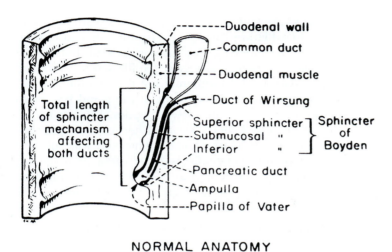

NORMAL ANATOMY

Figure 62–8. The duodenal wall and submucosal sphincter of Boyden together make up the constrictor mechanism of the major ampulla.

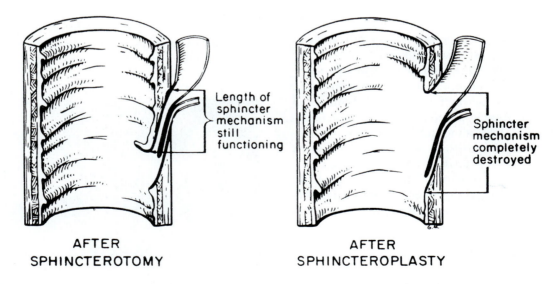

AFTER
SPHINCTEROTOMY

AFTER
SPHINCTEROPLASTY

Figure 62–9. The difference between sphincterotomy and sphincteroplasty, according to Jones. The portion of the sphincter remaining after sphincterotomy is made incompetent by sphincteroplasty.

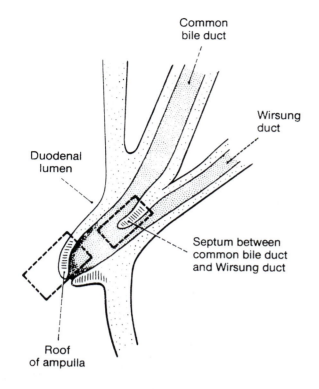

Figure 62–10. Abnormality of the septum between the common bile duct and the pancreatic duct may contribute to pancreatic duct obstruction in some patients. Sphincterotomy or sphincteroplasty of the choledochal (roof) portion of the ampulla may be inadequate.

perience, correlated with accessory papillary stenosis and with subsequent response to sphincteroplasty.

There is no medical treatment of accessory papillary stenosis. We have found oral pancreatic enzymes and spasmolytic drugs to be ineffective. Small numbers of patients have been treated with a variety of these endoscopic techniques, including balloon dilation, papillotomy, and stenting, but the overall experience has been disappointing. Analysis of collected anecdotes suggests that the attempted cannulation often is not possible, that pancreatitis follows the manipulations fairly frequently, that relief of symptoms is exceptional, and that restenosis is the rule. Furthermore, we have treated cases of stenosis of the minor papilla in which the stent has created a stricture of the dorsal duct 2 to 3 cm from its orifice, thereby creating an obstructive pancreatitis that cannot be treated by sphincteroplasty and may require pancreaticoduodenectomy.

Surgical sphincteroplasty of the accessory papilla also has been advocated. Although results vary and some observations are negative, it is difficult to discount the good results. We have performed the operation on 130

patients, not including those with changes suggestive of chronic pancreatitis. Of those patients who have been followed for >2 years, 80% were judged at operation to have a stenotic accessory papilla, and 85% of these have had a favorable response to the papillotomy. Only 15% who were judged to have a stenotic papilla have not had lasting benefit from the operation.

Most reported cases of pancreas divisum and pancreatitis have had acute recurrent disease without fibrosis or duct dilation. Changes of chronic pancreatitis may be seen in patients with pancreas divisum, but a causal relationship with accessory papilla stenosis has not been established. Confinement of the chronic fibrotic changes to the dorsal segment of the gland has been shown convincingly in a few exceptional instances. In any event, when there is established chronic pancreatitis, sphincteroplasty is inadequate and will fail. Resection of the pancreatic head or distal drainage by pancreaticojejunostomy has been advocated, and the decision depends on the degree of duct dilation.

TECHNIQUE OF TRANSDUODENAL SPHINCTEROPLASTY

The operation may be performed through a right subcostal or midline incision. The duodenum is mobilized from the bile duct to the superior mesenteric vessels by an extensive Kocher maneuver.

If a cholecystectomy or common duct exploration is being performed, a small catheter may be passed down the cystic or common duct through the major papilla to identify its location along the length of the duodenum. The papilla of Vater is usually easy to palpate between the fingers, in the groove between the second portion of the duodenum and the pancreas. The duodenum is opened

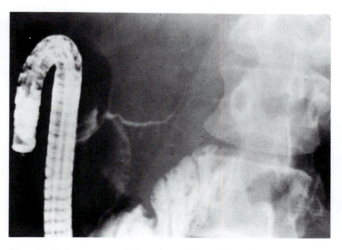

Figure 62–11. Pancreatogram via the major ampulla and duct of Wirsung, showing typical pancreas divisum. The duct is short (2 to 3 cm) and ends in a fine tapered arborization.

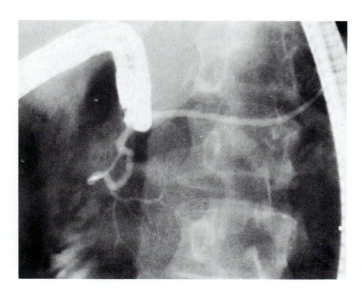

Figure 62–12. Pancreatogram showing a dominant dorsal duct. The dorsal duct in this case drains the entire pancreas, including the head. There is no duct of Wirsung.

transversely opposite the papilla. Silk sutures are preplaced at either end of the incision, to elevate the duodenum and to limit the duodenotomy, to keep it from extending too close to the pancreas for safe closure.

The orifice of the major papilla is cannulated with lacrimal duct probes and, if possible, a 5-Fr pediatric feeding catheter. The secretions that fill the tube identify whether it is in the bile duct or pancreatic duct. If the bile duct cannot be entered, it may be safer to pass a catheter or instrument from above for identification of the orifice, rather than to persist blindly from below. If ampullary obstruction is caused by an impacted stone, it is easy to cut down on it through the anterosuperior aspect of the papilla, opposite the pancreatic duct orifice and therefore, not endangering that structure. This procedure will release the stone.

Jones has advocated that the sphincteroplasty should be carried upward until the diameter of the stoma is equal to that of the largest diameter of the common duct. The entire sphincter mechanism, including the components derived from the intrinsic musculature of the duodenal wall, is thereby incapacitated (Fig 62–8). The sphincteroplasty may be up to 30 mm long and may reach the pancreatic substance outside the duodenal wall. Jones' argument is that such a complete elimination of the sphincter will maximize the freedom of bile drainage and minimize the chances for retention of missed stones, perhaps in the hepatic ducts, or formation of new primary common duct stones because of bile stasis (Fig 62–9).

The sphincteroplasty is carried out with sequential clamping and division and suture approximation of the duodenal mucosa and the bile duct mucosa (Fig 62–13). We prefer 4-0 synthetic absorbable sutures and carry the sphincteroplasty superiorly 2 to 3 cm to the end of

the intramural segment. The pancreatic duct characteristically opens onto the anteromedial aspect of the ampulla (commonly described as the 5 o'clock position on the back wall) within a few millimeters of the lip, but it may be at, or even outside, the lip of the ampulla. Secretin (1 U/kg) given intravenously may be helpful in identifying the orifice. A probe is passed into the pancreatic duct, the septum between the bile duct and pancreatic duct is incised, and the edges are sutured with interrupted fine synthetic absorbable sutures. The incision is carried far enough to produce a free flow of pancreatic secretions, generally 5 to 8 mm. We prefer to leave a 5-Fr pediatric feeding catheter in the duct to ensure against impedance of flow by postoperative edema (Fig 62–14). The catheter exits through the wall of the duodenum and the abdomen and is removed after 10 days.

Accessory papillary sphincteroplasty follows most of the same principles (Fig 62–14). The accessory papilla lies 2 to 3 cm proximal and 1 cm anterior to the major papilla. It often is best identified by palpation against the duodenal mucosa and by administration of secretin. It courses perpendicularly through the duodenal wall, in contrast to the oblique path of the duct of Wirsung. The papilla is short and opens into the vestibule of the duct within a few millimeters. The papillotomy needs to be no longer than 7 to 9 mm.

RESULTS OF SPINCTEROPLASTY

Adverse consequences of the operation should be minimal. Postoperative hyperamylasemia is common, but clinical pancreatitis has occurred in only 1% of patients. Mortality should be <1%. We have had one death in over 300 cases. Late restenosis is rare after sphincteroplasty of the major papilla, although it has occurred in

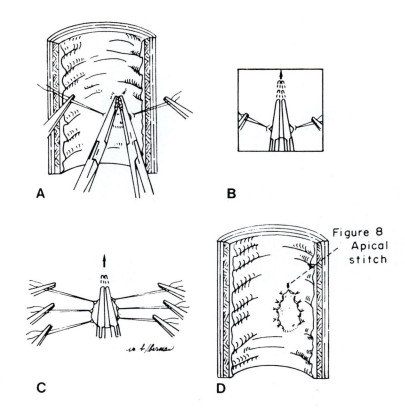

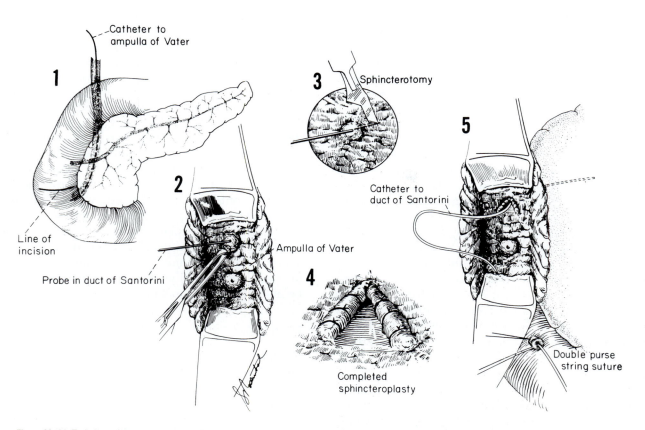

Figure 62–13. Technique of transduodenal sphincteroplasty; the roof of the ampulla is opened by serial clamping, division, and suture approximation of the common duct and duodenal walls until the opening created equals the maximum diameter of the intrapancreatic common bile duct.

Figure 62–14. Technique of accessory papilla sphincteroplasty. Note the 5-Fr catheter left in the pancreatic duct for postoperative drainage.

approximately 6% of our patients after accessory papillotomy. Cure of clinical symptoms by the operation will depend largely on the accuracy with which patients are selected for surgery. Our current cure rate is approximately 80%.

LOCAL EXCISION OF AMPULLARY TUMORS

Local excision is suitable treatment for certain small tumors (<2cm) arising from the ampulla of Vater or in the pancreatic or biliary duct within 2 cm of the ampulla. Some small adenomas (<1cm) may even be removed endoscopically with stenting of the biliary and pancreatic duct orifice to allow healing without stenosis. These tumors include carcinoid tumors, islet cell tumors, tubulovillous adenomas, and occasionally, small villous adenomas. In cases where there is a reasonable likelihood of malignancy, such as with villous adenomas, the risk of recurrent tumor and missed opportunity for cure must be balanced against the complications of a pancreaticoduodenectomy. It has been our preference to opt for a pancreaticoduodenectomy whenever there is a suspicion of malignancy. Since recurrence rates are close to 100% when local resections are performed for malignancy, patients must be taken to the operating room with preparation for a pancreaticoduodenectomy, if frozen section evaluation of the resected ampullary lesion demonstrates malignancy. Finally, the surgeon must recognize that the absence of malignancy on frozen section may not withstand a more rigorous evaluation on permanent section analysis. This situation is particularly true with respect to villous adenomas in which malignancy is found in >50%

of cases, even when biopsies have shown only a benign component. Notwithstanding these cautions, local resection may be an excellent treatment for benign lesions of the ampulla.

A transverse or a vertical duodenotomy can be used to expose the ampulla. A generous Kocher maneuver is essential to allow the second portion of the duodenum to be elevated into the wound. Normal duodenal mucosa 5 to 10 mm from the visible border of the tumor is tattooed with cautery to map out the margins of resection. A suture then is placed through the ampulla to provide traction. As the excision progresses, this suture can be replaced with an Allis clamp (Fig 62–15). The cautery is used to incise the mucosa circumferentially. One then works centripetally in a submucosal plane until the pancreatic and biliary ducts are encountered and transected. As this occurs, it can be helpful to place traction sutures in the duct margins to prevent retraction (Fig 62–16). Placing catheters in the ducts also can aid in their dissection. The tumor then is lifted off the muscular layers of the medial wall of the duodenum. Maintenance of hemostasis during resection is critical to ensure good visualization and accurate dissection.

With the specimen resected, one must reconstruct the defect. The superior wall of the pancreatic duct is sutured to the inferior wall of the bile duct with fine interrupted synthetic absorbable sutures, thereby forming a common channel. The duodenum and cloacal neoampulla then are joined with interrupted full-thickness 4-0 synthetic absorbable sutures to create a mucosa-to-mucosa anastomosis of the ducts to the duodenal wall (Fig 62–17). If the ducts are not dilated, the orifices of

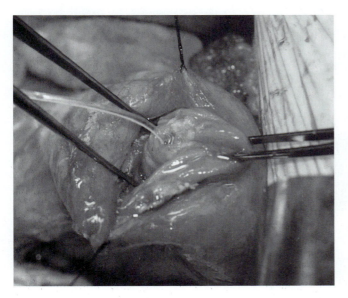

Figure 62–15. Early stage of the local resection of an ampullary carcinoid tumor. Stent is in the pancreatic duct and traction on the tumor is provided by an Allis clamp.

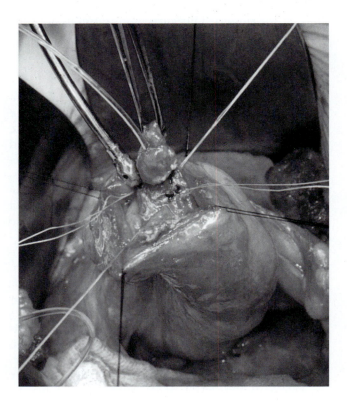

Figure 62–16. The ampullary tumor is dissected free centripetally in a submucosal plane.

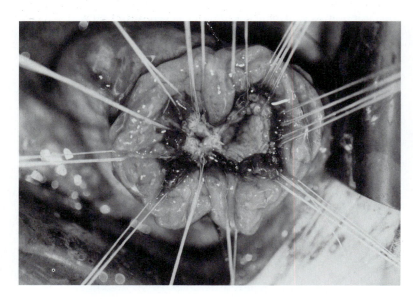

Figure 62–17. Anastomosis of the bile duct and pancreatic duct to the duodenal wall following local resection of an ampullary tumor.

each duct can be enlarged by incising along one wall proximally, as in a sphincteroplasty. Stents may be placed and brought out through the common duct, the third portion of the duodenum, or both. These stents remain in place at least 10 days. The duodenotomy is closed transversely.

After local resection of ampullary tumors, follow-up endoscopy is performed 6 to 12 months postoperatively to assess local recurrence. Patients who develop pancreatitis or jaundice months to years following local resection of ampullary tumors must be suspected of having local recurrence and should undergo repeat endoscopy with ERCP.

SELECTED READINGS

Anderson TM, Pitt HA, Longmire WP Jr. Experience with sphincteroplasty and sphincterotomy in pancreatobiliary surgery. *Ann Surg* 1985;20:399

Asbun HJ, Rossi RL, Munson JL. Local resection of ampullary tumors. Is there a place for it? *Arch Surg* 1993;128: 515–520

Bar-Meir S, Geenen JE, et al. Biliary and pancreatic duct pressures measured by ERCP manometry in patients with suspected papillary stenosis. *Dig Dis Sci* 1979;24:209

Blair AJ, Russell RC, Cotton PB. Resection for pancreatitis in patients with pancreas divisum. *Ann Surg* 1984;200:590

Boyden EA. The anatomy of choledochoduodenal junction in man. *Surg Gynecol Obstet* 1957;104:641–652

Branch CD, Bailey OT, Zollinger R. Consequences of instrumental dilatation of the papilla of Vater, experimental study. *Arch Surg* 1939;38:358

Brugge WR, Brand DL, Atkins HL et al. Gallbladder dyskinesia in chronic acalculous cholecystitis. *Dig Dis Sci* 1986;31: 461–467

Carey LC. Misplaced pancreatic duct orifice as a cause of recurrent acute pancreatitis. *Am J Surg* 1987;153:165

Cotton PB. Congenital anomaly of pancreas divisum as a cause of obstructive pain and pancreatitis. *Gut* 1980;21:105–114

Cotton PB. Pancreas divisum: Curiosity or culprit? *Gastroenterology* 1985;89:1431

Davidson BR, Neoptolemos JP, Carr-Locke DL. Endoscopic sphincterotomy for common bile duct calculi in patients with gallbladder in situ considered unfit for surgery. *Gut* 1988;29:114

Delhage M, Engelholm L, Cremer M. Pancreas divisum: congenital anatomic variant or anomaly? *Gastroenterology* 1985; 89:951

Dimagno EP, Malagaleda JR, Go VLW. The relationship between pancreatic ductal obstruction and pancreatic secretion in man. *Mayo Clin Proc* 1979;54:157–162

Farouk M, Niotis M, Branum GD, et al. Indications for and the technique of local resection of tumors of the papilla of Vater. *Arch Surg* 1991;126:650–652

Fuji T, Amano H, et al. Pancreatic sphincterotomy and pancreatic endoprosthesis. *Endoscopy* 1985;17:69

Geenen JE, Toouli J et al. Endoscopic sphincterotomy: follow-

up evaluation of effects on the sphincter of Oddi. *Gastroenterology* 1984;87:754

Geenen JE, Hogan WJ, Dodds WJ, et al. Intraluminal pressure recording from the human sphincter of Oddi. *Gastroenterology* 1980;76:317–324

Geenen JE, Hogan WJ, Dodds WJ, et al. The efficacy of endoscopic sphincterotomy after cholecystectomy in patients with sphincter of Oddi dysfunction. *N Engl J Med* 1989;320: 82–87

Geenen JE, Toouli J, Hogan WJ, et al. Endoscopic sphincterotomy: Follow-up evaluation of effects on the sphincter of Oddi. *Gastroenterology* 1984;87:754–758

Glaser J, Hogemann B, et al. Sonographic imaging of the pancreatic duct: new diagnostic possibilities using secretin stimulation. *Dig Dis Sci* 1987;32:1075

Gregg JA, Carr-Locke DL. Endoscopic pancreatic and biliary manometry in pancreatic, biliary and papillary disease, and after endoscopic sphincterotomy and surgical sphincteroplasty. *Gut* 1984;25:1247

Griffin CA. Diagnosis of papillary stenosis by calibration. Follow-up 15 to 25 years after sphincteroplasty. *Am J Surg* 1982;143:717–720

Guelrud M, Mendoza S, Rossiter G, et al. Effect of nifedipine on sphincter of Oddi motor activity: studies in healthy volunteers and patients with biliary dyskinesia. *Gastroenterology* 1988;95:1050–1055

Guelrud M, Siefel JH. Hypertensive pancreatic duct sphincter as a cause of pancreatitis: successful treatment with hydrostatic balloon dilation. *Dig Dis Sci* 1984;29:225

Habib FI, Corazziari E, et al. Manometric measurement of human sphincter of Oddi length. *Gut* 1988;29:121

Jones SA, Steedman RA, et al. Transduodenal sphincteroplasty (not sphincterotomy) for biliary and pancreatic disease: indications, contraindications and results. *Am J Surg* 1969;118:292

Keith RG, Shapero TF, Saibel FG. Treatment of pancreatitis associated with pancreas divisum by dorsal duct sphincteroplasty alone. *Can J Surg* 1982;25:622–626

Marshall JB, Eckhauser ML. Pancreas divisum: a cause of chronic relapsing pancreatitis. *Dig Dis Sci* 1985;30:582

Misra DC Jr, Blossom GB, Fink-Bennett D, et al. Results of surgical therapy for biliary dyskinesia. *Arch Surg* 1992;126: 957–960

Moody FG, Becker JM, Potts JR. Transduodenal sphincteroplasty and transampullary septectomy for postcholecystectomy pain. *Ann Surg* 1983;197:627

Nardi GL, Michelassi F, Zannini P. Transduodenal sphincteroplasty: 5 to 25 year follow-up of 89 patients. *Ann Surg* 1983;198:453

Nardi GL, Acosta JM. Papillitis as a cause of pancreatitis and abdominal pain. *Ann Surg* 1966;164:611–618

Nussbaum MS, Warner BW, Sax HC, et al. Transduodenal sphincteroplasty and transampullary septotomy for primary sphincter of Oddi dysfunction. *Am J Surg* 1989;157:38–42

Ponchon T, Berger F, Chavaillon A, et al. Contribution of endoscopy to diagnosis and treatment of tumors of the ampulla of Vater. *Cancer* 1989;64:161–167

Raddawi HM, Geenen JE, Hogan WJ, et al. Pressure measurements from biliary and pancreatic segments of sphincter of Oddi. *Dig Dis Sci* 1991;36:71–74

Ricci JL. Carcinoid of the ampulla of Vater: local resection or pancreaticoduodenectomy. *Cancer* 1993;71:686–690

Russell RC, Wong NW, Cotton PB. Accessory sphincterotomy (endoscopic and surgical) in patients with pancreas divisum. *Br J Surg* 1984;71:954

Ryan DP, Schapiro RH, Warshaw AL. Villous tumors of the duodenum. *Ann Surg* 1986;203:301–306

Sarles H, Sarles JC, et al. Observations of 205 cases of acute pancreatitis, recurring pancreatitis, and chronic pancreatitis. *Gut* 1965;6:545

Satterfield ST, McCarthy JH, et al. Clinical experience in 82 patients with pancreas divisum: preliminary results of manometry and endoscopic therapy. *Pancreas* 1988;3:248

Shaffer EA, Hershfield NB, Logan K, et al. Cholescintographic detection of functional obstruction of sphincter of Oddi: effect of papillotomy. *Gastroenterology* 1986;90: 728–733

Sherman S, Ruffolo TA, Hawes RH, et al. Complications of endoscopic sphincterotomy. *Gastroenterology* 1991;101:1068–1075

Sobol S, Cooperman AM. Villous adenoma of the ampulla of Vater: an unusual cause of biliary colic and obstructive jaundice. *Gastroenterology* 1978;75:107–109

Soehendra N, Kempeneers I, et al. Endoscopic dilatation and papillotomy of the accessory papilla and internal drainage in pancreas divisum. *Endoscopy* 1986;18:129

Staritz M, Meyer zum Buschenfelde KH. Elevated pressure in the dorsal part of pancreas divisum: the cause of chronic pancreatitis? *Pancreas* 1988;3:108

Tanaka M, Ikeda S, et al. Manometric diagnosis of sphincter of Oddi spasm as a cause of postcholecystectomy pain and the treatment by endoscopic sphincterotomy. *Ann Surg* 1985;202:712

Tanaka M, Ikeda S, Nakayama F. Nonoperative measurement of pancreatic and common bile duct pressure with a microtransducer catheter: Effects of duodenoscopic sphincterotomy. *Dig Dis Sci* 1981;26:545–552

Tanaka M, Ikeda S, Nakagama F. Change in bile duct pressure response after cholecystectomy: loss of gallbladder as a pressure reservoir. *Gastroenterology* 1984;87:1154–1159

Thomas MJ, Pellegrini CA, Way LW. Usefulness of diagnostic tests for biliary obstruction. *Am J Surg* 1982;144:102

Toouli J. Clinical relevance of sphincter of Oddi dysfunction. *Br J Surg* 1990;77:723–724

Toouli J. What is sphincter of Oddi dysfunction? *Gut* 1989;30: 753–761

Toouli J, Roberts-Thomson IC, et al. Manometric disorders in patients with suspected sphincter of Oddi dysfunction. *Gastroenterology* 1985;88:1243

Toouli J, Roberts-Thomson IC, et al. Sphincter of Oddi motility disorder in patients with idiopathic recurrent pancreatitis. *Br J Surg* 1985;72:859

Toouli J, Roberts-Thompson IC, Dent J, et al. Spincter of Oddi motility disorders in patients with idiopathic recurrent pancreatitis. *Br J Surg* 1985;72:859–863

Venu RP, Geenen JE. Diagnosis and treatment of diseases of the papilla: *Clin Gastroenterol* 1986;15:439–457

Warshaw AL. The relationship between pancreas divisum and pancreatitis: surgical aspects. In: *Disorders of the Pancreas* Burns GP, Banks S (eds), New York, NY: McGraw-Hill; 1992: 159–171

Warshaw AL. Pancreas divisum: a case for surgical treatment. In: Tompkins RK, Cameron JL, et al (eds), *Advances in Surgery*. vol 21. Chicago, IL: Year Book Medical; 1987:93–109

Warshaw AL, Simeone JF, Schapiro RH, et al. Evaluation and treatment of the dominant dorsal duct syndrome (pancreas divisum redefined). *Am J Surg* 1990;159:59–66

Warshaw AL, Richter JM, Schapiro RH. The cause and treatment of pancreatitis associated with pancreas divisum. *Ann Surg* 1983;198:443

Warshaw AL, Simeone J, et al. Objective evaluation of ampullary stenosis with ultrasonography and pancreatic stimulation. *Am J Surg* 1985;149:65

Warshaw AL, Simeone J, Schapiro RH, et al. Objective evaluation of ampullary stenosis with ultrasonography and pancreatic stimulation. *Am J Surg* 1985;149:65–71

White TT, Waisman H, Hopton D, et al. Radiomanometry, flow rates and cholangiography in the evaluation of common bile duct disease. *Am J Surg* 1972;123:73–78

Yamaguchi K, Enjoji M, Kitamura K. Endoscopic biopsy has limited accuracy in diagnosis of ampullary tumors. *Gastrointest Endosc* 1990;36:588–592

63

Recurrent Pyogenic Cholangitis

S.T. Fan ▪ *John Wong*

Recurrent pyogenic cholangitis (RPC) is characterized by repeated attacks of bacterial infection of the biliary tract. This name was introduced by Cook, in 1954, to describe a disease that is prevalent in Hong Kong and other parts of Southeast Asia in which cholangitis occurred primarily in the bile ducts with subsequent pigment stone and stricture formation. This entity is in contrast to the cholangitis seen in Western countries that arises from gallstones, iatrogenic strictures, and tumor obstruction.

Although rarely seen outside Southeast Asia in the past, ease of travel and migration have meant that this condition is now encountered in Western countries more regularly. Unlike gallstone disease seen in Western countries, which affects well-nourished women in their 40s and 50s, RPC typically afflicts a younger group of patients, with a peak age of 20 to 40 years. Men and women are equally susceptible, with those of the lower socioeconomic class more at risk. A decline in the incidence of this disease during the last decade and a shift of the peak age incidence to an older age group have been noted in the more developed countries of this region. Thus, in Hong Kong, in the last ten years, the peak age incidence was in the seventh decade. These elderly patients were those afflicted by the disease when young, survived the attacks of acute cholangitis, had one or more biliary operations and presented again to the clinicians with recurrent acute cholangitis, biliary cirrhosis, or liver failure. On the contrary, patients who presented for the first time in their life were often young immigrants from China or Vietnam.

The exact etiology of RPC is not yet defined but the pathogenesis and pathology are now well documented. Careful studies of its clinical course have allowed a more rational approach to its surgical treatment.

▪ ETIOLOGY

Many hypotheses have been advanced for the cause of RPC; most are difficult, if not impossible, to prove. The balance of available evidence firmly indicates that the initiating process is the establishment of enteric flora, via the portal venous system, in the intrahepatic biliary radicals. The reasons for the breakdown of normal host defense mechanisms may be (1) the organisms are particularly virulent, (2) the bowel wall is injured (eg, by enteric infection), thus allowing a larger than normal load of organisms of ordinary virulence to enter the bloodstream, (3) the metabolic activities of the hepatocytes have been altered (eg, by malnutrition) to produce bile that lacks or is reduced in bactericidal properties, or that is increased in lithogenicity, and (4) the biliary tree is damaged by the presence of parasites (eg, *Clonorchis sinensis, Ascaris lumbricoides*) to increase its susceptibility to infection. There are little data to support the first possibility, and RPC is found in countries where parasitic infestation is not endemic. Even in countries where both RPC and infestation are present, only a minority of patients (<25%) with RPC show infestation. Therefore, the most likely cause is the establishment of bowel organisms (of ordinary virulence and perhaps in greater dose) in the liver and biliary tract of a compromised host. However, this theory does not explain one of the main pathologic features of RPC, ie, the significant preponderance of left lobe involvement. It is likely that such anatomic factors as size, angulation, and branching of the intrahepatic ducts may have functional consequences, such as changes in flow rate and physicochemical properties, that are also important determinants of the pattern of the disease.

■ PATHOGENESIS

Once the organisms are established in the liver, an intense acute inflammatory reaction develops in the liver parenchyma and in the portal triad. This reaction is evidenced by neutrophil infiltration in the sinusoids of the lobules. Infection probably spreads from the cholangioles to the larger ducts as the process continues. Bile is altered by infection. There is deconjugation of bilirubin diglucuronide by β-glucuronidase, combination of deconjugated bilirubin with calcium to form insoluble calcium bilirubinate, and formation of microcalculi. These microcalculi may be discharged through the sphincter of Oddi into the duodenal lumen, but if the attack does not resolve quickly, or if there are frequent and recurrent attacks, the microcalculi (in addition to live or dead parasites) become niduses for large stones. These stones may fail to pass downward, especially if strictures also are present. Strictures probably are formed by the perpetuation of the normal healing process excited by transmural ductal injury from infection and the destruction of the surrounding liver parenchyma. In some patients, the stricture is a relative one; the diameter of the narrowed part is no smaller than a normal duct at the corresponding level, but the proximal ducts are grossly dilated and give the appearance of obstruction. This relative or functional obstruction has the same pathologic outcome, resulting in stagnation, inadequate drainage, stone formation, and cholangitis, regardless of the absolute size of the narrowed segment. The most common organisms isolated from blood and bile cultures are *Escherichia coli, Klebsiella, Streptococcus faecalis, Bacteroides fragilis,* and *Clostridium.* Mixed infections, including uncommon organisms, also are encountered frequently.

■ PATHOLOGY

Biopsy specimens of the liver taken at emergency operation show infiltration of hepatic sinusoids by neutrophils. Since neutrophils rarely are seen in sinusoids in cholangitis resulting from other causes, this finding lends support to the hypothesis that the pathogenic or-

ganisms arrive by the hematogenous route. The hepatocyte and Kupffer cells usually appear normal. However, in severe cases, toxic vacuolation is seen in the hepatocytes, and the Kupffer cells are stained with bile pigments.

In the acute stage, neutrophils infiltrate the portal triad and also are found in the small bile ducts. Continuing infection leads to destruction of these small ducts and adjacent liver parenchyma, leading to microabscesses formation. These microabscesses may continue to enlarge and coalesce into multiple pyogenic abscesses. Subsidence of the infective process is accompanied by fibrosis and chronic inflammatory cell infiltration of the portal tract that, in severe and persistent cases, results in bridging fibrous bands developing between portal tracts. Ultimately, replacement of the liver by fibrous tissue and liver atrophy occurs. Portal hypertension with its manifestation of splenomegaly, ascites, and bleeding varices may occur. In long-standing cases, dysplastic changes of ductal mucosa leading to cholangiocarcinoma have been observed.

The early ductal changes in RPC have been documented by endoscopic retrograde cholangiopancreatography (ERCP). There is excessive branching, "arrowhead" formation or abrupt termination of the proximal ducts, loss of parallelism of the walls of the larger ducts, and dilation of the first and second order hepatic duct (Figs 63–1, 63–2, and 63–3). Stricture formation is not a

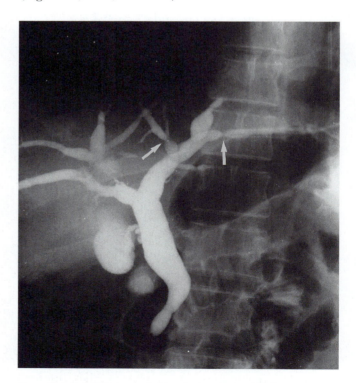

Figure 63–1. Early RPC changes. Left hepatic duct showing mild dilation with intrahepatic strictures (*arrows*). Stones are absent in the bile ducts and gallbladder. The ampulla of Vater is patulous.

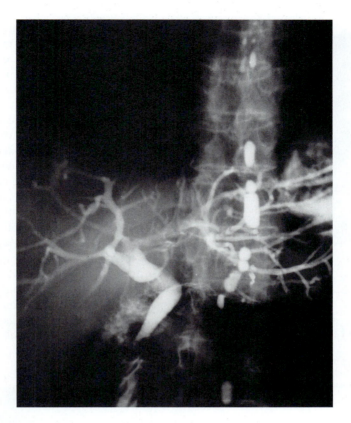

Figure 63–2. Extensive branching of left intrahepatic bile ducts in early RPC changes. Previous myelogram is noted.

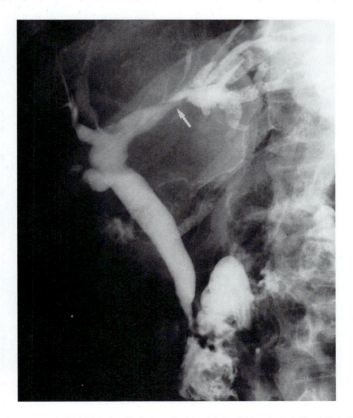

Figure 63–3. Intrahepatic stones are seen in the left intrahepatic duct proximal to a tubular stricture (*arrow*). The right duct is only minimally affected.

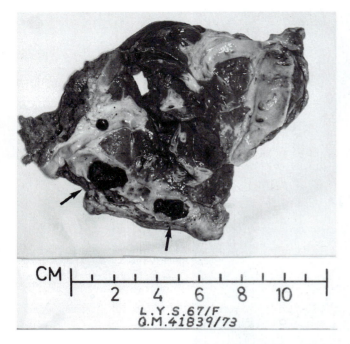

Figure 63–4. Specimen of a resected left lobe of liver affected by RPC. The intrahepatic ducts are thickened and dilated, and some are filled with pigmented stones (*arrows*). There is still residual liver parenchyma, which is traversed with fibrotic bands.

feature in the early stages of the disease but becomes the sine qua non in established disease.

Examination of the resected liver shows thickened and dilated ducts that contain many pigmented stones (Fig 63–4). Sometimes the stones and thick biliary mud form a cast of the biliary tree.

The surface of the affected duct has patchy, congested, or hemorrhagic areas, and the mucosal lining may be incomplete. Strictures have a predilection for the origin of the left hepatic duct but also may be present in segmental or subsegmental ducts, often at the ductal confluences (Figs 63–5 and 63–6). The right duct origin is rarely the only site of stricture. Most strictures in the larger ducts are short, and in the smaller ducts they may be tubular (Fig 63–3).

When the disease process is severe, liver parenchyma is destroyed and the left or right lobe of the liver is little more than a fibrous sac containing dilated ducts and stones (Fig 63–4). In these circumstances, there is compensatory hypertrophy of the contralateral lobe, which may be to such an extent as to distort normal anatomic relationships. When stones are present, the common hepatic and bile ducts may become grossly thickened and dilated (up to 10 cm; average 2 to 3 cm); thus, the ducts do not return to their normal size even when the mud and stones have been completely removed (Figs 63–7 and 63–8). Because these ducts do not drain ef-

fectively, they act as a sump that predisposes to further stone formation. Strictures also may occur in the extrahepatic ducts; they are usually diaphragmatic in appearance and are more likely to be located near the lower end of the common bile duct (Figs 63–9 and 63–10A).

The sphincter of Oddi is usually patulous and large dilators pass through without resistance. Pressure necrosis from a stone impacted at the lower end of the common bile duct may lead to a spontaneous choledochoduodenostomy above the major papilla, allowing air to enter the biliary tree.

Stones are found in 90% of patients with RPC, and the most common sites of occurrence are the common hepatic or bile ducts (50%). In 25% of all patients with RPC, stones are found only in the intrahepatic ducts, with a 4 to 1 preponderance of left to right. Thus, if stones are present in the right duct, they are very likely to be found in the left duct, as well. Even when stones are present in both ducts, the left is usually more severely affected. Only 15% of patients with RPC have

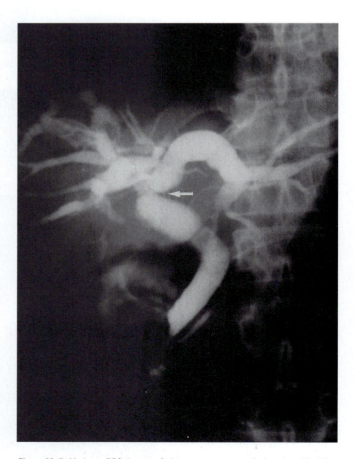

Figure 63–5. Moderate RPC changes. Strictures are present at the junction of both hepatic ducts with the common hepatic duct (*arrow*), with dilation, excessive branching, and "arrowhead" formation of the intrahepatic ducts. Stones are present in the intrahepatic and extrahepatic ducts.

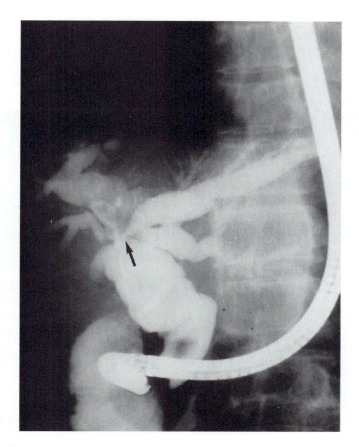

Figure 63–6. Severe RPC changes. Tight strictures are seen at the confluences of the right and left hepatic ducts (*arrow*), with dilation of the intrahepatic ducts. Stones are present in the right duct and in the common bile duct.

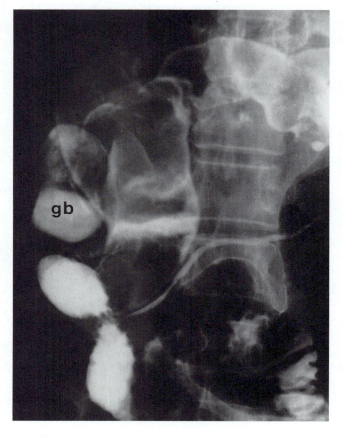

Figure 63–7. Severe RPC changes. The grossly dilated extrahepatic duct is completely filled with soft stones and thick biliary mud. The intrahepatic ducts are dilated and contain similar debris. The gallbladder (gb) was found to be normal at operation.

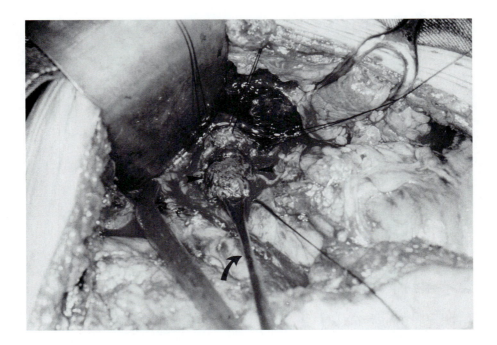

A

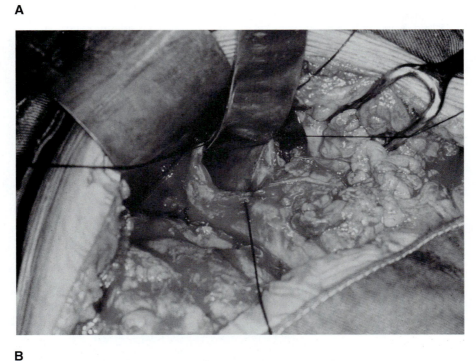

B

Figure 63–8. A. Operative finding of patient whose cholangiogram is seen in Fig 63–7. The common bile duct is opened, and a scoop (*curved arrow*) is used to evacuate the thick biliary mud through the choledochotomy (*arrow*). **B.** After mud, debris, and soft stones have been removed from the thickened and dilated common bile duct, a retractor is placed in the duct to allow direct visual inspection and digital examination. A choledochojejunostomy is the operation of choice.

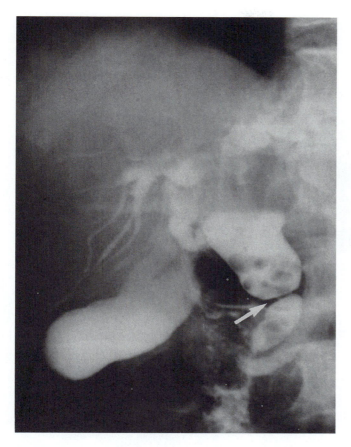

Figure 63–9. A diaphragmatic stricture (*arrow*) in the intrapancreatic portion of the common bile duct with stones above and below the stricture. The ducts proximal to the stricture are dilated, and the gallbladder is free of stones.

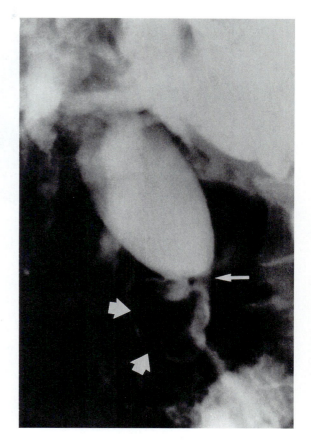

A

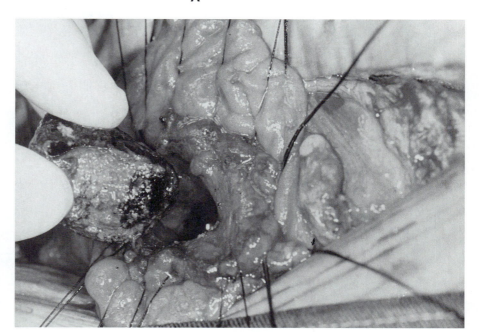

Figure 63–10. A. A stricture (*arrow*) in the intrapancreatic portion of the common bile duct is seen above a large stone (*short arrows*), which fills the distal bile duct completely. **B.** At operation, a soft pigmented stone, measuring 2.5 cm in length, is removed after a large sphincteroplasty is performed; the edges of the sphincteroplasty are indicated by the stay sutures.

B

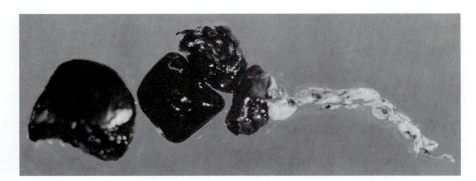

Figure 63–11. A dead *A lumbricoides* in the bile duct is the nidus for the development of stones. (Courtesy of C A Arcilla).

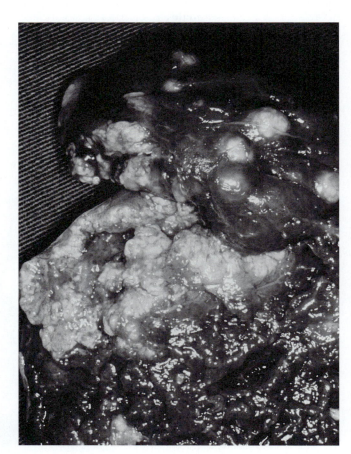

Figure 63–12. Chronic liver abscesses in a cholangitic liver. Resection is the only method for eradication of this persistent source of infection or to differentiate it from a tumor.

stones in the gallbladder, all of whom also have stones elsewhere in the biliary tree.

The stones found in RPC are pigmented and faceted; they have a brown, earthy appearance and are soft and friable. Inside, the color is usually yellow or orange (Fig 63–10B). When stone forceps are gently applied, the stones fragment. The pigment is bilirubinate, and layers of this pigment are deposited on top of each other over a central nidus, which may be a dead parasite, such as *C sinensis* or *A lumbricoides,* desquamated epithelium, or inspissated bile, mucus, or pus (Fig 63–11). The laminated nature of some stones bears testimony to the recurrent nature of this condition. Chemical analysis reveals the constituents of stones to be 24.7% bilirubin, 5.9% cholesterol, and 0.5% calcium; the rest are insoluble residue, accounting for their radiolucency.

An abscess in the left lobe may rupture into the peritoneal cavity or into the pericardium, leading to cardiac tamponade. A right lobe abscess may rupture through the diaphragm and cause thoracic empyema, or if it ruptures into the lung, a bronchobiliary fistula. A chronic abscess may render distinction from a tumor difficult (Fig 63–12).

Thrombophlebitis of the hepatic veins rarely gives rise to pulmonary emboli and pulmonary hypertension.

■ CLINICAL FEATURES

Patients are typically young, thin, and sometimes malnourished. Most have had previous episodes of cholangitis. The frequency and severity of attacks usually increase with the passage of time.

The chief complaints are right upper quadrant or epigastric pain, fever, and passing tea-colored urine. The pain is described as distending, sharp, cutting, or gnawing and often radiates to the back and right shoulder; this pain may last for hours or days and is usually unremitting. Only rarely is the pain colicky. Fever is continuous and is between 38.0°C and 39.5°C but is seldom above 40°C, which suggests septicemia. Often the fever is associated with chills and is preceded by rigors. Nausea is present with pain, but vomiting is rare.

Jaundice is mild and just perceptible clinically, since biliary obstruction is usually incomplete. For this reason the stool is not pale, and pruritus is not a complaint. More characteristically, the patient notices that the urine is tea-colored.

Physical examination shows a restless patient who not infrequently bears the scars of previous surgery. There is tenderness in the right upper quadrant or epigastrium. If the latter is marked, a left lobe abscess must be suspected. However, in 14% of patients, tenderness is absent; these patients are usually old and jaundiced and may not have fever or chills.

The liver is enlarged in 60% of patients, but this finding may be masked by abdominal guarding; the gallbladder is palpable in 30% and the spleen in 25% of patients. Acute pancreatitis is associated with RPC in 10% of patients. Signs of generalized peritonitis are present in 5% of patients, and this may be caused by rupture of a diseased gallbladder or liver abscess, or because of severe acute pancreatitis. These complications are associated with shock, which becomes rapidly fatal unless surgery is immediately undertaken.

■ LABORATORY FINDINGS

Routine laboratory tests do not show any diagnostic pattern specific to RPC, and the findings are those expected in obstructive jaundice and infection. Thus, there is a leukocytosis with a left shift, an elevated serum alkaline phosphatase, gamma-glutamyl-transpeptidase (the level depending on the severity and duration of obstruction), and an elevation of serum transaminases if there is associated hepatocellular damage. Since the biliary obstruction is incomplete, urinary urobilinogen is present, in addition to bile pigments. Blood cultures for aerobic and anaerobic organisms are taken for all patients in an acute attack.

Serum amylase is elevated 20% of the time. In 50% of patients, it exceeds 1000 U/L. In these patients, a stone impacted at the lower end of the common bile duct must be suspected. Stool examination for parasites should be performed. Although the incidence of infestation in RPC is not different from that in other hospital patients, treatment is given to those with positive results.

■ INVESTIGATIONS

The diagnosis of RPC is usually not in doubt because the clinical features are quite typical. Investigations are still necessary to define the exact location of all stones and strictures before definitive treatment.

Ultrasonography is noninvasive and is of particular value in providing objective evidence during an acute attack, especially when therapeutic intervention is likely. It may show features of biliary obstruction, stones in the biliary system, pneumobilia, liver abscesses, or pancreatitis. Intrahepatic stones usually are recognized on ultrasonography; however, some stones in RPC may not cast sonic shadowing or may form casts within the intrahepatic ducts, leading to the stones being missed by ultrasonography.

Computed tomography (CT) of the upper abdomen can provide much the same information as ultrasonography, with the advantage of less interference by bowel gas, surgical scars, and observer bias. In addition, CT

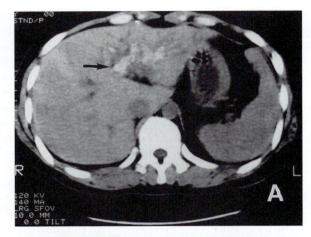

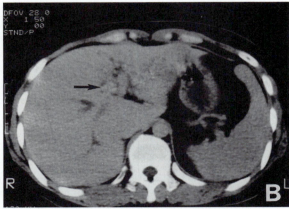

Figure 63–13. A. Noncontrast CT scan showing stones (*arrow*) inside left lateral segment. **B.** Contrast CT scan showing that the stone is less conspicuous after parenchymal enhancement.

can accurately differentiate intrahepatic stones from pneumobilia; provides accurate topographic localization for drainage of liver abscess, determines the degree of atrophy of the affected part of the liver and the compensatory hypertrophy of the unaffected part, which is sometimes necessary before liver resection as a therapeutic procedure is undertaken; and detects segmental or subsegmental ductal involvement when cholangiography fails to visualize these ducts because of complete obstruction. In interpreting CT scans in RPC, it is mandatory to examine noncontrast films first because intrahepatic stones may become less conspicuous after parenchymal enhancement (Fig 63–13).

In situations where biliary obstruction is complete, both ERCP and PTC are complementary in outlining the entire biliary system. ERCP is performed best a few days after the resolution of the acute attack. It is a safe investigation and usually provides visualization of all the bile ducts, a prerequisite before surgical intervention. The optimal surgical procedure can be planned only

when the exact locations of stones and strictures are known. In patients with previous sphincteroplasties or choledochoduodenal fistulae, visualization can be enhanced by the use of a balloon catheter that prevents injected contrasts from escaping.

Rarely, a chronic abscess develops requiring hepatic arteriography and CT-guided aspiration to distinguish it from a tumor or other mass lesion. Peritoneoscopy also may provide additional information in the unusual patient with RPC.

■ MANAGEMENT

INITIAL TREATMENT

After admission to the hospital for acute cholangitis, most patients improve on conservative therapy. Treatment involves intravenous fluid replacement, nasogastric aspiration, analgesics, and administration of broad-spectrum antibiotics, usually a second generation cephalosporin.

About 70% of the patients respond to this regimen. Resolution of the acute attack is evidenced by a reduction in abdominal tenderness and restoration of normal vital signs and temperature. If this does not occur within 2 or 3 days, or if the condition of the patient deteriorates, urgent surgery should be considered. An important feature of RPC is that a transient rise in blood pressure may be observed before the appearance of shock; this phenomenon should not be taken as a sign of improvement.

The principles of emergency surgery are decompression of the obstructed bile duct by a limited exploration of the bile duct and insertion of a T tube. Stones that can be extracted easily are removed. Irrigation should not be vigorous, since infected material may be forced into the blood, exacerbating the sepsis. Any tight strictures in the left or right hepatic duct should be dilated by graduated sound until there is free flow of infected bile. A stone impacted at the lower end of the common bile duct can be removed by transduodenal sphincteroplasty, choledochoscopic basket, or after fragmentation by electrohydraulic lithotripsy under choledochoscopic guidance. A large, solitary abscess in the liver is drained externally. Small multiple abscesses are not drained; they usually respond to antibiotic treatment and biliary decompression.

The gallbladder is left alone unless it is very distended, gangrenous, or contains pus. Cholecystostomy is performed if cholecystectomy is unsafe. A large T tube is inserted into the common duct at the end of exploration. If right or left hepatic ductal strictures are present, a transhepatic tube is inserted. It must be realized that emergency operations are usually inadequate, in terms of stone clearance. The type and the duration of the operation are limited by the stability of the patient.

Even if vital signs are stable intraoperatively, surgeons are frequently unable to perform optimal procedures because of insufficient knowledge of the location of stones and strictures. Detailed information of biliary abnormalities are obtained by postoperative cholangiography after the patient recovers, allowing adequate treatment by choledochoscopy.

When surgical intervention is required for patients failing conservative treatment, the operative mortality rate is 12% and the complication rate is 35%. Endoscopic or radiological approaches have been employed as alternative treatment. In a prospective randomized trial, endoscopic papillotomy and nasobiliary drainage were shown to be beneficial in reducing mortality in a series of patients with acute cholangitis, some of whom were suffering from RPC but were without intrahepatic stones. The radiological approach is percutaneous transhepatic biliary drainage. These nonoperative treatments would be effective for simple cases of RPC but may not be efficient in the presence of multiple stones or strictures within the intrahepatic ducts. It is also essential to emphasize that the drainage tubes used in nonoperative procedures are of narrow caliber and thus, blockage by the thick bile found in RPC is common.

The reasons why conservative treatment is successful in some patients but fails in others are unknown. A retrospective analysis suggested that conservative treatment is more likely to fail when there was obstruction at the common bile duct rather than isolated segmental duct. In other words, sepsis owing to obstruction of the entire biliary tract appears to be more virulent than segmental obstruction.

DEFINITIVE SURGERY

Principles of elective definitive surgery comprise (1) the complete removal of intrahepatic and extrahepatic stones, and (2) the establishment of satisfactory drainage of the affected segment of the biliary tree.

As mentioned previously, stones and strictures can occur extrahepatically, intrahepatically, or at both locations. Treatment of stones and strictures in the extrahepatic ducts is usually straightforward, since they can be approached directly. Treatment of intrahepatic pathology presents the most challenge to surgeons. Intrahepatic stones are found in 50% and strictures in intrahepatic or extrahepatic ducts in 35% of patients with RPC.

A definitive operation starts with a common bile duct exploration and choledochoscopy. The common bile duct and the main and segmental intrahepatic ducts are examined carefully. The locations of stones and strictures, as shown by preoperative investigations, are confirmed.

Consideration should be given as to whether liver resection is to be performed. Preoperative studies usually supply sufficient information to make the decision. If operative findings confirm that the disease is localized to one lobe or segment of the liver, the involved part of liver is atrophic (Fig 63–14 A, B), and the remaining liver is of normal size or hypertrophied, liver resection should be performed. Occasionally, two isolated segments separated by normal liver are involved. Separate excision of the segments can be performed. Table 63–1 shows the types of liver resection performed for RPC.

The technique of liver resection is no different from that for other diseases and may be easier, since liver transection does not involve a substantial amount of liver parenchyma. However, inflow and outflow vascular control may be difficult in about 50% of cases owing to severe perihepatic adhesions from previous surgery or recurrent infection. To avoid injury to the hepatic or portal veins, it may be advisable to abandon attempts at extrahepatic control of hepatic vasculature and proceed directly to parenchymal transection. Pringle's maneuver can be used, if difficulty is encountered. The segmental branches of the portal vein, hepatic artery and hepatic veins can be safely ligated within the liver parenchyma. The operative mortality of liver resection for RPC is 2% and the postoperative complication rate is 32%. The majority of complications are infections and are probably related to the high incidence of infected bile and liver abscesses in RPC. Biliary fistulae may complicate hepatic resection in RPC. Contrary to hepatic resection in a normal or cirrhotic liver, small bile ducts at the transected surface may remain open for a longer time because of chronic inflammation, if not sutured. The long-term prognosis after liver resection is good. Recurrence of stones occurs in about 16% of patients.

If liver resection is not indicated, common bile duct exploration is continued. Stones in the common bile duct are removed first. Stone forceps, scoops, and irrigation are used. Stones in the right and left hepatic ducts also can be removed with these instruments, but stones in the segmental ducts usually require removal with wire baskets or biliary balloon catheters under choledochoscopic guidance. The choledochotomy can be extended into the right or left hepatic duct to facilitate removal of stones impacted at the confluence of the hepatic ducts or within the intrahepatic ducts. Before extension of the choledochotomy, care is taken to avoid damaging the hepatic artery that may course near the bifurcation.

Stones in segmental bile ducts that cannot be retrieved easily may require electrohydraulic lithotripsy. The shocks are delivered by a 1.68-mm diameter electrode introduced through the irrigation channel of the choledochoscope. Care should be taken to extend the tip of the electrode at least 1.5 cm beyond the choledochoscope, to avoid damage to the choledochoscope. Electrohydraulic shock waves usually can fragment

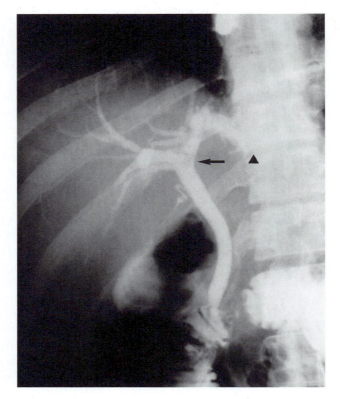

A

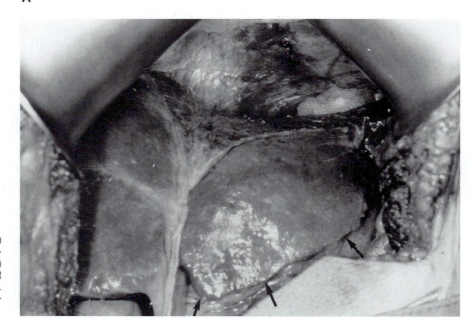

Figure 63–14. A. Cholangiogram of a 37 year–old man showing a stone (*arrow*) at confluence of bile duct and incomplete filling of left lateral segmental ducts (*short arrows*) owing to intrahepatic stones. **B.** Atrophic and scarred left lateral segment (*arrows*) in RPC identified at laparotomy. Left lateral segmentectomy is the best treatment in this situation.

B

TABLE 63-1. PARTS OF THE LIVER RESECTED IN RPC IN 113 PATIENTS

	Number
Left lateral segment	79
Left lobe	24
Right lobe	1
Right anterior segment	7
Right posterior segment	1
Left lateral segment and right anterior segment	1

large stones that either can be flushed out or removed with basket retrievers.

The incidence of residual intrahepatic stones after surgery remains high (50%). A small number of stones are missed during the operation. A large number, however, are left behind because of the practical limits of choledochoscopy during surgery, which are (1) repeated retrieval causes mucosal edema and bleeding, making further viewing difficult, and (2) the stones may be too numerous and complete eradication would necessitate a prolonged period of general anesthesia. The removal of the residual stones will depend on postoperative choledochoscopy.

MANAGEMENT OF BILIARY STRICTURES

Optimally, the biliary strictures should be identified and the corrective procedures planned before the operation. The procedures for extrahepatic strictures are sphincteroplasty and hepaticojejunostomy.

Sphincteroplasty is indicated (1) when there is *ampullary* stricture or (2) when a duct is dilated (1.5 to 2.5 cm) and thickened, and there is a previous history of bile duct surgery for stones. Sphincteroplasty usually is performed transperitoneally. In patients who have undergone multiple previous biliary operations, an extraperitoneal approach through a flank incision can be used. Using either approach, the second part of the duodenum is exposed and opened vertically. The sphincter of Oddi is divided at the 11 o'clock position. The division is extended to the most dilated part of the common duct, which may be 2 cm or more from the ampullary opening. The edges of the common bile duct and the duodenum are approximated with fine absorbable sutures. After complete removal of stones, the duodenum is closed longitudinally with continuous fine absorbable sutures.

The limitation of the extraperitoneal approach is that the common bile duct cannot be explored through a separate choledochotomy and other additional intraperitoneal procedures cannot be carried out. In the intraperitoneal approach, a choledochotomy usually is made to facilitate the sphincteroplasty.

The complication rate of sphincteroplasty in RPC patients is 10% and the mortality rate is 4%. Common

postoperative complications are septicemia and pancreatitis. The long-term results of sphincteroplasty are good, with 16% of patients having recurrent symptoms and about half of these requiring reoperation. Recurrent symptoms occur because of stricture of the sphincteroplasty or recurrent cholangitis owing to retained or reformed stones.

Strictures of the *common duct* are best treated by hepaticojejunostomy. This procedure is also indicated when the common duct is extremely dilated (>2.5 cm) and fibrotic.

Hepaticojejunostomy is constructed by a Roux-en-Y, end-to-side method using a 40-cm jejunal limb; the anastomosis is one layer of interrupted fine absorbable sutures. The jejunal limb is placed in the retrocolic position, and intestinal continuity is restored with an end-to-side jejunojejunostomy. A transanastomotic stent is brought out either through the jejunum or transhepatically. The location of the hepaticojejunal anastomosis depends on the site of the stricture of the common duct and the ease of exposure of the bile duct. It can be constructed at the common bile duct, common hepatic duct, left hepatic duct or the left lateral segmental duct (Fig 63–15).

Intrahepatic strictures are treated by dilation using a balloon or Gruntzig catheter or by resection of the involved liver segment. Intrahepatic strictures are occasionally diaphragm-like and located close to the confluence of the right and left hepatic ducts. These strictures are treated best by ductoplasties (Fig 63–16). The choledochotomy is extended to the orifice of the involved hepatic duct to expose the stricture. The diaphragm is excised and the ducts are reconstructed by approximating the cut edges of the mucosa together with fine absorbable sutures. Strictures that are deep inside the liver require balloon dilation.

HEPATICOCUTANEOUS JEJUNOSTOMY

When a need for postoperative choledochoscopy exists, the end of jejunal limb may be exteriorized as a stoma, forming access to the biliary tract (hepaticocutaneous jejunostomy) (Fig 63–17). After clearance of stones and adequate dilation of strictures by postoperative choledochoscopy, the cutaneous stoma can be closed and buried in the subcutaneous tissue.

The hepaticocutaneous jejunostomy is useful as a percutaneous access to the biliary tract when there is recurrence of stones or strictures. The buried end of the jejunal limb is opened under local anesthesia and the stoma reconstructed for choledochoscopy. Hepaticocutaneous jejunostomy is recommended for patients with known retained intrahepatic stones or when recurrent intrahepatic stones is thought likely. In practice, whenever a hepaticojejunostomy is indicated, consideration

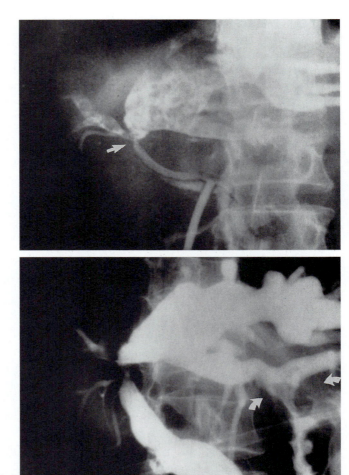

Figure 63–15. Stricture of hepatic duct confluence (*arrow*) treated by segment-III hepatico-jejunostomy, before (*top*) and after (*bottom*) the bypass. *Curved arrows* indicate the site of bilioenteric anastomosis.

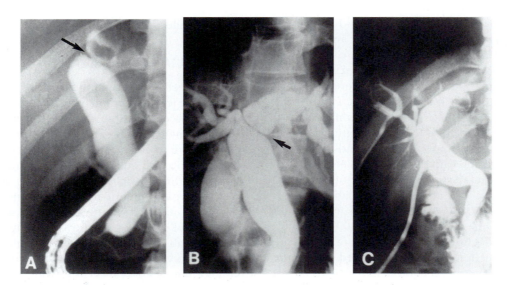

Figure 63–16. A and **B.** Cholangiograms showing diaphragmatic stricture of the left hepatic duct (*arrow*). **C.** Appearance after excision of diaphragm and reconstruction of duct.

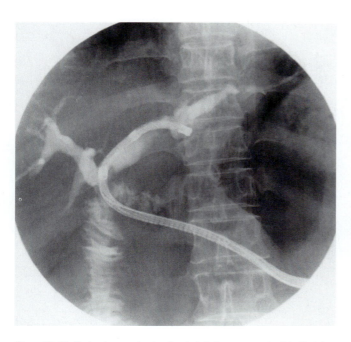

Figure 63–17. Cholangiogram showing the choledochoscope passing into the intrahepatic bile duct via a jejunal loop.

is given to lengthening the blind end of the jejunal limb to the subcutaneous level. If immediate postoperative choledochoscopy is not required, the blind end of the jejunal loop is implanted subcutaneously and its location marked by metal clips for future identification.

The complication rate of hepaticocutaneous jejunostomy is 10%. There was no mortality in our recent series of 41 patients having this procedure. The major morbidities are septicemia, wound sepsis, and biliary fistulae.

The long-term result of hepaticocutaneous jejunostomy has recently been analyzed. Of the 41 patients having this procedure, 12 patients developed recurrent symptoms. Reconstruction of the cutaneous stoma and flexible choledochoscopy helped to resolve the acute cholangitis in four patients and to eradicate recurrent stones in all cases. Hepaticocutaneous jejunostomy was also beneficial in the management of three patients who experienced recurrence of symptoms. Repeat laparotomy was required in only one patient who underwent a second bilioenteric anastomosis for a nondilatable left hepatic duct stricture.

POSTOPERATIVE CHOLEDOCHOSCOPY

Stones that are left behind or missed during the operation are removed postoperatively by choledochoscopy. These stones are localized by postoperative cholangiography. The T tube is left in place for about 6 weeks, af-

ter which it can be removed and the tract used for the introduction of the choledochoscope. In anticipation of the necessity for postoperative choledochoscopy, a large T tube is used to drain the common duct. The tube is brought out direct, and kinking is avoided. A 5.2-mm choledochoscope can readily pass through the tract of a 5.32-mm T tube. If the tract is not large enough, dilation can be performed by putting in slightly larger catheters through the tract in succession; each catheter is left in the tract for 2 or 3 days.

The biliary tract is thoroughly examined. Stones are removed by basket retrievers and biliary balloon catheters. Electrohydraulic shock waves may be required to break up large stones located behind relative strictures, and within sharply angulated segmental ducts that are inaccessible to the choledoscope. If all the stones cannot be removed in one session, the tract can be splinted with a catheter and repeat choledochoscopy performed in 2 or 3 days.

The removal of retained stones from the common bile duct is uniformly successful, with usually one session being sufficient. In contrast, the success rate for retained intrahepatic stones without electrohydraulic lithotripsy is about 85%. With the addition of electrohydraulic lithotripsy, the retained-stone rate has been reduced to 5%. An average of four sessions is required for complete eradication of all intrahepatic stones. Stones that cannot be removed are usually small and buried in blind pouches of subsegmental ducts. Generally, choledochoscopy via the T tube tract is not painful; some patients experience pain at the skin entry site or when large stones are pulled through the T tube tract.

If hepaticocutaneous jejunostomy has been constructed, postoperative choledochoscopy can be performed via the cutaneous stoma and the jejunal loop. Unlike choledochoscopy via the T tube tract, it can be performed soon after the surgery, usually about 2 weeks later, when the hepaticojejunal anastomosis is healed. It is also a more comfortable procedure than choledochoscopy via T tube tract and is free from the risk of permanent loss of percutaneous access to the biliary tract. When all stones are eradicated and all strictures are adequately dilated, the stoma can be closed and buried in the subcutaneous tissue under local anesthesia. However, closure should not be performed prematurely because of the technical difficulty arising from inflammation in the early stage and the risk of early recurrence of stones. Before the stoma is closed, loss of bile and irritation of skin may be a problem. Skin excoriation can be prevented by applying stomahesive around the stoma. A plastic flange is applied for easy change of the collecting bag. This flange also can be utilized during choledochoscopy to avoid wetting of the patient by the irrigating fluid (Fig. 63–18).

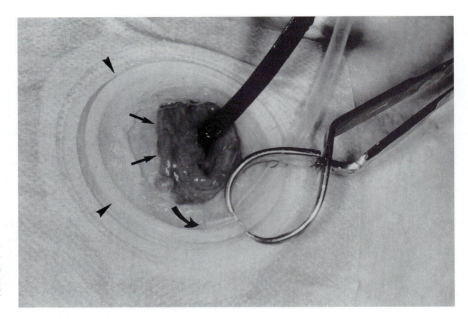

Figure 63–18. Picture showing a choledochoscope passing into a cutaneous stoma (*arrows*) that is protected by a stomahesive. A suction catheter (*curved arrow*) is clipped to the flange (*short arrows*) of stomahesive to suck away irrigating fluid escaping from the stoma so that wetting of the patient during the procedure could be avoided.

■ RESULT

Overall treatment results for RPC are satisfactory. Many complicated cases can be managed by partial hepatectomy together with hepaticocutaneous jejunostomy followed by postoperative choledochoscopy. The incidence of recurrence of stones and strictures is about 16%. This rate is likely to be higher if patients are observed for longer periods of time. Although the management of recurrent stones is facilitated by hepaticocutaneous jejunostomy, there remains a small group of patients who will develop portal hypertension and biliary cirrhosis and may require liver transplantation.

Recurrent pyogenic cholangitis exhibits a clinical syndrome that is characteristic, with the diagnosis seldom in doubt. Although most patients can expect a favorable outcome from appropriate treatment, in the acute attack, and also after definitive surgical treatment, a few may develop life-threatening complications. The conventional surgical repertoire can deal with extrahepatic disease safely and adequately. Failures are owing primarily to recurrent or retained stones, particularly in the intrahepatic site. Another major therapeutic problem is intrahepatic ductal stricture. Technical advances have enabled these strictures to be identified, and relief by surgical drainage is possible. The long-term results of these procedures are, however, less well defined. Hepatic resection offers the only cure and should be performed whenever indicated. Construction of hepaticocutaneous jejunostomy offers a readily available access to the biliary tract, if patients develop recurrence, and should be considered whenever biliary drainage is performed on these patients.

SELECTED READINGS

Chau EMT, Chan FL, Leong LLY. Recurrent pyogenic cholangitis: ultrasound evaluation compared with endoscopic retrograde cholangiography. *Clin Radiol* 1983;38:79

Choi S, Choi TK, et al. Intraoperative flexible choledochoscopy for intrahepatic and extrahepatic biliary calculi. *Surgery* 1987;101:571

Choi TK, Fok M, et al. Postoperative flexible choledochoscopy for residual primary intrahepatic stones. *Ann Surg* 1986; 203:260

Choi TK, Lee NW, et al. Extraperitoneal sphincteroplasty for residual stones—an update. *Ann Surg* 1982;196:26

Choi TK, Wong J, et al. Partial hepatectomy for intrahepatic stones. *World J Surg* 1986;10:281

Choi TK, Wong J, et al. Late result of sphincteroplasty in the treatment of primary cholangitis. *Arch Surg* 1981;116:1173

Choi TK, Wong J, et al. The surgical management of primary intrahepatic stones. *Br J Surg* 1982;69:86

Choi TK, Wong J, et al. Choledochojejunostomy in the treatment of primary cholangitis. *Surg Gynecol Obstet* 1982;155:43

Cook J, Hou PC, et al. Recurrent pyogenic cholangitis. *Br J Surg* 1954;42:188

Digby KH. Common-duct stones of liver origin. *Br J Surg* 1930;17:578

Fan ST, Choi TK, et al. Role of computed tomography in the management of recurrent pyogenic cholangitis. *Aust NZ J Surg* 1990;60:599

Fan ST, Choi TK, et al. Treatment of hepatolithiasis: improvement of results by a systematic approach. *Surgery* 1991; 109:474

Fan ST, Lai ECS, et al. Acute cholangitis secondary to hepatolithiasis. *Arch Surg* 1991;126:1027

Fan ST, Mok FPT, et al. Appraisal of hepaticocutaneous jejunostomy in the management of hepatolithiasis. *Am J Surg* 1993;165:332

Fan ST, Lai ECS, et al. Hepatic resection for hepatolithiasis. *Arch Surg* 1993;128:1070

Federle MP, Cello JP, et al. Recurrent pyogenic cholangitis in Asian immigrants: use of ultrasonography, computed tomography and cholangiography. *Radiology* 1982;143:151

Fung J. Liver fluke infestation and cholangio-hepatitis. *Br J Surg* 1961;48:404

Lam SK, Wong KP, et al. Recurrent pyogenic cholangitis: a study by endoscopic retrograde cholangiography. *Gastroenterology* 1978;74:1196

Lai ECS, Mok FPT, et al. Endoscopic biliary drainage for severe acute cholangitis. *N Engl J Med* 1992;326:1582

Maki T. Pathogenesis of calcium bilirubinate gallstone: role of *E coli*, β-glucuronidase and coagulation by inorganic ions, polyelectrolytes and agitation. *Ann Surg* 1966;164:90

Nakayama F, Soloway RD, et al. Hepatolithiasis in East Asia: retrospective study. *Dig Dis Sci* 1986;31:21

Ong GB. A study of recurrent pyogenic cholangitis. *Arch Surg* 1962;84:199

Ong GB, Adiseshiah M, et al. Acute pancreatitis associated with recurrent pyogenic cholangitis. *Br J Surg* 1971; 58:891

Ong GB, Lam KH, et al. Acute pancreatitis in Hong Kong. *Br J Surg* 1979;66:398

Teoh TB. A study of gall-stones and included worms in recurrent pyogenic cholangitis. *J Pathol Bacteriol* 1963;86:123

Wong J. Recurrent pyogenic cholangitis. In: Okuda K (ed), *International Association for the Study of the Liver/Asian Pacific Association for the Study of the Liver-Postgraduate Course*. Hong Kong: 1982

Wong J, Choi TK. Recurrent pyogenic cholangitis. In: Okuda K, Nakayama F, Wong J (eds), *Intrahepatic Calculi. Progress in Clinical and Biological Research*. vol 152. New York, NY: Alan R. Liss; 1984:175–192

64

Sclerosing Cholangitis

Steven A. Ahrendt ■ *Henry A. Pitt*

Sclerosing cholangitis is a cholestatic liver disease characterized by fibrotic strictures involving the intrahepatic and extrahepatic biliary tree. In most cases, the etiology of sclerosing cholangitis is unclear. However, a strong association exists between chronic ulcerative colitis and primary sclerosing cholangitis. Recent studies suggest that genetic and immunologic factors are important in the pathogenesis of this disorder and may partially explain the relationship between ulcerative colitis and primary sclerosing cholangitis.

Prior to 1980, sclerosing cholangitis was considered a rare disorder with fewer than 100 reported cases.[1] However, the introduction of endoscopic retrograde cholangiopancreatography and percutaneous transhepatic cholangiography, in the 1970s, has led to an increase in the identification of patients with the characteristic cholangiographic findings of sclerosing cholangitis. The diagnosis of *primary sclerosing cholangitis* requires the presence of multifocal strictures and beading of the intrahepatic and/or extrahepatic biliary tract in the absence of other precipitating causes. In cases where the biliary tract disease is caused by acute cholangitis, common bile duct stones, operative trauma, or other toxic agents, the term *secondary sclerosing cholangitis* is used.

The clinical course of patients with sclerosing cholangitis is highly variable. In some patients diagnosed with primary sclerosing cholangitis during an evaluation of abnormal liver function tests, the disease may remain asymptomatic for years, whereas in others the obliterative biliary tract changes may progress rapidly to secondary biliary cirrhosis and liver failure. Endoscopic,

radiologic, and surgical therapies are directed at improving biliary drainage and relieving symptoms of jaundice, pruritus, and cholangitis. When these methods fail or when cirrhosis develops, liver transplantation remains the only effective treatment for patients with sclerosing cholangitis.

■ PATHOPHYSIOLOGY

ETIOLOGY

The cause of primary sclerosing cholangitis remains unknown, despite many proposed etiologies (Table 64–1). A number of agents can produce injury to the biliary tract resulting in diffuse strictures similar to primary sclerosing cholangitis. These agents include bacteria and viruses, chemicals and drugs, and ischemia. No specific means exist to distinguish primary sclerosing cholangitis from sclerosing cholangitis secondary to these other causes. Any proposed etiology must explain the close association between ulcerative colitis and primary sclerosing cholangitis.[2] Recent studies have focused on genetic and immune factors as the most likely etiologic agent in these patients.

Primary sclerosing cholangitis is more common in certain HLA haplotypes. In a study of 25 patients, Chapman and associates found a close association between the HLA-B8 haplotype and primary sclerosing cholangitis, with 60% of patients with primary sclerosing cholangitis having the HLA-B8 haplotype as compared

TABLE 64–1. POSSIBLE ETIOLOGIES OF SCLEROSING CHOLANGITIS

| Autoimmune |
| Bacterial |
| Congenital |
| Copper |
| Drug-induced |
| Histiocytosis X |
| Viral |

to only 25% of the control group.[3] Schrumpf and associates also found a higher frequency of the HLA B8/DR3 haplotype in patients with primary sclerosing cholangitis when compared with controls,[4] and Prochazka and his associates have identified the HLA-DRw52a antigen on the DR3 locus in all 29 patients undergoing liver transplantation for primary sclerosing cholangitis at the University of California at Los Angeles.[5] Thus, the development of primary sclerosing cholangitis involves a strong genetic predisposition that appears to be closely linked to the HLA-DRw52a antigen.

The HLA haplotype B8/DR3 also is commonly associated with a number of autoimmune diseases. This haplotype occurs with high frequency in insulin-dependent diabetes mellitus, dermatitis herpetiformis, Graves' disease, Sjögren's syndrome, myasthenia gravis, celiac disease, and chronic active hepatitis.[5,6] Thus, primary sclerosing cholangitis may be an immunologically mediated disease occurring in genetically susceptible individuals.

A number of studies suggest that immunological factors also may play an important role in the pathogenesis of primary sclerosing cholangitis. Patients with primary sclerosing cholangitis have several abnormalities in cellular immunity including low values of circulating suppressor T cells as well as an increase in the number of suppressor T and helper T cells in the portal tracts.[7,8] Chapman and associates also have demonstrated the aberrant expression of HLA-DR antigens on the biliary epithelium in each of 10 patients with early primary sclerosing cholangitis.[9] However, aberrant expression of HLA-DR also was seen in patients with extrahepatic biliary obstruction and primary biliary cirrhosis. Although this aberrant HLA-DR expression may be secondary to cholestasis and inflammation, this factor may play a role in the immunologically mediated bile duct injury that occurs with primary sclerosing cholangitis.

Further support for an autoimmune etiology comes from several studies demonstrating humoral immune abnormalities in patients with primary sclerosing cholangitis. Increased levels of circulating immune complexes are present in the blood of patients with primary sclerosing cholangitis.[10] Increased levels of antineutrophil nuclear antibody in the serum of patients with primary sclerosing cholangitis and inflammatory bowel disease have

been demonstrated.[11] Recently, specific antineutrophil antibodies have been detected using Western blotting that may be helpful in the serological diagnosis of primary sclerosing cholangitis.[12,13] Current evidence suggests that primary sclerosing cholangitis is an immunologically mediated disease triggered in genetically susceptible individuals, perhaps by entry of infectious or toxic agents that may pass through the colonic mucosal barrier in patients with inflammatory bowel disease.[2]

Several other potential etiologic agents including bacteria and viruses are known to produce injury to the biliary epithelium that can produce cholangiographic and pathologic changes consistent with sclerosing cholangitis. Severe bacterial cholangitis can result in damage to the biliary epithelium and fibrous obliteration of the bile ducts and ductules.[14] Recently, several studies have reported a number of patients with fibrotic strictures involving both the intrahepatic and extrahepatic biliary tree in patients with advanced acquired immunodeficiency syndrome (AIDS).[15,16] The majority of these patients have either active cytomegalovirus infection or cryptosporidiosis at the time of presentation, suggesting a role for these opportunistic pathogens in the development of sclerosing cholangitis.[15,16]

Toxic and ischemic insults to the biliary tree also can result in injury. Treatment of echinococcal cysts with formalin has resulted in cases of sclerosing cholangitis.[17] Hepatic arterial infusion of 5-fluorodeoxyuridine in the management of colorectal cancer metastatic to the liver has resulted in hepatic arteriolar occlusion and sclerosing cholangitis in 17% of treated patients.[18] Finally, cholangiographic findings of sclerosing cholangitis have been observed with chronic rejection after hepatic transplantation. Whether this phenomenon is a result of a direct immunologically mediated injury to the biliary epithelium or is due, in part, to an ischemic insult to the biliary ductules following intimal thickening in the hepatic arterioles remains unclear.[19]

PATHOLOGY

The histologic findings on liver biopsy in primary sclerosing cholangitis are important in determining long-term prognosis and are essential in selecting the appropriate management.[20–22] However, the biopsy findings are often nonspecific and may be indistinguishable from the histologic features seen with primary biliary cirrhosis or other types of biliary obstruction.[23] Chapman and associates observed histologic findings diagnostic of sclerosing cholangitis in only 36% of 29 patients with the disease.[23] Nevertheless, for accurate staging, a liver biopsy should be obtained in any patient with the cholangiographic features of primary sclerosing cholangitis. This information is also essential for determining long-term prognosis.[20,21]

TABLE 64–2. PATHOLOGICAL STAGES IN PRIMARY SCLEROSING CHOLANGITIS

Stage 1 (portal stage)	Portal hepatitis or bile duct abnormalities or both, with little or no periportal fibrosis. The portal tracts are not enlarged.
Stage 2 (periportal stage)	Periportal fibrosis with or without periportal hepatitis, or prominent enlargement of portal tracts with seemingly intact newly formed limiting plates. Proliferation of bile ductules.
Stage 3 (septal stage)	Septal fibrosis and/or bridging necrosis. Bile ducts are often severely damaged or absent.
Stage 4 (cirrhotic stage)	Biliary cirrhosis

(Adapted from Ludwig J. Small-duct primary sclerosing cholangitis. Semin Liver Dis *1991;11:11)*

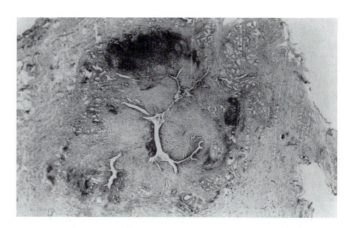

Figure 64–1. Cross-section of common bile duct in a patient with sclerosing cholangitis.

Ludwig and associates have described a staging system for primary sclerosing cholangitis based on the extent of inflammation and fibrosis on liver biopsy (Table 64–2).[24,25] These four histologic stages have been used to create a mathematical model useful in predicting survival in patients with sclerosing cholangitis.[20] In stage 1, inflammation and fibrosis are confined to the portal triad. Portal tracts are visually enlarged, and portal edema may be present. Hepatic parenchymal changes are mild or absent. Stage 2 is characterized by periportal fibrosis with or without periportal hepatitis. Portal tracts are enlarged with intact, newly formed limiting plates. Blood vessels and bile ducts appear small in the enlarged portal tracts, and focal ductopenia may coexist in the same specimen with portal tracts with proliferating bile ducts.

Progression to stage 3 disease is characterized by portal-to-portal bridging with the formation of fibrous septae. Bile ducts are severely damaged or absent, and cholestatic changes are prominent in periportal and periseptal hepatocytes. Copper-protein complexes are present within lipolysosomes adjacent to the nucleus in damaged hepatocytes. Eventually, biliary cirrhosis (stage 4) develops with true nodular regeneration. In stage 4 the number of interlobular bile ducts is markedly decreased, and the histologic changes are difficult to distinguish from primary biliary cirrhosis. Only in the early stages of the disease, when fibrous obliterative cholangitis is present, can primary sclerosing cholangitis be reliably differentiated histologically from primary biliary cirrhosis.

Occasionally, inflammatory changes involving interlobular bile ducts are present in biopsies obtained from patients without large duct involvement on cholangiography.[25] These changes usually occur in patients with ulcerative colitis and an elevated serum alkaline phosphatase. The prognosis in these cases of small-duct sclerosing cholangitis (formerly called "pericholangitis") remains unclear.

Grossly, the extrahepatic biliary tree appears thickened and may be surrounded by inflammatory adhesions and enlarged lymph nodes. The duct wall may be up to eight times normal thickness on cross-section (Fig 64–1). Microscopically, the extrahepatic bile duct contains monotonous layers of connective tissue with a chronic inflammatory infiltrate.

■ ASSOCIATED DISEASES

INFLAMMATORY BOWEL DISEASE

Numerous diseases have been associated with sclerosing cholangitis (Table 64–3). The strongest association exists between inflammatory bowel disease, primarily ulcerative colitis, and sclerosing cholangitis. The incidence of ulcerative colitis in patients with sclerosing cholangitis ranges from 60% to 72% in most series.[23,26] In addition, Crohn's disease occurs in approximately 8% of patients with sclerosing cholangitis.[27] Aadland and associates diagnosed inflammatory bowel disease in all 45 patients with sclerosing cholangitis submitted to ileocolonoscopy and biopsy, suggesting that the incidence of inflammatory bowel disease may depend on how aggressively the diagnosis is sought.[28] Conversely, the prevalence of sclerosing cholangitis in patients with ulcerative colitis ranges from 2.5% to 7.5%.[27,29] Rabinovitz and associates have demonstrated a higher male/female ratio (2.3:1) in patients with both inflammatory bowel disease and primary sclerosing cholangitis compared to those patients with primary sclerosing cholangitis alone (0.7:1). The observation supports the idea that two subsets of primary sclerosing cholangitis patients exist: those with and those without inflammatory

TABLE 64–3. DISEASES ASSOCIATED WITH SCLEROSING CHOLANGITIS

Disease	Frequency
Ulcerative colitis	60% to 75%
Pancreatitis	15% to 25%
Cholangiocarcinoma	5% to 10%
Crohn's disease	5% to 10%
Diabetes mellitus	5% to 10%
Peptic ulcer disease	5% to 10%
Acquired immunodeficiency syndrome	Rare
Angioimmunoblastic lymphadenopathy	Rare
Histiocytosis X	Rare
Hypertrophic osteoarthropathy	Rare
Retroperitoneal fibrosis	Rare
Rheumatoid arthritis	Rare
Riedel's thyroiditis	Rare
Sarcoidosis	Rare
Sicca complex	Rare

bowel disease.[30] Similarly, ulcerative colitis patients with primary sclerosing cholangitis are more likely to be male than those without primary sclerosing cholangitis.[29]

Symptoms of ulcerative colitis usually predate the development of sclerosing cholangitis. However, primary sclerosing cholangitis may present before, concurrently with, or after the diagnosis of inflammatory bowel disease.[2] The activity of either disease does not affect the activity of the other. The extent of colitis may differ in ulcerative colitis patients with or without primary sclerosing cholangitis. Ulcerative colitis in patients with primary sclerosing cholangitis almost always involves the entire colon, whereas left-sided colitis is more common in patients without sclerosing cholangitis.[29] Nevertheless, the colitis may be mild or in remission for long periods in patients with primary sclerosing cholangitis.

Patients with both ulcerative colitis and primary sclerosing cholangitis also may be at a greater risk of developing colon cancer than those patients with ulcerative colitis alone. Broomé and associates followed 72 patients with ulcerative colitis with surveillance colonoscopy for 15 years.[31] Patients with DNA aneuploidy, dysplasia, and/or carcinoma on surveillance biopsies were significantly more likely to have primary sclerosing cholangitis (5 of 17) than patients without any dysplastic changes (0 of 55).[31] Using multivariate analysis, the presence of sclerosing cholangitis and the duration of the ulcerative colitis were independent risk factors associated with the development of dysplasia and/or DNA aneuploidy. Since the risk for colon cancer may be increased in patients with sclerosing cholangitis and the colitis may be present in an undiagnosed mild form, annual colonoscopic examination is recommended for all patients with both ulcerative colitis and sclerosing cholangitis.

Several features of the hepatobiliary disorder also may differ between patients with and those without ulcerative colitis. Patients with inflammatory bowel disease often are diagnosed at an asymptomatic stage (59% versus 29% in noninflammatory bowel disease patients) during an evaluation of abnormal liver function tests.[30] Several studies have demonstrated a difference in the distribution of the cholangiographic lesions with inflammatory bowel disease patients more likely to have involvement of the entire biliary tree.[30] In patients with ulcerative colitis, the risk of cholangiocarcinoma is increased 30-fold versus the general population. However, the risk of developing cholangiocarcinoma does not appear to be greater in sclerosing cholangitis patients with ulcerative colitis than in those without it.[30,32] Finally, the course and prognosis of the hepatobiliary disease is not influenced by the presence or absence of inflammatory bowel disease.[30]

The operative management of either the ulcerative colitis or the sclerosing cholangitis does not significantly alter the course of the other disease. Cangemi and associates followed 45 patients with ulcerative colitis, of whom 20 had undergone proctocolectomy and were unable to demonstrate any effect of proctocolectomy on the biochemical, histologic, or radiographic features of sclerosing cholangitis.[33] Therefore, proctocolectomy should be avoided, unless clearly indicated in patients with advanced liver disease, because of the troublesome occurrence of stomal variceal hemorrhage. Recently, ileal pouch–anal anastomosis has been performed safely in patients with concomitant ulcerative colitis and primary sclerosing cholangitis.[34] However, the incidence of perioperative bleeding complications and the long-term risk of pouchitis were higher in patients with sclerosing cholangitis. On the other hand, bleeding complications from stomal varices were avoided and were not common from the region of the ileoanal anastomosis.

Liver transplantation remains the only treatment for patients with cirrhosis secondary to sclerosing cholangitis. In the largest series of liver transplant for sclerosing cholangitis, the presence of inflammatory bowel disease decreased long-term survival slightly, although this decrease did not achieve statistical significance.[35] The chronic immunosuppression administered following liver transplant may improve the severity of the associated ulcerative colitis.[36] Finally, the long-term risk of colon cancer following liver transplant in patients with ulcerative colitis remains unclear.

CHOLANGIOCARCINOMA

Patients with sclerosing cholangitis are at increased risk of developing cholangiocarcinoma. Between 10% and 30% of patients undergoing liver transplant have un-

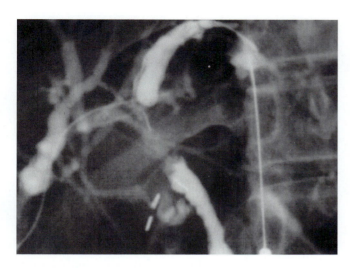

Figure 64–2. Cholangiogram demonstrating a perihilar cholangiocarcinoma in a patient with long-standing sclerosing cholangitis.

suspected cholangiocarcinoma in the hepatectomy specimen.[37,38] Patients who present with cholangiocarcinoma prior to liver transplant usually have a rapid deterioration in their clinical status with increasing jaundice, weight loss, and abdominal discomfort.[39]

In a series of 30 patients with cholangiocarcinoma complicating sclerosing cholangitis, <5% of the tumors were resectable for cure.[39] The median survival following the diagnosis of cholangiocarcinoma was only 5 months. The occurrence of cholangiocarcinoma was not related to the duration or the histological stage of the sclerosing cholangitis. Thirty percent of patients presented with both diseases simultaneously, and 71% of the cases of cholangiocarcinoma occurred before the progression of the sclerosing cholangitis to cirrhosis (stage 4).[39] The cancers were most often extrahepatic, and commonly occurred near the hepatic duct bifurcation (Fig 64–2). This site is also a common position for dominant benign strictures in primary sclerosing cholangitis, making the cholangiographic differentiation of benign and malignant lesions difficult.[22,39]

The anatomic distribution of these cancers, the presence of additional benign strictures, and the low sensitivity of imaging modalities in identifying these tumors all make early diagnosis very difficult. Recently, the use of serum and bile tumor markers has been shown to improve the early detection of cholangiocarcinoma in patients with primary sclerosing cholangitis.[40–42] The use of both serum carcinoembryonic antigen (CEA) and carbohydrate antigen 19-9 levels together has been shown to have a sensitivity of 66% and a specificity of 100% in diagnosing occult cholangiocarcinomas in patients with primary sclerosing cholangitis.[40] Nakeeb and associates have demonstrated that a biliary CEA level greater than 35 ng/mL resulted in a 79% sensitivity, a 100% specificity, and a 100% positive predictive value in differentiating sclerosing cholangitis and cholangiocarcinoma.[42]

■ NATURAL HISTORY

The natural history of patients with primary sclerosing cholangitis is highly variable, with some patients progressing rapidly to hepatic failure and others remaining asymptomatic for years. Predicting the prognosis of an individual patient is important in selecting a rational therapeutic approach. A number of studies have examined the natural history of sclerosing cholangitis in a large group of patients.

In a series of 174 patients from the Mayo Clinic, followed for a mean of 6 years, disease progression was noted in over 50% of patients.[43] Liver-related mortality was 31%, an additional 10% of patients underwent liver transplant, and 19% of patients developed cholangiocarcinoma. The median survival from the time of diagnosis was 11.9 years—significantly less than the age-matched United States population. In a subgroup of patients with asymptomatic sclerosing cholangitis reported separately, Porayko and associates demonstrated disease progression in 76% over a similar 75 month follow-up period.[44] Thirty-one percent of the asymptomatic patients developed liver failure resulting in death or referral for liver transplant. Similar rates of survival and progression to liver failure have been reported from King's College. In a group of 126 patients followed 70 months, 16% and 6% of the patients died of liver failure and cholangiocarcinoma, respectively, while 21% of the patients underwent liver transplant.[45] Median survival was 12 years.

Lower rates of disease progression and improved survival have been reported from several centers. Helzberg and associates documented progressive disease in only 17% of 42 patients followed for 56 months.[26] Liver-related mortality was only 12%, and only one patient received a liver transplant. Patients who were asymptomatic at presentation had a considerably improved survival when compared to symptomatic patients, after a 56 month follow-up. However, a recent larger series from this group has concluded that asymptomatic patients may have improved early survival, but that the long-term incidence of death or liver transplant is similar between symptomatic and asymptomatic patients.[46]

Predicting the survival of an individual patient from an analysis of larger series is difficult given the variability in disease progression. Several investigators have attempted to define variables that might improve the ability to predict survival.[43,45] In a recent multicenter survival analysis, Cox proportional-hazards regression was em-

TABLE 64–4. MAYO MODEL FOR SCLEROSING CHOLANGITIS

RISK SCORE (R)[a]

$R = (0.535 \times \log_e B) + (0.486 \times stage) + (0.041 \times age) + (0.705 \times M)$

SURVIVAL FUNCTION[b]

t(yr)	1	2	3	4	5	6	7
$S_0(t)$	0.951	0.915	0.871	0.844	0.779	0.752	0.741

[a]B = serum bilirubin (mg/dL), stage = histologic stage (see Table 64–2), age = age in years, M = presence (1) or absence (0) of splenomegaly

[b]$S_0(t)$ gives the estimated survival probabilities for a patient with risks core 3.326, which is the risk score of the average patient reported by Dickson and associates. To calculate the survival of a given patient, use the following equation: $S(t) = S_0(t)^{\exp(R-3.326)}$, where R is the risk score calculated above.

(Adapted from Dickson ER, Murtaugh PA, et al. Primary sclerosing cholangitis: refinement and validation of survival models. Gastroenterology 1992;103:1893)

ployed to identify the variables most useful in predicting survival in primary sclerosing cholangitis.[20] Serum bilirubin, histological stage on liver biopsy, age, and the presence of splenomegaly were independent predictors of a high risk of dying. A mathematical model to predict survival using these variables was created and validated (Table 64–4). This model may be useful in determining when patients should be activated for liver transplant or in evaluating the response of patients to other medical, radiologic, and/or resective therapies.[20,21]

■ DIAGNOSIS AND EVALUATION

The mean age at presentation for patients with primary sclerosing cholangitis ranges from 40 to 45 years of age.[20] Two-thirds of patients with primary sclerosing cholangitis are male, largely owing to the male predominance in patients with both ulcerative colitis and sclerosing cholangitis. Primary sclerosing cholangitis occurs in all races.

SIGNS AND SYMPTOMS

Patients present either with signs and symptoms of cholestatic liver disease or with abnormal serum liver function tests (Table 64–5). Approximately 75% of patients will be symptomatic at presentation.[26] The majority of these patients will have painless jaundice and pruritus.[20,26] Other common symptoms include right upper quadrant abdominal pain and fatigue. Symptoms of bacterial cholangitis (pain, fever, and jaundice) are uncommon, especially without preceding biliary tract manipulations. A small percentage of patients will present with signs and symptoms of advanced liver disease, including ascites, variceal bleeding, and/or splenomegaly.

A minority of patients will have abnormal serum biochemistries in the absence of other symptoms. Usually,

this situation occurs in patients being followed with inflammatory bowel disease. In this setting endoscopic retrograde cholangiopancreatography (ERCP) should be used to confirm the diagnosis of primary sclerosing cholangitis.

LABORATORY FINDINGS

Elevations of serum alkaline phosphatase and gamma glutamyl transferase are the most common laboratory findings and occur in essentially all patients with primary sclerosing cholangitis.[26] Serum alanine and aspartate aminotransferases also are modestly elevated in most patients. Serum bilirubin is less commonly elevated early in the course of sclerosing cholangitis. However, as the disease progresses, bilirubin levels often vary considerably. Serum albumin and prothrombin time are often normal until late in the course of the disease.

To date no specific serologic markers have proven useful in diagnosing sclerosing cholangitis. Tests for antinuclear antibody, antismooth muscle antibody, and antimitochondrial antibody are negative in the vast majority of patients.[26] Recently, antineutrophil nuclear antibodies have been detected in the sera of the majority of patients with both sclerosing cholangitis and ulcerative colitis.[11–13,47] However, the role of these antibodies in diagnosing primary sclerosing cholangitis remains unclear.

RADIOLOGIC FINDINGS

Primary sclerosing cholangitis is a cholangiographic diagnosis that is best made using ERCP. ERCP is technically easier than percutaneous methods in patients with sclerosing cholangitis owing to difficulties in percutaneously accessing the narrowed intrahepatic ducts. In addition, ERCP offers the advantage of visualizing the pancreatic duct.

Diffuse multifocal strictures are most commonly found in both the intrahepatic and extrahepatic bile ducts in patients with primary sclerosing cholangitis

TABLE 64–5. SYMPTOMS AND SIGNS IN PRIMARY SCLEROSING CHOLANGITIS

Symptom or Sign	Percent at Presentation
Jaundice	45 to 55
Pruritus	40 to 50
Pain	45 to 50
Weight loss	25 to 30
Anorexia	35 to 40
Cholangitis	20 to 25
Asymptomatic	20 to 25
Hepatomegaly	50 to 60
Splenomegaly	30 to 35

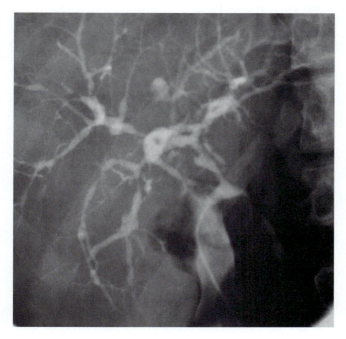

A

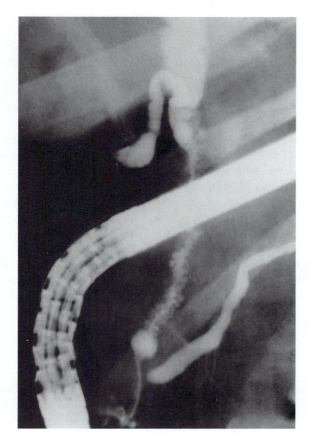

B

Figure 64–3. A. Cholangiogram demonstrating diffuse involvement of the intrahepatic and extrahepatic bile duct. **B.** Cholangiogram demonstrating sclerosing cholangitis confined to the common bile duct.

(Fig 64–3A).[1] Involvement of the extrahepatic ducts alone, without intrahepatic duct involvement, occurs in 5% to 10% of patients with primary sclerosing cholangitis (Fig 64–3B).[1,26] Strictures limited to the intrahepatic ducts are even less common, occurring in <5% of patients.[1] In addition, MacCarty and associates, in a series of 86 patients with primary sclerosing cholangitis, found disease limited to the intrahepatic and proximal extrahepatic ducts in just 20% of patients.[1] Despite the presence of diffuse disease in the majority of patients with sclerosing cholangitis, the hepatic duct bifurcation is often the most severely strictured segment of the biliary tree.[22,48] Cameron and associates found this anatomic pattern of ductal involvement in 24 of 36 patients undergoing hepatic bifurcation resection.[48] In addition, pancreatic duct abnormalities have been reported in 8% to 50% of patients with primary sclerosing cholangitis.[1,49]

Characteristic strictures are short (1 to 2 cm) and annular, alternating with normal caliber segments of bile duct to yield a "beaded" appearance on cholangiograms.[1] In advanced cases of primary sclerosing cholangitis, very long tapered confluent strictures occur, giving a pruned-tree appearance. Other typical findings include very short (1 to 2 mm) band-like strictures alternating with protruding, diverticulum-like outpouchings, usually in the extrahepatic bile duct.[1]

Ultrasound and computed tomography have not proven to be particularly useful in diagnosing sclerosing cholangitis. However, cholescintigraphy may be a noninvasive means of diagnosing sclerosing cholangitis. Technetium (Tc)-DISIDA scans demonstrate multiple hot spots corresponding to the areas of segmental dilatation between strictures, in patients with sclerosing cholangitis.[50] The degree of obstruction also can be estimated on the basis of the delay in hepatic clearance. Thus, cholescintigraphy may be a useful noninvasive means of monitoring the response to medical therapy.

DIFFERENTIAL DIAGNOSIS

The differential diagnosis of patients with sclerosing cholangitis includes all of the causes of cholestasis and bile duct obstruction. When the diagnosis is not clear, an ERCP should be performed. In most cases, the cholangiographic picture will be sufficiently clear to establish a diagnosis of sclerosing cholangitis. However, if the intrahepatic ducts are not adequately filled, the cholangiogram can be overinterpreted as representing sclerosing cholangitis. A significant problem can exist, however, in differentiating localized sclerosing cholangitis from cholangiocarcinoma, especially when the stricture is in the perihilar region. In these patients, resection with careful pathologic examination of the entire specimen may be necessary to establish a final diagnosis. Conversely, patients with cholangiocarcinoma and bacterial cholangitis may have a cholangiographic picture that mimics sclerosing cholangitis. Again, resection of the dominant stricture may be necessary to establish a diagnosis.

■ MANAGEMENT

MEDICAL MANAGEMENT

Medical therapy for primary sclerosing cholangitis has been disappointing, to date. To be effective, medical therapy must be instituted early in the course of the disease, prior to the development of cirrhosis or extensive bile duct destruction. The prolonged course of the disease, characterized by spontaneous remissions and exacerbations, makes the evaluation of efficacy of a drug difficult.[51] Most agents examined to date in randomized trials have been either anti-inflammatory or immunosuppressive drugs. Corticosteroids, penicillamine, azathioprine, and colchicine all have proven to be ineffective in the management of primary sclerosing cholangitis.[51,52] Initial results of a randomized trial comparing cyclosporine to placebo also have demonstrated no beneficial therapeutic effect for cyclosporine in this disease.[53] On the other hand, recent trials of ursodeoxycholate and methotrexate have demonstrated some encouraging results.[54,55]

Ursodeoxycholate has been examined in several trials in patients with primary sclerosing cholangitis. O'Brien and associates administered 10 mg/kg/day of ursodeoxycholate to 12 patients during 30 months and demonstrated significant decreases in serum alkaline phosphatase, gamma glutamyl transferase, alanine aminotransferase, and aspartate aminotransferase.[54] Symptoms of pruritus and fatigue improved although not significantly. Beuers and associates randomly allocated 14 patients to ursodeoxycholate (13 to 15 mg/kg/day) or placebo and reported similar biochemical improvements.[56] Despite the decrease in biochemical parameters, no symptomatic improvement occurred, and no significant improvement in posttreatment histologic score was identified. Ursodeoxycholate also has been reported to have improved the cholangiographic appearance of multiple intrahepatic strictures in at least one case of sclerosing cholangitis.[57] Unfortunately, the histologic progression to cirrhosis was not reversed in this case.

Low-dose methotrexate also has been shown to decrease serum alkaline phosphatase, alanine transferase, and aspartate aminotransferase.[55] In addition, symptomatic improvement occurred in 6 of 10 patients treated with methotrexate. A decrease in the histologic activity index also was seen with methotrexate in seven of nine patients undergoing liver biopsy. However, a randomized placebo-controlled trial of methotrexate failed to demonstrate any improvement in liver histology, cholangiographic appearance, or outcome in patients taking methotrexate.[58]

Despite encouraging initial results with ursodeoxycholate, the long-term effect in patients with primary sclerosing cholangitis remains unknown. Longer trials are necessary before it will be known whether initial biochemical improvements will translate into a delay in the progression of the inflammatory bile duct injury to cirrhosis.

■ NONOPERATIVE INTERVENTION

ENDOSCOPIC BALLOON DILATATION

Dominant extrahepatic and hilar strictures can be managed endoscopically with balloon dilatation and stenting. Lee and associates reported 53 patients with sclerosing cholangitis in whom endoscopic dilatation of biliary strictures was attempted.[59] Endoscopic sphincterotomy was performed and strictures were dilated with an 8 mm balloon and a stent was left in for three months, if the dilatation was not dramatically effective. The procedure was technically possible in 86% of the patients. However, after a mean follow-up of 31 months, only 56% of the patients had improvement in their symptoms, and cholangiograms improved in only 36% of them.

A similar approach also has been reported by Johnson et al.[60] Thirty-five symptomatic jaundiced patients with primary sclerosing cholangitis were managed with endoscopic dilatation. The endoscopic dilatation then was repeated at 6 months and annually thereafter. An endoprosthesis were inserted in 11 of 35 patients in whom residual strictures were present after dilatation. Mean serum bilirubin fell from 10 mg/dL pretreatment to 4 mg/dL after balloon dilatation and remained constant for the duration of follow-up (mean 24 months). Complications included hemorrhage, pancreatitis, and cholangitis. Three patients died during follow-up, including one patient with cholangiocarcinoma.

The endoscopic dilatation of extrahepatic and hilar strictures in primary sclerosing cholangitis offers several advantages over operative and percutaneous methods.[60] Endoscopic dilatation can be performed under intravenous sedation without a general anaesthetic at the time of the initial diagnostic procedure and avoids an operative dissection of the porta hepatis prior to hepatic transplantation. Both the right and left hepatic ducts may be approached simultaneously via the endoscopic route. In addition, external stents are not necessary after the endoscopic procedure. Although early re-

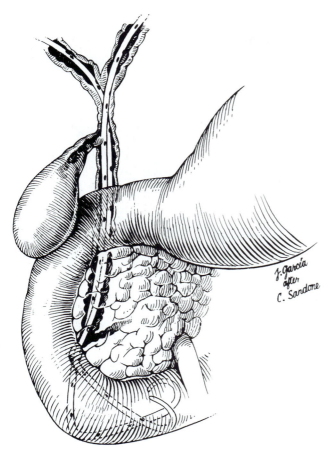

Figure 64–4. Management of sclerosing cholangitis with percutaneous transhepatic Ring catheters. (From Cameron JL. *Atlas of Surgery*, vol 1. Philadelphia, PA: BC Decker; 1990)

sults appear promising, longer follow-up is necessary before endoscopic results can be compared with the results of operative biliary decompression.

PERCUTANEOUS BALLOON DILATATION

Dilatation of biliary strictures associated with primary sclerosing cholangitis also can be performed percutaneously (Fig 64–4). Intrahepatic strictures can be dilated after percutaneous transhepatic cholangiography; however, this approach may be less effective than endoscopic dilatation. Mueller and associates reported 17 patients followed three years after a single session of percutaneous balloon dilatation of biliary strictures in sclerosing cholangitis.[62] Recurrent jaundice occurred in 58% of these patients. The percutaneous approach also may be beneficial both preoperatively as well as following surgical resection of the extrahepatic biliary tree. Recurrent intrahepatic or anastomotic strictures can be percutaneously dilated at the time of transhepatic stent change.

■ OPERATIVE MANAGEMENT

Traditionally, the operative management of patients with primary sclerosing cholangitis included cholecystectomy, operative cholangiography, choledochotomy, common bile duct dilatation, and placement of a T tube for long-term biliary drainage.[6] Currently, the diagnosis is made nonoperatively with ERCP, and the initial management is often with ursodeoxycholate or endoscopic dilatation. Patients who remain symptomatic with persistent jaundice, despite endoscopic attempts at balloon dilatation, are candidates for surgical therapy. A liver biopsy should be obtained preoperatively and is useful in guiding therapy.[22] If cirrhosis is present, the patient should become a candidate for hepatic transplantation. If cirrhosis is not present and a dominant extrahepatic stricture is present, the patient should be considered for resection of the hepatic duct bifurcation and the placement of transhepatic biliary stents. In addition, patients in whom a cholangiocarcinoma can not be excluded also should be explored.

SURGICAL RESECTION

Most patients with primary sclerosing cholangitis have involvement of both the intrahepatic and extrahepatic biliary tree. However, a significant proportion of patients have a dominant hilar stricture or primary involvement of the extrahepatic bile ducts. In 1983, Cameron and associates reported 11 patients managed with resection of the extrahepatic biliary tree, including the bifurcation, dilatation of the left and right hepatic ducts, and prolonged transhepatic stenting with Silastic catheters.[63] Ten of these patients had persistent jaundice preoperatively (mean bilirubin 15.3 mg/dL), and all 11 had narrowing at the hepatic duct bifurcation. One patient died postoperatively, and 9 of the 10 patients responded with a decrease in serum bilirubin to 2.9 mg/dL. Since 1980, this approach has been used at the Johns Hopkins Hospital to manage 50 patients with primary sclerosing cholangitis and persistent jaundice (bilirubin greater than 5 mg/dL for 3 months) or recurrent cholangitis.[22,64,65]

Preoperatively, Ring catheters are inserted percutaneously into both the left and right hepatic ducts. These catheters are not used solely for preoperative biliary drainage, but also to aid the surgeon in identifying the left and right hepatic ducts intraoperatively. Patients are explored through either a midline or a right subcostal incision.[61] The abdomen is thoroughly explored to exclude the presence of a disseminated cholangiocarcinoma. A cholecystectomy is performed to improve access to the hepatic duct bifurcation and to prevent the development of acute cholecystitis associated with a chronic indwelling stent. Next, the

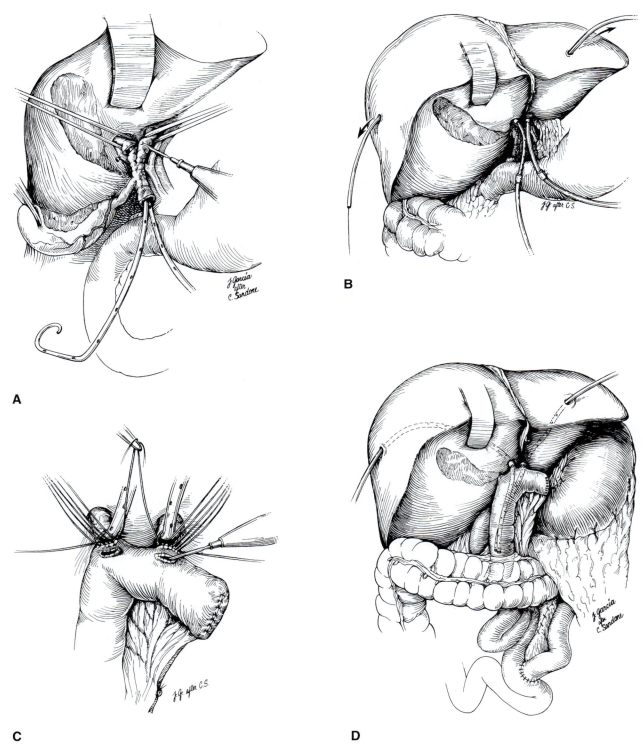

Figure 64–5. A. Resection of extrahepatic bile ducts and gallbladder. Note the preoperatively placed transhepatic stents. **B.** Passage of progressively larger Coudé catheters over guidewires. **C.** Bilateral hepaticojejunostomies with transhepatic stents. **D.** Completed, retrocolic Roux-en-Y hepaticojejunostomies with stents in place. (From Cameron JL. *Atlas of Surgery*, vol 1. Philadelphia, PA: BC Decker; 1990)

distal common bile duct is encircled with a vessel loop and then divided (Fig 64–5A). The distal common duct stump then is closed with interrupted 3-0 silk sutures.

The extrahepatic biliary tree then is dissected off the portal vein and hepatic artery by reflecting the bile duct and Ring catheters in a cephalad direction. Once the bifurcation is reached, the left and right hepatic ducts are easily identified by palpating the Ring catheters. Once dissected free, the left and right hepatic ducts are encircled and divided removing the extrahepatic biliary tree and hepatic duct bifurcation from the operative field.

Next, the intrahepatic biliary tree is dilated by suturing progressively larger Coudé catheters to the Ring catheters and withdrawing them out of the top of the liver (Fig 64–5B). A 12-French (Fr) catheter initially is sutured to the 8.3-Fr Ring catheter and pulled up into the intrahepatic biliary tree. A 14-Fr Coudé catheter is then sutured to the 12-Fr catheter, followed by a 14- to 16-Fr Coudé catheter and finally, the 16- or 18-Fr Silastic transhepatic stent. The dilatation is performed over a guidewire so that in case a catheter or suture breaks the track is not lost.

Transhepatic catheters are placed in both the right and left hepatic ducts in most patients. A Roux-en-Y jejunal loop then is constructed and passed in a retrocolic position into the subhepatic space. Bilateral hepaticojejunostomies then are constructed using interrupted 4-0 absorbable suture (Fig 64–5C). The transhepatic Silastic catheters extend 15 cm into the jejunum and are positioned so that the side holes are present in both the intrahepatic and jejunal portions of the catheter (Fig 64–5D). Closed-suction drains are positioned adjacent to the hepaticojejunostomies and in the subphrenic space.

Cameron and associates managed 31 patients with sclerosing cholangitis using the above approach.[22] Operative mortality was 9.7% overall, but only 3.7% in the noncirrhotic patients. Serum bilirubin fell from 9.9 mg/dL preoperatively to 3.4 mg/dL 12 months after the procedure. At 5 years, mean serum bilirubin remained low at 4.3 mg/dL. Actuarial 5 year survival was 77% in the noncirrhotic patients. Two of the twenty-six initially noncirrhotic patients have undergone subsequent liver transplant for progressive hepatic failure. Four of the five cirrhotic patients died during the follow-up period while one underwent liver transplant and was alive 80 months after her initial biliary reconstruction.

More recently, 146 patients with primary sclerosing cholangitis managed with operative resection, endoscopic dilatation, percutaneous stenting, and/or liver transplant have been reported from the Johns Hopkins Hospital.[64,65] Patients managed with resection and with

TABLE 64–6. OVERALL SURVIVAL BY TREATMENT METHOD

	n	Risk score	Actuarial Survival in Years (%)		
			1 year	3 year	5 year
All patients					
Surgical Resection	50	3.75 ± 0.15	86	84	76
Endoscopic Dilatation	35	3.66 ± 0.24	91	80	68
Percutaneous Stenting	19	4.08 ± 0.39	84	79	60
Combined nonoperative	54	3.80 ± 0.20	86	76	64
Liver transplant	21	5.28 ± 0.15	81	81	—
All patients	138	3.74 ± 0.13	86	81	71
Noncirrhotic patients					
Surgical Resection	40	3.36 ± 0.12	95	92	85
Endoscopic Dilatation	26	3.13 ± 0.27	88	72[a]	58[a]
Percutaneous Stenting	17	3.59 ± 0.28	87	79	63
Combined nonoperative	43	3.27 ± 0.21	87	74[b]	59[b]
Liver transplant	1	3.34 ± 0.00	100	—	—
Cirrhotic patients					
Surgical Resection	10	5.11 ± 0.17	50	38	38
Endoscopic Dilatation	9	4.73 ± 0.19	100	100	—
Percutaneous Stenting	2	6.05 ± 0.17	50	—	—
Combined nonoperative	11	4.95 ± 0.20	92	92	—
Liver transplant	20	5.30 ± 0.15	80	80	—

[a] p<0.01 versus resection
[b] p<0.05 versus resection
(Adapted from Ahrendt SA, Pitt HA, et al. Primary sclerosing cholangitis: resect, dilate or transplant? Gastroenterology 1995;108:A1211 and Ahrendt SA, Pitt HA, et al. Management of primary sclerosing cholangitis in the 1990s. Hepatology 1995;22:107A)

nonoperative dilatation or stenting had similar risk scores before treatment.[20] Overall survival was significantly longer in the noncirrhotic patients with primary sclerosing cholangitis managed with surgical resection than in the group of patients managed nonoperatively (Table 64–6).[64,65] Similarly, patients without cirrhosis managed with resection survived significantly longer before needing a liver transplant than patients managed nonoperatively (Table 64–7).[64,65]

HEPATIC TRANSPLANTATION

Primary sclerosing cholangitis is a progressive disease that eventually results in biliary cirrhosis. Once cirrhosis develops, nonoperative biliary dilatations or operative resection have little role in patient management and are associated with high morbidity and mortality.[22,64] Complications of portal hypertension, such as variceal bleeding, ascites, hepatic encephalopathy, and recurrent cholangitis, are clear indications for liver transplantation. The operative mortality of liver transplantation can be improved significantly by transplanting patients prior to the development of the life-threatening complications of end-stage liver disease. Several prognostic models have been developed to help predict which patients with primary sclerosing cholangitis are likely to have

TABLE 64–7. TRANSPLANT-FREE SURVIVAL BY TREATMENT METHOD[a]

	n	Risk score	Actuarial Survival in Years (%)		
			1 year	3 year	5 year
ALL PATIENTS					
Surgical Resection	50	3.75 ± 0.15	86	81	71
Endoscopic Dilatation	35	3.66 ± 0.24	76	55[c]	36[b]
Percutaneous Stenting	19	4.08 ± 0.39	84	61	49
Combined nonoperative	54	3.80 ± 0.20	78	57[c]	40[b]
Liver transplant	21	5.28 ± 0.15	81	81	—
NONCIRRHOTIC PATIENTS					
Surgical Resection	40	3.36 ± 0.12	95	92	82
Endoscopic Dilatation	26	3.13 ± 0.27	83	56[b]	42[b]
Percutaneous Stenting	17	3.59 ± 0.28	87	64[c]	51[c]
Combined nonoperative	43	3.27 ± 0.21	85	59[b]	46[b]
Liver transplant	1	3.34 ± 0.00	100	—	—
CIRRHOTIC PATIENTS					
Surgical Resection	10	5.11 ± 0.17	50	38	25
Endoscopic Dilatation	9	4.73 ± 0.19	56	56	—
Percutaneous Stenting	2	6.05 ± 0.17	50	—	—
Combined nonoperative	11	4.95 ± 0.20	58	47	—
Liver transplant	20	5.30 ± 0.15	80	80	—

[a]Data adapted from Ahrendt, et al. [64,65]
[b]$p < 0.01$ versus resection
[c]$p < 0.05$ versus resection

rapidly progressive disease in order to assist in selecting them for liver transplant.[21,43]

Survival following orthotopic liver transplant for primary sclerosing cholangitis is similar to that following liver transplant for other causes of end-stage liver disease.[66] In the combined University of Pittsburgh and Mayo Clinic experience, actuarial 1 and 5 year survival were 86% and 73%, respectively.[35] The survival following transplant exceeded the predicted survival without transplant, using the Mayo model, at 6 months and continued to surpass it throughout the 5 year follow-up period.[35] Patients who had had previous portal and/or biliary tract surgery do not have increased hospital mortality, but they tend to have a lower 5 year survival following transplantation, although this difference did not achieve statistical significance.[35,67]

The development of cholangiocarcinoma prior to liver transplantation significantly affects long-term outcome. Unsuspected cholangiocarcinoma was present in 11 of 216 hepatectomy specimens in the largest series to date of liver transplantation for sclerosing cholangitis.[35] Survival in this group of 11 patients was only 47% at 2 years.[35] Preoperative diagnosis of cholangiocarcinoma prior to liver transplantation remains difficult because endoscopic brushings for cytology have a low yield.[68] A concomitant cholangiocarcinoma should be suspected in patients with a rapid onset of persistent jaundice, pruritus, and weight loss associated with a marked rise in the serum bilirubin and alkaline phosphatase immediately prior to transplantation.[69] Cholangiography also may demonstrate dilated intrahepatic ducts with an associated cholangiocarcinoma.[69]

The incidence of recurrent primary sclerosing cholangitis following liver transplantation remains unclear. Several cases of histological changes similar to sclerosing cholangitis have been reported in transplanted livers.[66,70] However, similar changes have been observed during graft rejection.[66] Longer follow-up will be required before the true incidence of recurrent primary sclerosing cholangitis is known, but it does not appear to affect early survival following liver transplantation.

REFERENCES

1. MacCarty RL, LaRusso NF, et al. Primary sclerosing cholangitis: findings on cholangiography and pancreatography. *Radiology* 1983;149:39
2. Chapman RW. Etiology and natural history of primary sclerosing cholangitis: a decade of progress? *Gut* 1991;32:1433
3. Chapman RW, Varghese Z, et al. Association of primary sclerosing cholangitis with HLA B8. *Gut* 1983;24:316
4. Schrumpf E, Fausa O, et al. HLA antigens and immunoregulatory T cells in ulcerative colitis associated with hepatobiliary disease. *Scand J Gastroenterol* 1982;17:187

5. Prochazka EJ, Terasaki PI, et al. Association of primary sclerosing cholangitis with HLA- DRw52a. *N Engl J Med* 1990;322:1842

6. Lillemoe KD, Pitt HA, et al. Primary sclerosing cholangitis. *Surg Clin North Am* 1990;70:1381

7. Lindor KD, Wiesner RH, et al. Lymphocyte subsets in primary sclerosing cholangitis. *Dig Dis Sci* 1987;32:720

8. Whiteside TL, Lasky S, et al. Immunologic analysis of mononuclear cells in liver tissues and blood in patients with primary sclerosing cholangitis. *Hepatology* 1985;5:468

9. Chapman RW, Kelly PMA, et al. Expression of HLA-DR antigens on bile duct epithelium in primary sclerosing cholangitis. *Gut* 1988;29:422

10. Bodenheimer HCJ, LaRusso NF, et al. Elevated circulating immune complexes in primary sclerosing cholangitis. *Hepatology* 1983;3:150

11. Snook JA, Chapman RW, et al. Antineutrophil nuclear antibody in ulcerative colitis, Crohn's disease and primary sclerosing cholangitis. *Clin Exp Immunol* 1989;76:30

12. Seibold F, Weber P, et al. Clinical significance of antibodies against neutrophils in patients with inflammatory bowel disease and primary sclerosing cholangitis. *Gut* 1992;33:657

13. Klein R, Eisenburg J, et al. Significance and specificity of antibodies to neutrophils detected by Western blotting for the serological diagnosis of primary sclerosing cholangitis. *Hepatology* 1991;14:1147

14. Thompson HH, Pitt HA, et al. Primary sclerosing cholangitis: a heterogeneous disease. *Ann Surg* 1982;196:127

15. Forbes A, Blanshard C, et al. Natural history of AIDS related sclerosing cholangitis: a study of 20 cases. *Gut* 1993;34:116

16. Cello JP. Acquired immunodeficiency syndrome cholangiopathy: spectrum of disease. *Am J Med* 1989;86:539

17. Teres J, Gomez-Moli J, et al. Sclerosing cholangitis after surgical treatment of hepatic echinococcal cysts: report of three cases. *Am J Surg* 1984;148:694

18. Kemeny MM, Battifora H, et al. Sclerosing cholangitis after continuous hepatic artery infusion of FUDR. *Ann Surg* 1985;202:176

19. Demetris AJ, Lasky S, et al. Pathology of hepatic transplantation: a review of 62 adult allograft recipients immunosuppressed with a cyclosporine/steroid regimen. *Am J Pathol* 1985;118:151

20. Dickson ER, Murtaugh PA, et al. Primary sclerosing cholangitis: refinement and validation of survival models. *Gastroenterology* 1992;103:1893

21. Wiesner RH, Porayko MK, et al. Selection and timing of liver transplantation in primary biliary cirrhosis and primary sclerosing cholangitis. *Hepatology* 1992;16:1290

22. Cameron JL, Pitt HA, et al. Resection of hepatic duct bifurcation and transhepatic stenting for sclerosing cholangitis. *Ann Surg* 1988;207:614

23. Chapman RW, Arborgh BA, et al. Primary sclerosing cholangitis: a review of its clinical features, cholangiography and hepatic histology. *Gut* 1980;21:870

24. Ludwig J, Barham SS, et al. Morphologic features of chronic hepatitis associated with primary sclerosing cholangitis and chronic ulcerative colitis. *Hepatology* 1981;1:632

25. Ludwig J. Small-duct primary sclerosing cholangitis. *Semin Liver Dis* 1991;11:11

26. Helzberg JH, Petersen JM, Boyer JL. Improved survival with primary sclerosing cholangitis: a review of clinicopathologic features and comparison of symptomatic and asymptomatic patients. *Gastroenterology* 1987;92:1869

27. Fausa O, Schrumpf E, et al. Relationship of inflammatory bowel disease and primary sclerosing cholangitis. *Semin Liver Dis* 1991;11:31

28. Aadland E, Schrumpf E, et al. Primary sclerosing cholangitis: a long-term follow-up study. *Scand J Gastroenterol* 1987;22:655

29. Olsson R, Danielsson A, et al. Prevalence of primary sclerosing cholangitis in patients with ulcerative colitis. *Gastroenterology* 1991;100:1319

30. Rabinovitz M, Gavaler JS, et al. Does primary sclerosing cholangitis occurring in association with inflammatory bowel disease differ from that occurring in the absence of inflammatory bowel disease? A study of sixty-six subjects. *Hepatology* 1990;11:7

31. Broomé U, Lindberg G, Löfberg R. Primary sclerosing cholangitis in ulcerative colitis—a risk factor for the development of dysplasia and DNA aneuploidy? *Gastroenterology* 1992;102:1877

32. Rosen CB, Nagorney DM. Cholangiocarcinoma complicating primary sclerosing cholangitis. *Semin Liver Dis* 1991;11:26

33. Cangemi JR, Wiesner RH, et al. Effect of proctocolectomy for chronic ulcerative colitis on the natural history of primary sclerosing cholangitis. *Gastroenterology* 1989;96:790

34. Kartheuser AH, Dozois RR, et al. Complications and risk factors after ileal pouch-anal anastomosis for ulcerative colitis associated with primary sclerosing cholangitis. *Ann Surg* 1993;217:314

35. Abu-Elmagd KM, Malinchoc M, et al. Efficacy of hepatic transplantation in patients with primary sclerosing cholangitis. *Surg Gynecol Obstet* 1993;177:335

36. Gavaler JS, Delemos B, et al. Ulcerative colitis disease activity as subjectively assessed by patient-completed questionnaires following orthotopic liver transplantation for sclerosing cholangitis. *Dig Dis Sci* 1991;36:321

37. Abu-Elmagd KM, Selby R, et al. Cholangiocarcinoma and sclerosing cholangitis: clinical characteristics and effect on survival after liver transplantation. *Transplant Proc* 1993;25:1124

38. Farges O, Malassagne B, et al. Primary sclerosing cholangitis: liver transplantation or biliary surgery. *Surgery* 1995;117:146

39. Rosen CR, Nagorney DM, et al. Cholangiocarcinoma complicating primary sclerosing cholangitis. *Ann Surg* 1991;213:21

40. Ramage JK, Donaghy A, et al. Serum tumor markers for the diagnosis of cholangiocarcinoma in primary sclerosing cholangitis. *Gastroenterology* 1995;108:865

41. Nichols JC, Gores GJ, et al. Diagnostic role of serum CA 19-9 for cholangiocarcinoma in patients with primary sclerosing cholangitis. *Mayo Clin Proc* 1993;68:874

42. Nakeeb A, Fox-Talbot K, et al. Biliary CEA levels are a marker for cholangiocarcinoma. *Am J Surg* 1996;171:147

43. Wiesner RH, Grambsch PM, et al. Primary sclerosing cholangitis: natural history, prognostic factors, and survival analysis. *Hepatology* 1989;10:430

44. Porayko MK, Weisner RH, et al. Patients with asymptomatic primary sclerosing cholangitis frequently have progressive disease. *Gastroenterology* 1990;98:1594

45. Farrant JM, Hayllar KM, et al. Natural history and prognostic variables in primary sclerosing cholangitis. *Gastroenterology* 1991;100:1710

46. Fiarman G, Garcia-Tsao, et al. Primary sclerosing cholangitis, a follow-up study of the Yale experience. *Hepatology* 1993;18:212A

47. Chapman RW. Role of immune factors in the pathogenesis of primary sclerosing cholangitis. *Semin Liver Dis* 1991;11:1

48. Cameron JL, Gayler BW, et al. Sclerosing cholangitis. Anatomical distribution of obstructive lesions. *Ann Surg* 1984;200:54

49. Muller EL, Miyamoto T, et al. Anatomy of the choledochopancreatic duct junction in primary sclerosing cholangitis. *Surgery* 1985;97:21

50. Ament AE, Bick RJ, et al. Sclerosing cholangitis. Cholescintigraphy with Tc-99m-labeled DISIDA. *Radiology* 1984;151:197

51. Kaplan MM. Medical approaches to primary sclerosing cholangitis. *Semin Liver Dis* 1991;11:56

52. LaRusso NF, Wiesner RH, et al. Prospective trial of penicillamine in primary sclerosing cholangitis. *Gastroenterology* 1988;95:1036

53. Wiesner RH, Steiner B, et al. A controlled trial evaluating cyclosporine in the treatment of primary sclerosing cholangitis. *Hepatology* 1991;14:63A

54. O'Brien CB, Senior JR, et al. Ursodeoxycholic acid for the treatment of primary sclerosing cholangitis: a 30-month pilot study. *Hepatology* 1991;14:838

55. Kaplan MM, Arora S, et al. Primary sclerosing cholangitis and low-dose oral pulse methotrexate therapy. *Ann Intern Med* 1987;106:231

56. Beuers U, Spenger U, et al. Ursodeoxycholic acid for treatment of primary sclerosing cholangitis: a placebo-controlled trial. *Hepatology* 1992;16:707

57. Lebovics E, Salama M, et al. Resolution of radiographic abnormalities with ursodeoxycholic acid therapy of primary sclerosing cholangitis. *Gastroenterology* 1992;102:2143

58. Knox T, Kaplan MM. A double-blind controlled trial of oral-pulse methotrexate therapy in the treatment of primary sclerosing cholangitis. *Gastroenterology* 1994;106:494–499

59. Lee JG, Schutz SM, et al. Endoscopic therapy of sclerosing cholangitis. *Hepatology* 1995;21:661

60. Johnson GK, Geenen JE, et al. Endoscopic treatment of biliary tract strictures in sclerosing cholangitis: a larger series and recommendations for treatment. *Gastrointest Endosc* 1991;37:38

61. Cameron JL. *Atlas of Surgery,* vol 1. Philadelphia, PA: BC Decker: 1990

62. Mueller PR, vanSonnenberg E, et al. Biliary stricture dilatation: multicenter review of clinical management of 73 patients. *Radiology* 1986;160:17

63. Cameron JL, Gayler BW, et al. Sclerosing cholangitis: biliary reconstruction with Silastic transhepatic stents. *Surgery* 1983;94:324

64. Ahrendt SA, Pitt HA, et al. Primary sclerosing cholangitis: resect, dilate, or transplant? *Gastroenterology* 1995;108:A1211

65. Ahrendt SA, Pitt HA, et al. Management of primary sclerosing cholangitis in the 1990s. *Hepatology* 1995;22:107A

66. Marsh JW, Iwatsuki S, et al. Orthotopic liver transplantation for primary sclerosing cholangitis. *Ann Surg* 1988;207:21

67. Narumi S, Roberts JP, et al. Liver transplantation for sclerosing cholangitis. *Hepatology* 1995;22:451

68. Strasser S, Sheil AGR, et al. Liver transplantation for primary sclerosing cholangitis versus primary biliary cirrhosis: a comparison of complications and outcome. *J Gastrohepatol* 1993;8:238

69. Miros M, Kerlin P, et al. Predicting cholangiocarcinoma in patients with primary sclerosing cholangitis before transplantation. *Gut* 1991;32:1369

70. Shaked A, Colonna JO, et al. The interrelation between sclerosing cholangitis and ulcerative colitis in patients undergoing liver transplantation. *Ann Surg* 1992;215:598

65

Benign Biliary Strictures

J.B. Matthews ■ *Leslie H. Blumgart*

Benign stenosis and strictures of the bile ducts occur in a number of conditions and may affect the intrahepatic or extrahepatic biliary tree. They may be single or multiple. Table 65–1 details the causes of benign bile duct strictures.

Imprecise treatment is associated with disastrous results, but early recognition and correct management can lead to a successful outcome with a good prognosis.

■ BILE DUCT INJURIES

Injury to the bile ducts may follow damage inflicted during upper abdominal operations or may be the result of blunt or penetrating abdominal injury. Injuries occurring during surgical operations are important, first, because they are preventable and second, because they increase mortality and morbidity rates far in excess of those recognized for the initial surgical procedure. The results may be particularly tragic because many of the patients so afflicted are young and in the most productive years of life.

Repair must be carried out in a precise and expert manner *at the first attempt,* because repeated operative intervention is associated with less satisfactory results.

POSTOPERATIVE BILE DUCT STRICTURES

Injuries to the main ducts are nearly always the result of misadventures during operation and are therefore a serious reproach to the surgical profession. They cannot be regarded as just an ordinary risk . . ., though I know only too well that even with all the care which may reasonably be expected of us, accidents will occasionally happen.[1]

It is impossible to be accurate regarding the incidence of operative injury to the biliary tract. The risk of injury varies with the operation being performed, and with the exception of injury at cholecystectomy, there are no studies that reflect the frequency of such damage. Many injuries are not reported at all or are not detected, the patient's ultimate illness being ascribed to some other cause, such as cholangiocarcinoma or sclerosing cholangitis, or to some other complication.

Although the great majority of injuries to the bile duct occur during cholecystectomy, with or without exploration of the common bile duct, a number also occur in association with other operations on either the stomach, the pancreas, or the liver, or during surgery for portal hypertension. Stricture of biliary-enteric anastomoses after reconstructive or bypass surgery in association with other operations, for example, pancreatico-duodenectomy, also occur. It is important that such strictures are not misinterpreted as recurrent carcinoma. In addition to injury to a normal biliary tree, damage also may follow operations performed on the diseased biliary tract, such as after excision of a choledochus cyst and after operation for the management of sclerosing cholangitis. Indeed, an abnormal bile duct may be injured during cholecystectomy, the pathologic state of the bile duct being unrecognized.

TABLE 65–1. CAUSES OF BENIGN BILE DUCT STRICTURES

I. Congenital strictures, biliary atresia[a]
II. Bile duct injuries
   A. Postoperative bile duct strictures
      1. Cholecystectomy and exploration of the common bile duct/
         laparoscopic cholecystectomy
      2. Other operative procedures
         Biliary enteric anastomosis of previously normal bile duct
         Operations on liver or portal vein
         Pancreatic operations
         Gastrectomy
         Variety of other operations, if any
   B. Stricture after blunt or penetrating injury
III. Postinflammatory strictures associated with:
   A. Cholelithiasis/Choledocholithiasis
   B. Chronic pancreatitis
   C. Chronic duodenal ulcer
   D. Abscess or inflammation in subhepatic region or in the liver
   E. Parasitic infection
   F. Recurrent pyogenic cholangitis
IV. Primary sclerosing cholangitis
V. Radiation-induced stricture
VI. Papillary stenosis[a]

[a]Not discussed in this chapter.

POSTCHOLECYSTECTOMY INJURIES

Unfortunately, injuries to the bile ducts are not rare and often turn out to be tragedies.[1]

Cholecystectomy is probably the most commonly performed elective abdominal operation and has a high degree of safety. The surgical mortality rate is <0.5% in patients younger than 65 years of age, although it is higher in elderly patients undergoing emergency operation and in patients with coincident disease. When exploration of the common bile duct is required, the mortality rate is higher, especially in the presence of jaundice or cholangitis. Nevertheless, it is important to remember that *cholecystectomy is a major operation* and should never be undertaken lightly. With the introduction of laparoscopic cholecystectomy, this concept is even more important because of the learning curve in mastering this procedure. Of those patients with continuing problems, only 5% will have severe symptoms such as jaundice, pancreatitis, or cholangitis, and a minority of patients will suffer damage to the biliary tree. Figures are available from studies carried out in Sweden, Finland, Germany, and France, and all suggest that the incidence of biliary injury is roughly 2 per 1000 open operations for gallstones. Kune and Sali suggested that the incidence is approximately 1 in 300 to 500 gallstone operations.[2] However, a series of 1200 consecutive open cholecystectomies from a major urban academic center, performed in the years immediately prior to the introduction of laparoscopic surgery, reported only two ductal injuries.[3]

Laparoscopic cholecystectomy is now established and is replacing the traditional open operation as the technique of choice for elective and, in selected patients, emergency operations.[4] The reported risk of bile duct injury with this approach appears to be considerably higher compared with historical series, in the order of 1 per 100 to 200 operations.[5] As experience with this technique grows and understanding of the mechanisms of injury accrues,[6] the risk of bile duct injury might be expected to decrease; however, with the increasingly liberal application of laparoscopic cholecystectomy for the more difficult, acutely inflamed gallbladder, the overall frequency of iatrogenic damage may not significantly change or may even increase. It has been predicted that the revolutionary technological advances made in gallbladder surgery over the past five years will be accompanied by a wave of new cases of iatrogenic biliary stricture.[6–8]

CAUSATIVE FACTORS AND PREVENTION

A number of factors relate to bile duct injury during cholecystectomy.

Anatomic Variations

There are a wide number of anatomic variations in the extrahepatic biliary tree and in the adjacent hepatic arteries and portal vein. These variations are so frequent that the surgeon must be acquainted with their range and should always expect the unusual.

The most common variation is in the junction between the cystic duct and the main biliary channel. The cystic duct may join the common hepatic duct at a very high point, almost at the hilus of the liver (Fig 65–1A). In approximately 25% of patients, the right hepatic duct as such is absent, and major ducts draining the anterior and posterior sectors of the right lobe of the liver join the left hepatic duct directly (Fig 65–1B and C). A right sectoral duct may run a prolonged extrahepatic course to join the common hepatic duct. The cystic duct may drain directly into such a duct (Fig 65–1D). Similarly, the cystic duct may be closely adherent to the common hepatic duct, running together with it in a common sheath before joining it at a low point. In some instances, the cystic duct is very short. In such cases, misinterpretation of the anatomy and of the operative cholangiography can occur easily, especially if a cannula has been advanced so far that it passes into the common bile duct. In this instance, if there is no distal obstruction, the contrast medium passes rapidly down the duct and into the duodenum, there being no display of the proximal ducts. The surgeon then can easily mistake the common bile duct for a long cystic duct, ligate it, and remove it along with the attached gallbladder. This situation should not be confused with the almost obliterated cystic duct found in longstanding chronic cholelithiasis and chronic cholecystitis (see below). Failure to appre-

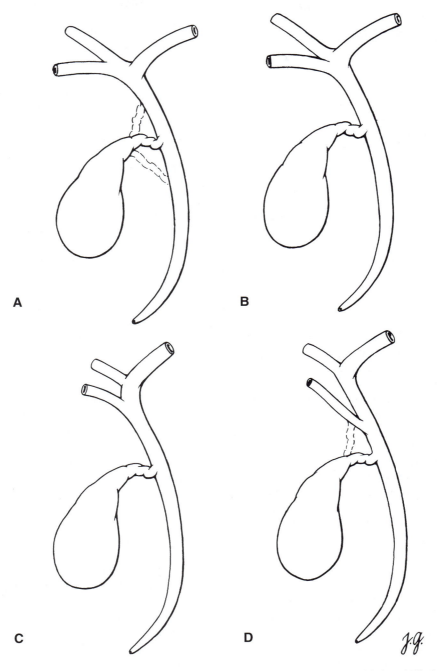

Figure 65–1. Representation of the manner of junction of the cystic duct with the hepatic duct. **A.** The cystic duct may join the main bile duct either very high, almost at the confluence of the hepatic ducts, or at a much lower level. Indeed, it may not join the common hepatic duct until almost at the ampulla. Note that in this figure the right hepatic sectoral ducts join to form a main right hepatic duct. **B.** The anterior and posterior sectoral ducts of the right lobe of the liver join the left hepatic duct at a common confluence. **C.** The right anterior and posterior sectoral ducts join the left hepatic duct independently. **D.** The anterior (or posterior) right sectoral duct joins the common hepatic duct at a much lower level. The cystic duct may, in fact, drain into such a sectoral duct. (From Blumgart LH, Bile duct strictures. In: Fromm D (ed), *Gastrointestinal Surgery*, vol 2. London, England: Churchill Livingstone; 1984:755).

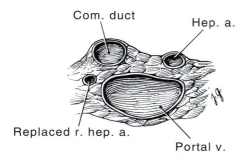

Figure 65–2. Cross-sectional view of duodenohepatic ligament. Note the position of the replaced hepatic artery lying posterolateral to the common bile duct. (Braasch JW. Unexpected findings at surgery of the biliary track. *Prob P Gen Surg* 1984;1:223)

ciate anatomical risk factors is also the major problem during laparoscopic cholecystectomy.[9] This is inherently riskier in laparoscopic cholecystectomy, since a decision to divide the ductal structure that is thought to be the cystic duct must be made before the gallbladder is dissected free of its bed. That is why many surgeons propose routine cholangiography in laparoscopic cholecystectomy (ie, to define the anatomy).

Anomalies of the vessels, in particular of the hepatic artery, are very frequent and occur in over 20% of patients. The most common abnormality is for the right hepatic artery to arise in whole or in part from the superior mesenteric trunk. The anomalous vessel usually runs up to the right of the portal vein and just posterolateral to the bile duct, running close to the cystic duct at the neck of the gallbladder, where it is prone to injury during cholecystectomy (Fig 65–2). During attempts to control bleeding, there may be coincident damage to the bile ducts, if clamps are blindly applied. The bleeding usually arises from the cystic artery or from the right hepatic arterial trunk, although injury to the common hepatic artery also occurs. In a series of 78 postcholecystectomy biliary strictures studied by Blumgart and associates at Hammersmith Hospital, London, selective celiac angiography was performed in 25 patients because of a history of vascular damage at operation before referral, hematemesis or melena, esophagogastric varices seen at endoscopy, or a palpable spleen.[10] Evidence of arterial damage or abnormality was noted in 14 cases and damage to the portal vein or one of its branches in five cases (Fig 65–3). In three patients, portal venous obstruction was accompanied by segmental or lobar atrophy. Esophagogastric varices were demonstrated in five patients and splenomegaly in nine. On occasion, not only is there a bile duct stricture or stenosis, but a hepatic artery aneurysm may form and erode into the biliary tree, producing hemobilia.

The microcirculation of the extrahepatic biliary tree has been described by Northover and Terblanche.[11] The blood supply of the bile duct runs in three columns, one posterior and two lateral, and damage to these vessels may result in ischemia to the bile duct with consequent necrosis and stricture. There is no firm evidence for this proposition, but it seems reasonable not to pursue extensive dissection of the common bile duct during cholecystectomy, as is taught in some centers. Transection of the bile duct disturbs the blood supply and, in particular, arterial flow arising from its lower end. Ischemia occurs in the upper transected duct and is probably responsible for the remarkable scarring and retraction of the stricture towards and into the hilus.

Pathologic Factors

Acute cholecystitis may be accompanied by extensive edema in the region of the porta hepatis and Calot's triangle, with considerable friability. During an open cholecystectomy, if dissection appears hazardous, cholecystectomy may be a safer option than cholecystectomy. During laparoscopic cholecystectomy, a decision to convert to open operation should be taken if the surgeon is faced with an obviously difficult and potentially hazardous situation.

Of undoubtedly greater significance is the small, contracted, fibrotic gallbladder with considerable surrounding inflammatory reaction, sometimes partly embedded in the liver tissue and obliterating Calot's triangle. In such instances, dissection of Calot's triangle, either laparoscopically or via an open procedure is impossible. There may already be preexisting benign stenosis consequent on the inflammation. Further, cholecystocholedochal fistula is not uncommon in longstanding disease. In any patient with gallstones, jaundice, and attacks of cholangitis who, at operation, has such a gallbladder, a cholecystocholedochal fistula should be suspected. In these circumstances, it is wiser to convert to an open procedure and to remove the greater part of the gallbladder wall and remove the stones. Such a partial cholecystectomy is a safe option and allows direct inspection of the depths of the gallbladder. If a fistula exists, then it frequently is associated with some degree of narrowing of the bile duct just distal to the fistula and is managed best by mobilizing the duodenum and carrying out a cholecystocholedochoduodenostomy (Fig 65–4). A variety of other techniques to close the defect also have been described.

Technical Factors

Some bile duct injuries occur after cholecystectomy is performed by inexperienced surgeons, but many occur after cholecystectomy done by experienced surgeons who find that they have damaged the bile duct during an easy cholecystectomy. As pointed out by Grey-Turner in 1944, injury might occur when in the hands of the highly skilled and experienced surgeon.[1]

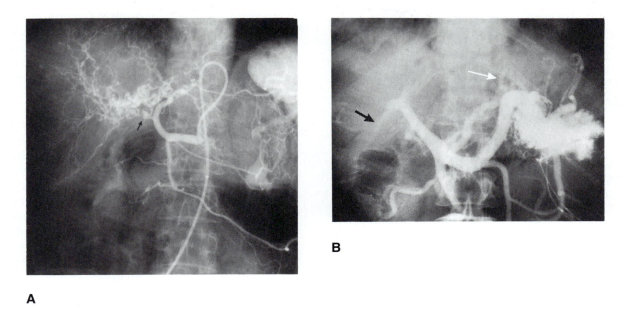

A

B

Figure 65–3. A. Selective hepatic arteriogram in a patient with high bile duct stricture. The study was carried out because of a history of hemobilia before referral. Note complete occlusion of the right hepatic artery (*arrow*) and the development of an extensive collateral circulation. **B.** Splenoportography in patient with benign bile duct stricture and history of vascular damage at time of initial operation. Patient had portal hypertension and bleeding esophageal varices. Note that only a portion of the right portal venous vasculature is outlined (*black arrow*). Note varices in the area of the gastric fundus (*white arrow*).

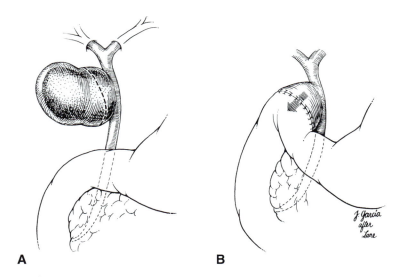

A   **B**

Figure 65–4. A. Obliteration of Calot's triangle (*curved arrow*) by the inflammatory process accompanying severe chronic cholecystitis. The gallbladder contains two large gallstones, one of which has eroded into the common hepatic duct, producing a cholecystocholedochal fistula. In such cases (which are usually associated with cholangitis and obstructive jaundice), there should be no attempt at cholecystectomy because this procedure is likely to be accompanied by biliary injury. Partial cholecystectomy (dotted line) can be performed with extraction of the calculi. **B.** Cholecysto-choledoch-duodenostomy can be carried out with safety and adequate drainage of bile. (From Blumgart LH, Bile duct strictures. In: Fromm D (ed), *Gastrointestinal Surgery*, vol 2. London, England: Churchill Livingstone; 1984:755).

TABLE 65–2. CAUSE OF BENIGN POSTCHOLECYSTECTOMY BILIARY STRICTURE IN 136 PATIENTS[a]

Condition	No. of Patients
Known duct injury	70
Massive bleeding at cholecystectomy	22
Contracted difficult bladder	12
Probably no injury	10
Ligature on duct	8
Followed gastrectomy	7
Acute cholecystitis	6
Duct narrowed around T tube	1
Total	136

[a]In 365 other patients in the series, no ascribable cause was found.
(Adapted from Cattell RB, Braasch JW. General considerations in the management of benign stricture of the bile duct. N Engl J Med 1959;261:929.)

The reason for error is often difficult to determine in any particular case (Table 65–2). It often is assumed that the hepatic duct or common bile duct has been mistaken for the cystic duct and has been partially excised or that a portion of the common biliary channel has been ligated along with the cystic duct. However, of 78 cases seen by us at the Royal Postgraduate Medical School, London, it was possible to incriminate one of these errors in only six cases. Cattell and Braasch had a similar experience (Table 65–2).[12] In the majority of cases, the high location of the injury suggested direct damage or ligation of the common hepatic duct.

Abdominal incisions must be adequate in length and appropriately situated. Early demonstration of the cystic artery and cystic duct is desirable. The cystic artery then should be ligated close to the gallbladder wall to avoid damage to the common hepatic artery or the right hepatic artery. The surgeon then can introduce a cystic duct cannula and perform operative cholangiography, which, in addition to its advantage of indicating the necessity for bile duct exploration, will, on occasion, reveal anatomic abnormalities. Of 72 patients with postcholecystectomy biliary strictures studied at Hammersmith Hospital, London, 71% did not have preoperative cholangiography at the time of initial cholecystectomy.[10] Although preoperative cholangiography is important, acceptance of poor cholangiographic pictures may mislead the surgeon, especially if the biliary tree is not fully demonstrated (Fig 65–5).

In patients with jaundice, preoperative cholangiography is advisable and may be obtained by means of percutaneous transhepatic cholangiography or endoscopic retrograde choledochopancreatography (ERCP).

Dense fibrosis in the area of Calot's triangle should lead to a change in policy. Thus, a partial cholecystectomy can be performed as described above. Alternatively, a dissection of the gallbladder from the fundus can be carried out slowly and cautiously while keeping close to the gallbladder wall. If difficulty is encountered as the neck of the gallbladder is approached, then the attempted total cholecystectomy should be abandoned in favor of a partial procedure. Excessive traction on the gallbladder during cholecystectomy should be avoided, since tenting of the common bile duct–common hepatic duct junction will occur and create a situation likely to result in excision of a segment of common duct. Some authors argue that the precise point of junction of the cystic duct with the common hepatic duct should be clearly demonstrated, and they consider it important to separate the cystic duct when it adheres to the common hepatic duct and to trace it to its termination. This precaution is unnecessary. There is no need to go to excessive lengths to display the entire cystic duct because such dissection might well lead to injury. The presence of cystic duct stones that require attention should have been demonstrated at operative cholangiography.

Bleeding that occurs during operation should be precisely controlled. Blood is removed by suction. Arterial hemorrhage can be controlled by pressure with the finger and thumb on the hepatic artery at the free edge of the lesser omentum, or by the application of a soft gastrointestinal clamp across this region. The offending vessels then are dissected and deliberately controlled.

When operative cholangiography reveals a very small common bile duct with a filling defect, indicating a possible small stone or stones within it, and in the presence of multiple small stones within the gallbladder, we and other surgeons advocate simple cholecystectomy without exploration of the common duct. Virtually all such stones will pass asymptomatically. Furthermore, operative exploration of such a small duct is difficult, often unrewarding, and more likely to result in damage to the biliary system than exploration easily carried out within a duct of normal size. The likelihood of further symptoms and of complications is almost certainly less if such a stone is left in situ rather than if a common bile duct exploration is attempted.

Exploration of the common bile duct should involve careful exposure of a sufficient length of duct to allow choledochotomy but no extensive dissection and stripping of the bile duct of its surrounding connective tissue. Exploration should be carried out with the gentle use of soft bougies, Fogarty-type balloon catheters, and choledochoscopy. Instruments should not be forced through the papilla of Vater. Should metal bougies, such as Bakes dilators, be passed downwards through the papilla into the duodenum, subsequent secondary postinflammatory stenosis of the papilla of Vater might occur. In addition, false passages may be created. The dilator may pass either into the pancreatic tissue or through the bile duct wall proximal to the papilla and into the duodenum, creating a choledochoduodenal

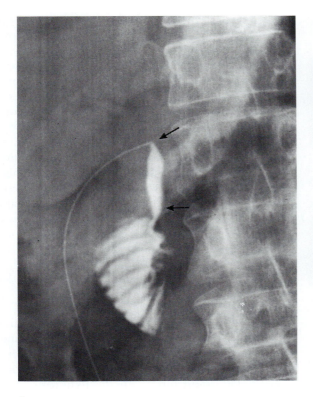

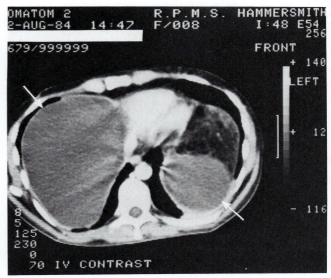

A

B

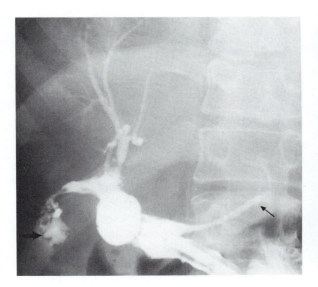

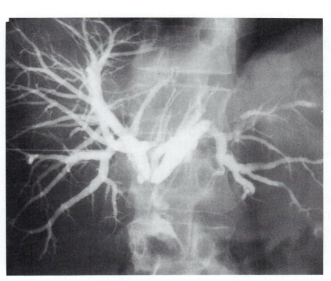

C

D

Figure 65–5. A. Operative cholangiogram obtained after cannulation of cystic duct. Note that the cannula has entered the common bile duct (*upper arrow*) and that the common hepatic duct has not been displayed at all. The surgeon proceeded with the cholecystectomy in the belief that he had cannulated the cystic duct. **B.** The patient became extremely ill after operation and on referral had jaundice, fever, and incipient renal failure. CT scan obtained on admission revealed intraperitoneal biliary collections (*arrows*). Operative drainage was instituted. **C.** Tubogram obtained after operative drainage revealed the presence of a fistulous tract with connections to both the right and left sides of the abdomen (*arrows*). A portion (right anterior sectoral duct) of the biliary tree is outlined. The patient was treated expectantly, and the fistula closed, but several weeks later, cholangitis and jaundice recurred. **D.** Percutaneous transhepatic cholangiogram obtained on patient's readmission to the hospital reveals a high stricture at the confluence of the hepatic ducts (Bismuth type 3). Repair was effected by hepaticojejunostomy Roux-en-Y loop with an approach to the left hepatic ductal system and extension of the dissection to the right.

fistula. Choledochoduodenal fistulas, either because of passage of an instrument or after an erroneously placed sphincteroplasty, may result in symptoms of jaundice, cholangitis, and pancreatitis. Passage of a dilator into the pancreas may result in postoperative pancreatitis, and secondary bile duct stricture may result. Stenosis or stricture of the peripapillary common bile duct also may follow surgical or endoscopic sphincteroplasty. Exploration of the common bile duct at the time of cholecystectomy usually should be carried out in a supraduodenal fashion. Sphincteroplasty is best reserved for patients with a stone impacted at the papilla of Vater.

In patients with multiple stones or primary stasis stones or those patients with distal obstruction such as might occur with stenosis of the papilla of Vater, a choledochoduodenostomy may be performed. This procedure generally should not be performed if the common bile duct is <15 mm in diameter and if a stoma of at least 2 cm cannot be created. If an adequate stoma is created, the results are good and late stenosis or cholangitis are rare. On the other hand, should choledochoduodenostomy be performed to a narrow common bile duct, then stenosis, perhaps associated with bile duct stricture, is more likely.

After exploration of the common bile duct, postexploratory cholangiography or choledochoscopy should be performed. Care must be taken in performing postexploratory cholangiography and in immediate re-exploration of the common bile duct to avoid damage to the duct by repeated suture around a T tube. We prefer the method of postexploratory cholangiography whereby a small Foley catheter is used to occlude the ducts, allowing proximal and distal cholangiography after exploration without the need to close the choledochotomy at the time of x-ray examination. In addition, good radiographs of the proximal and distal duct are obtainable.

Some series of laparoscopic cholecystectomy have suggested that injuries to the common bile duct tend to occur in the earlier operations,[5] but the uncomfortable fact is that this has not uniformly been the case.[13]

Injury with either the laparoscopic or traditional approach is more likely to occur if the surgeon is attempting to operate without adequate assistance. Proper trochar position for laparoscopic surgery is essential, and, occasionally, additional trochar sites should be used to allow adequate exposure. Early demonstration of the cystic artery and cystic duct is desirable. The cystic artery should be divided close to the gallbladder wall to avoid damage to the right hepatic or common hepatic artery.

Although data regarding the patterns of ductal injury with laparoscopic cholecystectomy are just beginning to accrue, certain technical factors are cited frequently. Some reports claimed that laser dissection is inherently more dangerous than electrocautery,[7,14] although large prospective series have failed to prove this point.[5] The use of the 0° viewing laparoscope does not afford as good a perspective of the anatomy of Calot's triangle as a 30° or 45° angled viewing laparoscope; this factor also has been implicated in bile duct injuries.[6]

Misidentification of the common bile duct for the cystic duct with resection of a portion of the common and hepatic ducts, often with associated right hepatic artery injury, appears to be the most common form of laparoscopic bile duct injury.[8] Extensive craniad traction on the fundus of the gallbladder causes significant distortion of Calot's triangle by aligning the cystic and common hepatic ducts, thus predisposing to this pattern of injury or to inadvertent clipping of the common bile duct. Gentle but adequate lateral and caudal traction on the neck of the gallbladder is essential to splay open Calot's triangle and restore easily recognizable anatomic relationships.[9]

PATHOLOGIC EFFECTS

Fibrosis

Biliary obstruction is associated with the formation of high local concentrations of bile salts at the canalicular membrane that initiate pathologic changes in the biliary system. An inflammatory exudate forms, leading to collagen deposition and eventually, to fibrosis and scarring around bile ducts and ductules. The fibrosis is accompanied by liver cell hyperplasia. These changes do not usually progress to true secondary biliary cirrhosis because the lobular structure of the liver is usually well preserved.[15a] This knowledge is important in planning therapy because many of the changes are potentially reversible and there may be a return to near normality of such a liver after relief of biliary obstruction.

Patients with biliary obstruction and secondary biliary fibrosis are at high risk, however (see below). Demonstration of liver fibrosis associated with portal hypertension usually requires 4 or 5 years, although it may be accomplished considerably earlier, especially if there is coincident liver atrophy. Major stigmata of hepatocellular dysfunction, such as spider nevi, ascites, and portal systemic encephalopathy, may develop. However, these changes are not common in benign biliary obstruction and should alert the clinician that there maybe associated parenchymal disease (eg, alcoholic cirrhosis). Changes also occur in the extrahepatic ducts, which are subject to fibrosis and upward retraction. These changes are accompanied by a sequence of mucosal atrophy, squamous metaplasia, inflammatory infiltration, and fibrosis in the subepithelial layers of the ducts that is seen especially in longstanding obstruction.

Atrophy

Quality and quantity of portal venous inflow are important in the maintenance of liver cell size and mass. Segmental or lobar atrophy results from a degree of portal

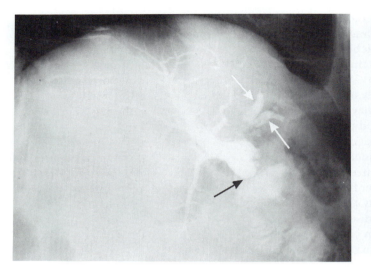
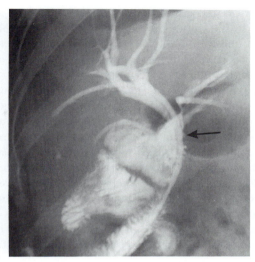

A

B

Figure 65–6. A. Percutaneous transhepatic cholangiogram in a patient with recurrent postcholecystectomy stricture after two previous attempts at creation of hepaticojejunostomy Roux-en-Y loop. The right hepatic ductal system is dilated, and there is a recurrent stricture (*black arrow*) of the common hepatic duct. The previous Roux-en-Y is faintly outlined. Note particularly (*white arrows*) the atrophic left hepatic ducts within a small left lobe. Intrahepatic calculi are present. HIDA scan in this patient failed to reveal any evidence of left lobe function at all. **B.** Cholangiogram obtained via transjejunal transanastomotic tube after refashioning of hepaticojejunostomy Roux-en-Y loop. A wide anastomosis (*arrow*) is shown. The stones have been removed from the left hepatic ductal system, and ducts are draining freely. The tube was removed 2 months after surgery.

venous occlusion or bile duct occlusion to that area of liver tissue. Unilobar atrophy is associated with hypertrophy of the contralateral lobe and may present diagnostic and operative difficulty. Changes of this nature are frequently found in benign stricture,[15] and may be associated with asymmetric stricture of lobar or sectoral hepatic ducts or with interference with the blood supply, particularly the portal venous supply. Additionally, they may be associated with decreased portal perfusion consequent on secondary fibrotic changes. In benign bile duct stricture, even though drainage of grossly dilated ducts within an atrophic segment may not be effective in relieving obstruction, the dilated ducts within the atrophic remnant are nearly always filled with infected bile. Continued cholangitis is therefore inevitable unless not only ducts in the hypertrophic area of liver tissue but also the ducts in the atrophic portion are drained (Fig 65–6). Liver atrophy and hypertrophy, in the presence of biliary obstruction, may be associated with the accelerated development of portal hypertension.[16]

DIAGNOSIS

The diagnosis requires confirmation of the suspicion that damage to the biliary tree has occurred, together with a precise demonstration of the level and extent of the stricture, particularly in its proximal portion. Any associated damage to adjacent blood vessels also should be shown.

Signs and Symptoms

Damage to the biliary tree may be recognized at operation; however, this is not usually the case. A biliary fistula or stricture usually becomes evident early in the postoperative period, or sometimes months later.

Excessive biliary drainage from the wound or drain sites in the early postoperative period may indicate a major injury to the bile ducts. In other patients, if localized or generalized peritoneal signs become evident and an intra-abdominal collection of bile is drained at a second operation, it then is clear that bile duct injury has occurred (Fig 65–5).

In some cases, a history of postoperative biliary drainage and fever, and perhaps even of a subphrenic or subhepatic abscess is evident, with the patient then being free of symptoms for some months before developing recurring bouts of pyrexia, rigors, and jaundice. In other patients, a steadily progressive obstructive jaundice may be the first sign of ductal injury. Although usually evident immediately after operation, this jaundice may come on weeks or even months after initial operation.

On physical examination, jaundice is usually present, although it may be intermittent in nature or even absent, depending on whether bile duct obstruction is complete or partial and whether or not a biliary fistula is present. Sometimes a patient with bile duct injury may have fever, but not jaundice, and in such cases, an internal or external biliary fistula may have been established or the stricture may involve only one sectoral duct. In the presence of recurring bouts of cholangitis or an established biliary fistula, weight loss and debility are invariable. The patient may complain of itching, with scratch marks evident on the limbs.

Hepatomegaly is frequently present and usually indicates longstanding obstruction. Splenomegaly may be the result of secondary liver fibrosis with associated portal hypertension, but the possibility of direct damage to, or thrombosis of, the portal vein must be considered. Splenomegaly, esophageal varices, or the presence of frank signs of liver failure such as spider nevi, a liver flap, or ascites should alert the clinician to the possibility of associated hepatocellular disease. Exclusion of this disease as a factor in the illness is of importance not only in planning management but also in a medicolegal context.

Laboratory Investigations

The majority of patients are jaundiced at presentation. The serum bilirubin level and the serum alkaline phosphatase level are raised. With incomplete or sectoral obstruction, the serum alkaline phosphatase level usually is elevated, even though the serum bilirubin level may be normal. Serum transaminase levels may be within normal limits or may be elevated, especially if there is cholangitis. In cases of prolonged obstruction, the serum albumin level may be depressed.

In patients with advanced secondary biliary fibrosis or associated hepatocellular disease or cirrhosis, it may be very difficult to distinguish the effects of stricture from those of hepatocellular dysfunction. Then, particularly if the patient is anicteric and the serum alkaline phosphatase level is raised, hepatic iminodiacetic acid (HIDA) scanning may be of value (see below).

Blood urea and serum creatinine levels should be measured as an index of renal function.

Radiologic Investigations

If an external fistula or a tube is in situ, contrast medium can be injected to outline the biliary ductal system (Fig 65–7). Because biliary infection is inevitable in such cases, it is wise to protect the patient with antibiotic prophylaxis against bacteremia that may follow fistulography.

Ultrasonography is an excellent means of demonstrating dilation of the intrahepatic ducts, but it is of little value in a precise demonstration of the extent of stricture and of no value if the ducts are not dilated. Percutaneous transhepatic cholangiography is the key investigation. Some investigators are wary of its preoperative use because of the risk of cholangitis and bile leakage, but the procedure has become much safer with the introduction of the fine needle and, provided antibiotic coverage is used and the ducts are not overfilled, cholangitis and leakage are uncommon. The biliary ductal system is entered in almost 100% of cases, and a

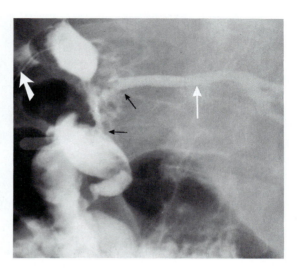

Figure 65–7. Complex biliary stricture and fistula after right hepatic lobectomy performed for hydatid cyst. A biliary fistula through the right side of the chest wall was demonstrated. X-ray film was obtained by injection of a tube within the fistulous tract. A cavity in the right side of the chest and another below the diaphragm were both outlined, and there was an associated right-sided empyema. The biliary ductal system (*black arrows*) is completely disrupted. The left hepatic duct in the liver remnant is shown (*white arrow*), with a fistula then filling the low common bile duct and the duodenum independently. The patient was managed by drainage of the right-sided empyema, antibiotics, and parenteral nutrition. Subsequently, repair of the duodenal fistula and creation of a hepaticojejunostomy Roux-en-Y loop to the exposed bile duct were successfully carried out.

successful cholangiogram will demonstrate the level and extent of the stricture (Figs 65–5 and 65–6). Great care must be taken to outline all branches of the intrahepatic biliary tree, particularly in cases of high bile duct stricture and recurrent stricture after previous reconstructive surgery. Films taken in a lateral projection may demonstrate posterior displacement of the hilus in cases with severe right lobe liver atrophy.

ERCP is seldom of value in the precise diagnosis of complete high bile duct stricture because there is usually discontinuity of the common bile duct, preventing display of the intrahepatic structures. However, the procedure is of value in demonstrating incomplete stricture (stenosis). In addition, it is important to carry out ERCP in any patient in whom there is a history of sphincteric damage at the time of initial exploration of the common bile duct, particularly if there is associated unexplained upper abdominal pain, because papillary stenosis and perhaps associated pancreatitis may be demonstrated. Furthermore, cholangitis may occur in association with stenosis of the high bile duct, since the infection is related to the presence of sphincteric incontinence consequent to surgical or endoscopic sphincterotomy or an associated choledochoduodenal fistula. This combination of high stenosis and low incontinence is easily misinterpreted.

If there has been excessive bleeding at the time of cholecystectomy or if there is any suspicion, either from the history, the presence of a palpable spleen, or endoscopic evidence of varices, that the patient has portal hypertension, then arteriography and splenoportography are necessary (Fig 65–3). The latter is usually obtainable by examination of late-phase films after splenic arterial injection of contrast medium.

It is of some importance to recognize associated liver atrophy (see above). Despite wide dilation of the ducts in such atrophic segments, the drainage of liver tissue into these ducts is not healthy. The radiologic signs of atrophy include crowding and irregularity of the smaller biliary radicles (Fig. 65–6) and arteries within the affected area. Isotope scanning may show what appears to be a filling defect in the related area or relatively poor function of an atrophic segment or lobe. Computed tomography (CT) scanning may reveal segmental liver atrophy and is probably the most easily interpreted imaging modality in this regard.

Isotopic scanning techniques may be of value in the assessment of bile duct strictures and, in particular, of the functional assessment of incomplete strictures and anastomoses carried out at previous reconstructive attempts. HIDA scanning methods allow a dynamic and quantitative assessment of liver function and of the clearance of bile across anastomoses and strictures (Fig 65–8). HIDA scanning may be of particular value in those cases where there is incomplete stricturing or restenosis and where ultrasonographic examination shows a nondilated ductal system. Similarly, in patients with hepatocellular disease, HIDA scanning may be of value in distinguishing the contribution of restricture to the biochemical and symptomatic problems, as distinct from the problem of liver disease. HIDA scanning is also valuable during follow-up of patients after surgical repair, because it is noninvasive and can demonstrate anastomotic patency and function in patients in whom no tube has been left across the anastomosis at the time of repair (Fig 65–9). Computer-assisted HIDA scans also may show quantitative changes in liver function over time.

Clinical Interpretation

It should be emphasized that discovery at cholangiography of an area of stenosis, or incomplete stricture, is not necessarily an indication for immediate operation. It is important not to "treat x-ray films." An established internal fistula may provide good long-term biliary drainage and allow a period of assessment before definitive treatment. Similarly, severe degrees of stenosis on cholangiography may be associated with few symptoms and with nearly normal liver function test results. It may be permissible in selected cases, especially in elderly patients, to accept a degree of obstruction or segmental obstruction if symptoms are minimal and easily controlled (for example, by intermittent administration of antibiotics). In a series of 78 patients, Blumgart chose conservative management in four patients based on this observation and successfully managed all of them for periods of 9 months to 5 years without resorting to operation.[17] Balloon dilation of benign strictures has been carried out recently and may be successful, but long-term results are not yet available. The results must be judged with caution, and balloon dilation resulting in incomplete relief of obstruction, especially, may be associated with relief of symptoms, but it also may be associated with progressive liver damage (see below). Regular observation is particularly important in all patients for whom operative treatment is not selected (or in whom dilation has been carried out), because progressive liver damage may be insidious and a persistently elevated alkaline phosphatase level may be the only index of incomplete obstruction.

CLASSIFICATION AND SEVERITY

The ease of management, operative risk, and ultimate prognosis of benign bile duct stricture vary considerably, and the factors influencing outcome have been discussed by many. In general, younger patients have a better prognosis than older patients. Patients with coincident disease such as cardiorespiratory disease have a worse outlook. The presence of hepatocellular disease or established secondary liver fibrosis and of portal hypertension are important adverse features. Also, it long

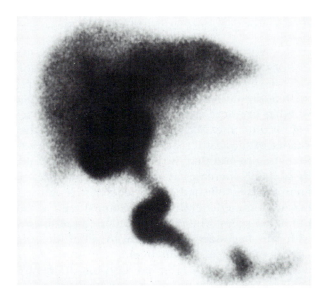

Figure 65–8. Anterior view of liver at 2 minutes after intravenous injection of 120 MBq (3 mCi)^{99m}Tc-HIDA in patient with hepaticojejunostomy for benign stricture. Illustration shows tracer in liver, major bile ducts, and also in upper portion of small bowel.

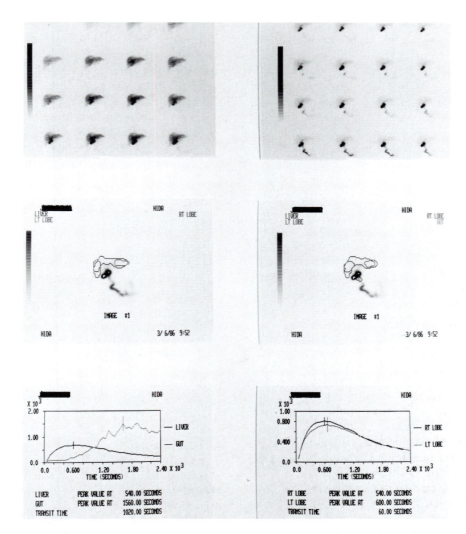

Figure 65–9. Upper images show 32 6.25-second sequential frames of the patient in Fig 65–8. Regions of interest have been selected over right and left lobes of the liver and over the gut (shown on central images). Time-activity curves (lower left and right) show prompt uptake of tracer and rapid clearance with a rising curve over the bowel. These findings are normal.

has been recognized that strictures involving the common bile duct or low common hepatic duct are easier to repair than higher strictures, which may compromise the confluence of the bile ducts. In recognition of these factors, Bismuth proposed an anatomic classification of bile duct strictures into five types[18] (Fig 65–10):

Type 1: Low common hepatic duct stricture; hepatic duct stump >2 cm

Type 2: Midcommon hepatic duct stump <2 cm

Type 3: High stricture (hilar), no hepatic duct; confluence intact (see also Fig 65–3)

Type 4: Destruction of hilar confluence; right and left hepatic ducts separated

Type 5: Involvement of sectoral right branch alone or with common duct

In addition, the presence of infection and especially whether or not reoperation has been done have a bearing on outcome. Many have commented that the best chance of successful repair of bile duct injuries is at the first attempt and that the risk of morbidity and mortality probably increases at each subsequent effort. Once an injury is established, then unless it is recognized and repaired immediately, the first repair should be carried out by a surgeon who is well versed in the problems and with the necessary experience to allow the highest chance of a successful outcome.

At Hammersmith Hospital, London, Blumgart and colleagues studied a number of preoperative indexes of outcome based on history and biochemical assessment in 78 cases of postcholecystectomy stricture.[10] Portal hypertension occurred more often in patients with

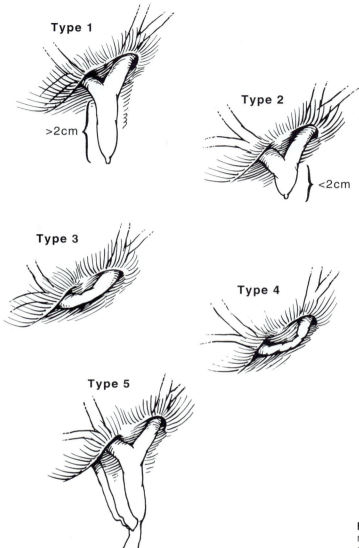

Figure 65–10. Classification of bile duct strictures based on the level of the stricture in relation to the confluence of the hepatic cuts. (From Bismuth H. Postoperative strictures of the bile duct. In: Blumgart LH (ed), *The Biliary Tract. Clinical Surgery International,* vol 5. Edinburgh, Scotland: Churchill Livingstone 1982;209–218)

prolonged duration of obstruction and with frequent episodes of cholangitis. Major infection was significantly more common in patients who had had more than one operation before referral. There was also a highly significant relationship between the postoperative mortality rate and the presence of liver fibrosis, a history of major infection, and a depressed serum albumin concentration. Similarly, patients with high strictures (Bismuth types 3 and 4) fared worse than patients in whom some part of the common hepatic duct was still intact. In essence, patients with multiple previous operations, with high strictures and particularly, with liver disease and portal hypertension fared badly, and infection was a major determinant in the progress of disease.

PREOPERATIVE MANAGEMENT

Except in the case of strictures recognized at the time of primary cholecystectomy or in patients in whom emergency operation is dictated by virtue of peritonitis, there is no hurry in proceeding to surgical reconstruction for bile duct stricture. The patient should be afforded full investigation and be brought to optimal condition for operation.

In the presence of recurrent cholangitis, the administration of antibiotics is important as a preliminary step to surgical treatment. The correct antibiotic can be selected on the basis of cultures obtained from aspiration of bile at percutaneous transhepatic cholangiography.

Although adequate surgical decompression is the only certain way of treating established cholangitis, preoperative antibiotics are important in managing recurrent attacks and in preventing infective complications.

Antibiotics regimens should take into account the frequent presence of anaerobic organisms and *enterococci* in cases of bile duct stricture.[19,20] Antibiotics should be commenced immediately preoperatively. Although there are no firm data to guide management, it is recommended that antibiotics be continued from 48 hours to 5 days postoperatively, depending on the extent of preoperative biliary infection and the presence of preoperative bacteremia.

Anemia should be corrected, if necessary, by blood transfusion; coagulation defects, usually a prolongation of the prothrombin time should be corrected by the administration of vitamin K. The nutritional status of patients with bile duct stricture is important. Some patients are anorexic and grossly malnourished. Although feeding through a fine-bore transnasal catheter may be successful in some cases, enterally administered nutrients often are not tolerated and parenteral nutrition is frequently necessary. However, weight gain is sometimes difficult to achieve in a patient with biliary tract obstruction, especially in the presence of chronic infection. If there is a significant external biliary fistula, the patient will lose electrolytes. Hyponatremia in particular is a risk. Fluid replacement and electrolyte repletion are important.

TREATMENT

Treatment of patients with benign bile duct stricture involves reconstruction of biliary enteric continuity. However, the management of such complications as biliary peritonitis, subphrenic and subhepatic abscess, and hematemesis owing either to erosive gastritis or to esophageal varices and the management of liver failure consequent on liver fibrosis are also important and often require treatment preliminary to biliary repair.

In general, drainage of abscesses and control of erosive gastritis take precedence and are carried out before definitive attempts are made to repair strictures. On the other hand, if sepsis arising from the obstructed biliary tree is a dominant feature, especially in erosive gastritis, or if bacteremia and renal failure are present, then immediate biliary drainage is essential. Drainage may be obtained at operation but, in such desperately ill patients, it may be preferable to attempt percutaneous transhepatic biliary drainage as a temporary measure to allow resuscitation. Management of portal hypertension occurring in association with stricture is discussed below. If a biliary fistula is present, it should, in general, be managed conservatively in the first instance (see below).

The operative management of biliary stricture depends on whether the injury is recognized at the time of the original operation, occurs in the postoperative period, or occurs as a late event.

Injury Recognized at Time of Operation

If injury to the extrahepatic biliary tree is recognized at the time of initial cholecystectomy, then the surgeon should immediately consider his experience and competence to deal with the situation. If a more experienced surgeon is available within the hospital or nearby, then advice should be sought. The situation is not an immediately desperate one, and there is always time to insert a pack, cover the wound, and wait a short time for another opinion.

The damaged area and the bile duct on either side require careful dissection to define the extent of injury. To accomplish this dissection without making matters worse, laparoscopic procedures must be converted immediately into full laparotomies, improved exposure must be obtained by extending incisions, and a call for additional assistance to aid in retraction must be made. Operative cholangiography may be helpful at this time. The injury may be high, close to the hilus of the liver, or lower in the supraduodenal area. The injury may be partial, with maintenance of mucosal continuity along one wall of the bile duct, or there may be complete transection or even excision of a length of common bile duct–common hepatic duct with loss of continuity.

Whether the lesion is high and close to the hilus of the liver or low, initial repair of injury *recognized at the time of cholecystectomy* should have two basic aims: (1) to maintain ductal length below the hilus and avoid sacrificing tissue, and (2) to effect a repair that does not result in postoperative biliary leakage.

Initial repair *may not* be the final definitive reconstruction. This is particularly true of injury to very small ducts, where repair may be difficult and the prime aims of preventing fistulation and maintaining length should guide the surgeon. It is probably preferable to provide external biliary drainage by means of a tube inserted proximally and then refer the patient for specialist treatment, rather than to complicate the situation by an attempted repair that causes further damage to the proximal ducts.

Unfortunately, the injury is almost always total and involves *transection or excision* of a length of bile duct. Occasionally, only a right sectoral duct is damaged (Bismuth type 5). Injury is particularly likely to occur if the common biliary channels are small. Thus, the repair also is likely to be difficult.

Several options are open to the surgeon. If the bile duct has been transected and the ends can be apposed without tension, then an end-to-end anastomosis may be feasible. The duodenum and head of the pancreas

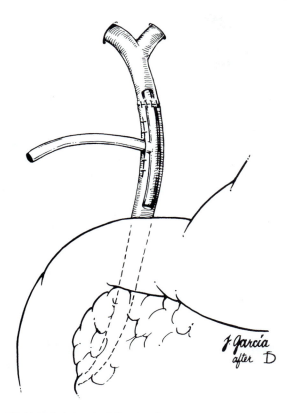

Figure 65–11. Method of repair of biliary ductal injury by end-to-end anastomosis over a T tube.

should be completely mobilized to minimize tension. An end-to-end anastomosis then is done with a single layer of interrupted fine chromic catgut sutures or other absorbable sutures (eg, Vicryl). Silk is not an alternative because silk sutures may come to lie within the bile duct lumen and act as a foreign body or a nidus for stone formation. The anastomosis is made over a T tube brought out of the bile duct lumen away from the anastomotic line (Fig 65–11). Because stricture may recur in 50% to 60% of such anastomoses (see below) and may be accompanied by some loss of length, it is preferable to avoid direct repair for high injuries where initial hepaticojejunostomy Roux-en-Y anastomosis is more likely to give good long-term results.

Lateral injuries without loss of length are unusual but important to recognize because it may be possible to effect repair by direct suture of the defect over a T tube. Longer lateral injuries that are not circumferential are much more difficult or impossible to suture transversely. Vein patches have been used to bridge gaps in the bile-ducts, and flaps of the cystic duct stump or pedicled flaps of jejunum have been used to close such defects. We have no experience in these techniques, but in this situation, a Roux-en-Y loop of jejunum can be pre-

pared and used as a serosal patch (Fig 65–12). A T tube is placed across the defect, and its long limb is led out across the Roux-en-Y loop and developed as a transjejunal tube to the skin. Such a repair has three advantages: (1) length is maintained, (2) the serosa of the jejunum is used to bridge the defect and suturing can be carried out with fine interrupted catgut sutures to the bile duct wall or adjacent connective tissue without attempting direct approaches to the ragged wall of a damaged bile duct, and (3) the T tube decompresses the biliary system across the jejunum, so that when it is removed, a fistula to the adjacent jejunum remains. Two patients managed in this manner remained well, with normal liver functions 4 and 6 years after operation, respectively. This method is occasionally most useful to the inexperienced surgeon caught in a difficult situation.

The frequency with which immediate repair of the common bile duct is effective and long lasting is difficult to ascertain. Although many injuries detected during the postoperative period (or later) are treated by specialists, injuries recognized at the time of operation may never come to the attention of referral centres and may not be documented. Some have suggested that the restricture rate is as high as 50%, but the evidence is not strong and there is almost certainly a considerable underestimate of the number of bile duct injuries and of immediate repair done in district hospitals.

Injuries Recognized in the Immediate Postoperative Period

Injuries not recognized at the time of operation may become apparent during the postoperative period in three ways.

First, there may be the formation of a *biliary fistula*. The essential management element in this situation is to *avoid early reoperation*. It is wiser to take stock of the situation, carry out fistulography, treat infection, nourish the patient, and wait. If fistulography reveals any continuity between the biliary system and the gastrointestinal tract, then a prolonged period of drainage, if well managed, may result in spontaneous closure of the fistula. Reoperation in such cases need never be hurried, because although eventual repair may be difficult, the patient often is not jaundiced and the adverse pathophysiologic features associated with cholestasis are not present. It is a mistake to think that immediate repair of such a fistula is a simple matter. Definitive exposure of healthy bile duct mucosa within a sufficiently dilated duct to permit good anastomosis can be very difficult and indeed, may be impossible. A cautious approach is preferable, because even ultimate closure of the fistula with the development of jaundice usually is associated with proximal ductal dilation and easier subsequent repair. Should fluid loss from the biliary fistula prove too heavy and too prolonged, then the external fistula can,

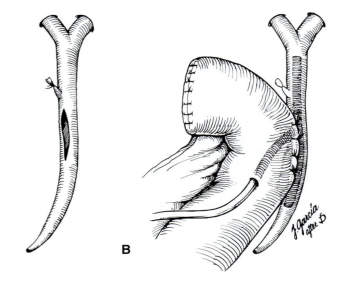

Figure 65–12. Method of repair of lateral biliary ductal injury. **A.** Lateral injury with loss of ductal wall over a considerable length. **B.** Roux-en-Y loop of jejunum is prepared and brought up. A T tube is placed within the injured bile duct, and the long limb is led out across the defect. (From Blumgart LH. Bile duct strictures. In: Fromm D (ed), *Gastrointestinal Surgery*, vol 2. London, England: Churchill Livingstone; 1984:755)

A   **B**

after some weeks or months, be converted to an internal fistula jejunostomy. Definitive repair, if necessary, then can be carried out at a later date. Some centers have now reported the use of endoscopic stenting across the defect to channel bile flow away from the external fistula, and some advocate early endoscopic sphincterotomy to decrease the relative resistance of transpapillary bile drainage to hasten closure of such fistulas.[21] However, while these approaches are occasionally useful, a waiting period of 2 to 3 weeks is recommended, since most cases will spontaneously close or significantly decrease after this interval. It is preferable to avoid the risks of endoscopic intubation, if possible. The majority of fistulas close spontaneously.[22]

Second, presentation in the postoperative period may be as *biliary peritonitis*. This situation is serious, and the patient is often desperately ill, especially if the bile is infected. However, in some patients with sterile bile, huge volumes may accumulate within the peritoneal cavity without overt signs of shock. Management of these cases demands closure of the biliary peritoneal fistula to prevent death. Definitive repair is seldom possible, since the bile ducts are collapsed and the tissues, deeply stained with bile, are friable. External drainage is the best initial approach. Such drainage may be carried out through a mobilized Roux-en-Y loop of jejunum, with the external drainage tube simply being led in a transjejunal fashion to the exterior. Such a procedure allows initial control, and the almost certain need for reoperation for stenosis at a later date should be accepted.

Finally, the patient may become progressively *jaundiced*. In this case, the injury should be managed as outlined below.

Injuries Presenting at an Interval After Initial Operation

The principles of management of late biliary stenosis and strictures are as follows:

1. Exposure of healthy proximal bile ducts draining all areas of liver
2. Preparation of a suitable segment of distal mucosa for anastomosis (usually a Roux-en-Y loop of jejunum)
3. Mucosa-to-mucosa suture anastomosis of the bile ducts to the intestinal mucosa

Although excision of the stricture and end-to-end anastomosis or repair of the damaged bile duct may be carried out in some cases, they have not been reported in most series. The disadvantage is that invariably there is loss of length as a result of fibrosis of the common hepatic duct and the common bile duct.

A staged procedure may be necessary because of the presence of abscesses, because of hematemesis, resulting, for example, from erosive gastritis or esophageal varices, or because of the poor general condition of the patient. It is unwise to attempt definitive repair of a stricture in the presence of severe local sepsis or if significant bleeding is in progress. In such cases, initial drainage procedures to evacuate pus or biliary collections and to establish external biliary flow are the only advisable procedures. Establishment of an external biliary fistula or drainage of pus allows the clinical condition to improve and the metabolic state to be brought under control before definitive management. Percutaneous transhepatic drainage techniques may be of value in such a staged approach, but there is scant published experience in this field. Similarly, in portal hypertension, sclerotherapy or initial portasystemic shunting may be required to control variceal bleeding (see below). Biliary repair is substantially more difficult in the presence of portal hypertension. In particular, dilated venous collateral channels lying within adhesions in the area of dissection are damaged easily, and intraoperative hemorrhage may be difficult to control. In such patients, radiologic interventional procedures may be used for the management of some benign strictures with the introduction of transhepatic percutaneously paced tubes draining the biliary tree and also allowing dilation of strictures. Although these methods also may lead to immediate complications, are difficult to use in the presence of a fibrotic liver with minimally dilated ducts, and may be entirely inappropriate if the obstruction is of multiple ducts or segmental in nature, they may be valuable in the treatment of patients with portal hypertension. Initial portosystemic shunting may be carried out, followed by later stricture repair; this course may be appropriate in some cases.

End-to-End Anastomosis

Excision of the stricture and end-to-end anastomosis may be carried out. Anastomosis establishes the repair with a normal anatomic status and drainage through an intact sphincter of Oddi. Cattell and Braasch reported such anastomosis, even for high strictures, after mobilization of the duodenum and lower common bile duct—if necessary with splitting of the pancreatic substance in an attempt to create a tension-free anastomosis to the proximal hepatic duct.[12] However, the procedure now is used only when the ends of the bile duct are close enough for anastomosis to be performed without any undue tension and where there is no appreciable discrepancy between the diameter of the proximal duct and that of the distal duct. The quality of the distal duct also must be satisfactory. These conditions are only rarely met in strictures at or near the hepatic hilus. A single row of interrupted fine chromic catgut or Vicryl sutures is used, with the anastomosis created over a T tube inserted at a separate point (Fig 65–11).

Biliary Enteric Repair Procedures

In the vast majority of cases, a biliary enteric repair procedure must be carried out to establish biliary drainage. There is abundant evidence that biliary intestinal anastomosis is superior to end-to-end anastomosis, and there should be little hesitation to abandon attempts at the latter if there is any difficulty.

For strictures of the retropancreatic portion of the common bile duct or of the immediate supraduodenal portion of the common bile duct, a choledochoduodenostomy, performed either side-to-side or end-to-side, is an ideal procedure. The procedure yields better results if the common bile duct is dilated. Low injuries suitable for this type of treatment are unusual after

cholecystectomy and are encountered more often after gastric operations (see below).

Treatment of strictures involving the common hepatic duct is more difficult, especially if such a stricture is close to the hilus of the liver. Hepaticojejunostomy is the best approach. When the stricture is of Bismuth type 1 or 2, then an approach to the common hepatic duct stump is usually not unduly difficult. When, however, the stricture involves the confluence of the right and left hepatic ducts (type 3), or extends so as to separate these ducts (type 4), the problem becomes much more complex and good results more difficult to obtain.

A variety of approaches to the proximal hepatic duct or ducts to expose ductal mucosa are described. The choice of approach depends on the height and extent of the lesion.

An important feature is early division of the falciform ligament right back to the diaphragm, thus freeing the liver from any adhesions. Dissection of the stricture should commence in the right subhepatic area, and it may be necessary to mobilize the hepatic flexure of the colon completely, starting from below and working upwards and medially. The duodenum is exposed and very frequency is adherent, as a result of previous surgery, to the posterior hilar structures and almost always in its upper part to the area of the structure. A fistula into the duodenum is sometimes found, or a hole may be made in the duodenum during dissection that must be repaired.

A search for the bile duct distal to the stricture is often difficult, may be dangerous and, in any event, is unnecessary because the surgeon will find that the distal duct is not suitable for anastomosis. The essential and most important point is identification of the bile duct proximal to the stricture. A systemic, careful, and patient approach is necessary.

It has been recommended that the area in the neighborhood of the hilus be explored and the bile duct that is lateral to the pulsation of the hepatic artery found. This approach is usually adequate for Bismuth type 1 lesions but is not preferable, especially for high strictures (see below): exposure is more reliable after incision at the base of the quadrate lobe and lowering of the hilar plate. This maneuver delivers the bile ducts and their confluence from the undersurface of the liver, making identification of the strictured area much easier (Fig 65–13).

Once the duct is prepared, anastomosis to a Roux-en-Y loop of jejunum usually is carried out, although some, in an attempt to obviate the subsequent duodenal ulceration that occasionally occurs, have suggested anastomosis to an interposed loop of jejunum between the exposed bile duct or ducts and the duodenum.

The suture technique employed is that describe by Voyles and Blumgart[23] and by Blumgart and Kelley[10] (Figs 65–14 through 65–17). Elevation of the posterior wall of the proximal bile duct from the underlying

Segment IV

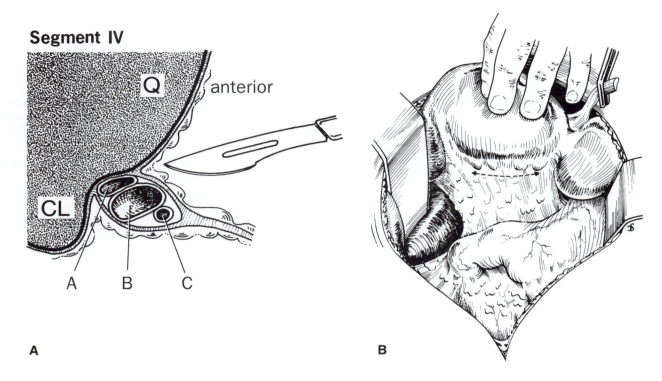

A

B

Figure 65–13. A. Sagittal section showing the relationship, in diagrammatic form, of the quadrate (Q) (segment IV) and caudate lobes (CL) to the left portal triad. A: bile duct. B: portal vein. C: hepatic artery. These structures are encased within a reflection of the lesser omentum, which fuses with Glisson's capsule at the base of the quadrate lobe. The knife indicates the point of incision for the dissection to the hilar plate. **B.** Initial line of incision for approach to the left hepatic duct by lowering of the hilar plane. The liver is elevated, and the quadrate lobe is retracted upward. The incision is made at the precise point at which Glisson's capsule reflects to the lesser omentum.

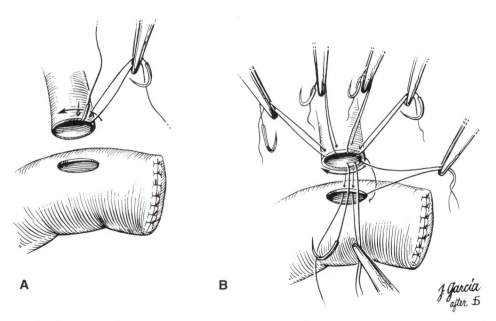

A

B

Figure 65–14. A. Initial step in creation of hepaticojejunostomy Roux-en-Y loop. The anterior layer of sutures on the bile duct is inserted first, and the sutures passed from the inside out commencing from the patient's left and working toward the right. The needles are retained, and the sutures kept in order. **B.** The anterior layer of sutures is elevated for the display of the posterior ductal wall. The posterior row of sutures is now placed again, with the surgeon working from left to right.

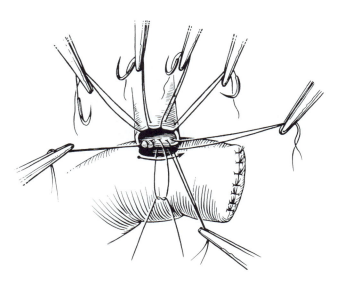

Figure 65–15. The posterior sutures are now held taut, and the jejunum is then "railroaded" upward into proximity with the bile duct. The posterior layer of sutures then is tied, with the surgeon working from right to left. Corner sutures are held; all other sutures are cut.

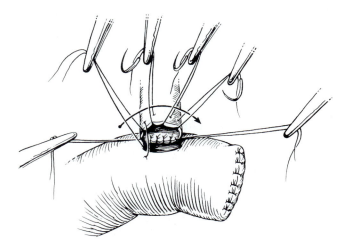

Figure 65–16. Working from the patient's right toward the left, the surgeon now passes the needles of the anterior layer through the jejunal wall from outside inward (to allow subsequent tying of the knots within). The entire anterior row of sutures is completed in this way but not yet tied.

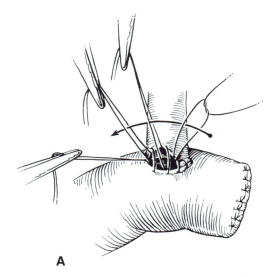

A

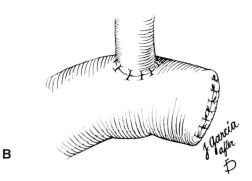

B

Figure 65–17. A. The left-hand stay is cut, and the anterior layer of sutures is now completed, with the surgeon working from the patient's left to right. **B.** Completed anastomosis. All knots are on the inside for accurate approximation of the mucosal surfaces of the bile duct and jejunum.

connective tissue, if it is difficult because of adhesions, may be only minimal. Suturing then is carried out posteriorly without undue difficulty.

Repair of high strictures (Bismuth types 2, 3, and 4) is much more demanding, and a variety of approaches may be used. In addition to the height and extent of the stricture, other complicating factors are the presence of secondary liver fibrosis and the presence of small ducts owing to incomplete obstruction or nondistensibility. In the vast majority of Bismuth types 2, 3, and 4 cases, adequate exposure of the bile ducts may be made by dissecting the left hepatic ductal system as described above (Fig 65–13). The approach, based on studies by Couinaud,[24,25] has been well described by Hepp and Couinaud,[26] and more recently, by Blumgart.[10] Occasionally, mobilization or even excision of the quadrate lobe may prove necessary in some Bismuth type 4 cases.

Although the vast majority of high strictures can be approached and dealt with as described above, it is occasionally very difficult to expose the left hepatic duct. This difficulty may be owing to dense adhesions. Bleeding may be encountered or the quadrate lobe may be large and may overhang the area of the left duct. Sometimes the extrahepatic length of the left duct may be so short as to make the approach difficult. In such instances, repair can be effected by dissection of the left hepatic duct within the umbilical fissure (*ligamentum teres approach*). This approach should not be used unless there is continuity at the hilus so that the whole biliary tree will be decompressed.[10,27a]

Smith described a method for treating the high stricture in which dissection at the area of the hilus is thought to be impossible and the ducts cannot be developed to reveal an adequate mucosa for anastomosis.[27,28] This mucosal graft procedure was hailed by some as an important advance in surgical technique. The object of the procedure is to utilize a transhepatic tube to draw the jejunal mucosa high up into the hepatic ducts and thus allow apposition for subsequent healing without fibrosis. The procedure is claimed to be an easier operation than formal anastomosis. The transhepatic tube is allowed to drain and a cholangiogram subsequently is performed. The tube is left in place, usually for 2 to 6 months, but may remain longer in very difficult cases.

Although the mucosal graft procedure originally was advocated for those cases in which suture anastomosis was thought to be impracticable, the procedure is by no means easy if the liver is densely fibrous or if secondary biliary cirrhosis is present. When the ducts are small, passage of a transhepatic tube may not be possible; moreover, it is easy to create false passages. Indeed, of a series of bile duct strictures treated by Smith, 8.4% were considered unsuitable for mucosal graft procedures as a result of liver fibrosis, secondary sclerosing cholangitis, sepsis, stones, or various combinations of these.[29] Furthermore, the method is a blind one without direct visualization, and the dome of mucosa pulled up into the hepatic ducts may block significant branches of the intrahepatic ductal system, thus occluding and isolating areas of liver tissue (Fig 65–18). Indeed, it is possible for the surgeon erroneously to "graft" only one sectoral duct, leaving the main stricture untouched. In addition, the mucosa may pull away postoperatively, and the whole jejunal loop may become detached and lie at a distance from the hilus. In an analysis of 22 cases with restricture after mucosal graft procedures, Blumgart found stricture at the site of the biliary enteric mucosal approximation in 15 cases.[30] In two cases, the right hepatic duct had been selectively occluded by the graft, and in two additional cases, the left hepatic duct was oc-

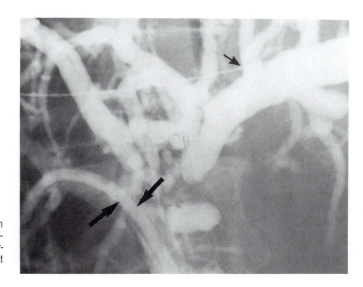

Figure 65–18. Combined tubogram and percutaneous transhepatic cholangiogram in complex case of high biliary stricture after two previous attempts at creation of hepaticojejunostomy Roux-en-Y loop with the use of the mucosal graft technique. *Large arrows* indicate tube. The graft is to one right sectoral duct only. The left hepatic duct (*small arrow*) is occluded.

cluded. Intrahepatic stones around and above the stent tube, causing obstruction and cholangitis, occurred in one case, and Roux-en-Y loop had pulled away from the hepatic duct in two cases.

Finally, doubts must be expressed about those cases in which it has been reported that dissection of bile duct mucosa for anastomosis is impossible. Such statements are based on misconceptions perpetuated by anatomic texts, by diagrams in the literature reporting the mucosal graft procedure, and by the experience of surgeons who approach the scarred fibrotic hilum directly. However, short segments of the right hepatic duct and up to 4 cm of the left hepatic duct are extrahepatic strictures and can be approached by lowering the hilar plate. Thus, in a series of 78 patients treated by Blumgart, many with complex high bile duct strictures and of whom 67 came to operation, mucosa-to-mucosa anastomosis was carried out in all but two, despite the fact that 20 had already been operated on previously by the mucosal graft technique. Similarly, Bismuth reported 180 consecutive cases, many of them of a serious nature, in which mucosal suture was possible and mucosal graft procedures were never necessary.[18]

Currently available evidence indicates that the approach rarely is indicated, has a significant failure rate, and is unlikely to stand the test of time.

Finally, we and other authors recommend that, in difficult strictures, hepaticojejunostomy be carried out over a transjejunal tube, which then is brought to the exterior across the blind end of jejunum. This portion of the jejunum is left long and is brought up subcutaneously (Fig 65–19) to allow easy subsequent interventional radiologic or choledochoscopic procedures (vide infra).

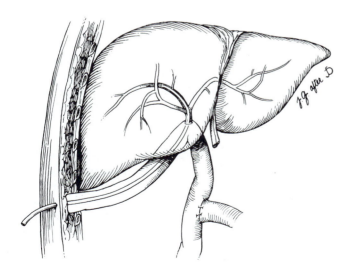

Figure 65–19. Method of hepaticojejunostomy used where surgeon desires to bring the jejunal loop to the abdominal wall to allow access for future instrumentation.

Liver Split Procedures and Mobilization of the Quadrate Lobe

Sometimes it is necessary to open the liver tissue by hepatotomy for adequate exposure of the bile ducts before repair. Wider exposure of the umbilical fissure for an approach to the segment III duct and exposure of the right hepatic ducts are the most frequent reasons for hepatotomy. This procedure is usually an extension of the subhepatic approach to the left duct, described above, and involves opening of the liver tissue in the line of the scar of the gallbladder fossa. In this situation, a liver split procedure, with opening of the umbilical fissure, allows upward mobilization of the entire quadrate lobe. These methods are usually necessary only for some type IV lesions, and especially where achieving access to the right hepatic ducts is difficult.

The liver tissue must be patiently divided, and the time required may result in some degree of hemorrhage. The technique should not be employed if exposure of the left hepatic duct is possible.

Liver Resection in Benign Stricture

Resection of liver tissue may be necessary for exposure of the bile ducts. In general, one of two forms of liver resection is used. First, excision of a part of the quadrate lobe may be carried out if mobilization of the quadrate lobe by opening the umbilical fissure and incising the bed of the gallbladder is not sufficient to allow adequate exposure of the hepatic ducts.

Second, and rarely, benign strictures of the bile ducts may be approached by means of intrahepatic hepatojejunostomy, as described by Longmire and Sandford.[31] In general, this procedure is difficult and can be dangerous in benign bile duct stricture because, if the operation is deemed necessary, the liver is always fibrous and resection of tissue is accompanied by hemorrhage. Furthermore, the bleeding vessels are in close proximity to the ducts required for anastomosis. However, the procedure can be valuable in exposing ducts for anastomosis where there is unilateral left-sided liver hypertrophy and generally is reserved for this situation. It can be valuable to develop a long jejunal loop that can be used for later interventional radiologic procedures in patients in whom a Longmire procedure is necessary.

Liver Atrophy and Hypertrophy: Influence on Approach to Repair

Segmental or lobar liver atrophy accompanied by compensatory hypertrophy and hyperplasia elsewhere in the liver may be encountered. If an entire half of the liver is affected, then the combination of atrophy and hypertrophy leads to distortion and difficulties in dissection and anastomosis (Fig 65–20).[15] The most common situation is gross hypertrophy of the left lobe accompanied by right lobe atrophy.

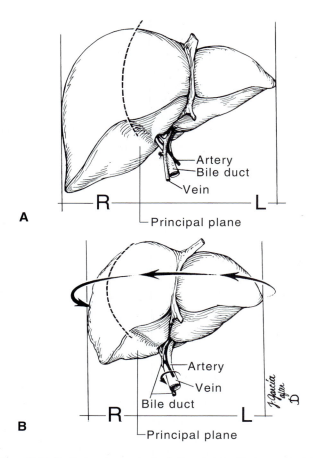

Figure 65–20. Atrophy-hypertrophy complex. **A.** Normal relationships between the right and left sides of the liver and of the hepatic artery, portal vein, and common bile duct. **B.** Gross atrophy of the right side of the liver and hypertrophy of the left side lead to rotation of the hilar structures, so that the portal vein comes to lie relatively more anteriorly and the common bile duct is rotated posterolaterally. The area of the hilus is displaced upward and to the right.

The approach to such lesions demands drainage of the entire liver substance (Fig 65–6). If, as is frequently the case, there is discontinuity of the right and left hepatic ducts at the hilus, then drainage of the left ductal system via the ligamentum teres approach or by the Longmire-Sandford operation will drain only the left side of the liver. This is usually unsatisfactory because the remaining obstructed area will continue to provide a focus of infection and a source of continued fever in the postoperative period. Anastomosis in the region of the hilus is still desirable but is always difficult. A *thoracoabdominal approach* to such strictures, in an effort to allow direct appreciation of the anatomy and access for suture repair, may be helpful. This approach, through the right side of the thorax after division of the diaphragm, allows rotation of the liver to the left and facilitates dissection. However, the problem of managing these serious lesions remains only partially solved.

PORTAL HYPERTENSION AND BILIARY STRICTURE

Portal hypertension may develop in about 14% to 20% of patients with biliary stricture and may be associated either with the development of secondary liver fibrosis or with direct damage to the portal vein. Sometimes there is coincident hepatocellular disease.

Bleeding esophageal varices occur commonly, and this complication, especially if accompanied by hypersplenism or ascites, renders the prognosis much worse. Furthermore, collateral venous channels in the subhepatic region and within vascular adhesions make dissection difficult and bloody. Finally, the patient in whom portal hypertension develops is also frequently the patient with a high stricture who has had multiple previous attempts at repair.

The development of techniques for balloon dilation of strictures by percutaneous means offers new possibilities but will seldom be a complete solution. In seriously ill patients with jaundice, portal hypertension, and a history of bleeding, it may be advisable to pass an initial percutaneous transhepatic drain or to treat the stricture, at least in the first instance, by means of percutaneous balloon dilation and then to assess the possibilities of late definitive repair.

If hemorrhage is encountered during the course of a stricture repair, then biliary drainage may be performed initially and a splenorenal shunt undertaken at a later date. Biliary repair carried out at the time of shunting procedures can be extremely difficult and, in any event, is best not performed at a time of severely compromised liver function. Some recommend that if profuse hemorrhage is encountered during attempted repair, the surgeon should carry out a three-stage procedure: hepaticostomy in the first instance, followed by a shunt some 3 weeks later, and then by reconstruction of the bile duct at a third operation when liver function is at an optimal level. This approach is now seldom necessary, however, if percutaneous drainage is used judiciously as a first stage, before attempted operation.

If a patient should have severe bleeding esophageal varices and established biliary obstruction at presentation, conservative measures should be tried in the first instance to control bleeding. The use of vasopressin infusions, the Sengstaken-Blakemore tube, and periesophageal injection of sclerosants into the varices are all reasonable first measures. If the bleeding does not stop, a two-stage operation is recommended—an immediate splenorenal shunt is performed in the first instance, and bile duct reconstruction at a later date.[32a] Percutaneous transhepatic drainage or balloon dilation may be used in association with the measures described above.

Occasionally, a patient has bleeding esophageal varices but no jaundice at presentation, owing to an inadequately repaired stricture at an earlier date. A portal systemic shunt may be indicated as an emergency measure, but it is preferable to postpone shunting until after initial conservative management of the bleeding. Experience with injection sclerotherapy in the management of this group of cases is very limited, but the treatment should be considered. However, there should be no hesitation in proceeding to shunting, if acceptable criteria are present. In general, the best and most convenient type of portosystemic shunt for these patients is a splenorenal shunt. Portocaval shunting would be technically difficult or impossible because of previous surgery in the hilar area.

There is some evidence, but no proof, that adequate biliary repair in patients with biliary stricture and portal hypertension is accompanied by slow improvement, with resolution of fibrosis and an eventual fall in portal pressure.

Finally, it should be emphasized that it is important to obtain liver biopsy specimens from patients with portal hypertension and benign bile duct strictures. Parenchymal liver disease, particularly alcoholic cirrhosis, may exist in association with iatrogenic bile duct stricture and can be a cause of confusion. Thus, in a series reported by Blumgart and associates, 2 of 11 patients with portal hypertension were found to have hepatocellular disease not consequent to obstruction.[10] It is important to emphasize that because many of these patients become subjects of medicolegal proceedings, precise documentation, to afford accurate assessment of the cause of symptoms and of the prognosis, is essential.

The prognosis for this group of patients is much worse than for patients without portal hypertension, and a hospital mortality rate approaching 40% to 80% is to be anticipated. In a series of 78 patients reported by Blumgart and associates, preoperative indices of prognosis were investigated.[10] It was found that portal hypertension was associated with a high mortality rate: 3 of 11 patients died in the hospital, and one of these patients died of uncontrolled variceal hemorrhage before any operation was undertaken. Portal hypertension was found more frequently with prolonged obstruction and recurrent episodes of cholangitis, which, in turn, were more frequent in patients who had had more than one operation before referral. There was a highly significant relationship between the presence of liver fibrosis and major infection.

NONOPERATIVE APPROACHES

It should be emphasized that the mere presence of an area of stenosis or stricture on cholangiography is not necessarily an indication for operation. An established internal fistula may provide good long-term biliary drainage, and impressive degrees of stenosis on cholangiography may produce little in the way of symptoms or altered liver chemistries. In selected cases, particularly for elderly or high-risk patients, it may be perfectly appropriate to accept a degree of obstruction, if symptoms are minimal and easily controlled by intermittent administration of antibiotics. The results of balloon dilation of benign strictures must be judged against no treatment at all.[32–36] Long-term results are not yet available, but early reports suggest a high restricture rate.[37] It is important to maintain close follow-up in all cases managed nonoperatively or by balloon dilation, since progressive liver damage may be insidious. A persistently elevated alkaline phosphatase may be the only index of incomplete obstruction.

COMBINED MODALITY APPROACHES

Standard surgical techniques of biliary reconstruction described above are suitable for the majority of cases. However, in the most complex and difficult strictures, and especially in the presence of intrahepatic strictures and stones, even optimal surgical management is met with a disappointingly high incidence of postoperative intrahepatic stone formation, cholangitis, and recurrent stricture. Interventional radiologic and endoscopic techniques used as primary therapy in this setting are likewise doomed to failure owing to recurrent cholangitis associated with stent occlusion, dislocation of the endoprosthesis, or recurrent stricture after balloon dilation. Often, these nonoperative approaches are technically impossible owing to the problem of safe access to the pathology.

Under these circumstances, hepaticojejunostomy may be carried out over a transjejunal tube that is then brought to the exterior across the blind end of the Roux limb, which is deliberately left long and secured subcutaneously or subperitoneally. This arrangement allows easy subsequent cholangiography and cholangioscopy. Via the tube tract, stricture dilation may be carried out in multiple postoperative sessions, if necessary (Fig 65–19). In the author's experience, the combined modality approach offers an excellent chance of definitive successful repair at the initial hospitalization. It also spares the patient the need for repeated major surgical intervention months or years later because of suspected restricture or recurrent stone formation.[38] The blind end of the Roux-en-Y limb may be reaccessed by percutaneous puncture under fluoroscopic guidance or via a small incision under local anesthetic for late diagnostic or therapeutic procedures, long after the transjejunal tube has been removed. It is generally unnecessary to add the morbidity of a formal stoma, although such an approach has been reported.[39]

RESULTS

A variety of factors influence the prognosis and outcome of bile duct stricture in patients admitted to the hospital (Table 65–3). *The main factors influencing a satisfactory stric-*

TABLE 65–3. FACTORS AFFECTING OUTCOME OF BILIARY STRICTURES

- Proximal biliary stricture (Bismuth types 2 and 4)
- Intrahepatic or multiple strictures
- Multiple prior attempts at repair
- Concurrent cholangitis or hepatic abscess
- Intrahepatic stones
- External or internal bile fistula
- Intra-abdominal abscess or bile collection
- Portal hypertension
- Hepatic parenchymal disease (cirrhosis or hepatic fibrosis)
- Liver lobe atrophy and/or hypertrophy (atrophy-hypertrophy complex)
- Advanced age or poor general medical condition

ture repair are the number of previous operations, the site of the stricture, and the type of repair, whereas those that influence mortality rates are the number of previous operations, whether there is a history of major infection, the site of the stricture, preoperative serum albumin concentration and particularly, whether liver fibrosis and portal hypertension are present.

The adequacy of surgical repair is of great importance in determining long-term prognosis. While untreated cases have a fatal outcome, surgical treatment that offers only partial relief of the biliary obstruction also results in progressive liver damage and, ultimately, death. Failure to drain all segments of the liver results in segmental liver atrophy.

Operative Morbidity and Mortality Rates

The morbidity rate after reconstructive surgery for bile duct stricture is high. Probably 1 patient in 10 will have one or more major nonfatal complications. However, some authors report higher figures, and more complications are to be expected from series that include a high proportion of reoperated cases. The common complications encountered are subphrenic, subhepatic, or pelvic infections, wound infections, cholangitis, bacteremic shock, secondary hemorrhage, biliary fistula, and pulmonary complications.

Mortality rates are very difficult to assess. First, some reports do not define operative death and whether it includes hospital death. Furthermore, some patients die before operation, and others die of infection, renal failure, or hematemesis because of variceal bleeding. Other features that make assessment of mortality rates difficult are failure to differentiate high strictures from low, to allow for the effects of multiple operations, and to differentiate clearly deaths associated with one operative procedure from deaths associated with another.

The operative mortality rate in patients with bile duct stricture is reported to be between 5% and 8%. The most common causes of death are uncontrolled hemorrhage, hepatic or renal failure, and a combination of

these features. Biliary fistula, bacteremia, and pulmonary complications are responsible for the remaining operative deaths. In the experience of Blumgart and associates the *overall* 30-day hospital mortality was 11.5%, including one death owing to bleeding esophageal varices before operation could be undertaken.[10] The operative mortality rate for *all procedures*, including surgery for drainage of abscesses, shunt procedures for control of bleeding, and biliary repair was 8.3%. There were no deaths among 58 patients treated by hepaticojejunostomy nor in 3 treated by choledochoduodenostomy. Two patients with complex high strictures were treated by mucosal apposition early in the series, and both died. Thus, in the 63 patients treated by stricture repair alone, there was an operative mortality rate of 3.2%. A total of 84 patients subjected to stricture repair alone were reported by Blumgart to have a 30 day mortality rate of 2.4% (two patients).[22] There were *no deaths among 82 consecutive patients treated by mucosa-to-mucosa suture.* This series has now been extended and updated.[40] Of 130 consecutive patients referred for the treatment of postcholecystectomy bile duct strictures over a 12 year period, 80 (61%) underwent multiple operative procedures before referral and 62% underwent at least one stricture repair. Seventy-eight patients (60%) had a stricture involving the confluence of the bile ducts (type III or type IV) and 18% had evidence of portal hypertension. Eight patients were treated nonoperatively and one of these died of variceal hemorrhage before any therapy could be effectively undertaken. A total of 122 (94%) patients underwent some form of operative treatment (Table 65–4). Two patients were treated early in the series by mucosal graft procedures and both died. Three of five patients in whom stricture repair and portal systemic shunt were attempted also died. Two of seven patients in whom operation but no stricture repair was carried out also died, both in the presence of portal hypertension. Therefore, the overall mortality

TABLE 65–4. POSTCHOLECYSTECTOMY BILE DUCT STRICTURE (n = 130)[a]

Operative	No. of Patients
Biliary repair only	106[b]
Longmire procedure	2
Mucosal grant	2
Portal shunt and repair	4
Portal shunt	1
Dilation and tube	2
Exploration drainage abscess	5
Total	122

[a]Data from Chapman WC, Halevy A, Benjamin IS, Blumgart LH. Postcholecystectomy bile duct strictures—management and outcome in 130 patients. In preparation, 1993
[b]Sutured anastomosis: 103 hepaticojejunostomy, 3 choledochoduodenostomy.

TABLE 65–5. POSTCHOLECYSTECTOMY BILE DUCT STRICTURES MORTALITY (IN-HOSPITAL/60 DAY) (n = 130)[a]

	Death (%)
Nonoperative (n = 8)	1
Operative	
Biliary repair (n = 106)	0
Longmire (n = 2)	0
Mucosal graft (n = 2)	2
Portosystemic anastomosis and repair (n = 5)	3
No biliary repair (abscess drainage intubation) (n = 7)	2
	8 (6.1%)

[a]Data from Chapman WC, Halevy A, Benjamin IS, Blumgart LH. Post-cholecystectomy bile duct strictures—management and outcome in 130 patients. *Arch Surg.* 1995; 130:597

was 6.1% (8 out of 130). However, it should be noted that there were *no deaths* among the 106 patients treated by mucosa-to-mucosa biliary enteric anastomosis, 97 of whom had hepaticojejunostomy via the left duct (Table 65–5).[41] In this series, factors influencing mortality included hypoalbuminemia and elevated serum bilirubin, the presence of liver disease, and portal hypertension. These results are comparable to those of Bismuth, who reported 186 patients operated on by hepaticojejunostomy, with a left hepatic duct approach, since the introduction of the technique in 1956.[22] Seventy percent of these patients had one or more operations before referral, and they had associated lesions that complicated operation and compounded the difficulty of biliary repair. The associated lesions were mainly intrahepatic stones above the stricture, biliary fistula, hepatic atrophy, and biliary fibrosis. Despite these complications, all patients were operated on by a mucosa-to-mucosa suture, and the left duct approach was possible in all but four. One patient was subjected to intrahepatic cholangiojejunostomy. The operative mortality rate, with operative death defined as that which occurs intraoperatively or immediately postoperatively, was 0.6%.

The safety of repair by an experienced surgeon, particularly in the uncomplicated case, needs to be appreciated and the results taken into account in assessing the newer techniques of transhepatic or transendoscopic biliary dilation.

Late Results

The late results of bile duct injury repair after cholecystectomy are difficult to evaluate. There is considerable variation in the criteria chosen to assess long-term results. Morbidity and mortality rates not associated with stricture repair must be taken into account, and the results of stricture repair in an uncomplicated case should be separable from those cases associated with liver disease, portal hypertension, or lobar atrophy. In many reports this is not possible. Similarly, there is scant in-

formation on relative mortality and morbidity rates according to the level of stricture. There is also variation in what is accepted as a satisfactory result. Thus, Braasch and associates accepted as a good result a patient's freedom from symptoms or the occurrence of only occasional attacks of cholangitis and jaundice 3 years after repair.[42] Other authors have defined a satisfactory repair as the absence of symptoms 2 years after operation. Bismuth suggested that a good result would be follow-up of at least 5 years, or preferably 10 years, during which the patient remains free of symptoms, with normal liver function test results and no restenosis.[22]

In a study reported by Blumgart and associates, it was found that Bismuth type 3 and type 4 strictures were associated with less satisfactory results. Similarly, Warren and Jefferson reported 958 patients reviewed at the Lahey Clinic, of whom 77 had strictures that were at, or proximal to, the common hepatic duct.[43] Although not differentiating type 3 and type 4 Bismuth strictures from type 2, this study also emphasized the difficulties in repairing ducts with higher strictures. In a literature survey, Warren and associates reported obtaining satisfactory results in only approximately 47% of patients (72% of those patients were followed for a suitable length of time), with an overall operative mortality rate of 8.3%.[44] Pitt and associates examined the factors influencing outcome of repair of benign strictures after cholecystectomy.[37] Better results are achieved in patients <30 years of age, with no previous attempted stricture repair, when a Roux-en-Y jejunal loop and transhepatic Silastic tubal splinting was used for longer than 1 month, extended to 9 months or more, with changeable Silastic splints in patients with difficult hilar strictures. Pellegrini and associates evaluated 50 consecutive patients with recurrent biliary stricture, all of whom had at least one previous repair, to determine the pattern of recurrence and the outcome of preoperative treatment.[45] Presenting features included cholangitis in 40% of patients, jaundice in 30%, and pain in 17%. The operative mortality rate was 4%, and 76% of patients had no further recurrence of symptoms. However, in 11 (22%) patients, recurrence developed, although six of these patients did well after yet another operation. Of four patients in whom a third recurrence developed, three were successfully treated at a fourth operation. Pellegrini and associates therefore concluded that two-thirds of recurrent strictures were evident by 2 years and 90% by 7 years. These authors calculated that the chance of recurrence was about 25% after retreatment of a first recurrent stricture, and they concluded that hepaticojejunostomy by direct suture is important and that prolonged stenting did not contribute to a good result.

Blumgart and associates reported that, in a series of 78 patients, a satisfactory result was achieved in 90% of cases treated by stricture repair only over a mean follow-up period of 3.3 years.[10] There were two late deaths within a year of surgery, one of which was caused by liver failure and the other in a patient in whom a coincidental cholangiocarcinoma developed.

Bismuth, in a series of 186 patients, chose a 10 year follow-up period.[18] Of 186 patients operated on by means of hepaticojejunostomy to the left duct, 141 were operated on between 1956 and 1972 and were assessed for late results. Fourteen (11%) patients were lost to follow-up. Seven died from nonbiliary causes, leaving 120 patients for reassessment at the 10 to 20 year period. Of these, 88% had an excellent result defined by the absence of any biliary troubles. Five percent had transitory trouble shortly after operation, probably related to the procedure itself, but did not require reoperation. Results were unsatisfactory in 7% of patients. Recurrent stenosis developed in three patients and required reoperation. Results were unsatisfactory in 7% of patients. Recurrent stenosis developed in three patients and required reoperation, and all three had a good outcome subsequently. Five patients, all with secondary biliary fibrosis, died.

These results are similar to those reported by Blumgart and associates from Hammersmith Hospital, London, and confirmed in a later extended series from the same institution.[10] In the latter series of 110 patients treated by stricture repair alone, 97 of whom had hepaticojejunostomy to the left duct, 82% had a good result with no biliary symptoms and no need for intervention during follow-up (mean 7.2 years). However, 18% of these patients required reoperation or interventional radiologic procedures for continued symptoms. Of these, 12 had subsequent biliary repair, while 4 were reoperated on to provide access for radiologic intervention. Two patients were operated on for pyloric stenosis consequent to a hepatic ulceration. Results of these procedures were good in only 50% of the patients. It is of interest that during the period of follow-up, 22 patients died—8 of unrelated cause but 14 of progressive liver failure. It is important to understand the gravity of bile duct injury and the prognosis over time; this is not always reported. Preoperative factors influencing failure of the stricture repair at long-term follow-up include discontinuity of the right and left ducts at the time of repair (Bismuth grade IV), and three or more previous attempts at operative repair before referral.[41]

Thus, Kune and Sali's estimate[2] that 85% of patients who have sustained an operative injury to the bile ducts will be restored to normal health if reconstruction is undertaken by an experienced surgeon is supported by recent experience from a number of specialist centers dealing with the problem.

Duodenal ulceration appears to develop in a small proportion of patients after Roux-en-Y biliary enteric repair and is an additional cause for later morbidity. The majority of cases will respond to the administration of H2 histamine receptor inhibitory agents.[46,47]

Late results for the mucosal graft procedure were reported by Smith.[48] Of 451 patients reviewed, 413 had mucosal graft procedures. At 2 years, 15% of those patients submitted to a mucosal graft procedure had continuing symptoms. In 4%, these symptoms were directly attributable to restenosis, although this figure may be considerably higher in the future. The remaining 11% were seriously compromised, having either liver disease, secondary sclerosing cholangitis, or severe sepsis with stones. Although patients with liver fibrosis, sclerosing cholangitis, sepsis, and stones were considered a high-risk group unlikely to derive lasting benefit from stricture repair and unsuitable for mucosal graft, in 11% of these patients actually submitted to a mucosal graft procedure, these features did, in fact, develop. Many patients (half of the patients reported to have had an excellent result) had a persisting elevation of the serum alkaline phosphatase level. This increase might be the result of segmental obstruction associated with the graft operation. The results reported appear to offer no advantage in the treatment of the complex case. The reason for the procedure—namely, that high strictures cannot be sutured—is open to question because precise direct anastomosis can be carried out with a very low mortality rate and excellent long-term follow-up results, even in patients with complex strictures who were previously submitted to mucosal graft operation.

Techniques of follow-up have varied from simple observation of the patient and measurement of liver function to the performance of transtubal cholangiography and HIDA scanning. Some patients will remain symptomless but yet have a persistently raised alkaline phosphatase level. Studies carried out by Blumgart and colleagues at the Royal Postgraduate Medical School, London, in which both HIDA scanning was done and alkaline phosphatase levels were measured, suggest that persistence of an elevated alkaline phosphatase level during a prolonged period is consequent either on an associated hepatocellular disease or on incomplete relief of obstruction. A result probably should not be regarded as excellent unless the alkaline phosphatase level returns to normal. This measurement is important in assessing late results of percutaneous transhepatic dilational techniques. A triad of criteria may be used to clarify results (Table 65–6), and this sort of system may prove useful in assessing the late results of both surgical repair and nonoperative techniques.[38]

The influence of long-term transanastomic tubal splinting on long-term patency has been debated. Transanastomic splinting has been used by many surgeons, and the length of time that the tube should be left in situ is still subject to controversy. Although one study suggested that better long-term results were ob-

TABLE 65–6. SUGGESTED CRITERIA FOR ASSESSMENT OF LATE RESULTS OF STRICTURE MANAGEMENT

Classification	Symptoms	Biochemistry*	Radiology[b]
Excellent	None	Normal	Normal
Good	None	+/− Elevated	+/− Abnormal
Fair	Improved	Elevated	Abnormal
Poor	Persistent or worse	Elevated	Abnormal

*Serum bilirubin and/or alkaline phosphatase
[b]HIDA scan and/or cholangiography.
*(From Blumgart LH, Matthews JB. Benign bile duct stricture. In: Blumgart LH (ed),
Surgery of the Liver and Biliary Tract, vol 2. Edinburgh, Scotland: Churchill Livingstone;
1993)*

tained in anastomoses splinted for longer than 12 months, 3 to 6 months is now generally considered to be the minimum period of splintage. The tube is left in place for 12 months in more difficult cases. The median duration of splintage in a study carried out at Hammersmith Hospital, London, by Blumgart and associates was only 4 months.[10] Some surgeons rarely use transanastomotic stenting and have obtained good results. It may well be that transanastomotic tubes are unnecessary for the average patient. We have recently omitted tubes altogether in a substantial series of uncomplicated cases, without noticeable problems. In complex cases, percutaneous transhepatic catheterization and dilation can be a useful maneuver. A planned combination surgical and interventional radiologic approach, as described above, also has been useful, especially if intrahepatic stones cannot be completely retrieved by the surgeon, or if repair is difficult or unsatisfactory and recurrent stricture is anticipated.

It should be emphasized that injury to the bile duct during cholecystectomy is a serious problem. Death, occurring both initially and late, is related to reoperative procedures, infection, and the evolution of secondary biliary fibrosis and to the development of portal hypertension. The following points summarize the problem:

1. Bile duct injury at cholecystectomy is inflicted as a result of imprecise dissection and poor visualization of anatomic structures.
2. Vascular damage to the hepatic artery, portal vein, or both is not uncommon.
3. A prolonged history of high stricture involving the hepatic ducts, multiple attempts at repair, infection, and the development of secondary liver fibrosis, together with a low preoperative serum albumin level, are adverse prognostic features.
4. Precise determination of the level of the stricture and demonstration of hepatic ducts before surgery are desirable.

5. Associated conditions such as abscess formation, gastrointestinal bleeding, fistula, and portal hypertension probably are treated best before stricture repair.
6. There is a place for conservative management or transhepatic percutaneous dilation in selected high-risk patients, especially in the presence of portal hypertension. However, nonoperative approaches should be used with care, because incomplete relief of a stricture may be dangerous in the long term and associated with development of insidious progressive liver damage. In any event, most strictures can be repaired safely by biliary-enteric anastomosis.
7. Interventional radiologic approaches may be used in an adjunctive manner with surgical repair, in selected cases. A percutaneous approach or the introduction of catheters along previously defined ductal tracts is used.
8. The majority of benign bile duct strictures can and should be managed by surgical restoration of biliary-enteric continuity, consisting of dissection of the left hepatic ductal system and confluence, followed by direct mucosa-to-mucosa anastomosis of the bile duct, usually to a Roux-en-Y loop of jejunum. For this approach and in the absence of liver disease, the operative mortality rate is probably <1%.
9. Mucosal graft techniques, hepatotomy, and left hepaticojejunostomy of the Longmire type have a limited indication only.
10. Investigations of this subject should examine prognostic indices and classification of bile duct strictures to allow comparison of results and assessment of new methods of treatment.
11. Repair of bile duct strictures is a specialist procedure, and the best results are obtained by adequate initial repair. Repeated attempts at anastomosis or intubation are associated with the development of high complex strictures and late liver disease, both of which are associated with poor long-term results.

■ BILE DUCT INJURY AFTER OPERATIONS OTHER THAN CHOLECYSTECTOMY

BILIARY OPERATIONS

Operations that involve biliary-enteric anastomosis may be complicated by postoperative stricture or fistula. Such procedures include reconstruction after pancreaticoduodenectomy,[49] after bile duct excision for tumors in its middle third, or after excision of a choledochal cyst. Typically, these procedures involve choledochoenteric or hepaticoenteric anastomosis. Late strictures after such procedures are most likely to occur when enteric anastomosis is performed to a normal caliber duct or when the duct itself is diseased, as after excision of choledochal cysts. Where biliary-enteric anastomosis has been carried out for long-standing biliary obstruction, the duct is dilated and thickened. The anastomosis is easy to construct, and late stenosis is rare. Stricture following pancreaticoduodenectomy for malignancy most often is attributed to recurrent disease rather than to a benign stenotic process.

Late stricture after side-to-side choledochoduodenostomy performed for choledocholithiasis or as a bypass procedure for chronic pancreatitis also may occur. This complication is rare if choledochoduodenostomy is performed to a sufficiently dilated duct (>1.5 cm) and if the anastomosis is sufficiently large (>1.5 cm).[50-52] The so-called "sump syndrome" after choledochoduodenostomy, in which particulate matter, stones, and food debris accumulate and stagnate in the distal "blind" end of the common duct, is an occasional cause of recurrent cholangitis that may develop with or without anastomotic stricture.[53] Endoscopic management, consisting of sphincterotomy with or without balloon dilation of the anastomosis has been reported for this condition.[39] However, this approach may not completely remove the thick, infected debris that often is densely adherent to the wall of the inflamed distal common bile duct. Restricture of the anastomosis is not infrequent. The authors prefer reoperation, with end-to-side hepaticojejunostomy Roux-en-Y, in order to prevent intestinobiliary regurgitation and to permanently eliminate the "sump."[53]

Recurrent cholangitis after biliary-enteric anastomosis is almost invariably attributed to anastomotic stricture; however, this assumption has been questioned.[54] Some patients develop repeated episodes of cholangitis despite apparently free drainage of bile through the anastomosis, in the absence of an overt stricture. In these more exceptional cases, there often is overlooked intrahepatic stricture or intrahepatic stone disease.[53]

POSTGASTRECTOMY BILIARY STRICTURE

Injury to the bile duct can occur during gastrectomy, particularly if, during the procedure, the pyloric region and first part of the duodenum are found to be grossly distorted or inflamed. The most common situation is biliary injury during the course of a Polya gastrectomy. Such injuries may become evident during the postoperative period in association with jaundice or a biliary fistula, and there may be difficulty in distinguishing the presentation from a leaking duodenal stump.

Blumgart has had experience with four bile duct strictures after gastrectomy (Table 65–7). Two were of the nature described, but the other two followed Billroth I gastrectomy. In the latter two cases, the surgeon carried out what was claimed to be an easy, straightforward Billroth I gastrectomy. In one case, the surgeon, after completing the operation, realized that he had removed the entire first and second part of the duodenum from the pancreatic head, thus exposing the bile duct and the pancreatic duct. In the second case, a precisely similar injury occurred, but the surgeon did not recognize the problem and closed the abdomen. A biliary-pancreatic fistula then became evident during the postoperative period. Surgical reexploration revealed the denuded pancreatic head.

Repair of a damaged bile duct after a Polya gastrectomy is usually not difficult. The stricture usually lies in close proximity to the duodenal stump, and it is a simple matter to identify the biliary tree and carry out a direct anastomosis at or near the blind end of the duodenum. Where the entire duodenal head is denuded, as described above, a Roux-en-Y loop of jejunum may be developed and brought up in a retrocolic fashion; the open end is used to envelop the pancreatic head.

OTHER PROCEDURES

In a series of 137 cases of benign bile duct stricture, one patient had late biliary stenosis after a portacaval shunt. In another case, a bile duct stricture occurred after irradiation of para-aortic nodes for testicular malignancy (Table 65–3).

Liver resection also may be complicated by biliary damage. In cases of hepatic injury, biliary damage may be associated with the original trauma or be inflicted during the subsequent operative treatment. It may be difficult or impossible to define precisely the cause of a subsequent evident biliary fistula or stricture. Biliary damage also may occur during liver resection for tumor or cyst and is more likely for lesions involving the hilus, where dissection renders the biliary tree more liable to injury (Table 65–7).

It is not necessary to insert a T tube into the common bile duct after partial hepatectomy. However, should a ductal injury be inflicted during operation, or if there is doubt as to the anatomy of the biliary tree at the time of surgery, then operative cholangiography can be valuable in displaying the anatomy. Opening the common bile duct with passage of fine, soft bougies into the right and left ducts may assist identification. If this procedure has been carried out, then a T tube should be inserted.

The management of injuries after partial hepatectomy can be extremely difficult; the problems are similar to those encountered in the atrophy-hypertrophy complex (Fig 65–7) (see above). It should be emphasized, however, that a biliary fistula occurring after partial hepatectomy should be treated expectantly for long

TABLE 65–7. OPERATIONS OR CONDITIONS ASSOCIATED WITH BENIGN BILIARY STRICTURE[a]

Operation or Condition	No. of Patients
Cholecystectomy	101
Choledocholithiasis	3
Penetrating injury	5
Blunt injury[b]	6
Pancreatitis	9
Gastrectomy	4
Operation for choledochus cyst	4
Periportal inflammation (including one after deep x-ray irradiation)	4
Portal shunt	1
Total	137

[a]Excludes peripapillary stricture, primary localized stricture (sclerosing cholangitis), and stricture owing to cholelithiasis or associated with the Mirizzi syndrome
[b]Five patients with liver injury.

periods. The surgeon should proceed with an operation only if the fistula fails to close after observation or if jaundice and cholangitis supervene.

■ BILE DUCT INJURY DUE TO BLUNT OR PENETRATING ABDOMINAL TRAUMA

The gallbladder or biliary tree may be damaged after closed abdominal injury or by penetrating stab or gunshot wounds. The latter, although common in some parts of the world, are generally an infrequent cause of biliary injury. In a series of 137 bile duct strictures treated by Blumgart, six occurred in association with blunt injury (five with associated liver injury) and five after stab wounds (Table 65–7).

Occasionally, late problems arise when prolonged fistulation occurs after a segment of the liver has been isolated by injury, so that the biliary product of a large portion of the liver is discharged through the fistulous tract. Management of such cases is difficult, and even prolonged observation may fail to detect closure of the fistula, especially in association with a distal stricture. When such fistulation occurs, management may be by one of three methods: First, resection of the isolated segment of liver tissue may be carried out. Such an approach can be difficult and is seldom warranted. Second, in rare instances, the fistula may be identified at operation and simply oversewn. Alternatively, a well-developed fibrous fistulous tract can be anastomosed either to a prepared loop of jejunum or to the gallbladder. Such an operation may produce a permanent cure, but late stenosis or stricture still may be a problem for which secondary repair must be carried out.

■ POSTINFLAMMATORY BILIARY STRICTURES

Bile duct stenosis and stricture may occur in association with any process that causes fibrosis of the common biliary channels or that causes a diffuse sclerotic process within the biliary tree. Such strictures may result from choledocholithiasis, granulomatous lymphadenitis, chronic pancreatitis, or recurrent pyogenic cholangitis. Additionally, these strictures may occur in association with parasitic disease, especially infection with *Echinococcus alveolaris*.

LONG-STANDING CHOLELITHIASIS

Long-standing cholelithiasis results in repeated attacks of cholecystitis. The gallbladder becomes progressively fibrosed, shrunken, and surrounded by inflammatory tissue. As this process proceeds, the Calot's triangle is obliterated until the gallbladder wall abuts against the common hepatic duct. In such instances, the inflammatory process may spread to involve the common hepatic duct, causing inflammatory stenosis and stricturing. Presentation usually includes jaundice and recurrent attacks of cholangitis (Mirizzi's syndrome). The surgeon who has proceeded to operation on the jaundiced patient without prior imaging of the biliary tree may discover that he has created a bile duct injury inadvertently during attempts to remove the gallbladder. Furthermore, as outlined above, a large stone in the region of Hartmann's pouch may erode into the common hepatic duct, causing a cholecystic-choledochal fistula. In such instances, the removal of the gallbladder results in an opening into the common hepatic duct or inadvertent removal of the portion of the common hepatic duct. This situation should be suspected in any patient with a long history of gallstones who has jaundice and cholangitis at presentation. Operation should never be performed in such cases without preliminary percutaneous transhepatic or endoscopic retrograde cholangiography to alert the surgeon to the operative problems that will be encountered.

Finally, the radiologic features of inflammatory strictures of the common hepatic duct in association with chronic cholelithiasis may be indistinguishable from those of cholangiocarcinoma (see Chapter 66).

CHRONIC PERIPAPILLARY DUODENAL ULCER

This type of ulcer can erode the entire papillary area, resulting in stricture or a choledochoduodenal fistula. Jaundice and cholangitis usually are present, and there is usually a prolonged history of duodenal ulcer. Management usually involves Polya gastrectomy and biliary bypass.

Granulomatous Lymphadenitis

Granulomatous lymphadenitis also may be responsible for stricture of the adjacent common hepatic or common bile duct. This condition may occur in association with tuberculosis. In such cases, there has almost always been long-standing obstruction to the bile ducts. Usually there is associated secondary biliary fibrosis and a degree of liver damage, which occasionally may be unilateral with liver atrophy. Treatment can be difficult because liver function is compromised and biliary drainage can be difficult to establish.

RECURRENT PYOGENIC CHOLANGITIS

Recurrent pyogenic cholangitis, as seen in Southeast Asia, is complicated by intrahepatic gallstones consisting of calcium bilirubinate. Intrahepatic bile duct strictures also occur. The best management of such intrahepatic strictures, particularly if they are unilateral, consists of a combination of Roux-en-Y hepaticojejunostomy and partial hepatectomy, including the affected ducts.

CHRONIC PANCREATITIS

Chronic pancreatitis also may result in bile duct stenosis and stricture. The characteristic stricture is long and narrow and occupies the retrohepatic portion of the common bile duct. However, other variants of stricture may occur and have been described in detail. Although this stricturing is more common in association with chronic alcoholism-related pancreatitis, it occasionally occurs in chronic pancreatitis unrelated to alcoholism. In addition to jaundice there may be associated pain, which is usually intermittent in character. Cholangitis and fever are unusual but also can occur.

Diagnosis is made either at endoscopic retrograde cholangiography or transhepatic percutaneous cholangiography, or sometimes at the time of operation. The radiologic appearance is of a long-standing stenosis in the retropancreatic portion of the common bile duct. However, because the fibrotic process, in association with inflammation of the pancreas, may affect the proximal duct, there may be very little dilation of the proximal bile duct. Stenosis may, however, be shorter or may involve only the immediate papillary area. Differentiation from carcinomatous obstruction may be very difficult. Although the long, tapering, narrow stricture of the bile duct is usually characteristic of chronic pancreatitis, especially in association with demonstrable pancreatic ductal abnormality at ERCP, carcinoma may still be present. Caution is therefore necessary.

Discovery of a bile duct stenosis or stricture in association with chronic pancreatitis is not an indication for therapy; relatively severe stenosis may be found in patients in whom results of liver function tests are absolutely normal and who have never been jaundiced. If, however, cholestasis or cholangitis occur, or if chronically elevated alkaline phosphatase exists, then biliary bypass is necessary. In addition, if an operation is to be carried out for the management of chronic pancreatitis itself, and if it is known that severe biliary stenosis is present, the surgeon may elect to perform a biliary bypass at the same time. Thus, in a series of 240 patients with chronic pancreatitis managed by the authors, 39 of whom came to surgery, nine had symptomatic biliary tract obstruction. Thirteen patients were subjected to some form of biliary enteric anastomosis, either alone or in association with excisional surgery for pancreatic disease.

While side-to-side choledochoduodenostomy may be employed in some cases, it is usually not the best procedure because the surrounding inflammatory reaction may render the duodenum rigid and therefore less mobile. Moreover, the common bile duct frequently is not grossly dilated. Roux-en-Y choledochojejunostomy is a preferable procedure in obstruction resulting from chronic pancreatitis and may be carried out as a side-to-side or an end-to-side procedure after division of the common bile duct. Cholecystojejunostomy should not be used in these circumstances, nor is transduodenal sphincteroplasty suitable, since the stricture is usually too long to allow this approach.

In patients with chronic pancreatitis in whom the primary presentation has been with cholestasis and in whom the pancreatic disease remains quiescent, biliary enteric anastomosis is an excellent operation with good, long-term relief of symptoms.

PARASITIC DISEASE

A number of parasitic infestations, including infestation with *Ascaris lumbricoides* and the various forms of echinococcal disease, may be associated with the development of bile duct strictures. *Echinococcus alveolaris*, in particular, produces dense strictures and also narrowing or obliteration of portal vessels and arteries. The severe distortion present, the density of the fibrosis, the vessel involvement, and the progressive nature of the disease make therapy difficult. Hepatic resection may be necessary.

Biliary stricture usually presents a complex problem in diagnosis and management. As such, it is a special abnormality demanding an experienced surgical team working in close collaboration with others and, in particular, having excellent diagnostic and interventional radiologic backup and facilities for endoscopic diagnosis and operative endoscopy, when indicated. Treatment decisions should be taken in consultation. Bile duct strictures, and in particular, high strictures and stenoses extending to the confluence of the bile ducts, should not be treated by the occasional operator.

REFERENCES

1. Grey-Turner RG. Injuries to the main bile duct. *Lancet* 1944;1:621

2. Kune GA, Sali A. Benign biliary strictures. In: *The Practice of Biliary Surgery*, 2nd ed. Oxford, England: Blackwell Scientific; 1981

3. Morgenstern L, Wong L, Gerci G. Twelve hundred open cholecystectomies before the laparoscopic era: a standard for comparison. *Arch Surg* 1992;127:400

4. Soper NJ, Stockman PT, Dunnegan DL, Ashley SW. Laparoscopic cholecystectomy: the new "gold standard"? *Arch Surg* 1992;127:917

5. The Southern Surgeon's Club. A prospective analysis of 1518 laparoscopic cholecystectomies. *N Eng J Med* 1991; 324:1073–1078

6. Rossi RL, Schirmer WJ, Braasch JW, et al. Laparoscopic bile duct injuries: risk factors, recognition, and repair. *Arch Surg* 1992;78:559

7. Moossa A, Easter DW, van Sonnenberg E, et al. Laparoscopic injuries to the bile duct: a cause for concern. *Ann Surg* 1992;215:203

8. Davidoff AM, Pappas TN, Murray EA, et al. Mechanisms of major biliary injury during laparoscopic cholecystectomy. *Ann Surg* 1992;215:196

9. Asbun HJ, Rossi RL, Lowell JA, Munson JL. Bile duct injury during laparoscopic cholecystectomy: mechanism of injury, prevention, and management. *World J Surg* 1993;17:545

10. Blumgart LH, Kelley CJ, Benjamin IS. Benign bile duct stricture following cholecystectomy: critical factors in management. *Br J Surg* 1984;71:836

11. Northover JMA, Terblanche I. Applied surgical anatomy of the biliary tree. In: Blumgart LH (ed), *The Biliary Tract, Clinical Surgery International*, vol 5. Edinburgh, Scotland: Churchill Livingstone; 1982:1–16

12. Cattell RB, Braasch JW. General considerations in the management of benign stricture of the bile duct. *N Engl J Med* 1959;261:929

13. Larson GM, Vitole GC, Casey J, et al. Multipractice analysis of laparoscopic cholecystectomy in 1983 patients. *Am J Surg* 1992;163:221

14. Easter DW, Moossa AR. Laser and laparoscopic cholecystectomy: a hazardous union. *Arch Surg* 1991;213:635

15a. Weinbren HK, Hadjis NS, Blumgart LH. Structural aspects of the liver in patients with biliary disease and portal hypertension. *J Clin Pathol* 1985;38:1013

15. Czerniak A, Søreide O, et al. Liver atrophy complicating benign bile duct strictures in surgical and interventional radiological approaches. *Am J Surg* 1986;152:294

16. Hadjis NS, Blumgart LH. Role of liver atrophy, hepatic resection and hepatocyte hyperplasia in the development of portal hypertension. *Gut* 1987;28:1022

17. Blumgart LH. Biliary tract obstruction: new approaches to old problems. *Am J Surg* 1978;135:19

18. Bismuth H. Postoperative strictures of the bile duct. In: Blumgart LH (ed), *The Biliary Tract, Clinical Surgery International*. vol 5. Edinburgh, Scotland: Churchill Livingstone, 1982:209–218

19. Blenkharn JI, Blumgart LH. Streptococcal bacteraemia in hepatobiliary operations. *Surg Gynecol Obstet* 1985;160:139

20. Thompson JE, Pitt HA, Doty JE, et al. Broad spectrum penicillin as an adequate therapy for acute cholangitis. *Surg Gynecol Obstet* 1990;171:275

21. Liguory C, Vitole GC, Lefebre JF, et al. Endoscopic treatment of postoperative biliary fistulae. *Surgery* 1991; 110(4):779

22. Blumgart LH. Benign biliary strictures. In: Blumgart LH (ed), *Surgery of the Liver and Biliary Tract*, vol 1. Edinburgh, Scotland: Churchill Livingstone; 1988;721–752

23. Voyles CR, Blumgart LH. A technique for the construction of high biliary-enteric anastomoses. *Surg Gynecol Obstet* 1983;154:885

24. Couinaud C. Les Heipato-cholangiostomies digestive. *La Presse Medicale* 1953;61:468

25. Couinaud C. Recherches sur la chirurgie du confluent biliaire superieur et des canaux hépatiques. *Presse Med* 1955; 63:669

26. Hepp J, Couinaud C. L'abord et l'utilisation du canal hépatique gauche dans les réparations de la voie biliaire principale. *Presse Med* 1956;64:947

27a. Soupault R, Couinaud CL. Sur un procédé nouveau de derivation biliaire intra-hépatique: les cholangiojejunostomies gauches sans sacrifice hépatique. *Presse Med* 1957;65:1157

27. Smith R. Strictures of the bile ducts. *Proc R Soc Med* 1969;62:131

28. Smith R. Obstructions of the bile duct. *Br J Surg* 1979; 69:317

29. Smith R. Injuries of the bile ducts. In: Lord Smith of Marlow, Dame Sheila Sherlock (eds), *Surgery of the Gallbladder and Bile Ducts*. 2nd ed. London, England: Butterworths; 1981;361

30. Blumgart LH, Imrie CW, McKay AJ. Surgical management of chronic pancreatitis. *J Clin Surg* 1982;1:229

31. Longmire WP Jr, Sandford MC. Intrahepatic cholangiojejunostomy for biliary obstruction: further studies—report of 4 cases. *Ann Surg* 1949;122:155

32a. Sedgwick CE, Poulantzas JK, Kune GA. Management of portal hypertension secondary to bile duct stenosis: review of 18 cases with splenorenal shunt. *Ann Surg* 1966;163:949

32. Toufanian A, Carey LC, Martin ET Jr. Transhepatic biliary dilatation: an alternative to surgical reconstruction. *Curr Surg* 1978;35:70

33. Teplick SK, Goldstein RC, et al. Percutaneous transhepatic choledochoplasty and dilatation of choledochoenterostomy strictures. *JAMA* 1980;244:1240

34. Molnar W, Stockum E. Transhepatic dilatation of choledochoenterostomy strictures. *Diagn Radiol* 1978;129:59

35. Schwarz W, Rosen RJ, Fitts WT Jr., et al. Percutaneous transhepatic drainage preoperatively for benign biliary strictures. *Surg Gynecol Obstet* 1981;152:466

36. Vogel SB, Howard RJ, Carid J, et al. Evaluation of percutaneous transhepatic balloon dilatation of benign biliary strictures in high-risk patients. *Am J Surg* 1985;149:73

37. Pitt HA, Kaufman SL, Coleman J, et al. Benign postoperative biliary strictures: operate or dilate? *Ann Surg* 1989; 210:417

38. Schweizer WP, Matthews JB, Baer HU, et al. Combined surgical and interventional radiological approach for complex benign biliary tract obstruction. *Br J Surg* 1991; 78:559

39. Baker EM, Winkler M. Permanent-access hepaticojejunostomy. *Br J Surg* 1985;71:188

40. Bloomgart LH, Matthews JB. Benign bile duct stricture. In: Blumgart LH (ed), *Surgery of the Liver and Biliary Tract,* vol 2. Edinburgh, Scotland: Churchill Livingstone; 1993

41. Chapman WC, Halevy A, Benjamin IS, Blumgart LH. Postcholecystectomy bile duct strictures—management and outcome in 130 patients. *Arch Surg* 1995;130:597

42. Braasch JW, Bolten JS, Rossi RL. A technique of biliary tract reconstruction with complete follow-up in 44 consecutive cases. *Ann Surg* 1981;194:635

43. Warren KW, Jefferson MP. Prevention and repair of strictures of the extrahepatic bile ducts. *Surg Clin North Am* 1973;53:423

44. Warren KW, Christophi C, Armendari ZR. The evolution and current perspectives of the treatment of benign bile duct strictures: a review. *Surg Gastroenterol* 1982;1:141

44a. Pitt HA, Miyamato T, et al. Factors influencing outcome in patients with post-operative biliary strictures. *Am J Surg* 1982;144:14

45. Pellegrini CA, Thomas MJ, Way LW. Recurrent biliary stricture: patterns of recurrence and outcome of surgical therapy. *Am J Surg* 1984;147:175

46. Sato Tm, Imamura M, et al. Biliary reconstruction and gastric acid secretion. *Am J Surg* 1982;144:599

47. Sato T, Mikio I, et al. Gastric acid secretion after biliary reconstruction. *Am J Surg* 1983;146:245

48. Smith EEJ, Bowley N, et al. The management of posttraumatic intrahepatic cutaneous biliary fistulae. *Br J Surg* 1982;69:317

49. Chadwick SJK, Dudley HAD. Stenosis at the choledochojejunostomy anastomosis following pancreaticoduodenectomy when the common bile duct is of normal calibre. *Ann R Coll Surg Engl* 1984;66:319

50. Degenshein GA, Hurwitz A. The technique of side-to-side choledochoduodenostomy. *Surgery* 1967;61:972

51. Degenshein GA. Choledochoduodenostomy: an 18 year study of 175 consecutive cases. *Surgery* 1974;76:19

52. Escudero-Fabre A, Escallon A, Sack J, et al. Choledochoduodenostomy: analysis of 71 cases followed for 5 to 15 years. *Ann Surg* 1991;145:450

53. Matthews JB, Baer HU, Schweizer WP, et al. Recurrent cholangitis with and without anastomotic stricture after biliary-enteric bypass. *Arch Surg* 1993;128:269

54. Goldman LD, Steer ML, Silen W. Recurrent cholangitis after biliary surgery. *Am J Surg* 1983;145;450

66

Tumors of the Gallbladder and Bile Ducts

Charles J. Yeo ▪ *John L. Cameron*

▪ TUMORS OF THE GALLBLADDER

Gallbladder carcinoma was first described by DeStoll in 1777.[1] The first hepatic resection for gallbladder cancer was performed by Keen in 1891,[2] and the association between gallbladder cancer and gallstones was made by Mayo in 1903.[3] The incidence of carcinoma of the gallbladder increases in frequency throughout life. As the population of the United States ages, the rates of gallbladder cancer have slowly increased. Currently, between 6000 and 7000 new cases of gallbladder cancer are diagnosed in the United States each year. The gender distribution of this malignancy favors women, with a 3:1 ratio of females to males. The incidence of gallbladder carcinoma is higher in the southwestern section of the United States, particularly among the Native American Indians, and also is higher in such countries as Israel, Chile, and Japan.

In autopsy series, gallbladder carcinomas account for up to 5% of all malignancies,[4] with many of these tumors being asymptomatic at the time of demise of the patient. Autopsy data from Chile have suggested that the risk of gallbladder carcinoma is seven times greater in the presence of chronic cholecystitis and cholelithiasis.[5]

▪ PATHOLOGY AND STAGING

Over 85% of gallbladder cancers are adenocarcinomas, the most common being papillary, nodular, or tubular variants, on histologic evaluation. Other types of gallbladder cancer include undifferentiated squamous cell and adenosquamous tumors, as well as such rare varieties as clear-cell adenocarcinoma, neuroendocrine tumors, small cell tumors, and giant cell tumors. The histologic grade of the carcinoma appears to have prognostic implications, since those tumors that are well differentiated are associated with a better prognosis than those tumors classified as poorly differentiated or undifferentiated. The histologic variants of papillary, tubular, and nodular patterns also have some implications regarding prognosis. In general, the papillary tumors are less likely to directly invade the liver, and they have a lower incidence of lymph node metastases.[6] Nodular forms are more likely to infiltrate early, invade the liver, and to have lymph node metastases. Tubular tumors appear to be intermediate with respect to these invasive characteristics.

The staging of gallbladder carcinoma, according to the American Joint Committee on Cancer (AJCC), is presented in Table 66–1. Survival is related to stages

TABLE 66–1. TNM STAGING FOR GALLBLADDER CANCER

	Tumor	Nodes	Metastases	5 yr Survival Postresection (%)
Stage 0	Tis	N0	M0	100
Stage I	T1	N0	M0	85
Stage II	T2	N0	M0	25–65
Stage III	T1–2	N1	M0	10
	T3	N0–1	M0	
Stage IV	T1–4	N2	M0	2
	T1–4	N0–2	M1	

Tis = Carcinoma in situ
T1 = Tumor limited to mucosa or muscularis
T2 = Tumor invades serosa
T3 = Tumor invades liver (<2 cm) or one adjacent organ
T4 = Tumor extends > 2 cm into liver or two or more adjacent organs

N0 = No nodal involvement
N1 = Metastases in cystic duct, bile duct or hilar lymph nodes
N2 = Metastases in other lymph nodes

M0 = No distant metastases
M1 = Distant metastases

both in this TNM system, and in a somewhat different classification system described by Nevin (Table 66–2).[7]

As with many other cancers, the DNA content of gallbladder cancer has been examined and found to correlate with prognosis. In recent reports,[8,9] the majority of patients with gallbladder carcinoma have been found to have aneuploid tumors, with a minority of patients having diploid tumors. Patients with aneuploid tumors were more likely to have poorly differentiated adenocarcinomas, invasion beyond the muscularis propria, a high mitotic index, and a poor overall prognosis.

As with other gastrointestinal malignancies, most notably colorectal carcinoma, an adenoma-carcinoma sequence has been proposed to be applicable to cancer of the gallbladder. Evidence has accumulated to suggest that adenomatous polyps of the gallbladder, as well as adenomyomatosis, should be considered premalignant lesions for gallbladder carcinoma. Cholesterol polyps and inflammatory polyps of the gallbladder appear to have no potential for malignant degeneration or transformation.

ETIOLOGY

Several factors have been associated with an increased risk of gallbladder cancer (Table 66–3). Among these factors, the presence of gallstones is observed most commonly, because of the high prevalence of cholelithiasis in the general population. Patients with choledochal cysts may have carcinoma developing anywhere in the biliary tree, with a percentage of these tumors arising in the gallbladder. The association between an anomalous pancreatic-biliary duct junction (APBDJ) and chole-

dochal cysts has been clearly demonstrated[10,11] and, in addition, there appears to be an association between APBDJ and gallbladder carcinoma.

DIAGNOSIS

Gallbladder carcinomas present most commonly in women more than 60 years of age. Abdominal pain is a common complaint in most of these patients, with more than one-half presenting with biliary colic or acute cholecystitis. Most patients who present with symptoms attributed to gallbladder cancer are found to be unresectable at the time of their initial diagnosis. A minority of patients can present with jaundice, which can be related to cholelithiasis and choledocholithiasis, or can represent tumor involvement of the extrahepatic biliary tree. A minority of patients present with hepatomegaly, a palpable gallbladder mass, or ascites. Incidental gallbladder cancers have been found on pathologic evaluation in up to 1% of all cholecystectomy specimens. In these patients the indication for cholecystectomy was the presence of symptomatic gallstones, and not the suspicion of malignancy.

Two serum tumor markers have been weakly associated with gallbladder carcinoma. These are carcinoembryonic antigen (CEA) and α-fetoprotein (AFP), which are common to other gastrointestinal malignancies. Unfortunately, because the incidence of elevated serum tumor markers in patients with gallbladder cancer is low, and the specificity of an elevated tumor marker for gallbladder cancer is poor, there are currently no accurate screening tests for gallbladder carcinoma.

The radiologic evaluation of patients with gallbladder carcinoma can include ultrasonography, computed tomography (CT), magnetic resonance imaging (MRI), cholangiography, and angiography. Unfortunately, most patients have coexisting gallstones, which can make the interpretation of ultrasonography, CT and cholangiography more difficult. Ultrasound examination is capable of identifying a mass either protruding into the gall-

TABLE 66–2. NEVIN CLASSIFICATION FOR STAGING OF GALLBLADDER CANCER

Stage	Depth of Tumor	5 yr Survival Postresection (%)
Stage I	Mucosa	70–97
Stage II	Muscularis	50–70
Stage III	Serosa	0–25
Stage IV	Liver invasion	0–20
Stage V	Adjacent organs or distant metastases	0–5

(From Nevin JE, Moran TJ, Day S, et al. Carcinoma of the gallbladder: staging, treatment, and prognosis. Cancer 1976;37:141–148)

TABLE 66–3. RISK FACTORS FOR GALLBLADDER CANCER

Cholelithiasis
Choledochal cysts
Anomalous pancreatic-biliary duct junction (APBDJ)
Carcinogens (azotoluene, nitrosamines)
Estrogens
Typhoid carriers
Porcelain gallbladder
Adenomatous gallbladder polyps

bladder or filling or replacing the gallbladder in approximately 50% of patients.[12] Some patients with gallbladder neoplasms are found, on CT scanning, to have an intraluminal gallbladder mass or a mass extending from the gallbladder into the liver (Fig 66–1). CT scanning is also reasonably accurate for discerning early hepatic invasion, liver metastases or dilatation of the biliary tree (Fig 66–2). The assessment of portal lymphadenopathy is less accurate by CT scanning. At the current time, the use of MRI does not appear to enhance the capability of diagnosing or staging gallbladder carcinoma. For patients who present with jaundice and who are found to have dilated intrahepatic ducts and a mass in the region of the gallbladder, both dynamic contrast-enhanced CT or MRI may provide a reasonably accurate assessment of invasion of the hepatic artery and portal venous structures. Better assessment of vascular invasion may be possible via angiography, with associated portal venous study.

Cholangiography has a well-defined role in diagnosing jaundiced patients with gallbladder carcinoma,[13] with both endoscopic retrograde cholangiopancreatography (ERCP) and percutaneous transhepatic cholangiogram (PTC) having been used (Fig 66–3). With each of these cholangiographic studies, the coexistence of gallstones may prevent adequate filling of the gallbladder and impair the ability to discern fine details of the gallbladder mucosa, thereby making it more difficult to identify the presence of an intraluminal gallbladder mass.

ASSESSMENT OF RESECTABILITY

When considering a patient for resection of gallbladder carcinoma, both patient- and tumor-related factors require consideration. Patient-related factors focus upon the age and general medical condition of the patient, and include evaluation of the cardiopulmonary status, the status of the liver and kidneys, overall nutritional status, and presence or absence of sepsis. Tumor-related factors focus upon the overall extent of tumor involvement, with particular attention to the vascular structures of the porta hepatis. In most situations, encasement or occlusion of the main portal vein or main hepatic artery preclude curative resection. However, en-

casement of the right portal vein or right hepatic artery do not prevent resection, if resection is planned to include a right hepatic lobectomy. Discontiguous bilobar metastatic liver involvement is considered a contraindication to resection, as is extensive involvement of adjacent organs such as invasion into the pancreas, duodenum, and colon. In carefully selected circumstances, limited local involvement of structures such as the duodenal wall or colon, in the absence of extensive portal node involvement, may be treated with en bloc resection. Distant metastases, to include peritoneal or extra-abdominal spread, are a strict contraindication to attempts at curative resection.

MANAGEMENT

Nonoperative Palliation

In patients whose preoperative assessment reveals them to be unacceptable risks for surgery, or reveals their tumor to be unresectable for cure, based on extensive local invasion or distant metastases, nonoperative palliation is appropriate therapy. Many of these patients will have obstructive jaundice that can be managed with either percutaneous transhepatic biliary stents or biliary endoprostheses. However, one potential problem with any form of palliative biliary stenting in these patients whose gallbladders remain in situ is the subsequent development of acute cholecystitis.[14]

In addition to jaundice, abdominal pain may require palliation. Appropriate narcotic therapy may provide adequate pain control in many patients. In those patients with disabling pain, either external beam radiation therapy or percutaneous celiac ganglion nerve block may be helpful in reducing the need for narcotics.

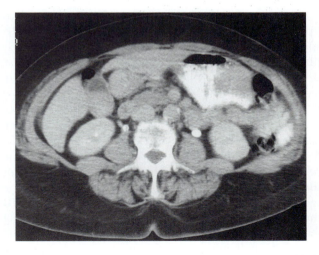

Figure 66–1. A CT scan in a patient with a gallbladder neoplasm showing a mass in the posterior wall of the gallbladder. (From Porter JM, Kalloo AN, Abernathy EC and Yeo CJ. Carcinoid tumor of the gallbladder: laparoscopic resection and review of the literature. *Surgery* 1992;112:100–105)

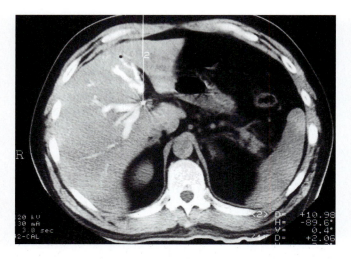

Figure 66–2. A CT scan in a patient with gallbladder carcinoma and extrahepatic biliary obstruction. The scan was performed immediately following endoscopic retrograde cholangiography. Contrast-filled dilated intrahepatic ducts are visualized in both lobes of the liver.

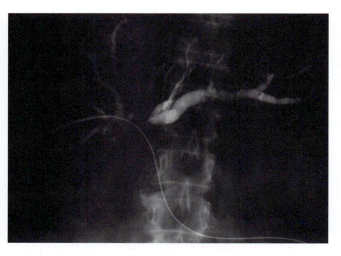

Figure 66–3. A percutaneous transhepatic cholangiogram in a jaundiced patient with extensive gallbladder cancer invading the portal hepatis. The cholangiogram shows obstruction at the level of the hepatic duct bifurcation, with a markedly dilated left hepatic ductal system. A guidewire has been placed through the right hepatic lobe, down the bile duct and into the duodenum.

The mean survival for the subset of patients who undergo nonoperative palliation for symptomatic gallbladder carcinoma is less than 6 months.

Operative Palliation

In patients who are candidates for exploration and believed to be resectable, but who are found at laparotomy to have unresectable disease, the goals of operative palliation include confirmation of a tissue diagnosis, removal of the gallbladder (if possible) to prevent acute cholecystitis, palliation of jaundice via one of several forms of biliary-enteric anastomosis, improvement or prevention of abdominal pain, and treatment or prevention of gastric outlet obstruction.

The operative palliation of jaundice is dependent upon the extent of hilar disease. In patients with widespread liver or peritoneal metastases, preoperatively placed percutaneous transhepatic stents or endoprostheses are commonly left in place, to provide continuing relief of jaundice for the limited duration of survival that is expected. Alternatively, locally unresectable tumors in the hilum may be stented with large-bore transhepatic Silastic catheters, and a Roux-en-Y choledochojejunostomy created to provide biliary decompression to a defunctionalized limb of jejunum. Further, if the hepatic hilum is invaded with tumor, a segment III bypass can be performed to the segment III duct found to the left of the falciform ligament (Fig 66–4). The segment III duct is identified by following the falciform ligament into the recess of the left hepatic lobe in the umbilical fissure. A biliary-enteric anastomosis between the segment III duct and a Roux-en-Y jejunal limb then is performed.

In patients with large bulky gallbladder cancers that invade into the hepatic hilum, with associated extensive periaortic and celiac adenopathy, the use of an intraoperative alcohol celiac nerve block[15] should be considered. Such a celiac splanchnicectomy has been shown in a prospective randomized trial to benefit patients with unresectable pancreatic cancer, and it seems reasonable to assume that the proven decrease in analgesic requirements will be observed in patients with unresectable gallbladder carcinoma.

Patients with tumors that invade into or toward the distal stomach, pylorus, or duodenum are at risk for gastric outlet obstruction and should undergo gastrojejunostomy for palliation. A vagotomy is not performed, and the patient is maintained on oral H2 receptor antagonists or omeprazole to decrease gastric acid secretion and to prophylax against the development of marginal ulceration.

Surgical Resection

Current recommendations for surgical therapy for gallbladder carcinoma are based on the pathologic staging of the tumor and the historical survival rates for the different tumor stages. Unfortunately, data from controlled prospective trials are lacking, and therefore, the recommendations are largely empiric.

In patients with TNM stage 0 tumors (carcinoma in situ), simple cholecystectomy alone is appropriate therapy, with a 100% 5 year disease-specific survival rate. Similarly, TNM stage I cancers (Nevin stages I and II) are also associated with high survival rates, and are treated with simple cholecystectomy alone. Although somewhat controversial, laparoscopic cholecystectomy

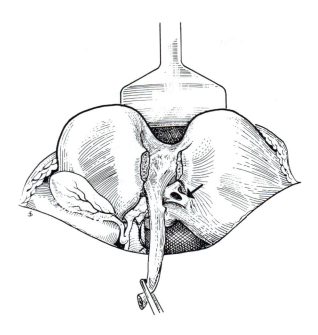

Figure 66–4. In patients with extensive tumor involvement of the porta hepatis, a segment III bypass to a Roux-en-Y jejunal limb can be performed for ductal decompression. Here the *arrow* depicts exposure of the segment III duct. (From Blumgart LH, Thompson JN. The management of malignant strictures of the bile duct. *Curr Probl Surg* 1987;24:69–127)

would appear to be adequate in patients with TNM stages 0, I, and II disease, as long as the gallbladder is removed in its entirety. There have been isolated reports of implantation of cancer cells in the laparoscopic port sites of patients treated via laparoscopic cholecystectomy; however, the risk of this occurrence in patients with early disease (stages 0, I and II) appears low.

In patients with TNM stages II and III disease (Nevin stages III and IV disease) the recommended surgical therapy is an extended cholecystectomy, which includes a wedge resection of the gallbladder bed and a lymph node dissection of the porta hepatis, hepatoduodenal ligament, and anterior and inferior peripancreatic lymph nodes. Typically, at least a 2 cm portion of the hepatic parenchyma is resected to include the gallbladder fossa, in an effort to insure a tumor-free margin, given the possibility of tumor infiltration along Glissen's capsule (Fig 66–5). A minority of authors advocate resection of hepatic segments V and IVb as part of the extended cholecystectomy. At this point, the most convincing data supporting extended cholecystectomy in patients with TNM stage II or III gallbladder carcinoma come from Japan,[16,17] where it has been reported that patients with T2 disease (tumor beyond the muscularis and into the serosa) may achieve a 5 year survival rate of >50% when treated with extended cholecystectomy. Recent American and European studies have also reported a survival advantage for extended cholecystectomy in this setting.[18,19] Whether this improvement in survival of TNM stages II and III disease (Nevin stages III and IV disease)

is related to the hepatic resection or the lymphadenectomy (or a combination of the two) remains unclear. The 30 day in-hospital mortality rate for extended cholecystectomy in most series has been acceptable at <5%.

The treatment of gallbladder carcinoma that has grossly invaded the liver or adjacent organs (TNM T3 or T4 disease or Nevin stage V disease) is controversial. In the past, radical resection of these advanced cancers was largely condemned because of the high rates of operative morbidity and mortality associated with such a large resection. Limited recent reports have suggested that long-term survival may be achievable with aggressive surgical resection in a small percentage of carefully selected patients with extensive local disease. For example, Nakamura and associates have reported a 23% 2 year survival and a 15% 5 year survival after aggressive surgery in patients with Nevin stage V disease.[17] Such aggressive surgery has included major liver resection plus lymphadenectomy, as well as pancreaticoduodenectomy, resection of extrahepatic bile ducts and portal vein, and resection of other adjacent adherent organs (including kidney and colon). Depending on the extent of hepatic involvement, liver resection may include wedge resection of the gallbladder fossa or segments V and IVb, central hepatectomy, extended right hepatic lobectomy, or even right trisegmentectomy. A formal right hepatic lobectomy is considered inadequate therapy for gallbladder carcinoma since the gallbladder fossa serves as the line of division between the right and left hepatic lobes.

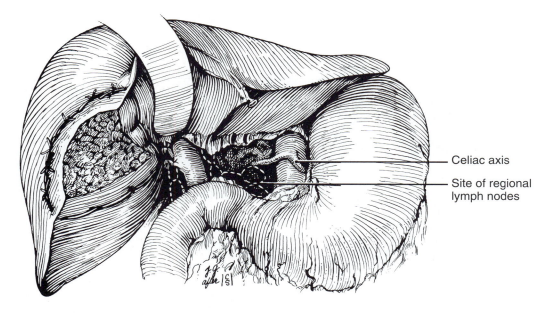

Celiac axis

Site of regional lymph nodes

Figure 66–5. In patients with TNM stage II or III gallbladder cancer the recommended surgical resection involves an extended cholecystectomy and lymph node dissection. The extended cholecystectomy includes a cholecystectomy plus a wedge resection of at least 2 cm of the hepatic parenchyma to include the entire gallbladder fossa. The regional lymph nodes from the bifurcation of the common hepatic duct down to the distal common bile duct, and medially along the hepatic artery over to the celiac axis are resected, along with the associated loose areolar tissue. (From Cameron JL. *Atlas of Surgery* vol I. Toronto, Canada: BC Decker; 1990:149)

Chemotherapy and Radiation Therapy

Chemotherapy. Chemotherapeutic options for the treatment of gallbladder carcinoma have remained limited because of a poor response to the currently available agents. 5-fluorouracil (5-FU) and mitomycin C have been used most frequently, with <20% of patients showing any demonstrable response. Most studies have shown a slight but nonsignificant improvement in survival in patients receiving chemotherapy.[20,21] In a recent study testing tumor explants in vitro, cis-platin was the most promising among eight anticancer agents tested.[22]

In patients who undergo presumed complete resection for early gallbladder carcinoma, the use of chemotherapy in the adjuvant setting has not been well studied. There is no universal agreement regarding the appropriate route of delivery for chemotherapy delivered in the adjuvant setting, nor is there agreement regarding the chemotherapeutic agent of choice.

Radiation Therapy. In patients who have unresected or incompletely resected gallbladder carcinoma, external beam radiation therapy has been used to help reduce abdominal pain and to relieve biliary obstruction. Because of the limited success of most external beam protocols, intraoperative radiation therapy also has been used at some centers.[23,24] Radiation therapy also has been used after a resection as an adjuvant.[25,26] In this

postoperative adjuvant setting, there has been no reproducible survival advantage observed in patients who received external beam radiation alone. Radiation sensitizers such as 5-FU may provide some benefit over radiation therapy alone in this adjuvant setting.

■ TUMORS OF THE BILE DUCTS

Like gallbladder cancer, the incidence of bile duct cancer increases with age. Bile duct malignancies have a more even distribution between men and women than do gallbladder malignancies. Overall, the annual incidence of bile duct cancer in the United States is approximately 1 per 100 000 people.[27] The annual incidence is increased in such countries as Israel and Japan, and in Native American Indians. In autopsy series, the incidence of bile duct cancer varies between 0.01% and 0.46%.[28]

Cancer of the bile ducts has been recognized for more than a century. Eighteen cases of primary extrahepatic bile duct cancer were reported in the literature in 1889 by Musser.[29] In 1940, Stewart and associates reviewed 306 cases of extrahepatic bile duct cancer reported in the literature,[30] and two decades later Sako and associates reviewed the literature from 1935 to 1954, and found 570 additional cases of extrahepatic bile duct cancer.[28] Malignancies of the intrahepatic and perihilar bile ducts have been described more recently, with Altemeier and associates reporting three cases of primary adenocarcinoma of the major intrahepatic bile ducts in 1957,[31] and Klatskin reporting 13 patients with cancers of the hepatic duct bifurcation in 1965.[32]

■ PATHOLOGY AND STAGING

Adenocarcinomas make up >95% of bile duct cancers, ranging from well-differentiated to poorly differentiated varieties. Many other histologic types of bile duct cancers have been reported including squamous, leiomyosarcoma, mucoepidermoid, carcinoid, cystadenocarcinoma, rhabdomyosarcoma, and granular cell carcinoma.[28,33–36] The distinction between reactive bile duct epithelium and malignancy is made more difficult in the settings of cholangitis, biliary obstruction, hepatolithiasis, and bile duct stenting. The diagnosis of bile duct cancer may be supported by positive findings in two of the following three indicators: (1) a positive reaction to CEA, (2) nuclear size variation, or (3) formation of distended intracytoplasmic lumina.[37] Neural invasion is another histologic finding that confirms the diagnosis of bile duct cancer.

Immunohistochemical and molecular biologic aspects of bile duct cancers have become more defined in recent years. In addition to CEA, many tumors also will stain positively for the carbohydrate antigens CA50 and CA19-9.[38,39] Some recent reports also have identified mutations in k-ras oncogenes in 60% to 70% of both intrahepatic and perihilar bile duct cancers.[40–42] Further studies have identified abnormalities on chromosomes 5 and 17,[43] documented the presence of C-erb oncogenes,[44] epidermal growth factors,[45] and proliferating nuclear antigens.[46]

The location of bile duct cancer within the biliary tree greatly influences the choice of treatment and eventual prognosis. In two reviews comprising more than 2000 extrahepatic bile duct cancers, the most common site for bile duct cancer was the common bile duct (33% to 40%), followed by the common hepatic duct (30% to 32%), the hepatic duct bifurcation (20%), and the cystic duct (4%).[47,48] Diffuse tumors and those not able to be anatomically classified accounted for up to 7% of the total. Other reports with more than 700 patients have subdivided bile duct tumors into upper-, middle-, and lower-third lesions.[49,50] Using this system, approximately 55% are upper-third tumors, 15% are middle-third tumors, and 20% are lower-third tumors, with 10% being classified as diffuse. This distribution is more in keeping with our most recent experience.

Bile duct cancer is staged in the United States according to the TNM classification[51,52] (Table 66–4).

ETIOLOGY

A number of etiologic factors have been linked to bile duct cancer in man (Table 66–5). Factors common to a number of these etiologic factors include stones, biliary stasis, and infection. Strong associations have been found between bile duct cancer and cystic dilatations of the biliary tree, hepatolithiasis, liver flukes, primary sclerosing cholangitis, ulcerative colitis, and the radiocontrast agent Thorotrast.

Cholelithiasis has been observed in many patients with cholangiocarcinoma.[53,54] However, as gallstones are not uncommon in the elderly population, a definite cause and effect relationship between gallstones and bile duct cancer has not been established. In contrast to cholelithiasis, hepatolithiasis is a definite risk factor for cholangiocarcinoma.[55–57] The association between bile duct cancer and congenital dilatation of the bile duct was first reported by Irwin and Morison in 1944.[58] Subsequently, numerous reports have linked cholangiocar-

---

TABLE 66–4. TNM STAGING FOR BILE DUCT CANCER

	Tumor	Nodes	Metastases
Stage I	T1	N0	M0
Stage II	T2	N0	M0
Stage III	T1–2	N1	M0
Stage IVA	T3	N0–1	M0
Stage IVB	T1–3	N0–1	M1

T1 = Tumor limited to mucosa or muscle layer
T2 = Tumor invades periductal tissue
T3 = Tumor invades adjacent structures

N0 = No nodal involvement
N1 = Metastases in regional lymph nodes

M0 = No distant metastases
M1 = Distant metastases

TABLE 66–5. RISK FACTORS FOR BILE DUCT CANCER

Cystic dilatation of the bile duct
  Choledochal cyst
  Caroli's disease
Gallstones
Hepatolithiasis
Clonorchis sinensis
Opisthorchis viverrini
Primary sclerosing cholangitis
Ulcerative colitis
Thorium dioxide (Thorotrast)
Radionuclides
Carcinogens (asbestos, dioxin, nitrosamines, polychlorinated biphenyls)
Oral contraceptives
Methyldopa
Isoniazid

cinoma to cystic abnormalities of the bile duct.[59–61] One anatomic explanation for the origin of choledochal cysts and for the subsequent formation of bile duct cancer involves the finding of an anomalous high entry of the pancreatic duct into the extrahepatic biliary tree (APBDJ).[62,63] This finding of an APBDJ suggests that reflux of pancreatic exocrine secretions into the bile duct epithelium may initiate or promote malignant transformation of the bile duct.

DIAGNOSIS

Patients with bile duct cancer are typically diagnosed between 50 to 70 years of age, with the average being between 60 and 65 years of age.[47,48] A slight male predominance has been reported, with a male to female ratio of 1.3:1.[46] More than 90% of patients present with jaundice. Less common presenting clinical features include pruritus, mild abdominal pain, anorexia, fatigue, and weight loss. Cholangitis is not a frequent presenting finding, but often develops after biliary manipulation by endoscopic or percutaneous techniques. Apart from jaundice, the physical examination typically is unrevealing. In distal bile duct tumors, a distended nontender gallbladder may be palpable. In patients whose tumors are located above the hepatic duct bifurcation, the biliary tree may be obstructed initially on only one side. These patients usually present with mild abdominal pain, unilobar hepatic enlargement, and elevations of the serum alkaline phosphatase or gamma glutamyl transferase, without elevations of serum bilirubin and without clinical jaundice.

At the time of presentation, most patients with bile duct cancers have an elevated total serum bilirubin. Marked elevations also are routinely observed in the markers of bile duct epithelial cell injury: alkaline phosphatase and gamma glutamyl transferase. Markers of hepatocyte injury such as alanine aminotransferase and aspartate aminotransferase usually are elevated, but only to a mild degree. Mild anemia may be seen in a minority of patients, and a prolonged prothrombin time may be a reflection of diminished hepatic synthetic function. The serum tumor markers CEA and AFP are usually normal.

The radiologic evaluation of patients with bile duct carcinoma is designed to localize the site of mechanical biliary obstruction, and to delineate the overall extent of the tumor, including the involvement of the bile ducts, liver, portal vessels, and to screen for distant metastases. An ordered sequence of tests usually will achieve these goals. The initial radiographic study consists of either abdominal ultrasound or CT scanning. The findings at ultrasound or CT scanning suggestive of a hilar bile duct cancer include a dilated intrahepatic biliary tree (Fig 66–6) with a normal collapsed gallblad-

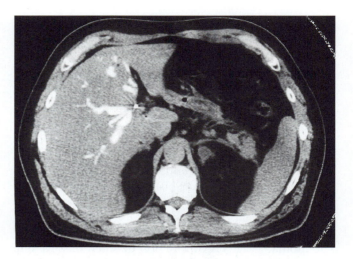

Figure 66–6. A CT scan in a patient with hilar bile duct cancer. The scan was performed immediately following an endoscopic retrograde cholangiogram and endoprosthesis placement. Note the dilated, contrast-filled intrahepatic ducts.

der and extrahepatic biliary tree. Findings suggestive of a common bile duct cancer include a dilated intrahepatic and extrahepatic biliary tree with a distended gallbladder. In addition to ultrasound and CT scanning, magnetic resonance imaging also may be used to diagnose bile duct tumors.[64,65] There appears to be no consistent advantage in preoperative tumor localization and staging afforded by the use of MRI.

The definition of biliary anatomy via cholangiographic means can be accomplished by either PTC or ERCP techniques. In tumors of the proximal biliary tree, PTC is favored because it defines the extent of the proximal tumor involvement at the hepatic hilus (Fig 66–7), and allows for the preoperative placement of percutaneous transhepatic catheters. These transhepatic catheters allow for assistance in the technical aspects of hilar dissection and facilitate the intraoperative placement of Silastic transhepatic stents.[66] Currently available data do not support the practice of preoperative biliary decompression in an effort to reduce operative mortality.[67–69] For distal tumors, the use of ERCP allows visualization of the uppermost extent of the tumor within the extrahepatic biliary tree, and may be followed by endoprosthesis placement.

Efforts to establish a tissue diagnosis can include percutaneous fine-needle aspiration biopsy, brush and scrape biopsy, and cytologic examination of bile.[70–72] If surgery is contemplated, a preoperative tissue diagnosis is not essential, and prolonged efforts at obtaining a preoperative tissue diagnosis are not indicated. Bile obtained from a percutaneous catheter may demonstrate malignant cells in one-third of cases.[71] This yield may be improved by brush cytologic techniques through transhepatic stents, or at the time of endoscopic procedures.

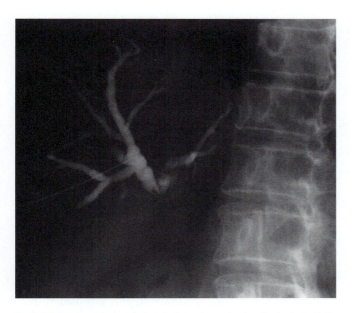

Figure 66–7. A percutaneous transhepatic cholangiogram in a jaundiced patient with hilar bile duct cancer. The cholangiogram reveals dilated intrahepatic ducts and complete obstruction at the level of the hepatic duct bifurcation.

The use of fine-needle aspiration can assist further in tissue diagnosis.[73] Fine-needle aspiration has better results than core biopsy techniques.

Differential Diagnosis (Table 66–6)

Many diseases can mimic bile duct cancer. In some cases, the distinction between bile duct cancer and another process will be possible on the basis of the clinical presentation and the results of imaging studies, particularly CT scanning and cholangiography. The entities that are most difficult to distinguish from bile duct cancer are strictures (related to chronic pancreatitis, sclerosing cholangitis, or prior operation) and other malignant tumors of the periampullary region or gallbladder, which can spread locally to the bile duct and give a cholangiographic appearance similar to that of bile duct carcinoma.

ASSESSMENT OF RESECTABILITY

Both patient-related and tumor-related factors must be considered when assessing the resectability of patients with bile duct cancers. These factors are similar to those outlined above for patients with gallbladder cancer.

A special consideration in patients with obstructive jaundice who are to undergo major surgical procedures relates to the numerous physiologic abnormalities associated with jaundice. These abnormalities include alterations in hepatic and pancreatic function, the gastrointestinal barrier, immune function, cardiopulmonary function, hemostatic mechanisms, renal

function, and wound healing. Obstructive jaundice further alters multiple aspects of hepatic metabolism such as hepatic mitochondrial respiratory function, hepatic protein synthesis, and hepatic reticuloendothelial function.[74,75] In addition, endotoxemia may contribute to the cardiac, pulmonary, and renal insufficiency sometimes observed in patients with sepsis from obstructive jaundice.[76]

Complete staging of patients with bile duct cancer usually is accomplished using a combination of CT scan, cholangiography, and visceral angiography.[77–81] CT scan findings such as bilobar peripheral hepatic metastases, or extrahepatic disease preclude curative resection. Findings by cholangiography such as extensive bilobar hepatic parenchymal involvement are also indicative of unresectability. The angiographic findings of tumor encasement or occlusion of the common hepatic artery or main portal vein also are considered a contraindication to resection, by most groups. Endosonography recently has been reported to be of some benefit in staging patients with extrahepatic bile duct cancer,[82] although the reported experience is limited.

MANAGEMENT

Nonoperative Palliation

When the preoperative assessment reveals that the patient is an unacceptable risk for surgery or reveals that the tumor is unresectable for cure, nonoperative palliation is appropriate. Prolonged biliary obstruction may result in hepatocellular dysfunction, progressive malnutrition, coagulopathy, pruritus, renal dysfunction, and cholangitis, supporting the need for some form of palliation. Minimally invasive techniques to restore bile duct patency are preferable to conventional surgical alternatives in these patients with limited life expectancy. Both endoscopic and percutaneous radiological approaches are available.

PTC and biliary drainage was first reported by Molnar and Stockum in 1974.[83] PTC is performed using sterile technique, with a 22-gauge flexible Chiba needle under fluoroscopic guidance. A right-sided approach is usually preferred, and a guidewire is advanced across the stricture allowing subsequent placement of a drainage catheter (Ring catheter) through the stricture, thereby establishing drainage.

Endoscopic decompression of the obstructed biliary tree utilizes diagnostic ERCP followed by deep cannulation of the bile duct with or without the assistance of a guidewire or sphincterotome. Precut sphincterotomy with a needle knife may be necessary in selected patients when deep cannulation cannot be achieved otherwise. A guidewire is manipulated above the stricture to the level of the right or left hepatic ductal system, the malignant stricture may be dilated by balloon or step dila-

TABLE 66–6. DIFFERENTIAL DIAGNOSIS OF BILE DUCT CARCINOMA

Congenital dilatation of the bile duct
    Choledochal cyst
    Caroli's disease
Non-neoplastic strictures
    Chronic pancreatitis
    Sclerosing cholangitis
    Inflammatory strictures (typically secondary to calculus disease)
    Postoperative strictures (typically secondary to cholecystectomy)
    Post-radiation strictures
    Chemotherapy-induced strictures
    Mirizzi's syndrome
    Strictures secondary to external trauma
    Retroperitoneal fibrosis
    Strictures related to AIDS
Neoplastic lesions
    Benign tumors of the bile duct
        Leiomyoma
        Carcinoid tumor
        Neuroma
        Hemangioma
        Papilloma
        Adenoma
        Cystic hepatobiliary neoplasms
        Granular cell myoblastoma
    Malignant tumors in proximity to the bile duct
        Periampullary tumors
            Pancreatic
            Ampullary
            Duodenal
        Islet cell tumors
        Gallbladder carcinoma
        Lymphoma
        Lymphosarcoma
        Metastases to porta hepatis or hepatic parenchyma
        Hepatocellular carcinoma
Infestations
    Clonorchis sinensis
    Ascaris lumbricoides

(From Yeo CJ, Pitt HA, Cameron JL. Bile duct carcinoma: diagnosis. In: Terblanche J (ed), Hepatobiliary Malignancy: Its Multidisciplinary Management. London, England: Edward Arnold; 1994:400)

tor, and then an endoprosthesis can be placed. In most cases, a stiff polyethylene Teflon-coated catheter is used.

A recent advance in endoprosthesis technology uses larger diameter expandable metal stents that can be placed either endoscopically or percutaneously. Stents such as the Palmaz device, the Strecker stent, the Gianturco Z-stent, and the Wallstent have all undergone trials[84] and appear to offer some advantages over standard polyethylene endoprostheses.

Operative Palliation

In good-risk patients without preoperative evidence of metastatic or locally unresectable disease, surgical exploration is indicated. In most series, approximately one-half of all patients undergoing surgical exploration are found to have intraperitoneal tumor dissemination or extensive tumor involvement of the porta hepatis, either of which preclude curative resection. Patients found to have widespread intraperitoneal tumor should undergo minimal operative intervention. In these cases, previously placed transhepatic biliary catheters or endoprostheses are left intact for palliation of biliary obstruction. Additionally, the gallbladder should be removed to prevent the subsequent development of acute cholecystitis from cystic duct obstruction related to the biliary stent or advancing tumor.

In patients with locally advanced unresectable tumors, several operative approaches are available for palliation of jaundice. Two commonly used options for perihilar tumors include (1) Roux-en-Y hepaticojejunostomy with intraoperative placement of Silastic transhepatic stents and (2) segment III bypass to the left intrahepatic ducts. The first approach to operative palliation of unresectable perihilar tumors begins with isolation of the extrahepatic biliary tree distal to the tumor. The common hepatic duct distal to the tumor mass is divided and the distal stump of the common bile duct is oversewn (Fig 66–8). The proximal extrahepatic biliary tree can be examined using intraoperative choledochoscopy, and biopsy specimens of the malignant stricture obtained to establish a tissue diagnosis. The bile duct then is dilated using progressively larger Coudé catheters, replacing the percutaneous transhepatic catheters with Silastic transhepatic stents.[66] A standard hepaticojejunostomy then is created to a Roux-en-Y limb of jejunum (Fig 66–9). The second approach to operative palliation in patients with unresectable hilar tumors is to decompress the liver through the segment III branch of the left hepatic duct above the tumor, as described in the previous section on tumors of the gallbladder.

In patients with distal bile duct tumors requiring operative palliation, the operation of choice is typically a biliary-enteric bypass using the upper part of the extrahepatic bile duct (choledochojejunostomy or hepaticojejunostomy), or the gallbladder (cholecystojejunostomy). If the gallbladder is to be used, it is essential to document that the cystic duct joins the common hepatic duct several centimeters above the site of biliary obstruction, to avoid recurrent jaundice. Although symptomatic gastroduodenal obstruction is uncommon at the initial diagnosis of distal common bile duct cancer, up to one-third of patients with unresectable tumors may have symptoms of gastroduodenal obstruction develop prior to their death. For this reason, prophylactic gastrojejunostomy should be considered. In our hands, this anastomosis is routinely performed in a retrocolic fashion, with a vanishingly low rate of obstruction of the anastomosis due to advancing tumor growth. Finally, in order to palliate abdominal and back pain that can develop in patients with unresectable bile duct cancer,

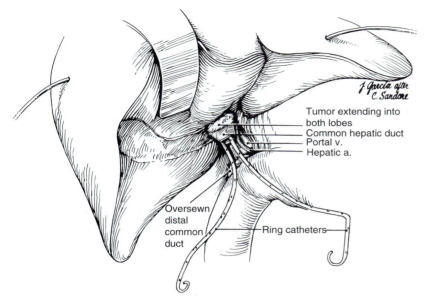

Figure 66–8. Illustration depicting an extensive unresectable hilar bile duct cancer involving both lobes of the liver. A portion of the distal extrahepatic biliary tree has been resected and the distal common bile duct has been oversewn. The previously-placed percutaneous transhepatic Ring catheters are shown exiting the proximal aspect of the biliary tree. (From Cameron JL. *Atlas of Surgery.* vol I. Toronto, Canada: BC Decker; 1990;87)

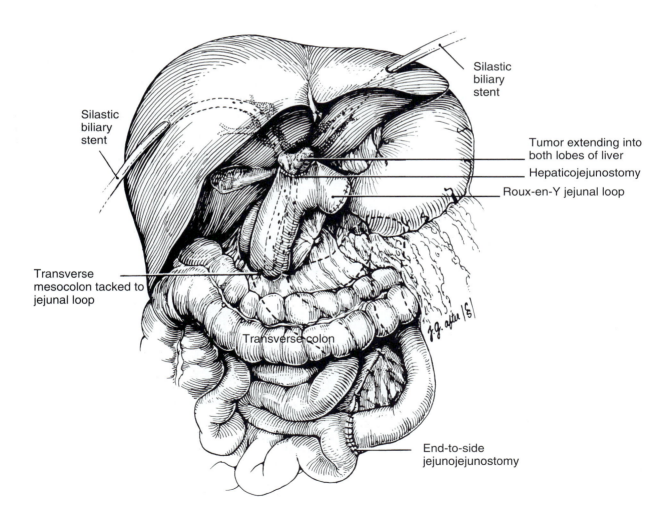

Figure 66–9. The completed palliative reconstruction showing the retrocolic Roux-en-Y hepaticojejunostomy and the operatively-placed Silastic transhepatic biliary catheters stenting the tumor at the bifurcation. (From Cameron JL. *Atlas of Surgery.* vol I. Toronto, Canada: BC Decker; 1990;93)

chemical splanchnicectomy, using 50% alcohol, can be performed intraoperatively, to improve postoperative pain control[15] and reduce narcotic requirements.

Surgical Resection

Resection of Proximal Bile Duct Cancer with Reconstruction via Bilateral Hepaticojejunostomy Using Silastic Transhepatic Biliary Stents. In patients with potentially resectable proximal bile duct cancers, it has been our practice to perform percutaneous cholangiography with insertion of transhepatic biliary catheters into the right and left hepatic ducts through the tumor, leaving the distal aspect of the biliary catheter either in the distal decompressed biliary tree or the duodenum. Exploration is performed via a right subcostal or midline incision, and the entire abdomen is explored for evidence of tumor dissemination. Two maneuvers that assist in exposure and dissection of the hepatic duct bifurcation are (1) early mobilization of the gallbladder and (2) early division of the distal common bile duct. Once the common bile duct has been divided distally, the dissection continues cephalad, dissecting the extrahepatic biliary tree off the portal vein up to the bifurcation of the hepatic duct (Fig 66–10). The right and left hepatic ducts subsequently are dissected and looped by vessel loops and divided above the tumor. The specimen then is removed (Fig 66–11), and the distal common bile duct margins, as well as the right and left hepatic ducts, are marked with sutures to aid the pathologist in evaluating the histologic status of the margins.

Next, both the right and left hepatic ducts are intubated with Silastic transhepatic stents that can be pulled into position by utilizing the previously placed percutaneous biliary catheters.[66] The biliary reconstruction is completed (Fig 66–12) by creating a 60-cm long Roux-en-Y jejunal loop, placing it in a retrocolic position, and performing bilateral one-layer hepaticojejunal anastomoses using interrupted sutures. Once both hepaticojejunostomies have been completed, the Roux-en-Y jejunal loop is tacked to the undersurface of the liver, and the transverse mesocolon is sutured to the Roux-en-Y loop. Each Silastic transhepatic biliary stent is brought out through a stab wound in the right or left upper quadrant, and sutured to the skin.

Resection of Proximal Bile Duct Cancer Plus Hepatic Resection with Reconstruction via Hepaticojejunostomy Using a Silastic Transhepatic Biliary Stent. A minority of patients with proximal bile duct cancer will have extensive tumor involvement of the right or left lobes of the liver, with sparing of the opposite lobe. In such cases, it is not infrequent to have a branch of the portal vein or hepatic artery on the side of tumor involvement encased or occluded by tumor. Such patients can undergo surgical resection if right or left hepatectomy is added to resection of the hepatic duct bifurcation.[77,85–88] The operative procedure commences as described in the immediately previous section. The gallbladder is mobilized early, and the distal common bile duct is divided. Once the hepatic duct bifurcation has been mobilized and dissected off the bifurcation of the portal vein, tumor extension into one lobe of the liver may be apparent. At this point, the hepatic duct of the uninvolved lobe is divided, and a standard liver resection of the involved lobe is performed including an en-bloc resection of the hepatic duct bi-

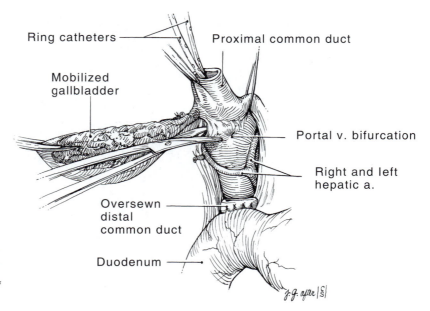

Figure 66–10. Following division of the common bile duct and mobilization of the gallbladder, the proximal extrahepatic biliary tree is dissected cephalad up to the bifurcation of the hepatic ducts. The distal common bile duct is shown oversewn. (From Cameron JL. *Atlas of Surgery.* vol I. Toronto, Canada: BC Decker; 1990;63)

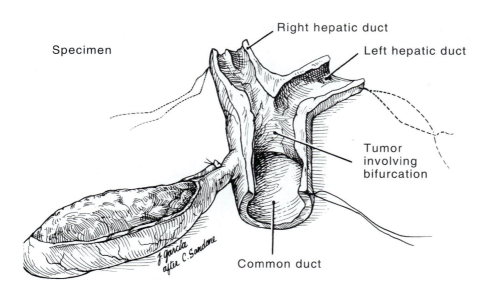

Specimen

Right hepatic duct

Left hepatic duct

Tumor involving bifurcation

Common duct

Figure 66–11. The resected specimen in a case of hilar bile duct cancer, including the right and left hepatic ducts, the entire common hepatic duct, the gallbladder and the proximal common bile duct. (From Cameron JL. *Atlas of Surgery*. vol I. Toronto, Canada: BC Decker, 1990:63)

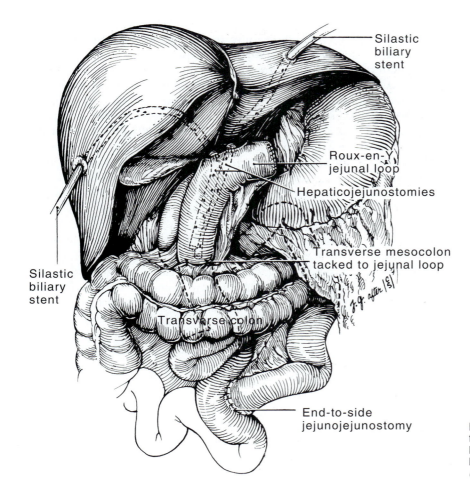

Silastic biliary stent

Roux-en-Y jejunal loop

Hepaticojejunostomies

Transverse mesocolon tacked to jejunal loop

Silastic biliary stent

Transverse colon

End-to-side jejunojejunostomy

Figure 66–12. The completed reconstruction following resection of a hilar bile duct cancer. Bilateral hepaticojejunostomies have been performed to a single Roux-en-Y limb, over right and left sided Silastic transhepatic stents. (From Cameron JL. *Atlas of Surgery*. vol I. Toronto, Canada: BC Decker, 1990:71)

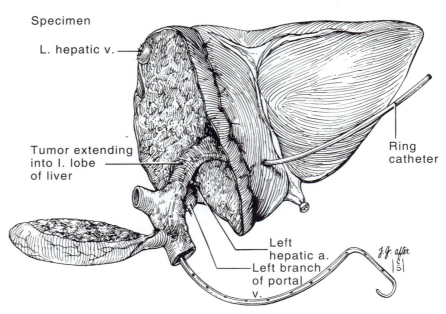

Specimen

L. hepatic v.

Tumor extending
into l. lobe
of liver

Ring
catheter

Left
hepatic a.
Left branch
of portal
v.

Figure 66–13. Illustration depicting a completed resection specimen from a hilar bile duct cancer involving the hepatic duct bifurcation and left hepatic lobe. An en bloc resection of the extrahepatic biliary tree, hepatic duct bifurcation and left hepatic lobe has been completed. (From Cameron JL. *Atlas of Surgery.* vol I. Toronto, Canada: BC Decker, 1990, page 81, Inset).

furcation (Fig 66–13). Utilizing the preoperatively placed biliary catheter exiting the hepatic duct in the retained lobe, a Silastic transhepatic biliary stent is pulled through the hepatic parenchyma and placed in position. A 60-cm long Roux-en-Y jejunal loop then is constructed, brought out in retrocolic fashion, and a standard hepaticojejunostomy is performed using one layer of interrupted suture. The appearance of a postoperative cholangiogram performed in this setting is shown in Fig 66–14.

Resection of Proximal Bile Duct Cancer Plus Segment I (Caudate Lobe) with Reconstruction via Bilateral Hepaticojejunostomies.

The proximity of the caudate lobe to the hepatic duct bifurcation results in the caudate lobe being involved by proximal bile duct cancer in a variable proportion of cases. In such circumstances, resection of the hepatic duct bifurcation combined with some form of hepatic resection, including segment I (caudate lobe), has been advocated. Typically, these resections involve either extended right or left hepatectomy. In rare cases, central liver resections have been performed.

Hepatic Resection for Peripheral Bile Duct Cancer.

The clinical presentation, radiographic findings, and operative treatment of patients with peripheral bile duct carcinoma differ from those of patients with proximal bile duct carcinoma. Peripheral bile duct carcinoma is approached surgically in a fashion similar to hepatocellular carcinoma, with standard hepatic resectional techniques involved. In these cases, no specialized reconstruction of the intrahepatic or extrahepatic biliary tree is necessary.

Resection of Distal Bile Duct Cancer via Pylorus-preserving Pancreaticoduodenectomy.

Patients with bile duct cancer arising within the distal common bile duct require pancreaticoduodenectomy for complete extirpation of the tumor. The abdomen is explored thoroughly to detect evidence of disseminated disease. Once tumor dissemination has been ruled out, the duodenum is extensively mobilized. The portal vein then is exposed posterior to the common bile duct, and the ventral aspect of the superior mesenteric vein is identified at the level of the third portion of the duodenum. The portal vein and superior mesenteric veins are cleared anteriorly, and then separated from the undersurface of the neck of the pancreas so that a connection is made anterior to these two venous structures. The first portion of the duodenum then is mobilized, preserving a 2-cm segment of duodenum distal to the pylorus. The duodenum is divided and the gastroduodenal artery is controlled and divided. If present, the gallbladder then can be dissected from the gallbladder fossa, and the common hepatic duct divided. The neck of the pancreas then is divided with the electrocautery, (Fig 66–15) and the uncinate process of the pancreas dissected from the portal and superior mesenteric veins. The proximal jejunum then is exposed and divided 10 to 20 cm from the ligament of Treitz. The proximal jejunal mesentery is controlled and divided, and the proximal jejunum is passed posterior to the superior mesenteric vessels to the right side of the abdomen. At this point, any remaining attachments of the uncinate process to the region of the superior mesenteric vein and the superior mesenteric artery are divided, and the specimen is removed from the opera-

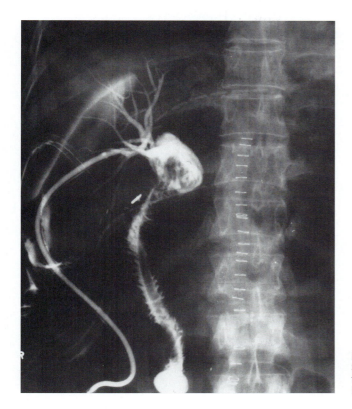

Figure 66–14. A postoperative cholangiogram obtained by contrast injection into a right-sided Silastic transhepatic catheter in a patient with hilar bile duct cancer, following en bloc resection of the hepatic duct bifurcation and left hepatic lobe. The visualized portions of the right hepatic ductal system appear normal, with good flow of contrast to the Roux-en-Y jejunal limb.

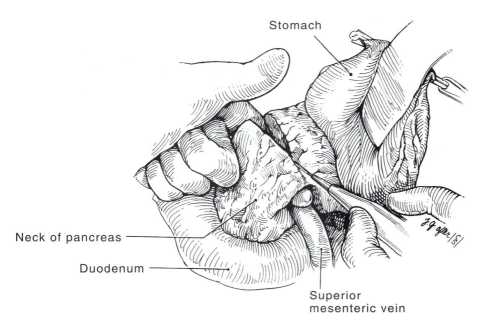

Stomach

Neck of pancreas

Duodenum

Superior
mesenteric vein

Figure 66–15. Division of the pancreatic neck using the electrocautery during the performance of a pancreaticoduodenectomy for a distal common bile duct cancer. (From Cameron JL. *Atlas of Surgery*. vol I. Toronto, Canada: BC Decker, 1990:393)

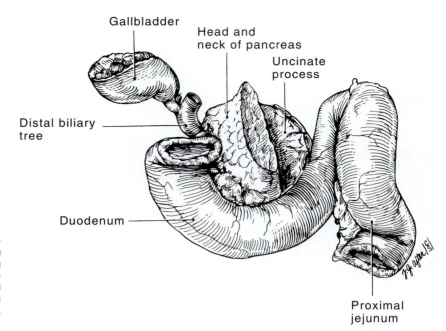

Figure 66–16. The resected specimen following pylorus-preserving pancreaticoduodenectomy for distal common bile duct cancer. The specimen includes the gallbladder, common bile duct, pancreas (head, neck, and uncinate process), duodenum (distal first portion and entirety of second, third and fourth portions) and several centimeters of proximal jejunum. (From Cameron JL. *Atlas of Surgery.* vol I. Toronto, Canada: BC Decker, 1990:399)

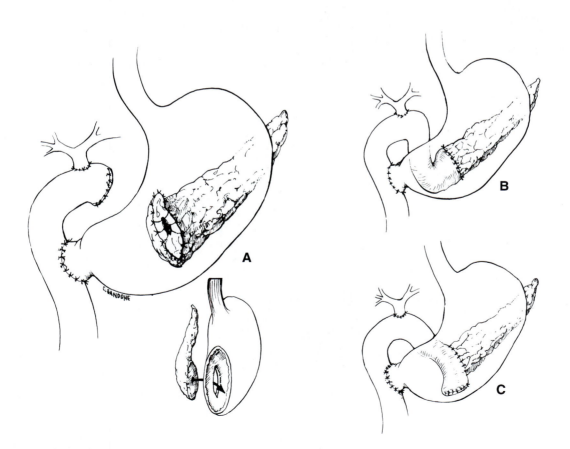

Figure 66–17. Three commonly-used options for reconstruction following pylorus-preserving pancreaticoduodenectomy. **A.** pancreaticogastrostomy; **B.** end-to-end pancreaticojejunostomy; and **C.** end-to-side pancreaticojejunostomy. The inset details the pancreaticogastrostomy, noting the posterior location of the gastrostomy. (From Yeo CJ, Cameron JL, Maher MM et al. A prospective randomized trial of pancreaticogastrostomy versus pancreaticojejunostomy following pancreaticoduodenectomy. *Ann Surg,* 222:580–592, 1995.).

tive field (Fig 66–16). Reconstruction of the gastrointestinal tract can be performed in one of several fashions (Fig 66–17). Our preference has been to perform an end-to-end pancreaticojejunostomy, followed by an end-to-side hepaticojejunostomy and conclude with an end-to-side duodenojejunostomy. More recently, the pancreaticoenteric anastomosis has been performed, in some cases, as a pancreaticogastrostomy.[89]

CHEMOTHERAPY AND RADIATION THERAPY

Chemotherapy

Chemotherapy alone, using 5-FU or other drugs has not been shown to improve survival in patients with either resected or unresected bile duct cancer. Whether hormonal manipulations will be helpful in malignancies of the biliary tract is unknown. Additionally, further investigation is required to see if CCK, CCK receptor antagonists, or somatostatin will influence the growth of these tumors.

Radiotherapy

Radiation therapy has been evaluated in patients with bile duct cancer using a variety of methods including external beam radiotherapy, intraoperative radiotherapy, internal radiotherapy, radioimmunotherapy, and charged particle irradiation. External beam radiotherapy has been delivered most frequently through multi-shaped portals using three or four fields with standard fractions (1.8 to 2.0 Gy/day) to a total dose of 45 to 60 Gy.[77,90–92] Intraoperative radiotherapy has been administered to a total dose of 5 to 20 Gy and is generally followed by additional external beam therapy.[93,94] Internal radiotherapy has been delivered through either percutaneous or endoscopically placed biliary stents using Iridium[192] or Cobalt[60] as the radiation source.[95,96] Radioimmunotherapy also has been used in the treatment of unresectable intrahepatic cholangiocarcinoma using ^{131}I-anti-CEA as a component of the therapy.[97]

To date, no prospective randomized trials of the use of radiotherapy have been reported in patients with bile duct carcinoma. One of the largest retrospective experiences comes from Johns Hopkins Hospital, where the use of radiotherapy postresection of hilar bile duct cancer did not improve survival.[98]

RESULTS

Hilar Bile Duct Cancer

In most series, the overall resectability rate for hilar bile duct cancer averages between 40% and 60%. Factors such as patient performance status at diagnosis, completeness of resection, histologic grade of tumor, status of nodal metastases, status of liver invasion, and the presence or absence of perineural invasion all influence survival. We currently lack sophisticated multivariate analysis of patients undergoing resection for hilar bile duct carcinoma, so the factors that are the most important in determining outcome cannot be determined.

Data from selected recent series reviewing potentially curative resection of hilar bile duct carcinoma reveal a mean survival of 22 months.[99] The percentages of patients alive at 1 year, 3 years, and 5 years following potentially curative resection of hilar bile duct cancer range between 67% and 80%, 25%, and 36%, and 11% and 21%, respectively.

A recent collective review of patients with resected hilar bile duct cancer compared the survival differences in patients undergoing local resection alone versus those treated by major liver resection.[100] In 201 patients undergoing local resection, the operative mortality was 8%, the mean survival was 21 months, and the percentages of patients alive at 1, 3 and 5 years were 76%, 21% and 7%, respectively. In contrast, in the 188 patients undergoing major liver resection for bile duct cancer, the operative mortality rate was doubled at 15%, the mean survival was 24 months, and the percentages of patients alive at 1, 3 and 5 years were 61%, 28%, and 17%, respectively. These results indicate that the mean survival was not improved by the addition of major liver resection to surgery for hilar bile duct cancer, although pathological staging of the tumors was not a controlled variable. Certainly, additional data are needed to determine the optimum treatment of patients with hilar bile duct cancer.

Distal Common Bile Duct Cancer

In most series, the resectability rate for distal common bile duct cancer exceeds 60%. The results of selected recent series of patients treated with potentially curative resection of distal common bile duct cancer (pancreaticoduodenectomy) show better outcomes as compared to patients with hilar bile duct carcinoma. Data from more than 221 patients reveal an average mean survival of 39 months, nearly double the mean survival following potentially curative resection of hilar bile duct cancer.[99] The percentage of patients alive at 1 year, 3 years and 5 years following potential curative resection of distal common bile duct cancer range between 50% and 70%, 28% and 53%, and 17% and 39%, respectively.

REFERENCES

1. DeStoll M. Rationis medenchi. In: Batavorum L (ed), *Nosocomio practico vendobonensi.* part 1. Honkoop, Hoak et Socios et A et J, 1788.

2. Sheinfeld W. Cholecystectomy and partial hepatectomy for carcinoma of the gallbladder with local liver extension. *Surgery* 1947;22:48–58

3. Adson MA. Carcinoma of the gallbladder. *Surg Clin North Am* 1973;53:1203–1216

4. Piehler JM, Crichlow RW. Primary carcinoma of the gallbladder. *Surg Gynecol Obstet* 1978;147:929–935

5. Aretxabala X, Roa I, Burgos L et al. Gallbladder cancer in Chile: a report on 54 potentially resectable tumors. *Cancer* 1992;69:60–65

6. Sumiyoshi K, Nagai E, Chijiiwa K et al. Pathology of carcinoma of the gallbladder. *World J Surg* 1991;15:315–321

7. Nevin JE, Moran TJ, Day S et al. Carcinoma of the gallbladder: staging, treatment and prognosis. *Cancer* 1976;37:141–148

8. Suto T, Sasaki K, Sugai T et al. Heterogeneity in the nuclear DNA content of cells in carcinomas of the biliary tract and pancreas. *Cancer* 1993;72:2920–2928

9. Sato Y, Tanaka J, Koyama K et al. Tumor DNA content in gallbladder carcinoma. *Hepatogastroenterology* 1993;40:375–379

10. Suda K, Miyano T, Konuma I et al. An abnormal pancreaticocholedochoductal junction in cases of biliary tract carcinoma. *Cancer* 1983;52:2086–2088

11. Kimura K, Ohto M, Saisho H et al. Association of gallbladder carcinoma and anomalous pancreaticobiliary ductal union. *Gastroenterology* 1985;89:1258–1263

12. Tsuchiya Y. Early carcinoma of the gallbladder: macroscopic features and US findings. *Radiology* 1991;179:171–175

13. McNulty JG. Preoperative diagnosis of carcinoma of the gallbladder by percutaneous transhepatic cholangiography. *AJR Am J Roentgenol* 1967;101:605–610

14. Lillemoe KD, Pitt HA, Kaufman SL et al. Acute cholecystitis occurring as a complication of percutaneous transhepatic drainage. *Surg Gynecol Obstet* 1989;168:348–352

15. Lillemoe KD, Cameron JL, Kaufman HS et al. Chemical splanchnicectomy in patients with unresectable pancreatic cancer: a prospective randomized trial. *Ann Surg* 1993;447–457

16. Ogura Y, Mizumoto R, Isaji S et al. Radical operations for carcinoma of the gallbladder: present status in Japan. *World J Surg* 1991;15:337–343

17. Nakamura S, Sakaguchi S, Suzuki S et al. Aggressive surgery for carcinoma of the gallbladder. *Surgery* 1989;106:467–472

18. Gagner M, Rossi RL. Radical operations for carcinomas of the gallbladder: present status in North America. *World J Surg* 1991;15:344–347

19. Gall FP, Kockerling F, Scheele J et al. Radical operations for carcinoma of the gallbladder: present status in Germany. *World J Surg* 1991;15:328–336

20. Morrow CE, Sutherland DER, Florack G et al. Primary gallbladder cancer: significance of subserosal lesions and results of aggressive surgical treatment and adjuvant chemotherapy. *Surgery* 1983;94:713–720

21. Falkson G, Macintyre JM, Moertel CG. Eastern cooperative oncology group experience with chemotherapy for inoperable gallbladder and bile duct cancer. *Cancer* 1984;54:965–969

22. Tsubono M, Nio Y, Tseng CC et al. Experimental chemotherapy for xenograft cell lines of human bile duct and gallbladder cancers in nude mice. *J Surg Oncol* 1992;51:274–80

23. Busse PM, Cady B, Bothe A et al. Intraoperative radiation therapy for gallbladder cancer. *World J Surg* 1991;15:352–356

24. Todoroki T, Iwasaki Y, Orii K et al. Resection combined with intraoperative radiation therapy (IORT) for stage IV gallbladder carcinoma. *World J Surg* 1991;15:357–366

25. Houry S, Schlienger M, Huguier M et al. Gallbladder carcinoma: role of radiation therapy. *Br J Surg* 1989;76:448–450

26. Bosset JF, Mantion G, Gillet M et al. Primary carcinoma of the gallbladder: adjuvant postoperative external irradiation. *Cancer* 1989;64:1843–1848

27. Miller BA, Ries LAG, Hankey BF et al. *SEER Cancer Statistics Review: 1973–1990.* (NIH publication No 93-2789). Bethesda, MD: National Cancer Institute; 1993

28. Sako S, Seitzinger GL, Garside E. Carcinoma of the extrahepatic bile ducts: review of the literature and report of six cases. *Surgery* 1957;41:416–422

29. Musser JH. Primary cancer of the gallbladder and bile ducts. *Boston Med Surg J* 1989;121:581–588

30. Stewart HL, Lieber MM, Morgan DR. Carcinoma of the extrahepatic bile ducts. *Arch Surg* 1940;41:662–668

31. Altemeier WA, Gall EA, Zinninger MM et al. Sclerosing carcinoma of the major intrahepatic bile ducts. *Arch Surg* 1957;75:450–455

32. Klatskin G. Adenocarcinoma of the hepatic duct at its bifurcation within the porta hepatis: an unusual tumor with distinctive clinical and pathologic features. *Am J Med* 1965;38:241–247

33. Dixon J, Lisehora GB, Lee YTM. Carcinoid tumor of the common bile duct. *Contemp Surg* 1992;41:37–40

34. Koo J, Ho J, Wong J et al. Mucoepidermoid tumor of the bile duct. *Ann Surg* 1982;196:140–6

35. Iemoto Y, Kondo J, Fukamachi S. Biliary cystadenocarcinoma with peritoneal carcinomatosis. *Cancer* 1981;48:1664–7

36. Farris FB, Faust BF. Granular cell tumors of the biliary ducts. *Arch Pathol Lab Med* 1979;103:510–5

37. Nakajima T, Kondo Y. Well differentiated cholangiocarcinomas: diagnostic significance of morphologic and immunohistochemical parameters. *Am J Surg Pathol* 1989;13:569–74

38. Wolber RA, Greene CA, Dupuis BA. Polyclonal carcinoembryonic antigen staining in the cytologic differential diagnosis of primary and metastatic hepatic malignancies. *Acta Cytol* 1991;35:215–20

39. Haglund C, Lindgren J, Robert PJ, et al. Difference in tissue expression of tumour markers CA19-9 and CA50 in hepatocellular carcinoma and cholangiocarcinoma. *Br J Cancer* 1991;63:386–9

40. Tada M, Omata M, Ohto M. Analysis of ras gene mutations in human hepatic malignant tumors by polymerase chain reaction and direct sequencing. *Cancer Res* 1990;50:1121–4

41. Levi S, Ispizua AU, Gill R et al. Multiple K-ras codon 12 mutations in cholangiocarcinomas demonstrated with a sensitive polymerase chain reaction technique. *Cancer Res* 1991;51:3497–3502

42. Tada M, Omata M, Ohto M. High incidence of ras gene mutation in intrahepatic cholangiocarcinoma. *Cancer* 1992;69:1115–8

43. Ding SF, Delhanty JDA, Bowles L et al. Loss of constitutional heterozygosity on chromosomes 5 and 17 in cholangiocarcinoma. *Br J Cancer* 1993;67:1007–10

44. Brunt EM, Swanson PE. Immunoreactivity for c-erbB-2 oncopeptide in benign and malignant diseases of the liver. *Am J Clin Pathol* 1992;97:S53–S61

45. Minote H, Inoue K, Higashide S et al. Immunohistochemical study on epidermal growth factor (EGF) receptor during carcinogenesis in the rat liver. *Nippon Geka Hokan* 1992;61:249–58

46. Roncalli M, Patriarca C, Gambacorta M et al. Expression of new phenotypic markers in cholangiocarcinoma and putative precursor lesions. *J Surg Oncol* 1993;3:173–4

47. Broe PJ, Cameron JL. The management of proximal biliary tract tumors. *Adv Surg* 1981;15:47–62

48. Sons HU, Borchard F. Carcinoma of the extrahepatic bile ducts: a postmortem study of 65 cases and review of the literature. *J Surg Oncol* 1987;34:6–12

49. Tompkins RK, Saunders K, Roslyn JJ et al. Changing patterns in diagnosis and management of bile duct cancer. *Ann Surg* 1990;211:614–621

50. Reding R, Buard JL, Lebeau G, et al. Surgical management of 552 carcinomas of the extrahepatic bile ducts: results of the French surgical association survey. *Ann Surg* 1991;213:236–41

51. Spiessl B, Beahrs OH, Hermanek P et al. *TNM Atlas.* Heidelberg, Germany: Springer-Verlag; 1989

52. Sobin L, Hermanek P, Hutter RVP. TNM classification of malignant tumors. *Cancer* 1988;61:2310–4

53. Longmire WP Jr, McArthur MS, Bastounis EA et al. Carcinoma of the extrahepatic biliary tract. *Ann Surg* 1973;178:333–40

54. Ross AP, Braasch JW, Warren KW. Carcinoma of the proximal bile ducts. *Surg Gynecol Obstet* 1973;136:923–8

55. Sheen-Chen SM, Chou FF, Eng HL. Intrahepatic cholangiocarcinoma in hepatolithiasis: a frequently overlooked disease. *J Surg Oncol* 1991;47:131–5

56. Fan ST, Lai EC, Wong J. Hepatic resection for hepatolithiasis. *Arch Surg* 1993;128:1070–4

57. Chijiiwa K, Ichimiya H, Kuroki S et al. Late development of cholangiocarcinoma after the treatment of hepatolithiasis: immunohistochemical study of mucin carbohydrates and core proteins in hepatolithiasis and cholangiocarcinoma. *Int J Cancer* 1993;55:82–91

58. Irwin ST, Morison JE. Congenital cyst of common bile duct containing stones and undergoing cancerous change. *Br J Surg* 1944;32:319–23

59. Aoki H, Sugaya H, Shimazu M. A clinical study on cancer of the bile duct associated with anomalous arrangements of the pancreaticobiliary ductal system: analysis of 569 cases collected in Japan. *J Bile Tract Pancreas* 1987;8:1539–51

60. Todani T, Tabuchi K, Watanabe Y et al. Carcinoma arising in the wall of congenital bile duct cysts. *Cancer* 1979;44:1134–9

61. Voyles CR, Smadja C, Shands WC et al. Carcinoma in choledochal cysts: age-related incidence. *Arch Surg* 1983;118:986–91

62. Babbitt DP. Congenital choledochal cyst: new etiological concept based on anomalous relationship of the common bile duct and pancreatic bulb. *Ann Radiol* 1969;12:231–40

63. Iwai N, Yanagihara J, Tokiwa K et al. Congenital choledochal dilatation with emphasis on pathophysiology of the biliary tract. *Ann Surg* 1992;215:27–30

64. Tani K, Kubota Y, Yamaguchi T et al. MR imaging of peripheral cholangiocarcinoma. *J Comput Assist Tomogr* 1991;15:973–8

65. Fan ZM, Yamashita Y, Harada M et al. Intrahepatic cholangiocarcinoma; spin-echo and contrast-enhanced dynamic MR imaging. *AJR Am J Roentgenol* 1993;161:313–7

66. Yeo CJ, Cameron JL. Transhepatic stents in high benign and malignant biliary tract obstructions. In: Nyhus LM, Baker RJ (eds), *Mastery of Surgery,* 2nd ed. Boston, MA: Little, Brown; 1992:960–967

67. Pitt HA, Gomes AS, Lois JF et al. Does preoperative percutaneous biliary drainage reduce operative risk or increase hospital cost? *Ann Surg* 1985;201:545–53

68. Pitt HA. The changing role of preoperative biliary decompression. *Perspect Gen Surg* 1990;1:113–26

69. Little JM. A prospective evaluation of computerized estimates of risk in the management of obstructive jaundice. *Surgery* 1987;102:473–6

70. Cope C, Marinelli DL, Weinstein JK. Transcatheter biopsy of lesions obstructing the bile ducts. *Radiology* 1988;169:555–60

71. Desa LA, Akosa AB, Lazzara S et al. Cytodiagnosis in the management of extrahepatic biliary stricture. *Gut* 1991;32:1188–91

72. Foutch PG, Kerr DM, Horlan JR et al. Endoscopic retrograde wire-guided brush cytology for diagnosis of patients with malignant obstruction of the bile duct. *Am J Gastroenterol* 1990;85:791–5

73. Earnhordt RC, McQuone SJ, Minasi JS et al. Intraoperative fine needle aspiration of pancreatic and extrahepatic biliary masses. *Surg Gynecol Obstet* 1993;177:147–52

74. Koyama K, Takagi Y, Ito K et al. Experimental and clinical studies on the effect of biliary drainage in obstructive jaundice. *Am J Surg* 1981;142:293–9

75. Katz S, Grosfeld JL, Grossk K et al. Impaired bacterial clearance and trapping in obstructive jaundice. *Ann Surg* 1984;199:14–9

76. Thompson JN, Cohen J, Moore RH et al. Endotoxemia in obstructive jaundice: observations on cause and clinical significance. *Am J Surg* 1988;155:314–21

77. Cameron JL, Pitt HA, Zinner MJ et al. Management of proximal cholangiocarcinoma by surgical resection and radiotherapy. *Am J Surg* 1990;159:91–8

78. Yamashita Y, Takahashi M, Kanazawa S et al. Parenchymal changes of the liver in cholangiocarcinoma: CT evaluation. *Gastrointest Radiol* 1992;17:161–6

79. Saeki M, Pitt HA, Tempany CM. Magnetic resonance imaging of hilar cholangiocarcinoma [Abstract]. In: *Proceedings of the International Hepatobiliary Pancreatic Association.* 1992:100A.

80. Lynn RB, Wilson JAP, Cho KJ. Cholangiocarcinoma: role of percutaneous transhepatic cholangiography in determination of resectability. *Dig Dis Sci* 1988;33:587–92

81. Dooley WC, Cameron JL, Pitt HA et al. Is preoperative angiography useful in patients with periampullary tumors. *Ann Surg* 1990;211:649–55

82. Tio TL, Cheng J, Wijers OB et al. Endosonographic TNM

staging of extrahepatic bile duct cancer: comparison with pathological staging. *Gastroenterology* 1991;100:1351–61

83. Molnar W, Stockum AE. Relief of obstructive jaundice through percutaneous transhepatic catheter: a new therapeutic method. *AJR Am J Roentgenol* 1974;122:356–360

84. LaBerge JM, Doherty M, Gordon RL, Ring EJ. Hilar malignancy: treatment with an expandable metallic transhepatic biliary stent. *Radiology* 1990;177:793–797

85. Bengmark S, Ekberg H, Evander A et al. Major liver resection for hilar cholangiocarcinoma. *Ann Surg* 1988; 207:120–5

86. Bismuth H, Nakache R, Diamond T. Management strategies in resection for hilar cholangiocarcinoma. *Ann Surg* 1992;215:31–8

87. Beazley RM, Hadjis N, Benjamin IS et al. Clinicopathological aspects of high bile duct cancer: experience with resection and bypass surgical treatments. *Ann Surg* 1984; 199:623–36

88. Fortner JG, Vitelli CE, Maclean BJ. Proximal extrahepatic bile duct tumors: analysis of a series of 52 consecutive patients treated over a period of 13 years. *Arch Surg* 1989;124:1275–9

89. Yeo CJ, Cameron JL, Maher MM, Sauter PK, Zahurak ML, Talamini MA, Lillemoe KD, Pitt HA. A prospective randomized trial of pancreaticogastrostomy versus pancreaticojejunostomy after pancreaticoduodenectomy. *Ann Surg* 1995;222:580–592.

90. Hayes JK Jr, Sapozink MD, Miller FJ. Definitive radiation therapy in bile duct carcinoma. *Int J Radiat Oncol Biol Phys* 1988;15:735–40

91. Verbeek PC, van Leeuwen DJ, van der Heyde MN et al. Does additive radiotherapy after hilar resection improve survival of cholangiocarcinoma: an analysis in sixty-four patients. *Ann Chir* 1991;45:350–4

92. Shiina T, Mikuriya S, Uno T et al. Radiology of cholangiocarcinoma: the roles for primary and adjuvant therapies. *Cancer Chemother Pharmacol* 1992;31(suppl):S115–S118

93. Busse PM, Stone MD, Sheldon TA et al. Intraoperative radiation therapy for biliary tract carcinoma: results of a 5-year experience. *Surgery* 1989;105:724–8

94. Monson JR, Donohue JH, Gunderson LL et al. Intraoperative radiotherapy for unresectable cholangiocarcinoma: the Mayo Clinic experience. *Surg Oncol* 1992;1:283–90

95. Ede RJ, Williams SJ, Hatfield ARW et al. Endoscopic management of inoperable cholangiocarcinoma using iridium-192. *Br J Surg* 1989;76:867–71

96. Koyama K, Tanaka J, Sato S et al. New strategy for treatment of carcinoma of the hilar bile duct. *Surg Gynecol Obstet* 1989;168:523–9

97. Stillwagon B, Order SE, Haulk T et al. Variable low dose irradiation (^{133}I-anti-CEA) and integrated low dose chemotherapy in the treatment of nonresectable primary intrahepatic cholangiocarcinoma. *Int J Rad* 1991;21:1601–5

98. Pitt HA, Nakeeb A, Abrams RA et al. Perihilar cholangiocarcinoma: postoperative radiotherapy does not improve survival. *Ann Surg* 1995;221:788–798.

99. Yeo CJ, Pitt HA, Cameron JL. Bile duct carcinoma: outcome, prognosis and followup. In: Terblanche J (ed), *Hepatobiliary Malignancy: Its Multidisciplinary Management.* London, England: Edward Arnold; 1994;480–484

100. Boerma EJ. Research into the results of resection of hilar bile duct cancer. *Surgery* 1990;108:572–80

67

Laparoscopic Cholecystectomy

R. David Rosin

No operation has exploded upon the surgical scene quite like laparoscopic cholecystectomy. It has rejuvenated general surgery and, in a very short time, has become the gold standard operation for conditions of the gallbladder. Born in secrecy and developed under an atmosphere of skepticism and hostility, laparoscopic cholecystectomy triumphed and was quickly accepted.

■ HISTORY

The first cholecystectomy performed was extremely well documented, unlike the first laparoscopic cholecystectomy. It was carried out by Langenbuch on July 15, 1882, in Berlin, on a male patient, 48 years of age, suffering from biliary colic for years.[1] The patient's pain was so severe that he had become addicted to morphine. Records indicate that he was given 5 days of enemas before the operation. He recovered so well that he was able to smoke a cigar on the first postoperative day. He became ambulatory on day 12, and was discharged after 6 weeks. The first laparoscopic cholecystectomy was performed by Muhe in 1985, 104 years later.[2] However, on presenting this operation to the German Surgical Congress the following year, Muhe was greeted with disbelief and outright hostility.

The first laparoscopic cholecystectomy recorded in the medical literature was performed in March, 1987 by Mouret, in Lyon, France.[3] The technique was perfected a year later, in March, 1988, by Dubois[4,5] in Paris, and later that year by Perrisat[6] in Bordeaux, France, and by Reddick[7] in Nashville, Tennessee. Within 5 years, laparoscopic cholecystectomy surpassed conventional cholecystectomy as the procedure of choice for anasthesia diseases of the gallbladder.

■ INDICATIONS

In our unit, laparoscopic cholecystectomy has been offered to all of our patients since the initial operation in March, 1990.[8] The only contraindications have been patients deemed unfit for general considerations and/or pregnancy.

In other units where laparoscopic cholecystectomy was started, criteria was established to determine which patients were suitable for this type of operation.[9,10] In some units, patients with thick-walled gallbladders on ultrasound, patients with large gallstones measuring >3 cm, and patients who had had previous upper abdominal incisions were excluded from this type of operation.

Patients with symptomatic gallstones causing biliary colic, acute cholecystitis, acalculus cholecystitis or gallstone pancreatitis were all submitted to laparoscopic cholecystectomy. The procedure also has been performed on patients with gallbladder polyps > 1 cm and on young people with asymptomatic gallstones. Patients with a history of jaundice, or those actually jaundiced at the time of admission, underwent endoscopic retrograde cannulation of the common bile duct and sphincterotomy, if indicated.

In every patient, preoperative investigations include an ultrasound of the gallbladder and common bile duct, and liver function tests. Occasionally, a HIDA scan may be indicated for a nonfunctioning gallbladder.

■ PREOPERATIVE PREPARATION

It is our practice to use thromboembolic deterrent (TED) stockings in all patients. Subcutaneous heparin is used in high-risk patients, especially those who have had a previous deep-vein thrombosis. Patients undergoing laparoscopic cholecystectomy may be at an increased risk for developing deep-vein thrombosis owing to the increased intra-abdominal pressure that accompanies the pneumoperitoneum and that may impede venous return. The reverse Trendelenberg position that is routinely used also may lead to a relative venous stasis in the pelvic and lower extremity veins. Two other factors that predispose to deep-vein thrombosis occur in female patients: obesity and the use of the contraceptive pill.

Before the procedure, fully informed consent must be obtained by the surgeon. Often with the aid of a diagram, the patient is informed that the gallbladder and stones will be removed. Additionally, consent for conversion to an open procedure must be obtained, although the patient should be reassured that conversion from one procedure to another does not suggest failure, since the operation still will be completed, and the two techniques differ only in terms of form of access to the gallbladder.

Patients usually are admitted on the day of the operation and are asked to void urine 1 hour before the operation. This will ensure an empty bladder, thus avoiding the need for catheterization.

■ EQUIPMENT

Compared with open cholecystectomy, laparoscopic cholecystectomy requires a vast amount of equipment that may be grouped into three categories: video equipment, laparoscopic instruments, and energy sources.

VIDEO EQUIPMENT

The explosion of laparoscopic surgery in recent years has undoubtedly been fueled by video technology. The greatest advance made in laparoscopic surgery occurred in 1986 with the development of the computer chip video camera that could be attached to the telescope. Thus began the era of video-guided surgery. Elaborate developments in the arena of video imaging have resulted in high-resolution video monitors that afford greater clarity and definition, as well as improved magnification of the operative field. As a result, fine dissection has become simpler to perform. With these developments, the surgeon and the entire team now can visualize the peritoneal cavity concurrently. Thus, assistance by other members of the operative team becomes possible.

The video equipment includes a telescope, light transmission cable, video camera, processing unit, an efficient light source (eg, Xenon) and high-resolution video monitor(s).

Telescopes come in a variety of sizes and optical configurations. For laparoscopic cholecystectomy, a 10-mm 0° wide angle is the most popular telescope used, although in certain circumstances, a 30° telescope may prove to be helpful.

The camera is either a single-chip camera that attaches to the telescope and easily fits into the palm of one's hand, or the more sophisticated model, which incorporates three chips in one head, thereby improving both color and resolution. These chips generate an electrical signal that is sent to the processing unit. The signal is manipulated and sent to the light source. It then travels to the video monitor, where it is viewed. Newer, three-dimensional cameras have been manufactured and will be helpful, particularly in training surgeons, since depth perception can be difficult when operating in a three-dimensional cavity while viewing a two-dimensional screen.

The light source is used to generate a high-intensity beam that is transmitted to the telescope via an optical cable. Sophisticated models incorporate an automatic iris function into the light source itself. The intensity of the signal sent from the camera processor to the light source is interpreted by the auto iris mechanism and the output of the light source is either dimmed or enhanced depending on the incoming intensity. This function becomes important in situations in which the telescope has to be routinely moved alternatively closer and farther from the object inside the peritoneal cavity. The video monitors must have high-resolution capabilities so that precise identification of anatomical structures can be made for accurate dissection.

LAPAROSCOPIC INSTRUMENTS

These include instruments used to create and maintain a pneumoperitoneum, those used for grasping, cutting, and dissecting tissues, those used for ligating, clipping or suturing vessels and other structures, and those used to maintain a clear field, such as suction and irrigation devices.

To establish pneumoperitoneum, the Veress needle, with its spring-loaded safety clip, is the most commonly used. Although the flow of carbon dioxide is limited using this needle, it affords the greatest safety in the initial blind puncture. The needle is connected to the insufflator, which has the capacity of achieving a high flow rate (4 to 12 L/min) while regulating the intra-abdominal pressure without exceeding the preset maximum limit. An insufflator that does not have the capacity to flow at 4 L/min or more is inadequate, and those that do not have automatic shut-off devices, when the preset pressure limit is reached, are unsafe.

Access ports can be reusable or disposable. The former are cheaper to use but in time the trochars will become blunt and there is no safety shield device. Reusable 10-mm ports also need reducing sleeves that are cumbersome to use and take more time to change. The long instruments used in this procedure must be capable of passing through the cannula used. Many instruments are incompatible with other manufacturer's ports. A basic set of instruments should include at least two grasping forceps, one or more angled dissecting forceps, scissors, clip appliers, and extraction forceps for removing the gallbladder from the peritoneal cavity. Conventional instruments to close the fascia and skin also should be available.

ENERGY SOURCE

Sources include endocoagulators, diathermy units, lasers, aquadissection instruments, the harmonic scalpel, and ultrasonic dissecting instruments.[11]

Endocoagulators achieve their effect by heating tissues to obtain coagulation, necrosis or denaturation of protein. Diathermy units are present in all operating rooms and are the cheapest to use. They cause warming, protein denaturation, coagulation, and necrosis by generating and passing an electrical current through the tissues. Diathermy units are available in either unipolar or bipolar modalities. The latter are considered safest, since the entire circuit within the patient exists between the electrodes at the tip of the hand-held instrument. Unipolar diathermy units have been known to cause arcing and burns to the organs.[12]

There are many different lasers available, each of which derives its name from the medium that was used to produce its specific wavelength of light. The most common laser used in laparoscopic cholecystectomy is the Nd:Yag contact-tip laser. The laser is precise, causes no adjacent tissue damage, produces less smoke, has no visual distortion, is safe, and has inherent tissue effects. The greatest danger using lasers in the peritoneal cavity is that of "overshoot."

■ OPERATING ROOM SET-UP

Laparoscopic cholecystectomy requires bulky operating room equipment. Thus, the operating room must be large enough to house comfortably this equipment

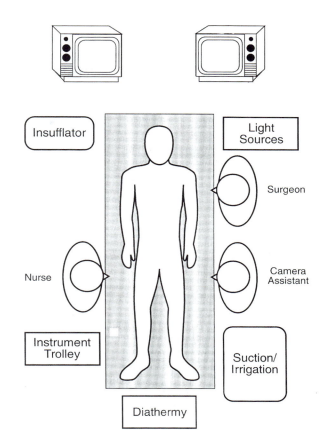

Figure 67–1. Diagrammatic representation of the position of the TV monitors, insufflator and other equipment in relation to the surgeon. The English/American set-up.

without obstructing the surgeon, anesthetist, or nursing staff. The anesthetist and his equipment are placed in the usual site at the head of the table. Since the surgeon must have an unobstructed view of the video monitor, the anesthetic equipment trolley must be placed in a position to allow for placement of the surgeon's video monitor trolley at, or near to, the right shoulder of the patient. The insufflator is located below this video screen to allow easy monitoring of the insufflation pressures throughout the operation, so that the surgeon can be aware instantly of any alterations that may prove hazardous to the patient (Fig 67–1).

An assistant usually is used as a camera operator and stands next to the surgeon. The scrub nurse or other assistant stands opposite the surgeon with the video monitor placed by the left shoulder of the patient. These monitors should be placed on custom built trolleys that also house the insufflator, light source, and camera equipment. The light source, camera, and video recording equipment may be placed on either trolley. If a laser is to be used, it is placed at the foot of the table, or behind the surgeon. Suction and irrigation machines should be placed in such a way that their tubing to the patient does not interfere with the movements of the operating team.

The positioning of the surgeon, assistant(s), and scrub nurse, as described, is that used in our unit. However, many surgeons, particularly in France and Germany, prefer to stand between the legs of the patient, using a split table approach. In this set-up, the camera person would be on the left side of the patient and to the right of the surgeon, and the scrub nurse would be to the right of the patient.

The operating table should be automatic, so that the anesthetist easily can change its position during the operation. It also should be capable of taking x-rays or preferably, an image intensifier. Although some surgeons turn off the operating room lights to reduce glare, it is our practice merely to dim them.

■ OPERATIVE TECHNIQUE

Laparoscopic cholecystectomy can be performed in various ways. It may be accomplished with as many as four persons at the operating table, or as few as two.

PREPARATION AND POSITIONING

The patient is anesthetized and placed in a supine position on the operating table. The abdomen is percussed to ensure that the bladder is not full; if the bladder is palpable, it is decompressed using a catheter which is then removed. An orogastric tube is inserted to decompress the stomach which, when distended, will obstruct visualization of the porta hepatis. This tube is removed at the end of the operation. The abdominal skin is prepared and towelled in the usual manner for abdominal surgery. The equipment tables and trolleys are placed in position and all device cables and tubing is routed properly. The operating team can be positioned as described (Figs 67–1 and 67–2), and all equipment is checked before beginning the procedure.

ESTABLISHING PNEUMOPERITONEUM

Pneumoperitoneum may be established by blind puncture, using a Veress needle or open laparoscopy.[13] In the blind puncture method, a spring-loaded Veress needle with a protective blunt tip is inserted through a small incision made at the umbilicus, since it is the thinnest portion of the abdominal wall and allows easy access. This incision should be 1 cm in length so that a 10-mm port can be inserted through it. The incision may be made in a transverse or vertical direction depending on the skin folds of the patient and the preference of the surgeon. A vertical incision in the umbilicus gives excellent cosmetic results. Before inserting the Veress needle, the patient is placed in a 15° Trendelenberg posi-

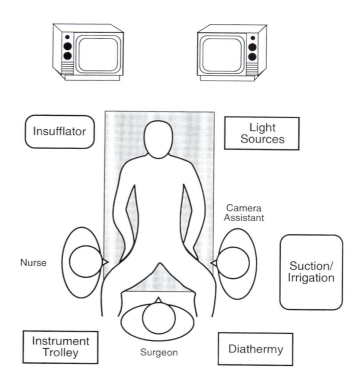

Figure 67–2. Diagramatic representation of the position of the TV monitors, insufflator and other equipment in relation to the surgeon. The French/European set-up.

tion, which moves the intestine upward and out of the path of the needle.

The anterior abdominal wall must be elevated during needle insertion. The entire thickness of the abdominal wall at the umbilicus must be elevated and this is done effectively by grasping the abdominal wall with one's hand. Although the needle can be inserted in any direction, it is our practice to pass it towards the sacral promontory, being careful of depth of penetration.

Confirmation of the intraperitoneal location of the needle tip is made by the saline drop test, in which saline is drawn into the peritoneal cavity by the negative pressure exerted. Once the needle is confirmed to be in the right position, the peritoneal cavity is insufflated, using carbon dioxide. The abdomen should become tympanitic and this generally takes between 2 and 4 L of gas. To prevent problems of venous return, the pressure should never exceed 15 mm Hg. When adequate distension has been obtained, the Veress needle is removed.

Open laparoscopy is probably the safest means of establishing pneumoperitoneum. The same incision is made in the umbilicus, and the abdominal wall is incised under direct vision. If the incision is just 1 cm in length, then a secure seal around the port should be obtained. The cannula is inserted without its trochar, under direct vision. If there have been previous incisions into the umbilicus, then an open laparoscopy technique, either just above or just below the umbilicus, can be used. With this method, stay sutures are placed in the fascia on either side of the wound and the rectus sheath is incised under direct vision. A specially designed cannula, the Hassan cannula, with its blunt-tipped obturator and external movable cone then is inserted while gentle upward traction is placed on the stay sutures. The external cone port is secured in position on the sheath and the stay sutures are tied to pleats on this sheath. This procedure should prevent leakage of carbon dioxide and therefore, loss of pneumoperitoneum.

PRIMARY PORT PLACEMENT

While elevating the abdominal wall manually to avoid injury to underlying viscera, a 10/11-mm port is inserted through the same incision used for the Veress needle. The trochar should not be angled too inferiorly, since this may result in it not penetrating the peritoneum and can lead to insufflation of the subcutaneous tissue or preperitoneal space. Insertion is safest if the index finger is placed along the sheath as the port is inserted. This positioning will help lower the depth of penetration of the sharp trochar. It is our practice to use disposable trochars with spring-loaded safety shields for the primary port, since they help prevent injury to underlying viscera.

PERITONEOSCOPY

The telescope is placed through this primary cannula and a peritoneoscopy is performed. This procedure should be done in the same methodical, careful manner used when performing a laparotomy. It is our practice to start by examining the pelvis, including the hernial orifices, and then moving along the right paracolic gutter and examine the cecum and ascending colon. The liver is inspected and the state of the gallbladder is noted. The falciform ligament and left lobe of the liver then is inspected, as well as the hiatus, stomach, and duodenum. If visible, the spleen is inspected followed by inspection of the splenic flexure, descending colon, and left paracolic gutter. The patient then is placed in a reverse Trendelenberg position and, if necessary, the table is tilted to the left to allow a clear view of the porta hepatis.

SECONDARY PORT PLACEMENT

At present, it is our practice to perform the operation with just three ports. However, if the gallbladder is difficult to dissect or very long and floppy, then a fourth port is inserted. A 5-mm port is placed under direct vision in the midclavicular line just below the right costal margin. The trochar and cannula are watched carefully as they come through the peritoneum, and the port

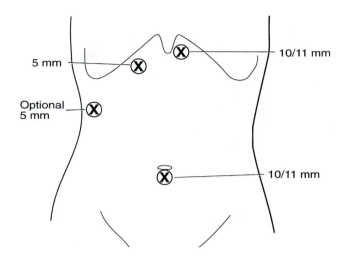

Figure 67–3. Diagram of the abdomen and port positions.

then is fixed with a grip, if this is available. An epigastric port then is placed in the midline, entering the peritoneal cavity again under direct vision to the right of the falciform ligament. This procedure is done by angling the trochar and cannula to the right during insertion. If a fourth port is to be used, a 5-mm port is inserted in the anterior axillary line just below the costal margin. The epigastric and two subcostal ports should be in a straight line so that should conversion to an open operation be necessary, these small incisions can be joined (Fig 67–3).

Some surgeons prefer to insert the 10/11-mm secondary port to the left of the falciform ligament lateral to the left rectus muscle because they feel that dissection is easier since it is further away from the operating field. If the ports are placed too close together, the instruments will clash (cross swords) with each other.

Once the secondary ports have been established, a grasping forceps is inserted and the gallbladder grasped halfway down through the 5-mm port. If a fourth port is utilized, a second 5-mm forceps is placed through it and the fundus of the gallbladder is grasped and elevated (Fig 67–4). Instruments used to perform the dissection are passed through the epigastric port.

DISSECTION OF THE TRIANGLE OF CALOT

Dissection of the triangle of Calot is the most dangerous part of the operation and the surgeon must proceed cautiously. Before any ligature or clip is applied, each structure in the triangle of Calot must be identified accurately. The safest approach involves commencing the dissection as close to the gallbladder as possible and working on the lateral (right) side of the cystic duct. Using a three-port technique, the forceps, through the 5-

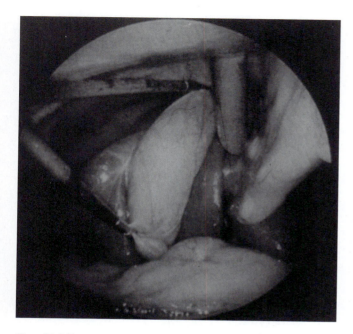

Figure 67–4. The gallbladder is elevated with the fundal grasper. Hartmann's pouch is held with a second grasping forceps.

mm port, are used to grasp the gallbladder at Hartman's pouch while a blunt dissector is passed through the epigastric port. It is our preference to use curved forceps and to break down the loose adhesions around the cystic duct (Fig 67–5). If adhesions are present to the gallbladder, these must be taken down first. This usually is performed most easily using scissors with diathermy attached. A thicker peritoneum also may be divided by scissors. The cystic duct is dissected out and secured close to the neck of the gallbladder with a clip. If the cystic artery is easily visible and can be dissected out, then this is doubly clipped, although not divided. The cystic duct then is incised with microscissors so that a cholangiogram can be performed. If cholangiography cannot be performed, the cystic duct is dissected down to its junction with the common hepatic duct, prior to any placement of clips. The cystic artery, if controlled, is not divided in case incision into the cystic duct is taken too far and it parts. By not dividing the cystic artery, it is easier to control the end of the cystic duct that, if the cystic artery has been divided, will spring apart.

CHOLANGIOGRAPHY

We strongly recommend the performance of routine cholangiography, first and most importantly, to familiarize oneself with the procedure so that when it becomes necessary to perform it will be easy to do.[14–16] It is also particularly useful in defining the anatomy and for evaluating the ductal system for any unsuspected calculi. Even though there has been great debate as to the need

for operative cholangiography, it is our opinion that the first two reasons given make it almost mandatory. Finally, routine cholangiography will facilitate laparoscopic exploration of the common bile duct, if the surgeon is experienced, when unsuspected calculi are discovered.

Two different methods are used: the portal technique and the percutaneous technique. Reddick and Olsen described using the most lateral port, or inserting an extra port, to introduce a specially designed clamp that both placed and secured the cholangiogram catheter in the cystic duct[7] (Fig 67–6). With this method, the remaining 5-mm grasping forceps has to be repositioned to maintain exposure. The radiopaque clamp is oriented so as not to obscure the ductal system during the x-ray (Fig 67–7). The second method, the percutaneous technique, was developed and popularized by Petelin, in 1990.[17] This technique employs a 14-French (Fr) gauge polythene sleeve inserted directly through the anterior abdominal wall, just medial to the midclavicular port. The cholangiogram catheter is inserted through the sleeve into the peritoneal cavity where it is grasped by forceps inserted via the epigastric port. Using the forceps, the catheter is manipulated into the cystic duct where it is se-

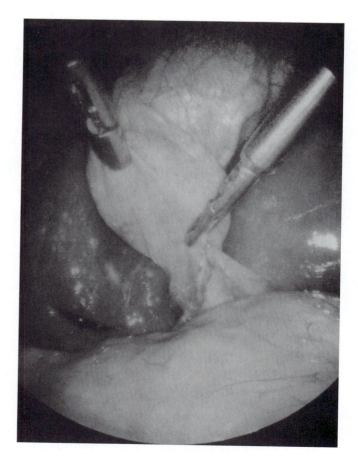

Figure 67–5. The cystic duct and artery are freed by blunt dissection.

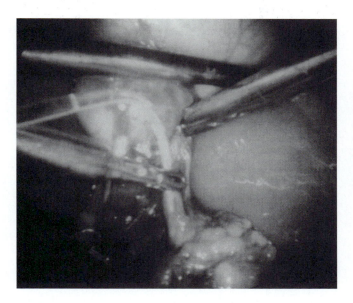

Figure 67–6. A clamp holds the cholangiogram catheter in the cystic duct.

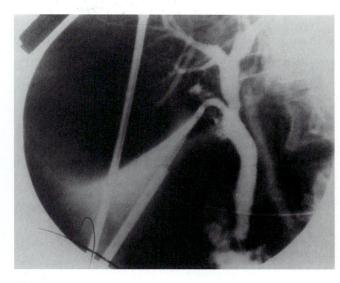

Figure 67–7. An operative cholangiogram using the Reddick clamp.

cured into position by placing a clip across the catheter and cystic duct (Fig 67–8). The surgeon secures the clip and simultaneously injects saline. When there is enough resistance to injection, the clip application is stopped. This procedure allows a watertight seal at the insertion site and still enables sufficient flow for contrast injection into the ductal system. After completion of the cholangiogram, the clip is removed easily and the catheter withdrawn from the duct. The advantage of this method over the portal method is that exposure is maintained and no specialized clamp is required. Also, the site of the partially applied clip is easily demonstrated on the x-ray and therefore allows the surgeon precise delineation of the cystic duct–common duct junction.

It is our practice to perform operative cholangiogram using an image intensifier so that no time is wasted. The intrahepatic, common hepatic, and common bile ducts are all visualized and free flow of contrast with no filling defects in the duct system should normally be obtained.

DISSECTION OF THE GALLBLADDER FROM ITS LIVER BED

Once the cholangiogram has been performed, the catheter is removed and the cystic duct is secured by placing two clips across it. Care is taken not to place these clips too close to its junction with the common hepatic duct. If the cytic duct is very large, it should be closed using a catgut endoloop, since the clips may not be large enough to close it. The cystic duct and artery are then divided. If there is a posterior branch to the artery, it will now be encountered and can be clipped prior to its division.

Following division of the cystic duct and artery, the gallbladder may be dissected from the liver bed (Fig 67–9). The energy source, the diathermy hook, dia-

thermy scissors, laser or harmonic scalpel, is passed through the epigastric port and dissection is started behind Hartmann's Pouch. If a laser is to be used, the laser fiber is inserted through the center of the suction irrigation cannula and then passed through the epigastric port. During dissection, gentle traction is applied to the gallbladder, moving it from side to side so that the loose areolar tissue, which is present in all but the most inflamed cases, can be demonstrated. As more of the gallbladder wall is detached from the liver, the midclavicular port forceps are moved closer to the line of dissection. This is often referred to as "walking down" the under surface of the gallbladder. The most difficult part of the gallbladder to detach is the fundus, since traction is difficult to maintain. The gallbladder should not be completely removed from its liver bed; by leaving the fundus attached, the liver can be elevated and the gallbladder fossa carefully inspected for accessory bile ducts and/or bleeding. Using irrigation and suction, the liver bed is closely scrutinized and dealt with, as necessary. The cystic duct stump and cystic artery also are inspected at this stage to ensure that the clips are in position.

EXTRACTION OF THE GALLBLADDER

Once the gallbladder is completely detached from the liver, it is our practice to pass it across to the epigastric port through which large grasping forceps can be inserted. The gallbladder is rotated so that the grasping forceps holds the neck of the gallbladder just above the clips. The other forceps then release the gallbladder, which then is extracted with the port through the epigastric incision. By removing it through the epigastrium, there is no need to change the camera from the umbilical

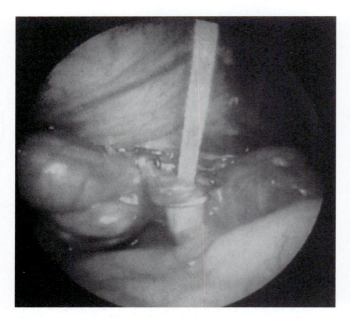

Figure 67–8. The Petelin method of performing operative cholangiography; the catheter is held in place using a snug clip across it and the cystic duct.

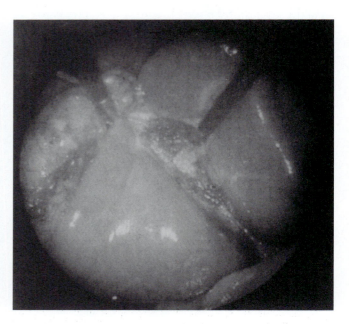

Figure 67–9. Dissection of the gallbladder from its liver bed.

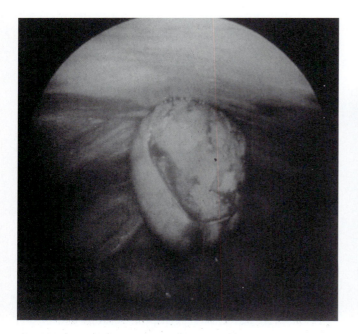

Figure 67–10. A tense gallbladder being taken through the anterior abdominal wall.

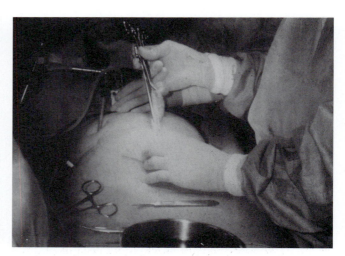

Figure 67–11. The gallbladder brought onto the abdominal wall surface.

port to the epigastric port. However, in very obese patients, it may be more sensible to remove the gallbladder through the umbilical incision, where the abdominal wall is thinnest. In this case, the grasping forceps are placed through the umbilical port and the camera is placed inside the epigastric port. If the gallbladder is tense (Fig 67–10) once the neck is brought out onto the surface (Fig 67–11), the gallbladder is opened and a sucker is placed inside to decompress it. If the stones are large, they can be crushed within the gallbladder or the incision can be enlarged before removing the gallbladder. This prevents the gallbladder from tearing during extraction and losing gallstones into the peritoneal cavity. In such cases, manual stone extraction is required, often necessitating considerable time and effort. If the gallbladder is very inflamed or there is a possibility of stones escaping, then it should be placed into a retrieval bag before removal from the peritoneal cavity. Once the gallbladder has been removed, the epigastric port is replaced into the peritoneal cavity and the gallbladder fossa is inspected once again and irrigated, if necessary. If there is no bleeding or bile leak, use of a drain is not necessary. However, if a laser is being used, a suction drain is inserted and left in situ for a few hours to extract the irritating laser smoke. We have devised an easy way of inserting a drain by placing a straight grasping forceps through the epigastric port and out through the 5-mm port onto the surface. The port then is removed and the suction drain grasped. It then is pulled into the peritoneal cavity and placed under the liver in the gallbladder fossa.

Prior to removal of the ports and expulsion of the carbon dioxide, it is our practice to instill 10 mm of bupivacaine (Marcaine) into the gallbladder fossa. The ports are removed slowly, under vision, to ensure there is no bleeding. The primary port incision also can be inspected by withdrawing the camera into the sheath and slowly removing the port while inspecting the tract made. The table is straightened and the gas is expelled from the peritoneal cavity through the incisions.

CLOSURE

It is our practice to close the fascia at the umbilicus and in the epigastrium with a 0 vicryl suture on a J shaped needle. If the patient is obese, these sutures can be placed with the laparoscope using a Grice needle (Meadox). The skin wounds are closed with subcuticular nylon or steristrips. These incisions are injected subcutaneously with 0.5% Marcaine to help alleviate postoperative wound discomfort.

As a matter of practice, one dose of Cefuroxime (750 mg) is given at induction of anesthesia and a votarol (Diclofenac) suppository is used for analgesia purposes following the procedure. Opiates are not used, since we have found them to be unnecessary in the postoperative period.

■ DIFFICULTIES ENCOUNTERED DURING THE OPERATION

The pneumoperitoneum may be difficult to create because of previous surgery with adhesions to the scars. An area that is clear of incisions should be selected for insertion of the Veress needle. Once the pneumoperitoneum is established, the peritoneal cavity is carefully inspected using the telescope from this site. Adhesions then can be visualized and taken down; if necessary, under direct vision, a secondary port can be placed in a safe area and adhesiolysis effected using scissors and a grasping instrument. For dense adhesions, the Nd:Yag laser is very effective.

The next problem may be dense adhesions around an inflamed gallbladder and these should be separated with care, keeping close to the gallbladder wall. If the gallbladder is very tense, it should be aspirated and if it has a very thick wall, special three-pronged grasping forceps (Weck) can be used to grasp it. If there is much inflammation around the triangle of Calot, a safe way to proceed is to dissect around the back of Hartmann's pouch and elevate this from its liver bed. One then can dissect carefully down the cystic duct which then is cannulated to delineate the anatomy. If this proves impossible, a direct puncture into the gallbladder and cholecystography may be carried out. On a few occasions, a Foley catheter has been placed laparoscopically into the gallbladder and sutured into place as a cholecystostomy tube. Some weeks later, after the inflammation has settled down, a laparoscopic cholecystectomy can be performed more easily.

The surgeon must be aware of the anatomical variations of the cystic duct, especially of the short cystic duct and the cystic duct draining directly into the right hepatic duct. There are many variations of the cystic artery and these must be known to the operating surgeon. A common mistake is to miss the posterior branch of the cystic artery which, when divided, leads to bleeding that may obscure the view. Bleeding from the liver bed should be controlled easily with diathermy, but if this does not control it, a swab may be inserted and pressure applied. The use of Surgicell is also useful on occasion. Finally, rupture of the gallbladder leading to escape of bile and stones will prolong the procedure, since these have to be retrieved. A large stone scoop or stone sucker is useful, although placement of the gallbladder and these stones into a bag is probably quicker and easier.

■ POSTOPERATIVE CARE

Patients are allowed to take fluids as soon as they have recovered from the anesthesia and to have food as soon as they can tolerate it. Most patients will tolerate a light

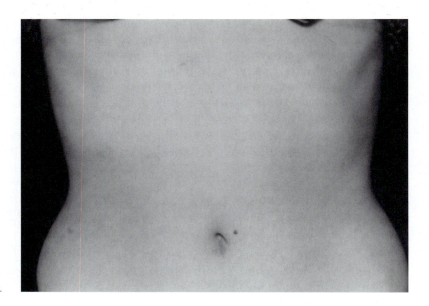

Figure 67–12. The abdominal incisions after removal of the sutures.

meal within 8 hours of surgery. We routinely administer a glycerine suppository within 8 hours after surgery since patients often will experience a slight feeling of distension that can be alleviated by a bowel movement.

Patients are allowed out of bed as soon as they are fit enough to walk and >85% of patients are discharged from the hospital within 36 hours. Fit patients who have been preoperatively selected may be operated on as day cases and can be safely discharged within 6 hours following surgery. Patients are evaluated 1 week following surgery and if sutures are present, they are removed (Fig 67–12). At this time, >95% of patients are back to a normal routine and most return to work immediately following their clinic visit.

■ EXPLORATION OF THE COMMON BILE DUCT

Although the thought of exploring the common bile duct under laparoscopic guidance seemed like sheer madness, this preconceived notion has been dispelled. The view of the porta hepatis is not only comparable to that obtained at open surgery, but it is, in fact, superior owing to the magnification afforded by the telescope and camera systems. In addition to the basic equipment necessary to perform laparoscopic cholecystectomy, a limited number of other instruments are required to facilitate common duct exploration. These include Fogarty embolectomy catheters, a flexible 3-mm choledochoscope with a separate light source, stone retrieval baskets and a standard T tube, if choledochotomy is performed. The duct can be explored in one of two ways: transcystic exploration, which may necessitate dilation of the cystic duct first, and choledochotomy.[8]

In most cases, laparoscopic common duct exploration may be accomplished through the cystic duct. The duct should be dilated to at least a 10-Fr diameter (approximately 3.3 mm) to allow insertion of the various instruments. If a single stone is present in the common bile duct, this often may be retrieved by passing a basket down into the common bile duct under an image intensifier and catching the calculus. However, if a flexible choledochoscope is available, this is a more efficient method of retrieving common bile duct stones, since the basket can be passed through the choledochoscope. Exploration via the cystic duct does not allow inspection of the common hepatic and intrahepatic bile ducts. The choledochoscope usually is passed through an extra 5-mm port placed between the epigastric and midclavicular secondary ports. If the common bile duct is large and contains many calculi, a choledochotomy is the preferred method of exploration. This offers the added advantage of easier access to the proximal extrahepatic-intrahepatic ductal system, since a flexible choledochoscope may be advanced in that direction through an opening in the common duct. Such access is impossible via the cystic duct. Once the duct has been cleared and checked by choledochoscopy, a T tube is inserted and the common bile duct closed over it, using 3/0 or 4/0 vicryl sutures. Only three or four sutures are usually needed to achieve closure over the T tube.

■ COMPLICATIONS

Complications include those of laparoscopy itself,[19] which usually occur at induction of the pneumoperitoneum, and complications of the cholecystectomy operation. It is imperative that surgeons be careful when creating the pneumoperitoneum, and inexperienced surgeons should probably use the open technique. The open technique also should be used if previous surgery is evident.

Although it has been speculated that the incidence of bile duct injuries has increased significantly, it is still quoted at approximately <1.5%.[20] In a large confidential audit by the Royal College of Surgeons of England, there was no statistical difference in bile duct injuries between conventional cholecystectomy and laparoscopic cholecystectomy.[21] In all of the large series reported, the injuries occurred mostly during the first 50 cases, indicating that there is a definite learning curve in mastering this operation.[22,23]

Difficulties in setting up clinical trials between conventional versus laparoscopic cholecystectomy have been highlighted by Neugebauer and associates.[24] Many patients included in this study, who specifically requested laparoscopic cholecystectomy, would certainly not have agreed to be randomized. However, by careful audit of large series, it has been shown that laparoscopic cholecystectomy has great advantages over open cholecystectomy. These include a shorter time in the hospital, far less pain, a quicker return to normal activities, and a shortened time off from work. The operation has been classified by Troidl as "patient-friendly."[25] We have certainly found this to be so with our patients and, although the initial cost in the operating room is slightly higher, the savings made in terms of shorter length of stay in the hospital more than compensates for this cost. Although this operation may take longer than conventional cholecystectomy, when the surgeon is unfamiliar with the procedure, the average time it takes to perform a laparoscopic cholecystectomy is approximately 40 minutes, which is the same as and, in some cases less than, the time needed for conventional cholecystectomy. Finally, it should be pointed out that wound infections and other wound-related complications virtually have been abolished by this procedure. Rapid postoperative mobilization means that common complications such as chest infections and deep vein thrombosis have been reduced greatly. Finally, laparoscopic cholecystectomy greatly diminishes contact with the patient's blood and other body fluids, which in turn reduce the risk of viral disease transmission.

REFERENCES

1. Langenbuch C. Ein fall von exstirpation der gallenblase wegen chronischer cholelithiasis: heilung berliner. *Klinische Wochenschrift.* 1882;48:725–727

2. Muhe E. Die erste cholezystektomie durch das laparoskop. *Langenbecks Arch Chir Kongerssband.* 1986;804

3. Mouret P. From the first laparoscopic cholecystectomy to the frontiers of laparoscopic surgery; the future prospectives. *Dig Surg* 1991;8:124–125

4. Dubois F, Icard P, Bethelot G, et al. Coelioscopic cholecystectomy: preliminary report of 36 cases. *Ann Surg* 1990;211:60–62

5. Dubois F, Bethelot G, Levard H. Laparoscopic cholecystectomy: historic perspective and personal experience. *Surg Laprosc Endosc* 1991;4:52–57

6. Perrisat J, Collet D, Belliard B. Gallstones; laparoscopic treatment; cholecystectomy; cholecystoscopy and lithotripsy. *Surg Endosc* 1990;4:1–5

7. Reddick E, Olsen D, Daniell J, et al. Laparoscopic laser cholecystectomy. *Laser Med Surg News Adv* 1989;3:38–40

8. Rosin RD, Hershman MJ. Laparoscopic laser cholecystectomy: our first 200 patients. *Ann R Coll Surg (Engl)* 1992;74:242–247

9. McKernan JB. Laparoscopic cholecystectomy. *Am Surg* 1991;57:311–312

10. Perrisat J. Laparoscopic cholecystectomy In: Rosin RD (ed), *Minimal Access General Surgery.* Radcliffe Medical; 1993:27

11. Beneveto A, Carcano G, Cuffari A, et al. New techniques in laparoscopic cholecystectomy; ultrasonography, CUSA and argon coagulator. *Br J Surg* 1993;80(suppl):543

12. McAnena OJ, Willson PD. Diathermy in laparoscopic surgery. *Br J Surg* 1993;80:1094–1096

13. Veress J. Neues instrument zur Ausfuhrung von Brust oder Bauch punktionen. *Dtsch Med Wochenschr.* 1938;41:1480–1481

14. Keane FBV, Tanner WA, Gillen P. Operative cholangiography and laparoscopic bile duct exploration. *Br J Surg* 1993;80:957–958

15. Paterson-Brown S, Garden OJ, Carter DC. Laparoscopic cholecystectomy. *Br J Surg* 1991;78:131–132

16. Sackier J, Berci G, Phillips E, et al. The role of cholangiography in laparoscopic cholecystectomy. *Arch Surg* 1991;126:1021–1026

17. Petelin J. The argument for contact laser laparoscopic cholecystectomy. *Clin Laser Monthly.* 1990;71–74

18. Petelin J. Laparoscopic approach to common duct pathology. *Am J Surg* 1993;165:487–491

19. Chamberlain GVP, Carron Brown JA. *Report of the Working Party of the Confidential Enquiry into Gynecological Laparoscopy.* London, England: R Coll Obstet Gynecologists: 1978

20. Moosa AR, Easter DW, Van Sonnenberg E, et al. Laparoscopic injuries to the bile duct; a cause for concern. *Ann Surg* 1992;215:203–208

21. Nair R, Dunn D, Fowler S, et al. Confidential comparative audit of 11 354 cholecystectomies. *Min Inv Ther* 1993;2:277

22. Cuschieri A, Dubois F, Mouiel J, et al. The European experience with laparoscopic cholecystectomy. *Am J Surg* 1991;161:385–387

23. Rosin RD. Training of surgeons in video-enhanced telescopic surgery. In: Rosin RD (ed), *Minimal Access General Surgery.* Radcliffe Medical; 1993:221

24. Neugebauer E, Troidl H, Spangenberger W, et al. Conventional versus laparoscopic cholecystectomy and the randomised controlled trial. *Br J Surg* 1991;78:150–154

25. Troidl H. The philosophy of patient-friendly surgery. In: Rosin RD (ed), *Minimal Access Medicine and Surgery, Principles and Techniques.* Radcliffe Medical; 1993:11

68

Choledochoduodenostomy

David L. Nahrwold

Choledochoduodenostomy has been performed since the latter part of the 19th century for a variety of diseases of the biliary tract and pancreas. The advances in interventional biliary endoscopy and interventional radiology have radically altered the diagnosis and management of biliary calculi and other disorders of the bile ducts and pancreas. Accordingly, the indications for choledochoduodenostomy have changed, and less invasive procedures now are indicated for many of the problems formerly treated by choledochoduodenostomy.

■ INDICATIONS

BILE DUCT STONES

Bile duct stones usually can be managed very successfully by endoscopic sphincterotomy and extraction of the stones.[1] After cholecystectomy, retained stones that are impacted or too large to traverse the incised sphincter can be fragmented by lithotripsy under direct vision. The stones then will pass spontaneously or may be extracted (Fig 68–1). Open surgical treatment is reserved for patients in whom endoscopic methods fail. Failure of endoscopic management may occur in patients with large stones, multiple stones, impacted stones, and multiple intrahepatic stones.

Large Stones
Stones >1.5 cm in diameter are difficult to extract endoscopically. The use of endoscopic sphincterotomy and a crushing stone basket (mechanical lithotripter) is essential.[2] When a T tube is in place in the common bile duct, the tract should be allowed to mature for approximately 6 weeks. An attempt then can be made to remove the stones through the T tube tract after temporary removal of the tube. A fiberoptic choledochoscope is introduced through the tract and into the duct system, where, under direct vision, stones are fragmented using the laser lithotripter. In addition to extraction with a basket, stones or fragments can be pushed into the duodenum, under direct vision. Catheters also can be placed through the tract into the duct and used for flushing the biliary tree with saline. Fewer options are available when a T tube is not present. Success has been achieved in approximately 75% of patients using extracorporeal shock-wave lithotripsy to fragment large stones.[3] Before lithotripsy, endoscopic sphincterotomy is carried out and a nasobiliary tube is placed with its tip adjacent to the stone for infusion of contrast medium during the lithotripsy procedure.

Open exploration should be performed when these nonoperative methods fail. If the stone is distal and cannot be removed through a choledochotomy, choledochoduodenostomy is indicated.

Multiple Stones
Patients with longstanding multiple stones usually have a dilated duct that is packed with calculi. If the stones are present at the time of cholecystectomy, choledochoduodenostomy should be considered. If the multiple stones are present at a time distant from the initial cholecystectomy, then endoscopic sphincterotomy and

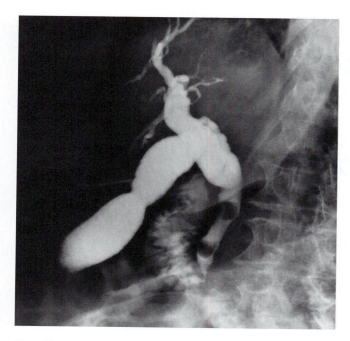

Figure 68–1. Two large stones in the common bile duct managed by sphincterotomy and extraction.

stone extraction should be attempted. However, if this maneuver is unsuccessful, a choledochoduodenostomy should be performed. As many stones as possible should be removed at operation. Fragmentation of large stones and removal of the fragments can be facilitated by operative choledochoscopy.

Impacted Stones

Impaction of stones occurs most often in the distal end of the common bile duct, where it traverses the pancreas and is most narrow (Fig 68–2). The surrounding duct and tissue are inflamed and edematous, exacerbating the impaction. Endoscopic sphincterotomy and passage of a nasobiliary catheter proximal to the stone, when possible, often facilitates resolution of the inflammation and edema. The second attempt to dislodge and extract the stone is often successful. If not, choledochoduodenostomy proximal to the impacted stone should be performed.

Multiple Intrahepatic Stones

This situation is a common problem in Asia and is associated with multiple intrahepatic strictures and continuing stone formation, if left untreated. Eventually, biliary cirrhosis and esophageal varices arise. Intrahepatic cholangiocarcinoma occurs in approximately 2% to 10% of these patients.[4] Because of the serious sequelae, hepatic lobectomy has been performed in patients in whom the disease is present in only one lobe.[5] Recently, patients in

whom a T tube has been placed previously have been treated with encouraging success by a series of nonoperative interventions that include stone extraction, balloon dilation of strictures, and temporary stenting of the intrahepatic ducts.[6] In the refractory case, choledochoduodenostomy is an alternative, albeit an unsatisfactory one, because a good result is dependent upon spontaneous passage of stones out of the intrahepatic ducts, into the extrahepatic ducts, and into the duodenum through the anastomosis. However, in Chile, only 4% of patients treated for intrahepatic stones had residual stones.[7] The etiology of the stones and the presence or absence of intrahepatic bile duct strictures clearly influence the outcome of surgical treatment.

STRICTURES

Strictures within the bile duct system predispose the patient to episodes of cholangitis, stone formation, and possibly biliary cirrhosis, esophageal varices, and death. Repeated episodes of cholangitis frequently cause fibrosis and narrowing of the bile ducts proximal to a stricture, making surgical reconstruction difficult. Accordingly, bile duct strictures associated with repeated episodes of cholangitis or persistently elevated bilirubin or alkaline phosphatase values should be treated. The long-term value of stenting and balloon dilation has not been established in patients who have normal bile ducts

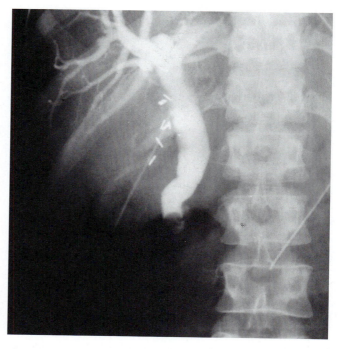

Figure 68–2. Stone impacted in the distal portion of the common bile duct. (From Sabiston DC Jr. *Textbook of Surgery. The Biological Basis of Modern Surgical Practice,* 14th ed. Philadelphia, PA: WB Saunders; 1991:1065)

except for the stricture and proximal dilation, and who have no significant risk factors for surgery.

Stricture Associated with Chronic Pancreatitis

Patients with chronic pancreatitis have a 5% to 10% incidence of a significant distal bile duct stricture.[8] The stricture results from chronic fibrosis within the pancreas, and external compression and scarring of the intrapancreatic portion of the common bile duct. The symptoms were first described by Snape and associates in 1976, and the condition is sometimes called Snape's syndrome.[9] The clinical manifestations are markedly elevated serum alkaline phosphatase and normal to mildly elevated serum bilirubin. Occasionally, patients develop upper abdominal pain or cholangitis. Ultrasonography often reveals a dilated proximal duct system, a finding confirmed by cholangiography (Fig 68–3). Apparent strictures also may result from temporary edema and compression of the distal common bile duct during and immediately after episodes of pancreatitis or pseudocyst formation. Surgical therapy should be undertaken only when the stricture is persistent. The distal location of the stricture makes it

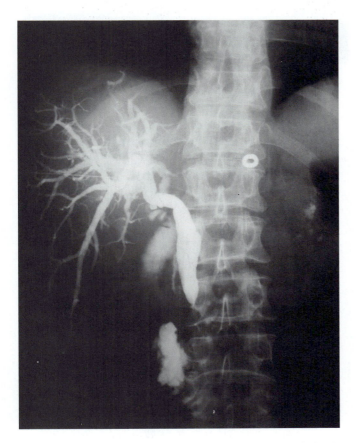

Figure 68–3. Distal common bile duct stricture due to chronic pancreatitis. Calcium is present in the body and tail of the pancreas. (From Moody FG, Carey LC, Jones RS, et al. *Surgical Treatment of Digestive Disease*, 1st ed. Chicago, IL: Year Book Medical; 1986:330)

ideal for successful treatment by choledochoduodenostomy. The procedure can be performed safely concomitant with internal drainage of pancreatic pseudocysts or lateral pancreaticojejunostomy, when necessary.[10]

Stricture from Stone Impaction

Patients who have had removal of an impacted stone from the distal common bile duct occasionally develop a short stricture in the area of impaction that is thought to result from mucosal destruction and bile duct inflammation associated with the presence of the stone. Subsequent fibrosis of the bile duct and surrounding tissue causes the stricture. These patients are ideal candidates for choledochoduodenostomy.

Iatrogenic Stricture

Strictures resulting from iatrogenic injury of the common bile duct distal to the cystic duct are rare, but are easily treated by end-to-side choledochoduodenostomy after complete mobilization of the duodenum and pancreas.

JUXTAPAPILLARY (PERIVATERIAN) DIVERTICULUM

Duodenal diverticula that are adjacent to the ampulla of Vater rarely cause symptoms. However, juxtapapillary diverticula are associated with an increased incidence of gallstones, both within the gallbladder and the bile duct system.[11,12] The presence of a juxtapapillary diverticulum may contraindicate the performance of endoscopic sphincterotomy for the removal of bile duct stones or the treatment of a dysfunctional sphincter, because of the risk of perforation of the diverticulum. In such rare instances, choledochoduodenostomy may be a useful alternative, especially in patients who have retained stones, multiple bile duct stones, primary bile duct stones, or intrahepatic stones (Fig 68–4).

IATROGENIC INJURIES

Bile duct injuries are most common during cholecystectomy. The incidence of injury is higher during laparoscopic than open cholecystectomy.[13] When an injury is recognized or thought to be likely, open exploration of the biliary tract should be performed. Injuries that are not circumferential often can be managed by suture and T tube stenting, but circumferential injuries or those in which loss of bile duct tissue has occurred must be treated by a biliary-enteric anastomosis. A tension-free end-to-side anastomosis of the common hepatic duct to the duodenum usually is not possible. However, when the duct is injured at or distal to the entrance of the cystic duct, an end-to-side choledochoduodenostomy is usually possible, especially if an extensive Kocher maneuver is carried out to eliminate tension on the anastomosis. The alternative procedure, Roux-en-Y choledochojejunostomy, takes longer and provides sim-

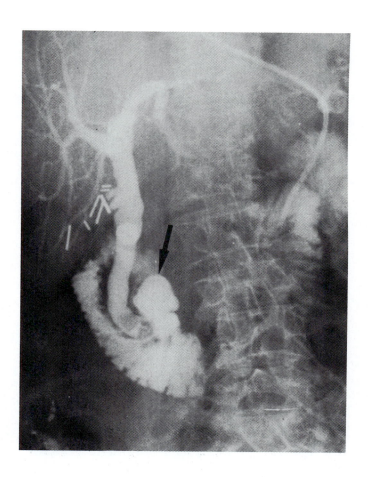

Figure 68–4. Cholangiogram in a patient after cholecystectomy with a juxtapapillary diverticulum (*arrow*) and stones in the distal duct.

ilar results. The latter procedure is almost always necessary for injuries proximal to the cystic duct.

MALIGNANT OBSTRUCTION

Prior to the introduction of bile duct stenting procedures, relief of obstructive jaundice from carcinoma of the head of the pancreas was provided by one of several biliary bypass operations. Cholecystojejunostomy, choledochojejunostomy, and choledochoduodenostomy were those used most frequently. Postoperatively, episodes of cholangitis are less frequent with choledochoenteric bypass than cholecystoenteric bypass,[14] but mortality and morbidity are lowest with choledochoduodenostomy. Furthermore, occlusion of the stoma by extension of the tumor is rare.[14,15]

■ TECHNIQUE

SIDE-TO-SIDE ANASTOMOSIS

Side-to-side choledochoduodenostomy is the procedure of choice for all indications except iatrogenic injuries and the controversial indication of malignant obstruction. Complete circumferential division of the common bile duct or the common hepatic duct compromises the blood supply to both ends of the duct and may predispose the anastomosis to an ischemic stricture. Therefore, end-to-side choledochoduodenostomy should be performed only when the side-to-side procedure is inappropriate or not possible. Many techniques have been described, most of which provide good results when performed meticulously. The main principles are to construct the anastomosis as large as possible and avoid leakage at the suture line. Most bile leaks close spontaneously when adequate drainage is provided, but the toxicity of bile acids to tissue and the potential for scarring and stricture cannot be ignored. The procedure described by Gliedman and Gold satisfies these principles[16] (Fig 68–5).

The duodenum and pancreas are mobilized by an extensive Kocher maneuver. The common bile duct is incised longitudinally with a scalpel, beginning at the point at which it traverses the duodenum posteriorly and extending proximally for 2.5 cm, an incision that often extends proximal to the entrance of the cystic duct. Any manipulations within the duct, such as stone removal or biopsy, should be completed at this time. Us-

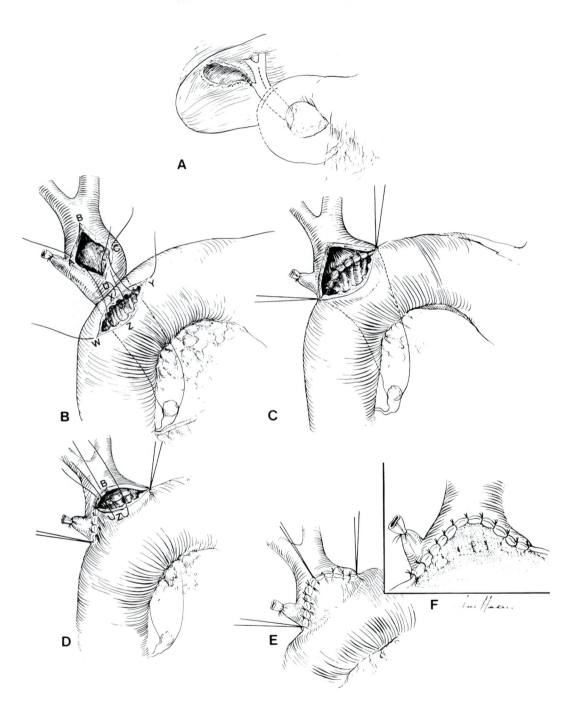

Figure 68–5. A. Dotted lines indicate placement of choledochal and duodenal incisions. **B.** Incisions have been made and corner sutures have been placed. **C.** Posterior row completed. **D.** Half of anterior row completed with knots on outside. **E.** Anterior row completed. **F.** Completed anastomosis. Funnel effect is visible.

ing cautery, the duodenum is incised longitudinally along its superior border for a distance of approximately 1.5 cm. A single layer anastomosis using 4-0 polypropylene sutures is accomplished by beginning posteriorly and positioning the knots on the outside of the anastomosis. Although a satisfactory anastomosis can be performed with the use of absorbable suture, we prefer the security of monofilament nonabsorbable sutures. The anterior portion of the anastomosis is performed using simple interrupted sutures. The sutures should be placed 1 to 2 mm apart, and they should be tied tightly to create a water-tight anastomosis. We prefer not to use a T tube, although it can be inserted proximally, if the anastomosis is unavoidably narrow. A closed-suction drain is placed in the area of the anastomosis but not in direct contact with it. The drain is removed on the second postoperative day, if the drainage is not bile stained.

A side-to-side anastomosis, done in one or two layers after incising the bile duct transversely and the jejunum longitudinally, is easier to perform, but the opening may not be as large as that formed by the Gliedman-Gold technique. Accordingly, it should be used only when the transverse diameter of the bile duct is >2 cm. The common bile duct is incised transversely along the anterior half of its circumference, placing the incision approximately 1 cm superior to the superior margin of the first portion of the duodenum. A 1-cm longitudinal incision is made in the superior aspect of the duodenum. The posterior portion of the anastomosis is performed using a single layer of monofilament polypropylene sutures placed 1 to 2 mm apart, with the knots positioned on the outside. The anterior portion of the anastomosis is performed in identical fashion. A two-layer anastomosis can be performed in the patient with a very large duct to ensure a water-tight seal. The initial posterior layer consists of seromuscular sutures of 4-0 polypropylene, which are reinforced with a running, interlocking suture of 4-0 polyglycolic acid, brought around the sides and continued anteriorly as an inverting Connell suture. The anterior portion of the anastomosis then is reinforced with interrupted seromuscular sutures of 4-0 polypropylene. Although both side-to-side methods are satisfactory, the method of Gliedman and Gold results in a larger anastomosis, and therefore is strongly recommended.

END-TO-SIDE ANASTOMOSIS

This method is used in cases of iatrogenic injury to the common bile duct or the distal common hepatic duct when mobilization of the pancreas and duodenum can result in a tension-free anastomosis. The distal portion of the transected duct is sewn closed with interrupted 4-0 polypropylene sutures. To perform a single-layer anas-

tomosis, a 1-cm longitudinal opening is made in the superior aspect of the duodenum, using the cautery. Beginning posteriorly, the anastomosis is performed using interrupted 4-0 polypropylene sutures placed 1 to 2 mm apart.

In patients with a dilated duct, the posterior portion of the anastomosis is begun with interrupted seromuscular 4-0 polypropylene sutures. The longitudinal incision in the duodenum then is performed and the posterior portion of the anastomosis is reinforced with a running interlocking 4-0 polyglycolic acid suture. This suture is continued anteriorly as an inverting Connell suture. The anterior portion of the anastomosis is reinforced with interrupted polypropylene sutures.

LAPAROSCOPIC CHOLEDOCHODUODENOSTOMY

Anastomosis of the common bile duct to the duodenum using laparoscopic techniques has been successfully performed in 11 patients in France.[17] Further development and refinement of laparoendoscopic techniques may lower mortality, morbidity, and length of stay to the extent that the use of palliative stenting procedures for pancreatic cancer should be reappraised.

■ COMPLICATIONS

BILE LEAK

Leakage of bile from the suture lines occurs in a small number of cases. The closed-suction drain should not be removed if the drainage is bile stained. All such leaks will eventually close with conservative management. If necessary, cholescintigraphy with technetium (^{99m}-TC) 99m-HIDA can be employed to demonstrate patency of the anastomosis. In the rare case of a persistent leak, a carefully placed transhepatic stent will hasten the closure by diverting bile through the stent. This procedure is particularly useful in patients with uncontrolled leaks.

STRICTURE

All biliary-enteric anastomoses are subject to stricture. Repeated episodes of cholangitis, including one or more of the symptoms of chills and fever, upper abdominal pain or jaundice is reason to perform upper gastrointestinal endoscopy and retrograde cholangiography. Persistently elevated serum alkaline phosphatase concentrations also should prompt cholangiography. ^{99m}-Tc-HIDA cholescintigraphy and sonography also have been used to evaluate the patency of choledochoenteric anastomoses,[18] but the ease of cholangiography in the presence of a choledochoduodenal anastomosis favors its use. When present, an anastomotic stricture can be treated first by balloon dilation. Re-

TABLE 68–1. RESULTS OF CHOLEDOCHODUODENOSTOMY PERFORMED FOR BENIGN DISEASE

Reference Number	Number of Patients	Operative Mortality (%)	Asymptomatic at Follow-up (%)
25	225	1.8	72
26	126	4.0	94
24	54	0	100
23	190	5.3	96
22	75	1.3	92

operation will be required if balloon dilation is not successful after several treatments.

Episodes of cholangitis do not occur in patients who have a large, patent anastomosis. Abdominal roentgenograms and barium studies of the upper gastrointestinal tract routinely demonstrate air and barium, respectively, in the biliary tract of completely asymptomatic patients with choledochoduodenostomy. These are rarely a problem, so long as the anastomosis is patent and the barium (as well as intestinal contents) are free to drain out of the duct.

THE SUMP SYNDROME

Food and debris may collect in the portion of the bile duct distal to a side-to-side choledochoduodenostomy, which is said to serve as a sump. Although cholangitis and symptoms of biliary obstruction can occur if the anastomosis is partially or completely obstructed by vegetable matter and debris, this appears to be a very rare complication, occurring in 0.14% to 1.30% of cases.[19] The mechanism by which debris in the bile duct distal to the anastomosis could produce symptoms is not clear; in fact, the very existence of the sump syndrome is in doubt.

■ RESULTS

MORTALITY AND MORBIDITY

The mortality in recently reported series of patients who have undergone choledochoduodenostomy for benign diseases of the biliary system ranges from 1.3% to 5.3% (Table 68–1). The early complications specific to the operation include bile leak, cholangitis, and intra-abdominal abscess, each of which occur in <5% of patients. The only significant long-term problems are the previously described sump syndrome and narrowing of the anastomosis, which sometimes causes episodes of cholangitis.[22–26]

A randomized trial conducted in France compared the results of choledochoduodenostomy with those of choledochojejunostomy, in a total of 130 patients.[27] All operations were performed for choledocholithiasis. There were no significant differences between the groups for postoperative mortality or morbidity rates. The incidence of cholangitis during a mean follow-up of 29 months was 10% in each group. The conclusions are that the operations are equally efficacious, but choledochoduodenostomy is preferred because it is easier to perform and, if problems develop later, the stoma is easily examined endoscopically.

Choledochoduodenostomy is an effective operation for strictures of the distal common bile duct and for complications associated with the presence of calculi in the bile duct system that are not amenable to treatment using endoscopic techniques. Mortality and morbidity are low and long-term results are excellent.

REFERENCES

1. Hawes RH, Cotton PB, Vallon AG. Follow up 6 to 11 years after duodenoscopic sphincterotomy for stones in patients with prior cholecystectomy. *Gastroenterology* 1990; 98:1008

2. Siegel JH, Ben-Zvi JS, Pullano WE. Mechanical lithotripsy of common duct stones. *Gastrointest Endosc* 1990;36:351

3. Bland KI, Jones RS, Maher JW, et al. Extracorporeal shock-wave lithotripsy of bile duct calculi. *Ann Surg* 1989; 209:743

4. Sheen-Chen SM, Chou FF, Eng HL. Intrahepatic cholangiocarcinoma in hepatolithiasis: a frequently overlooked disease. *J Surg Oncol* 1991;47:131

5. Fan ST, Lai ECS, Wong J. Hepatic resection for hepatolithiasis. *Arch Surg* 1993;128:1070

6. Sheen-Chen SM, Chou FF, Lee CM, et al. The management of complicated hepatolithiasis with intrahepatic biliary stricture by the combination of T tube tract dilation and endoscopic electrohydraulic lithotripsy. *Gastrointest Endosc* 1993;39:168

7. Yarmuch J, Csendes A, Diaz JC, et al. Results of surgical treatment in patients with "Western" intrahepatic lithiasis. *Hepatogastroenterology* 1989;36:128

8. Frey CF, Suzuki M, Isaji S. Treatment of chronic pancreatitis complicated by obstruction of the common bile duct or duodenum. *World J Surg* 1990;14:59

9. Snape WJ, Long WB, Trotman BW, et al. Marked alkaline phosphatase elevation with partial common bile duct obstruction due to calcified pancreatitis. *Gastroenterology* 1976;70:70

10. Pereira LL, Kalil AN, Wilson TJ. Surgical treatment of chronic pancreatic cholangiopathy. *Br J Surg* 1989;76: 1129

11. Lotoeit T, Foss OP, Osnes M. Biliary pigment and cholesterol calculi in patients with and without juxtapapillary duodenal diverticula. *Scand J Gastroenterol* 1981;16:241

12. Kennedy RH, Thompson MH. Are duodenal diverticula associated with choledocholithiasis? *Gut* 1988;29:1003

13. Deziel DJ, Millikan KW, Economou SG, et al. Complica-

tions of laparoscopic cholecystectomy: a national survey of 4 292 hospitals and an analysis of 77 604 cases. *Am J Surg* 1993;165:9

14. Potts JR, Broughan TA, Hermann RE. Palliative operations for pancreatic carcinoma. *Am J Surg* 1990;159:72
15. Birkenfeld S, Serour F, Levi S, et al. Choledochoduodenostomy for benign and malignant biliary tract diseases. *Surgery* 1988;103:408
16. Gliedman ML, Gold SM. Choledochoduodenostomy. In: Schwartz SI, Ellis H (eds), *Maingot's Abdominal Operations,* 9th ed. Stamford, CT: Appleton and Lange; 1989: 1915–1918
17. Farello GA, Cerofolini A, Bergmaschi G, et al. Choledochal anastomosis by laparoscopy. *J Chir* 1993;130: 226
18. Wilson SR, Toi A. Sonography accurately detects biliary obstruction in patients with surgically created biliary-enteric anastomosis. *Am J Roentgenol* 1990;155:789
19. Escudero-Fabre A, Escallon A Jr, Sack J, et al. Choledochoduodenostomy: analysis of 71 cases followed for 5 to 15 years. *Ann Surg* 1991;213:635
20. Miros M, Kerlin P, Strong R, et al. Postcholedochoenterostomy sump syndrome. *Aust NZJ Surg* 1990;60:109
21. Eaton MC, Worthley CS, Toouli J. Treatment of post choledochoduodenostomy symptoms. *Aust NZJ Surg* 1989; 59:771
22. Rizzuti RP, McElwee TB, Carter JW. Choledochoduodenostomy: a safe and efficacious alternative in the treatment of biliary tract diseases. *Surgery* 1987;53:22
23. Baker AR, Neoptolemos JP, Leese T, et al. Choledochoduodenostomy, transduodenal sphincteroplasty and sphincterotomy for calculi of the common bile duct. *Surg Gynecol Obstet* 1987;164:245
24. Berlatzky Y, Freund HR. Primary choledochoduodenostomy for benign obstructive biliary tract disease. *J Clin Gastroenterol* 1990;12:420
25. Parrilla P, Ramirez P, Sanchez-Bueno F, et al. Long-term results of choledochoduodenostomy in the treatment of choledocholithiasis: assessment of 225 cases. *Br J Surg* 1991;78:470
26. Deutsch AA, Nudelman I, Gutman H, et al. Choledochoduodenostomy: an important surgical tool in the management of common bile duct stones. A review of 126 cases. *Eur J Surg* 1991;157:531
27. Panis Y, Fagniez PL, Brisset D, et al. Long-term results of choledochoduodenostomy versus choledochojejunostomy for choledocholithiasis. The French Association for Surgical Research. *Surg Gynecol Obstet* 1993;177:33

69

Common Bile Duct Exploration

Alfred Cushierei

Ductal calculi may originate from migration of stones from the gallbladder or develop de novo in the ductal system. They carry a significant morbidity and usually require active intervention. Ductal calculi may be asymptomatic or cause nonspecific dyspepsia, but the majority present with complications—pancreatitis, jaundice or cholangitis. The latter is the most serious complication and is associated with a significant morbidity.[1]

The options for management of ductal calculi in patients with symptomatic gallstones are:

- Endoscopic sphincterotomy and stone extraction followed by laparoscopic cholecystectomy
- Open cholecystectomy and common duct exploration
- Laparoscopic cholecystectomy and ductal clearance

In the view of this author, the correct treatment in the individual patient depends on five factors: the clinical setting, the condition of the patient, the caliber of the common duct, extent of stone load, level of local expertise in endoscopic treatment, and the experience of the surgeon in laparoscopic biliary surgery. Irrespective of the surgical approach to common bile duct exploration, conventional open surgery, or laparoscopic surgical management, the same surgical principles apply in the treatment of patients with ductal calculi.

In patients with retained stones, the orthodox management is endoscopic sphincterotomy. However, in patients with an indwelling T tube, percutaneous extraction via the T tube tract is a viable and safe alternative.[2]

■ PREOPERATIVE WORK-UP AND PREPARATION

Regardless of the surgical approach, open or laparoscopic, the standard preoperative work-up includes ultrasound examination and liver function tests (bilirubin, transaminase, alkaline phosphatase). Patients with a history of jaundice or acute pancreatitis and those who exhibit abnormalities of the liver function tests or suggestive ultrasound features should be considered likely to harbor ductal calculi or other organic disease of the extrahepatic biliary tract. A preoperative endoscopic retrograde cholangiogram (ERC) should be considered for these patients. Others maintain the view that ERC is not necessary for those patients in whom surgery is intended at the time of laparoscopic cholecystectomy, since cholangiographic documentation is obtained during surgery. These surgeons restrict ERC to those patients in whom preoperative stone extraction by endoscopic sphincterotomy is contemplated. Although this policy appears logical and cost effective, it overlooks a small but significant cohort of patients who have organic ductal disease (cancer or otherwise) rather than calculi or, indeed, dual ductal pathology. Regrettably, most instances of hilar cholangiocarcinoma are first diagnosed during cholecystectomy and exploration of the common bile duct because an ERC was omitted in the preoperative work-up.

Jaundiced patients require correction of the prolonged prothrombin time by the intramuscular injection of vitamin K analogs. They also need special prophylactic measures, including perioperative antibiotic therapy and intravenous hydration (crystalloids) with forced diuresis (osmotic or loop diuretic) to prevent infectious complications and renal failure, respectively. The urinary output should be measured hourly by an indwelling catheter from the time of surgery until ambulation, in all of these patients. Since the majority of patients with ductal calculi are elderly, chemoprophylaxis with heparin and antithrombosis graduated elastic stockings are advisable.

■ ROLE OF ERC AND INTERVENTIONAL FLEXIBLE ENDOSCOPY

There is a definitive and important role for ERC and interventional flexible endoscopy in the management of patients undergoing biliary surgery for gallstone disease. ERC with or without endoscopic intervention may be required for

- Preoperative detection of ductal calculi
- Extraction of ductal calculi: preoperative, intraoperative, and postoperative
- Investigation and management of biliary complications

PREOPERATIVE DETECTION OF DUCTAL CALCULI

The detection of ductal calculi and abnormal bile duct anatomy in patients undergoing biliary surgery remains problematic. Certainly, there is no justification for ERC in all patients undergoing cholecystectomy since the yield from such an approach is low and the risk-benefit ratio is high. In one prospective study of 264 patients who had ERC prior to laparoscopic cholecystectomy, a normal bile duct system was observed in 227 (86%), atypical bile duct anatomy in eight and stones in 29 patients (11%).[3] The consensus policy is to confine preoperative ERC to those patients who are likely to harbor duct calculi on the basis of recognized clinical (history of jaundice or acute pancreatitis), ultrasound (duct dilation and suspicious calculi), and biochemical risk factors (abnormal liver function tests). Unfortunately, these criteria overestimate the incidence of ductal calculi. In one prospective study of patients undergoing laparoscopic cholecystectomy, 25 patients were identified in the high-risk group; preoperative ERC identified stones in only six patients (24%).[4] Experienced endoscopists recommend and practice selective use of ERC in the preoperative work-up of these patients in the certain knowledge that in the few patients in whom ductal stones are missed, these can be treated endoscopically during or after the cholecystectomy.[5] Aside from the detection of calculi, the selective use of ERC will identify occult disease, particularly hilar cholangiocarcinoma in patients.

■ TREATMENT OF DUCTAL CALCULI IN PATIENTS UNDERGOING LAPAROSCOPIC CHOLECYSTECTOMY

The management of ductal calculi in patients undergoing laparoscopic cholecystectomy depends on several factors: stones may be detected during the preoperative work-up, at the time of laparoscopic cholecystectomy when unsuspected stones are identified in 3% to 4%[6,7] of patients when routine intraoperative cholangiography (IOC) is practiced, or declare themselves after the intervention because of renewed symptoms or complications such as jaundice or cholangitis.

The issue of management of ductal calculi is best addressed by reference to the time of detection of the ductal calculi in relation to surgery and to the clinical state of the patient. In the preoperative situation, there is no question that if the patient is ill with jaundice and cholangitis, then endoscopic sphincterotomy and stone extraction is the appropriate treatment. The situation is perhaps less certain in patients who harbor ductal calculi but do not have significant jaundice or cholangitis. The predominant practice is endoscopic stone extraction followed by laparoscopic cholecystectomy during the same admission.[8] The results of this well-established approach have been good. The alternative management in these patients is single-stage treatment with laparoscopic stone extraction either through the cystic duct[9–11] or by direct supraduodenal exploration of the common bile duct.[12–14] The transcystic wire basket approach is applicable to small (<1.0 cm) distal calculi but is effective in 80% to 90% of these cases.[15] Following ductal clearance, the cystic duct stump is ligated. The cystic duct approach has the merit that both the common bile duct and the choledochal sphincter are left intact.

Direct common bile duct exploration which can be performed by the open or the laparoscopic approach is reserved for large stone load and proximal calculi in patients with a dilated common bile duct. In this respect, direct exploration of a narrow bile duct (<0.8 mm) by either approach is inadvisable because of the enhanced risk of stricture at the choledochotomy site. These patients are best managed with endoscopic sphincterotomy and stone extraction before or after surgery. Laparoscopic direct common bile duct exploration requires considerable experience in laparoscopic biliary surgery and in endoscopic suturing, otherwise the risk of bile duct damage and stricture is high. If such expertise is not available, the procedure should be performed by the open conventional approach.

The single-stage laparoscopic management of patients undergoing laparoscopic cholecystectomy who harbor ductal calculi may have cost benefit and other advantages over the current two-stage management of endoscopic stone extraction followed by laparoscopic cholecystectomy. However, there are no hard data comparing the relative merits of these two approaches and definitive conclusions must await the results of the prospective randomized trial currently being conducted by the European Society for Endoscopic Surgery. Currently, the recommendation regarding the management of these patients must depend on the local expertise available; since there are more trained interventional endoscopists than trained laparoscopic biliary tract surgeons, the majority of these patients are likely to have their ductal stones extracted endoscopically, which is best performed before the laparoscopic cholecystectomy.

For stones encountered during laparoscopic surgery, unsuspected or otherwise, the options include transcystic extraction or direct supraduodenal laparoscopic bile duct exploration for large or proximal stones. A recent promising alternative is endoscopic stone extraction during the cholecystectomy after the insertion of a catheter guide down the bile duct and through the papilla into the duodenum. This considerably facilitates the sphincterotomy, which is otherwise difficult in the supine patient and ensures correct orientation of the cut.[16]

There are situations when surgeons without experience of laparoscopic ductal clearance or facilities for intraoperative guided endoscopic sphincterotomy encounter unsuspected nonoccluding ductal calculi during laparoscopic cholecystectomy. In these patients, the cholecystectomy should be completed and reliance placed on postoperative ERC and sphincterotomy, which is successful in the vast majority of patients.[17,18] The insertion of a cystic duct drainage catheter is very useful in this situation,[19] since it permits a postoperative cholangiogram that may demonstrate that the stone or "contrast shadow" has disappeared. The presence of the cystic duct cannula enables the insertion of a guide-wire through the papilla into the duodenum and guarantees successful endoscopic sphincterotomy in all of these patients.

■ INTRAOPERATIVE FLUOROCHOLANGIOGRAPHY DURING BILIARY SURGERY

One of the few residual controversial issues relating to biliary surgery is the need or otherwise of routine intraoperative cholangiography (IOC) during cholecystectomy. The controversy has intensified since the advent of laparoscopic cholecystectomy. Following the French lead, some rely on preoperative intravenous cholangiography and dispense with IOC.[20] Others recommend its routine performance in every case,[21–25] whereas many recommend the selective use based on clinical, biochemical, and intraoperative criteria.[26–31]

There are a number of considerations relating to this controversy. In the first instance, different groups base their adjudication without reference to the technology used. The proponents for routine IOC have repeatedly stressed the need for modern portable C-arm digitized fluorocholangiography with image processing facilities and acknowledge that blind static cholangiography with portable x-ray machines should be abandoned because of poor diagnostic yield, inadequate exposure, and length of time to perform the procedure.[21–25] An audit of routine intraoperative cholangiography in a consecutive series of 496 patients undergoing laparoscopic cholecystectomy has demonstrated that cannulation of the cystic duct was possible in 483 (97%) patients. The use of portable digitized C-arm fluorocholangiography was vastly superior to the use of mobile x-ray machine and static films in terms of reduced time to carry out the procedure and total abolition of unsatisfactory radiological exposure of the biliary tract. Repeat of the procedure was necessary in 22% of patients when the mobile x-ray equipment was used. Aside from the detection of unsuspected stones in 18 (3.9%) patients, routine intraoperative cholangiography identified four (0.8%) patients whose management would have been undoubtedly disadvantaged if intraoperative cholangiography had not been performed.[25]

The endpoints used for the performance of IOC during laparoscopic cholecystectomy vary from report to report. Furthermore, conclusions drawn from studies performed in relation to open cholecystectomy may not apply to laparoscopic cholecystectomy. In one prospective randomized clinical trial in patients undergoing open cholecystectomy, 280 out of 475 patients had none of the predefined clinical criteria for ductal calculi and were randomized during surgery to IOC and non-IOC groups. The results of this study showed that there were no residual stones in either group on follow-up.[32] However, the arguments for the routine performance of digitized fluorochlolangiography during laparoscopic cholecystectomy do not center on the detection of unsuspected stones. The main reason for IOC in laparoscopic cholecystectomy is in the detection of abnormal anatomy and on the selection of the appropriate point for ligature or clipping of the medial end of the cystic duct. The cystic duct–common bile duct junction is not often clearly visualized during laparoscopic cholecystectomy and the upward and lateral retraction of the gallbladder often results in tenting of the junction such that partial or total occlusion of the bile duct is a possibility. Routine use is needed for the surgeons to become proficient in cannulation of the cystic duct and in the interpretation of fluorocholangiographic appearances. The selective policy for IOC during laparoscopic cholecystectomy does not provide the necessary experience and thus, when a cholangiogram is needed, the chances are that it is performed inexpertly and possibly interpreted incorrectly.

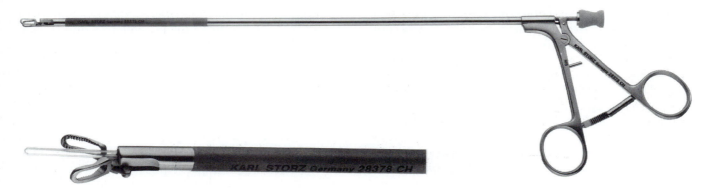

Figure 69–1. Cholangiograsper used for intraoperative cystic duct cholangiography during laparoscopic cholecystectomy (Storz, Tuttlingen).

TECHNIQUES OF INTRAOPERATIVE CHOLANGIOGRAPHY

The standard technique for IOC, *if the gallbladder is to be removed,* is by means of cannulation of the cystic duct, both during open and laparoscopic surgery. The other method, which does not commit the surgeon to cholecystectomy, is by direct puncture of the gallbladder prior to any dissection.

Cystic Duct Cholangiography

This procedure entails preliminary dissection of the structures in the triangle of Calot. The cystic duct is mobilized and its distal end (near the gallbladder neck) is ligated or clipped. A small incision is made on the anterosuperior wall of the cystic duct and a cannula or catheter then is introduced into the common bile duct through the cystic duct and secured in place. There is a large variety of catheters and cannulae used for cystic duct cholangiography both during open and laparoscopic surgery. What is important is familiarization with one specific type and technique.

During laparoscopic surgery, the author finds the use of the cholangiograsper (Fig 69–1) most useful for expediting the procedure. The cholangiograsper is loaded with a Cook ureteric catheter and following the insertion of the catheter into the duct, the jaws of the cholangiograsper are closed on the duct and catheter (Fig 69–2).

There are certain rules which must be observed during the performance of cystic duct cholangiography (laparoscopic or open). The important ones include

- The system must be primed such that air bubbles are excluded—this entails a three-way tap connected by suitable tubing to saline and contrast (sodium diatrizoate) containing syringes.
- On no account must aspiration be applied since this sucks up duodenal air into the bile duct.
- The patient must be placed in a slight head

down position and the table rotated slightly to the right to remove the overlapping spinal column and transverse processes of the vertebrae.
- All radiopaque objects, cables, and instruments must be removed from the fluoroscopic field.
- The contrast medium must be injected slowly during fluoroscopy. The early filling phase is crucial for the detection of small distal calculi.
- The entire biliary tract, including the proximal intrahepatic ducts, must be displayed.

Good quality and reliable radiological documentation will be obtained if these simple rules are followed (Fig 69–3A and B). With experience and if performed routinely, cystic duct fluorocholangiography should not take more than 10 minutes to complete. At the end of the procedure, the catheter is removed and the cystic duct ligated with absorbable material. Ligation is far better than clipping for two reasons. In the first instance, the risk of slippage and postoperative bile leakage from the cystic duct stump is considerably reduced.[33,34] Secondly, instances of internalization of metal clips into the common bile duct are well documented after both open and laparoscopic cholecystectomy.[35–41]

During laparoscopic cholecystectomy, the safest technique of closure of the cystic duct stump is by ligature in continuity[42,43] using dry catgut with an external Roeder slip knot (Fig 69–4). This method has been employed in over 1400 cases of laparoscopic cholecystectomies, including 43 patients with acute cholecystitis, without a single instance of postoperative bile leakage. The alternative is to secure the duct with a preformed catgut endoloop (Fig 69–5).

Cholecystocholangiography

This procedure entails direct puncture of the gallbladder followed by injection of contrast medium. It is primarily indicated when the decision to remove the

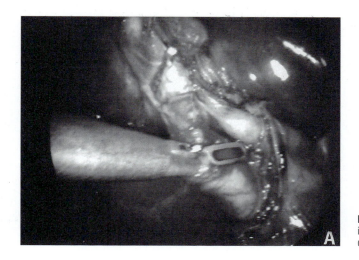

Figure 69–2. The cholangiograsper is loaded with a Cook ureteric catheter and following the insertion of the catheter into the duct, the jaws of the cholangiograsper are closed on the duct and catheter.

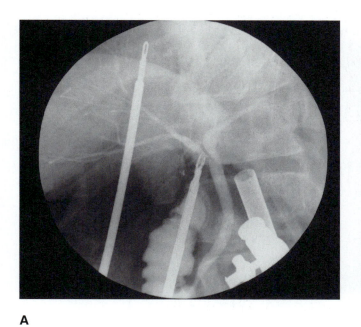

A

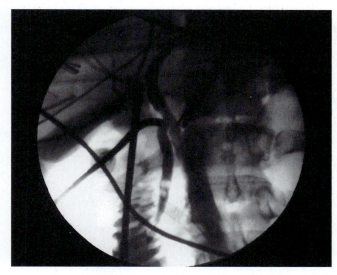

B

Figure 69–3. A. Normal cystic duct cholangiogram during laparoscopic cholecystectomy. **B.** Cystic duct cholangiogram showing ductal calculi.

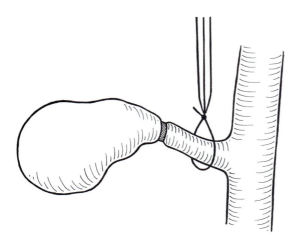

Figure 69–4. The safest technique of closure of the cystic duct stump during laparoscopic cholecystectomy is by ligature in continuity using dry chromic catgut with an external Roeder slip knot.

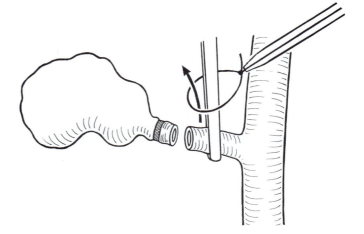

Figure 69–5. Alternative safe method of securing the cystic duct during laparoscopic cholecystectomy by means of a preformed catgut endoloop.

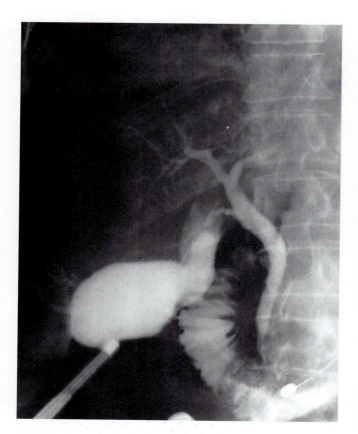

Figure 69–6. Technique of cholecystocholangiography during laparoscopic cholecystectomy. The Veress needle is used to puncture the gallbladder fundus along the long axis of the organ.

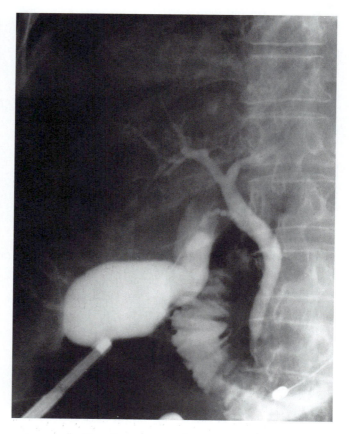

Figure 69–7. Normal cholecystocholangiogram.

gallbladder has not been made. It also is used when cholecystojejunostomy is contemplated as a palliative procedure in patients with large bile duct obstruction owing to an inoperable carcinoma of the head of the pancreas. In this situation, it ensures that there is a good distance (at least 1.5 cm) between the termination of the cystic duct and the upper limit of the tumor. Effective relief of jaundice will not be obtained if the tumor encroaches on the cystic–common duct junction and, in these cases, choledochojejunostomy is required for effective and lasting palliation. The risk of cholecystocholangiography in patients with multiple small gallstones is dislodgement of some of these into the common duct, especially in the presence of a dilated cystic duct. This risk is the main reason for not advocating its routine use during cholecystectomy.

When performed laparoscopically, the best instrument for carrying out a cholecystocholangiogram is the Veress needle which is used to puncture the gallbladder fundus along the long axis of the organ (Fig 69–6). A much larger volume of contrast is needed than in the case of cystic duct cholangiography since the gallbladder has to be filled before the contrast medium enters the bile ducts. Thus, a 50 mL syringe loaded with sodium diatrizoate is connected to the system. Otherwise, the same precautions as for cystic duct cholangiography are adopted. Again, with meticulous technique and attention to detail, good quality cholecystocholangiograms can be obtained (Fig 69–7). On completion, the gallbladder is aspirated before the Veress needle is withdrawn. The small perforation in the fundus of the gallbladder is closed by a Z suture.

■ TECHNIQUE OF OPEN EXPLORATION OF THE COMMON BILE DUCT

Exploration of the common duct is performed after the cholangiogram has confirmed the presence of common duct stones and before removal of the gallbladder. The cystic duct is ligated before the common bile duct exploration is commenced. This step obviates the risk that manipulation of the gallbladder will force small stones down the cystic duct and into the common duct after the latter has been explored.

The decision to explore the common duct having been made, the area of the free edge of the lesser omentum is exposed by suitable position of packs, retractors, and the assistant's hand. The essential steps are the retraction of the right lobe of the liver upward, displacement of the duodenum downward, and retraction of the stomach to the left. The peritoneum over the anterolateral surface of the common bile duct is divided, and the duct is exposed by clearing away any overlying fatty tis-

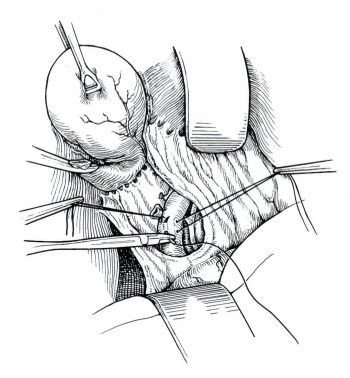

Figure 69–8. Open exploration of the common duct; insertion of stay sutures. After RN Lane.

sue. A small pledget (peanut swab) held in a long artery forceps is invaluable for this maneuver.

Before the duct is opened, a sample of bile is taken by needle aspiration and is sent for bacteriological examination. Two 3-0 stay sutures (coated vicryl or PDS [Ethicon] or Polysorb [USSC]) are placed on the anterior surface of the duct approximately 1.0 to 2.0 cm above the superior border of the duodenum (Fig 69–8) and the duct opened longitudinally between them with a scalpel (Fig 69–9). The incision initially is enlarged to about 1.5 cm. Any escaping bile is removed by aspiration. If the initial incision exposes calculi, they should be removed immediately.

With the margins of the incision held open by stay sutures, the biliary tract is explored by means of a biliary balloon catheter. Proximal exploration is carried out first. The catheter is passed sequentially into the common hepatic, and the right and left hepatic ducts. In each case, once the tip of the catheter cannot be advanced further, the balloon is inflated with air and then the catheter is "trawled" to extract any stones. This technique is much less traumatic than extraction by means of a Dejardin's forceps and is therefore preferable.

After exploration of the proximal ducts, the lower system, including the choledochal sphincter, is explored in a similar manner by the use of the biliary balloon catheter. If it is suspected that the lower reaches of

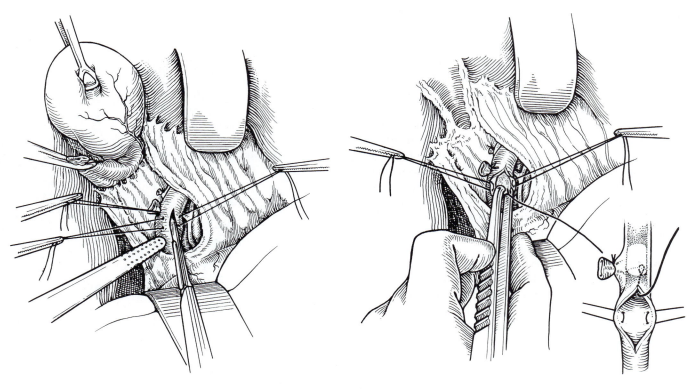

Figure 69–9. Open exploration of the common duct. The duct is incised between the stay sutures. Note the sucker, to remove escaping bile. After RN Lane.

Figure 69–10. Open exploration of the common duct, insertion of small swab into the common hepatic duct. When the lower duct is thought to contain small stones and debris, this maneuver is useful in preventing the passage of small stones up into the proximal duct. Note the stay suture attached to the swab. After RN Lane.

the common bile duct may contain multiple stones, it is wise to insert a small tagged pledget into the common hepatic duct to prevent stones passing up toward the liver during subsequent manipulations. A marker length of suitable ligature material must be attached to this swab, with care to see that it is removed at the end of the procedure (Fig 69–10).

For clearance of the lower duct, the biliary balloon catheter is passed down to the lower choledochal sphincter. The balloon is dilated before the catheter is withdrawn, thereby dislodging the stones up to the choledochotomy, from where they are removed. During common bile duct exploration, the number of stones removed should match those identified on the operative cholangiogram. Following complete clearance and in the absence of any obstructed lower choledochal sphincter, the surgeon should be able to pass the deflated biliary balloon catheter into the duodenum. When the balloon is inflated, it should be easily palpable through the duodenal wall. The inflated balloon cannot be negotiated through the normal sphincter. However, after minimal deflation, the balloon slips through into the ampullary region, where it is inflated fully again before it is trawled.

COMPLETION CHOLEDOCHOSCOPY

This procedure is nowadays considered an essential step of exploration of the common bile duct since its regular use reduces the incidence of retained or missed stones to negligible levels.[44] The flexible fiber-optic choledochoscope attached to a saline Fenwell pressure irrigation system is inserted through the choledochotomy and the stay sutures crossed over the instrument to minimize the leakage of irrigation fluid.

The choledochoscope is held in the left hand with the thumb controlling the angulation lever, while the right hand manipulates the shaft of the instrument within the ducts, using the thumb in opposition to the index and middle fingers. The entire length of the common bile duct, including the narrower intramural portion of the lower end down to the papilla, is inspected. The papilla has the appearance of a rosette of mucosal folds. Sometimes, the papillary channel may be seen to open and close as the irrigation fluid passes into the duodenum, and the duodenal mucosa is visualized through the patent lower sphincter. After establishing that the lower ductal system is clear, the choledochoscope is withdrawn and reinserted proximally to inspect the hepatic ducts.

Since these are supported by the surrounding liver tissue, viewing is much easier. The bifurcation of the right and left ducts should be identified in all cases, and higher up, the secondary and sometimes tertiary ducts can usually be visualized, especially in patients with obstructive jaundice and a dilated extrahepatic ductal system.

Throughout the inspection, any stones that are identified are extracted under vision using a Dormia basket which is introduced through the operating channel of the choledochoscope. The basket is positioned distal to the stone before the wires are opened, the stone trapped with the right amount of closure to secure the stone without crushing it, and removed by withdrawing the instrument and basket "en masse." Good team work and coordination between the surgeon and his assistant is necessary during this process since the closure and entrapment of the stone by the basket has to be carried out by the assistant. This procedure is therefore much smoother and easier if a CCD camera is attached to the choledochoscope so that both the surgeon and the assistant can visualize the proceedings on a television monitor.

DRAINAGE OF COMMON BILE DUCT AND CLOSURE OF CHOLEDOCHOTOMY

Although there are a few surgeons who close the choledochotomy without drainage,[45] this practice is unwise since temporary edema and obstruction at the lower end of the bile duct is inevitable and lasts several days after exploration of the common duct.[46] The orthodox manner is drainage by the insertion of a T tube. There are a number of important practical points regarding the technique of T tube drainage. In the first instance, the tube should be composed of latex rubber, its size should not be smaller than 14 French (Fr) and the site of insertion through the abdominal wall should be lateral in the right flank such that the tube runs in a smooth curve from the parieties to the choledochotomy. These measures greatly facilitate extraction of any retained stones through the T tube tract.[47] The limbs of the T should be cut short, each limb being approximately 1.0 cm in length (Fig 69–11). The T tube should be brought out at the lower extremity of the choledochotomy (Fig 69–12) that is closed above it with interrupted 3-0 absorbable sutures (coated Vicryl or PDS or Polysorb).

Another technique of common duct drainage is via the cystic duct stump, using a special cystic duct drainage catheter (size 7.5 or 8.5 Fr). This catheter is passed through the cystic duct into the common bile duct and then secured to the cystic duct stump by two catgut ligatures. In this instance, the choledochotomy wound is closed completely with interrupted 3-0 absorbable sutures (Fig 69–13).

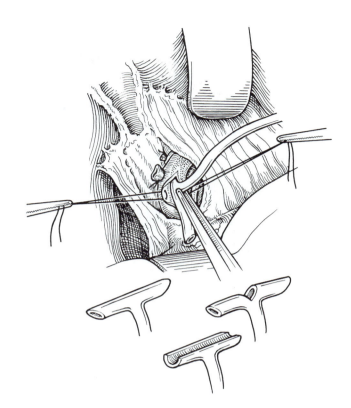

Figure 69–11. Open exploration of the common duct; insertion of T tube. Insert shows the various types of T tubes available. Maingot's split tube (top left) is the most commonly used, and is the easiest to insert. Before inserting the tube, its patency should be tested by flushing it with saline. After RN Lane.

COMPLETION CHOLANGIOGRAPHY

It is the author's opinion that completion choledochoscopy dispenses with the need for completion cholangiography, although many surgeons are reluctant to dispense with it. A difficulty that is encountered often with the execution of completion cholangiography is the removal of air bubbles from within the common bile duct. To effect this, the T tube is flushed with normal saline, first to check that a water-tight closure has been obtained (Fig 69–14) and then to wash all the bubbles from the duct. Once this is achieved (often impossible), contrast medium (sodium diatrizoate) is injected from a 50 mL syringe as the ducts are visualized by fluoroscopy.

Apart from the problem of the presence of air bubbles, the interpretation of the fluoroscopy findings after ductal exploration is further complicated by the fact that failure to demonstrate flow of contrast into the duodenum is common and is the result of edema or spasm. In this situation, entry of contrast medium into the duodenum can be achieved by the intravenous administration of spasmolytic drugs (glucagon, secretin, nitrites, ceuletide etc.) but in any event, the only reliable indication of a residual stone is a filling defect (Fig 69–15).

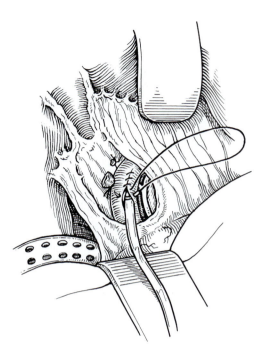

Figure 69–12. Open exploration of the common duct; closure of the duct with 3/0 synthetic absorbable sutures around the emergent T tube. Note that the tube protrudes from the lower end of the incision. A subhepatic drain also is inserted. After RN Lane.

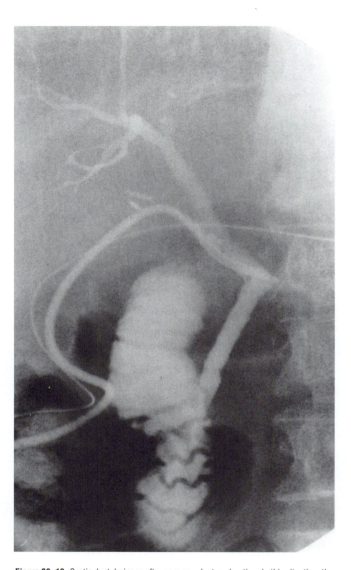

Figure 69–13. Cystic duct drainage after common duct exploration. In this situation, the choledochotomy is closed completely.

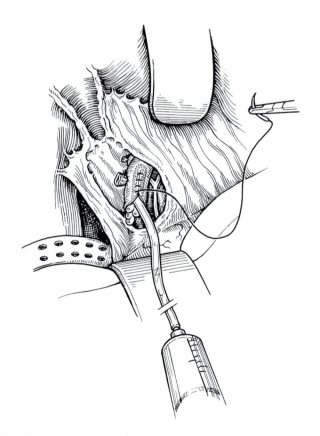

Figure 69–14. Completion cholangiography. To remove bubbles from the duct, the T tube is flushed with saline at intervals during closure of the duct. After RN Lane.

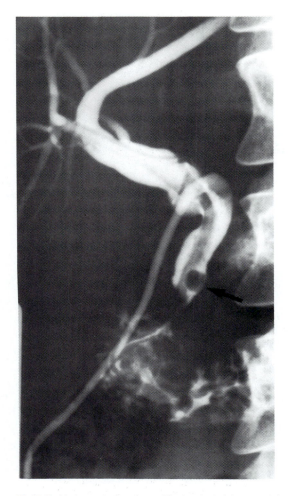

Figure 69–15. Residual stone in the common bile duct (*arrow*) demonstrated on the completion T tube cholangiogram.

SUBHEPATIC DRAIN

Since some bile leakage is inevitable during the first few days after exploration of the common bile duct, a subhepatic drain leading to a closed drainage collecting system is recommended and is routinely used by the author.

MANAGEMENT OF IMPACTED STONES

If stones are impacted in the lower end of the common bile duct, several measures are possible:

1. Kocherization of the duodenum and head of the pancreas and massage of the lower duct and impacted stone with two fingers, one placed behind the head of the pancreas and the other anteriorly. This procedure may require simultaneous grasping of the stone with a Dejardin's forceps introduced through the choledochotomy.

2. Disintegration of the stone either by electrohydraulic lithotripsy using a probe attached to a spark generator (Calcutript, Storz, Germany) or dye laser. The most useful is stone fragmentation by visually guided (choledochoscopic) electrohydraulic lithotripsy using a 2.7-Fr probe. This maneuver requires accurate placement of the tip of the probe on the stone away from the duct wall, otherwise a small perforation may be induced when the electric spark is generated. Other methods of fragmentation, such as pulse dye laser (504 nm) transmitted through a thin quartz fiber (300 to 400 μ) can be used.[48,49] The laser operates at 60 mJ/pulse at 10 Hz and achieves stone fragmentation within 1 to 2 minutes. Resulting large fragments are extracted, and small (<2.0 mm) fragments are flushed through the ampulla.

3. Transduodenal sphincteroplasty (vide infra)

■ SURGICAL DRAINAGE OF THE COMMON BILE DUCT

Regardless of the approach used, open or laparoscopic, there are patients in whom ductal clearance of stones provides inadequate treatment since these patients have distal benign stenotic disease of the lower choledochal sphincter. These patients require ductal drainage in addition to removal of the calculi. This subgroup of patients can be identified by the following features:

- Grossly dilated duct (>2.0 cm)
- Large multiple pigment stones filling the common bile duct

If identified preoperatively, these patients should have endoscopic sphincterotomy. When encountered during surgery, the options are choledochoduodenostomy or sphincteroplasty.

TRANSECTION CHOLEDOCHODUODENOSTOMY

This procedure is traditionally performed as a side-to-side anastomosis. However, this operation has a number of intrinsic problems, including inadequate drainage, the development of the inspissated sump syndrome and a tendency to recurrent cholangitis. For this reason, the transection choledochoduodenostomy that involves closure of the lower end of the bile duct and reimplantation of the proximal common duct into the duodenum is preferred.[50]

The procedure of transection choledochoduodenostomy commences by complete mobilization of the lower end of the common bile duct above the duodenum and head of the pancreas. The duct is then completely transected low down and the distal, or pancreatic, end

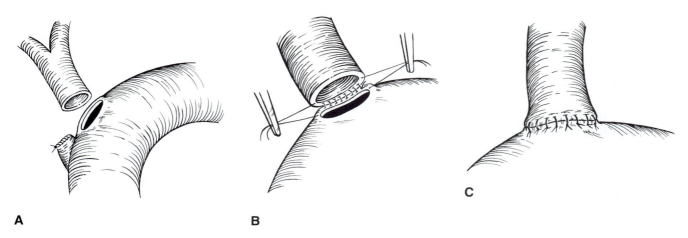

A

B

C

Figure 69–16. Transection choledochoduodenostomy. **A.** Following mobilization, the duct is then completely transected low down and the pancreatic end closed with a running 3-0 absorbable suture. **B.** Following complete mobilization of the duodenum, the proximal end is anastomosed end-to-side to the duodenum at the junction of the first with the second part of this organ. The posterior walls of the anastomosis are approximated by a running suture. **C.** The anterior walls are closed by interrupted sutures tied externally.

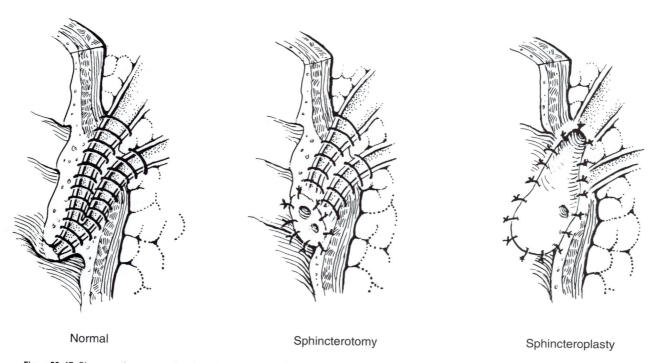

Normal   Sphincterotomy   Sphincteroplasty

Figure 69–17. Diagrammatic representation of the difference between the operations of sphincterotomy and sphincteroplasty. In the operation of sphincterotomy, the greater part of the intraduodenal portion of the sphincteric musculature surrounding the lower end of the common bile duct is divided, but a significant portion remains undisturbed. Sphincteroplasty involves division of the whole length of the sphincter and, of necessity, involves an incision through the full thickness of the posteromedial wall of the duodenum.

closed with a running 3-0 absorbable suture (Fig 69–16A). Following complete mobilization of the duodenum, the proximal end is anastomosed end-to-side to the duodenum at the junction of the first with the second part of this organ. This anastomosis is carried out using a single-layer technique with 4-0 PDS or coated vicryl suture. Following the insertion of two corner stay sutures, the posterior walls of the anastomosis are approximated by a running suture (Fig 69–16B). The anterior walls are approximated by interrupted sutures that are tied externally (Fig 69–16C).

SPHINCTEROPLASTY

This procedure is a viable alternative to choledochoduodenostomy and is favored by some biliary surgeons. The entire length of the musculature (lower, middle, and upper choledochal sphincters) surrounding the lower end of the common bile duct is divided (Fig 69–17) with mucosal approximation at the cut edges by interrupted sutures. The operation is described fully in Chapter 60. In essence, sphincteroplasty is a form of internal choledochoduodenostomy.

■ TECHNIQUE OF LAPAROSCOPIC CLEARANCE OF DUCTAL CALCULI

Laparoscopic clearance of ductal calculi usually is undertaken in patients undergoing laparoscopic cholecystectomy, although there have been instances, in our experience, when laparoscopic common bile duct exploration was performed in patients who had had a previous cholecystectomy. These cases are much more difficult technically and should not be attempted by the laparoscopic approach unless the surgeon has considerable experience with laparoscopic technique. Even so, the threshold for conversion to open surgery should be low.

PATIENT POSITIONING AND LAYOUT

The same position as that for laparoscopic cholecystectomy is used: supine with a moderate head-up tilt. The skin of the abdomen from the lower chest to the suprapubic region is prepared with medicated soap and then disinfected with the antiseptic of choice. A vented nasogastric tube is passed for deflation of the stomach and duodenal bulb, an essential measure for adequate laparoscopic visualization of the common bile duct.

The surgeon operates from the left side of the operating table. Unless a telescope holder is used, the camera person stands on the same side, with the first assistant and the scrub nurse on the opposite side of the operating table. Dual monitor display is essential and a "picture in picture" video set-up is desirable. The light source, camera unit, insufflator, electrosurgical unit and suction/irrigation are placed on a stack behind the surgeon. The instrument trolley is placed beyond and behind the nurse on the right side. A separate sterile trolley is used for the flexible endoscope(s), guidewires, selection of Dormia baskets, balloon extraction catheters, angioplasty dilation catheters, T tube and cystic duct drainage catheters (Cook, USA).

In addition to the basic set, the following instruments are needed: portable C-arm fluorocholangiographic unit, cholangiograsper (for cholangiography), pair of 5.0-mm needle holders, flexible narrow operating endoscope (for visually guided transcystic extraction), flexible choledochoscope (common duct exploration) and a selection of Dormia baskets (3- to 5-Fr), guidewires, and balloon catheters. Laparoscopic clearance of ductal stones is considerably facilitated by use of the 30° forward-oblique telescope. The following consumables are also required: 4-0 atraumatic absorbable sutures mounted on endoski needles (Polysorb, coated vicryl), 14-Fr T-tube (common duct exploration), Cuschieri cystic duct drainage catheter and chromic catgut (1.5-m lengths) mounted on push rods or preformed catgut endoloops.

■ TRANSCYSTIC CLEARANCE

Cystic duct clearance is applicable to small calculi (up to 1.0 cm) in the distal common duct. It is unsuitable for proximal stones and multiple large occluding calculi where laparoscopic supraduodenal bile duct exploration is indicated. Cystic duct clearance can be performed under radiological control or by direct visual guidance. *Irrespective of technique, the procedure must be performed before the cystic duct continuity is disrupted and before dissection of the gallbladder from the liver bed is commenced.*

PORTS

Usually no extra ports to those used in the conduct of laparoscopic cholecystectomy are needed for laparoscopic transcystic extraction of ductal calculi. However, in cases where there is a floppy quadrate lobe, an extra 5.5-mm cannulla below and to the right of the xiphoid is used for retraction. This extra cannula also is advisable for the introduction of the flexible choledochoscope during direct exploration of the common bile duct (vide infra).

RADIOLOGICALLY CONTROLLED TECHNIQUE

This technique has been popularized by Hunter.[9] It is quicker than the endoscopically guided method and avoids the need for dilation of the cystic duct. Multiple stone evacuation per single basket passage constitutes a further advantage. The radiologically guided technique necessitates the availability of modern real-time fluoro-cholangiography. In this respect, we have found the "road mapping" mode of the OEC Diasonics C-arm Unit particularly useful since it shows the basket against the contrast background and filling defects caused by the calculi in relief and with remarkable clarity.

The procedure consists of the following steps:

1. Initial cholangiogram. An opening is made by the curved microscissors on the anterosuperior walls of the dissected cystic duct. The cholangiography catheter (5-Fr Cook ureteric catheter or substitute) loaded inside the cholangiograsper is introduced into the cystic duct for a distance of 1.0 cm and the jaws of the cholangiograsper are closed, gripping the cystic duct walls over the cholangiocatheter. The fully primed system is connected by a three-way tap to saline- and contrast-filled syringes (sodium diatrizoate). Resistance to the passage of the catheter tip may be owing to the mucosal folds (Heister valve), or a small calculus in the cystic duct. When encountered, gentle saline injection assists in catheter insertion. If this measure fails, a cystic duct calculus should be suspected. In this case, the cystic duct should be massaged gently between the jaws of an atraumatic grasper in a mediolateral direction. This maneuver will dislodge the stone which then appears in the cystic duct opening and is removed before the cholangiography catheter is re-introduced. If small distal calculi are encountered, warm saline irrigation, together with the intravenous administration of a spasmolytic agent (glucagon or secretin), may result in passage of the stones into the duodenum. If not, transcystic extraction is carried out.

2. Insertion of Dormia basket and stone capture. The cholangiogram catheter is replaced by a 4-Fr Dormia or Segura basket, preferably with filiform tip. Under screening control, the basket (in the closed position) is passed down the cystic duct into the distal common bile duct such that its floppy tip lies in the duodenum.

3. Trawling and extraction of the stones. When this position is achieved, the wire basket is opened just above the lower choledochal sphincter and pulled back along the distal common bile duct into the cystic duct where the basket is closed over the stones caught in the trawl. If the stones are larger than the cystic duct lumen, the basket is closed as it reaches the cystic duct to achieve crushing. The trawling process is repeated until ductal clearance of all discernible

stone fragments is obtained. Alternatively, the stones, once trapped inside the basket, can be delivered into the duodenum where they are released or crushed by full closure of the basket. This method is quick and effective but must be limited to one, or at most, two passages, otherwise the risk of postoperative pancreatitis is increased. The other possible complication of this technique is impaction of the basket in the sphincter. It is less often used than transcystic extraction because of these perceived risks.

4. Flushing and completion cholangiography. The Dormia basket is withdrawn and replaced by the cholangiocatheter. The biliary tract is flushed gently and filled with saline. This technique washes out any debris and removes air bubbles. High-pressure injection must be avoided to reduce the risk of cholangiovenous reflux. The cholangiogram then is repeated and if ductal clearance is confirmed, the cholangiocatheter is removed and the cystic duct ligated in continuity with catgut or transected and then secured with a preformed catgut endoloop.

5. Insertion of cystic duct drainage cannula. If the completion cholangiogram is equivocal (usually debris in the distal duct), the safest measure consists of the insertion of a cystic duct drainage catheter through the cystic duct into the common bile duct. A specially designed catheter is now available for this purpose (Cook, USA) in two sizes (7.5 Fr, 8.5 Fr). The catheter has a terminal S-configuration that facilitates insertion and minimizes the risk of subsequent dislodgement (Fig 69–18). The catheter is secured to the cystic duct stump by two catgut ligatures. The cystic duct catheter, aside from providing drainage, permits the performance of postoperative cholangiography (Fig 69–19). Further management is based on the findings of this investigation. In most instances, the postoperative cholangiogram proves to be normal.

VISUALLY GUIDED TECHNIQUE

This technique was pioneered by Dubois in France and subsequently popularized by Phillips and associates and Petelin in the United States.[51–54] It necessitates the dilation of the cystic duct followed by the introduction of a narrow flexible operating endoscope (Fig 69–20) attached to a CCD camera for visually guided transcystic extraction of the ductal calculi. The endoscope has a functional length of 30 cm, an outer diameter of 3.4 mm and an instrument channel of 1.2 mm. Finer endoscopes are available and can be used, but these must have an instrument channel of at least 1.0 mm, other-

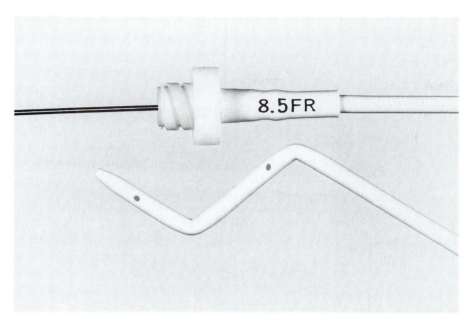

Figure 69–18. Cuschieri cystic duct drainage catheter (Cook, USA). This catheter has a terminal S shaped configuration that facilitates insertion and minimizes the risk of subsequent dislodgement.

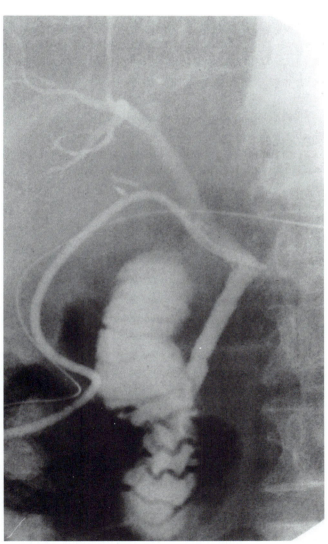

Figure 69–19. Postoperative cholangiogram performed through cystic duct drainage catheter.

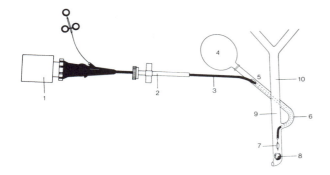

A

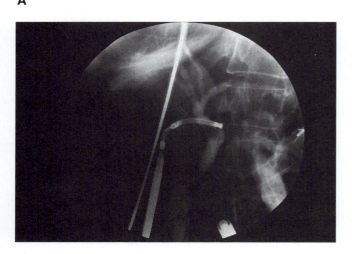

B

Figure 69–20. Visually guided transcystic laparoscopic extractiion of ductal calculi. **A.** Diagrammatic representation. **B.** Fluoroscopic appearance.

wise irrigation is impossible once the basket is introduced. The other items of equipment needed are angioplasty 3/4-Fr Dormia or Segura baskets, balloon dilators and guidewires. The balloon dilators should be 6- to 7-Fr gauge with a balloon length of 40 mm that is capable of achieving maximal dilation of 5.0 mm. They are insufflated with saline through a customized pressure gauge using a special syringe. Torque guidewires with soft pliable tips or J wires which fit the balloon catheters are used.

1. Initial cholangiogram. This procedure is performed as previously outlined.
2. Insertion of guidewire. The guidewire is inserted under fluoroscopic control through the cholangiocatheter into the common bile duct and, if possible, into the duodenum. The cholangiocatheter then is removed and replaced by the balloon catheter, which is threaded over the guidewire.

3. Dilation. If the common bile duct is dilated, the balloon is positioned under fluoroscopic control across the choledochal sphincter and then inflated. Following dilation of the sphincter, the balloon is deflated and the catheter withdrawn until the balloon lies in the cystic duct where it is re-inflated to dilate this structure. The dilation of the choledochal sphincter is omitted if the common bile duct is not dilated. At this stage, an antispasmodic agent that relaxes the sphincter of Oddi is administered intravenously. This step is followed by irrigation of warm saline through the deflated balloon catheter in an attempt at flushing small calculi into the duodenum. The effect of this maneuver is ascertained by fluoroscopy and injection of contrast medium.
4. Insertion of endoscope. If unsuccessful, the guidewire is re-inserted through the lumen of the balloon catheter into the common duct and the catheter then removed. The flexible endoscope connected to the irrigation system (Fenwall pressure cuff) and a CCD camera is inserted through the midclavicular cannula and threaded over the guidewire into the common duct. The guidewire then is replaced by the Dormia basket which is used to trap and remove the stones under direct vision, either through the cystic duct or into the duodenum. A completion cholangiogram is performed to establish stone clearance. The cystic duct then is ligated in continuity with chromic catgut using a Roeder slip knot or by means of a preformed catgut endoloop. If the completion cholangiogram is equivocal, a cystic duct drainage cannula is inserted as described previously.

■ LAPAROSCOPIC EXPLORATION AND CLOSURE OF THE COMMON BILE DUCT

This technique is indicated if the common duct diameter is larger than 1.0 cm, in the presence of a large or occluding stone load, and in patients with proximal stones. The dipping endoretractor (Storz) is useful for elevating the quadrate lobe ahead of the optic and thereby provides excellent exposure of the common bile duct (Fig 69–21). If not available, the quadrate lobe and central part of the liver are elevated using the falciform/round ligament sling.[55] The use of the 30° forward-oblique telescope is essential. The insertion of the flexible choledochoscope is best achieved through an extra 5.5 mm cannula placed below and to the right of the xiphoid process in line with the common bile duct. The author's technique of laparoscopic bile duct exploration has changed during the past two years, and he

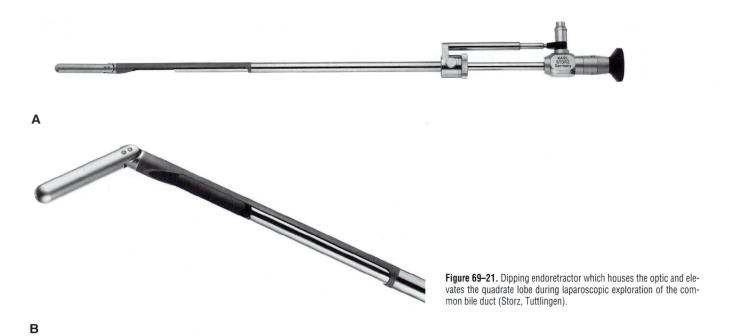

A

B

Figure 69–21. Dipping endoretractor which houses the optic and elevates the quadrate lobe during laparoscopic exploration of the common bile duct (Storz, Tuttlingen).

now dispenses with the visual extraction under endoscopic control with Dormia baskets. Although undoubtedly effective, this method can be very time consuming and is unnecessary since the vast majority of ductal calculi encountered during laparoscopic cholecystectomy can be readily dislodged and brought to the choledochotomy by ductal massage, mild suction, or blind trawling using embolectomy or biliary balloon catheters inflated with air.

1. Dissection of the common bile duct and choledochotomy. The catheter used for the cholangiogram is left in situ. Minimal dissection of the common duct is needed since only the anterior wall needs to be exposed. Stay sutures are unnecessary and use up ports. The incision of the anterior wall of the common bile duct is made low down in a verticle oblique fashion and should initially not exceed 1.0 cm in length. It may require extension if the stone is large, but in practice, we have observed that choledochotomy wounds (by virtue of the high elastin content of the bile duct) can be stretched to allow delivery of stones 30% to 50% longer than the size of the wound. Bleeding from the cut edges is controlled by precise soft electrocoagulation. Saline is injected forcibly through the cystic duct cannula. This procedure may result in escape of the stone which then is picked by the spoon forceps and retrieved.

2. Suction extraction. The next step consists of insertion of a suction device just inside the choledochotomy, with the tip of the instrument pointing towards the choledochal sphincter. Low suction is applied and used to adhere the stone to the tip of the suction instrument. Following delivery through the choledochotomy, the stone is transferred to a spoon forceps and removed. Complete ductal clearance often can be achieved by this simple technique.

3. Duct massage. Two round-ended atraumatic graspers are used to straddle the common duct, which is massaged between the two instruments in a proximal direction starting at the lower end. Once the stone has reached the choledochotomy, one of the graspers is used to compress the bile duct anteroposteriorly above the choledochotomy and the other is used to ease it out of the choledochotomy. We have found this technique to be useful for large calculi.

4. Extraction by biliary balloon catheters. If the above methods fail, a biliary balloon catheter is inserted through a large Medicut cannula into the common bile duct and through the sphincter into the duodenum. After the balloon is inflated with air, the catheter is withdrawn gently until the resistance caused by the sphincter is encountered. The balloon is partially deflated while gentle traction is maintained until it negotiates the sphincter and then the balloon is re-inflated rapidly and the catheter used to trawl the stones to the choledochotomy wound.

5. Visually guided extraction with choledochoscope. In our experience, the above three methods used in the sequence outlined above result in successful ductal clearance within 30 minutes, in 80% of patients. In these cases, the flexible choledochoscope is inserted to conduct a completion inspection. In the other 20% of patients, visually guided Dormia basket extraction is performed. The flexible choledochoscope connected to the irrigation system (Fenwall) and the CCD camera is introduced through a separate 5.5-mm cannula below and to the right of the xiphoid in line with the common bile duct. After placement of the distal 1.0 cm of the choledochoscope inside the bile duct lumen, the walls of common bile duct are gathered around the flexible endoscope by an atraumatic forceps and irrigation is commenced. The entire biliary tract is inspected (proximally and distally) and any stones are trapped and removed under vision through the choledochotomy, by means of a Dormia basket. Once outside the bile duct, the stones are transferred on each occasion to a spoon forceps and retrieved. After clearance is achieved, repeat choledochoscopic inspection of the biliary tract is performed.

6. Common duct drainage. As previously mentioned, drainage of the bile duct is advisable after supraduodenal bile duct exploration, since obstruction owing to edema is encountered for several days after this procedure. In addition, the drainage tube provides a ready access for postoperative cholangiography as a final check against retained stones. As in open exploration of the common bile duct, there are two techniques that can be used to provide biliary drainage: insertion of a T tube and cystic duct drainage.

T TUBE METHOD

This procedure is the standard technique. The horizontal limb of a 14-Fr latex tube is trimmed to a total length that does not exceed 1.5 cm and is filleted. These modifications greatly facilitate the insertion of the horizontal part inside the common bile duct. The tube is inserted into the peritoneal cavity through a stab wound in the right flank, such that the long limb runs a straight course to the choledochotomy. This straight alignment of the long limb of the T tube is important should any residual stones be discovered postoperatively since a straight tube tract facilitates percutaneous stone extraction by this route. In this respect, it is a mistake to use one of the cannula sites for the insertion of the T tube since, more often than not, these sites do not provide the ideal location. Once the tube is in the peritoneal cavity, its short horizontal limbs are compressed together by means of an atraumatic forceps and then fed into the common bile duct, when the forceps is released. When the T tube is in place, saline is instilled to irrigate the extrahepatic biliary tract.

CYSTIC DUCT DRAINAGE

We now prefer this technique because it results in a quicker recovery of the patient. It provides adequate drainage (average 300 mL/day) and excellent access for postoperative cholangiography.

The cholangiocatheter is replaced by cystic duct drainage cannula. This cannula is introduced in the right flank via a peel-away sheath and then is inserted through the cystic duct wall into the common bile duct. The cystic duct then is tied over the cannula in continuity using a Roeder catgut slip knot. A second Roeder knot is applied a few millimeters further laterally but medial to the clip on the gallbladder end of the cystic duct. The cystic duct then is divided with hook scissors between the lateral ligature and the clip. Saline is infused through the cystic duct cannula to ensure patency.

SUTURE CLOSURE OF THE COMMON BILE DUCT

The incision in the common bile duct is closed by 2 to 3 interrupted 4-0 absorbable sutures (Polysorb, coated vicryl). If a T tube is placed, the choledochotomy is closed above the long limb with then comes to lie at the bottom of the closed incision. If cystic duct cannula drainage is used, primary complete closure of the choledochotomy is performed. In either case, when the suturing has been completed, saline is injected through the cystic duct cannula or T tube to ensure a watertight seal.

A completion contrast study to ensure ductal clearance is advisable in all cases undergoing laparoscopic exploration of the common bile duct. A subhepatic drain is inserted routinely in these patients. This drain is introduced though the midclavicular cannula and placed in the subhepatic pouch close to the choledochotomy. The drain is connected to a closed drainage system. Thereafter, the peritoneum is desufflated and the drain and T tube or cystic duct cannula are fixed by sutures to the skin.

■ POSTOPERATIVE MANAGEMENT

GENERAL MEASURES

These measures apply to all patients whether they are treated by open surgery or by the laparoscopic approach. The nasogastric tube is removed after recovery from anesthesia or the next day since postoperative ileus is not commonly encountered in these patients. In the presence of jaundice, hourly monitoring of the urinary output is maintained for the first few days after surgery.

Prophylactic antibiotics are administered for 24 hours after surgery. In patients with bacterbilia (shown on culture or gram stain of the common bile duct bile), a full 5 day course of antibiotics is recommended.

The subhepatic drain usually is removed on the second day after establishing that there is no bile leakage.

MANAGEMENT OF PATIENTS WITH T TUBES

The T tube is left on free closed drainage for 4 to 5 days when a postoperative cholangiogram is performed. If this is satisfactory and the patient is fully ambulant with return of bowel function, the T tube is spigoted and covered with an occlusive dressing and the patient is allowed to go home. This stage is usually reached 4 days after laparoscopic common bile duct exploration and 6 to 8 after the equivalent open procedure. A sufficient period of time must be allowed (minimum of 10 days) for maturation of the T tube tract before the T tube is removed in an outpatient setting. In elderly, immunosuppressed, or diabetic patients, a longer period is advisable (3 weeks) before T tube removal.

MANAGEMENT OF PATIENTS WITH CYSTIC DUCT DRAINAGE

These patients progress more rapidly and have usually undergone laparoscopic ductal clearance (transcystic or direct common bile duct exploration). The cystic duct catheter is left on free closed drainage for 24 hours and a postoperative cholangiogram is performed on the second postoperative day. If this is satisfactory, the cystic duct drainage cannula is sealed and covered by an occlusion dressing. The patient usually is allowed to go home on day 3 and returns some 10 days later for catheter removal.

MANAGEMENT OF COMPLICATIONS

Patients should recover rapidly after common bile duct exploration, whether this is carried out by the open conventional technique or the laparoscopic approach. However, the surgeon should be on the alert for possible complications. The clinical features that require medical attention and investigation during the postoperative period are

- Persistent fever and leucocytosis
- Persistent pain—beyond 24 hours
- Bile leakage through the drain
- Jaundice and rigors

Biliary Complications

Biliary leakage and bile duct injury declare themselves in the postoperative period by pain and fever, with or without abnormal liver function tests and jaundice. Other manifestations include external discharge of bile, if a subhepatic drain has been placed, or biliary ascites.[56] The initial investigation of these patients should include ultrasound or CT examination for the detection of fluid collections. Biliary scintigraphy is useful in the detection of biliary leakage and bile flow obstruction in the early postoperative period.[57–59] Minor collections in the presence of an intact extrahepatic biliary tract can be treated by percutaneous drainage under radiological guidance. If the patient improves, no further action is needed. However, in the presence of a major leak, jaundice, cholangitis, or any suspicion of iatrogenic bile duct trauma, an ERC is mandatory since this is the definitive method of establishing the presence, extent, and severity of bile duct injury.

If the ERC demonstrates bile duct leakage, most commonly from the cystic duct owing to a slipped titanium clip, and much less frequently from the gallbladder fossa, endoscopic management involves nasobiliary stenting or endoscopic sphincterotomy or both.[60–62] However, in patients who develop this complication after laparoscopic surgery, the author favors re-laparoscopy with suction of extravasated bile and ligature of the cystic duct stump by a catgut endoloop. If the leakage is from the gallbladder fossa, then suture ligation of the small duct of Luschka is carried out. A subhepatic drain is left in situ for a few days. The laparoscopic approach appears to be more direct and definitive and avoids the risk, albeit small, of endoscopic sphincterotomy and stenting.

If ERC confirms a ductal injury in the early postoperative period, then the best management is referral to a center with the necessary expertise for dealing with these problems. Outcome is dependent on the expertise of the surgeon undertaking the remedial reconstruction.[63] If the patient is ill with cholangitis, then a period of drainage (usually percutaneous transhepatic) with appropriate antibiotics should precede surgical intervention. Partial injuries may declare themselves several months to years later as recurrent jaundice with attacks of cholangitis.

Retained Stones

Active intervention is advisable, if retained stones are diagnosed on the postoperative cholangiogram, even if the patient is not jaundiced, in view of the pathogenic potential of ductal calculi. Exception is made to this policy if the patient's general condition is poor because of comorbid disease. The options are (1) endoscopic sphincterotomy and stone extraction. (2) Extraction via the T tube tract in patients with an indwelling T tube.

Endoscopic Sphincterotomy and Stone Extraction. This technique is the most generally favored technique and provided it is performed by an experienced interventional endoscopist, its success rate exceeds 90%. In patients with a cystic duct drainage cannula, insertion of a guidewire under radiological control through the cannula into the common bile duct, and then into the duodenum, virtually guarantees success of the procedure in all patients.

Percutaneous Extraction via the T Tube Tract. This combined radiological and flexible endoscopic approach is applicable to patients with an indwelling T tube and is successful in the majority of cases. Its main disadvantage is the long period (minimum of 4 weeks) before the procedure can be attempted safely. This delay is necessary to enable maturation of the T tube tract since otherwise the tract can be perforated during the manipulations. The procedure entails insertion of a guidewire under radiological control into the common bile duct, after which the T tube is removed. The flexible choledochoscope then is threaded over the guidewire into the common bile duct through the choledochotomy. Extraction of the stone is carried out by means of a Dormia basket.

REFERENCES

1. Boey JH, Way LW. Acute cholangitis. *Ann Surg* 1980; 264–270
2. Mason RR. Percutaneous extraction of retained gallstones via the T tube tract—British experience of 131 cases. *Clin Radiol* 1980;1:497–499
3. Neuhaus H, Feussner H, Ungeheuer A, et al. Prospective evaluation of the use of endoscopic retrograde cholangiography prior to laparoscopic cholecystectomy. *Endoscopy* 1992;24:746–749
4. Clair DG, Carr-Locke DL, Becker JM, et al. Routine cholangiography is not warranted during laparoscopic cholecystectomy. *Arch Surg* 1993;128:551–554
5. Cotton PB. Endoscopic retrograde cholangiopancreatography and laparoscopic cholecystectomy. *Am J Surg* 1993; 165:474–478
6. Bruhn EW, Miller FJ, Hunter JG. Routine fluoroscopic cholangiography during laparoscopic cholecystectomy: an argument. *Surg Endosc* 1991;5:111–115
7. Sackier JM, Berci G, Phillips E, et al. The role of cholangiography in laparoscopic cholecystectomy. *Arch Surg* 1991;126:1021–1025
8. Vitale GC, Larson GM, Wieman TJ, et al. The use of ERCP in the management of common bile duct stones in patients undergoing laparoscopic cholecystectomy. *Surg Endosc* 1993;7:9–11
9. Hunter JG. Laparoscopic transcystic common bile duct exploration. *Am J Surg* 1992;163:53–56
10. Appel S, Krebs H, Fern D. Techniques for laparoscopic cholangiography and removal of common duct stones. *Surg Endosc* 1992;6:134–137
11. Ido K, Kimura K, Kawamoto C, et al. Preliminary experience using laparoscopic trancystic cholangioscopy for the treatment of common bile duct stones. *Endoscopy* 1992; 24:750–753
12. Shapiro SJ, Gordon LA, Daykhovsky L, et al. Laparoscopic exploration of the common bile duct in 16 selected patients. *J Laparosc Surg* 1991;1:33–41
13. Stoker ME, Leveillee RJ, McCann JC Jr, et al. Laparoscopic explanation of common bile duct *J Laparosc Surg* 1991;1: 287–293
14. Ferzli GS, Massaad A, Ozuner G, et al. Laparoscopic exploration of the common bile duct. *Surg Gynecol Obstet* 1992;174:419–421
15. Hunter JG, Soper NJ. Laparoscopic management of bile duct stones. *Surg Clin North Am* 1992;72:1077–1097
16. Deslandres E, Gagner M, Pomp A, et al. Intraoperative endoscopic sphincterotomy for common bile duct stones during laparoscopic cholecystectomy. *Gastrointest Endosc* 1993;39(1):54–58
17. Boulay J, Schellenberg R, Brady PG. Role of ERCP and therapeutic endoscopy in association with laparoscopic cholecystectomy. *Am J Gastroenterol* 1992;87:837–842
18. Traverso LW, Kozarek RA, Ball TJ, et al. Endoscopic retrograde cholangiopancreatography after laparoscopic cholecystectomy. *Am J Surg* 1993;165:581–586
19. Shimi S, Banting S, Cuschieri A. Transcystic drainage after laparoscopic exploration of common bile duct. *Minim Inv Ther* 1992;1:273–276
20. Joyce WP, Keane R, Burke GJ, et al. Identification of bile duct stones in patients undergoing laparoscopic cholecystectomy. *Br J Surg* 1991;78:1174–1176
21. Handy JE, Rose SC, Nieves AS, et al. Intraoperative cholangiography: use of portable fluoroscopy and transmitted images. *Radiology* 1991;181:205–207
22. Flowers JL, Zucker KA, Graham SM, et al. Laparoscopic cholangiography: results and indications. *Ann Surg* 1992; 215:209–216
23. Cuschieri A, Berci G. In: *Laparoscopic Biliary Surgery*, 2nd ed. Blackwells: Oxford, 1992;155–169
24. Phillips EH: Routine versus selective intraoperative cholangiography. *Am J Surg* 1993;165:505–507
25. Cuschieri A, Shimi S, Banting S, et al. Intraoperative cholangiography during laparoscopic cholecystectomy: routine versus selective policy. *Surg Endosc* 1994;6: 302–305
26. Huguier M, Bornet P, Charpak Y, et al. Selective contraindications based on multivariate analysis for operative cholangiography in biliary lithiasis. *Surg Gynecol Obstet* 1991;172:470–474
27. Lillemoe KD, Yeo CJ, Talamini MA, et al. Selective cholangiography: current role in laparoscopic cholecystectomy. *Ann Surg* 1992;215:669–674
28. Pace BW, Cosgrove J, Breuer B, et al. Intraoperative cholangiography revisited. *Arch Surg* 1992;127:448–450
29. Chattopadhyay TK, Kumar A, Kapoor VK. Preoperative cholangiogram—routine or selective results of a prospective study. *Trop Gastroenterol* 1992;13:75–77
30. Carlson MA, Ludwig KA, Frantzides CT, et al. Routine or

selective intraoperative cholangiography in laparoscopic cholecystectomy. *J Laparoendosc Surg* 1993;3:27–33

31. Clair DG, Carr-Locke DL, Becker JM, et al. Routine cholangiography is not warranted during laparoscopic cholecystectomy. *Arch Surg* 1993;128:551–554

32. Hauer-Jensen M, Karesen R, Nygaard K, et al. Prospective randomised study of routine intraoperative cholangiography during open cholecystectomy: long-term follow-up and multivariate analysis of predictors of choledocholithiasis. *Surgery* 1993;113:318–323

33. Branum G, Schmitt C, Biallie J, et al. Management of major biliary complications after laparoscopic cholecystectomy. *Ann Surg* 1993;217:532–540

34. Walker AT, Shapiro AW, Brookes DC, et al. Bile duct disruption and biloma after laparoscopic cholecystectomy: imaging evaluation. *Am J Surg* 1992;158:785–789

35. Raoul JL, Bretagne JF, Siproudhis L, et al. Cystic duct clip migration into the common bile duct: a complication of laparoscopic cholecystectomy treated by endoscopic biliary sphincterotomy. *Gastrointest Endosc* 1992;38:608–611

36. Dhalla SS, Duncan AW. Endoscopic removal of a common bile duct stone associated with a Ligaclip. *Can J Surg* 1992;35:344–345

37. Janson JA, Cotton PB. Endoscopic treatment of a bile duct stone containing a surgical staple. *Hepatobil Surg* 1990;3:67–71

38. Brutvan FM, Kampschroer BH, Parker HW. Vessel clip as a nidus for formation of common duct bile stone. *Gastrointest Endosc* 1982;28:222–223.

39. Mansvelt B, Harb J, Farkas B, et al. "Clip-stone" formation within the biliary tract. *Hepatobil Surg* 1993;6:185–188

40. Hemmi P, Diaz D, Steffen A, et al. Ictere tardiff apres cholecystectomie par laparoscopie, du a un clip endocholedocien. *Gastroenterol Clin Biol* 1992;16:725–726

41. Matsuura T, Kanisawa Y, Sato T, et al. Migration of "endoclips" into common bile duct after laparoscopic cholecystectomy. *Lancet* 1992;340:306

42. Nathanson LK, Easter DW, Cuschieri A. Ligation of the cystic duct pedicle during laparoscopic cholecystectomy. *Am J Surg* 1991;161:350–354

43. Nathanson LK, Shimi S, Cuschieri A. Laparoscopic cholecystectomy, the Dundee technique. *Br J Surg* 1991;78:155–159

44. DenBesten L, Berci G. The current status of biliary tract surgery: an international study of 1072 consecutive cases. *World J Surg* 1986;10:116–122

45. Sawyers JL, Herrington JL, et al. Primary closure of the common bile duct. *Am J Surg* 1965;109:107

46. Holdsworth RJ, Sadek SA, Ambikar S, et al. Dynamics of bile flow through the human choledochal sphincter following exploration of the common bile duct. *World J Surg* 1989;13:300–306

47. Cuschieri A, Berci G. *Common Bile Duct Exploration*. Boston, MA: Martinus Nijhoff; 1984

48. Berci G, Hamlin JA, Daykhovsky L, et al. Common bile duct lithotripsy. *Gastrointest Endosc* 1990;36:137–139

49. Shapiro SJ, Gordon LA, Daykhovsky L, et al. Laparoscopic exploration of the common bile duct. *J Laparosc Endosc* 1991;1:333–341

50. Cushieri A, Wood RAB, Metcalf MJ, et al. Long-term experience with transection choledochoduodenostomy. *World J Surg* 1983;7:502–504

51. Cuschieri A, Dubois F, Mouiel J, et al. The European experience with laparoscopic cholecystectomy. *Am J Surg* 1991;161:385–387

52. Sackier JM, Berci G, Paz-Partlow M. Laparoscopic transcystic choledocholithotomy as an adjunct to laparoscopic cholecystectomy. *Am Surg* 1991;53:323–326

53. Sackier J, Berci G, Phillips E, et al. The role of cholangiography in laparoscopic cholecystectomy. *Arch Surg* 1991;126:1021–1026

54. Petelin JB. Laparoscopic approach to common duct pathology. *Surg Laparosc Endosc* 1991;1:33–41

55. Bantin S, Shimi S, Vander Velpen G, et al. Abdominal wall lift: low pressure pneumoperitoneum laparoscopic surgery. *Surg Endosc* 1993;7:57–59

56. Rossi RL, Schirmer WJ, Braasch JW, et al. Laparoscopic bile duct injuries: risk factors, recognition and repair. *Arch Surg* 1992;127:596–601

57. Estrada WN, Zanzi I, Ward R, et al. Scintigraphic evaluation of postoperative complications of laparoscopic cholecystectomy. *J Nucl Med* 1991;32:1910–1911

58. Pasmans HL, Go PM, Gouma DJ, et al. Scintigraphic diagnosis of bile leakage after laparoscopic cholecystectomy: a prospective study. *Clin Nucl Med* 1992;17:697–700

59. Gentili A, Gilkeson RC, Adler LP. Scintigraphic detection of bile duct leaks after laparoscopic cholecystectomy. *Clin Nucl Med* 1993;18:1–6

60. Howell DA, Bosco JJ, Sampson LN, et al. Endoscopic management of cystic duct fistulas after laparoscopic cholecystectomy. *Endoscopy* 1992;24:796–798

61. Yau MP, Tsai C CH, Liu R CH, et al. Diagnostic and therapeutic interventions in post-laparoscopic cholecystectomy biliary complications. *Hepatogastroenterology* 1993;40:139–144

62. Weber J, Adamek HE, Riemann JF. Endoscopic stent placement and clip removal for common bile duct stricture after laparoscopic cholecystectomy. *Gastrointest Endosc* 1992;38:181–182

63. Blumgart LH, Kelley CJ, Benjamin IS. Benign bile duct stricture following cholecystectomy: critical factors in management. *Br J Surg* 1990;125:1028–1032

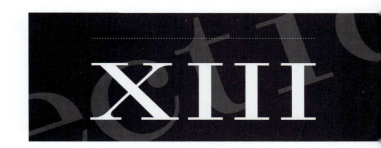

XIII

PANCREAS

70

Acute Pancreatitis

John H.C. Ranson

In 1579, Ambrose Pare, the French surgeon, provided an early description of acute and chronic pancreatitis. During the next two centuries, a number of anecdotal descriptions of pancreatic disease were published and, in 1856, Ancelet prepared a pathologic description of acute pancreatitis, pancreatic gangrene and abscess from a review of the reports existing at that time. Clinical and pathologic descriptions of the various forms of acute pancreatitis were made by Nicholas Senn, a Chicago surgeon, in 1886, and by Reginald Fitz, a Boston physician, in 1889.

Acute pancreatitis is currently defined as pancreatic inflammation that may be followed by clinical and biologic restitution of the gland, if the primary cause is eliminated. It includes a spectrum of clinical illness that ranges from mild self-limiting symptoms to rapid deterioration and death. The initiating etiologic factors are multiple and diverse and the pathologic findings may range from pancreatic edema to hemorrhagic infarction. Therefore, although acute pancreatic inflammation of all types has certain common features, it is important to recognize that multiple disease entities are included in this term and the management of patients must be highly individualized.

■ ETIOLOGY

Etiologic associations of acute pancreatitis have been identified primarily on the basis of epidemiologic evidence. Approximately 80% of patients either have gallstones or a history of sustained alcohol abuse. The relative frequency of these two associations depends on the prevalence of alcoholism in the population studied. Other factors that have been implicated in the etiology of acute pancreatitis are listed in Table 70–1.

METABOLIC FACTORS

Alcohol

Clinical pancreatitis is recognized in 0.9% to 9.5% of alcoholic patients. Symptoms are usually first noted only after an 11 to 18 year period of heavy alcohol ingestion. Studies by Sarles have shown that chronic alcohol administration leads to changes in pancreatic exocrine secretion, with development of precipitates within the pancreatic ducts. It is postulated that these precipitates may lead to ductal obstruction and inflammation.

Other

Pancreatitis is associated with hyperlipoproteinemia, especially Frederickson types I, IV, or V, with hypercalcemia and with the bite of the black scorpion of Trinidad. In addition, a causal relationship generally is accepted between the administration of adrenal corticosteroids, thiazide diuretics, estrogens, azathioprine, and furosemide and the occurrence of pancreatitis. It also may occur as an unexplained familial illness.

TABLE 70–1. ETIOLOGIC FACTORS IN ACUTE PANCREATITIS

METABOLIC
    Alcohol
    Hyperlipoproteinemia
    Hypercalcemia
    Drugs
    Genetic
    Scorpion venom
MECHANICAL
    Cholelithiasis
    Postoperative
    Pancreas divisum
    Post-traumatic
    Retrograde pancreatography
    Pancreatic duct obstruction: pancreatic tumor, ascaris infestation
    Pancreatic ductal bleeding
    Duodenal obstruction
VASCULAR
    Postoperative (cardiopulmonary bypass)
    Periarteritis nodosa
    Atheroembolism
INFECTION
    Mumps
    Coxsackie B
    Cytomegalovirus
    Cryptococcus

MECHANICAL FACTORS

Cholelithiasis

Gallstones are present in approximately 60% of nonalcoholic patients with acute pancreatitis. Their causative role is further indicated by the finding that, if stones are allowed to persist, 36% to 63% of patients will develop recurrent acute pancreatitis. This risk can be reduced to 2% to 8% by surgical correction of biliary lithiasis. Studies of the stools of patients recovering from gallstone pancreatitis have demonstrated gallstones in 85% to 94% of cases. It has been proposed that obstruction of a common biliary and pancreatic channel at the ampulla of Vater may lead to reflux of bile into the pancreas and the initiation of pancreatitis. Although reflux of dye into the pancreatic duct during cholangiography is more frequent in patients with pancreatitis, it is not clear whether pancreatitis is secondary to reflux or to simple calculous obstruction of the pancreatic duct.

Postoperative Pancreatitis

Acute pancreatitis has been recognized following 0.8% to 17% of surgical operations on the stomach and 0.7% to 9.3% of biliary operations. In these patients, it is probable that direct injury to the pancreas, or to its blood supply or obstruction of the pancreatic duct at the duodenum, is responsible. Acute pancreatitis also occurs in

patients following cardiopulmonary bypass or major vascular surgery, and ischemic injury to the pancreas is probably a major factor in this setting.

Other Mechanical Factors

Acute pancreatitis occurs in approximately 6% of patients who sustain blunt or penetrating injuries to the pancreas. The injection of dye into the pancreatic duct during endoscopic retrograde pancreatography is followed by clinically obvious pancreatitis in about 1% of such studies. Obstruction of the pancreatic duct owing to tumor or parasitic infestation occasionally leads to pancreatitis. In rare instances, bleeding into the pancreatic duct causes pancreatitis. In patients with failure of communication between the dorsal and ventral ducts (pancreas divisum), it has been proposed that the relative obstruction to flow may lead to recurrent pancreatitis. The frequency with which the association occurs is uncertain.

VASCULAR FACTORS

Pancreatitis has been demonstrated in association with atheromatous emboli to the pancreatic vessels and in patients with periarteritic nodosa. It also occurs following periods of profound hypoperfusion.

INFECTIOUS FACTORS

Viral infection of the pancreas has been implicated in the pathogenesis of pancreatitis observed during mumps or coxsackievirus infections.

■ PATHOLOGY AND PATHOPHYSIOLOGY

The mildest pathologic change observed in the pancreas during acute pancreatitis consists of edema of the gland. This may be accompanied by infiltration of the intralobular septa by inflammatory cells. Microscopic examination also may show areas of fat necrosis in the pancreas and in surrounding tissues. If such necrosis is more extensive, it becomes grossly recognizable as characteristic whitish-yellow plaques. Finally, vascular thrombosis or disruption may result in pancreatic necrosis or gross hemorrhagic infarction. Increased levels of active pancreatic enzymes have been observed within the pancreas, in the peritoneal exudate, and in the bloodstream of patients with pancreatitis and usually are implicated in the multiple systemic and local complications of this disease.

FLUID AND ELECTROLYTE CHANGES

Circulating blood volume frequently is reduced markedly owing to losses from the intravascular space, primarily of plasma. These losses occur both systemically and into the retroperitoneum. Additional fluid and electrolyte losses occur following vomiting or nasogastric suction. Hypocalcemia and hypomagnesemia are frequent. In many instances, decreased total calcium levels are a reflection of hypoalbuminemia, but decreases in ionized calcium levels also occur and usually are attributed to binding of calcium in areas of fat necrosis.

CARDIOVASCULAR FAILURE

Hypotension, tachycardia, increased total peripheral resistance, and decreased cardiac output are well-recognized sequelae of hypovolemia and are observed frequently in patients with acute pancreatitis. In some patients with severe pancreatitis, hemodynamic evaluation demonstrates a high cardiac output and low peripheral vascular resistance. These findings, which are similar to those observed in sepsis or hepatic cirrhosis, have been attributed to circulatory vasoactive substances. In such patients, hypotension may persist despite restoration of a functional intravascular volume.

RESPIRATORY COMPLICATIONS

Arterial hypoxemia is a frequent early feature of acute pancreatitis, and arterial oxygen tensions <66 mm Hg are observed in 38% of patients during the initial 48 hours of treatment. Early pulmonary function studies have shown decreases in inspiratory lung volume, with decreased pulmonary compliance and decreased diffusing capacity. Early pathologic changes in the lung are increased lung weight with pulmonary congestion, microatelectasis, and infarction.

Early respiratory failure often resolves as pancreatitis subsides, but patients with severe or unresolving pancreatitis may develop progressive pulmonary insufficiency, infiltrates, and pleural effusions. Factors that have been implicated in the pathogenesis of pulmonary complications in acute pancreatitis include abdominal distension and elevation of the diaphragm, alteration in the lecithin of pulmonary surfactant by circulating pancreatic lecithinase, pulmonary thromboembolism, circulating free fatty acids, and circulating products of the proteolytic cleavage of complement.

RENAL FAILURE

In the past, impaired renal function was a major factor in deaths from pancreatitis. In most instances, renal failure was principally the result of hypovolemia. Nonetheless, renal impairment occurs in normovolemic patients and histologic studies have shown deposits of fibrin and fibrinogen within the glomeruli.

OTHER SYSTEMIC FEATURES

Abnormal liver function, with elevations of serum bilirubin, alkaline phosphatase, and transaminase levels, occurs and has been attributed to biliary obstruction, hepatic parenchymal necrosis, and pericholangitis.

Early intravascular thrombosis, with decreased platelet counts and fibrinogen levels, is well documented and is usually attributed to the effects of pancreatic proteolytic enzymes. Early changes may be followed by marked thrombocytosis and hyperfibrinogenemia.

LOCAL SEQUELAE

The intra-abdominal complications of acute pancreatitis include paralytic ileus and duodenal or biliary obstruction. In most patients, these are attributable to pancreatic inflammation and enlargement. Release of pancreatic enzymes also may lead to enzyme-rich peripancreatic fluid collections and to destruction of tissues adjacent to the pancreas. The accumulation of fluid in the general peritoneal cavity and in the tissues around the pancreas is common. It is rarely associated with demonstrable gross disruption of the pancreatic ductal system and is usually self-limited. In approximately 1% of patients with acute pancreatitis, a persistent chronic pseudocyst may evolve. In severe acute pancreatitis, extensive destruction of tissues in and around the pancreas may result in secondary infection. Infected pancreatic necrosis occurs in 1% to 9% of patients, and the organisms involved are usually enteric. Extension of local necrosis to involve the colonic wall occurs in about 1% of patients. It leads to colonic perforation, usually in the left transverse colon or splenic flexure.

NATURAL HISTORY

The natural history of acute pancreatitis ranges widely, from mild, self-limiting symptoms to a fulminant rapidly lethal disease. Approximately 80% of patients recover without life-threatening complications. The remaining 20% of patients develop serious cardiopulmonary or septic complications. In the past, overall mortality was in the 15% to 20% range and approximately 75% of deaths were related to early cardiovascular and respiratory complications. Following improvements in early supportive care, overall mortality has fallen to the 5% to 10% range, and most deaths are related to the septic complications of pancreatic and peripancreatic necrosis.

PROGNOSTIC ASSESSMENT

Because the natural history of this disease is so varied, a rational approach to treatment requires the early identification of those patients who have a high risk of developing life-threatening complications. Clearly, treatment that in itself has little risk or morbidity can be

TABLE 70–2. EARLY OBJECTIVE PROGNOSTIC SIGNS THAT CORRELATE WITH THE RISK OF MAJOR COMPLICATIONS OR DEATH IN ACUTE PANCREATITIS

AT ADMISSION OR DIAGNOSIS
- Age over 55 years
- White blood cell count over 16,000/mL
- Blood glucose level over 200 mg/dL (10 mmol/L)
- Serum lactic dehydrogenase concentration >350 IU/L
- Serum glutamic oxaloacetic transaminase >250 sigma-Frankel units/dL

DURING INITIAL 48 HOURS
- Hematocrit decrease >10%
- Blood urea nitrogen increase >5 mg/dL
- Serum calcium level <8 mg/dL (2 mmol/L)
- Arterial Po_2 <60 mm Hg (8 kPa)
- Base deficit >4 mEq/L (4 mmol/L)
- Estimated fluid sequestration >6000 mL

applied to all patients with pancreatitis. However, many of the monitoring and therapeutic measures that may be helpful to patients with severe pancreatitis are associated with risks and morbidity that make them inappropriate or unduly hazardous for patients with mild disease. In the past, identification of "severe" pancreatitis has usually been based upon findings such as failure to respond to treatment, the severity of abdominal signs, or the appearance of the pancreas at operation. Most of these findings are impossible to quantify and are, therefore, influenced by observer variation.

Statistical analysis of multiple early laboratory and clinical measurements in patients with pancreatitis has led to the identification of the eleven early prognostic signs shown in Table 70–2. Figure 70–1 shows the relationship between the number of these signs that were present in individual patients and the risk of death or complications requiring more than 1 week of treatment in an intensive care unit. Clearly, not every patient with three, four, or even five positive signs has severe pancreatitis. The signs serve only to identify groups of patients with increased risk of major complications.

The APACHE II illness grading system (acute physiology and chronic health evaluation) has been applied to prognostic assessment of pancreatitis. Reports indicate that the accuracy of this system is comparable to that of specific multiple prognostic criteria. APACHE II is more complex but has the advantage that it may be applied at periods of time other than at diagnosis.

McMahon and associates have reported a correlation between prognosis and the color and volume of fluid obtained by paracentesis. This method has the advantage of early assessment of prognosis but the disadvantage of invasiveness and potential for visceral injury. Relationships have been described between early he-

modynamic measurements, coagulation factors, complement levels, antiproteases, and C reactive protein and severity of pancreatitis. In some instances, early levels do not differ in severe and mild groups, thus limiting their prognostic, as opposed to diagnostic, values.

NECROSIS AND SEPSIS

In recent years, the availability of noninvasive methods for imaging the pancreas and peripancreatic retroperitonem by ultrasound and computed tomography (CT) has renewed interest in the morphologic classification of acute pancreatitis. The usual morphologic classification of acute pancreatitis involves edematous or interstitial and necrotizing forms of the disease (Fig 70–2). The majority of patients with life-threatening complications have the necrotizing form of disease and considerable efforts have been expended in trying to identify patients in this group. Most such efforts have been diagnostic rather than prognostic. Correlations have been reported between α1 protease inhibitor, α2 macro proteins, complement factors C3 and C4, and C reactive protein and the presence of necrotizing pancreatitis. Most intriguing has been the use of contrast-enhanced CT. Radiographic enhancement of the pancreas following contrast injection has been interpreted as evidence of tissue viability. Failure of enhancement has been interpreted as evidence of tissue necrosis. Estimations of pancreatic necrosis using CT have been reported to correlate well with operative estimates of the extent of pancreatic necrosis. The timing of these studies relative to the onset of symptoms of pancreatitis is not, however, always reported. Therefore, the prognostic, as opposed to diagnostic, value of this study is uncertain. Furthermore, identification of the presence of necrosis is only of value if this is shown to be associated with specific complications or overall morbidity. In our studies and those of Bradley, approximately 70% of patients who had nonenhancement on early CT went on to develop infection of devitalized pancreatic and peripancreatic tissue. However, approximately 30% of patients escaped this complication. In our own experience, the risk of pancreatic infection in patients with early normal pancreatic enhancement was only 8.5%. Therefore, although nonenhancement is a finding of ominous prognostic significance, in terms of infection, its overall sensitivity and specificity are limited.

A study of the prognostic value of CT findings, not based on enhancement following contrast administration, was reported in 1985. Early CT findings were grouped into five categories: (1) normal, (2) peripancreatic enlargement alone, (3) inflammation confined to the pancreas, (4) one peripancreatic fluid collection, and (5) two or more fluid collections. The frequency of these findings in our population of patients was (1)

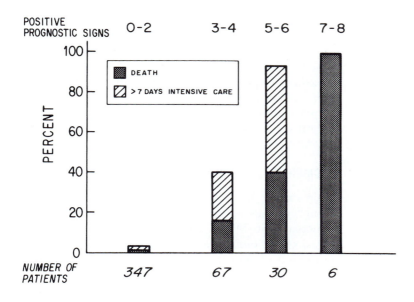

Figure 70–1. The relationship between the number of positive early prognostic signs recorded and the morbidity and mortality in 450 patients with acute pancreatitis. (From Ranson JHC. The role of peritoneal lavage in acute pancreatitis. *Ann Surg* 1978;187:565–575)

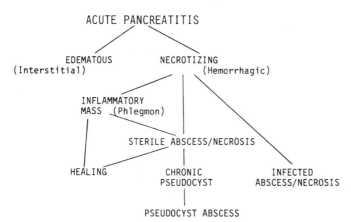

Figure 70–2. The morphologic classification of acute pancreatitis. (From Ranson JHC. Acute Pancreatitis. In Braasch JW, Tompkins RK (eds), *Surgical Diseases of the Biliary Tract and Pancreas, Multidisciplinary Management.* St. Louis, MO: Mosby Year-Book, 1995)

14.5%, (2) 22.9%, (3) 20.5%, (4) 14.5%, and (5) 27.7%. There was a weak relationship between the grade of CT finding and overall morbidity, but this was of little clinical value. However, CT findings did provide a valuable guide to the risk of late pancreatic sepsis. In patients with CT grades A or B, the incidence of infection was 0%. In those with grades C or D, it was 11.8% and 16.7%, respectively, and in those with grade E, it was 60.9%. It should be stressed that, among those patients with one or more fluid collection on initial CT scan, these collections resolved without specific treatment in 54% of cases. The value of CT findings in predicting late sepsis can be increased if they are combined with the prognostic criteria listed in Table 70–2.

■ CLINICAL MANIFESTATIONS AND DIAGNOSIS

The initial symptoms and signs of acute pancreatitis are varied and may closely mimic those of acute myocardial or other intra-abdominal disease. Nonetheless, in most patients, diagnosis depends primarily on careful clinical evaluation. Abdominal pain is usually the dominant initial complaint and is present in 85% to 100% of cases. Characteristically, the pain is upper abdominal and constant. It radiates to the back in approximately 50% of patients and may be severe. The pain often starts after a heavy meal or during a drinking binge. It increases rapidly in intensity, but its onset is less sudden than that of the pain resulting from a perforated ulcer.

The second most prominent symptoms are nausea and vomiting, which are noted in up to 92% of patients. Vomiting may be repeated but usually is not copious in volume. The vomitus is primarily gastric and duodenal contents and is not feculent.

The findings on physical examination are variable. The patient may be restless, with a rapid pulse and respiratory rate. Arterial hypotension may be present but transient hypertension also occurs. The abdomen usually is moderately distended and may exhibit a characteristic epigastric fullness. Tenderness may be generalized but is usually most marked over the upper abdomen. Moderate muscle spasm is usual but true rigidity is infrequent. Grey Turner sign or a grey-green discoloration of the flank may be present in patients with peripancreatic hemorrhage.

LABORATORY FINDINGS

Determination of serum amylase level is the most widely used laboratory test for the diagnosis of pancreatic disease. Elevated levels are observed at hospital admission in 95% of patients with acute pancreatitis and in only 5% of patients with other acute intra-abdominal conditions. The most common nonpancreatic intra-abdominal conditions associated with elevated serum amylase levels are perforated peptic ulcer, biliary lithiasis, intestinal obstruction, and mesenteric infarction. Clearly, a normal initial serum amylase level does not exclude acute pancreatitis, and this is particularly true in patients with hypertriglyceridemia and lactescent serum. Routine determination of serum amylase in these patients often yields normal results, and dilution of the serum is necessary to demonstrate hyperamylasemia.

Elevated serum lipase levels also are observed in acute pancreatitis. They appear to be somewhat more specific than amylase levels but are more difficult to measure. Hyperglycemia or glycosuria may occur in patients with acute pancreatitis but is nonspecific. Hypocalcemia is a well-recognized feature of acute pancreatitis, but also may occur in patients with perforated peptic ulcer.

RADIOGRAPHIC FINDINGS

Plain radiographs of the chest and abdomen demonstrate findings that may support a diagnosis of acute pancreatitis in 79% of patients. The most common findings are segmental small bowel ileus or a "sentinel loop" in the left upper quadrant, dilatation of the transverse colon, increased epigastric soft tissue density, and obscured psoas muscle margins. Although these findings are nonspecific, they may be valuable in the overall clinical evaluation. When simpler studies are equivocal, radiographic evaluation of the upper gastrointestinal (GI) tract, using water soluble contrast media, may be helpful. Occasionally, duodenal edema or pancreatic enlargement may be demonstrated, but even when positive evidence of pancreatitis is absent, such studies help to reduce the possibility of overlooked upper GI obstruction or perforation. In the rare patient in whom life-threatening obstructive biliary disease must be excluded, percutaneous transhepatic cholangiography (PTC) is a valuable method for demonstrating biliary anatomy.

Abdominal ultrasonography is helpful in evaluating the presence or absence of associated cholelithiasis, but early demonstration of the pancreas is often incomplete in patients with acute pancreatitis owing to gas within the GI tract. CT provides better definition of pancreatic anatomy but may show little or no abnormality in the early phase of mild acute pancreatitis.

PARACENTESIS

The character of the peritoneal fluid in patients with pancreatitis is variable and, unless clear evidence of GI perforation or infarction is found, paracentesis has not proved to be a reliable method for differentiating acute pancreatitis from conditions requiring urgent surgical correction.

DIAGNOSTIC LAPAROTOMY

In most patients, careful clinical, radiographic, and biochemical evaluation, combined with observation of the response to treatment, permits differentiation of acute pancreatitis from other acute intra-abdominal diseases. Life-threatening extrapancreatic pathology cannot, however, always be excluded by nonoperative measures, and approximately 5% of patients require early laparotomy to exclude or treat possible mesenteric infarction, gangrenous cholecystitis, or other conditions requiring urgent surgical correction.

When uncomplicated pancreatitis is found, the exploration should be complete and establish the diagnosis beyond question. If gallstones are present and pancreatitis is mild, definitive biliary surgery usually can be completed safely at this time. In patients with severe pancreatitis, it is probably safer to limit operative intervention. Pancreatic drains should be avoided.

■ TREATMENT

NONOPERATIVE THERAPY

Measures that have been proposed for the treatment of patients with acute pancreatitis may be classified as those that are intended to limit the severity of pancreatic inflammation or to interrupt the pathogenesis of complications and those that are intended to support the patients and treat specific sequelae (Table 70–3).

Nasogastric suction usually is initiated to reduce vomiting and abdominal distension. It also has been suggested that aspiration of gastric acid may reduce pancreatic exocrine secretion by reducing secretin release. Small unstratified controlled clinical trials have failed to demonstrate significant improvement in the course of mild acute pancreatitis by nasogastric suction. We continue, however, to recommend nasogastric suction in most patients because of the symptomatic improvement that often follows and the occasional reduction in pancreatic inflammation, which is apparent. Although the role of nasogastric suction is controversial, it has been clearly shown that early oral feedings may increase the severity of pancreatic inflammation and it is important that such feedings be withheld until abdominal pain and tenderness, fever, and leukocytosis have all subsided.

Attempts to inhibit pancreatic secretion by a variety of drugs, hypothermia, or pancreatic irradiation have been recommended on the basis of experimental studies or anecdotal clinical experience. The administration of anticholinergic drugs, glucagon, cimetidine, somatostatin, and calcitonin has been evaluated in prospective clinical studies, and all have been found ineffective in reducing morbidity.

TABLE 70–3. NONOPERATIVE MEASURES PROPOSED FOR THE TREATMENT OF ACUTE PANCREATITIS

TO LIMIT SEVERITY OF PANCREATIC INFLAMMATION
Inhibition of pancreatic secretion
    Nasogastric suction
    Pharmacologic: anticholinergics, glucagon, 5-fluorouracil, acetazolamide, cimetidine, propylthiouracil, calcitonin, somatostatin
    Hypothermia
    Pancreatic irradiation
Inhibition of pancreatic enzymes
    Aprotinin, epsilon-aminocaproic acid, soybean trypsin inhibitor, insulin, snake antivenom, gabexate mesilate, camostate, FFP, chlorophyll, xylocaine
Corticosteroids
Prostoglandins

TO INTERRUPT THE PATHOGENESIS OF COMPLICATIONS
Antibiotics
Antacids, cimetidine
Heparin, fibrinolysin
Low molecular weight dextran
Vasopressin
Peritoneal lavage

TO SUPPORT THE PATIENT AND TREAT COMPLICATIONS
Restoration and maintenance of intravascular volume
Electrolyte replacement
Respiratory support
Nutritional support
Analgesia
Heparin

The inhibition of pancreatic enzymes has been proposed, but the agent that has been most extensively studied is aprotinin, an extract of bovine parotid glands that inhibits trypsin and kallikrein. Large trials have failed to demonstrate clinical benefit from this drug. Trials of other protease-inhibitors also have failed to establish therapeutic benefit.

Adrenal corticosteroids have been recommended because of their antiinflammatory effects, but there is no clinical evidence to support their administration.

Controlled clinical studies have shown no benefit from the administration of ampicillin to patients with mild, alcoholic pancreatitis. The efficacy of antibiotics in patients with gallstone-associated pancreatitis is not known, but we continue to give broad-spectrum antibiotics to these patients. A controlled trial has demonstrated decreased infectious complications in patients with necrotizing pancreatitis receiving inipenem.

GI bleeding from gastroduodenal ulceration is a frequent complication of severe pancreatitis. It may be reduced greatly by monitoring of gastric pH and administration of antacids to maintain a pH >5. In some patients, cimetidine may help to maintain a satisfactory intragastric pH.

Intravascular coagulation occurs during acute pancreatitis, and it has been suggested that administration of anticoagulants may be beneficial. Experimental evaluation of the efficacy of heparin has led to variable results. Our limited clinical experience has, however, indicated that heparin administration during the first few days of pancreatitis may be associated with extensive retroperitoneal hemorrhage and should be avoided whenever possible. Although the early administration of heparin may be hazardous, marked hypercoagulability occurs after the first week of treatment of some patients with severe pancreatitis. Pulmonary emboli are a frequent problem in these patients. Coagulation factors should, therefore, be monitored, and in patients with marked thrombocytosis or hyperfibrinogenemia, we recommend constant intravenous administration of heparin, 750 to 1000 units per hour, depending on the partial thromboplastin time. Heparin administration is begun only after the first 2 weeks of treatment.

Experimental studies support that attempts to improve pancreatic blood flow using low molecular weight dextran or vasopressin may be beneficial. Clinical data are not available.

Intravascular Volume Management

Assessment of intravascular volume and cardiovascular function depends upon regular measurements of pulse rate and blood pressure. In most patients, a central venous catheter should be introduced and an indwelling urethral catheter placed for monitoring of central venous pressure, venous blood gases, and hourly urine output. Further monitoring of pulmonary arterial pressures by a Swan-Ganz catheter may be essential in those patients with associated cardiovascular disease, massive fluid requirements, or respiratory failure.

In most patients, intravascular volume can be satisfactorily restored and maintained using crystalloid solutions. Blood transfusion may be required to maintain a satisfactory hematocrit, and albumin may be given to correct early hypoalbuminemia.

Electrolyte Management

Hypokalemia is frequent and potassium administration is usually required once adequate urinary output has been established. The intravenous administration of calcium and magnesium has been recommended. In many patients, decreased calcium levels in acute pancreatitis are related to hypoalbuminemia, with normal circulating levels of ionized calcium. Since hypercalcemia has been implicated in the genesis of pancreatitis, calcium should be administered with caution.

Renal Failure

Renal failure is a well-recognized complication of severe acute pancreatitis, but it is usually secondary to hypovolemia and hypoperfusion. It may be largely prevented by adequate restoration and maintenance of the intravascular volume and cardiovascular function. In those patients in whom renal function does not respond to these measures, dramatic improvement sometimes may be observed following the introduction of peritoneal lavage.

Respiratory Monitoring and Support

Since early respiratory failure occurs in patients who do not have severe disease by the usual clinical criteria and who may not have any obvious clinical evidence of pulmonary insufficiency, it is essential that arterial blood gas values be determined at diagnosis and at intervals of not less than 12 hours for the initial 48 to 72 hours of treatment in every patient.

In most patients with early arterial hypoxemia, the only necessary management is close monitoring and administration of oxygen. In patients with progressive respiratory failure, it has been proposed that the volume of fluid administered intravenously should be decreased and the urinary output maintained or increased by the administration of diuretic drugs. There is usually no clinical or radiographic evidence of fluid overload in these patients, but improvement of respiratory function may be observed following such management. In those patients with severe pulmonary insufficiency, endotracheal intubation and positive end–expiratory pressure ventilation should be instituted early.

Analgesia

The pain associated with acute pancreatitis may be extremely severe. It is traditional to administer meperidine rather than morphine because of the spasm of the ampulla of Vater that is associated with morphine. Splanchnic block or continuous epidural anesthesia has been recommended because they do not cause ampullary spasm and may increase pancreatic blood flow. They have not, however, been widely used.

Nutritional Support

Marked nutritional depletion has been well documented in patients with severe acute pancreatitis. In those with mild pancreatitis, oral feedings usually can be resumed after a short time. Patients with severe pancreatitis cannot accept oral feedings for substantial periods, and intravenous alimentation should be instituted in this group as soon as practical. The safety of intravenous lipids in this setting has been controversial. Available data indicate that it is well tolerated by most patients.

OPERATIVE MANAGEMENT

Surgical intervention in patients with acute pancreatitis may be required for diagnostic, therapeutic, or preventive reasons (Table 70–4).

TABLE 70–4. OPERATIVE MEASURES PROPOSED FOR THE MANAGEMENT OF ACUTE PANCREATITIS

DIAGNOSTIC LAPAROTOMY

TO LIMIT THE SEVERITY OF PANCREATIC INFLAMMATION
  Biliary procedures

TO INTERRUPT THE PATHOGENESIS OF COMPLICATIONS
  Pancreatic drainage
  Pancreatic resection
  Pancreatic debridement
  Peritoneal lavage

TO SUPPORT THE PATIENT AND TREAT COMPLICATIONS
  Drainage of pancreatic infection
  Feeding jejunostomy

TO PREVENT RECURRENT PANCREATITIS

Diagnosis

In the majority of patients, a reasonably certain diagnosis of acute pancreatitis can be reached on the basis of careful clinical, laboratory, and radiographic evaluation. A small proportion of patients, however, require surgical exploration of the abdominal cavity to exclude or treat acute extrapancreatic pathology. In this regard, it is important to remember that nonpancreatic disease may closely mimic acute pancreatitis and also can occasionally occur coincidentally with pancreatitis. Thus the presence of strong evidence of pancreatitis does not exclude the possibility of coexistent gangrenous cholecystitis, mesenteric infarction, or other intra-abdominal catastrophe.

When diagnostic laparotomy is undertaken, abdominal exploration must be complete and thorough. If uncomplicated acute pancreatitis is found, the choice of surgical procedure should be determined by specific therapeutic goals. If cholelithiasis is present and pancreatitis is very mild, definitive correction of biliary disease usually may be undertaken to prevent subsequent episodes of pancreatitis. However, early biliary surgery does not reduce the morbidity of the acute episode of pancreatitis and it may be hazardous in the presence of severe pancreatitis. If, therefore, severe gallstone pancreatitis is found at diagnostic laparotomy or if the severity of pancreatitis is unclear, it is our present practice to limit biliary surgery to cholecystostomy and cholangiography. There is no evidence that cholecystostomy improves the course of these patients. However, severe pancreatitis is often associated with high fevers and jaundice and the subsequent management is simplified by the presence of established biliary drainage and access to the biliary tree for radiographic study.

Peritoneal lavage appears to ameliorate the early complications of acute pancreatitis and therefore, soft Silastic catheters may be placed into the lesser omental sac and pelvis for postoperative lavage. More extensive procedures such as pancreatic debridement or resection should be avoided at this time. Furthermore, soft rubber or sump drains in the area of the pancreas are, in our experience, associated with a substantially increased incidence of late pancreatic sepsis and should not be placed.

Early Therapeutic Operations

Pancreatic Drainage. Early operative drainage of the pancreas was recommended at the beginning of this century and has recently received renewed attention. A small controlled trial of early sump drainage of the pancreas in patients with severe pancreatitis demonstrated a marked increase in frequency of intra-abdominal sepsis and in severity of respiratory complications in those patients who underwent early operation.

Pancreatic Resection. In 1963, Watts reported survival of a patient with pancreatitis who was treated by pancreatectomy approximately 48 hours after the onset of symptoms. Since that report, there has been extensive interest, especially in Europe, in the possibility that early removal of all or part of the pancreas may decrease the devastating systemic and local sequelae of severe acute pancreatitis. In most reports of pancreatic resection, assessment of the severity of pancreatitis has depended primarily on the interpretation of the operative findings by the surgeon, and those reports therefore have been difficult to evaluate.

Kivilaakso and associates have reported a controlled trial in which early pancreatic resection was compared with formal celiotomy and placement of catheters for postoperative peritoneal lavage. In that study, the mortality following pancreatic resection was 22%, comparing favorably with that following celiotomy and peritoneal lavage, which was 47%. However, this difference did not achieve statistical significance. The average number of positive prognostic signs in the resected patients was only 3.7 (range 2 to 6) and in the lavaged patients 3.9 (range 2 to 7). Thus, a significant number of patients may have been included in this study who had a low risk of life-threatening complications of pancreatitis. The data certainly can be interpreted as favoring pancreatic resection in patients in whom severe pancreatitis is found at celiotomy. An important flaw was the absence of a group of patients who were managed without celiotomy.

This flaw was overcome by a subsequent study by the same group. This study compared early pancreatic resection with nonoperative peritoneal lavage. Only 21 patients were included and although there was no significant difference in overall mortality, three resected patients died (27%) compared to one lavaged patient (10%). The mean period of intensive-care treatment was reduced from 26 days in the resected group to 16 days in the lavage patients, and overall hospital stay was significantly longer with pancreatic resection.

Experimental studies have shown that the mortality among dogs treated by total pancreatectomy 24 hours after induction of pancreatitis is twice as great as that among animals treated by intravenous fluid administration alone. Evaluation of the influence of the timing of resection on survival suggests that mortality is reduced only if resection is carried out with 30 minutes of induction of experimental pancreatitis.

At the present time, formal early pancreatic resection does not appear beneficial compared to nonoperative early management.

Biliary Procedures. In patients with acute pancreatitis associated with gallstones, it has been suggested that early biliary surgery or endoscopic intervention may ameliorate the severity of pancreatic inflammation. Recommendations have included cholecystectomy and endoscopic sphincterotomy.

Evaluation of the efficacy of early biliary intervention has been confused by difficulty in determining the diagnosis and estimating the severity of pancreatitis. Up to 75% of patients with acute abdominal pain, gallstones, and elevated serum amylase levels have no gross evidence of significant pancreatitis at early operation or autopsy. In such patients, early definitive treatment of biliary disease usually may be undertaken safely with prompt subsidence of biliary symptoms. Among patients who have clear evidence of pancreatitis, approximately 80% have mild disease. In this group, early surgery can often be undertaken safely but does not ameliorate the course of pancreatitis. In a controlled clinical trial by Kelly, however, biliary surgery during the initial 48 hours in patients with severe pancreatitis was followed by 82.6% morbidity and 47.8% mortality. If biliary surgery was deferred until signs of pancreatitis had subsided, morbidity fell to 17.8%, and mortality was 11.8%. It is clear, therefore, that early biliary surgery should be avoided, if possible.

Endoscopic retrograde cholangiography and sphincterotomy for extraction of common duct stone has been advocated in recent years. A controlled clinical evaluation of this approach from Hong Kong indicates that it is associated with a significant reduction in biliary complications. Morbidity related to pancreatic inflammation was not reduced significantly. Since endoscopic manipulation of the ampulla of Vater is able to initiate pancreatitis, this approach should be applied cautiously and requires a highly skilled endoscopist.

Debridement of Necrotic Tissue. Beger and his associates have proposed necrosectomy or debridement of necrotic pancreatic and peripancreatic tissue in patients with severe pancreatitis. Debridement was followed by postoperative lavage of the operative field. The timing of surgical intervention varied but was, on average, day 8 of treatment for pancreatitis. Patients were selected by clinical criteria or the finding of significant volumes of nonperfused pancreas on contrast-enhanced computed tomography (CT). The average number of positive prognostic signs (Table 70–2) was 4.5, and overall mortality was 8.1%. Thirty-nine percent of patients had pancreatic infection at the time of surgery, and mortality was 13.8% in this group. Sixty-one percent of patients did not have demonstrated pancreatic infection at surgery, and in this group mortality was 4.4%. It is, at present, impossible to judge how many of this latter group might have survived without intervention. Reported results indicate that this approach requires further evaluation.

It has been our overall experience that early intra-abdominal surgery, whether a biliary procedure, pancreatic drainage, or pancreatic resection, does not ameliorate the morbidity and mortality of acute pancreatitis in any group of patients. Occasionally, operation is followed by a dramatic improvement in cardiovascular function. This improvement is unfortunately greatly outweighed by increased respiratory complications and late pancreatic sepsis.

Peritoneal Lavage. By contrast with formal intra-abdominal operations, peritoneal lavage by catheters introduced percutaneously appears to be associated with immediate clinical improvement without increased respiratory or septic complications.

We consider any patient experiencing a first or second episode of acute pancreatitis and who has three or more positive prognostic signs to be a candidate for lavage. Because bowel distension is common in severe pancreatitis, the lavage catheter should be introduced through an open incision about 4 to 5 cm in length, with direct visualization of the peritoneum to reduce the risk of visceral injury. The incision is placed in the midline below the umbilicus, using full sterile technique and local infiltration anesthesia. In patients with previous abdominal incisions, an area remote from these incisions is selected. Our preferred lavage catheter is a soft but noncollapsible Silastic tubing. The incision is tightly closed about the catheter.

The lavage fluid is an approximately isotonic, balanced electrolyte solution containing 15 gm/L of dextrose (Dianeal). Potassium (4 mmol), heparin (500 USP units), and a broad-spectrum antibiotic usually are added to each liter of lavage fluid. In general, 2 L of fluid are run into the peritoneal cavity under gravity during about 15 minutes, remain intraperitoneally once about 30 minutes, and then are drained out by gravity. This cycle is repeated hourly. Lavage should be instituted during the initial 48 hours of treatment and continued for 48 hours to 7 days, depending upon the clinical course of the patient.

In addition to the risk of visceral injury, there are two important hazards of peritoneal lavage. First, respiratory failure is frequent in severe pancreatitis and adding 2 L of fluid to the peritoneal cavity may lead to significant decrease in ventilation. Respiratory status must, therefore, be closely monitored, and it is often necessary to reduce the volume and timing of the lavage cycle to avoid undue respiratory impairment. Second, the tonicity of the lavage fluid is maintained with glucose. Since impaired glucose tolerance is a feature of severe pancreatitis, serum glucose levels must be measured and insulin administered as needed.

In our own initial studies, the maximum duration of peritoneal lavage was limited to 4 days because of fear that longer lavage would result in an increased risk of intra-abdominal infection. While lavage for periods of 2 to 4 days was associated with dramatic early improvement, overall mortality was not significantly affected because late pancreatic infection was not reduced. A controlled clinical trial of peritoneal lavage by Stone and Fabian, in 1980, confirmed the early improvement in clinical status that we had observed in patients treated by peritoneal lavage. A further multicenter controlled trial, reported by Mayer in 1985, did not demonstrate any change in overall mortality nor in the cause or timing of death.

A chance observation in 1979 led to a further study of the duration of peritoneal lavage, which was reported in 1990. At that time, we reported a prospective controlled clinical trial that compared 15 patients who underwent peritoneal lavage for periods of 2 days with 14 patients who underwent peritoneal lavage for a period of 7 days. All patients had three or more positive prognostic signs. As shown in Table 70–5, there was a striking reduction in the incidence of pancreatic infection and of death from this cause. Fig 70–3 shows our overall experience with patients who had three or more positive prognostic signs and who were managed initially by nonoperative measures. In this analysis, 20 patients managed by long (7 day) lavage were compared to 16 short-lavage (2 days) patients combined with previously reported patients who received nonoperative lavage for 2 to 4 days (17 patients) or were managed by nonoperative measures without lavage (58 patients). The patients who died within the first few days of treatment without developing sepsis are not included.

The overall frequency of pancreatic sepsis in the two groups is approximately equal, although deaths from sepsis were reduced from 13% to 5% by long lavage. These findings are, however, related to the relatively

TABLE 70–5. INCIDENCE OF PANCREATIC INFECTION AND DEATH AFTER LAVAGE

	STUDY GROUP RESULTS		
	Positive Prognosis Signs		
	>3	3–4	>5 Signs
LONG LAVAGE (7 DAYS)			
Patients	14	4	10
Deaths	2 (14%)	0	2 (20%)
Abscess	3 (21%)	0	3 (30%)
Abscess death	0	0	0 [a]
SHORT LAVAGE (2 DAYS)			
Patients	15	8	7
Deaths	3 (20%)	0	3 (43%)
Abscess	6 (40%)	2 (25%)	4 (57%)
Abscess death	3 (20%)	0	3 (43%)[a]

[a]$P = .051$

small number of long-lavage patients with only three or four positive signs. In the three or four sign group, long lavage reduced the incidence of sepsis and death from sepsis from 13% and 5%, respectively, to 0%. In patients with five or more positive prognostic signs, long lavage reduced the incidence of sepsis from 40% to 27% ($P = 0.03$) and of death from this cause from 30% to 7% ($P = 0.08$).

Studies of peritoneal lavage in the treatment of pancreatitis in dogs, guinea pigs, and rats have shown immediate improvement and reduced mortality. It is not clear why prolonged lavage reduces late pancreatic in-

LONG LAVAGE (LL) vs. ALL OTHER NONOPERATIVE TREATMENT (OT)

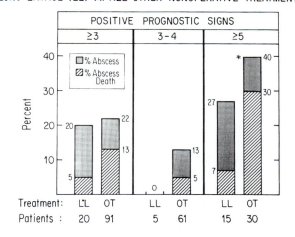

Figure 70–3. The incidence of pancreatic sepsis and death from pancreatic sepsis in patients treated by 7 day lavage compared to all other nonoperative treatments. (From Ranson JHC, Berman RS. Long peritoneal lavage decreases pancreatic sepsis in acute pancreatitis. *Ann Surg* 1990;211:708–716)

fection. However, lavage is reported to have reduced necrosis of the pancreas and peripancreatic fat, in some experimental studies.

In our initial studies, peritoneal lavage was usually associated with a marked improvement in the early systemic manifestations of severe pancreatitis. In non-lavaged patients, approximately 40 percent of all deaths occur during the first 10 days of treatment and are primarily due to respiratory and cardiovascular failure. Peritoneal lavage has been an extremely effective adjunct to the management of these complications and has been associated with almost complete prevention of early deaths.

It is usually presumed that the efficacy of lavage is due to removal of toxic factors present in the peritoneal exudate rather than to improvement in fluid and electrolyte status or removal of dialyzable substances from the blood. However, attempts to remove toxic substances by plasma pheresis or by hemofiltration have also been promising in preliminary reports.

OPERATIVE MANAGEMENT OF LOCAL COMPLICATIONS

The most common local sequelae of acute pancreatitis are paralytic ileus, acute sterile peripancreatic fluid collection, and duodenal or biliary obstruction. These complications usually resolve as pancreatitis subsides, and they rarely require specific treatment. Chronic pseudocysts occur in approximately 1% of patients.

Fluid collections seen on ultrasound or CT are common following acute pancreatitis. Most of these resolve without specific treatment. If they are asymptomatic and not increasing in size, no form of intervention usually is required.

A mature pseudocyst with an identifiable fibrous wall may, if symptomatic, require drainage. This may be accomplished either by percutaneous catheter placement or by operation. If surgery is undertaken and the cyst walls are not well established, or if substantial amounts of necrotic material are present, treatment should be by debridement and external operative drainage. Uncomplicated mature cysts are well treated surgically by cystgastrostomy or cystduodenostomy, if the stomach or duodenum form part of the cyst wall. Other cysts may be drained into a defunctionated jejunal loop.

Percutaneous catheter drainage of pseudocysts under radiologic control has been reported. The population in whom this technique has been applied is not always clearly defined and the relative morbidity in terms of fistula and infection remains unclear.

The most common local complication that requires surgical treatment is the development of infection in peripancreatic fluid and devitalized tissues.

■ INFECTED PANCREATIC NECROSIS

INCIDENCE

Pancreatic infection occurs in up to 9% of patients but the frequency is related to the severity of the underlying pancreatitis. It occurs in 2.7% of patients with less than three positive early prognostic signs and in 34% of those with more severe disease. Pancreatic sepsis occurs in 3.6% or 6.6% of patients with alcoholic- or gallstone-associated pancreatitis and in 14.8% of those with other etiologies. It is much more common in patients in whom postoperative pancreatitis is diagnosed, occurring in 39% of this group. Finally, pancreatic infection is increased in patients who undergo early laparotomy and should be anticipated in this group.

CLINICAL DIAGNOSIS

Peripancreatic sepsis may occur at any time during the course of acute pancreatitis, but it is most commonly recognized after the first 2 weeks of treatment. The clinical and laboratory features are listed in Table 70–6. The cardinal clinical features are persistent or recurrent fever and leukocytosis, usually with abdominal distension and a palpable mass after 14 to 21 days of treatment. The occurrence of positive blood cultures without another source is also strong evidence for pancreatic infection.

RADIOGRAPHIC DIAGNOSIS

Plain radiographic examination of the abdomen is rarely helpful in the diagnosis of pancreatic infection. However, when contrast studies of the upper gastrointestinal tract are possible, they demonstrate displacement of the stomach or duodenum in 76% of cases. Unfortunately, similar displacement may occur secondary to uninfected peripancreatic fluid or pancreatic enlargement. Radiographic demonstration of gas outside the gastrointestinal tract provides clear evi-

TABLE 70–6. PERCENT INCIDENCE OF CLINICAL AND LABORATORY FEATURES IN PATIENTS WITH INFECTED PANCREATIC NECROSIS

Fever >101°F	100
Abdominal distension	94
Abdominal mass	71
Hypotension (BP <90 mm Hg)	39
Pneumonia or effusion	89
Renal failure	39
Coma	28
Elevated serum amylase	28
Leukocytosis (>10,000/mm^3)	78

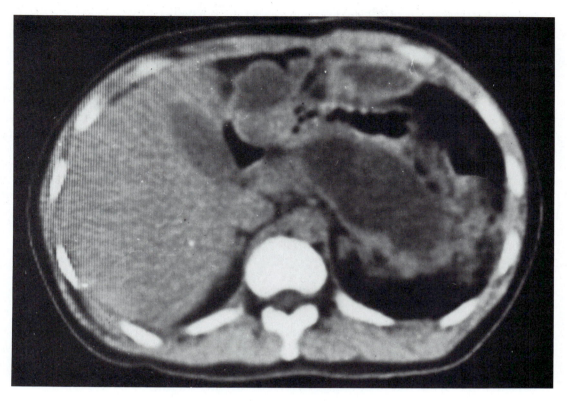

Figure 70–4. CT scan showing an abscess involving the pancreatic tail. (From Ranson JHC. Necrosis and abscess. In: Bradley E (ed), *Complications of Pancreatitis.* Philadelphia, PA: WB Saunders; 1982:83)

dence of sepsis and was documented in 16% of our patients.

Abdominal ultrasonography has, in our experience, been of limited value in the diagnosis of pancreatic infection, possibly because of the presence of marked intestinal gaseous distension in these patients. CT has been far more accurate, demonstrating a peripancreatic fluid collection in 85% of our patients (Fig 70–4).

It should be emphasized, however, that approximately 50% of fluid collections identified on CT early in pancreatitis resolve without any specific therapy. Hence, demonstration of fluid collection is not by itself an indication of infection. If gas is identified within the peripancreatic retroperitoneum, this finding indicates infection and the need for drainage, in most patients.

Because of the difficulty in evaluating possible infection, percutaneous aspiration of the pancreas under CT guidance with gram stain and culture has been described as a means for the evaluation of pancreatic inflammatory masses. Experience with this diagnostic approach is encouraging and advocates report that this step leads to earlier drainage in patients with infection, while avoiding intervention in those with sterile pancreatitis.

TREATMENT

As indicated in Table 70–6 patients with pancreatic sepsis are usually critically ill. This is owing not only to the infection but also to the fact that infection occurs in patients with severe underlying pancreatitis. Supportive management must therefore be vigorous. This includes antibiotic administration, as indicated by operative and drain cultures, and meticulous attention to respiratory care, nutritional support, and prevention of gastrointestinal hemorrhage. The most essential feature of treatment is, however, to provide adequate drainage of the infection.

Percutaneous drainage by catheters placed under radiographic control has been described. In most cases, however, contents of the abscess include semisolid infected tissue that cannot be evacuated except by surgical debridement and placement of large drains.

Since these patients are severely ill, there is a tendency to limit the surgical procedure to identification of the most obvious abscess and provision of external drainage. Full exploration and thorough debridement of necrotic material is, however, required.

The approach we have favored for debridement of

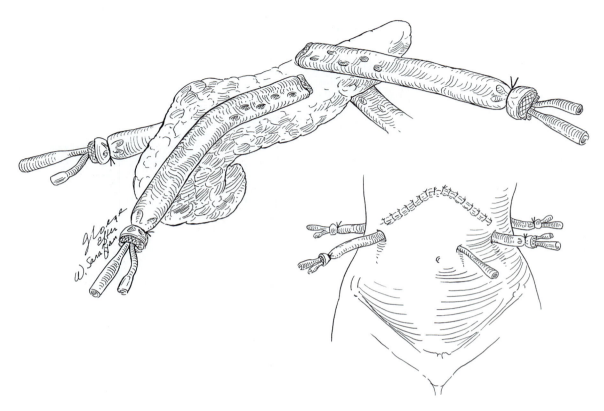

Figure 70–5. The technique of wide sump drainage of the peripancreatic retroperitoneum in patients with infected pancreatic abscess. (From Ranson JHC. Necrosis and abscess. In: Bradley E (ed), *Complications of Pancreatitis.* Philadelphia, PA: WB Saunders; 1982:88)

infected pancreatic necrosis is illustrated in Fig 70–5. It involves systematic exploration of the whole peripancreatic retroperitoneum and the institution of prolonged sump drainage. The patient is placed supine, with the left side elevated approximately 15 degrees. The arms are widely abducted to allow exposure of the flanks. A long, bilateral subcostal incision is made from the anterior axillary line on the right to the midaxillary line on the left. The lesser omental sac is opened widely by dividing the gastrocolic omentum, and the entire anterior surface of the pancreas is explored, including the pancreatic head. Fat overlying the pancreas may appear remarkably normal, and it should be opened to expose the pancreas itself. The duodenum is mobilized anteriorly, and the area posterior to the pancreatic tail is explored by dissection carried posteriorly at the inferior margin of the distal one-third of the pancreas. The areas posterior to the ascending and descending colon and the root of the small bowel mesentery are examined closely. As much necrotic material as possible is debrided. Penrose and soft sump drains are placed anterior and posterior to the head, body, and tail of the pancreas. We have used a sump catheter (Fig 70–6).

Continuous irrigation and suction of the drains is maintained in the postoperative period.

We have treated 36 patients with infected necrosis by radical debridement and sump drainage during a recent period. Hospital mortality was 13.9%, and 58.3% of patients required only one operative procedure.

An alternative surgical approach has been to debride and pack the pancreatic bed. The essential features of this approach, as advocated by Bradley, are to debride necrotic tissue and cover the viscera with nonadherent porous gauze followed by packing of the wound with moist laparotomy pads. The dressings are changed under general anesthesia every 2 or 3 days until sufficient granulation has formed to permit changes on the ward. Redebridement is carried out at each dressing change. A mortality rate of 10.7% has been achieved with this approach in 28 patients reported by Bradley in 1987. Since this method of treatment is not necessary in every patient and is associated with the morbidity of repeated anesthesia and the risk of bleeding and intestinal fistulas, we have not accepted it as a routine approach. It does have the advantage that a required debridement can not be deferred.

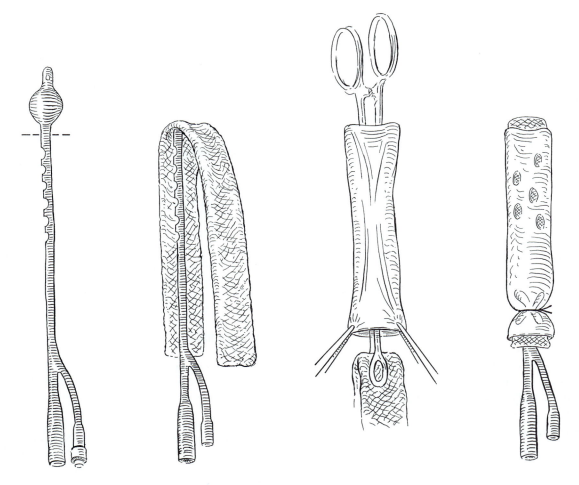

Figure 70–6. Method of construction of a large soft catheter used for drainage of pancreatic abscesses. A 24 Foley catheter is covered by two to three layers of sympathectomy packing and placed in a 1 1/2 inch Penrose drain. (From Ranson JHC. Necrosis and abscess. In: Bradley E (ed), *Complications of Pancreatitis.* Philadelphia, PA: WB Saunders; 1982:89)

OTHER LOCAL COMPLICATIONS

Severe peripancreatic necrosis may extend to involve the colon and small bowel. Colonic necrosis is best treated by resection of the involved bowel, with colostomy and mucous fistula formation. Massive hemorrhage may occur because of necrosis of major blood vessels or their erosion by drains placed during drainage of pancreatic abscesses. Bleeding may be extremely rapid; however, immediate surgical intervention will usually lead to control. Angiography and embolisation may be valuable in some cases of bleeding.

PROTRACTED PANCREATITIS

In a small group of patients, acute pancreatitis does not subside completely with nonoperative management. These patients usually do not have evidence of severe pancreatitis and respond well initially to nonoperative measures. When attempts are made to reintroduce oral feedings, however, pain, fever, and hyperamylasemia recur. These findings resolve with the reintroduction of nasogastric suction but recur when oral feedings are reinstituted. When this course repeats itself over several weeks, a mechanical local cause must be sought, by exploratory operation if necessary. The most common cause, in our experience, has been biliary calculi that were too small to visualize with current cholangiographic techniques. Small pseudocysts or pancreatic ductal obstruction also may cause this clinical picture. It should be emphasized that this group forms <2% of patients.

■ PREVENTION OF RECURRENT PANCREATITIS

In patients who survive one episode of acute pancreatitis, every effort must be made to prevent recurrent disease. This involves the identification and correction of remediable etiologic associations such as hyperlipoproteinemia or cholelithiasis. Patients in whom gallstones are demonstrated radiographically traditionally have been advised to wait 4 to 6 weeks before undergoing correction of cholelithiasis. For most patients, this delay is unnecessary and exposes them to the risk of recurring bouts of pancreatitis. There is no evidence that the risk of definitive biliary surgery is increased once acute pancreatitis has subsided. It is, therefore, our usual practice to correct cholelithiasis during the same hospitalization as soon as signs of pancreatitis have subsided. In the occasional patient who has a large pancreatic phlegmon, it is advisable to postpone surgery for a further period.

TABLE 70–7. SUMMARY OF CURRENT MANAGEMENT OF ACUTE PANCREATITIS

ALL PATIENTS:
- Nasogastric suction
- No oral feedings until pancreatitis subsides
- Monitoring and maintenance of intravascular volume
- Respiratory monitoring and support: measure Po_2, diuretics, PEEP
- Antibiotics (selective)
- Early laparotomy: only for diagnosis
- Estimate prognosis by early signs

IF 3 OR MORE POSITIVE PROGNOSTIC SIGNS:
- Peritoneal lavage
- Nutritional support
- Suspect and treat pancreatic sepsis
- Late heparin (after 14 days) if hypercoagulable

PEEP = Positive end-expiratory pressure.

■ CURRENT MANAGEMENT

The major features of our current treatment of patients with acute pancreatitis are summarized in Table 70–7. Since no single therapeutic measure has been clearly demonstrated to limit the severity of pancreatitis itself, management is directed primarily at avoiding pancreatic stimulation and support of the patient. Nonetheless, the approach described is associated with an overall survival of 95%.

SELECTED READINGS

Acosta JM, Pellegrini CA, et al. Etiology and pathogenesis of acute biliary pancreatitis. *Surgery* 1980;88:118–125

Balldin G, Ohlsson K. Demonstration of pancreatic protease-antiprotease complexes in the peritoneal fluid of patients with acute pancreatitis. *Surgery* 1979;85:451

Beger HG, Buchler M, Bittner R, et al. Necrosectomy and postoperative local lavage in patients with necrotizing pancreatitis: results of a prospective clinical trial. *World J Surg* 1988;12:255–62

Bradley EL (ed). *Complications of Pancreatitis.* Philadelphia, PA: WB Saunders; 1982

Bradley EL, Murphy F, Ferguson C. Prediction of pancreatic necrosis by dynamic pancreatography. *Ann Surg* 1990; 210:495–503

Coppa GF, LeFleur R, Ranson JHC. The role of Chiba-needle cholangiography in the diagnosis of possible acute pancreatitis with cholelithiasis. *Ann Surg* 1981;193;393–398

Corfield AP, Williamson RCN, McMahon MJ, et al. Prediction of severity in acute pancreatitis: prospective comparison of three prognostic indices. *Lancet* 1985;403–407

Fan S-T, Lai ECS, Mok FPT, et al. Early treatment of acute biliary pancreatitis by endoscopic papillotomy. *N Engl J Med* 1993;328:228–232

Gerzoff SG, Banks PA, Robbins AH, et al. Early diagnosis of pancreatic infection by computed tomography-guided aspiration. *Gastroenterology* 1987;93:1315–1320

Imrie CW, Fergus JC, Murphy D, Blumgart LH. Arterial hypoxia in acute pancreatitis. *Br J Surg* 1977;64:185–188

Imrie CW, Whyte AS. A prospective study of acute pancreatitis. *Br J Surg* 1975;62:490

Kelly TR, Wagner DS. Gallstone pancreatitis: a prospective randomized trial of the timing of surgery. *Surgery* 1988;104:600–605

Kivilaakso E, Lempinen M, Makelainen A, et al. Pancreatic resection versus peritoneal lavation for acute fulminant pancreatitis. *Ann Surg* 1984;199:426–431

Kivilaakso E, Fraki O, Nikki P, Lempinen M. Resection of the pancreas for acute fulminant pancreatitis. *Surg Gynecol Obstet* 1981;151:493–8

Mayer DA, McMahon MJ, Corfield AP, et al. Controlled clinical trial of peritoneal lavage for the treatment of severe acute pancreatitis. *N Eng J Med* 1985;312:399–404

McMahon MJ, Playforth MJ, Pickforth IR. A comparative study of methods for the prediction of severity of attacks of acute pancreatitis. *Br J Surg* 1980;67:22–25

Ranson JHC, Spencer FC. The role of peritoneal lavage in severe acute pancreatitis. *Ann Surg* 1978;187:565–575

Ranson JHC: Acute pancreatitis. *Curr Probl Surg* 1979;16:1

Ranson JHC, Balthazar E, Caccavale R, Cooper M: Computed tomography and the prediction of pancreatic abscess in acute pancreatitis. *Ann Surg* 1985;201:656–663

Ranson JHC, Berman RS. Long peritoneal lavage decreases pancreatic sepsis in acute pancreatitis. *Ann Surg* 1990;211:708–716

Sarles H. Chronic calcifying pancreatitis—chronic alcoholic pancreatitis. *Gastroenterology* 1974;66:604–616

Schroeder T, Sainio V, Kivisaari L, et al. Pancreatic resection versus peritoneal lavage in acute necrotizing pancreatitis. *Ann Surg* 1991;214:663–666

Stone HH, Fabian TC. Peritoneal dialysis in the treatment of acute alcoholic pancreatitis. *Surg Gynecol Obstet* 1980;150:878–882

Stone HH, Fabian TC, Dunlop WE. Gallstone pancreatitis: biliary tract pathology in relation to time of operation. *Ann Surg* 1981;194:305–312

Warshaw AL, Imbembo AL, Civetta JM, Dag WM. Surgical intervention in acute necrotizing pancreatitis. *Am J Surg* 1974;127:484–490

Wilson C, Heath DI, Imrie CW. Prediction of outcome in acute pancreatitis: a comparative study of APACHE II, clinical assessment and multiple factor scoring systems. *Br J Surg* 1990;77:1260–1264

71

Pancreatic Cysts, Pseudocysts, and Fistulas

Andrew L. Warshaw ▪ *Carlos Fernández-del Castillo* ▪ *David W. Rattner*

Hidden by its retroperitoneal location, the pancreas has, in the past, been a somewhat mysterious organ. The rapid development of noninvasive imaging techniques has led to a much better understanding of pancreatic disease and pathology. This has generated new enthusiasm and widespread interest in pancreatic diseases. Many small lesions, previously concealed by the relative inaccessibility of the pancreas, are now detected, occasionally in asymptomatic patients. Cysts of the pancreas, once considered rare, are now recognized with increasing frequency (Table 71–1).

The common pancreatic cysts are of two types: true cysts lined by epithelial cells and encapsulated fluid collections consequent to pancreatitis (ie, pseudocysts). The tendency to assume that a cystic lesion of the pancreas is a pseudocyst is all too prevalent but should be condemned. The failure to recognize a cystic neoplasm, mistreating it as a pseudocyst, can have disastrous consequences. On the other hand, some true cysts are benign and of little clinical consequence. If they can be diagnosed preoperatively, unnecessary surgical procedures may be avoided. In some parts of the world, hydatid (echinococcal) cysts occur with greater frequency and must be considered in the practical differential diagnosis.

A better understanding of the natural history of inflammatory masses (phlegmons) and fluid collections accompanying acute pancreatitis also has been acquired. A spectrum of changes, including peripancreatic effusions, acute pseudocysts, and pancreatic necrosis, can now be differentiated. The ability to study these lesions noninvasively at multiple points in time has allowed the distinction between acute and chronic pseudocysts, two seemingly similar entities with quite different natural histories and treatment requirements. Endoscopic retrograde pancreatography (ERCP) has been critical in the improved understanding and operative results achieved in the treatment of many pancreatic diseases. In perhaps no instance is ERCP more valuable than in planning treatment of pancreatic fistulas. Since pancreatic fistulas are essentially noncontained variants of pseudocysts, their management will also be discussed in this chapter.

■ CONGENITAL TRUE PANCREATIC CYSTS

SOLITARY CYSTS

Solitary true pancreatic cysts are extremely rare, with only 10 cases reported in the literature. Congenital cysts are believed to result from anomalous development of the pancreatic ducts. Persistence or sequestration of primitive ducts during organogenesis may give rise to isolated nests of ductal epithelium that secrete fluid to create a cyst. Grossly, the cysts usually are enclosed in a thin fibrous capsule and are filled with mucoid or serous fluid.

TABLE 71–1. CYSTIC LESIONS OF THE PANCREAS

I.	CONGENITAL	IV.	NEOPLASTIC
	Cystic fibrosis		Serous cystadenoma
	Polycystic disease		Mucinous cystic neoplasm
	Enteric duplication		(cystadenoma-cystadeno-
	Intrapancreatic choledochal cyst		carcinoma)
	Simple (dysgenic) cyst		Mucinous ductal ectasia
			Papillary cystic tumor
II.	PSEUDOCYSTS		Cystic islet cell tumor
	Postinflammatory		Acinar cystadenocarcinoma
	Posttraumatic		Cystic teratoma
	Associated with tumor necrosis		Lymphangioma
			Hemangioma
			Paraganglioma
III.	RETENTION	V.	PARASITIC
	Chronic pancreatitis		*Echinococcus*
	Pancreatic cancer		Amoebic
	Ascariasis		Cysticercosis
	Clonorchis sinensis		

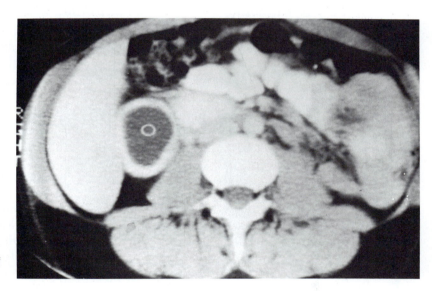

Figure 71–1. CT scan of a patient with a congenital cyst (*marker*) of the head of the pancreas. The cyst has a thick wall.

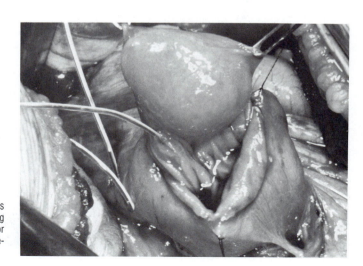

Figure 71–2. Intraoperative photograph of a congenital cyst of the head of the pancreas (same patient as in Fig 71–1). The cyst, pedunculated within the duodenal lumen, is being withdrawn from the opened duodenum. A catheter has been placed through the major papilla, which is adjacent. The cyst, which communicated with the pancreatic duct, was resected. The patient's recurrent pancreatitis was cured.

The cysts are lined by a smooth glistening membrane. Conclusive identification of a particular cyst as congenital sometimes can be difficult. An intact epithelial lining, the sine qua non for congenital cysts, may show preservation of squamous or low columnar epithelium or may not be seen because of obliteration by infection or inflammation. The cyst fluid need not be rich in amylase because communication with acinar tissue may be interrupted during development or by inflammation.

A true congenital cyst generally presents in infancy as an abdominal mass. Symptoms may be produced by compression of the duodenum, stomach, or bile duct. Physical examination, upper gastrointestinal series, and ultrasound examinations can aid in diagnosis. Because of their symptomatic nature, solitary congenital cysts should be completely excised, when possible. Lesions in the head of the pancreas can be drained into the duodenum or intestine as long as the surgeon can exclude the possibility that the cyst is neoplastic.

Unilocular serous cysts in adults now are thought more likely to be serous cystadenomas rather than simple congenital or dysgenic cysts. Resection is preferred for symptomatic and indeterminate cysts.

ENTEROGENOUS CYSTS

Enteric duplication cysts are common throughout the gastrointestinal tract; only two cases have been reported in the pancreas, however. These cysts contain both smooth muscle and an epithelial lining. In contrast to simple cysts, the two reported cases have occurred in adults. It is not possible to differentiate these cysts from neoplastic lesions preoperatively. Therefore, the optimal treatment is complete cyst excision (Figs 71–1, 71–2, and 71–3).

DERMOID CYSTS

Dermoid cysts (also known as cystic teratomas) of the pancreas also have been reported and contain the usual epidermal elements. Again complete excision is the treatment of choice.

MULTIPLE CONGENITAL PANCREATIC CYSTS

Multiple congenital pancreatic cysts generally occur in conjunction with cysts of the kidney, liver, lungs, or central nervous system. Many of these patients die in the neonatal period. Fifty percent of patients with von Hippel-Lindau syndrome (cerebellar and retinal hemangioblastoma) have multiple pancreatic cysts, at least some of which are serous cystadenomas. Polycystic kidney disease, which may present in adolescence or adulthood, also is associated with cysts of the liver and pancreas. The pancreatic cysts in these conditions are generally <5 cm and are lined by cuboidal epithelium. They are rarely problematic and almost never require surgical treatment.

FIBROCYSTIC DISEASE OF THE PANCREAS

Cystic fibrosis is the most common lethal genetic disease in Caucasians, estimated to occur in 1 of 2000 live births. The disease is the most common cause of pancreatic insufficiency in children and was initially thought to involve only the exocrine pancreas. Although the basic defect in cystic fibrosis has not been identified, pancreatic secretion is markedly diminished. The pathologic changes in the pancreas resemble chronic pancreatitis with fibrosis, loss of pancreatic parenchyma, and multiple cystic spaces filled with inspissated secretions. Recurrent pancreatitis is seen in cystic fibrosis patients who have not

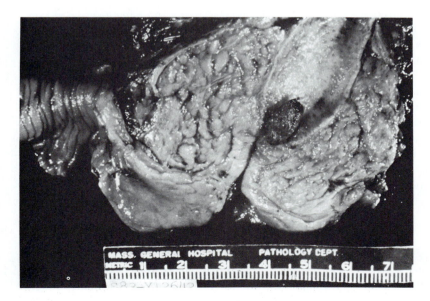

Figure 71–3. Intrapancreatic duplication cyst. The patient, a 16 year–old girl, presented with unremitting pancreatitis. She was cured by pancreaticoduodenectomy. Note the concretion in the cyst cavity.

yet developed signs of pancreatic insufficiency. This is presumably owing to obstruction of the pancreatic duct by viscous secretions. Surgical intervention for complications of acute pancreatitis in these children is rarely needed.

■ ACQUIRED TRUE PANCREATIC CYSTS (RETENTION CYSTS)

Retention cysts of the pancreas are associated with diseases that lead to chronic obstruction of the pancreatic ducts, such as chronic pancreatitis or pancreatic carcinoma. These epithelial-lined cysts are formed by progressive dilatation of pancreatic ducts proximal to an obstruction. Sarles found that one-fourth of his patients with chronic calcific pancreatitis had what he called retention cysts. Clinically, these cysts are virtually impossible to distinguish from chronic pancreatic pseudocysts. Since presentation and treatment requirements are identical, the management of retention cysts is considered in the subsequent section on pseudocysts.

■ NEOPLASTIC CYSTS

Neoplastic cysts of the pancreas are estimated to account for at least 10% of pancreatic cysts. The prevalence may be increasing owing to the serendipitous finding of asymptomatic lesions in patients being imaged for other purposes. These cysts always have an epithelial lining and never resolve spontaneously. In the past, cystic tumors of the pancreas were considered as a group, without distinguishing subtypes, and thus the understanding of their biology, behavior, and malignant potential was confused. The current classification of these lesions, based on the original work of Compagno and Oertel, clearly defines neoplasms of different biology and with different treatment imperatives.

The most common group of cystic neoplasms are the mucinous family, benign and malignant. Next in frequency are the serous cystadenomas, often called microcystic adenomas because of the numerous small locules that characterize their morphology. These are almost invariably benign. Papillary cystic epithelial neoplasms are low-grade malignancies found primarily in young women. Other rare cystic neoplasms include lymphangioma, hemangioma, angiosarcoma, rapidly growing ductal adenocarcinoma with central necrosis, and cystic neuroendocrine tumors.

SEROUS CYSTADENOMA

Although only 400 cases of serous (microcystic) cystadenoma have been reported in the literature, there has been an increased recognition of this lesion in recent years. They comprise 27% and 18%, respectively, of the cystic tumors reported from the Massachusetts General and Johns Hopkins Hospitals. Serous cystadenomas are seen almost exclusively after 35 years of age and 82% occur after 60 years of age. There is a strong female predominance with a sex ratio of 2:1. These tumors occur in association with extrapancreatic neoplasms in up to 20% of patients. A predisposition to formation of serous cystadenomas may be present in von Hippel-Lindau syndrome (8 of 15 patients in the original report had cystadenomas).

The most common presenting symptom is vague abdominal pain. Back pain also may be present. Adenomas in the head of the gland may compress the common bile duct, causing jaundice in as many as 10% of patients. Compression of the pancreatic duct causes pancreatitis in >5%. The gradual onset of abdominal pain and weight loss may mimic the presentation of pancreatic adenocarcinoma. Compression of the duodenum and stomach may produce symptoms of partial gastric outlet obstruction. A palpable epigastric mass is present in nearly two-thirds of patients. However, nearly one-third of microcystic adenomas produce no symptoms and may be discovered radiologically, at laparotomy, or at autopsy as incidental findings.

Serous cystadenomas are generally solitary lesions, although rarely, multiple cysts may be present. Many are located in the head of the pancreas. Serous cystadenomas average 7 cm in diameter, with ranges from 1 to 25 cm reported. The tumors are generally spherical or ovoid with a smooth glistening surface. On cut section, most are composed of multiple smaller cysts containing clear fluid that gives the tumor a honeycombed appearance (Fig 71–4). Microscopically, one sees multiple cystic spaces lined by cuboidal epithelium. The cytoplasm in these cells is rich in glycogen. Mucin is not present. Intermediate varieties of cystadenomas with features of both microcystic adenoma and mucinous cystadenomas occasionally are encountered, making diagnosis less definitive than currently stated in the literature. In these instances, it is hard to exclude malignancy. True microcystic adenomas, however, are almost always benign lesions. Although they may become densely adherent to adjacent organs, malignant transformation, that is serous cystadenocarcinoma or metastases, has been reported only twice.

MUCINOUS CYSTIC NEOPLASMS

Like serous cystadenomas, mucinous cystadenomas occur more frequently in females (4:1) although at a slightly younger age. The mean age in Compagno's series was 48 years and 59 years at the Massachusetts General Hospital. Women tend to present almost 20 years younger than males (47 yrs vs 66 yrs). Mucinous cystic

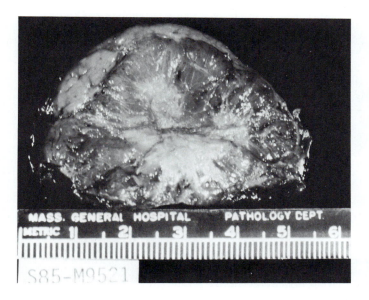

Figure 71–4. Microcystic serous cystadenoma of the head of the pancreas, resected by pancreaticoduodenectomy. The tumor has a honeycomb appearance.

neoplasms are not associated with extrapancreatic neoplasms. These lesions are symptomatic in the majority of cases, particularly when malignant transformation has occurred. Most patients present with abdominal pain. Weight loss is present in 40% and is more commonly seen with carcinoma. An abdominal mass is palpable in 60% to 75% of patients, and jaundice or symptoms of partial gut obstruction can be produced by compression or invasion of adjacent organs. These tumors are most commonly located in the body and tail of the pancreas. The average diameter is 6 cm (Fig 71–5). The external surface is often smooth and glistening with large vessels commonly coursing over the outside of the cyst, but some are densely adherent to surrounding structures. On cut section, they are either unilocular or multilocular and contain mucoid fluid. The internal lining frequently has papillary projections and the cyst wall tends to be thick and fibrous. Microscopically, these cysts are lined by columnar epithelium containing mucin-rich goblet cells.

All mucinous cystic neoplasms are potentially malignant. The larger the lesion the more likely it is to be a carcinoma. While normal epithelium may be present in some sections of the cyst wall, extensive histologic sectioning frequently will identify foci of carcinoma. Eighty percent of these cysts contain either obviously atypical epithelium or frank carcinoma. In Compagno's series, the only cysts containing solely benign epithelium were either very small or incidentally discovered at autopsy. The variability of the epithelium and the consequent uncertainty of whether a given mucinous tumor is truly benign, borderline, or early malignancy has given rise to the new usage of the term mucinous cystic neoplasm instead of mucinous cystadenoma.

It is commonly taught that cystic tumors are slow growing and easily cured. They may, in fact, remain indolent for many years, but mucinous cystic neoplasm are capable of sudden transformation into a high-grade, aggressive, rapidly progressing mucinous cystadenocarcinoma, without warning. This transformation coincides with the appearance of increased mitoses, pseudostratification of the epithelium, cytologic atypia, and genetic changes expressing the tumor antigens CA72-4 and CA15-3, and overexpression of the epidermal growth factor receptor (EGFR). Once they reach this phase, life expectancy is short, and survival parallels that of the more common ductal adenocarcinoma of the pancreas.

MUCINOUS DUCTAL ECTASIA

In recent years a new category of mucin-producing pancreatic tumor has been distinguished from the mucinous cystic neoplasm, which it resembles in some respects. This entity has been called ductectatic mucinous cystadenoma, intraductal mucin-secretory neoplasm, and mucinous ductal ectasia, among other apellations. In contrast to mucinous cystic neoplasms, which are related to peripheral ducts, mucinous ductal ectasia involves the main pancreatic duct, usually in the head of the gland. It is characterized by dilation and filling of the main pancreatic duct and its side branches with thick, viscid mucus (Fig 71–6).

The hyperplastic epithelium of the duct is arranged in papillary projections, probably similar to those lesions called intraductal papillomas or papillary adenomas and a precursor to papillary carcinoma of the pancreas. The epithelium may range from a normal ap-

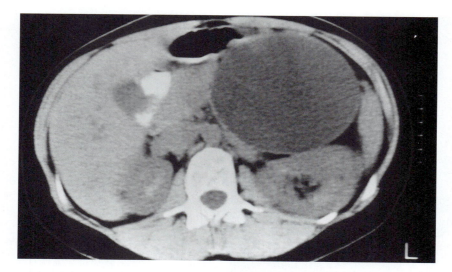

Figure 71–5. CT scan showing a unilocular mucinous cystadenoma of the pancreas. The radiographic characteristics may be indistinguishable from those of a cystadenocarcinoma or a pseudocyst.

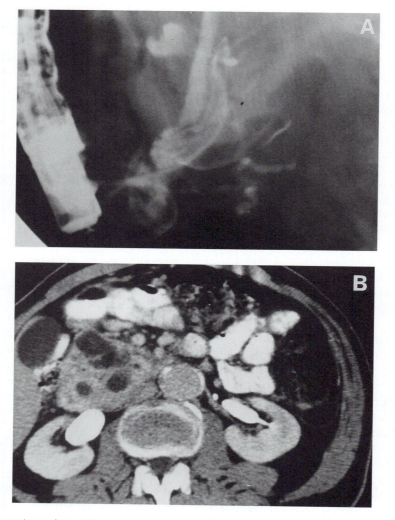

Figure 71–6. A. Endoscopic pancreatogram demonstrating the dilated pancreatic duct filled with viscid mucus in the head of the gland. **B.** CT scan showing the cystic dilatation of the pancreatic ducts.

pearance, through severe atypia and carcinoma in-situ, to infiltrating carcinoma. Characteristically, the tumor grows along the duct before invading the parenchyma, but invasion of the duodenum and bile ducts, as well as lymph node metastases, has been recorded.

Patients often present with recurrent acute pancreatitis or symptoms that mimic chronic pancreatitis, including steatorrhea and diabetes. The pathogenesis relates to ductal obstruction caused by inspissated mucus. The striking finding on endoscopic examination is that of mucus extruding from a patulous ampulla. Computed tomography (CT) shows dilation of the main pancreatic duct in the tail and clusters of cysts (mucus-filled ducts) in the head of the pancreas.

PAPILLARY CYSTIC NEOPLASM

Papillary cystic neoplasm, also synonymously known as "solid and cystic tumor" and "solid and papillary neoplasm of the pancreas," was first described in 1970 by Hamoudi. Since then more than 50 cases have been reported in the English literature and another 60 from Japan. This is almost exclusively a disease of young women; 95% of the cases thus far reported have been in women with a mean age of 23 years, and 85% fall between 15 and 35 years. These patients present with either an abdominal mass and/or with abdominal pain. The diagnosis is usually not suspected until the time of laparotomy when a large, partially cystic mass originating from the pancreas is encountered. The tumors are highly vascular. Bombi reported a case that presented with spontaneous intra-abdominal hemorrhage and the only reported operative mortality occurred from exsanguination following attempted biopsy of the neoplasm wall.

These tumors have a distinctive gross and microscopic appearance. They are typically encapsulated hemorrhagic masses with areas of necrosis. The cystic component can predominate or be minor. Microscopically, they are composed of solid and papillary epithelium, and microcysts with little mitotic activity. The monomorphic features of the solid areas closely resemble neuroendocrine tumors, with which they can be confused easily, especially on frozen section. Invasion of the cyst capsule is common, but invasion of adjacent tissue or metastases are not. Nonetheless the tumor has definite malignant potential and Warren has reported a case with liver metastases.

CYSTIC ISLET-CELL TUMORS

Endocrine (islet-cell) tumors of the pancreas are usually solid but rarely may undergo cystic degeneration and, thus, have to be differentiated from other pancreatic cystic neoplasms. Most will be nonfunctioning, but we have seen a functioning cystic insulinoma with very high insulin concentrations in the cyst fluid. Cystic islet cell tumors are nonetheless distinct from the other pancreatic cystic neoplasms that often contain prominent neuroendocrine elements. One-third of the reported cystic islet-cell tumors have been considered malignant, but long-term survival has been described even in the presence of distant metastases.

OTHER CYSTIC TUMORS OF THE PANCREAS

Ductal adenocarcinoma may undergo degeneration and cyst formation or induce formation of a pseudocyst by duct obstruction. Although this has been uncommon in our experience, 6 of 50 cystic tumors reported by Talamini from John Hopkins were pseudocysts associated with adenocarcinoma.

Other tumors that may have cystic components or a cystic appearance on scans include acinar cell carcinoma, paraganglioma, hemangioma, and lymphangioma.

DIAGNOSIS AND TREATMENT OF CYSTIC NEOPLASMS

There is a tendency among physicians and surgeons to assume that a cyst discovered in the pancreas is a pseudocyst and to treat it accordingly. In Warshaw's series, one-third of the patients with neoplastic cysts who were referred to a tertiary medical center initially had been diagnosed and treated for pseudocysts. This error is fostered by the similarity of many cystic tumors to pseudocysts on CT scans. Thus, one must consider the possibility of neoplasia to make the diagnosis (Table 71–2). Pseudocysts usually occur in patients with either a history of acute pancreatitis or in the setting of chronic pancreatitis, often owing to alcoholism. They occur more frequently in males, whereas cystic tumors are more frequent in females without those antecedent factors. The serum amylase is elevated in 50% to 75% of patients with pseudocysts, but it is almost always normal in cystic tumors.

Ultrasound and CT scans are the most useful imaging studies. Frequently, both the cystic and solid component of the mass may be identified (Fig 71–7). Internal septa

TABLE 71–2. DISTINGUISHING CHARACTERISTICS OF PRINCIPAL PANCREATIC CYSTIC NEOPLASMS

	Serous Cystadenoma	Mucinous Cystic Neoplasms	Papillary Cystic Neoplasms	Mucinous Ductal Ectasia
Age	50–80	40–60	20–30	50–80
Sex ratio (F:M)	2:1	4:1	14:1	1:4
Predominant location	Head	Body + Tail	Body + Tail	Head
Malignant potential	None	High	Moderate	Moderate

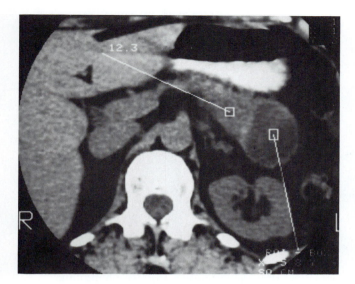

Figure 71–7. This CT scan demonstrates an apparent pseudocyst of the tail of the pancreas with thickening of the adjacent parenchyma. Biopsy of the cyst wall showed an epithelial lining, and this proved to be a mucinous cystadenocarcinoma.

or multiloculated cysts should raise the suspicion of tumor (Fig 71–8). Focal or "rim" calcifications also may be seen in the wall of neoplastic masses especially when malignant. Arteriography will show hypovascularity and displacement of vessels by a pseudocyst whereas cystic tumors, especially if there is a significant solid component or malignancy, may be hypervascular. Encasement of neighboring vessels is a sure sign of cancer.

ERCP also may be valuable in determining the nature of a cystic lesion of the pancreas. Most, but not all, pseudocysts communicate with the pancreatic duct, whereas most neoplastic cysts do not originate from the ductal system and therefore do not communicate with it. In our experience, nearly half of the benign tumors had a normal pancreatogram; half had draping or distortion of the duct by the tumor; 5% had communication with cyst cavity; and none were obstructed. In contrast, 25% of the malignant tumors had obstructed ducts and none communicated.

The precise diagnosis of a pancreatic cystic lesion may be impossible by radiologic means alone. Even the combination of CT, ultrasound, ERCP, and angiography may not be able to distinguish with certainty a pseudocyst from a cystic tumor, serous from mucinous neoplasms, or benign from malignant forms. That differential may be unnecessary in practical terms because symptoms mandate surgical intervention, in most cases. However, when the type of operation or the need for operation is in question or when the status of the patient leaves the decision uncertain, percutaneous aspiration of the cyst to sample its contents may be invaluable. The viscosity of the fluid may indicate its mucinous nature and cytologic

examination will be conclusive in half the cases. Several tumor markers have proven to be of particular value in differential diagnosis, notably CEA, CA15-3, CA72-4, and EGFR (Table 71–3). CA19-9 is of no value in this setting, nor are the serum levels of any of these indices. Needle aspiration should not be used indiscriminately in light of the theoretical concern that malignant cells could be disseminated by the needling (although we have yet to observe that happening).

At the time of laparotomy, gross findings usually suffice to differentiate neoplastic lesions from pseudocysts. Pseudocysts tend to adhere to adjacent viscera and the surrounding pancreas is indurated. Neoplastic cysts usually have a thin glistening wall and the pancreas adjacent to the cyst has a normal texture. Biopsy of the cyst wall can clinch the diagnosis because the presence of an epithelial lining means the cyst is neoplastic. The absence of an epithelial lining on a limited biopsy, however, does not exclude the possibility of a neoplasm as this lining is often discontinuous and may be absent from more than half of the lining surface.

Attempts to drain neoplastic cysts internally are misguided and ill conceived. Internal drainage will inadequately control symptoms, may lead to infection, and will fail to cure cancer. A pseudocyst adequately drained either externally or internally collapses within 1 to 3 weeks. The finding of a persistent cavity after decompression should raise concern that a stiff neoplastic wall is present. This may be a late key to the diagnosis of malignancy.

The cornerstone of treatment of cystic pancreatic neoplasms is complete excision. There is no valid role for internal or external drainage of these cysts. Lesions in the body and tail of the pancreas can be treated by distal pancreatectomy with or without splenectomy. Lesions located in the head of the gland require a pancreaticoduodenectomy. Total pancreatectomy generally is not required unless there is diffuse involvement of the gland by multiple cysts. Under favorable conditions, the presence of metastases is not an absolute contraindication to resection and, in fact, excision of isolated synchronous liver metastases may be curative. In our series of >100 cystic tumors of the pancreas, 45% were malignant: three-fourths of the malignant tumors were resectable for cure and two-thirds were cured (overall cure rate, 50%). No patients survived 5 years with a proven cystadenocarcinoma in the absence of complete excision. The role of chemotherapy is unknown. The role of intraoperative radiation therapy currently is being investigated.

In the past, the high morbidity and mortality rates associated with major pancreatic resections were a deterrent to an aggressive surgical approach in these lesions. However, recent reports have demonstrated that pancreaticoduodenectomy can be safely carried out by ex-

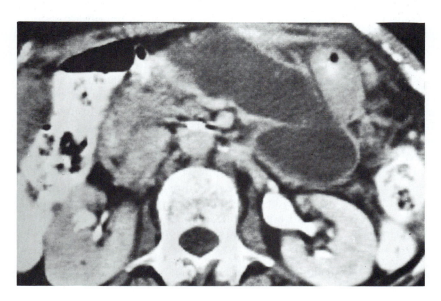

Figure 71–8. Cystic tumor of the pancreatic body and tail. In this case, the internal septae clearly indicate the likelihood of a neoplastic process.

TABLE 71–3. CYST FLUID INDICES USEFUL IN DIFFERENTIAL DIAGNOSIS OF PANCREATIC CYSTS

Type of Cystic Lesion	Viscosity	CEA	CA 125	CA 15-3	CA 72-4	Amylase	Cytology
Pseudocyst	Low	Low	Low	Low	Low	High	Negative
Serous cystadenoma	Low	Low	Low	Low	Low	Variable	Negative
Benign mucinous cystic neoplasms	Usually high	High	Low	Low	Low	Variable	Usually positive
Mucinous cystadenocarcinoma	High	High	High	High	High	Variable	Usually positive

perienced surgeons with mortality rates of <3%. Compagno and Alpert have argued that because the serous cystadenoma is a benign lesion, it need not be resected in older patients. There is certainly merit to this point of view when the patient presents a high operative risk, the symptoms are minor, and the diagnosis can be established preoperatively. If the diagnosis cannot be made with confidence, or if there are symptoms sufficient to warrant relief, there may be no reasonable alternative to surgical removal. Relatively few cystic tumors will meet the criteria for passive treatment.

■ PSEUDOCYSTS OF THE PANCREAS

ETIOLOGY

Pancreatic pseudocysts are the most common cystic lesions of the pancreas. They are distinguished from other types of pancreatic cysts by their lack of an epithelial lining. Pseudocysts are localized collections of pancreatic juice occurring as a result of pancreatic inflammation, trauma, or duct obstruction. Their walls are composed of fibrous and granulation tissue derived from peritoneum, retroperitoneal tissue, or the serosal surface of adjacent viscera.

Pancreatic pseudocysts were once thought to be an unusual complication of pancreatitis. With the development of improved imaging techniques, such as ultrasound and computerized tomography, they are being recognized in over 10% of cases of pancreatitis. Acute pseudocysts arise in association with a discrete episode of pancreatic inflammation. The pathway by which they are formed often follows a progression including diffuse peripancreatic effusions, pancreatic necrosis, liquefaction, swelling (phlegmon), acute pseudocyst, and finally, encapsulation (maturation). Cysts arising in the setting of chronic pancreatitis, most often without a determinate antecedent flare of acute pancreatitis, are referred to as chronic pseudocysts and generally have a mature wall on presentation. The management of acute and chronic pseudocysts is therefore different.

Acute pseudocysts may occur after acute pancreatitis of any etiology, including acute flares of chronic pancreatitis. This pathogenesis is via duct disruption with leakage of pancreatic juice into the surrounding tissues, presumably as a consequence of the necrotizing effect of pancreatitis. Since there is no natural barrier to the dissection of this fluid either cephalad or caudad in the retroperitoneum, acute pseudocysts may locate anywhere from the mediastinum to the scrotum. They are found most often in the lesser sac or anterior pararenal space. In contrast, traumatic pancreatic pseudocysts are caused by duct disruption secondary to blunt trauma. The duct is usually injured where it crosses the vertebral column, and therefore these cysts tend to occur anterior to the body of the gland. Frequently, the original injury goes unappreciated so that traumatic cysts may be more mature at the time of presentation than those arising in the setting of acute pancreatitis.

In chronic pancreatitis, it appears that the initiating event is duct rupture owing to inspissated proteins, stones, or strictures with subsequent blow out of the pancreatic duct. Because the pancreatic parenchyma is firm and fibrotic, chronic pseudocysts commonly are located within the substance of the gland. Chronic pseudocysts are virtually impossible to distinguish clinically from pancreatic retention cysts which are formed by progressive dilatation of a pancreatic duct distal to an obstruction and also arise in the setting of chronic pancreatitis. The widespread use of CT scans has lead to increasing detection of asymptomatic cysts in patients with chronic pancreatitis, many of which are probably retention cysts. For practical purposes, the only difference between pseudocysts and retention cysts is the presence of an epithelial lining in the retention cyst. Even this lining, however, may become flattened or destroyed by inflammation and high intracystic pressure, further blurring the distinction between these two entities.

DIAGNOSIS

Pancreatic pseudocysts should be suspected in patients with acute pancreatitis whose symptoms fail to resolve within 7 to 10 days or in patients with chronic pancreatitis who complain of persistent pain, nausea, or vomiting. According to Crass and Becker, epigastric pain is the presenting complaint in 90% of patients. Nausea and vomiting are present in nearly half of the patients and weight loss is present in 40%. As many as 60% of patients have an epigastric mass and fever and jaundice may also be part of the presentation. The absence of a mass does not exclude the diagnosis of pseudocysts, since even large pseudocysts can be hidden by the costal margin. While persistent hyperamylasemia following an attack of acute pancreatitis is a clue to the presence of pseudocyst formation, it is present only 50% of the time. There is no other laboratory test that is helpful in the diagnosis of pseudocysts. The most reliable way of making the diagnosis is by ultrasound or CT scanning. Hessel found ultrasound to be 90% accurate and 98% specific when the pancreas could be visualized. Unfortunately, gas obscures the pancreas in nearly one-third of patients with pancreatitis. CT scans have increased sensitivity and specificity and provided additional information about retroperitoneal extension of fluid collections and the relationship between cysts and adjacent enteric lumen that is not available from ultrasound. Therefore, CT scanning is the preferred initial test for detection of pseudocysts. Ultrasound is less costly and does not expose the patient to ionizing radiation. Therefore, it is more practical for follow-up.

Endoscopic retrograde cholangiopancreatography (ERCP) demonstrates abnormalities of the pancreatic duct in up to 90% of the patients with pseudocysts. Nearly two-thirds of pseudocysts communicate with the pancreatic duct. Obstruction of the pancreatic duct, compression of the duct by the cyst, or changes consistent with chronic pancreatitis are frequently noted. ERCP is very helpful in managing chronic pseudocysts arising in the setting of chronic pancreatitis. Finding a dilated pancreatic duct or multiple pseudocysts leads to alteration of the surgical procedure in as many as 25% of cases. Jaundiced patients also should undergo preoperative ERCP to assess potential obstruction of the distal common bile. Since ERCP adds little to the management of acute cysts in nonalcoholics, it should not be employed routinely in these patients. ERCP is an invasive procedure that potentially can aggravate pancreatitis or introduce infection into the pseudocyst in spite of the use of prophylactic antibiotics. Thus, some have proposed that if ERCP is to be used, especially in patients with large pseudocysts, it should be performed within 48 hours of a planned drainage procedure.

Angiography is generally not useful for diagnosis of pseudocysts nor should it be necessary in the preoperative evaluation of pseudocysts. However, in patients who have had bleeding complications from pseudocysts or those who have portal hypertension, it may provide valuable information that can alter the surgical approach. The finding of splenic vein thrombosis with left-sided portal hypertension is an indication for splenectomy in patients undergoing operation for drainage of pseudocysts. The therapeutic use of angiography to control bleeding from pseudocysts is discussed below.

NATURAL HISTORY

Understanding the natural history of pancreatic pseudocysts requires an appreciation of the spectrum of peripancreatic fluid collections seen during the course of pancreatitis. The distinction between peripancreatic edema, lesser sac effusion, and acute pseudocysts often cannot be made with certainty early in the course of pancreatitis. The inflammatory process is dynamic and consequently the morphologic alterations detected by ultrasound and CT scans change as the underlying pancreatitis progresses or resolves. Confusing terminology and attempts to rigidly classify fluid collections have led to some misconceptions about the likelihood of resolution and the indications for percutaneous or surgical intervention.

More than 50% of patients with moderately severe acute pancreatitis have associated fluid collections. Early fluid collections may be seen as blister-like projections protruding from the anterior surface of the pancreas or may occupy the lesser sac, left pararenal space, subhepatic space, mediastinum or retroperitoneum. Only when a collection persists beyond 3 weeks should it be considered a true pseudocyst. Studies involving serial ultrasound or CT examinations have shown that some of these collections will resolve spontaneously. When Bradley followed acute fluid collections in 24 patients with symptoms of 1 week duration or less, 42% of the collection resolved. Other authors have reported rates of resolution between 8% and 85%. These widely divergent results are owing to problems differentiating pseudocysts from peripancreatic fluid collections, as well as the inclusion of patients in these series with chronic pancreatitis whose pseudocysts are unlikely to resolve. As experience has been accumulated with CT scans in acute pancreatitis, certain findings have proved helpful in differentiating fluid collections that will resolve from pseudocysts that will not. Collections with an indistinct interface between fluid and adjacent organs, irregular contours with segments of pancreatic wall that are concave and convex, and collections with changing size, contour, and location, are most likely to resolve. Spherical or ovoid collections with sharp margins, especially in association with pancreatic calcifications, are likely to persist. In general, the closer to the onset of acute pancreatitis a fluid collection is detected, the more likely it is to resolve. Fluid collections may resolve by spontaneous transperitoneal reabsorption, decompression of the collection into the pancreatic duct, or erosion of a cyst into a hollow viscus with subsequent cyst-enteric fistula formation (Fig 71–9) or, rarely, by free rupture into the peritoneal cavity.

Once a truly cystic collection is formed, certain features indicate that it is unlikely to resolve spontaneously. Cysts larger than 4 to 6 cm are less likely to resolve than smaller cysts. Likewise, cysts that fail to show a decrease in size or those that show an increase in size during a 3 to 4 week period of observation are unlikely to resolve. Patients with multiple cysts are unlikely to reabsorb all of them. Chronic pseudocysts, especially those which are not associated with an identifiable flare of pancreatitis, are extremely unlikely to resolve. Since traumatic cysts tend to be more mature at the time of diagnosis, these, too, are less likely to resolve than acute pseudocysts.

COMPLICATIONS

Acute pancreatic pseudocysts that fail to resolve spontaneously and chronic pseudocysts require drainage or excision. Left untreated, they are liable to cause complications such as infection, obstruction, bleeding, or rupture. The risk of complications was said to increase with the duration of observation. In Bradley's prospec-

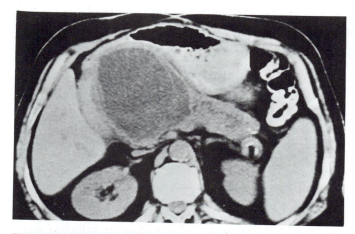

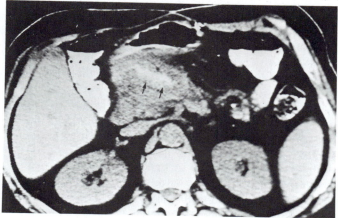

Figure 71–9. The CT scan in the top panel demonstrates a large pseudocyst in the head of the pancreas following a severe bout of acute pancreatitis. A CT scan 1 week later (*bottom*), just before a planned surgical decompression, shows the disappearance of the pseudocyst. Notice the contrast in the collapsed cavity (*arrows*). Presumably rupture of the pseudocyst into the duodenum created a spontaneous cystenteric fistula that was curative.

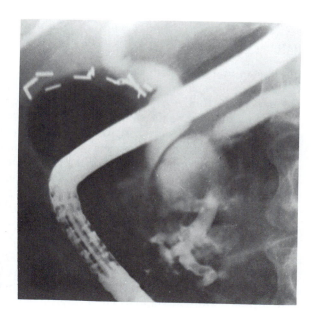

Figure 71–10. ERCP apparently demonstrating obstruction of the distal common bile duct by a pseudocyst. Drainage of the pseudocyst, in this instance, did not relieve the biliary obstruction, which was actually due to a common duct stricture from chronic pancreatitis. Note the dilated pancreatic ducts as well.

tive study, complications occurred in 21% of cysts within 6 weeks of diagnosis and increased to 57% in cysts observed for more than 6 weeks. Likewise Becker and Pratt reported a 42% complication rate in patients awaiting surgery. However these older studies were predicated on patients who were identified because of symptoms. At present, when many asymptomatic pseudocysts are being diagnosed by scans, it has become apparent that asymptomatic cysts, especially if smaller, are unlikely to develop complications and can be safely followed and observed.

Other than pain, infection is the most common complication. Secondary infection of a pancreatic pseudocyst frequently can be distinguished from a pancreatic abscess by the presence of a thick wall and absence of large amount of necrotic material in the cavity. There are, however, intermediate situations where the difference between these two entities, particularly occurring late in the course of pancreatitis, is primarily semantic. The diagnosis of secondary infection can frequently be made from clinical parameters. The appearance of fever, leukocytosis, and abdominal pain in a previously stable patient is highly suggestive of infection. Differentiating infection, in an immature pseudocyst, from ongoing pancreatitis, however, is not possible on clinical parameters alone. Gerzof found that in this situation, percutaneous aspiration can detect accurately the presence of infection. Any collection found to be infected must be drained to avoid extension of the septic process with erosion of vascular structures in the retroperitoneum. In general, surgical drainage is preferable to percutaneous approaches because it allows for removal of all infected necrotic debris frequently found in these pseudocysts (see below). Unsuspected infection of pseudocysts determined by cultures taken at operation has been reported in 14% to 78% of cases. The highest reported infection rate was noted by O'Connor in a series of patients who all had preoperative ERCPs. If, at the time of laparotomy, the cyst fluid is nonpurulent and there are no preoperative signs of sepsis, the finding of bacteria in pseudocyst fluid is unlikely to be clinically significant and the cyst can be internally drained if the wall is mature.

Obstruction of the duodenum and common bile duct occur in up to 10% of patients with pseudocysts. Duodenal obstruction is always relieved by cyst decompression, but jaundice is not. Many of these patients have fibrosis in the head of the pancreas causing distal common bile duct obstruction. After the cyst believed to be responsible for bile duct obstruction is drained, it is important to perform a cholangiogram, since a biliary bypass may still be necessary to relieve persisting distal common bile duct obstruction from fibrosis (Fig 71–10).

Bleeding associated with pancreatic pseudocysts is a life-threatening complication. There are several causes of bleeding. Bleeding may occur secondary to erosion of gut mucosa by an impending cyst-enteric fistula. In these cases, there is clear cut evidence of GI bleeding. More ominous is the direct erosion of a major visceral vessel or one of its branches. The action of activated pancreatic enzymes, particularly elastase, creates pseudoaneurysms that are the precursors of vessel rupture. Rupture of the pseudoaneurysm leads to intracystic hemorrhage, that can be massive. Because of the communication between the pseudocyst and the pancreatic duct, the hemorrhage may vent via the duct into the duodenum. Blood also may escape into the peritoneal cavity causing severe abdominal pain and hypotension. Major hemorrhage from an arterial source is most common when there is ongoing acute pancreatitis with extensive regional necrosis, especially when infected. Direct arterial erosion by pseudocysts has a mortality rate of 40% to 80%. Since most cysts arise in the body and tail of the pancreas, the splenic artery is the most commonly involved vessel but colonic arteries and the gastroduodenal artery are also vulnerable. Management of this complication has been greatly facilitated by the aggressive use of arteriography to delineate the site of bleeding (Fig 71–11). Transcatheter occlusive techniques are frequently successful in providing temporary control of bleeding to allow restoration of hemodynamic stability and convert an emergency operation into a safer semi-elective procedure. However, unless the ongoing necrotizing process that was responsible for erosion of the vessel is controlled by surgical debridement and drainage, angiographic control may not be permanent.

Rupture of pseudocysts can occur in several fashions. Cysts that erode into the gastrointestinal (GI) tract form cyst-enteric fistulas, frequently leading to decompression and resolution of the cyst. Continuing leakage from a pancreatic pseudocyst that has ruptured into the peritoneal cavity or the pleural space can lead to pancreatic ascites or a pancreatic-pleural fistula (see below). The most dramatic and serious presentation, albeit rare, is sudden intraperitoneal rupture of a pseudocyst. These patients present with sudden onset of acute abdominal pain and tenderness mimicking a duodenal perforation, and urgent operation with cyst drainage is necessary. Experimental work by Bradley suggests that enzymatic digestion with thinning of the cyst wall, rather than hydrostatic force, is responsible for cyst rupture in such cases. He suggests that this is consistent with the observation that complications are more likely to occur in cysts observed for long periods of time.

MANAGEMENT

Since not all fluid collections are pseudocysts and not all pseudocysts have the same natural history, one must in-

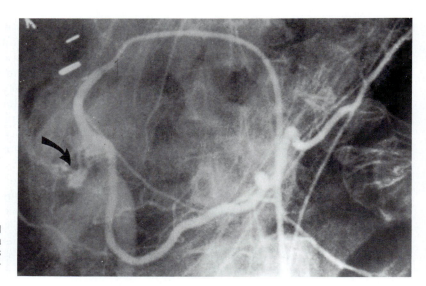

Figure 71–11. Selective arteriographic injection of the gastroduodenal artery demonstrating extravasation from a vessel in the wall of a pseudocyst. Selective embolization or other angiographic techniques for producing arterial occlusion can provide temporary control of bleeding to permit a safer definitive operation.

dividualize management of these patients. The desire to allow time for spontaneous resolution to occur must be balanced against the risk of complications while awaiting cyst wall maturity. Several generalizations can be made. Chronic pseudocysts can be drained immediately upon diagnosis and one can expect to find a mature cyst wall capable of holding sutures for internal drainage. Clinically infected pseudocysts, on the other hand, require external drainage without delay. More judgment is required in the management of acute cysts. If operation is performed too early, the cyst wall will be friable and unsuitable for anastomosis. External drainage with its attendant higher morbidity and mortality will be necessary. Experimental studies by Warren in a canine model showed that 6 weeks were required for formation of a mature cyst wall. This study and accumulated surgical experience has led to a consensus that a waiting period of 4 to 6 weeks from the time of diagnosis of an acute cyst is needed for cyst wall maturity to occur. Nonetheless, Grace and Shatney were able to perform internal drainage procedures in a large percentage of patients within three weeks of diagnosis, but many of these patients may have had chronic cysts. Warshaw and Rattner have reported that a form of pancreatic isoamylase called "old amylase" was a reliable marker for cyst wall maturity in a small series of patients.

PERCUTANEOUS DRAINAGE

With the rise of ultrasound and CT-guided percutaneous procedures, it has become fashionable to treat pseudocysts by percutaneous means. There is no question that percutaneous sampling of pancreatic fluid collections provides valuable information regarding the presence or absence of infection. Attempts to provide definitive therapy with catheters, however, are often hampered by their inability to provide egress for necrotic material that may be contained in the cyst, if it is a consequence of acute pancreatitis. On the other hand, chronic pseudocysts may have arisen because of obstruction of the duct downstream. It is, therefore, no surprise that simple aspiration of pseudocysts carries a 70% recurrence rate. To have a chance for success there must be repeated aspiration or placement of indwelling catheters, but long-term catheter drainage is, in many respects, equivalent to external surgical drainage. In uncomplicated pseudocysts that do not contain solid debris, the results are comparable. Success rates of 67% to 85% have been reported by van Sonnenberg and Torres. A permanent fistula along the catheter tract will occur if there is no prograde drainage route open (Fig 71–12). This ultimately may require resection of the isolated pancreatic tail in a situation that otherwise could have been treated with a simpler internal drainage of the pseudocyst.

ENDOSCOPIC DRAINAGE

Chronic pseudocysts impinging on the gastric or duodenal wall may be drained endoscopically by creating a cyst-enteric fistula. After puncturing the cyst through the gut wall, diathermy is used to create a 1 to 2 cm opening. Acute cysts should not be endoscopically drained because it is difficult to be certain that the cyst is adherent to the gut. Furthermore these cysts usually contain necrotic material that requires debridement. Not surprisingly the most frequent complications of this procedure are bleeding from the cyst wall or leakage of cyst fluid into the peritoneal cavity.

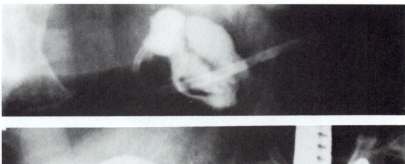
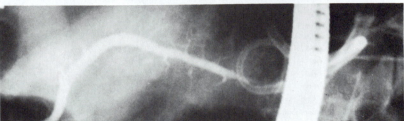

Figure 71–12. External percutaneous catheter drainage of a pancreatic pseudocyst involving the tail of the pancreas (*top*). This resulted in a nonhealing external pancreatic fistula. Retrograde pancreatography showed an obstruction of the pancreatic duct just proximal to the cyst cavity (*bottom*), resulting in isolation of the pancreatic tail and failure of the percutaneous attempt at treating the pseudocyst. The fistula was cured by resection of the pancreatic tail.

The results are not as good as surgically performed internal drainage procedures, although many of the endoscopically treated patients are poor surgical candidates. It is crucial, as noted earlier, to be sure that the cystic structure to be drained is truly a pseudocyst and not a cystic neoplasm before cutting a window between the cyst cavity and the GI tract. An important application of percutaneous sampling of the cyst contents may be for precise diagnosis to determine appropriate therapy if endoscopic methods are being contemplated.

SURGICAL PROCEDURES

There is no one surgical procedure appropriate for all pseudocysts. Drainage procedures generally are preferred over resection because they preserve pancreatic function, are technically easier, and have a lower mortality rate. Internal drainage is the preferred method of decompression because both the complication rate (68% vs 32%) and the mortality rate (11% vs 5%) are lower than with external drainage. It is not clear whether the choice of internal versus external drainage affects the recurrence rate, although fistula formation is certainly higher following external drainage.

DISTAL PANCREATIC RESECTION

Pseudocysts in the tail of the pancreas involving the spleen are the most suitable lesions for distal resection (Fig 71–13). ERCP in these situations may provide valuable information about the proximal pancreatic duct, helping to define the extent of resection. Pancreatic duct closure distal to an obstruction is likely to lead to recurrent pain, pancreatitis, or fistula. Properly per-

formed, however, the recurrence rate following distal resection is <3%. Some traumatic pseudocysts associated with the body of the gland, if operated upon early, may be most expeditiously obliterated by distal pancreatectomy also.

EXTERNAL DRAINAGE

Although external drainage of pseudocysts has the highest morbidity, mortality, and recurrence rate of the various surgical options, it remains an extremely useful and lifesaving operation. Many of the deaths following this procedure are not the result of the operative procedure per se but rather are the result of underlying ongoing pancreatitis and its complications. Most of the patients who report undergoing external drainage are operated upon urgently. This carries a six- to seven-fold increase in mortality over elective operations. Under elective circumstances, it is likely that mortality following external drainage procedures would be similar to internal drainage. Twelve to twenty percent of patients undergoing external drainage develop either a pancreatic fistula or a recurrent pseudocyst. This is generally owing to an underlying injury to the pancreatic duct. A controlled external fistula is an acceptable goal of external drainage of a pseudocyst in the acute situation. Seventy to eighty percent of these fistulas will close without further surgery, although this may take several months. When fistulas fail to close owing to proximal pancreatic duct obstruction, distal pancreatectomy, or Roux-en-Y drainage of the fistula may be necessary (Fig 71–14).

External drainage is the procedure of choice for grossly infected cysts, cysts associated with hemorrhage or free rupture necessitating emergency laparotomy, and those cysts with a soft wall which will not hold sutures. The procedure is performed by breaking into the

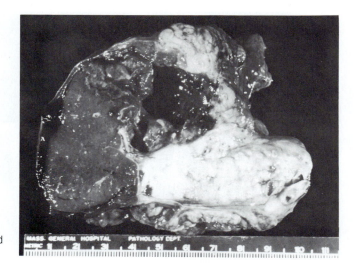

Figure 71–13. Splenectomy and distal pancreatectomy. The pseudocyst has partially eroded into the spleen.

cyst wall in as dependent a location as possible and placing large closed-suction drains into the cavity. Debridement of any necrotic material in the cyst cavity should be carried out, and the cavity can be packed with gauze-filled penrose drains to tamponade bleeding from the wall.

INTERNAL DRAINAGE

In patients with a mature cyst wall, internal drainage is the best surgical option. Cystenterostomy should have mortality rates as low as 2% and recurrence rates of under 5%. Mature cysts can be drained into the stomach, duodenum, or small bowel. The choice of surgical procedure depends on the locale of the pseudocyst and the local topography.

Cysts adherent to the stomach are ideally drained by a cystgastrostomy. After ascertaining that the cyst is firmly adherent to the stomach, an anterior gastrotomy is made. The contiguity of the pseudocyst is confirmed by needle aspiration and as long an incision as possible is made through the posterior gastric wall into the pseudocyst. A small ellipse of the common posterior gastric and cyst wall is excised and sent for frozen section examination to exclude neoplasia. If several contiguous pseudocysts are found, it may be possible to break up the septa between them and create one large cyst. The stoma should be large enough to allow transgastric debridement of the pseudocyst cavity. Hemostasis along the cut edges is achieved with closely spaced interrupted nonabsorbable sutures to approximate the gastric wall

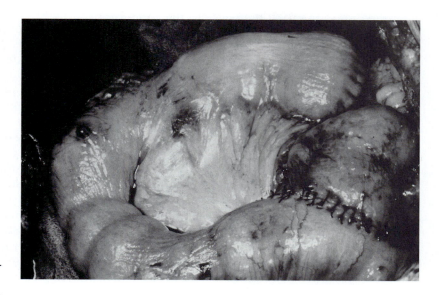

Figure 71–14. Use of a Roux-en-Y loop of jejunum to channel a pancreatic fistula back into the intestine.

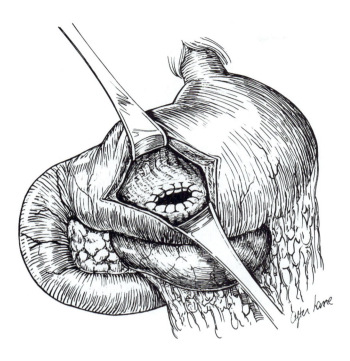

Figure 71–15. Transgastric cystogastrostomy. This is the most popular operation for a chronic pseudocyst that is firmly adherent to the posterior wall of the stomach.

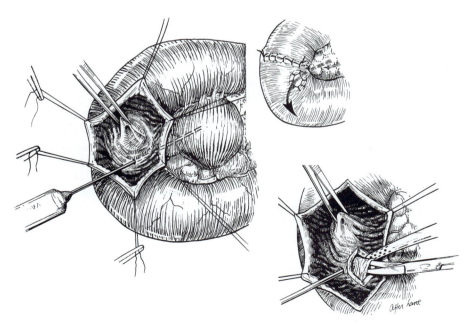

Figure 71–16. Transduodenal cystoduodenostomy for a pseudocyst at the head of the pancreas. The proximity of the pseudocyst to the duodenal wall and an estimation of the intervening distance is made by needle aspiration. The opening into the pseudocyst is made as large as safely possible. Injury to the bile duct and pancreatic duct must be avoided. The margins of the cyst wall are sutured to the full thickness of the second portion of the duodenum with a series of closely applied nonabsorbable sutures.

and the pseudocyst (Fig 71–15). Failure to carefully suture the cystgastrostomy leads to serious anastomotic bleeding in 10% to 50% of cases. After completing the cystgastrostomy, the anterior gastrotomy is closed. Occasionally, giant pseudocysts or lesser sac collections are encountered. Although it is tempting to drain these into the stomach, there is a tendency for gastric and pancreatic secretions to pool in the dependent portion of these large cavities and form an abscess. Therefore, giant pseudocysts are drained best externally or dependently into a loop of jejunum. Cystjejunostomy generally is employed for cysts in the body and tail of the pancreas which are not adherent to the stomach. It is also useful in patients with chronic pancreatitis who have a dilated main pancreatic duct that can be drained concomitantly. Combining lateral pancreaticojejunostomy with cyst drainage may greatly improve the outcome without increasing the morbidity and mortality of the procedure. Drainage into a Roux-en-Y limb is preferable to a loop cystjejunostomy. Some cysts may be anastomosed through the transverse mesocolon, but in many situations the Roux limb needs to be brought into the lesser sac, particularly if lateral pancreaticojejunostomy is being performed. When this is done, the blind end of the Roux limb should be oriented toward the tail of the pancreas. Should biliary obstruction secondary to fibrosis occur later in the disease process, the common bile duct can be anastomosed to the same Roux limb.

Cystduodenostomy should be performed for pseudocysts in the head of the pancreas that impinge on the duodenal wall. The technique is quite similar to cystgastrostomy (Fig 71–16). It is important to avoid the intrapancreatic portion of the common duct and the gastroduodenal artery when fashioning the cystduodenostomy. It is also important to provide a stoma sufficiently large for drainage. If there is a wide rim of pancreatic parenchyma between the cyst and the duodenal mucosa, this procedure should not be performed.

■ PANCREATIC FISTULAS

Disruption of a major duct with ongoing leakage leads to formation of a pancreatic fistula. When this occurs following surgery or percutaneous drainage of a collection, an external fistula is formed. When pancreatic duct disruption owing to chronic pancreatitis or rupture of a pseudocyst occurs, an internal fistula is formed resulting in either pancreatic ascites, pancreatic pleural fistula, or a fistula into the gastrointestinal tract. A classification of the varieties of fistulas is offered in Table 71–4. Since the etiology, natural history, and treatment of internal and external fistulas differ, they will be discussed separately (Table 71–3).

TABLE 71–4. CLASSIFICATION OF PANCREATIC FISTULAS

INTERNAL
Open
    Pancreaticoperitoneal
    Pancreaticopleural
    Pancreaticopericardial
    Pancreaticobronchial
Closed
    Pancreaticoenteric

EXTERNAL
Simple (pancreaticocutaneous)
    Low output (<200 mL/day)
    High output (>200 mL/day)
Complex (pancreaticoentericcutaneous)

INTERNAL FISTULAS

Although the clinical presentation of pancreatic pleural effusions and pancreatic ascites differ, their etiology is similar. In fact, as many as one-third of patients with pancreatic ascites have pancreatic pleural effusions. It is important to distinguish these two entities from the fluid collections seen early in the course of acute pancreatitis. Left-sided pleural effusions in acute pancreatitis are usually sympathetic effusions secondary to subdiaphragmatic inflammation. Consequently, they resolve as the underlying pancreatitis subsides. Likewise, free peritoneal fluid accumulates in acute pancreatitis, but is reabsorbed as the disease process wanes. Internal fistulas are rarely associated with a definable attack of pancreatitis. Cameron and Zuidema noted that a history of acute abdominal pain is almost always absent in these patients. Internal fistulas usually occur in patients with alcoholic chronic pancreatitis and most do not resolve without specific therapy. The underlying etiology of internal fistulas is duct disruption secondary to chronic pancreatitis. This may occur as a direct blowout of the pancreatic duct into the peritoneal cavity or retroperitoneum, or as a slow leak from a pancreatic pseudocyst (Fig 71–17). Anterior duct disruption produces pancreatic ascites. Since there is little, if any, acute inflammation, the enzymes are not activated and acute chemical peritonitis does not ensue. If the duct ruptures posteriorly into the retroperitoneum, the fluid tracts cephalad through the aortic or esophageal hiatus, or posterior to the diaphragmatic attachments into the mediastinum. In the mediastinum, it may form a pseudocyst or may erode into the pleural space to form an effusion. Rarely, internal fistulas can erode into the pericardium or bronchial tree.

Patients with pancreatic ascites most commonly present with an insidious increase in abdominal girth, often

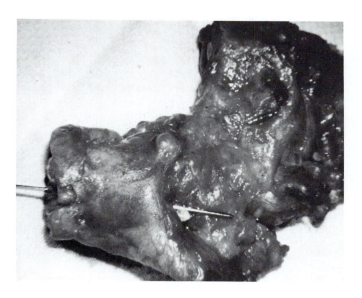

Figure 71–17. Resected distal pancreas and part of the wall of ruptured pseudocyst from a patient with pancreatic ascites. Just below the probe in the pancreatic duct is a stone that obstructed it. We presume that the pseudocyst formed because of this obstruction and then ruptured to cause an internal pancreatic fistula.

without abdominal pain. Nine percent of patients in a series from Cameron and Donowitz also had skin lesions which proved to be subcutaneous fat necrosis. The ascites may be massive enough to cause respiratory embarrassment. Since almost all these patients are alcoholics, the ascites initially is attributed to cirrhosis. But, unlike cirrhosis, most patients have elevated serum amylase due to reabsorption of amylase rich fluid from the peritoneal cavity. Paracentesis reliably differentiates pancreatic ascites from other causes because the amylase content of the ascitic fluid in pancreatic ascites is always markedly elevated. The protein content is usually >3 gm/dL, unless severe malnutrition coexists.

Pancreatic pleural effusions present exclusively with respiratory symptoms. Most patients complain of dyspnea, cough, or chest pain. Since there are no abdominal complaints, the diagnosis is rarely suspected until a thoracentesis is performed which demonstrates an elevated amylase. Although the majority of pancreatic pleural effusions are left-sided, ≤25% are bilateral, and as many as 12% to 20% may be associated with pancreatic ascites.

The differential diagnosis of pancreatic ascites is really quite limited. The major consideration is to exclude abdominal carcinomatosis. Cameron has pointed out that, in the presence of active inflammation, cytology may be falsely positive and thus an aggressive work-up should be pursued irrespective of the cytological results. Occasionally, pleural effusions associated with a primary thoracic malignancy may have elevated amylase content. However, the degree of elevation is usually minimal and generally an associated chest x-ray abnormality is present.

CT scans in these patients usually demonstrate a pseudocyst in addition to the previously recognized ascites or pleural effusion. In Pottmeyer's series, nine of ten patients with internal fistulas had pseudocysts demonstrated by CT scans. ERCP is essential in planning an operative approach to internal fistulas (Fig 71–18). When it cannot be performed preoperatively, an intraoperative pancreatogram should be performed. Sankaran and Walt demonstrated that knowledge of the pancreatic ductal anatomy based on a pancreatogram reduced the incidence of recurrence from 53% to 0%. ERCP usually demonstrates a pancreatic pseudocyst, but the leak from the cyst is less commonly seen. This may be owing to failure to completely fill the cyst with contrast or to rapid dilution of contrast material. Rapid disappearance of contrast from a pseudocyst is considered diagnostic evidence of a leaking pseudocyst by Sankaran. Other intraductal abnormalities that may alter the surgical procedure are seen frequently. These include strictures, dilatation, stones, and other pseudocysts. The absence of ductal dilatation does not exclude the possibility of ductal obstruction, because the duct is decompressed by the leak. Furthermore, the duct distal to the pseudocyst, or blow out, frequently cannot be evaluated by a retrograde approach. Careful gross inspection of the distal pancreas at the time of surgery is therefore essential.

Once the diagnosis of an internal pancreatic fistula is established, the initial treatment should be nonoperative. Since many of these patients are malnourished and because between one-quarter and one-half of internal fistulas will close nonoperatively, a trial of medical therapy generally is indicated. The goals of medical therapy are to minimize pancreatic secretion and remove ascites or pleural fluid so that peritoneal or pleural surfaces can appose to seal the leak or fistula.

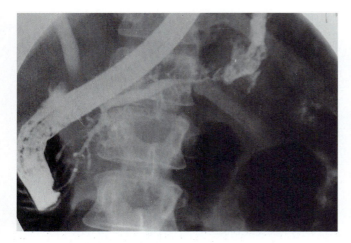

Figure 71–18. ERCP demonstrating a fistula from the distal pancreatic duct into a cavity. This leak was the origin of pancreatic ascites. Note the changes of chronic pancreatitis in the duct configuration.

Therefore, the patient is fasted and total parenteral nutrition is given to minimize pancreatic secretion. Anticholinergic agents and carbonic anhydrase inhibitors have been administered to decrease pancreatic secretion in the past, but there is no evidence that they are more effective than total parenteral nutrition alone. Long-acting somatostatin analogue (octreotide) has been shown to reduce pancreatic secretion and fistula outputs significantly, but there is not yet conclusive evidence of enhanced fistula healing. Daily paracentesis or tube thoracostomy should be performed to drain accumulated pancreatic juice. Cameron successfully managed 7 of 17 patients with pancreatic ascites nonoperatively. However, there were four deaths in this group, three of which occurred after 2 weeks of medical therapy. Furthermore, Sankaran and Walt reported a 22% mortality in medically treated patients. Therefore, if medical therapy is unsuccessful after 2 weeks, surgery should be undertaken.

The medical treatment of pancreatic pleural effusion appears, at first glance, to be slightly more successful. Fifty percent of patients with pancreatic pleural effusions treated by Pottmeyer were successfully treated medically. However, 40% of the successfully treated patients subsequently required surgery for treatment of a pseudocyst or complication of chronic pancreatitis. As with pancreatic ascites, octreotide has a logical role in reducing pancreatic secretion in hopes of fistula closure. Low-dose pancreatic irradiation may be given to patients who fail to respond to standard medical therapy and are very high operative risks. Gambil, Kavin, and Morton have reported successful use of external beam radiation to shut off pancreatic secretion in patients who were not candidates for surgery.

When surgery is indicated, the choice of operation is dictated by the pancreatic ductal anatomy and findings at laparotomy. In 10% of cases, a ruptured duct will be found without a pseudocyst. In this situation, a Roux-en-Y limb of jejunum should be anastomosed to the duct. More frequently, however, a small pseudocyst is found. If located in the tail of the gland, a distal pancreatectomy can be performed provided there is no proximal duct disease. If proximal duct disease is present, it is necessary to drain the pancreatic remnant into a Roux-en-Y limb in order to avoid a blowout of the stump closure, with resulting pseudocyst, abscess or recurrence of ascites. In cases where there is proximal duct dilatation or multiple pseudocysts, it may be wise to combine resection with a lateral pancreaticojejunostomy (Fig 71–19). If the leak originates from a large pseudocyst or one located in the head of the pancreas, a cyst-enterostomy is indicated. External drainage of the fistula should not be performed, since it is likely to become a persistent external fistula and require reoperation. Operative treatment of pancreatic pleural effusions follows the same principles. Thoracoabdominal incisions are unnecessary unless the fistula penetrates the lung as bronchus. Correction of the underlying pancreatic pathology will cure the fistula into the pleural space. When the sinus tract to the mediastinum can be identified, it should be ligated (Fig 71–19); however partial pancreatic resection or Roux-en-Y drainage will generally either disrupt the fistula or sufficiently divert pancreatic secretions so as to allow healing. The results of surgical therapy for pancreatic internal fistulas based on knowledge of the anatomy of the pancreatic duct are excellent, with extremely low mortality and recurrence rates reported by multiple authors.

EXTERNAL FISTULA

External pancreatic fistulas usually result from complications of pancreatic surgery or pancreatic trauma. They are most common following external drainage of pancreatic pseudocysts or debridement of pancreatic necrosis, but may complicate local excision of pancreatic tumors, pancreatic biopsies, pancreaticoenteric anastomoses or operative injury to the pancreas during splenectomy, gastrectomy, or other upper abdominal operation. As indicated in Table 71–4, we categorize fistulas not involving an enteric component as *simple,* and those in which there is also discontinuity of the GI tract, such as at a disrupted pancreaticojejunal anastomosis as *complex.* The latter are far more dangerous and liable to become complicated by sepsis and hemorrhage.

Simple external fistulas generally are described as high output (>200 cc/day) or low output (<200 cc/day). In Zinner's study done prior to the widespread use of total parenteral nutrition and ERCP, nearly two-thirds of fis-

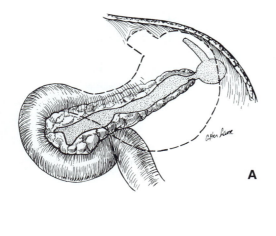
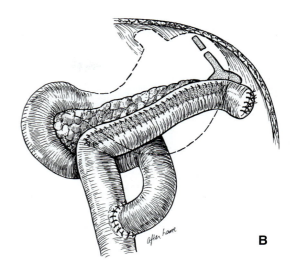

Figure 71–19. When a pancreatic fistula is present in combination with dilation of the pancreatic duct, and especially if the patient has significant pain from chronic pancreatitis, closure or redirection of the fistula can be combined efficiently with a lateral pancreaticojejunotomy (modified Puestow procedure).

tulas closed spontaneously. A more recent report by Pederzoli reported a 93% closure rate. The likelihood of closure for low-output fistulas appears to be better, and high-output fistulas also take longer to close and are more frequently associated with complications. The most common complication is local sepsis in and around the fistula tract. Since the drainage may contain activated digestive enzymes, erosion of adjacent viscera or vessels may lead to hemorrhage. Skin irritation is also a major problem. Loss of protein and bicarbonate-rich pancreatic juice from high-output fistulas can lead to electrolyte abnormalities and malnutrition. Treatment of the fistula requires correction of these problems.

Pancreatic fistulas will not close in the presence of distal obstruction, sepsis, tumor, or foreign body. In the absence of these factors, however, nonoperative therapy is likely to be successful. One of the cornerstones of nonoperative therapy is diminishing pancreatic secretion. Bowel rest and total parenteral nutrition will diminish pancreatic secretion while, at the same time, correcting nutritional and electrolyte deficits. Low-output fistulas do not require restriction of diet as long as the secretions are adequately channeled and sepsis is well drained. In high-output fistulas, a variety of pharmacologic agents have been used to minimize pancreatic secretion, but only octreotide (long-acting somatostatin analogue) is effective enough to have significant potential. When proximal obstruction of the pancreatic duct is present, however, the fistula will not heal (Fig 71–12). Therefore, ERCP or fistulograms can be very helpful in determining how long to persist with nonoperative therapy. If pancreatic duct obstruction is the cause of the persistence of the fistula, operation should not be delayed needlessly.

Fistulas arising in the body and tail of the pancreas are treated optimally by distal resection, especially if there is significant pain related to partial obstruction of the distal pancreatic duct and consequent recurrent or persistent pancreatitis. Fistulas arising in the head of the pancreas can be problematic. If the fistula arises from an area of injury in the proximal duct, anastomosis of a Roux-en-Y limb to the origin of the fistula is the preferred treatment. Resection of the pancreatic head in the setting of severe inflammation is difficult and hazardous, but may be needed occasionally, especially when there is intolerable pain from chronic pancreatitis.

Complex pancreaticocutaneous fistulas involve the enteric lumen as well as the pancreas. These may be caused by breakdown of a pancreaticoenteric anastomosis or by injury to the intestinal or gastric walls as a consequence of severe pancreatitis. Complex fistulas are particularly dangerous because of the higher likelihood of sepsis and hemorrhage from the fistula site, perhaps owing to the portal of entry for bacteria and the activation of pancreatic proteases by intestinal enterokinase.

Anastomotic breakdown is rare after operations to decompress dilated ducts in chronic pancreatitis. After pancreaticoduodenectomy and reconstruction, however, pancreatic anastomotic leaks have been reported in up to 70% and are considered the major cause of morbidity and mortality after that operation. Recent statistics suggest a marked reduction in the incidence of this dreaded complication. The threshold for reoperation should be low: if there are substantial signs, it is unwise to wait until sepsis or hemorrhage become life-threatening. The surest means of cure is completion pancreatectomy and closure of the intestinal segment.

Necrosis of a segment of the duodenum, colon, stom-

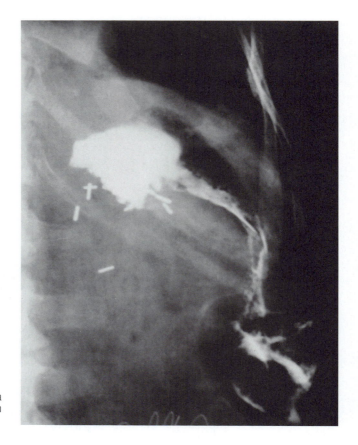

Figure 71–20. Complex pancreaticocutaneous fistula with gastric perforation caused by a pancreatic abscess. Because of sepsis and hemorrhage from the fistula tract, reoperation for partial gastrectomy and closure became necessary.

ach, or jejunum, as a consequence of necrotizing pancreatitis and abscess, leads to a particularly lethal variant of complex pancreatic fistula. It usually is heralded by the appearance of bilious or fecal material in the discharge after debridement and drainage of pancreatic necrosis or abscess. A gastric perforation (Fig 71–20) should be suspected if the drainage has an acidic pH. Because of the great potential for life-threatening complications during conservative nonoperative management, surgical treatment, including resection and stomas to divert enteric flow from the damaged bowel segment, is warranted in most cases of complex pancreatic fistula.

SELECTED READINGS

Adams DB, Anderson MC. Percutaneous catheter drainage compared with internal drainage in the management of pancreatic pseudocyst. *Ann Surg* 1992;215:571

Agha F. Spontaneous resolution of acute pancreatic pseudocysts. *Surg Gynecol Obstet* 1984;158:22

Ahearne PM, Baillie JM, et al. An endoscopic retrograde cholangiopancreatography (ERCP)-based algorithm for the management of pancreatic pseudocysts. *Am J Surg* 1992;163:111

Albores-Saavedra J, Gould EW, et al. Cystic tumors of the pancreas. *Pathol Annu* 1990;25:19

Aldridge MC, Hittinger R, et al. Natural history of acute peripancreatic fluid collections. *Gut* 1991;32:A343

Alles AJ, Warshaw AL, et al. Expression of CA 72-4 (TAG72) in the fluid contents of pancreatic cysts: a new marker to distinguish malignant from benign pancreatic neoplasms and pseudocysts. *Ann Surg* 1994;219:131–134

Barkin JS, Reiner DK, et al. Sandostatin for control of catheter drainage of pancreatic pseudocyst. *Pancreas* 1991;6:245

Bastid C, Bernard JP, et al. Mucinous ductal ectasia of the pancreas: a premalignant disease and a cause of obstructive pancreatitis. *Pancreas* 1991;6:15

Bradley EL. A clinically based classification system for acute pancreatitis: summary of the International Symposium on Acute Pancreatitis, Atlanta, GA, September 11 through 12, 1992. *Arch Surg* 1993;128:586

Bradley EL, Vito RP. Mechanisms for rupture of pancreatic pseudocysts. *Ann Surg* 1984;200:51

Bresler L, Boissel P, et al. Major hemorrhage from pseudocysts and pseudoaneurysms caused by chronic pancreatitis: surgical therapy. *World J Surg* 1991;15:649

Buchler M, Friess H, et al. Role of octreotide in the prevention of postoperative complications following pancreatic resection. *Am J Surg* 1992;163:125

Capellari JO, Geisinger KR, et al. Malignant papillary cystic tumor of the pancreas. *Cancer* 1990;66:193

Compagno J, Oertel, JE. Mucinous cystic neoplasms of the pancreas with overt and latent malignancy (cystadenocarcinoma and cystadenoma): a clinicopathologic study of 41 cases. *Am J Clin Pathol* 1978;69:573

Compagno J, Oertel JE. Microcystic adenomas of the pancreas (glycogen-rich cystadenomas). A clinicopathologic study of 34 cases. *Am J Clin Pathol* 1978;69:289

Compagno J, Oertel JE, et al. Solid and papillary epithelial neoplasm of the pancreas, probably of small duct origin: a clinicopathologic study of 52 cases. *Lab Invest* 1979; 40:248

Crass RA, Way LW. Acute and chronic pancreatic pseudocysts are different. *Am J Surg* 1984;142:660

Cremer M, Deviere J, et al. Endoscopic management of cysts and pseudocysts in chronic pancreatitis: long-term follow-up after 7 years of experience. *Gastrointest Endosc* 1989;35:1

Criado E, DeStefano AA, et al. Long term results of percutaneous catheter drainage of pancreatic pseudocysts. *Surg Gynecol Obstet* 1992;175:293

Davtyan H, Nieberg R, et al. Pancreatic cystic endocrine neoplasms. *Pancreas* 1990;5:230

D'Egidio A, Schein M. Percutaneous drainage of pancreatic pseudocysts: a prospective study. *World J Surg* 1991;16:141

Fielding GA, McLatchie GR, et al. Acute pancreatitis and pancreatic fistula formation. *Br J Surg* 1989;76:1126

Gazelle GS, Mueller PR, et al. Cystic neoplasms of the pancreas: evaluation with endoscopic retrograde pancreatography. *Radiology* 1993;188:633

Gerzof SG, Banks PA, et al. Early diagnosis of pancreatic infection by computed tomography guided aspiration. *Gastroenterology* 1987;93:1315

Gerzof SG, Johnson WC, et al. Percutaneous drainage of infected pancreatic pseudocysts. *Arch Surg* 1984;119:888

Ihse I, Lindstrom E, et al. The value of preoperative imaging techniques in patients with chronic pancreatic pleural effusions. *Int J Pancreatol* 1987;2:269

Ishikawa O, Ohigashi H, et al. Concomitant benefit of preoperative irradiation in preventing pancreas fistula formation after pancreatoduodenectomy. *Arch Surg* 1991;126:885

Johnson LB, Rattner DW, et al. The effect of size on giant pancreatic pseudocysts on the outcome of internal drainage procedures. *Surg Gynecol Obstet* 1991;173:171

Kawarada Y, Yano T, Yamamoto T, et al. Intraductal mucin-producing tumors of the pancreas. *Am J Gastroenterol* 1992; 87:634

Kozarek RA, Ball TJ, et al. Endoscopic transpapillary therapy for disrupted pancreatic duct and peripancreatic fluid collections. *Gastroenterology* 1991;100:1362

Kozarek RA, Bryako CM, et al. Endoscopic drainage of pancreatic pseudocysts. *Gastrointest Endosc* 1985;31:322

Lewandrowski KB, Southern JF, et al. Cyst fluid analysis in the differential diagnosis of pancreatic cysts: a comparison of pseudocysts, serous cystadenomas, mucinous cystic neoplasms, and mucinous cystadenocarcinoma. *Ann Surg* 1993; 217:41

Lewandrowski KB, Warshaw AL, et al. Macrocystic serous cystadenoma of the pancreas: a morphologic variant differing from microcystic adenoma. *Hum Pathol* 1992;23:871

Lewis G, Krige JEJ, et al. Traumatic pancreatic pseudocysts. *Br J Surg* 1993;80:89

Lipsett PA, Cameron JL. Internal pancreatic fistula. *Am J Surg* 1992;163:216

Mann JS, Aranha GV, et al. Simultaneous treatment of chronic pancreatitis and pancreatic pseudocyst. *Arch Surg* 1987;12:662

Mares AJ, Hirsch M. Congenital cysts of the head of the pancreas. *J Pediatr Surg* 1977;12:547

Nealon WH, Townsend CM, et al. Preoperative endoscopic retrograde cholangiopancreatography (ERCP) in patients with pancreatic pseudocyst associated with resolving acute and chronic pancreatitis. *Ann Surg* 1989;209:532

Neumann HPH, Dinkel E, et al. Pancreatic lesions in the von Hippel-Lindau syndrome. *Gastroenterology* 1991;101:465

Newell KA, Liu T, et al. Are cystgastrostomy and cystjejunostomy equivalent operations for pancreatic pseudocysts? *Surgery* 1990;108:635

Nguyen BLT, Thompson JS, et al. Influence of the etiology of pancreatitis on the natural history of pancreatic pseudocysts. *Am J Surg* 1991;162:527

Ohta T, Nagawaka T, et al. The "duct-ectatic" variant of mucinous cystic neoplasm of the pancreas: clinical and radiologic studies of seven cases. *Am J Gastroenterol* 1992; 87:300

Pederzoli P, Bassi C, et al. Conservative treatment of extended pancreatic fistulas with parenteral nutrition alone or in combination with continuous intravenous infusion of somatostatin, glucagon or calcitonin. *Surg Gynecol Obstet* 1986; 163:428

Pottmeyer EW, Frey CF, et al. Pancreatic pleural fistulas. *Arch Surg* 1987;122:648

Prinz PA, Pickleman J, et al. Treatment of pancreatic cutaneous fistulas with a somatostatin analogue. *Am J Surg* 1988;155:36

Pyke CM, van Heerden JA, et al. The spectrum of serous cystadenoma of the pancreas. *Ann Surg* 1992;215:132

Rubin D, Warshaw AL, et al. Expression of CA 15-3 protein in the cyst contents distinguishes benign from malignant pancreatic mucinous cystic neoplasms. *Surgery* 1994;115:52–55

Sahel J, Bastid D, et al. Endoscopic cystoduodenostomy of cysts of chronic calcifying pancreatitis: a report of 20 cases. *Pancreas* 1987;2:447

Schmidt J, Rattner DW, et al. Surgical treatment of pancreatic fistulas: Rationale, timing, and techniques. In: Pederzoli P, Bassi C, Vesentini S (eds), *Pancreatic Fistulas*. Heidelberg, Germany: Springer-Verlag; 1992:176

Schulze S, Baden H, et al. Pancreatic pseudocysts during the first attack of acute pancreatitis. *Scand J Gastroenterol* 1986; 21:1221

Smith CD, Sarr MG, et al. Completion pancreatectomy following pancreaticoduodenectomy: Clinical experience. *World J Surg* 1992;15:521

Stamm B, Burger H, et al. Acinar cell cystadenocarcinoma of the pancreas. *Cancer* 1987;60:2542

Talamini MA, Pitt HA, et al. Spectrum of cystic tumors of the pancreas. *Am J Surg* 1992;163:117

van Sonnenberg E, Wittich GR, et al. Percutaneous drainage of infected and noninfected pancreatic pseudocysts: experience in 101 cases. *Radiology* 1989;170:757

Vitas GJ, Sarr MG. Selected management of pancreatic pseudocysts: Operative versus expectant management. *Surgery* 1992;111:123

Waltman AC, Luers PA, et al. Massive arterial hemorrhage in patients with pancreatitis: complementary roles of surgery and transcatheter occlusive techniques. *Arch Surg* 1986; 121:439

Warshaw AL. Inflammatory masses following acute pancreatitis. *Surg Clin North Am* 1974;54:621

Warshaw AL. Mucinous cystic tumors and mucinous ductal ectasia of the pancreas. *Gastrointest Endosc* 1991;37:199

Warshaw AL, Compton CC, et al. Cystic tumors of the pancreas: new clinical, radiologic, and pathologic observations in 67 patients. *Ann Surg* 1990;212:432

Warshaw AL, Lee K-H. Aging changes of pancreatic isoamylases and the appearance of "old amylase" in the serum of patients with pancreatic pseudocysts. *Gastroenterology* 1980; 1246

Warshaw AL, Rattner DW. Fact and fallacies of common bile duct obstruction by pancreatic pseudocyst. *Ann Surg* 1980;192:33

Warshaw AL, Rattner DW. Timing of surgical drainage for pancreatic pseudocyst. *Ann Surg* 1985;202:720

Warshaw AL, Rutledge PL. Cystic tumors mistaken for pancreatic pseudocysts. *Ann Surg* 1987;205:393

Wood D, Silberman AW, et al. Cystadenocarcinoma of the pancreas: neoadjuvant therapy and CEA monitoring. *J Surg Oncol* 1990;43:56

Yamaguchi K, Hirakata R, et al. Papillary cystic neoplasm of the pancreas: radiological and pathological characteristics in 11 cases. *Br J Surg* 1990;77:1000

Yoshimi N, Sugie S, et al. A rare case of serous cystadenocarcinoma of the pancreas. *Cancer* 1992;69:2449

Zinner MJ, Baker RR, et al. Pancreatic cutaneous fistulas. *Surgery* 1974;138:710

72

Chronic Pancreatitis

Howard A. Reber

Chronic pancreatitis is an inflammatory disease of the pancreas characterized by destruction of its exocrine and endocrine tissue and by their replacement with fibrous scar. In the United States, the majority of cases are caused by chronic alcoholism. The process is almost always progressive, even when patients stop drinking. Most of these individuals suffer chronic abdominal and back pain, and it is for this problem more than any other that they seek surgical help. Other common indications for surgery include the development of chronic pseudocysts and obstruction of the common bile duct.

Gallstone pancreatitis is not thought to result in such widespread parenchymal destruction, even in patients who experience multiple attacks. Indeed, when such an attack of acute pancreatitis induced by gallstones subsides, the pancreas is believed to return to normal, both functionally and structurally. It is this difference in the ability of the pancreas to recover that is the basis for the classification of pancreatitis into acute and chronic varieties (Table 72–1).

It is important to distinguish between alcoholic (chronic) and gallstone (acute) pancreatitis in each patient because of the obvious implications in regard to long-term management and prognosis. However, it should be stressed that people with chronic pancreatitis often suffer episodes of acute pancreatic inflammation that are indistinguishable clinically from an attack of gallstone acute pancreatitis (or acute pancreatitis from other causes). Indeed, the treatment of such acute episodes is identical.

■ ETIOLOGY

ALCOHOLIC PANCREATITIS

In the United States, alcoholism causes about 75% of all cases of chronic pancreatitis. The disease may take one of several clinical forms. An episode of binge drinking may precipitate an attack typical of acute pancreatitis. This usually occurs in a patient who is a chronic alcoholic. In this setting, the pancreas probably has already been permanently damaged by alcohol, even though there might not be any other evidence of pancreatic disease (eg, pancreatic exocrine insufficiency, diabetes). The other clinical presentation also occurs in chronic alcoholics in whom there was no acute episode of inflammation. These individuals have chronic abdominal and/or back pain, often with steatorrhea and diabetes from pancreatic exocrine and endocrine insufficiency.

Pancreatic calcifications occur in at least one-third of patients. Weight loss is common since food often aggravates the pain and intake is voluntarily restricted. The patients may be addicted to the narcotics necessary for pain relief. The usual age at onset is in the mid 30s and men are affected more commonly than women.

Alcoholic pancreatitis is generally diagnosed after patients consume alcohol for at least 2 years and usually, between 6 to 10 years. It probably makes no difference whether the ethanol is consumed as wine, beer, or spirits, but the daily consumption averages 100 to 150 gm of ethanol/day. There is evidence that the diet of alco-

TABLE 72–1. CLASSIFICATION OF PANCREATITIS (MARSEILLES—1984)

Classification	Characteristics	
	Clinical	*Morphologic*
ACUTE PANCREATITIS Both exocrine and endocrine functions are impaired to a variable extent for a variable duration. *But, if the primary cause and complications such as pseudocysts are eliminated, clinical, morphologic, and functional restitution to normal occurs. Only rarely does acute pancreatitis lead to chronic pancreatitis.*	Acute abdominal pain, with increased pancreatic enzymes in blood, urine, or both; usually a benign course but may be severe and prove fatal; may be a single episode or may recur.	Gradation of lesions from mild (peripancreatic fat necrosis, interstitial edema) to severe (peripancreatic and intrapancreatic fat necrosis, pancreatic parenchymal necrosis, hemorrhage); may be little correlation between clinical features and morphologic findings.
CHRONIC PANCREATITIS *In chronic pancreatitis (except obstructive chronic pancreatitis), the irreversible morphologic changes in the pancreas may lead to a progressive or permanent loss of exocrine and endocrine pancreatic function. In obstructive chronic pancreatitis, both structural and functional changes tend to improve when the obstruction is removed.*	Recurrent or persistent abdominal pain, although pain may not be present; evidence of pancreatic insufficiency, eg, steatorrhea or diabetes, may be present.	Irregular sclerosis, with destruction and permanent loss of exocrine parenchyma that may be either focal, segmental, or diffuse; may be varying degrees of dilatation of the duct of Wirsung or its small ducts or both; all types of inflammatory cells, as well as edema and focal necrosis, may be present; cysts and pseudocysts, with and without infection, which may or may not communicate with ducts, are common; calculi are common; the islets of Langerhans are relatively well preserved, compared to the degree of acinar destruction. A distinct morphologic form of chronic pancreatitis is obstructive chronic pancreatitis; here the ductal system is dilated proximal to the occlusion of one of the major ducts (eg, by tumor or scars), and there is diffuse atrophy of the acinar parenchyma and uniform, diffuse fibrosis; calculi are uncommon.
The first manifestation of alcoholic chronic pancreatitis may be an episode of clinically acute pancreatitis. In the early phases of alcoholic chronic pancreatitis, exacerbations closely resemble attacks of acute pancreatitis.		

holic patients who develop pancreatitis is richer in fat and protein than other alcoholics who do not. It is estimated that about 10% to 15% of individuals who consume such large amounts of alcohol eventually develop pancreatitis; a similar number develop cirrhosis of the liver. The factors that govern individual susceptibility are unknown.

Early studies suggested that ethanol caused pancreatitis by inducing spasm of the sphincter of Oddi, thereby creating an obstruction to the outflow of pancreatic juice. Experimentally, secretion in the face of similar obstruction has caused acute pancreatitis, but this cannot be the full explanation. Ethanol is also a cellular metabolic poison, and it has deleterious effects on the synthesis and secretion of digestive enzymes by the pancreatic acinar cells. This causes an increase in the concentration of enzyme protein in pancreatic juice, and the eventual precipitation of this protein in the pancreatic ducts. Calcium, normally soluble in pancreatic juice, then may precipitate within the matrix of these protein plugs. This creates multiple points of ductal obstruction randomly scattered throughout the pancreas. Further damage follows continued secretion in the face of this widespread obstruction. Another effect of ethanol is to increase the permeability of the pancreatic ducts. This allows pancreatic enzymes, normally contained within the ducts, to leak out into the surrounding tissue. If the enzymes are active, damage to the pancreas results. Finally, there is evidence that alcohol significantly depresses pancreatic blood flow for several hours after ingestion. This may cause ischemic injury to the gland.

DUCT OBSTRUCTION

Obstruction to the secretion of pancreatic juice is a less commonly primary cause of chronic pancreatitis. It may be particularly important to establish obstruction as the cause since, unlike other forms of chronic pancreatitis, there is evidence that some morphologic and functional recovery of the pancreas can occur if the obstruction is

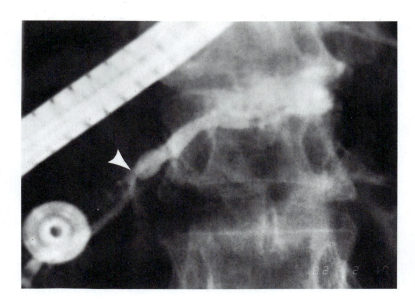

Figure 72–1. ERCP reveals ductal stricture (*arrow*) with dilated pancreatic duct proximally. The duct is normal in caliber past the stricture. (From Reber HA. Chronic pancreatitis: etiology, pathology, and diagnosis. In: Howard JM, Jordan GL Jr, Reber HA (eds), *Surgical Diseases of the Pancreas.* Philadelphia, PA: Lea and Febiger; 1987:479)

removed. Of course when the process is advanced, significant recovery is not possible. Obstruction as a cause of chronic pancreatitis occurs in a variety of clinical settings.

Congenital or Acquired Strictures of the Pancreatic Duct

When fusion of the ventral and dorsal pancreatic ducts occurs during fetal life, an area of narrowing up to 2 cm long may persist at the point of fusion. When this is seen on ERCP, it is only thought to have pathological significance if there is ductal dilatation proximal to it. Chronic pancreatitis has been reported in patients with severe strictures at this point. Strictures also occur in other areas of the main pancreatic duct and are probably the result of scarring after trauma or acute pancreatitis from any cause (Fig 72–1).

Pancreas Divisum

This entity has been most commonly associated with recurrent episodes of acute pancreatitis (see Chapter 70). Nevertheless, chronic pancreatitis may occur when the outflow obstruction is severe and persistent over a period of years. In a number of reported cases in which pancreatic resections were performed, the changes of chronic pancreatitis were confined to that part of the pancreas that drained through the minor papilla (dorsal pancreas). The ventral pancreas that drained through the papilla of Vater with the bile duct was normal. In patients with established chronic pancreatitis and pancreas divisum, therapy directed toward relief of obstruction at the minor papilla is ineffective. However, endoscopic or surgical sphincteroplasty may help in the clinical setting, when the patient is experiencing recurrent episodes of acute pancreatitis.

Duct Obstruction from Tumors

Microscopic areas of chronic pancreatitis almost always surround a cancer in the head of the pancreas. At operation, it is also common to find an abnormally firm, even hard, pancreas with a dilated pancreatic duct proximal to the malignant obstruction. Nevertheless, clinically significant chronic pancreatitis is unusual in this setting. Occasionally, with some slowly growing cancers, the symptoms may be present for several years and be indistinguishable from those of chronic pancreatitis. In such cases, pain and steatorrhea are prominent, and episodes of acute pancreatitis occur. The patients are usually older than those with alcoholic pancreatitis. A high index of suspicion is necessary to make the correct diagnosis early.

Inflammation of the Papilla of Vater

Acute and chronic inflammation of the papilla of Vater with obstruction of the duct of Wirsung is rare. In most cases, the inflammation is probably caused by the passage of common duct stones through the papilla. In others, there is no apparent explanation. There are probably some cases of chronic pancreatitis that are secondary to the outflow obstruction caused by this process. Nevertheless, the clinician must be extremely cautious about attributing the diagnosis of chronic pancreatitis to this entity. In any case, as with pancreas divisum, treatment directed toward the relief of papillary obstruction is ineffective.

PROTEIN MALNUTRITION

Children with severe protein calorie malnutrition may develop Kwashiorkor and a specific type of chronic pancreatitis. Treatment with adequate diet rapidly restores pancreatic function to normal, provided that parenchymal fibrosis is not too extensive, pancreatic calcification is absent and episodes of abdominal pain are infrequent. Another variety of chronic pancreatitis, possibly related to malnutrition, occurs only in certain tropical and subtropical countries (eg, Nigeria). It begins in childhood, and is associated with abdominal pain, pancreatic calcification, steatorrhea, and diabetes, in most cases. The pancreatic ducts are usually dilated and obstructed. Adequate nutrition does not reverse the process.

CYSTIC FIBROSIS

Pancreatic insufficiency occurs in 80% to 85% of patients with cystic fibrosis; the remainder have well preserved pancreatic function. Occasionally, individuals in this latter group develop acute recurrent or chronic pancreatitis. Pancreatic calcifications, steatorrhea, diabetes, and abdominal pain have been described. The surgical management is the same as in patients with pancreatitis from other causes.

HYPERCALCEMIC STATES

Hypercalcemic states, most commonly hyperparathyroidism, may cause acute and chronic pancreatitis. The mechanism is unclear, but hypercalcemia may favor the intraductal precipitation of calcium stones which are seen in up to half of these patients. Calcium also influences the activation of certain pancreatic enzymes and a variety of acinar cell synthetic and secretory events. Acute hypercalcemia increases the permeability of pancreatic ducts, perhaps allowing enzymes to leak from them.

HEREDITARY PANCREATITIS

Chronic pancreatitis can occur as a genetic condition, probably transmitted as a Mendelian dominant trait. The condition is rare, but more than 250 patients have been reported. Symptoms appear in most patients between 12 and 14 years of age, and are typical of acute pancreatitis. Relentless progression of the process is usual, with recurrent attacks of acute inflammation. Eventually, many patients develop the typical manifestations of chronic pancreatitis, including calcifications (32%), diabetes (19%), and steatorrhea from exocrine insufficiency (15%). An increased incidence of pancreatic carcinoma has been noted in these patients. In most of the reported cases where ERCP has been performed, the ducts have been dilated and the pancreas amenable to decompression by lateral pancreaticojejunostomy (Fig 72–2).

IDIOPATHIC PANCREATITIS

Twenty to thirty percent of cases of chronic pancreatitis have no apparent cause. There is recent evidence that this form of the disease is more likely to be free of pain

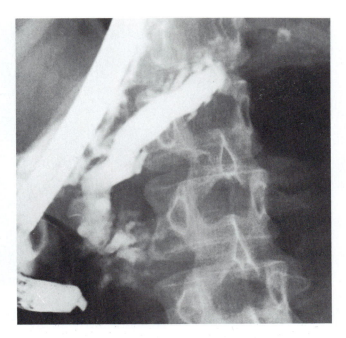

Figure 72–2. ERCP in a 23 year–old man with hereditary pancreatitis and onset of attacks at 16 years of age. It shows marked dilatation of the main duct, without stones, extending almost to the duodenum. (From Elliott DW: Familial pancreatitis. In: Howard JM, Jordan GL Jr, Reber HA (eds), *Surgical Diseases of the Pancreas.* Philadelphia, PA: Lea and Febiger; 1987:319)

as compared to the alcoholic variety (up to 50% painless vs 5%). Nevertheless, pancreatic calcifications, and exocrine and endocrine insufficiency are common. It is to be anticipated that the number of cases labeled idiopathic will decrease as our understanding of the causes of the disease improves.

● PATHOLOGY

GROSS

Early in the disease the pancreas may be grossly normal in appearance and ERCP may reveal a normal duct. As the disease progresses, the pancreas may become enlarged, indurated, and edematous from recent attacks of acute inflammation. The duct may still be normal, or there may be slight dilatation of the main duct and one or two of its tributaries. When the disease is far advanced, the pancreas is usually small and may be reduced to a contracted cord no more than 2 to 3 centimeters in diameter. Its edges are characteristically rounded; it may have a rubbery consistency or it may be rock hard. Pancreatography at this stage usually shows some degree of ductal dilatation, but in some cases the duct may be narrow and distorted. However, even then the duct may look completely normal. Ductal stones are

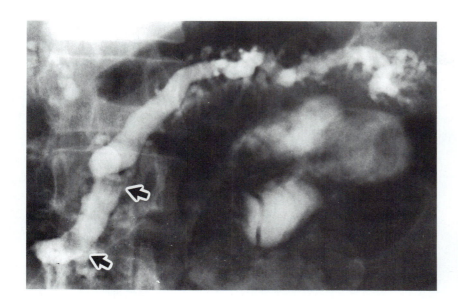

Figure 72–3. ERCP reveals the main pancreatic duct and its side branches to be dilated and tortuous. Two large pancreatic calculi are seen as filling defects in the main duct (*arrows*). (From Ariyama J. Endoscopic evaluation of pancreatic disease. In: Howard JM, Jordan GL Jr, Reber HA (eds), *Surgical Diseases of the Pancreas.* Philadelphia, PA: Lea and Febiger; 1987:128)

frequently present. They vary in size from less than a millimeter to more than a centimeter in diameter (Figs 72–3 and 72–4). It should be noted that all pancreatic calcifications are actually intraductal in location. Thus, the size of a stone seen on a plain abdominal film provides information about the minimal diameter of the pancreatic duct in which it must reside. In patients with large dilated ducts, the duct often can be palpated at operation as a longitudinal soft depression on the anterior surface of the gland. In a normal pancreas, its position is closer to the posterior surface in most cases, and it cannot be palpated.

MICROSCOPIC

Chronic calcific pancreatitis is most frequently the result of chronic alcoholism, but it is pathologically similar to pancreatitis secondary to hypercalcemic states and hereditary pancreatitis. Early in the disease, the lesions are spotty and affect one or more lobules, which are surrounded by normal parenchyma. The lesions show partial or complete dilatation of the acini with both intralobular and perilobular fibrosis. Some of the ducts are obstructed by deposits of protein, which later calcify to form stones. In advanced stages, fibrosis extends throughout the gland, but the lobules are still variably affected and some remain normal. In the most advanced stages, the pancreas is almost entirely replaced with fibrous tissue (Figs 72–5 and 72–6). Cysts are found where the duct epithelium has been destroyed. The islets of Langerhans appear to survive and look hyperplastic. Nevertheless, since many such patients are diabetic by the time this stage of the disease has been reached, the islets probably do not function normally. Recent studies on the intrapancreatic nerves in chronic

pancreatitis suggest that they are preserved in number while the surrounding tissue is destroyed and the gland shrinks. The effect is that they are more densely distributed throughout the pancreas when the disease is advanced. The perineural sheath also appears to be destroyed, possibly allowing noxious substances to reach the nerve fibers and irritate them. This could be one cause of the pain so common in the disease.

The lesions of chronic pancreatitis secondary to obstruction of the main duct are more diffuse than those just described. They are evenly distributed and all lobules are equally affected. The ducts are moderately dilated and stenotic areas are less common. Protein plugs and calcifications are unusual. Nevertheless, when the process is far advanced, the pathological picture is similar regardless of etiology.

EXTRAPANCREATIC INVOLVEMENT

Common Bile Duct Obstruction

Jaundice is seen in up to one-third of patients with chronic calcific pancreatitis at some point during the course of the disease. This is most often the result of transient obstruction of the intrapancreatic portion of the common bile duct during an episode of acute pancreatic inflammation. It subsides when the acute process resolves. However, as many as 10% of patients develop persistent common duct obstruction from fibrous constriction of the duct in the head of the gland. The radiographic characteristics are described as a diffuse, longitudinal, symmetrical stricture (Fig 72–7). The common duct proximal to the stricture usually is moderately dilated. The gallbladder and cystic duct also may be distended. The obstruction is almost never complete. This is different than the obstruction caused by pancre-

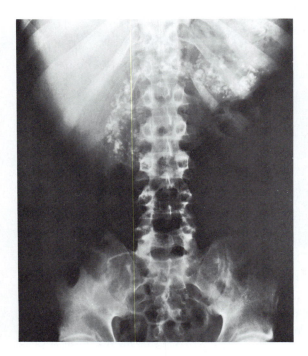

Figure 72–4. An abdominal roentgenogram shows multiple pancreatic calcifications secondary to chronic pancreatitis. (From Gooding GAW. Conventional radiography of the pancreas. In: Howard JM, Jordan GL Jr, Reber HA (eds), *Surgical Diseases of the Pancreas*. Philadelphia, PA: Lea and Febiger; 1987:72)

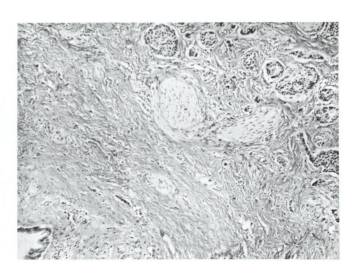

Figure 72–5. Advanced pancreatitis. Note prominence of nerve bundles that are encased in dense hyalinized collagen. Observe the close relationship of the islets of Langerhans to these nerve bundles. The interlobular duct is lined by cuboid epithelial cells with abundant mucin. Hematoxylin and eosin (X70). (From Reber HA. Chronic pancreatitis: etiology, pathology, and diagnosis. In: Howard JM, Jordan GL Jr, Reber HA (eds), *Surgical Diseases of the Pancreas*. Philadelphia, PA: Lea and Febiger; 1987:487)

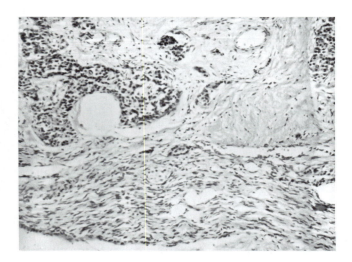

Figure 72–6. Advanced pancreatitis. Saccularly dilated main duct demonstrates irregular peripheral distribution of elastic fibers disrupted by inflammatory infiltrate. van Gieson-Verhoeff (X28). (From Reber HA. Chronic pancreatitis: etiology, pathology, and diagnosis. In: Howard JM, Jordan GL Jr, Reber HA (eds), *Surgical Diseases of the Pancreas*. Philadelphia, PA: Lea and Febiger; 1987:487)

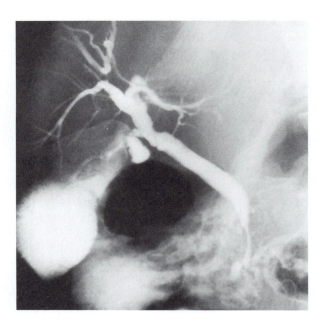

Figure 72–7. Stenosis of the common bile duct caused by chronic pancreatitis. ERCP shows a long smooth stricture of the common bile duct with slight dilatation above. Calcification is seen in the head of the pancreas. (From Ariyama J. Endoscopic evaluation of pancreatic disease. In: Howard JM, Jordan GL Jr, Reber HA (eds), *Surgical Diseases of the Pancreas*. Philadelphia, PA: Lea and Febiger; 1987:129)

atic cancer where the stricture is more often shorter in length, assymetric, and complete. When the obstruction is caused by chronic pancreatitis, and the duct is freed surgically from the constricting pancreas, it often expands to relieve the obstruction.

Duodenal Obstruction

Less than 1% of patients with chronic pancreatitis develop persistent duodenal obstruction caused by the inflammation in the adjacent pancreatic head. Duodenoscopy shows marked narrowing of the second or third portion of the duodenum with intact mucosa. The differential diagnosis includes pancreatic cancer, peptic ulcer, and rare conditions such as duodenal diverticulitis and annular pancreas. The correct diagnosis may only be possible at operation. Gastrojejunostomy is effective treatment.

Colonic Obstruction

A recent review listed 34 patients with pancreatitis and colon obstruction. In 80% to 90% of these patients, the transverse colon and/or splenic flexures were involved. The hepatic flexure was narrowed in 15% of cases. In 80% of patients, the obstruction was partial. When an episode of acute pancreatic inflammation was part of the clinical presentation, the obstruction often resolved with conservative therapy. When it was not, operation was required for relief. Carcinoma of the colon generally can be ruled out by preoperative colonoscopy because benign strictures are associated with an intact mucosa. Colon resection with end-to-end anastomosis is satisfactory.

■ DIAGNOSIS

CLINICAL MANIFESTATIONS

In 95% of patients with chronic pancreatitis, the principal symptom is **abdominal pain.** The intensity of the pain is often great. It has been described as cramping, boring, dull, and aching in nature. It usually is located in the epigastrium, with radiation to either subcostal area. In more than half the cases, it also is felt in the back. During an episode of acute inflammation, the pain is the same as it is in a patient with an attack of acute pancreatitis. In between such episodes, patients experience recurrent pain that may last several days to several weeks, separated initially by several months or more. Typically, the pain-free intervals become shorter and the painful attacks last longer, so that pain eventually occurs every day. When the disease is so far advanced that most of the exocrine function is lost, approximately one-third of patients experience spontaneous pain relief. Another 10% to 20% have temporary remissions of pain that last 1 to 3 years. Some pain relief is typically obtained when the patients sit with the knees flexed and a pillow pressed to the abdomen. Or they may lie in bed on their side in a fetal position. Eating may increase the pain, so many patients avoid food and lose weight. Most require analgesic drugs and many become addicted to narcotics.

Assessment of the severity of pain is often difficult because many of these patients are addicted to alcohol and/or narcotics and have unstable personalities. Thus, secondary gain may be a factor leading to an exaggeration of symptoms.

The mechanism of the pain is uncertain. In patients with dilated ducts, intraductal pressures are generally elevated to 30 to 50 cm of water (up to 20 cm of water is normal). Pancreatic interstitial pressures are also high (20 to 30 cm of water). Operations designed to drain the ducts (which also decrease the intraductal and interstitial pressures) reliably relieve the pain. Although it is not known whether the ductal pressures are elevated in patients with pain and small duct disease, recent data indicates that pancreatic tissue pressures are elevated in such cases. In general, tissue pressures correlate well with ductal pressures. There is evidence that the pancreas afflicted with chronic pancreatitis behaves as if it were the site of a compartment syndrome. The pancreatic blood flow is severely restricted, suggesting that the pain may have an ischemic basis. Operations that drain the dilated ducts and relieve pain also return pancreatic blood flow to normal.

Variable weight loss occurs in 75% of patients with chronic pancreatitis. As already indicated, this is because food usually aggravates the pain, and intake is voluntarily restricted. Significant weight loss from malabsorption is less common. Even when malabsorption occurs, most patients who are able to eat maintain their weight by eating more.

Significant exocrine insufficiency does not occur until 90% of the secretory capacity of the pancreas is lost. This can be the result of either progressive parenchymal destruction or obstruction of the major ducts which prevents the pancreatic digestive enzymes from reaching the duodenum. In either case, it is a late development. The major consequences are steatorrhea and creatorrhea, which is excessive loss of fat and protein in the stools. Carbohydrate digestion is not impaired because amylase also is produced by the salivary glands. The patients may complain of bulky, offensive, fatty, or oily stools.

About two-thirds of patients with chronic pancreatitis have abnormal glucose tolerance and half of these have diabetes mellitus. In them, some degree of malabsorption is also present, since exocrine and endocrine insufficiency usually develop in parallel. The diabetes usually is controlled easily with insulin, but hypoglycemia may be a problem in alcoholics with irregular eating habits.

As a rule, most patients with chronic pancreatitis have failed to adapt to the stresses of society and have inadequate personalities. The additional stresses created by the disease often result in depression and anxiety. These personality traits are important in evaluating these patients, as well as in choosing specific types of therapy.

Most patients with chronic pancreatitis have few physical findings. There may be some epigastric tenderness. There may be evidence of weight loss and occasionally jaundice is evident. If a mass is palpable, it is most likely to be a pancreatic pseudocyst.

LABORATORY FINDINGS

These are not especially helpful in making the diagnosis of chronic pancreatitis. Early in the disease, the serum amylase and lipase concentrations are elevated during episodes of acute inflammation. As the disease becomes more advanced, they often remain normal even during such acute episodes. Possible explanations for the failure of the enzyme levels to increase in the serum are that (1) the progressive destruction of the acinar cells limits the amount of enzyme available for release, and (2) the chronic fibrosis limits the permeability of the ducts to the enzymes that normally leak out of them into the capillaries during acute inflammation.

About two-thirds of patients with alcoholic pancreatitis have abnormal liver function. Mild elevations of serum concentrations of bilirubin (2 to 4 mg/dL), alkaline phosphatase, and SGOT, and mild depression of serum albumin concentration may occur.

Pancreatic exocrine function is impaired in almost all patients, but there is a wide range of normal values for bicarbonate and enzyme secretion and volume flow in response to standard secretory stimuli (secretin and cholecystokinin). For this reason, mild abnormalities may not be apparent. Pancreatic function tests are rarely indicated in patients with overt pancreatic disease (chronic pancreatitis or pancreatic cancer). Although they would confirm the presence of pancreatic insufficiency, they (1) rarely influence therapeutic decisions and (2) cannot distinguish between pancreatitis and cancer. They are of greater value in patients with vague complaints in whom the presence of pancreatic disease is suspected but for which no direct evidence exists. In that setting, these tests are 90% sensitive to detect functional abnormalities. Thus, a normal test along with one or two other studies that are also normal (eg, ERCP or computer-assisted tomography (CAT) scan) reliably rules out pancreatic disease. The newer simplified function tests that do not require intubation and collection of pancreatic juice (eg, oral N-benzoyl-L-tyrosyl-p-aminobenzoic acid, bentiromide) are even less sensitive and specific for the detection of pancreatic insufficiency.

RADIOLOGIC FEATURES

In 30% to 50% of patients with chronic pancreatitis, plain x-rays of the abdomen reveal pancreatic calcifications (Fig 72–4). Indeed, when calcifications are present, the diagnosis of chronic pancreatitis is certain even if there is no clinical evidence of pancreatic disease.

With early chronic pancreatitis, and even in some patients with advanced disease, ductal abnormalities demonstrated by ERCP may be minimal. However in the majority of patients with advanced disease, the main duct may be dilated up to one centimeter or more in diameter with intermittent points of obstruction (Fig 72–8). Strictures, cysts, and ductal calculi may be seen (Figs 72–9 and 72–10). The common bile duct also is opacified by this technique, and any distortion of its anatomy is evident. Chronic pancreatitis characteristically produces angulation of the distal common duct with a smooth, tapered narrowing of its intrapancreatic portion (Fig 72–7). Most patients with chronic pancreatitis who are being considered for surgical intervention should undergo ERCP examination. The study provides important information about ductal anatomy that may influence a decision for surgery. For example, a patient with pain and a widely dilated duct may be a candidate for a pancreaticojejunostomy. If the duct were not dilated, pancreatic resection might be indicated instead (Fig 72–11). Occasionally, a preoperative ERCP may not be possible to obtain. If a pancreatogram is required, it can be done at operation by cannulating the duct in the head or the tail of the pancreas, or by puncturing it directly through the anterior surface of the gland (Fig 72–12).

CAT scans also may provide useful information about ductal anatomy. When the duct is grossly dilated, it usually can be seen running the length of the gland (Fig 72–13). In that situation, an ERCP may be unnecessary, since pseudocysts and cystic communications with the ductal system are evident (Fig 72–13). Biliary dilatation and the level of bile duct obstruction are defined clearly. CAT scans provide the most precise information about the size and configuration of the pancreas. This may be useful in decisions regarding possible pancreatic resection. For example, in a patient with pain and an enlarged head of the pancreas seen on CAT scan, a pancreaticoduodenectomy might be the best choice (Fig 72–14).

DIFFERENTIAL DIAGNOSIS

Usually the diagnosis of chronic pancreatitis is straightforward. Most patients are chronic alcoholics with recurring episodes of abdominal pain, diabetes, weight loss, pancreatic calcifications, and some evidence of malabsorption. Occasionally, the distinction between

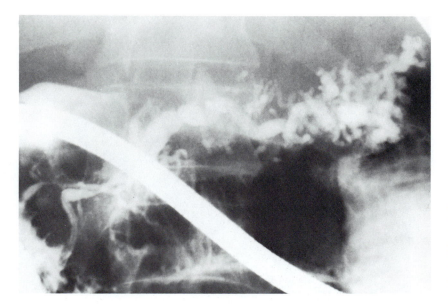

Figure 72–8. ERCP demonstrates the dilatation and irregularity of the pancreatic duct system that is characteristic of advanced chronic pancreatitis. Intermittent points of ductal narrowing and dilatation have been described as having a "chain-of-lakes" appearance. (From Ariyama J. Endoscopic evaluation of pancreatic disease. In: Howard JM, Jordan GL Jr, Reber HA (eds), *Surgical Diseases of the Pancreas*. Philadelphia, PA: Lea and Febiger; 1987:126)

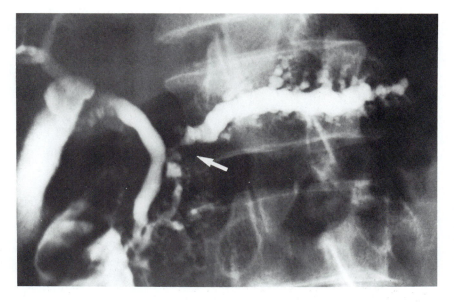

Figure 72–9. ERCP shows stenosis of the main pancreatic duct (*arrow*) in chronic pancreatitis. The main duct and side branches proximal to the stenosis are dilated and irregular. (From Ariyama J. Endoscopic evaluation of pancreatic disease. In: Howard JM, Jordan GL Jr, Reber HA (eds), *Surgical Diseases of the Pancreas*. Philadelphia, PA: Lea and Febiger; 1987:126)

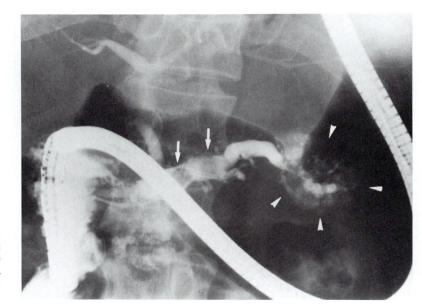

Figure 72–10. Two calculi are seen in the main pancreatic duct (*arrows*) in this ERCP. A large communicating pseudocyst is seen in the tail of the pancreas (*arrowheads*). (From Ariyama J. Endoscopic evaluation of pancreatic disease. In: Howard JM, Jordan GL Jr, Reber HA (eds), *Surgical Diseases of the Pancreas*. Philadelphia, PA: Lea and Febiger; 1987:128)

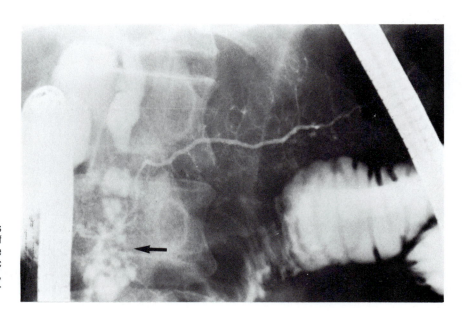

Figure 72–11. ERCP showing the main pancreatic duct and its side branches to be narrowed and irregular, manifestations of chronic pancreatitis. Pancreatic calcification is present in the head of the pancreas (*arrow*). (From Ariyama J. Endoscopic evaluation of pancreatic disease. In: Howard JM, Jordan GL Jr, Reber HA (eds), *Surgical Diseases of the Pancreas*. Philadelphia, PA: Lea and Febiger; 1987:127)

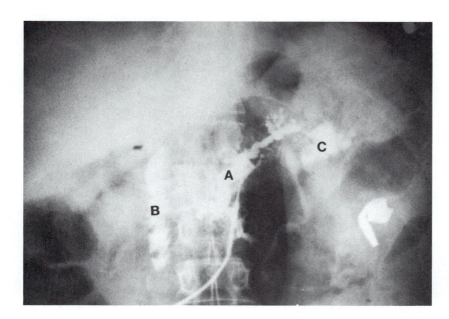

Figure 72–12. This radiograph of an operative pancreatogram shows the dilated pancreatic duct (A), contrast material outlining the duodenum (B), and a pseudocyst in the tail of the pancreas (C), which had not been suspected. The duct was punctured with a needle that can also be seen on the x-ray picture.

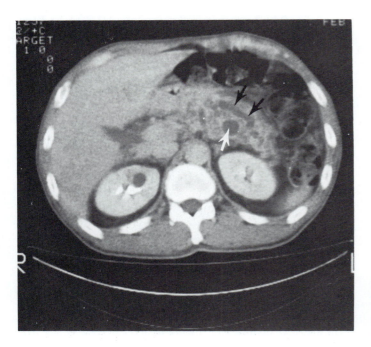

Figure 72–13. A computerized tomograph shows an enlarged pancreatic duct (*arrows*) and a small pseudocyst in the tail of the pancreas (*white arrow*) in a patient with chronic pancreatitis. (From Gooding GAW. Computerized tomography of the pancreas. In: Howard JM, Jordan GL Jr, Reber HA (eds), *Surgical Diseases of the Pancreas*. Philadelphia, PA: Lea and Febiger; 1987:95)

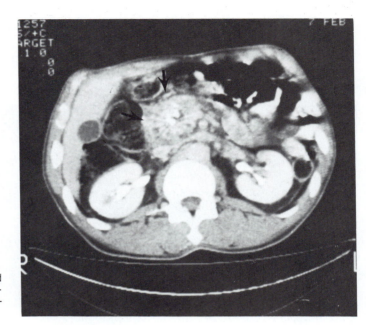

Figure 72–14. At another level in the same patient as in Fig 72–13, the pancreatic head is enlarged (*arrows*) and has calcifications. (From Gooding GAW. Computerized tomography of the pancreas. In: Howard JM, Jordan GL Jr, Reber HA (eds), *Surgical Diseases of the Pancreas.* Philadelphia, PA: Lea and Febiger; 1987:95)

chronic pancreatitis and pancreatic cancer may be difficult. This may occur when there is no previous history of pancreatitis, when the patient presents with jaundice, pain is not a prominent part of the picture, and weight loss is significant. In such circumstances, operation may be necessary to make the diagnosis.

■ TREATMENT

MEDICAL

The medical treatment of an episode of acute pancreatic inflammation is the same as the treatment of any episode of acute pancreatitis. The medical management of malabsorption, diabetes, and chronic pain will be reviewed.

Pancreatic Insufficiency

Pancreatic insufficiency affects fat absorption more than that of protein or carbohydrate, because protein digestion is aided by gastric pepsin and carbohydrate digestion by salivary amylase. The diet should supply 3000 to 6000 kcal a day, emphasizing carbohydrate (400 gm or more) and protein (100 to 150 gm). Patients with steatorrhea may or may not have diarrhea, and dietary restriction of fat is important, mainly to control diarrhea. Patients with diarrhea may be restricted to 50 gm/day of fat and the amount increased until diarrhea appears. Permissible fat intake averages 100 gm/day, distributed equally throughout 4 meals. Pancreatic enzyme replacement may be accomplished with pancreatic extracts (eg, Cotazym, Ilozyme, Pancrease MT-16, Viokase) containing at least 30 000 units of lipase given with each of 4 daily meals. An hourly dosage regimen probably has no advantage. If enzymes alone do not improve the malabsorption enough, the problem is probably the result of the destruction of lipase by gastric acid. Then an H2 receptor blocking agent should be added to the regimen.

It is important to realize that the malabsorption of fat can never be eliminated entirely. Nevertheless the diarrhea should cease and patients should be able to regain weight with the proper combination of diet, enzyme replacement, and (in some cases) acid antisecretory drugs.

Diabetes Mellitus

In patients with diabetes from chronic pancreatitis, ketoacidosis is rare, even if blood glucose levels are quite high. However even small amounts of subcutaneous insulin may induce a profound hypoglycemia. This is probably because there is also a deficiency of glucagon, the islet hormone that normally corrects hypoglycemia by converting liver glycogen to glucose. Thus, the patient must be instructed thoroughly on the dangers of hypoglycemia, its symptoms, and management. Mild elevations in blood sugar do not require treatment, but fasting elevations in excess of 250 mg/dL should be managed with insulin. Frequently only 20 to 30 units a day are required. Rigid control of blood sugar is not advisable, and it is reasonable to maintain the fasting level around 200 mg/dL. Oral agents are almost never successful.

In those patients who are not yet diabetic and who are to undergo pancreatic resection, the chance for the development of diabetes is related to the amount of pancreas removed. Most patients with abnormal glucose tolerance before operation will require insulin after a resection of 50% or more.

Pain

The medical management of pain in patients with chronic pancreatitis should include the cessation of all alcohol intake. Although it is difficult to predict the effect in an individual case, as many as 50% of patients experience some pain relief when they stop drinking. Pain relief may be more likely in those with early disease and relatively well preserved pancreatic function. In those with pain who already have severe pancreatic insufficiency, pain is likely to persist.

There is some evidence that pancreatic secretion, especially when the gland is still capable of synthesizing significant amounts of digestive enzymes, may exacerbate the pain. This notion has led to certain dietary recommendations with the goal of minimizing the stimuli to secretion. Thus, patients may be advised to consume semisolid or liquid diets instead of solids; carbohydrates have been stressed rather than fats or proteins. Antacids or H2 receptor antagonists also have been used. Nevertheless, the efficacy of all of these regimens is unproved.

Another approach attempts to take advantage of the phenomenon of negative feedback inhibition of pancreatic secretion. Normally, the presence of endogenous pancreatic enzymes within the lumen of the small intestine decreases the subsequent synthesis and secretion of additional enzymes. Thus, patients with chronic pancreatitis and pain may be treated with oral pancreatic enzyme supplements in order to suppress their own pancreatic synthetic and secretory activity. Although several studies have indicated significant pain reduction with such treatment, most clinicians have been disappointed with the results. A recent trial of a parenteral somatostatin analogue to inhibit pancreatic secretion also appeared to relieve pain in some patients, but larger studies are needed.

The analgesic management of these patients should begin with small doses of oral medications such as codeine derivatives, either alone or combined with acetaminophen. If more potent narcotic analgesics are required, especially for prolonged periods of time, serious consideration must be given to surgery for pain relief. All too often these patients are denied surgical treatment until they have become addicted to narcotics and are severely disturbed psychologically as a result of living with constant pain. In the opinion of the author, operation earlier in the course of the disease (at least in patients with dilated ducts amenable to pancreaticojejunostomy) appears indicated in many. In patients who would require a major pancreatic resection, a more conservative approach still seems appropriate.

SURGICAL TREATMENT

The indications for surgery for pain relief in these patients are impossible to state in precise terms. When the pain interferes substantially with the quality of life, surgery should be considered. Pertinent issues include obvious effects on health and well-being, such as weight loss and malnutrition, need for frequent hospitalization, inability to maintain employment, depression, deterioration of family life, and impending or actual narcotic addiction.

All patients who are being evaluated for surgery should undergo an abdominal CT scan and (usually) an ERCP, in addition to the standard preoperative assessment for a major abdominal procedure. Angiography may be helpful for those in whom pancreatic resection is being considered, but most pancreatic surgeons have not performed this routinely. Indeed, the newer spiral CT scans also provide detailed information about vascular anatomy. Psychiatric evaluation is appropriate in many. These studies are important to provide information about the type of surgical procedure that may be indicated, as well as whether any procedure is appropriate at all. Although decisions for surgery are always the result of a risk vs benefit assessment, that is particularly so in this group of patients. Thus, even in an individual with narcotic addiction and severe depression who has a widely dilated pancreatic duct, a pancreaticojejunostomy may be indicated. It could be done with very low morbidity and operative mortality rates, and with virtually no risk of creating diabetes. If the same patient had a narrowed or normal size duct (not amenable to pancreaticojejunostomy), a major pancreatic resection might be contraindicated because of the likelihood of the appearance of diabetes postoperatively. Such a patient might not be able to manage safely the dietary and insulin requirements that would ensue. Therefore, in a given patient with clear indications for surgery, a decision for or against operation might well be made on the basis of information derived from such an evaluation.

Operations to relieve pain in patients with chronic pancreatitis take one of two forms. The first are the so-called drainage operations that attempt to drain more adequately a dilated ductal system that is presumed to be obstructed. The second are the pancreatic resection operations that remove diseased pancreatic tissue, usually in situations where the pancreatic ducts are normal or narrowed in size. Sphincterotomy or sphincteroplasty of the sphincter of Oddi has no place in the treatment of pain in patients with this disease.

TABLE 72–2. OPERATIVE MORTALITY FROM LONGITUDINAL PANCREATICOJEJUNOSTOMY FOR CHRONIC PANCREATITIS

Author	Patients	Deaths	Percent
Prinz and Greenlee (1981)	96	3	3
Arnesjo (1975)	8	0	0
Sato (1975)	24	0	0
Warshaw (1980)	10	0	0
Howard (1981)	42	1	2
White (1973)	50	1	2
White (1979)	52	3	6
Potts (1981)	10	0	0
Adson (1979)	2	0	0
Williams (1982)	3	0	0
Puestow (1958)	21	0	0
Jordan (1977)	24	0	0
Proctor (1979)	9	0	0
Silen (1963)	15	0	0
Leger (1974)	45	2	4
Taylor (1981)	22	0	0

(Adapted from Howard JM: Surgical treatment of chronic pancreatitis. In: Howard JM, Jordan GL, Reber HA (ed), Surgical Diseases of the Pancreas. Philadelphia, PA: Lea & Febiger; 1987:503

Drainage Operations (Pancreaticojejunostomy, Puestow Procedure)

The main pancreatic duct has a normal diameter of approximately 4 to 5 mm in the head, 3 to 4 mm in the body, and 2 to 3 mm in the tail of the gland. When the diameter in the head and body increases to 7 to 8 mm or larger, a pancreaticojejunostomy is technically feasible and is likely to be effective in producing lasting pain relief. If the operation is done in a pancreas with a normal size duct, both short- and long-term results are poor, perhaps because the anastomosis strictures closed, in most cases.

The operative mortality rate of longitudinal pancreaticojejunostomy averages about 4% (Table 72–2), and the morbidity is minimal. Diabetes does not result from the operation; indeed, there is some evidence that exocrine and endocrine function may even improve slightly after pancreaticojejunostomy. Nevertheless, some patients will eventually require insulin, since the destruction of the pancreas often continues. Pancreatic fistula is an uncommon complication of the operation, probably because the fibrous pancreas holds sutures quite well. Nevertheless, with a drain in place, it is not a serious complication and will almost certainly close spontaneously. Although pancreatic enzymes can now empty freely through the pancreaticojejunostomy, there is rarely any clinical improvement in the degree of malabsorption. Nevertheless, patients may gain weight because eating no longer produces pain, and they eat more. Pain is relieved completely or substantially in 80% to 85% of patients for the first several years after the operation. Unfortunately, it recurs in a considerable number of cases, so that by the time 5 years have passed, only about 60% to 70% still report good pain relief (Table 72–3). In some patients, recurrence of pain may be owing to stenosis of the pancreaticojejunal anastomosis, which can be proved by

TABLE 72–3. RESULTS OF OPERATION FOR CHRONIC PANCREATITIS

Operation and Author	5-year Results			Functional Results of Survivors (%)		
	Patients (No.)	Deaths[a] (No.)	Alive (%)	Failed	Fair	Good
DISTAL PANCREATECTOMY						
Leger	71	15	79	21	11	68
Taylor	40	—	—	—	—	60
Frey	114	30	74	13	7	80
PANCREATICOJEJUNOSTOMY						
Leger	45	5	89	37	15	48
Taylor	22	—	—	—	—	50
Silen	24	6	75	25	37	38
Howard	33	5	85	38	6	56
PANCREATICODUODENECTOMY						
Leger	16	8	50	12	12	75
Taylor	29	—	—	—	—	60
Guillemin	57	20	65	12	14	74
Howard	9	0	100	0	33	67

[a]Includes operative deaths.
(Adapted from Howard JM. Surgical treatment of chronic pancreatitis. In: Howard JM, Jordan GL, Reber HA (eds), Surgical Diseases of the Pancreas. Philadelphia, PA: Lea & Febiger; 1987:504)

TABLE 72–4. ENDOCRINE FUNCTION IN PATIENTS WITH CHRONIC PANCREATITIS AFTER DUODENUM-PRESERVING RESECTION OF HEAD OF PANCREAS

Status	Preoperative Status (128 Patients)		Early Postoperative Status[a] (127 Patients)		Late Postoperative Status (109 Patients)	
	Ratio	Percent	Ratio	Percent	Ratio	Percent
Normal	80:128	62.5	77:127	60.6	62:109	56.9
Latent	23:128	17.9	24:127	18.9	20:109	18.3
Insulin-dependent	25:128	19.5	25:127	20.5	27:109	24.8

Final Results (%)

Improved	6
Deteriorated	13
Unchanged	81

[a]Early results are within 3 months of operation; late results are after that time, with a median time at evaluation of 3.6 years.
(From Beger HG: Personal communication.)

ERCP. Then reconstruction of the anastomosis may be beneficial. In the majority of cases, there is no apparent cause for the recurrence of pain, and other forms of treatment, including pancreatic resection, must be considered.

A variation of the longitudinal pancreaticojejunostomy in which the head of the pancreas is "cored out," has been described by Frey. It may be done in patients with a dilated pancreatic duct, in whom the head of the pancreas is enlarged (4 to 5 cm antero-posterior diameter), and contains calcifications and cystic dilatations of the pancreatic duct. Such patients might otherwise have been considered candidates for a pancreaticoduodenectomy, but this operation is associated with lower short- and long-term morbidity and mortality than the Whipple resection. Pain relief is at least as effective as the standard Puestow operation.

Pancreatic Resections (Pancreaticoduodenectomy, Pylorus-Preserving Pancreaticoduodenectomy, Pancreatic Head Resection, 95% Pancreatectomy, Distal Pancreatectomy)

Pancreatic resection should be considered for pain relief when the pancreatic duct is narrow or normal in diameter, when a previous pancreaticojejunostomy has failed, or when the pathologic changes in the pancreas particularly involve one part of the gland, and the rest is less diseased. Common examples of the latter are (1) when the head of the pancreas is especially enlarged, compresses the bile duct, contains multiple cysts and calcifications, and the body and tail are less involved, and (2) when the pancreas is only minimally diseased up to the point of a stricture in the body of the gland, but the disease is severe past the stricture in the tail. In the first situation, some form of resection of the head of the pancreas may be appropriate; in the second, a distal pancreatectomy beginning at the stricture might be indicated.

Pancreaticoduodenectomy. When pancreaticoduodenectomy is to be performed for chronic pancreatitis and there is little concern about the presence of pancreatic cancer, the resection itself may proceed with minimal delay. Nevertheless, a complete abdominal exploration must be performed, and any findings suspicious for the diagnosis of cancer must be pursued. The surgeon must be alert to the fact that the distinction between chronic pancreatitis and pancreatic cancer may be exceedingly difficult. Indeed, in some patients with chronic pancreatitis, the inability to rule out the presence of pancreatic cancer may be the main indication for operation.

Pylorus-preserving Pancreaticoduodenectomy. A modification of the standard Whipple operation is the pylorus-preserving pancreaticoduodenectomy. The entire stomach, pylorus, and first 3 to 4 cm of duodenum are preserved. The theoretical advantage of this is that it preserves gastric function and may avoid some of the nutritional disturbances that can follow the standard

TABLE 72–5. LATE RESULTS AFTER DUODENUM-PRESERVING RESECTION OF HEAD OF PANCREAS[a]

	Status	Patients	Percent
Abdominal pain	Free	84:109	77
	Seldom	13:109	12
	Frequent	12:109	11
Professional rehabilitation	Complete	68:101	67
	Unemployed	13:101	13
	Retired	20:101	20
Consumption of alcohol	None	59:109	54
	Occasional	31:109	29
	Frequent	19:109	17

[a]Duration of follow-up of 109 patients (96%): 6 mo–1 y (20%), 1–2 y (15%), 2–3 y (15%), 3–16y (50%).
(From Beger HG. Personal communication)

TABLE 72–6. OPERATIVE MORTALITY FROM PANCREATICODUODENECTOMY FOR CHRONIC PANCREATITIS

Author	Patients	Deaths	Percent
Proctor (1979)	7	1	14
Leger (1974)	16	1	6
Sarles (1982)	23	2	9
Guillemin (1971)	63	1	2
Gall (1981)	49	4	8
Frey (1976)	19	1	5
Taylor (1981)	29	2	7
White (1979)	18	1	6
Traverso (1979)	5	0	0
Stefanini (1972)	5	1	20
Howard (1987)	14	0	0
Adson (1979)	7	0	0
Mercadier (1967)	21	1	5
Fre (1981) (collected)	286	26	9
Cohen (1983) (collected)	334	16	5
Cuilleret (1985) (collected)	1000	50	5

(Adapted from Howard JM. Surgical treatment of chronic pancreatitis, In: Howard JM, Jordan GL, Reber HA (ed), Surgical Diseases of the Pancreas. Philadelphia, PA: Lea & Febiger; 1987:501)

pancreaticoduodenectomy. It also is said that the pylorus-preserving Whipple operation is technically easier to perform, and that it can be done more quickly with less blood loss. However, the few comparisons that have been made so far have failed to prove that preservation of the pylorus confers significant benefit. The incidence of delayed gastric emptying in the early postoperative period may be increased after the pylorus-preserving operation.

Pancreatic Head Resection. Beger and his colleagues from Germany have described an operation in which the head of the pancreas is resected, and the entire stomach and duodenum are preserved. The body and tail of the pancreas as well as a thin rim of pancreatic tissue in the C loop of the duodenum also remain. The theoretical advantages of the procedure include the preservation of gastroduodenal and biliary continuity and function and a low likelihood of the development of diabetes, because the body and tail of the pancreas are preserved. The procedure has been done in patients where most of the pathologic changes involved the head of the pancreas, with duodenal compression in about half, common bile duct compression in two-thirds, and compression of the portal vein in one quarter of the cases.

The results in over 100 operated patients are presented in Tables 72–4 and 72–5. Although they appear promising both from the point of preservation of endocrine function and the relief of pain, longer follow-up and confirmation of these results in other centers will be important.

Ninety-five Percent Distal Pancreatectomy. Ninety-five percent distal pancreatectomy entails the removal of the spleen and all of the pancreas except for a thin rim of tissue that lies within the C loop of the duodenum. Because the spleen is sacrificed and all of the patients require insulin after this operation, it is not done frequently. Nevertheless if the entire pancreas is uniformly and severely diseased, and especially if lesser operations have failed to provide relief, it may be considered. Total pancreatectomy is rarely done today because of the uniform requirement for insulin and the significant alterations in digestive and absorptive functions that follow. The 95% pancreatectomy that preserves normal gastrointestinal and biliary continuity is often preferred in situations where such a major resection is indicated.

Distal Pancreatectomy. Distal pancreatectomy is an imprecise term that describes resection of variable amounts of the tail, or body and tail, of the pancreas, in which the head of the gland is preserved. Examples of clinical sit-

TABLE 72–7. OPERATIVE MORTALITY FROM DISTAL PANCREATECTOMY FOR CHRONIC PANCREATITIS

Author and Percent Resection	Patients	Deaths	Percent
Proctor (1979)			
40–80	17	0	0
95	1	0	0
Leger (1974)	71	5	7
With pancreaticojejunostomy	(39)		
Without pancreaticojejunostomy	(32)		
Sarles (1982)			
40	22	3	14
Frey (1976)			
40–80	53	1	2
80–95	77	1	1
Grodsinsky (1980)			
60–80	19	0	0
95	11	0	0
Taylor (1981)	40	0	0
White (1979)	50	2	4
40–80	(35)		
80–95	(15)		
Traverso (1979)			
40–80	7	1	14
80–95	8	1	13
Trapnell (1978)			
95	15	0	0
Mercadier (1967)			
90	15	1	7
50	32	1	3
Howard (1987)			
40–60	27	0	0
Frey (1981) (collected)	538	24	4

(Adapted from Howard JM. Surgical treatment of chronic pancreatitis, In: Howard JM, Jordan GL, Reber HA (eds), Surgical Diseases of the Pancreas. Philadelphia, PA: Lea & Febiger; 1987:501)

TABLE 72–8. CAUSES OF DEATH IN CHRONIC PANCREATITIS

Author	Number of Patients	Original Operation	Progressive Pancreatitis	Sudden Unexplained	Cardiac	Cirrhosis or Alcohol	Other
PANCREATICODUODENECTOMY							
Guillemin	63	1		5	6	8	—
Gall	49	4		—	1	7	2
Leger	16	1	4[a]	—	—	2	2
DISTAL PANCREATECTOMY							
Leger	71	5	13	2	2	10	1
PANCREATICOJEJUNOSTOMY							
Leger	45	2	6	—	—	4	5
Prinz	100	4	4	—	19	8	15
TOTAL PANCREATECTOMY							
Braasch	26	0			5[b]	—	2
Gall	68	14[c]			2	2	3

[a]Includes insulin shock in two patients.
[b]Two from marginal ulcer, 3 from diabetes or insulin complications.
[c]Six from diabetes or insulin complications.
(Adapted from Howard JM. Surgical treatment of chronic pancreatitis. In: Howard JM, Jordan GL, Reber HA (eds), Surgical Diseases of the Pancreas. *Philadelphia, PA: Lea & Febiger;
1987:506)*

uations in which distal pancreatectomy may be done are (1) recurrent episodes of pancreatitis requiring repeated hospitalization, with multiple pseudocysts in the tail of the pancreas and splenic vein thrombosis, and (2) recurrent episodes of pancreatitis with a stricture in the main duct in the body of the pancreas, and a dilated duct past that point. In most instances, a splenectomy is also part of the pancreatic resection, even if the splenic vein is patent. This is because of the difficulty often encountered in separating the splenic vein from the adherent pancreatic parenchyma.

The operative mortality rates for pancreaticoduodenectomy and subtotal resections of the pancreas are summarized in Tables 72–6 and 72–7. Experienced surgeons can perform a pancreaticoduodenectomy today with an operative mortality rate of about 5%. Complications specific to the operation include pancreaticojejunal and choledochojejunal fistulas. The mortality rates for varying degrees of distal pancreatectomy also have usually been less than 5%, and several series had rates of 0% to 2%. A specific complication includes injury to the common bile duct when the resection is extended to 95%.

Pain is relieved in about 85% of the patients in the first several years after the operation. Unlike patients who have undergone longitudinal pancreaticojejunostomy where pain recurs in some, this initial good result is more likely to be permanent after resection (Table 72–3). Thus after 5 years, about 80% of the survivors continue to experience relative freedom from pain as compared to 60% to 70% in the drainage group. It should be stressed that these figures repre-

sent data from the few studies in which reasonable periods of follow-up have been reported. However, no controlled studies have been done that compare the results of different operations done for pain in this patient population.

Destruction of the Celiac Ganglia

Nonsurgical destruction of the celiac ganglia may have a place in the management of patients with severe pain from chronic pancreatitis. In those in whom the surgeon wishes to avoid or delay pancreatic resection, percutaneous injection of the ganglia with absolute ethanol may provide some relief for a period of time. Consultation with an anesthesiologist interested in pain management may be helpful. Although permanent pain relief is unusual with this technique, the experience may be useful for patient and surgeon alike. Thus, a better rapport may be established and a better understanding of the commitment of the patient to a treatment program may be gained. In a few cases, spontaneous improvement in the pain may even occur.

Pancreatic Transplantation

In an effort to avoid diabetes, autografts of the body and tail of the pancreas have been done in a small number of patients who were subjected to total or near-total pancreatectomy. The technique involves preservation of the splenic artery and vein for anastomoses to the iliac or femoral vessels. The pancreatic duct has usually been ligated or obliterated with a polymer. The Lahey Clinic group recently reported their results in 11 patients at a median follow-up of 62 months. Six patients (3 after 90% to 95% resection, 3 after total pancreatectomy) required no insulin. Five patients required insulin. Islet cell function seems to decrease with time.

Another technique involves pancreatic islet cell autotransplantation via the portal vein into the liver. In patients with extensive pancreatic fibrosis, the recovery of adequate amounts of functional islet cells is a problem. More experience will be required before these approaches can be recommended widely.

■ PROGNOSIS

In patients with alcoholic chronic pancreatitis, it is of interest to review mortality statistics unrelated to surgical intervention for complications of the disease. In general, life expectancy is reduced by 10 to 15 years, and the mean age at death in several series was about 50 years. The principal causes of death include upper respiratory malignancies (most patients are heavy cigarette smokers), malnutrition, complications of diabetes, and suicide. Abuse of ethanol and/or drugs often is contributory. Recent studies reveal a 2 to 5 times increase in the incidence of pancreatic cancer in patients with chronic pancreatitis from a variety of causes. Presumably, this is owing to the repeated episodes of inflammation and repair, and is similar to the increased incidence of cancer in other chronic inflammatory gastrointestinal conditions (eg, colon cancer in ulcerative colitis). In spite of the relationship between chronic pancreatitis and pancreatic cancer, the likelihood of malignant change is not great enough to justify prophylactic pancreatic resection. Table 72–8 outlines the causes of late death after the various operations in a number of centers.

SELECTED READING

Aldridge MC, Williamson RCN. Distal pancreatectomy with and without splenectomy. *Br J Surg* 1991;78:976–979

Alvarez C, Widdison L, Reber HA. New perspectives in the surgical management of chronic pancreatitis. *Pancreas* 1991; 6:576–581

Ammann RW, Akovbiantz A, Largiader F, Schueler G. Course and outcome of chronic pancreatitis: longitudinal study of a mix medical-surgical series of 245 patients. *Gastroenterology* 1984;86:820–828

Aranha GV, Prinz RA, Freeark RJ, Greenlee HB. The spectrum of biliary tract obstruction from chronic pancreatitis. *Arch Surg* 1984;119:595–600

Beger HG, Buchler M. Duodenum-preserving resection of the head of the pancreas in chronic pancreatitis with inflammatory mass in the head. *World J Surg* 1990;14:83–87

Beger HG, Buchler M, Bittner RR, et al. Duodenum-preserving resection of the head of the pancreas in severe chronic pancreatitis. *Ann Surg* 1989;209:273–278

Beger HG, Buchler M, Bittner R, Uhl W. Duodenum-preserving resection of the head of the pancreas—an alternative to Whipple's procedure in chronic pancreatitis. *Hepatogastroenterology* 1990;37:283–289

Beger HG, Kratzberger W, Bittner R, et al. Duodenum-preserving resection of the head of the pancreas in patients with severe chronic pancreatitis. *Surgery* 1985;97:467–473

Bockman DE, Buchler M, Malfertheiner P, Beger HG. Analysis of nerves in chronic pancreatitis. *Gastroenterology* 1988;94:1459–1469

Bradley EL. Long-term results of pancreaticojejunostomy in patients with chronic pancreatitis. *Am J Surg* 1987;153:207–213

Bradley EL, Clements JL. Idiopathic duodenal obstruction: an unappreciated complication of pancreatitis. *Ann Surg* 1981;193:638–648

Cooper MJ, Williamson RCN, Benjamin IS, et al. Total pancreatectomy for chronic pancreatitis. *Br J Surg* 1987;74:912–915

Cotton PB, Sarner M. International workshop on pancreatitis, Cambridge, March 1983. In: Gyr KE, Singer MV, Sarles H (eds), *Pancreatitis, Concepts and Classification.* Amsterdam, Netherlands: Elsevier Science; 1984:xxiii–xxv.

Devaux MA, Lechene de la Porte P, Johnson C, Sarles H. Structural and functional effects of long-term alcohol administration on the dog exocrine pancreas submitted to two different diets. *Pancreas* 1990;5:200–209

Dlugosz J, Folsch UR, Czajkowski A, Gabryelewicz A. Feedback regulation of stimulated pancreatic enzyme secretion during intraduodenal trypsin perfusion in man. *Eur J Clin Invest* 1988;18:267–272

Easter DW, Cuschieri A. Total pancreatectomy with preservation of the duodenum and pylorus for chronic pancreatitis. *Ann Surg* 1991;214:575–580

Ebbehoj N, Borly L, Bulow J, et al. Pancreatic tissue fluid pressure in chronic pancreatitis: relation to pain, morphology, and function. *Scand J Gastroenterol* 1990;25:1046–1051

Ebbehoj N, Borly L, Madsen P, Matzen P. Comparison of regional pancreatic tissue fluid pressure and endoscopic retrograde pancreatographic morphology in chronic pancreatitis. *Scan J Gastroenterol* 1990;25:756–760

Ebbehoj N, Borly L, Madsen P, Matzen P. Pancreatic tissue fluid pressure during drainage operations for chronic pancreatitis. *Scand J Gastroenterol* 1990;25:1041–1045

Farney AC, Najarian JS, Nakhleh RE, et al. Autotransplantation of dispersed pancreatic islet tissue combined with total or near-total pancreatectomy for treatment of chronic pancreatitis. *Surgery* 1991;110:427–439

Frey CF, Smith GJ. Description and rationale of a new operation for chronic pancreatitis. *Pancreas* 1987;2:701–707

Frey CF, Suzuki M, Isaji S, Zhu Y. Pancreatic resection for chronic pancreatitis. *Surg Clin North Am* 1989;69(3):499–528

Gall FP, Gebhardt C, Zirngibl H. Chronic pancreatitis: results of 116 consecutive and partial duodenopancreatectomies combined with pancreatic duct occlusion. *Hepatogastroenterology* 1982;29:115–119

Go VLW, DiMagno EP, Gardner JD, et al. (eds), *The Pancreas; Biology, Pathobiology, and Diseases,* 2nd ed. New York, NY: Raven; 1993

Greenlee HB, Prinz RA, Aranha GV. Long-term results of side-to-side pancreaticojejunostomy. *World J Surg* 1990;37: 295–300

Gross JB, Hereditary pancreatitis. In: Go VLW, Gardner JD, Brooks FP, et al. (eds), *The Exocrine Pancreas: Biology, Pathobiology and Disease.* New York, NY: Raven; 1986:193–211

Gullo L, Barbara L, Labo G. Effect of cessation of alcohol use on the course of pancreatic dysfunction in alcoholic pancreatitis. *Gastroenterology* 1988;95(4):1063–1068

Howard JM, Zhang Z. Pancreaticoduodenectomy. (Whipple resection) in the treatment of chronic pancreatitis. *World J Surg* 1990;14:77–82

Howard J, Jordan G, Reber HA (eds). *Surgical Diseases of the Pancreas.* Philadelphia, PA: Lea & Febiger; 1987

Jalleh RP, Aslam M, Williamson RCN. Pancreatic tissue and ductal pressures in chronic pancreatitis. *Br J Surg* 1991; 78:1235–1237

Kalthoff L, Layer P, Clain JE, DiMagno EP. The course of alcoholic and nonalcoholic chronic pancreatitis. *Dig Dis Sci* 1984;29:953

Kalvaria I, Bornman PC, Marks IN, et al. The spectrum and natural history of common bile duct stenosis in chronic alcohol-induced pancreatitis. *Ann Surg* 1989;110:608–613

Karanjia ND, Singh SM, Widdison AL, et al. Pancreatic ductal and interstitial pressures in cats with chronic pancreatitis. *Dig Dis Sci* 1992;37:268–273

Karanjia ND, Widdison AL, Leung FW, et al. The effect of decompression of the main pancreatic duct (PPD) on pancreatic blood flow (PBF) in chronic pancreatitis (CP). *Pancreas* 1990;5:713

Karanjia ND, Widdison AL, Leung FW, et al. Compartment syndrome in experimental chronic obstructive pancreatitis: effect of decompressing the main pancreatic duct. *Br J Surg* 1994;81:259–264

Keith RG, Saibil FG, Sheppard RH. Treatment of chronic alcoholic pancreatitis by pancreatic resection. *Am J Surg* 1989; 157:156–162

Konomi K, Funakoshi A, Kimura T, et al. Prognosis of pancreatic endocrine function in chronic pancreatitis. *Fukuoka Acta Med* 1990;81(11):348–354

Lambert MA, Linehan IP, Russell RCB. Duodenum-preserving total pancreatectomy for end-stage chronic pancreatitis. *Br J Surg* 1987;74:35–39

Lankisch PG, Cretzfeldt W. Therapy of exocrine and endocrine pancreatic insufficiency. In: Creutzfeldt W (ed), *Clinics in Gastroenterology.* Philadelphia, PA: WB Saunders; 1984:985–999

Layer P, Jansen JBMJ, Cherian L, et al. Feedback regulation of human pancreatic secretion. *Gastroenterology* 1990;98: 1311–1319

Littenberg G, Afroudakis A, Kaplowitz N. Common bile duct stenosis from chronic pancreatitis: A clinical and pathologic spectrum. *Medicine (Baltimore)* 1979;58:6

Mannell A, Adson MA, McIlrath DC, Ilstrup DM. Surgical management of chronic pancreatitis: long-term results in 141 patients. *Br J Surg* 1988;75:467–472

McFadden D, Reber HA. Chronic pancreatitis. In: Braasch JW,

Tompkins RK (eds), *Surgical Diseases of the Biliary Tract and Pancreas, Multidisciplinary Management.* Chicago, IL: Mosby Year-Book; 1994

Morel P, Mathey P, Corboud H, et al. Pylorus-preserving duodenopancreatectomy: long-term complications and comparison with the Whipple procedure. *World J Surg* 1990;14: 642–647

Mossner J, Secknus R, Meyer J, et al. Treatment of pain with pancreatic extracts in chronic pancreatitis. *Gastroenterology* 1991;100:A290

Nealon WH, Townsend CM, Thompson JC. Operative drainage of the pancreatic duct delays functional impairment in patients with chronic pancreatitis. *Ann Surg* 1988; 208:321–399

Patel A, Toyama MT, Alvarez C, et al. Pancreatic interstitial pH in human and feline chronic pancreatitis. *Gastroenterology* 1995;109:1639–1645

Patel A, Toyama MT, Ashley SW, Reber HA. Pancreaticojejunostomy restores normal pancreatic interstitial pH and pancreatic blood flow in chronic pancreatitis. *Am J Surg* 1994;167:447

Pitchumoni CS, Jain NK, Lowenfels AB, DiMagno EP. Chronic cyanide poisoning: unifying concept for alcoholic and tropical pancreatitis. *Pancreas* 1988;3:200–222

Pitchumoni CS. "Tropical" or "Nutritional Pancreatitis" an update. In: Gyr KE, Singer MV, Sarles H (eds), *Pancreatitis, Concepts and Classification.* Amsterdam, Netherlands: Elsevier Science; 1984:359–363

Prinz RA. Pancreatic duct drainage in chronic pancreatitis. In: Beger H, Buchler M, Malfertheiner R (eds), *Standards in Pancreatic Surgery.* Berlin, Germany: Springer-Verlag; 1993: 364–371

Prinz RA, Greenlee HB. Pancreatic duct drainage in chronic pancreatitis. *Hepatogastroenterology* 1990;37:295–300

Prinz RA, Aranha GV, Greenlee HB. Redrainage of the pancreatic duct in chronic pancreatitis. *Am J Surg* 1986;151: 150–156

Rao R, Prinz RA. Surgical therapy in chronic pancreatitis. *Curr Opinion in Gen Surg* 1993;287–293

Reber HA, Roberts C, Way LW. The pancreatic duct mucosal barrier. *Am J Surg* 1979;137(1):128–134

Reber HA, Karanjia ND, Alvarez C, et al. Pancreatic blood flow in cats with chronic pancreatitis. *Gastroenterology* 1992;103: 652–659

Rossi RL, Soeldner JS, Braasch JW, et al. Long-term results of pancreatic resection and segmental pancreatic autotransplantation for chronic pancreatitis. *Am J Surg* 1990;159: 51–57

Sarles H, Adler G, Dani R, et al. The pancreatitis classification of Marseille-Rome 1988. *Scand J Gastroenterol* 1989;24(6): 641–642

Sarles H, Barnard JP, Chonson C. Pathogenesis and epidemiology of chronic pancreatitis. *Annu Rev Med* 1989;40: 453–468

Singh SM, Reber HA. The pathology of chronic pancreatitis. *World J Surg* 1990;14:2–10

Stahl TJ, Allen MMO, Ansel HJ, Vennes JA: Partial biliary obstruction caused by chronic pancreatitis. *Ann Surg* 1988; 207:26–32

Sugerman HJ, Barnhart GR, Newsome HH. Selective drainage

for pancreatic, biliary, and duodenal obstruction secondary to chronic fibrosing pancreatitis. *Ann Surg* 1986;203:558–567

Taylor SM, Adams DB, Anderson MC. Duodenal stricture: a complication of chronic fibrocalcific pancreatitis. *South Med J* 1991;84:338–341

Trede M, Schwall G, Saeger HD. Survival after pancreatoduodenectomy. *Ann Surg* 1990;211:447–458

Warshaw AL, Schapiro RH, Ferrucci JT Jr, Galdabini J. Persistent obstructive jaundice, cholangitis, and biliary cirrhosis due to common bile duct stenosis in chronic pancreatitis. *Gastroenterology*. 1976;70:562–567

Warshaw AL, Jin G, Ottinger LW. Recognition and clinical implications of mesenteric and portal vein obstruction in chronic pancreatitis. *Arch Surg* 1987;122:410–415

Warshaw AL. Conservation of the spleen with distal pancreatectomy. *Arch Surg* 1988;123:550–553

Widdison AL, Alvarez C, Karanjia ND, Reber HA. Experimental evidence of beneficial effects of ductal decompression in chronic pancreatitis. *Endoscopy* 1991;23(3):151–154

Widdison AL, Alvarez C, Reber HA. The influence of ethanol on pancreatic blood flow in cats with chronic pancreatitis. *Surgery* 1992;112:202–210

73

Endocrine Tumors of the Pancreas

R. Daniel Beauchamp ■ *James C. Thompson*

Endocrine tumors of the pancreas belong to a broad group of neuroendocrine tumors that are located in a variety of locations. When associated with the pancreas, these tumors likely arise from the neuroendocrine stem cells located in pancreatic ductules from which pancreatic islet cells arise. These cells are members of a diffuse neuroendocrine system that ultimately includes about 40 different endocrine cell types that produce a number of different peptide hormones as well as bioactive amines. These tumors share a number of morphological and biochemical features. Histologically, endocrine tumors of the pancreas cannot be differentiated from carcinoid tumors that are located elsewhere in the gastrointestinal tract. These tumors are composed of monotonous sheets of small round cells with uniform nuclei and cytoplasm. Mitotic figures are rare and there are no histologic factors that distinguish benign from malignant tumors. In addition to the ability for amine precursor uptake and decarboxylation, these cells also produce neuron specific enolase, a glycolytic enzyme that was first recognized in brain tissue. These tumors have the potential to produce a number of different hormonally-active peptides commonly found in the gut, pancreas, central nervous system, and peripheral nerves. The cells have specific electron microscopic characteristics that include dense core granules containing the bi-

ologically active peptides characteristically produced by these tumors. The islet cell types, with their predominant endocrine agents and the syndromes associated with neoplasia, are shown in Table 73–1. The widespread nature of the neuroendocrine system and its involvement in the development of endocrine tissues have important implications in the multiple endocrine neoplasia (MEN) syndromes that can involve diverse and anatomically remote endocrine organs.

■ HISTORY

Langerhans first described islands of pancreatic cells in 1969. The relationship of the islet cells to glucose metabolism was first suggested by Mincowsky in 1889 when he observed glycosuria in dogs after pancreatectomy. The concept of humoral products regulating physiologic processes was introduced in 1902 by Bayliss and Starling with the discovery of secretin. The discovery of insulin was reported by Banting and Best in 1921. Later in the same decade, the first successful operation for removal of an insulinoma was performed by Roscoe Graham and reported by Howard and colleagues in 1929. An extract from this tumor was proven, by Professor Best, to contain insulin. In 1935, Allen Whipple reviewed the subject of hyperinsulin and described the classic triad for clinical diagnosis of insulinoma.

The first pancreatic islet cell tumor (insulinoma) was described by Nicholls in 1902. The first intentional op-

This work is supported by grants from the National Institutes of Health (5P01 DK35608, 5R37 DK15241), the John Sealy Memorial Endowment Fund (2508-92), and Shriners Hospitals for Cripple Children (15860).

TABLE 73–1. PANCREATIC ISLET CELL TUMORS

Alpha cell	Glucagon	Glucagonoma
Beta cell	Insulin	Insulinoma
Delta cell	Somatostatin	Somatostatinoma
Delta-two cells	Vasoactive intestinal peptide (VIP)	WDHA
G cell	Gastrin	Zollinger-Ellison syndrome

(From Marx M, Newman JB, Guice KS, et al. *Gastrointestinal Endocrinology*. New York, NY: McGraw-Hill; 1987:414)

eration performed for an endocrine tumor was in 1926 by WJ Mayo, who resected an insulinoma. By 1974, Stephanni and colleagues had collected, from the literature, more than 1000 cases of insulinoma that had been treated surgically. Tseng in Beijing had a personal series of 104 patients diagnosed and treated between 1955 and 1985.

Despite the frequency with which endocrine tumors of the pancreas appear in the literature, they remain rare in patients. Overall incidence is estimated at between 1 and 10 per 1 million population who present for treatment. The most interesting features of the pancreatic endocrine tumors are the associated clinical syndromes that occur because of the secretion of active peptide hormones. Numerous clinical syndromes associated with these tumors have been identified since the original description of a diagnostic triad observed in patients with insulinoma and described by Whipple and Frantz in 1935. This triad includes (1) symptoms caused by fasting or exercise, (2) hypoglycemia (<45 mg/dL), and (3) relief of symptoms by administration of glucose.

Insulinoma is the most common endocrine tumor of the pancreas. The second most common endocrine tumor of the pancreas causing a clinical syndrome is *gastrinoma*. The syndrome associated with gastrinoma was described in 1954 by Zollinger and Ellison, who operated on two patients with massive hypersecretion of gastric acid, peptic ulcers of the jejunum, and islet cell tumors of the pancreas. Gastrin subsequently was found to be the biologically active peptide hormone that caused the clinical syndrome since known as Zollinger-Ellison syndrome. Additional clinical syndromes caused by functioning endocrine tumors of the pancreas have been defined, although none are as common as insulinomas or gastrinomas. These include *VIPoma* (also known as the Verner-Morrison or watery diarrhea, hypokalemia, and alkalosis [WDHA] syndrome), the *glucagonoma* syndrome, and the *somatostatinoma* syndrome. In addition, endocrine tumors of the pancreas may present with a *carcinoid-type* syndrome (crampy abdominal pain, diarrhea, weight loss, periodic flushing).

Tumors have been identified that secrete primarily pancreatic polypeptide, neurotensin, and, with less frequency, a number of other biologic amines or hormone peptides that include serotonin, adrenocorticotropic hormone (ACTH), growth hormone releasing factor (GRF), calcitonin, growth hormone or growth hormone-releasing hormone, and parathyroid hormone. The presenting clinical syndrome usually results from the overproduction of a single peptide hormone; however, some of these tumors have been found to produce and secrete two or more hormones or combinations of hormones and amines. Approximately 15% of all islet cell tumors secrete no detectable hormones and may remain clinically silent until detected at an unresectable stage, with symptoms owing to mass effect of the tumor or to metastatic disease, usually to the liver.

■ INSULINOMA

INCIDENCE AND PATHOPHYSIOLOGY

Insulinomas occur with approximately equal distribution among men and women. Almost all insulinomas occur in the pancreas, with approximately equal distribution in the head, body, and tail. About 2% to 3% of reported insulinomas are ectopic, usually in the duodenum, hilum of the spleen, or gastrocolic ligament. There are rare reports of ectopic fibrotic tumors that secrete insulin or insulin-like substances. Insulinomas usually occur in patients between 20 to 75 years of age, with the average age of presentation 44 to 46 years. The reported incidence of insulinomas ranges from 0.8 to 0.9 persons per million population per year. Tumors vary in size from minute dots that are hard to find to huge masses over 1500 gm. The average size is 10 to 15 mm, but approximately 30% are >1 cm in diameter. These tumors usually are encapsulated, firm, yellow-brown nodules and histologically are composed of cords and nests of well-differentiated β cells that do not differ from those of the normal islet. On electron microscopy, the insulinoma cells exhibit the dense core granules typical of endocrine cells. Insulin can be detected in these cells by immunohistochemistry. Nearly 10% of insulinomas are malignant. Histologically, the malignant tumors display little evidence of anaplasia and are impossible to differentiate from benign tumors unless they show local invasion of surrounding tissue, which is a rare occurrence. The diagnosis of malignancy is based upon the presence of metastasis or local invasion beyond the substance of the pancreas. Most insulinomas occur as single tumors, but about 10% are multicentric. Whenever multiple tumors are found, chances are high that the patient has the multiple endocrine neoplasia type-1 (MEN-1) syndrome. Between 4% to 10% of patients with insulinoma have been found in association with MEN-1.

The syndrome associated with insulinoma is caused by excess levels of circulating insulin. Proinsulin is formed within the rough endoplasmic reticulum of the β cells. Proteolytic enzymes convert proinsulin molecules into insulin by cleaving a portion of the proinsulin peptide. This process results in release of an associated peptide called C-peptide (C = connecting) that has 31 amino acids and comprises the major part of the connection between the α and the β chain of the proinsulin molecule. C-peptide is stored in the β cell granules and is normally released in equimolar concentrations with insulin. Insulinoma tumor cells release both insulin and C-peptide inappropriately under conditions of fasting, in which circulating blood sugar values are low. Low blood sugar levels suppress normal insulin release.

DIAGNOSIS AND EVALUATION

Signs and Symptoms

The clinical symptoms are primarily neurologic, and result from acute and chronic episodes of hypoglycemia; they may persist for years prior to diagnosis. A rapid fall in blood sugar causes the release of catecholamines from the autonomic nervous system, which yields symptoms of trembling, sweating, palpitations, nervousness, and hunger. Catecholamine release (along with the release of glucagon) stimulates glycogenolysis, which may terminate the attack. Frequently, patients learn to control or anticipate these attacks and avoid them by eating frequent meals. (Patients may gain weight.) When a drop in blood sugar occurs more slowly, there are more symptoms related to cerebral dysfunction, since the brain is dependent upon glucose for its energy requirements. The symptoms include apathy, dizziness, cloudy sensorium, behavioral disorders, coma, or even seizures. Patients with insulinoma may exhibit bizarre behavioral disorders or decreased mental capacity as a result of prolonged periods of hypoglycemia that can result in permanent neurologic deficits. Several early cases of insulinoma were uncovered in patients who had been consigned to mental hospitals.

Laboratory Findings

A standard test to confirm the diagnosis of insulinoma syndrome is a 72 hour fast, during which the patient should be under close observation. More than 95% of cases can be diagnosed on the basis of response to a 72 hour fast (Table 73-2). During this test, serial glucose and insulin levels are obtained until the patient becomes symptomatic (Fig 73-1, A, B). To judge the effectiveness of the fast, the blood sugar must reach a level of <50 mg/dL in men and <40 mg/dL in women. Si-

TABLE 73-2. DIAGNOSIS OF INSULINOMA

1. Whipple's triad precipitated with fasting
    symptoms of hypoglycemia
    low (<40 mg) blood sugar
    relief of symptoms with glucose
2. Inappropriately high level of circulating insulin (and C-peptide)

multaneous measurement of insulin levels revealing an inappropriately high insulin level for the measured levels of glucose confirms the diagnosis of insulinoma. Symptoms of hypoglycemia with blood sugar levels <45 mg/dL can be precipitated by a 12 hour fast in 37% of patients with insulinoma, in 73% by a 24 hour fast, and in 95% by a 72 hour fast. This test is important because the absolute insulin level is not elevated in all patients with insulinomas and a normal level does not rule out the disease. A fasting insulin level of >24 μU/mL is found in 50% of patients with insulinoma, and values of insulin >7 μU/mL after a prolonged fast in which the blood glucose is <40 mg/dL are highly suggestive of insulinoma. An insulin to glucose

$$\left(\frac{\mu U/mL}{mg/dL} \right)$$

ratio of >0.3 has been found in virtually all patients proven to have insulinoma or other islet cell disease causing organic hyperinsulinism. In some normal obese individuals, the fasting ratio of plasma insulin to glucose may be elevated because of increased insulin levels owing to insulin resistance that can mimic the pattern in insulinoma. A distinguishing characteristic in these patients is a fasting glucose level that does not decrease below 55 mg/dL, even during prolonged fasting.

Measurements of proinsulin and C-peptide also may be helpful in the diagnosis of patients suspected of having organic hypoglycemia. More than 90% of patients with insulinoma will have a circulating proinsulin concentration that accounts for >24% of the total circulating insulin immunoreactivity. Levels of proinsulin >40% of circulating immunoreactivity are frequently found in malignant islet cell tumors. Measurement of C-peptide concentrations in the blood further aids in the diagnosis, since changes in the level of C-peptide reflect β cell activity. Commercial insulin preparations contain no C-peptide, and low levels of C-peptide combined with high insulin levels confirm the diagnosis of insulin self-administration. The C-peptide suppression test can be useful in equivocal cases. Commercial insulin is infused into the patient to produce hypoglycemia. When the blood glucose levels reach 40 mg/dL or less, normal individuals will have a 50% to 70% reduction in endogenous insulin and C-peptide secretion. Patients with insulinoma do not suppress the secretion of the C-

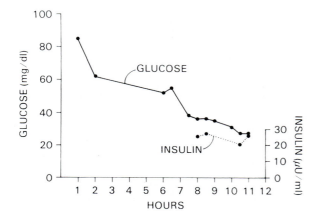

A

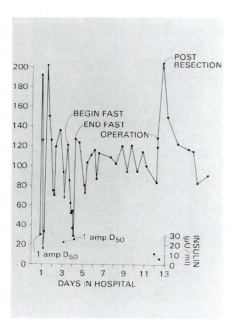

B

Figure 73–1. A. Simultaneous circulating glucose and insulin levels in a fasting patient with insulinoma. Although glucose levels fall, insulin levels remain constant, demonstrating a relative hyperinsulinemia. **B.** Periodic glucose determinations in a patient with insulinoma. The first major fall was spontaneous and the patient became comatose but was resuscitated with an ampule of 50% glucose. On the second occasion, the patient was fasted on purpose. Glucose increased to 200 and then decreased gradually and remained between 90 and 120.

peptide. C-peptide levels >1.2 μg/mL are observed in most patients with insulinoma when the blood glucose is 40 mg/dL or less. The tests described above, if performed carefully, will be diagnostic in >95% of patients.

Provocative testing may help identify patients for whom the fasting tests were negative or equivocal. Intravenous infusion of calcium gluconate (15 mg/kg, elemental calcium ion) during the course of 4 hours will cause hyperinsulinemia and hypoglycemia in >90% of

patients with insulinoma. In normal subjects, calcium infusion has no effect on blood glucose. Another provocative test is the administration of tolbutamide (1 gm after an overnight fast) which produces hypoglycemia of <50 mg/dL of glucose in 97% of patients and hyperinsulinemia (>20 μU/mL) in 85% of patients with insulinoma, at 150 minutes. Normal subjects have a similar, but less pronounced, insulin and glucose response to tolbutamide; however, values usually return to normal within 1 hour. Other provocative tests include using glucagon or L-leucine as an infusion. Patients undergoing any of these fasting or provocative tests should be monitored closely since they can induce profound hypoglycemia that, if untreated, can result in devastating neurologic injury. For this reason, the tolbutamide test has been nearly abandoned.

LOCALIZATION

Once the diagnosis of hyperinsulinism is biochemically confirmed, the next step is localization of the source of excessive insulin production. With insulinoma, successful localization can be achieved in approximately 90% of patients in whom a clinical and biochemical diagnosis is confirmed. Most of these tumors are small and not detectable by CT scan or ultrasonography. CT scan is useful, however, in identifying large malignant tumors and liver metastases. However, dynamic CT scanning has been reported to localize up to 66% of primary insulinomas. If no tumor is seen by CT scan, an arteriogram with digital subtraction should be performed since it has the potential of determining the location of highly vascular insulinomas as small as 5 mm in size. Often there is a characteristic blush on angiography (Fig 73–2). If the insulinoma is not identified by angiography, insulin measurements from blood obtained by selective sampling of the pancreatic veins are often helpful in localizing the region (head, body, or tail) of the pancreas in which the insulinoma may be found. Transhepatic portovenous sampling has a ~90% success rate in localizing the region of the pancreas in which the insulinoma resides.

Recently, an innovative method that is simpler than selective portovenous sampling has been described. This method involves selective intra-arterial injection of calcium (0.01 to 0.25 mEq Ca^{++}/kg) into the superior mesenteric artery and celiac plexus branches with simultaneous hepatic venous sampling of the insulin concentration. Another experimental method that may prove useful in selected cases is intraoperative selective portal venous sampling with rapid radioimmunoassay of insulin levels. Endoscopic ultrasonography also has been evaluated for the localization of pancreatic endocrine tumors, most of which are insulinomas. Endoscopic ultrasonography was found to be more sensitive

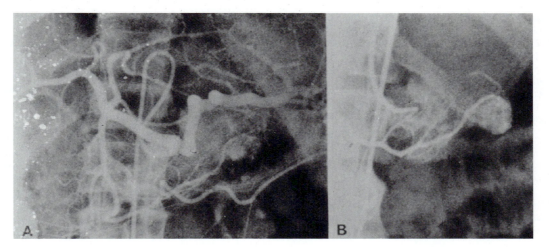

Figure 73–2. Arteriogram of insulinoma. **A.** Injection in the celiac artery reveals a 2-cm adenoma in the tail of the pancreas. **B.** Solution injected into the dorsal pancreatic artery shows better definition of the tumors.

than angiography for localization of lesions not detected by transabdominal ultrasound or CT. When the technique becomes more widely available, it may replace angiography in the work-up of small tumors of the pancreas.

The studies described above can localize 90% or more of insulinomas before operation; however, these tumors may be quite small and difficult to identify by visual inspection or direct palpation of the pancreas. Intraoperative ultrasonography in experienced hands has been useful in precise localization of insulinomas. Once the tumor is localized, we proceed to operation. In one study, the combined use of local exploration, palpation and intraoperative ultrasonography localized 100% of insulinomas in patients in whom preoperative localization procedures had failed. Intraoperative ultrasonography has particular value in patients with MEN-1, who may have multiple insulinomas. The sequence of work-up of insulinoma that we currently follow is shown in Table 73–3. The majority of tumors are located by palpation at operation.

TREATMENT, MANAGEMENT, AND ADJUVANT THERAPY

Surgical resection is usually curative since most insulinomas are small (<2 cm), benign (80% to 90%) and solitary. The clinical and biochemical diagnosis of insulinoma should be secure before an operation is performed. Preoperative management involves the prevention of severe hyperglycemic attacks and assessment and management of concurrent diseases. It may be necessary to treat the patient with diazoxide on a short-term basis. Diazoxide is a smooth-muscle relaxant, antihypertensive agent that suppresses insulin release from β cells. Diazoxide should be started at a dose of

3 mg/kg/day in two to three divided doses. The dose may be increased to a maximum of 600 to 800 mg/day. Patients who are refractory to diazoxide may require continuous intravenous glucose infusion. In the preoperative period before resection of an insulinoma, an intravenous infusion of glucose should, in all cases, be started before the diet is stopped, and maintained until well after the operation.

At operation, the entire abdomen is explored to exclude extrapancreatic tumors. Particular attention should be paid to the liver. Even after a tumor is identified, the entire pancreas should be inspected and palpated because of the ~10% incidence of multiple tumors. Details for operative procedures of the pancreas are provided in Chapter 75. Isolated benign insulinomas usually can be removed by enucleation. Injury to the main pancreatic duct should be avoided. Intraoperative ultrasonography is useful in order to localize a solitary insulinoma or multiple tumors and to identify the pancreatic ducts.

Most insulinomas not localized preoperatively can be found by experienced surgeons by combined palpation and intraoperative ultrasonography. Surgical exploration is clearly indicated in patients in whom a firm biochemical diagnosis of insulinoma has been established, even when all attempts at preoperative localization have failed. Empiric (blind) resection of the tail and body of the pancreas should rarely be necessary. Blind resection of the pancreatic head (pancreaticoduodenectomy) is not warranted, in our opinion, because of the potential morbidity from the procedure.

In the 10% to 15% of insulinomas that are malignant, the patient usually will have a larger tumor (mean size, 6 cm), with bowel invasion, lymph node metastases, or distant metastases (usually hepatic or

TABLE 73–3. DIAGNOSIS AND LOCALIZATION OF INSULINOMA

- Supervised 72 hr fast, demonstrating Whipple's triad and insulin/glucose ratio of >0.3
- Dynamic CT of the abdomen
- Selective arteriogram with intra-arterial calcium injection and hepatic venous insulin sampling
- Transhepatic transportal selective pancreatic vein sampling
- Surgical exploration and intraoperative ultrasound

peritoneal). Resection of peripancreatic lymph nodes may be curative when there is moderate spread. Debulking of the primary tumor mass may provide effective palliation, even in the presence of residual metastatic deposits, because not all metastases retain secretory function. Approximately 4% to 10% of patients with insulinomas are found to have MEN-1, and most of these patients have multiple islet cell tumors. A more aggressive surgical approach that includes subtotal pancreatectomy along with enucleation of any tumors identified in the pancreatic head may render these patients normoglycemic, whereas local resection is likely to fail.

Patients with malignant insulinoma have a median survival of 5 years after primary resection. Resection of primary and metastatic insulinoma tumors should be attempted, when possible. The somatostatin analog, octreotide, may be effective for controlling the symptoms of hypoglycemia through its ability to inhibit insulin secretion. Adjuvant chemotherapy may delay tumor growth and provide significant palliation, but responses are unpredictable. Streptozotocin is the most effective single chemotherapeutic agent available and, in combination with 5-fluorouracil (5-FU), a 63% objective response rate has been reported.

■ ZOLLINGER-ELLISON SYNDROME (ZES)

In 1955, Zollinger and Ellison described a syndrome of severe peptic ulcer disease, hypersecretion of gastric acid and non-β islet cell tumor of the pancreas. They postulated the ulcerogenic agent to be a hormonal factor that was secreted by the pancreatic tumor. This ulcerogenic factor was subsequently identified as gastrin by Gregory and colleagues, and the tumors are called gastrinomas.

Gastrinomas, like all functional endocrine tumors, are uncommon, with an annual incidence of 1 in 2.5 million people. Estimates of prevalence vary from 0.5 to 1.2 times as common as insulinomas. ZES may occur from childhood into old age with a mean age of 50.5 years. There is a slight (60%) male predominance.

PATHOPHYSIOLOGY

Gastrin is a polypeptide that is normally produced and released by G cells located in the antral mucosa. It is released from G cells by direct contact of amino acids and peptides with antral mucosa, and by mechanical distention of the antrum. The release of gastrin normally is inhibited by exposure of the antral G cells to relatively high concentrations of gastric acid (suppression is initiated at pH 3.0 and is complete at pH 1.5). Secretin released from the duodenum also inhibits release of gastrin. In contrast, gastrin that arises from the gastrinoma is not inhibited by antral acid, and is released, paradoxically, by intravenous administration of secretin. Gastrin stimulates acid secretion from parietal cells, increases gastric mucosal blood flow, and acts as a growth hormone for fundic and duodenal epithelium.

The clinical manifestations of ZES result from hypersecretion of gastric acid owing to elevated levels of gastrin. Approximately 60% of gastrinomas are malignant, 35% are benign adenomas, and 5% represent islet cell hyperplasia. Malignancy is determined by metastatic behavior or aggressive bowel invasion and cannot be determined histologically, as with all neuroendocrine tumors. Metastases primarily involve the liver, but also may be found in peripancreatic lymph nodes or in more distant locations such as the lungs. Approximately 90% of gastrinomas are found in the so-called gastrinoma triangle identified by Stabile and Passaro (Fig 73–3), the boundaries of which are defined by the cystic duct, the junction of the second and third portions of the duodenum, and the junction of the neck and body of the pancreas. Approximately 20% of patients with ZES have MEN-1. The most commonly associated abnormality in patients with gastrinoma and MEN-1 is hyperparathyroidism. Gastrinomas tend to occur at a younger age in the MEN-1 syndrome and more frequently occur as multiple tumors.

In addition to gastrin, gastrinomas may secrete other biologically active peptides such as insulin, glucagon, somatostatin, ACTH, or pancreatic polypeptide (PP). These secondary peptides may alter the clinical presentation dramatically.

DIAGNOSIS AND EVALUATION

Peptic ulcers occur in >90% of patients with ZES. Most patients have ulcers in the duodenal bulb, but multiple ulcers or ulcers in atypical locations (postbulbar) are common in ZES. Most patients have epigastric pain. Other common complaints include GI bleeding (~50%) that may produce either melena or hematemesis, diarrhea (~35%), weight loss, nausea and vomiting. The severe secretory diarrhea may be the only complaint in 7% to 10% of patients with ZES. The symptoms of ZES may be present from months to years be-

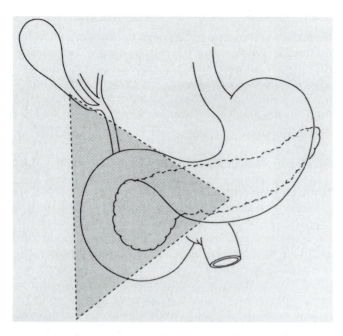

Figure 73–3. The anatomic triangle in which ~90% of gastrinomas are found. (From Stabile BE, Morrow DJ, Passaro E. The gastrinoma triangle: operative implications. *Am J Surg* 1984;147:26)

fore the diagnosis is made. Jejunal ulcer perforation may occur in up to 7% of ZES patients. Secretion of other peptides, either from other adenomas as part of the MEN-1 syndrome or from the gastrinoma, is not uncommon. Hyperparathyroidism in gastrinoma patients with MEN-1 may result in skeletal disease, nephrolithiasis, or other manifestations of hyperparathyroidism. ACTH overproduction may cause Cushing's syndrome. One of our patients with metastatic gastrinoma died with Cushing's syndrome when her tumor suddenly began producing massive amounts of ACTH.

ZES should be suspected in any patient with complaints of peptic ulcer and diarrhea, with familial ulcer disease, atypical or multiple peptic ulcers, or peptic ulcer disease refractory to treatment, especially ulcers that recur after acid-reducing operations. These patients often have peptic ulcers that fail to heal with conventional doses of histamine type-2 (H2) receptor antagonists and may be referred for surgical management. Any patient with peptic ulcer disease that requires surgical intervention should have a fasting serum gastrin determination by radioimmunoassay (RIA). We try to have three measurements. The upper limit of normal for fasting serum gastrin is 100 to 150 pg/mL. Patients with ZES usually have increased gastrin levels, ranging from 200 to >1000 pg/mL.

Patients who have an elevated fasting serum gastrin level should have gastric acid analysis. An elevated basal acid output (BAO, 15 mEq/hr or more in patients not previously subjected to an acid-reducing procedure) is necessary to confirm that the elevation in gastrin is not owing to hypochlorhydria or achlorhydria. A gastric pH of ≥3 in the absence of medication or prior acid-reducing operation virtually excludes ZES.

Serum gastrin levels may be elevated in the absence of gastrinoma under several conditions. High gastrin levels and low or absent acid output may be found in patients with atrophic gastritis, pernicious anemia, renal failure, and in patients on H2 receptor antagonists or omeprazole. ZES can be excluded if there is no acid production in association with elevated gastrin levels. High gastrin levels and high acid production can be found in patients with gastric outlet obstruction, G cell hyperplasia, and retained gastric antrum after incomplete antrectomy and gastrojejunostomy.

The secretin test is of great help in confirming the diagnosis of gastrinoma. The test is performed in the fasting state. The patient is given pure secretin (2 IU/kg) in 10 mL of normal saline as an intravenous bolus during 30 seconds. Two blood samples should be obtained before the secretin injection and at 2 minute intervals three times, and then at 5 minute intervals for 30 minutes afterward. An increase in serum gastrin level of >200 pg/mL (or a >50% increase in gastrin levels) after secretin injection is considered a positive test. Gastrin levels have been shown to increase by 200 pg/mL in 87% and by more than 50% in 85% of patients with ZES.

Intravenous infusion of calcium has been used to provoke gastrin release. However, this procedure is not as reliable as the secretin test and has been largely abandoned.

LOCALIZATION

Upper endoscopy and barium upper gastrointestinal radiographs often reveal the consequences of hypergastrinemia and acid hypersecretion. These studies may reveal a single peptic ulcer, multiple peptic ulcers, atypical ulcer locations, large gastric rugal folds, edema of the mucosa of the duodenum and upper jejunum, and jejunal hypermotility. A greatly enlarged stomach is common. Several techniques may be helpful in localizing gastrinoma or for making the diagnosis of metastatic disease. CT scanning is ~50% accurate in detecting primary gastrinoma and metastatic disease. Unfortunately, it is incapable of detecting primary tumors <1 cm and detects only 30% of tumors 1 to 3 cm in diameter. Primary gastrinomas in the duodenum (from 6% to 31% of primaries) are usually <1 cm in diameter and are usually missed by CT scan. CT scan generally is more accurate for detecting pancreatic gastrinomas and hepatic metastases than for detecting extrahepatic and extrapancreatic tumors. Approximately 21% to 65% of gas-

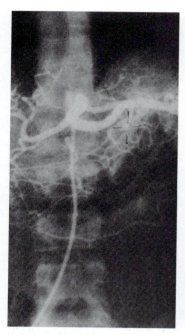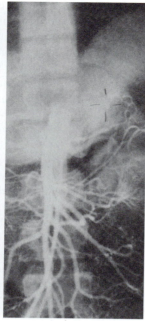

A   **B**

Figure 73–4. Patient with Zollinger-Ellison syndrome. **A.** Selective celiac arteriogram. **B.** Superior mesenteric arteriogram. Both views show the small isolated tumor that was found in the midportion of the tail of the pancreas. (From Thompson JC, Reeder DD, Villar HV, et al. Natural history and experience with diagnosis and treatment of the Zollinger-Ellison syndrome. *Surg Gynecol Obstet* 1975;140:721–739)

trinomas are found in the pancreas. Magnetic resonance imaging (MRI) has recently been found to be more accurate than CT for identifying metastatic gastrinoma in the liver, although it offers no advantage over CT for identifying the primary tumor. Unfortunately, most tumors that can be localized by CT or MRI are easily located at operation. What is greatly needed is a technique to localize tumors that are too small, or too deeply embedded, to be felt.

Selective visceral angiography (Fig 73–4) can detect some primary gastrinomas and a higher percentage of hepatic metastases, and is more accurate for localizing tumors in the pancreatic head and body than elsewhere. The combination of angiography and CT scan detects a very high percentage of liver metastases. Selective transhepatic portal venous sampling is considerably less useful for localizing gastrinoma as compared with insulinoma, and probably offers no advantage over imaging studies. Selective intra-arterial injection of secretin with hepatic vein sampling has been used extensively in Japan and Europe and is technically simpler and more accurate than selective portal venous sampling. Endoscopic ultrasonography is a newer technique that may prove useful in the preoperative localization of small gastrinomas. However, experience to date is limited.

Intraoperative localization procedures that may be helpful are ultrasonography and endoscopic transillumination. Palpation plus intraoperative ultrasonography can detect most pancreatic gastrinomas but somewhat fewer extrapancreatic tumors. Use of intraoperative endoscopic transillumination has been useful in localizing small gastrinomas in the submucosa of the duodenum.

TREATMENT, MANAGEMENT, AND ADJUVANT THERAPY

Many patients with ZES will have incurable disease because of metastasis from the gastrinoma, at the time of diagnosis. Until overwhelming metastatic disease occurs, most of the symptoms from gastrinoma are the result of hypersecretion of gastric acid. Nonoperative control of gastric acid production often can be accomplished with H2 receptor antagonists (eg, cimetidine, ranitidine, famotidine) or omeprazole. The doses of H2 receptor antagonist that are required may be substantially higher (two- to three-fold) than in peptic ulcer disease not associated with gastrinoma. Omeprazole is an agent that inhibits $H^{\pm}K^{\pm}ATPase$ in parietal cells and is approved for use in gastrinoma patients. The treatment failure rate is <10% with this agent; the drug is the drug of choice for treatment of gastric hypersecretion in patients with ZES. Doses that are two- to three-fold higher than required for routine peptide ulcer disease may be required in ZES patients. The efficacy of these drugs (H2 blockers or omeprazole) in suppressing gastric acid secretion should be demonstrated by gastric acid analysis of BAO in each patient. The dosage should be adjusted so that gastric acid secretion is <10 mEq/hr for three hours before the next dose of medication, in patients who have not had a previous acid-reducing procedure, and to <5 mEq/hr in patients who have had a previous acid-reducing procedure. Octreotide, the somatostatin analog, can reduce gastrin release and gastric acid secretion and may be used in conjunction with other antisecretory agents.

Operative treatment of patients with ZES is for one of three potential indications: (1) to cure resectable gastrinoma, (2) as palliative reduction of tumor burden, and (3) rarely, as treatment of gastric hypersecretion. Patients with gastrinoma and no known metastases should have operative exploration with an attempt at curative resection of the gastrinoma. At operation, if no gastrinoma is readily located by palpation and intraoperative ultrasonography of the pancreas, then a careful search in the gastrinoma triangle should be performed. Endoscopic transillumination of the duodenum, along with duodenotomy and careful transmural palpation of the duodenum between the thumb and index fingers, will often localize the gastrinoma in patients with sporadic ZES. Solitary gastrinomas in the liver should be re-

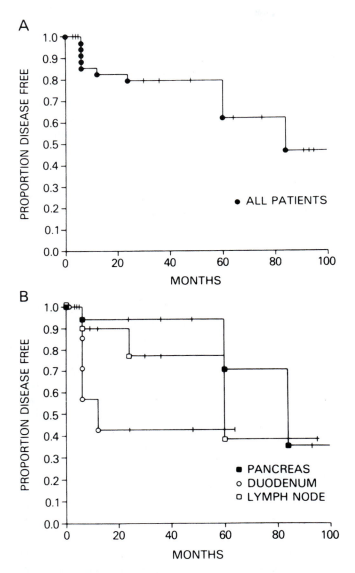

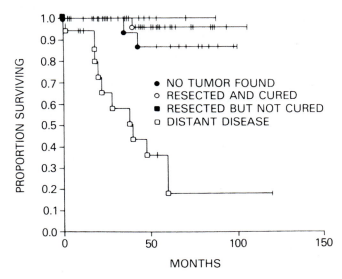

Figure 73–5. Time to recurrence of Zollinger-Ellison syndrome in patients initially disease free by surgery. **Top:** The Kaplan-Meier plot of the time to recurrence for all patients (n = 42) who were disease-free of Zollinger-Ellison syndrome at the initial (either 3 or 6 month) postoperative follow-up. Disease-free is defined as no evidence of gastrinoma on imaging studies, normal fasting gastrin concentration, and negative secretin and calcium provocative tests. Recurrent disease has developed in few patients. **Bottom:** Kaplan-Meier plot of the time to recurrence of Zollinger-Ellison syndrome of patients who were rendered disease-free of Zollinger-Ellison syndrome at the initial postoperative follow-up, divided by primary disease site: duodenum (n=12), pancreas (n=19), and lymph node (n=10). One patient with the primary ovarian gastrinoma is excluded. Patients with primary duodenal gastrinomas had a significantly shorter disease-free interval than patients with pancreatic gastrinomas ($P < .01$). The differences between patients with duodenal gastrinomas and those with lymph node–only gastrinomas were not significant ($P = .1$). The median disease-free survival for patients with duodenal, pancreatic, or lymph node primary gastrinomas was 12, 84, and 60 months, respectively. (From Norton JA, Doppman JL, Jensen RT. Curative resection in Zollinger-Ellison syndrome. *Ann Surg* 1992;215:8–18

Figure 73–6. Survival of patients with Zollinger-Ellison syndrome from the day of diagnosis. Patients were divided into four groups based on preoperative evaluation, operative findings, and initial postoperative evaluation: patients who had biopsy confirmation of bulky metastatic gastrinoma on initial evaluation (n=18, *open squares*); patients who had no tumor found during surgery (n=16, *closed circles*); patients who had all tumor resected and were functionally disease free (cured) at initial postoperative evaluation (n=42, *open circles*); and patients who had all tumor resected but were functionally not disease-free (cured) (n=15, *closed squares*). There were no significant differences seen among the three groups who did not have metastatic gastrinoma. However, the group with distant disease survived for a significantly shorter time than all other patient groups ($P < .001$). (From Norton JA, Doppman JL, Jensen RT. Curative resection in Zollinger-Ellison syndrome. *Ann Surg* 1992;215:8–18)

sected. Localized disease is treated best by local excision. Enucleation is a curative procedure for small solitary gastrinomas and is the technique of choice for lesions in the pancreatic head. Distal pancreatectomy may be required for lesions in the body and tail of the pancreas. Pancreaticoduodenectomy may be required for locally invasive lesions in the pancreatic head or uncinate process when metastatic disease is absent, but should be performed only by surgeons who have extensive experience. Pancreatic resection should not be performed blindly in an attempt to resect a gastrinoma that cannot be localized. Norton and associates found that among 73 patients who had surgical exploration, 58% had normalized serum fasting gastrin levels and negative provocative tests in the early (3 to 6 month) postoperative period. With a median follow-up of 45 months, 10 of these 42 patients developed recurrence. The Kaplan-Meier plot of the data (Fig 73–5) suggests that ~50% will have recurrence by 5 years.

As with other neuroendocrine tumors, removal of all resectable tumors even with metastases may provide significant palliation of hypersecretory symptoms, and may prolong survival. One of Dr. Zollinger's original patients lived >20 years with an hepatic metastasis. We have a patient who had seven different tumors excised (including metastatic tumor to a lymph node) who is alive and well 12 years after operation, which consisted of removal of all visible tumor tissues and total gastrectomy.

Medical management of gastric acid hypersecretion is successful in almost all ZES patients who are compliant. Total gastrectomy is effective therapy and can be accomplished with low morbidity and low mortality by experienced surgeons. This procedure should be offered to those patients who cannot comply with medical treatment.

Treatment with chemotherapeutic agents (eg, streptozotocin, 5-FU, doxorubicin), antihormonal response modifiers (eg, octreotide), and biological response modifiers (eg, interferon) have been reported, but responses are not uniform. None of these agents provide proven survival benefit for metastatic disease. Patients who present with bulky metastasis diagnosed on preoperative evaluation have a <20% 5-year survival, whereas patients with no evidence of metastatic disease at initial preoperative and operative evaluation, even with evidence of residual functional gastrinoma, have a mean 5-year survival of 90% (Fig 73–6).

■ VIPoma

The VIPoma syndrome, characterized by watery diarrhea, hypokalemia and achlorhydria (WDHA), was first described by Verner and Morrison in 1958. Barbezat and Grossman suggested vasoactive intestinal peptide (VIP) as a cause of the WDHA syndrome in 1971. In 1973, Bloom and colleagues demonstrated elevated levels of VIP in both the plasma and tumors of patients with the syndrome. The syndrome is caused by excessive release of VIP. This peptide is normally found in brain, gastrin cells, adrenal medulla, gut mucosal cells, pancreatic neurons, and D cells of the pancreatic islets.

The VIPoma syndrome is even less common than insulinoma or ZES. It is quite rare. There is a bimodal age distribution with 11% occurring in patients <10 years of age, and the remainder occurring in middle-aged adults. In children, the VIP syndrome usually arises from ganglioneuroma, whereas in adults, 80% to 90% of VIPomas arise from the pancreas. The tumors are predominantly solitary, with 75% located in the body or tail of the pancreas. Nearly two-thirds of VIPomas are malignant, as defined by the presence of metastases. The histology of these tumors is typical for neuroendocrine tumors, except that most are positive for VIP immunostaining. Malignancy is defined by behavior and not histology.

VIP is clearly the major mediator of the syndrome. Plasma VIP levels are consistently elevated (>150 pg/mL). VIP acts on receptors on intestinal epithelial cells and causes adenylate cyclase activation. The resultant increase in intracellular cyclic adenosine monophosphate (AMP) results in secretory diarrhea. VIP causes reversal of the normal absorptive process in intestinal epithelial cells along with inhibition of sodium absorption and stimulation of chloride secretion against an electrochemical gradient.

The chief complaint of patients with the VIPoma syndrome is a profuse watery iso-osmotic secretory diarrhea that occurs independently of food ingestion. There are no inflammatory cells, blood or fat in the stool. The diarrhea is described as having the appearance of weak tea and persists during fasting, even with continuous nasogastric aspiration, which differentiates it from diarrhea associated with the ZES. A volume of diarrhea <700 gm/day usually excludes the diagnosis of VIPoma. In association with the diarrhea, patients with VIPoma uniformly have weight loss, electrolyte abnormalities, especially hypokalemia, dehydration, and metabolic acidosis. Approximately 70% to 75% of patients have hypochlorhydria or achlorhydria. Abdominal cramping pain occurs in more than half of patients with VIPoma.

There is a long list of disorders that present with classical features of secretory diarrhea, including ZES, laxative abuse, carcinoid, medullary carcinoma of the thyroid, hyperthyroidism, and others. The biochemical diagnosis of VIPoma is made by demonstrating an elevated fasting level of VIP in the plasma in a patient with secretory diarrhea. Localization of these tumors has been accomplished by CT scan, selective angiography (Fig 73–7), and intraoperative ultrasonography.

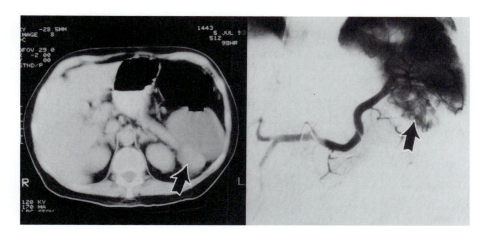

Figure 73–7. CT and selective digital subtraction angiographic images of a large VIPoma in the pancreatic tail. Arrows denote mass arising with pancreatic tail extending into splenic hilum. (Photograph courtesy of Courtney M Townsend Jr, MD)

The treatment of these patients requires aggressive rehydration and correction of electrolyte and acid-base abnormalities even before the diagnosis is confirmed. The best agent for decreasing the volume of diarrhea is octreotide (Sandostatin), which decreases circulating VIP levels, decreases stool volume and simplifies correction of fluid and electrolyte abnormalities. The starting dose should be 50 to 100 mg three times daily, but some patients may require much higher doses. Concomitant administration of glucocorticoids with octreotide may be effective in patients that do not respond to octreotide alone.

Surgical resection of the VIPoma is the treatment of choice, when possible. These tumors are often invasive and simple enucleation is probably inadequate. Partial pancreatic resection is recommended. Unfortunately, only one-third of patients with VIPoma are cured by operation, with the exception of VIP-producing ganglioneuroblastoma, in which 78% of patients are cured. Aggressive resection of metastatic disease has been advocated as effective palliation; however, the reported experience is small.

■ GLUCAGONOMA

The first description of a pancreatic islet cell tumor associated with cutaneous rash and other signs and symptoms of glucagonoma was in 1942 by Becker and associates. McGavran and associates described a similar patient in 1966; however, the clinical syndrome was not recognized fully until 1974 when Mallinson and associates reported on nine patients who had the syndrome, comprised of migratory necrolytic dermatitis, stomatitis, glossitis, and mild glucose intolerance, in association with a glucagon-producing tumor of the pancreas.

Glucagonoma is a rare tumor, similar in prevalence to VIPoma. The tumor is more common in women than in men, with a 2:1 to 3:1 ratio. Glucagonoma tends to be large at the time of diagnosis, with an average size of 5 to 10 cm. Almost all glucagonoma tumors occur in the pancreas and are distributed mostly in the pancreatic body and tail (65% to 75%), similar to the normal pancreatic α cell distribution.

Between 50% and 80% of glucagonomas are malignant, as defined by metastatic spread or invasion of adjacent tissues. Metastases occur most frequently to the liver and regional lymph nodes, but may be found more distantly.

The histology of the tumor is typical for the entire class of neuroendocrine tumors. The distinguishing characteristic is the production and release of large quantities of glucagon. Glucagon acts primarily on the liver where it causes glycogenolysis, gluconeogenesis, and ketogenesis, in contrast to the effects of insulin. Glucagon also inhibits glycolysis and lipogenesis. The glycogenolysis and gluconeogenesis result in mild hyperglycemia and decreased amino acid levels in blood, muscle, and liver. Increased lipolysis leads to depletion of fat stores, weight loss, and deficiencies of fat soluble vitamins.

The catabolic effects of glucagon cause numerous clinical manifestations of glucagonoma (Table 73–4). Virtually all patients have hypoaminoacidemia. Approximately 85% have a normochromic normocytic anemia. Glucose intolerance occurs in 83% of patients but is rarely of clinical significance. The most striking clinical feature is the skin lesion, a migratory necrolytic dermatitis that occurs in two-thirds of patients (Fig 73–8). The lesions begin as erythematous patches in intertriginous areas and in areas around the mouth, vagina, or anus. The lesions spread in an annular and serpiginous pattern to confluence and involve the trunk, extremities and face. Bullae develop centrally, then slough, leaving crusting necrotic areas. There is a tendency toward central healing as the lesions continue to spread readily.

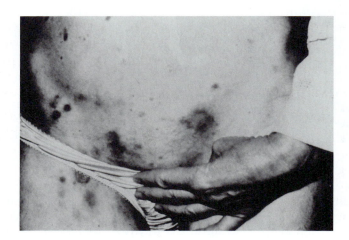

Figure 73–8. Characteristic skin rash associated with glucagonoma. This figure shows the migratory necrolytic dermatitis in a woman, 42 years of age, who had been symptomatic for 16 years. The rash had spread to involve the entire body. Note the central clearing. (Photograph courtesy of Hugo V Villar, MD)

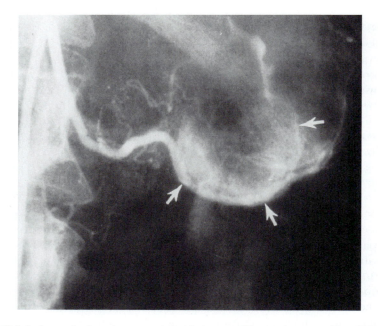

Figure 73–9. Angiogram showing a glucagonoma in the tail of pancreas (Photograph courtesy of Hugo V Villar, MD)

TABLE 73–4. GLUCAGONOMA SYNDROME

- Necrotyzing dermatitis (dermatitis necrolysis migrans)
- Diabetes mellitus
- Anemia
- Weight loss
- Elevated glucagon levels

Fungal superinfection of the skin lesions may occur. Upon healing, in 2 to 3 weeks, there is often hyperpigmentation. Biopsy of the healing edge of the lesion will reveal the characteristic superficial spongiosis and necrosis between the stratum corneum and malpighian layer. The skin lesion is thought to occur because of hypoaminoacidemia. Intravenous amino acid administration has been shown to clear the dermatitis. The lesions are so common and so characteristic to the experienced eye that the great majority of glucagonoma patients are identified by dermatologists.

Other manifestations of glucagonoma are weight loss (60%), stomatitis or glossitis (34%), thromboembolism (30%), diarrhea (15%) and vulvovaginitis (12%).

The diagnosis of glucagonoma usually is not made until the cutaneous manifestations occur, and these may be late events. The diagnostic finding is an elevated fasting plasma glucagon level. Preoperative localization studies are more successful than for other functional endocrine tumors of the pancreas because of their large size. CT of the abdomen is the best single imaging study since it is accurate, sensitive and relatively noninvasive. CT alone detects most hepatic metastases. Angiography is helpful in localizing tumors that are not seen with CT since these tumors tend to be highly vascular (Fig 73–9).

Medical therapy should be instituted before operation to stabilize the patient. Hyperalimentation can help reverse the catabolic state. Subcutaneous injections of octreotide (starting dose, 50 to 100 mg tid) can significantly reduce the levels of circulating glucagon and may improve nutrition. The dosage should be adjusted according to the degree of symptomatic relief, and doses up to 1000 mg have been well tolerated in humans, except for pain on injection. Octreotide can be palliative in patients with incurable disease. Perioperative subcutaneous heparin administration is recommended to prevent thromboembolic complications.

The treatment of choice is surgical excision. Most glucagonomas are large and malignant and, since they are usually located in the body or tail of the pancreas, distal pancreatectomy is required. Enucleation is not recommended because of the malignant potential of these tumors. Resection is recommended even for large or metastatic tumors because the tumors tend to grow slowly and resection may provide prolonged palliation.

■ SOMATOSTATINOMA

Somatostatinomas are extremely rare tumors with fewer than 100 patients reported. The tumors were first described in 1977, in two separate reports. The full syndrome, characterized by steatorrhea, diabetes mellitus, hypochlorhydria and cholelithiasis, was characterized by Krejs in 1979. The syndrome is caused by a somatostatin-producing neuroendocrine tumor that may be found in the pancreas (68%) or in extrapancreatic locations such as the duodenum (19%) or small bowel (3%). The tumors are usually large (1.5 to 10 cm) and solitary. When found in the pancreas, most are located in the head of the gland. Histologically, these tumors are well differentiated and have typical secretory granules that are found in pancreatic D cells. Immunohistochemistry reveals somatostatin-like immunoreactivity. Metastases of pancreatic and intestinal somatostatinomas are so common as to be the rule; metastatic sites are the liver and regional lymph nodes.

Somatostatin is a hormone that inhibits many endocrine and exocrine functions of the gastrointestinal tract and is the basis for the pathophysiology observed in somatostatinoma syndrome. Somatostatin inhibits release of many hormones of the gut and pancreas, such as gastrin, secretin, cholecystokinin, motilin, VIP, pancreatic polypeptide (PP), insulin, and glucagon. It inhibits gastrin and secretin and pancreatic exocrine secretion, and is an inhibitor of gut and gallbladder smooth muscle contraction.

The clinical presentation consists of a constellation of problems, none of which are specific. The mean age of presentation is 51 to 53 years. Diabetes mellitus occurs in most patients with pancreatic tumor but in fewer than one-third of patients with intestinal tumors. Cholelithiasis, steatorrhea, hyperchlorhydria, and weight loss each occur in more than half of patients with pancreatic tumors but in less than half of patients with primary tumors of the intestine.

The diagnosis of somatostatinoma is seldom made until the tumor is found coincidentally during laparotomy for cholecystectomy or during radiologic work-up of abdominal pain, diarrhea, or jaundice. The diagnosis of somatostatinoma is confirmed by an elevated fasting plasma somatostatin level. The optimal treatment is surgical resection, if possible, since this modality offers the only chance for cure. The large size and possibility of malignancy necessitate resection rather than enucleation of pancreatic tumor. Metastasis should be excluded before major resection (for example, a Whipple procedure) is performed. Smaller duodenal tumors may be treated by local excision. Metastasis excludes the chance for cure in most patients who present with somatostatinoma.

■ OTHER FUNCTIONAL PANCREATIC ENDOCRINE TUMORS

Pancreatic endocrine tumors that secrete growth hormone-releasing factor (GRF), neurotensin, and adrenocorticotropic hormone (ACTH) with resultant endocrine syndromes have been reported. Tumors that secrete GRF may originate in the lung (53%), pancreas (30%), small intestine (10%), or adrenal gland. These tumors are invariably associated with MEN-1; 40% of patients with GRF-secreting tumors have the ZES syndrome and 40% also have Cushing's syndrome. In a review of 30 cases, metastases were found in association with 30% of pancreatic GRF tumors and in 2 of the 3 patients with primary tumors of the intestine. Patients with GRF tumors often are seen first with acromegaly and often have additional symptoms caused by other endocrinopathies, such as the ZES syndrome or Cushing's disease.

Pancreatic endocrine tumors that secrete neurotensin have been described. The syndrome in patients with neurotensinomas includes hypokalemia, weight loss, cyanosis, hypotension, flushing, and diabetes mellitus. It is not clear which of these signs and symptoms is the result of neurotensin since these tumors may produce other biologically active peptides, such as gastrin or VIP, and amines such as serotonin. Pancreatic endocrine tumors that cause Cushing's syndrome have been described. The Cushing's syndrome results from ectopic ACTH production by these tumors. Cushing's syndrome occurs in 5% of all patients with ZES syndrome and in 19% of patients with both ZES syndrome and MEN-1.

■ PPomas AND NONFUNCTIONAL PANCREATIC ENDOCRINE TUMORS

These tumors are grouped together because they are associated with no detectable endocrinopathy syndrome. PPomas are associated with high circulating levels of the hormone, pancreatic polypeptide (PP), while nonfunctioning endocrine tumors have no associated elevation of peptide hormones. Most PPomas are clinically indistinguishable from nonfunctioning tumors, but there are reports of PPomas associated with WDHA-like syndrome or skin rash. Patients with these tumors often are seen late, and most tumors are ≥5 cm in diameter at diagnosis. Except when associated with MEN-1, tumors are usually solitary and are found predominantly in the head of the pancreas, although they may arise anywhere in the gland. Most are malignant, as defined by invasiveness or metastasis at the time of diagnosis. The initial symptoms are often owing to mechanical or mass effects of the tumor. Abdominal pain or jaundice are common initial complaints. In the absence of distinguishing symptomatology, it is not surprising that most PPomas and nonfunctioning tumors are diagnosed incidentally by cytologic or histologic examination of a suspected exocrine pancreatic tumor. When possible, surgical resection should be attempted for cure.

Because of delay in the appearance of any symptoms, >60% of these tumors are metastatic at the time of diagnosis. In contrast to the exocrine pancreatic cancers, prolonged survival is possible even with incurable disease (60% at 3 years and 44% at 5 years).

■ PANCREATIC ENDOCRINE TUMORS AND MEN-1 SYNDROME

The multiple endocrine neoplasia syndrome type I, (MEN-1), was initially named for Werner, who first described the familial syndrome that consists of pancreatic endocrine and pituitary gland tumors and hyperplasia of the parietal glands. MEN-1 is inherited as an autosomal dominant trait and is the result of genetic defect localized to the large arm of chromosome 11.

The first signs and symptoms of MEN-1 characteristically occur in the third and fourth decades of life. The disease occurs with equal frequency among men and women. The clinical presentation in descending order of frequency is hypercalcemia, nephrolithiasis, peptic ulcer disease, hypoglycemia, headaches, visual field loss, hypopituitarism, acromegaly, galactorrhea and Cushing's syndrome. More than 90% of patients have hyperparathyroidism. Islet cell tumors of the pancreas occur in more than 80% of these patients, the stated order of frequency being PPomas (80% to 100%), gastrinomas (54%), insulinomas (21%), glucagonomas (3%), VIPomas (1%), and other islet cell tumors. Pituitary adenomas occur in 54% to 80% of patients with MEN-1.

The pancreatic involvement in MEN-1 results in multicentric and diffuse hyperplasia of the islets in addition to discrete tumors that also tend to be multicentric and malignant. MEN-1 is found in 20% of all patients with ZES syndrome. The Zollinger-Ellison syndrome is the most commonly associated endocrinopathy in MEN-1 (54%). Patients who have elevated gastrin and gastric acid hypersecretion along with hyperparathyroidism and who undergo successful parathyroidectomy have better responses to medical therapy of gastric acid hypersecretion. Therefore, parathyroidectomy should be performed before any acid-reducing procedure. There is no proof that attempted surgical resection of gastrinomas associated with MEN-1 prolongs survival, and normalization of gastrin levels rarely occurs. Surgical resection in these patients is controversial and probably should be attempted only when preoperative studies reveal a well-demarcated lesion in a location that favors resection. Our experience is that, while impossible to cure, patients with the ZES and MEN-1 have long life expectancies.

The next most common islet tumor found in MEN-1 patients is insulinoma. Conversely, MEN-1 is reported in 4% to 10% of patients with insulinoma. In contrast to gastrinoma, aggressive surgical resection of insulinoma, even when multiple, in patients with MEN-1 is warranted. There are even fewer MEN-1 patients with VIPoma. Although they may present as multiple tumors, VIPomas are usually solitary tumors. The symptoms that occur from high circulating levels of insulin or VIP are disabling and difficult to manage medically. Surgical resection of these tumors has a reasonable chance for success and should be attempted when possible.

Any endocrine cell in the pancreas may give rise to a benign or malignant tumor. One tumor, the gastrinoma, arises from cells that are not present in the normal adult pancreas. Histologically, all tumors are similar and can be differentiated by immunocytochemistry, by their circulating products, and by the signs and symptoms they produce. The criterion for malignancy is the presence of metastases.

Many tumors produce multiple active agents. Thus, they are known by the name of the agent that produces the predominant symptoms. The only cure of the tumors is surgical, but as with carcinoid tumors, which they may closely resemble, distant metastases may be compatible with a long life expectancy.

SELECTED READINGS

Banting FG, Best CH. The internal secretion of the pancreas. *J Lab Clin Med* 1922;7(5):256

Bayliss WM, Starling EH. The mechanisms of pancreatic secretion. *J Physiol (Lond)* 1902;28:325

Becker S, Kahn D, Rothman S. Cutaneous manifestations of internal malignant tumors. *Arch Dermatol Syphilis* 1942;45:1069

Bloom S, Polak J. Glucagonoma syndrome. *Am J Med* 1987;92:25

Bloom S, Polak J, Pearse A. Vasoactive intestinal peptide and watery diarrhea syndrome. *Lancet* 1973;ii:14

Carty SE, Jensen RT, Norton JA. Prospective study of aggressive resection of metastatic pancreatic endocrine tumors. *Surgery* 1992;112:1024

Caruso DR, O'Dorisio TM, Mazzaferri EL. Multiple endocrine neoplasia. *Curr Opin Oncol* 1991;3:103

Cherner JA, Doppman JL, Norton JA, et al. Selective venous sampling for gastrin to localize gastrinomas. A prospective assessment. *Ann Int Med* 1986;105:841

Cherner JA, Sawyers JL. Benefit of resection of metastatic gastrinoma in multiple endocrine neoplasia type I. *Gastroenterology* 1992;102:1049

Demeure MJ, Klonoff DC, Karam JH, et al. Insulinomas associated with multiple endocrine neoplasia type I: The need for a different surgical approach. *Surgery* 1991;110:998

Doherty GM, Doppman JL, Shawker TH, et al. Results of prospective strategy to diagnose, localize, and resect insulinomas. *Surgery* 1991;110:989

Doppman JL. Pancreatic endocrine tumors—the search goes on. *N Engl J Med* 1992;326:1770

Ermak TH, Grendell JH. Anatomy, histology, embryology, and developmental anomalies. In: Sleisenger MH, Fordtran JS (eds), *Gastrointestinal Disease. Pathophysiology, Diagnosis, Management*, 4th ed. Philadelphia, PA: WB Saunders; 1989:1765

Evers BM, Ishizuka J, Townsend CM Jr, et al. Expression of neurotensin messenger RNA in a human carcinoid tumor. *Ann Surg* 1991;214:448

Frucht H, Howard JM, Slaff JI, et al. Secretin and calcium provocative tests in the Zollinger-Ellison syndrome: a prospective study. *Ann Int Med* 1989;111:713

Goletti O, Chiarugi M, Buccianti P, et al. Resection of liver gastrinoma leading to persistent eugastrinemia: case report. *Eur J Surg* 1992;158:55

Harris GJ, Tio F, Cruz AB Jr. Somatostatinoma: a case report and review of the literature. *J Surg Oncol* 1987;36:8

Howland G, Campbell W, Maltby E, et al. Dysinsulinism: Convulsions and coma due to islet cell tumor of the pancreas with operation and cure. *JAMA* 1929;93:674

Jensen R. Zollinger-Ellison syndrome: current concepts and management. *Ann Intern Med* 1983;98:59

Kahan R, Perez-Figaredo M, Neimanis A. Necrolytic migratory erythema: distinctive dermatosis of the glucagonoma syndrome. *Arch Dermatol* 1977;113:792

Ko TC, Flisak M, Prinz RA. Selective intra-arterial methylene blue injection: a novel method of localizing gastrinoma. *Gastroenterology* 1992;102:1062

Krejs G. VIPoma syndrome. *Am J Med* 1987;82:37

Krejs GJ, Orci L, Conlon JM, et al. Somatostatinoma syndrome: biochemical, morphologic and clinical features. *N Engl J Med* 1979;301:285

Lamers CBH, van Tongeren JHM. Comparative study of the value of the calcium, secretin, and meal stimulated increase in serum gastrin to the diagnosis of the Zollinger-Ellison syndrome. *Gut* 1977;18:128

Larsson L-I, Holst JJ, Hakanson R, et al. Distribution and properties of glucagon immunoreactivity in the digestive tract of various mammals: an immunohistochemical and immunochemical study. *Histochemistry* 1974;44:281

MacGavern M, Unger R, Recant L, et al. A glucagon-secreting alpha-cell carcinoma of the pancreas. *N Engl J Med* 1966;274:1408

Mallinson CN, Bloom SR, Warin AP, et al. A glucagonoma syndrome. *Lancet* 1974;ii:1

Maton PN, Miller DL, Doppman JL, et al. Role of selective angiography in the management of patients with Zollinger-Ellison syndrome. *Gastroenterology* 1987;92:913

Mozell E, Stenzel P, Woltering EA, et al. Functional endocrine tumors of the pancreas: clinical presentation, diagnosis, and treatment. *Curr Probl Surg* 1990;27:302

Nagorney DM, Bloom SR, Polak JM, et al. Resolution of recurrent Verner-Morrison syndrome by resection of metastatic VIPoma. *Surgery* 1983;93:348

Norton JA, Cromack DT, Shawker TH, et al. Intraoperative ultrasonographic localization of islet cell tumors: a prospective comparison to palpation. *Ann Surg* 1988;207:160

Norton JA, Levin B, Jensen RT. Cancer of the endocrine system. In: DeVita VT Jr, Hellman S, Rosenberg SA (eds), *Can-*

cer: *Principles and Practice of Oncology,* 4th ed. Philadelphia, PA: JB Lippincott; 1993:1333

Norton JA, Shawker TH, Doppman JL, et al. Localization and surgical treatment of occult insulinomas. *Ann Surg* 1990; 212:615

Parekh D, Ishizuka J, Townsend CM Jr, et al. Characterization of a human pancreatic carcinoid in vitro: morphology, amine and peptide storage and secretion. *Pancreas* 1994;9:83–90

Pasieka JL, McLeod MK, Thompson NW, et al. Surgical approach to insulinomas: assessing the need for preoperative localization. *Arch Surg* 1992;127:442

Pearse A. 5-Hydroxytryptophan uptake by dog thyroid "C" cells and its possible significance in polypeptide hormone production. *Nature* 1966;211:598

Pearse A. Common cytochemical and ultrastructural characteristics of cells producing polypeptide hormones (the APUD series) and their relevance to thyroid and ultimobranchial C cells and calcitonin. *Proc R Soc Lond (Biol)* 1968;170:71

Pisegna JR, Doppman JL, Norton JA, et al. Prospective comparative study of ability of MR imaging and other imaging modalities to localize tumors in patients with Zollinger-Ellison syndrome. *Dig Dis Sci* 1993;38:1318

Pisegna JR, Norton JA, Slimak GG, et al. Effects of curative gastrinoma resection on gastric secretory function and antisecretory drug requirement in Zollinger-Ellison syndrome. *Gastroneterology* 1992;102:767

Rosch T, Lightdale CJ, Botet JF, et al. Localization of pancreatic endocrine tumors by endoscopic ultrasonography. *N Engl J Med* 1992;326:1721

Sloan DA, Schwartz RW, Kenady DE. Surgical therapy for endocrine tumors of abdominal origin. *Curr Opin Oncol* 1993; 5:100

Sugg SL, Norton JA, Fraker DL, et al. A prospective study of intraoperative methods to diagnose and resect duodenal gastrinomas. *Ann Surg* 1993;218:138

Thom AK, Norton JA, Axiotis CA, et al. Location, incidence, and malignant potential of duodenal gastrinomas. *Surgery* 1991;110:1086

Thompson JC, Hirose FM, Lemmi CAE, et al. Zollinger-Ellison syndrome in a patient with multiple carcinoid-islet cell tumors of the duodenum: effect of tumor extract on isolated gastric mucosa. *Am J Surg* 1968;115:177

Thompson JC, Lewis BG, Wiener I, et al. The role of surgery in the Zollinger-Ellison syndrome. *Ann Surg* 1983;197: 594

Thompson JC, Reeder DD, Bunchman HH. Clinical role of serum gastrin measurements in the Zollinger-Ellison syndrome. *Am J Surg* 1972;124:250

Thompson JC, Reeder DD, Villar HV, et al. Natural history and experience with diagnosis and treatment of the Zollinger-Ellison syndrome. *Surg Gynecol Obstet* 1975;140:721

Udelsman R, Yeo CJ, Hruban RH, et al. Pancreaticoduodenectomy for selected pancreatic endocrine tumors. *Surg Gynecol Obstet* 1993;177:269

Verner J, Morrison A. Islet cell tumor and a syndrome of refractory watery diarrhea and hypokalemia. *Am J Med* 1958; 25:374

Vinik AI, Delbridge L, Moattari R, et al. Transhepatic portal vein catheterization for localization of insulinomas: a ten-year experience. *Surgery* 1991;109:1

Vinik AI, Moattari R. Treatment of endocrine tumors of the pancreas. *Endocrinol Metab Clin North Am* 1989;18:483

Whipple AO, Frantz VK. Adenoma of islet cells with hyperinsulinism: a review. *Ann Surg* 1935;101:1299

Zollinger R, Ellison E. Primary peptic ulcerations of the jejunum associated with islet cell tumors of the pancreas. *Ann Surg* 1955;142:709

74

Pancreatic and Periampullary Carcinoma

Keith D. Lillemoe ▪ *John L. Cameron*

Periampullary cancers include a group of malignant neoplasms arising at or near the ampulla of Vater. The location of these tumors produces their primary symptom, obstructive jaundice. Because of their common location they require similar management for both curative resection (pancreaticoduodenectomy) and palliation. In the vast majority, these tumors are adenocarcinomas arising from the head of the pancreas, ampulla of Vater, distal common bile duct, or duodenum. Although other malignant cell types may present as a periampullary neoplasm, they seldom present with the unrelenting jaundice from bile duct obstruction seen with adenocarcinomas. Often, distinguishing malignant biliary obstruction from fibrosing chronic pancreatitis is a more common clinical problem.

The first successful resection of a periampullary tumor was performed by Halsted in 1899. The tumor was resected locally and reconstruction was performed by reimplanting the pancreatic and biliary ducts into the duodenum. The first successful pancreaticoduodenectomy was performed by Kausch in 1912. However, pancreaticoduodenectomy was not popularized until 1935 with the report of Whipple and colleagues of a successful two stage en bloc resection of the head of the pancreas and the duodenum.[1] Over the next decade, a number of modifications and technical refinements were made in the procedure, including the first one-stage pancreaticoduodenectomy, reported in the United States by Trimble in 1941. Despite technical advances, until the 1980s, pancreaticoduodenectomy was associated with formidable operative morbidity and mortality rates. Furthermore, the poor prognosis associated with pancreaticoduodenectomy for pancreatic carcinoma led to an overall grim picture associated with this disease. Yet, during the last decade, significant advances have been made in our understanding of the pathogenesis of pancreatic and periampullary carcinoma, our ability to diagnose and stage these diseases adequately, and the efficacy of surgical and nonsurgical approaches to their treatment.

▪ INCIDENCE

Pancreatic and periampullary carcinoma are major public health concerns throughout the world. Pancreatic cancer, by far the most common periampullary malignancy, is the ninth most common cancer and is the fourth and fifth leading cause of cancer death in men and women, respectively, in the United States.[2] Over 27 000 people die from pancreatic cancer in this country each year. The incidence of pancreatic and periampullary carcinoma rose dramatically from the 1930s until the mid 1970s, nearly doubling during this time period. Since 1973, the incidence in the United States has remained stable at 8 to 9 per 100 000 population. The incidence in Western Europe is similar to the

United States and also has remained stable during the last two decades. In Japan, however, a dramatic increase has been observed during the last two decades, although their overall incidence is still less than in the United States and Great Britain. The lowest incidence worldwide is seen in India and in parts of the Middle East.

The incidence of pancreatic and periampullary carcinoma increases steadily with age, with over 80% of patients seen in the sixth, seventh, or eighth decade of life. There is a slight male predilection; however, the incidence and mortality rate in women has increased in the last two decades while remaining constant in men. Blacks are more commonly affected than whites with black males having the highest overall incidence in the United States.

■ PATHOLOGY

The sight of origin of a periampullary malignancy often can be difficult to determine. Frequently, the clinical presentation, preoperative imaging studies, and findings at laparotomy do not allow differentiation of the specific site of origin. Pathologic examination of resected specimens showed that adenocarcinomas of the head of the pancreas (40% to 60%), ampulla of Vater (20% to 40%), distal common bile duct (10%), and duodenum (10%) account for the vast majority of periampullary neoplasms. Since these data represent resected specimens, the incidence of ampullary, distal bile duct, and duodenal carcinomas is somewhat higher owing to these tumors often having a greater rate of resectability than tumors arising in the head of the pancreas. Therefore, overall, carcinoma of the pancreas is the likely site of origin in up to 90% of cases.

Ductal adenocarcinoma is by far the most common malignant histologic type of pancreatic carcinoma with more than two-thirds of these tumors arising in the pancreatic head, neck, or uncinate process. Rare cell types include acinar, squamous, islet cell tumors, or tumors of nonepithelial origin. Islet cell tumors, or neuroendocrine tumors, may be either histologically benign or malignant and may be functional with excessive hormone production resulting in clinical manifestations. Nonfunctional islet cell tumors produce no recognizable hormonal manifestations and usually are detected due to their space-occupying characteristics. Obstructive jaundice is uncommon, with benign islet cell tumors seen in the head of the pancreas, but it can occur with malignant lesions. Cystic neoplasms of the pancreas also arise from the exocrine pancreas and are classified as either benign serous cystadenomas, potentially malignant mucinous cystadenomas, or malignant mucinous cystadenocarcinomas. These cystic neoplasms are much less common than ductal adenocarcinoma, tend to occur in women, and can be found throughout the entire gland. Malignant cystic neoplasms of the head of the pancreas also can produce obstructive jaundice, but less commonly than ductal carcinoma. Various sarcomas, including the fibrosarcomas, leiomyosarcomas, hemangiopericystomas, and histiocytomas, also may arise in the pancreas. Similarly, lymphomas can occur in and around the pancreas. These so-called pancreatic lymphomas may present with obstructive jaundice, are usually quite large on CT scan, and have less well-defined margins than does a typical adenocarcinoma.[3] Finally, the pancreas and periampullary region can be the site of metastasis from other tumors. In fact, although rarely of clinical significance, autopsy studies show that metastatic involvement of the pancreas is more common (by approximately 4-fold) than primary malignancy. The sites of origin, in decreasing frequency include breast, lung, malignant melanoma, stomach and colon.

■ ETIOLOGY

The etiology of pancreatic and periampullary carcinoma is unknown. The frequency of these tumors and their dismal prognosis has led to sophisticated investigations into the associated risk factors and the molecular genetic basis of these conditions. It is the hope that these investigations will develop strategies for earlier diagnosis and improved survival.

ENVIRONMENTAL RISK FACTORS

Cigarette smoking is the only environmental risk factor that has been consistently associated with pancreatic cancer. The estimates of risk associated with current smoking are generally a 2- to 3-fold increase for both males and females.[4] The risk increases with the number of cigarettes smoked and risk levels 10 to 15 years after smoking cessation. An elevated risk also has been associated with pipe and cigar smoking. The mechanism by which tobacco products cause pancreatic cancer appears to be related to tobacco-specific nitrosamines that reach the pancreas either through the blood or bile that is in contact with the pancreatic duct. Alternatively, smoking can elevate blood lipids, which also may increase the risk of pancreatic cancer. Pancreatic tumors can be induced experimentally in animals by the administration of tobacco-specific nitrosamines, either in the water or parenterally.

A second proposed risk factor associated with pancreatic cancer is diet. A high intake of animal fat or meat has been linked to the development of pancreatic carcinoma. Japanese studies have shown that daily consumption of meat increased the risk of developing pancreatic cancer by 1.5 times, perhaps suggesting the adaptation of a Western diet had contributed to the recent increase of pancreatic cancer in that country. It is felt that diets high in fat stimulate cholecystokinin (CCK) release, which may induce pancreatic ductal hyperplasia and hypertrophy of pancreatic acinar cells. Increased protein intake associated with meat consumption also may affect pancreatic enzyme output. Increased trypsin in the intestinal lumen leads to further increased CCK release, while excess protease secretion may damage ductal epithelium and promote carcinogenesis through the increased cell proliferation of the repair process. High intake of fresh fruits and vegetables and increased dietary fiber have been sighted as protective factors against pancreatic cancer. The report of an increased risk of pancreatic cancer associated with coffee intake generated a significant deal of scientific and public controversy. A number of studies have dealt with this issue but a recent comprehensive review analyzing 30 epidemiologic studies concluded that although a possible increased risk has been suggested by some, there has been no confirmed statistically significant association and therefore no causal association can be drawn.[5] Similarly, there has been no confirmed relationship between tea consumption and pancreatic carcinoma. Finally, extensive review of the relationship between alcohol consumption and pancreatic cancer has concluded that there is insufficient epidemiologic evidence of a causal relationship.

Pancreatic cancer, as well as bile duct cancer, has been associated with occupational exposure to various chemicals including naphthylamine and benzidine, and in individuals working in chemical plants, refineries, and other chemical-related industries. There has been no consistent evidence supporting radiation exposure as a risk factor for pancreatic cancer.

PREDISPOSING MEDICAL CONDITIONS

A strong positive association exists in the development of pancreatic cancer in patients with a history of previous gastrectomy for peptic ulcer disease; such individuals have a five to seven times greater risk of pancreatic cancer. It has been proposed that increased production of N-nitroso compounds by bacteria that proliferate in the hypoacidic stomach could be responsible for both the development of gastric and pancreatic cancers. Similarly, detoxification of substances metabolized in the small intestine may be less efficient after gastrectomy. The growth of pancreatic cancers in animal models tends to be promoted by exogenous cholecystokinin. Increased endogenous production of this hormone can be seen in patients following cholecystectomy, which has also been associated with an increase in the risk of

pancreatic cancer. Previous tonsillectomy and certain allergic diseases have been associated with a protective effect for pancreatic cancer, suggesting the role of immunologic factors in pancreatic carcinogenesis.

Chronic pancreatitis has been suggested as a risk factor for pancreatic cancer because of the frequent association between the two conditions. This relationship, however, remains unresolved.[6] It would appear more likely that the association with pancreatitis is, rather, the result of the pathologic changes caused by ductal obstruction by the carcinoma rather than a true risk factor. Furthermore, a patient occasionally may present with acute pancreatitis as the first manifestation of pancreatic cancer. As with chronic pancreatitis, diabetes mellitus and pancreatic carcinoma have been associated. Although no other malignancy is increased in diabetics, experimentally the diabetic state enhances the growth of pancreatic carcinoma. The literature is inconsistent with respect to the epidemiologic association of pancreatic cancer with diabetes; much of this association appears to be the result of the destruction of pancreatic tissue owing to the obstructing pancreatic cancer and the resultant endocrine insufficiency. Therefore, as with chronic pancreatitis, the development of diabetes in the patient after 40 years of age should be considered a clue to the diagnosis of pancreatic cancer.

MOLECULAR GENETIC FACTORS

The most dramatic association with periampullary malignancy and a hereditary disorder is the association of familial polyposis of the colon and Gardner's syndrome. In both conditions, preexisting adenomatous polyps of the duodenum or ampulla predispose to the development of carcinoma. The increase in periampullary malignancy in these patients may be 200 times that of the normal population. There are several hereditary disorders also associated with pancreatic cancer, including hereditary pancreatitis, von Hippel-Lindau's syndrome, Lynch's syndrome II, and ataxiatelangiectasia. These diseases however are rare disorders and generate little concern with respect to pancreatic cancer on the large scale. Population-based case control studies have suggested that there is an increased association with a positive family history of pancreatic cancer or any cancer in a close relative among patients with pancreatic cancer. The molecular genetic substantiation of a primary genetic base for this disease, however, has not been established.

A number of genetic alternatives have been recently identified to be associated with pancreatic cancer. Molecular abnormalities include a mutant K-ras gene on codon 12 (up to 85%) and a mutation of the p53 gene on chromosome 17 (50% to 70%) have been discovered in a large percentage of patients with pancreatic cancer.[7] Similarly, an over-expression of the EGF receptor and production of EGF-α have been found in pancreatic cancer specimens. Currently, the rate of advance in this field is tremendous and it can be anticipated that further descriptions of this area will be forthcoming. The clinical importance of these investigations in the areas of risk assessment, early diagnosis, therapy, and prognosis only can be anticipated at present.

■ DIAGNOSIS AND PREOPERATIVE EVALUATION

The diagnosis of pancreatic and periampullary carcinoma is made on the basis of clinical presentation, laboratory data, and radiologic work-up. Although in some situations a preoperative tissue diagnosis may be available, treatment should not be delayed by attempts to obtain histologic confirmation of malignancy.

CLINICAL PRESENTATION

The early symptoms of periampullary carcinoma are usually vague and include anorexia, weight loss, abdominal discomfort, and nausea. Unfortunately, the nonspecific nature of these symptoms often contributes to delay in diagnosis by both the patient and physician. Specific symptoms usually develop only after invasion or obstruction of a nearby structure. Since a periampullary carcinoma, by definition, arises near the distal biliary tree, obstructive jaundice is the hallmark presentation. Jaundice is progressive and often is associated with significant pruritus. Pain of moderate intensity may be present as a result of obstruction of either the biliary or pancreatic ducts. This pain, often described as dull and located in the epigastrium, may be accompanied by back pain and is often worse in a supine position and relieved by sitting forward.

In patients with carcinoma of the head of the pancreas, more intense pain can be caused by invasion of the tumor into the splanchnic plexus and the retroperitoneum as well as by obstruction of the pancreatic duct. Although intractable pain frequently is associated with pancreatic carcinoma, it is seldom an early manifestation. Recent studies suggest that less than one-third of patients presenting with pancreatic carcinoma described moderate to severe pain.[8] Duodenal obstruction, with nausea and vomiting, is usually a late manifestation of periampullary carcinoma. Duodenal and ampullary carcinomas may bleed intermittently. Both exocrine and endocrine pancreatic insufficiency may be observed in patients with periampullary carcinoma, especially when the tumor originates in the pancreas. New onset diabetes is observed in 15% to 20% of patients with pancreatic cancer during the two years before tumor diagnosis.[9] Finally, an unexplained attack of pancreatitis in an older patient must be investigated thoroughly once the acute attack has subsided, because this presentation may be a rare first manifestation of a periampullary tumor.

In many patients, physical findings are absent, especially early in the course. The development of jaundice is often the first physical finding that is apparent as the tumor obstructs the biliary tree. An enlarged liver or palpable gallbladder is present in 25% to 30% of patients. In more advanced stages, a palpable mass or ascites may be observed. Occult fecal blood loss may be found in those patients with periampullary cancers that can bleed into the intestinal lumen, such as duodenal and ampullary tumors.

Laboratory Data

There are no specific diagnostic laboratory tests for periampullary carcinoma. Virtually all patients present with liver function test abnormalities, including increased levels of total bilirubin, alkaline phosphatase, and transaminases. Because of the obstructive nature of these tumors, the alkaline phosphatase is generally more elevated than the transaminases. Anemia may be present with any periampullary carcinoma, although patients with ampullary or duodenal carcinomas are more likely to experience significant gastrointestinal bleeding and marked anemia.

The tumor-associated antigen, CA 19-9, has a sensitivity and specificity approaching 90% for tumors arising in the pancreas.[10] The levels of CA 19-9 are frequently normal in the early stages of pancreatic cancer and with other periampullary neoplasms. Therefore, it is not considered suitable as a screening technique. The finding of an elevated CA 19-9 may be useful in differentiating benign from malignant conditions. Furthermore, after resection, if the CA 19-9 level falls, the antigen may be useful for prognosis and follow-up surveillance. Recently, the glycoprotein antigen CA 494 has shown early promise as a marker for pancreatic cancer. Because of a higher specificity, CA 494 may better differentiate chronic pancreatitis from pancreatic cancer.[11]

Imaging Studies

Early diagnosis of periampullary carcinoma requires a high index of suspicion and appropriate aggressiveness in pursuing the diagnosis. The prompt evaluation of a patient with jaundice, however, offers the opportunity for early diagnosis. Any patient presenting with jaundice should promptly undergo diagnostic imaging with either ultrasound or computed tomography (CT). Both tests confirm the obstructive nature of jaundice by demonstrating dilated intrahepatic and extrahepatic bile ducts. Conventional ultrasonography is an easy and safe examination, does not entail radiation exposure,

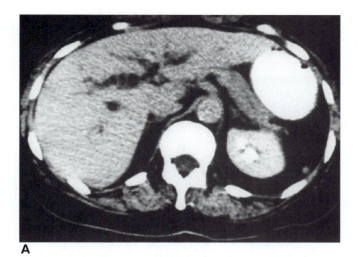

A

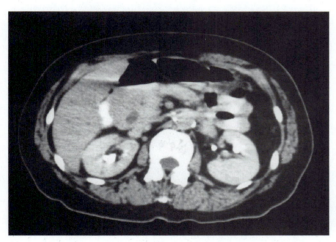

B

C

Figure 74–1. CT scan of a patient with obstructive jaundice due to pancreatic cancer. **A.** Scan shows dilated intrahepatic ducts. **B.** Scan demonstrates a mass in the head of the pancreas surrounding the dilated common bile duct. **C.** Scan taken 1 cm inferiorly shows persistence of the pancreatic mass but the absence of the dilated common bile duct, representing complete obstruction of the duct by tumor. (From Lillemoe KD. Current management of pancreatic carcinoma. *Ann Surg* 1995;221:133)

and is relatively inexpensive. This technique is much more sensitive for detecting gallstones than other modalities but suffers from being technically suboptimal in up to 25% of patients. CT is generally considered more useful in defining the level of obstruction, demonstrating the presence of pancreatic mass (as small as 1 cm in size), and detecting liver metastases or local vascular invasion (Fig 74–1).[12] Currently, the use of intravenous and oral contrast-enhanced spiral CT offers the best form of imaging of the pancreas. Magnetic resonance imaging (MRI) has no apparent advantage over CT.

Once biliary obstruction has been confirmed by imaging studies, the next step in the evaluation of the jaundiced patient is cholangiography. Either the endoscopic or percutaneous approach is appropriate with the choice of technique depending on local expertise[12] (Fig 74–2). Using the endoscopic approach, ampullary and duodenal carcinomas can be visualized and biopsied. In addition, a pancreatogram may be obtained that may be important if the differential diagnosis includes chronic pancreatitis. In most cases of pancreatic cancer, the ductal system will be obstructed with no distal filling of the duct. The percutaneous approach is usually technically easier with a dilated biliary tree and offers the advantages of defining the proximal biliary system that will be used in reconstruction.

A biliary stent can be placed through the obstructing lesion in the bile duct by either the endoscopic or percutaneous approach to alleviate jaundice. The use of biliary stents preoperatively in an attempt to improve the overall operative risk has been addressed by a number of prospective randomized studies with mixed results. In a study by Pitt and colleagues, percutaneous biliary decompression preoperatively did not affect morbidity and mortality while increasing total hospital stay.[13] In contrast, Lygidakis and his group in Amsterdam, using preoperative endoscopic biliary drainage, significantly reduced operative morbidity and mortality.[14] It appears likely, therefore, although not indicated routinely, that in selected patients with advanced malnutrition, sepsis, and/or correctable medical conditions, preoperative biliary drainage is useful. Theoretically, internal drainage of biliary secretions may also provide an immunologic basis for decreased perioperative septic complications. Finally, the percutaneous biliary catheter can be useful during the operative management for either resection or palliation, especially in reoperative cases.

A tissue diagnosis of a periampullary cancer can be confirmed by several methods preoperatively. Duodenal or ampullary cancers can be biopsied easily by endoscopy and cytologic brushings obtained. A biopsy of a periampullary mass showing invasive adenocarcinoma will be diagnostic in virtually all cases, however, the histologic finding of a benign villous adenoma with or without dysplasia can not reliably rule out malig-

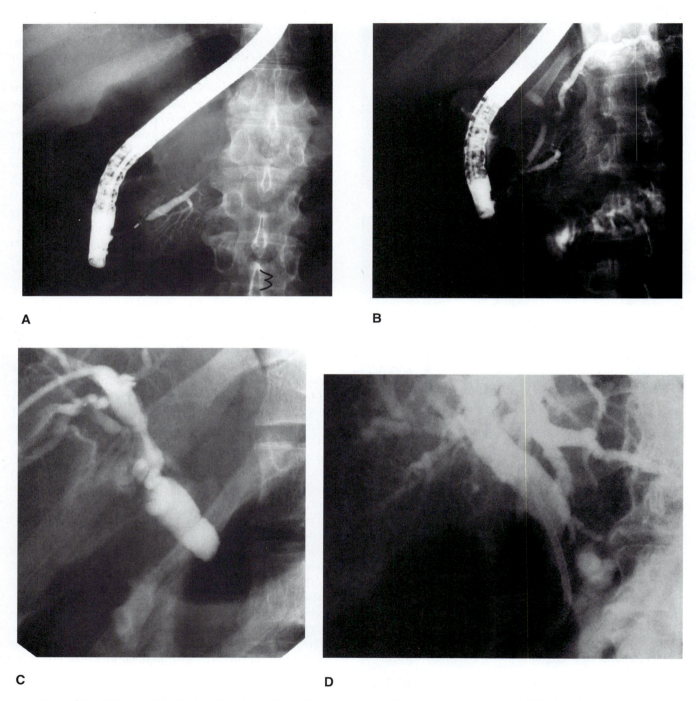

A

B

C

D

Figure 74–2. A. ERCP of a patient with pancreatic carcinoma with cut-off of main pancreatic duct owing to pancreatic carcinoma. **B.** ERCP of a patient with pancreatic carcinoma with partial obstruction of both the main pancreatic duct and common bile duct. **C.** Percutaneous transhepatic cholangiogram of patient in part B showing dilated proximal biliary tree with complete obstruction at the "knee" of the common bile duct. **D.** Completion cholangiogram after endoscopic placement of an endo-prosthesis. (From Lillemoe KD. Current management of pancreatic carcinoma. *Ann Surg* 1995;221:133)

nancy. A number of clinical reports have documented a false-negative rate approaching 50% in this scenario. If a pancreatic tumor can be demonstrated by CT, a fine-needle aspiration can be performed percutaneously to gain material for cytologic diagnosis. Although this technique is very accurate, with a sensitivity greater than 90% and a specificity of virtually 100%, it is of limited use in patients in whom surgical exploration for attempted resection or palliation is planned. There are two reasons for not using fine-needle aspiration for potentially resectable lesions. First, even after repeated sampling, a negative result cannot exclude malignancy; in fact, it is the smaller and more likely curable tumors that are most likely to be missed by this technique. A second concern is seeding of the tumor, either along the needle tract or with intraperitoneal spread. The primary indication for percutaneous biopsy is therefore in those patients with periampullary or pancreatic carcinoma who would appear not to be surgical candidates because of either extent of disease or medical contraindications. Percutaneous biopsy may be useful if the CT picture suggests pancreatic lymphoma, which is best managed nonoperatively.

PREOPERATIVE STAGING

The goal of preoperative staging of pancreatic or periampullary carcinoma is to determine the feasibility of surgery and the optimal treatment for each individual patient. In general, preoperative staging is more useful for pancreatic tumors than for other forms of periampullary cancer, since resectability for the latter lesions is usually significantly higher at the time of pre-

sentation than it is for pancreatic cancer. In many patients, dynamic spiral CT with oral and intravenous contrast will provide all the information necessary by demonstrating liver metastases or major vascular invasion (Fig 74–3). The extent of further staging to be performed is dependent upon the individual patient and the preference of the surgeon. If the surgeon's philosophy is to pursue surgical treatment for all patients, either in order to attempt resection or to provide palliation, further staging is unnecessary. However, if the findings at staging could preclude an operation and lead to nonoperative palliation, these efforts are worthwhile.

Local invasion of adjacent visceral vessels precludes resection in a significant number of patients explored for periampullary carcinoma. Of the periampullary malignancies, major vessel involvement is far more common in tumors originating in the head of the pancreas. Preoperative visceral angiography with arterial injection of the celiac and superior mesenteric arteries with venous phase studies provides the best demonstration of vascular anatomy and major vessel encasement or occlusion (Fig 74–4). In a review of this technique in patients with periampullary carcinomas identified by CT scan at The Johns Hopkins Hospital, 77% of patients without evidence of major visceral vessel occlusion or encasement were resectable.[15] Major vessel encasement indicated a lower resectability rate (35%). Furthermore, in all patients with major vessel occlusion, the tumor was found to be unresectable at operation. Finally, visceral angiography also will detect anatomic variations, such as a replaced right hepatic artery or atherosclerotic stenosis or occlusion of the celiac axis, that may alter opera-

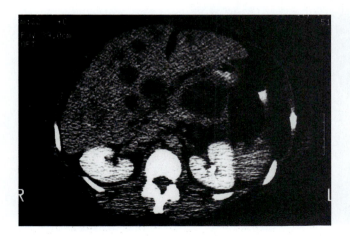

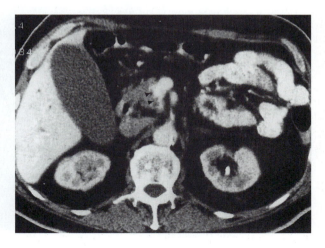

A   **B**

Figure 74–3. A. CT scan demonstrating a cystic tumor of the body of the pancreas and multiple liver metastases. **B.** Superior mesenteric vein involvement is demonstrated by tumor-vessel contiguity by spiral CT scan. Abnormal enhancement of the medial border of the head and uncinate process of the pancreas is seen (*arrowheads*).

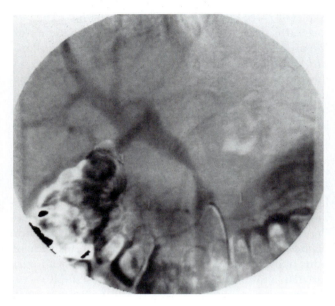
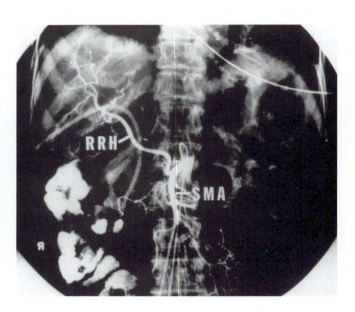

A   **B**

Figure 74–4. A. Venous phase of superior mesenteric artery injection demonstrates encasement of the SMV and portal vein owing to an unresectable pancreatic carcinoma. **B.** Superior mesenteric artery (SMA) injection demonstrating a replaced right hepatic artery (RRH). (From Dooley WC, Cameron JL, Pitt HA, et al. Is preoperative angiography useful in patients with periampullary tumors? *Ann Surg* 1990;211:649).

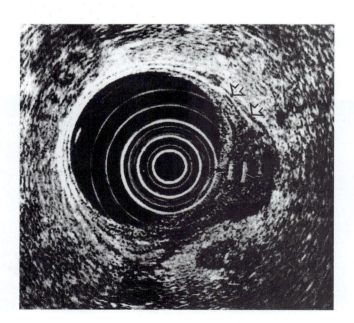

Figure 74–5. Endoscopic ultrasound of ampullary tumor represented by a hypoechoic area on right. An endoprosthesis (*small black arrows*) can be seen running through the center of the tumor. The tumor clearly infiltrates beyond the muscularis propria (*open arrows*) into the pancreas.

tive management. In patients with tumors of the body or tail of the pancreas, involvement including occlusion of the splenic artery and vein is common. This finding does not preclude resection. Angiography is indicated, however, in these patients to rule out involvement of the superior mesenteric and portal vein and/or the celiac axis.

Endoscopic ultrasonography is a minimally invasive technique in which a high-frequency transducer is placed in the gastric and duodenal lumen in close proximity to the pancreas and adjacent organs. The main usefulness of this technique is to detect small pancreatic lesions (<2 cm) and also lymph node and vascular involvement. This technique is also particularly useful in the evaluation of ampullary tumors with respect to invasion of the duodenal wall and pancreas (Fig 74–5). A recent study in preoperative patients suggested that endoscopic ultrasound examination was superior to conventional sonography, CT, and angiography in assessing resectability.[16] Experience with this technique, which is operator-dependent, is still limited, precluding its widespread use.

Liver metastases and peritoneal implants are the most common sites of spread of periampullary carcinoma. Once distant metastases are present, survival is so limited that a conservative approach is indicated. Liver metastases greater than 2 cm can generally be detected by CT, but approximately 30% of metastases are smaller and therefore not routinely detected. Furthermore, peritoneal and omental metastases are usually only 1 to 2 mm in size and frequently can be detected only by direct visualization. The technique of diagnostic laparoscopy, before the patient is subjected to laparotomy, has been used by several groups as an additional staging modality for the evaluation of patients with pancreatic and periampullary malignancies. In one such series, 40% of patients without demonstrable extrapancreatic involvement on the basis of CT scan were found at laparoscopy to have small liver or peritoneal metastases, precluding resection.[17] In addition, at the time of laparoscopy, irrigation of the peritoneal cavity can be performed, with washings analyzed cytologically for evidence of shed cells. Although this technique offers advantages, especially in patients in whom neo-adjuvant therapy is planned, published reports suggest a laparoscopy does not improve the resectability rate in comparison with other less invasive forms of evaluation. Therefore, it is not recommended as a routine preoperative staging procedure.

The information gained from preoperative staging provides a basis for planning for each individual patient. If preoperative staging with CT, angiography, and laparoscopy is normal, resectability rates may approach 90% for tumors of the head of the pancreas.[18] Preoperative staging, therefore, results in a considerable improvement from previous resectability rates of less than 25%, and thus eliminates the need for an unnecessary operation in a large number of patients.

■ TREATMENT OF PANCREATIC AND PERIAMPULLARY CARCINOMA

Surgical resection currently provides the only opportunity for cure for patients with pancreatic and periampullary carcinoma. Although in selected patients a lesser operation may be appropriate, in most patients, pancreaticoduodenectomy is the preferred technique.

SURGICAL TREATMENT FOR AMPULLARY CARCINOMA

In 1899 Halsted described the local resection of an ampullary carcinoma. Although the operation was technically successful and short-term results satisfactory, the patient died of recurrent carcinoma. Since popularized in 1935, most periampullary carcinomas, including carcinoma of the ampulla, have been managed with pancreaticoduodenectomy. During the last decade, however, several reports have surfaced advocating local ampullary resection for patients with benign and premalignant tumors and for selected patients with malignant lesions. In many such cases, preoperative biopsies have suggested a benign villous tumor and attempt at local resection would appear appropriate. However, it must be remembered that owing to sampling error of endoscopic biopsies, the ultimate diagnosis of malignancy cannot always be determined accurately by this technique.

The technique for ampullectomy begins with a generous Kocher maneuver. If the gallbladder is in place, a cholecystectomy is performed and the cystic duct can be catheterized with a Fogarty biliary balloon catheter, which is useful for identification of the ampulla. The duodenum then is opened longitudinally over either the palpable mass or balloon catheter. The cautery or scalpel is used to excise the lesion in an effort to obtain a clear gross margin around the lesion. As the tumor is excised, the orifices of the common bile duct and pancreatic duct are visualized. A sphincteroplasty of the common bile duct is made by incising the anterior common bile duct wall. A similar septoplasty can be performed on the pancreatic duct. In both cases, the duct is sutured to the duodenal mucosa with fine interrupted absorbable sutures. The duodenotomy is usually closed transversely to avoid narrowing. After local excision, the specimen should be carefully examined by pathologists and frozen sections performed (Fig 74–6). If evidence of invasive carcinoma exists, a pancreaticoduodenectomy should be performed unless the patient's age and/or overall medical status will not allow the proce-

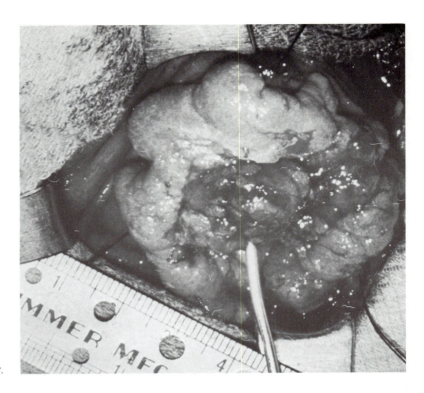

Figure 74–6. A primarily excised polypoid ampullary tumor.

dure. However, if the lesion is benign or shows only evidence of carcinoma in situ and margins are negative, the ampullectomy as described should be adequate treatment. However, it is not uncommon that, in such cases when permanent pathologic examination is completed, evidence of invasive carcinoma may exist. At that time, the surgeon must face the difficult decision of returning to the operating room to complete a pancreaticoduodenectomy versus simple follow-up. This decision is based primarily on the extent of the invasion and the overall age and medical status of the patient.

PANCREATICODUODENECTOMY FOR PANCREATIC AND PERIAMPULLARY CARCINOMA

In 1935 Whipple and associates described a technique for radical excision of a periampullary carcinoma.[1] The operation was performed in two stages, with a cholecystogastrostomy performed to decompress the obstructing biliary tree and a gastrojejunostomy performed to relieve gastric outlet obstruction in the first stage. The second stage was performed several weeks later when the jaundice had resolved and nutritional status was improved. During the second stage, an en bloc resection of the second portion of the duodenum and a small wedge of the head of the pancreas was performed without reestablishing pancreaticoenteric continuity. Although earlier attempts at pancreaticoduodenal resection had been described, the report by Whipple and

colleagues began the modern era of the treatment of periampullary carcinoma.

Since Whipple's original description, pancreaticoduodenal resection has undergone numerous modifications and technical refinements. Unfortunately, during most of the original 50 years that the procedure was performed, the reported morbidity and mortality rates were unacceptably high and long-term survival rates were disappointing. During the late 1960s and 1970s, the high operative morbidity and mortality and the poor long-term survival led some authors to suggest that the Whipple procedure be abandoned.[19-21] However, during the last decade, a number of reports have documented both improved operative results and better long-term survival rates for patients with periampullary tumors following the Whipple procedure, leading to a resurgence in its popularity.

OPERATIVE TECHNIQUE OF PANCREATICODUODENECTOMY

Much of the improvement in operative results and long-term survival following pancreaticoduodenectomy have come from centers reporting large series of patients undergoing this procedure. This fact strongly suggests that this operation should be performed by surgeons who are experienced in the surgical management of periampullary carcinoma. This management consists of two phases: first, assessing tumor resectability and then, if the tumor is resectable, completing a pancreaticoduodenectomy with reconstruction. The operative technique has been described in detail elsewhere and will be discussed here briefly.[22]

The determination of resectability is based both on preoperative evaluation and operative findings. In many cases, the former complements the latter. Specifically, evidence of major vascular encasement on preoperative arteriography, although not definitive evidence of unresectability, should certainly warrant special attention to this area. The abdomen should be explored through an upper midline or bilateral subcostal incision. A careful search for tumor outside the limits of a pancreaticoduodenal resection should be begun. The liver and peritoneal surfaces are inspected and palpated, with suspicious lesions biopsied and submitted for frozen section examination. Regional lymph nodes are evaluated for the presence of tumor involvement. Tumor present in the periaortic lymph nodes of the celiac axis indicates that the tumor is beyond the limits of normal resection. However, the presence of tumor-bearing lymph nodes that normally would be incorporated within the resection specimen do not constitute a contraindication to resection, since long-term survival may be possible.

Once distant metastases have been excluded, an assessment is made as to whether the primary tumor is resectable. Local factors that preclude pancreaticoduodenal resection include retroperitoneal extension of the tumor to involve the inferior vena cava or aorta, or direct involvement or encasement of the superior mesenteric artery, superior mesenteric vein (SMV), or portal vein. The technical aspects of determining local resection begin with a Kocher maneuver and mobilizing the duodenum and the head of the pancreas from the underlying inferior vena cava and aorta (Fig 74–7). Once the duodenum and head of the pancreas are mobilized sufficiently, the surgeon's hand can be placed under the duodenum and the head of the pancreas in order to palpate the relationship of the tumor mass to the superior mesenteric artery. The inability of the surgeon to identify a plane of normal tissue between the mass and the arterial pulsation indicates direct tumor involvement of the superior mesenteric artery, eliminating the possibility of complete tumor resection.

The final step to determine resectability involves dissection of the superior mesenteric and portal vein to rule out tumor invasion. Identification of the portal vein can be greatly simplified if the common hepatic duct is divided and reflected early in the dissection. In the past, most surgeons have left the biliary tree intact and retracted it medially while identifying the portal vein. However, since the hepatic duct can be used for palliation via the performance of a hepaticojejunostomy if the patient is unresectable, the division of this structure at this time facilitates exposure of the portal vein. Once

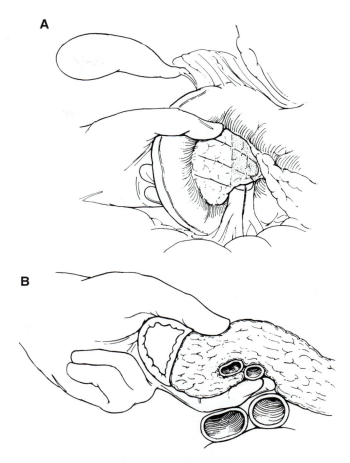

Figure 74–7. A and **B.** The uncinate process, head of the pancreas, and superior mesenteric artery are palpated between the thumb and index finger. This maneuver enables the surgeon to determine whether the tumor has extended into the uncinate process to involve the superior mesenteric artery. (From Crist DW, Cameron JL. The current status of the Whipple operation for periampullary carcinoma. *Adv Surg* 1992;2J:21)

the hepatic duct has been divided, the posteriorly located portal vein can be identified easily. Furthermore, this step untethers the first portion of the duodenum so it can easily be retracted, allowing further dissection under direct vision of the anterior surface of the portal vein from the posterior aspect of the first portion of the duodenum and the neck of the pancreas. Not only does this improve the exposure for dissection but, in the process, eliminates blind dissection with the risk of substantial bleeding.

Once the anterior surface of the portal vein is dissected posterior to the neck of the pancreas, the next step is to identify the SMV and to dissect its anterior surface (Fig 74–8). This is done most easily by extending the Kocher maneuver past the second portion of the duodenum to include the third and fourth portion of the duodenum. During this extensive Kocher maneuver, the first structure that one encounters anterior to the third portion of the duodenum is the SMV. The an-

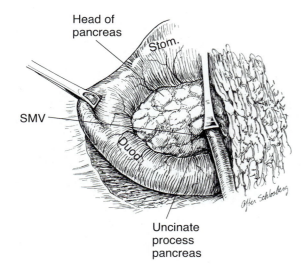

A

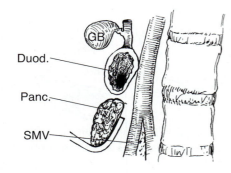

B

Figure 74–8. If one extends the Kocher maneuver of the duodenum along the third portion, the first structure one encounters anterior to the duodenum is the SMV. It can be cleaned quickly and visualized under direct vision from the posterior aspect of the pancreas (insert), and the dissection can be connected to that of the portal vein from above. Stom: stomach; Duod: duodenum; GB: gallbladder.

terior surface of the vein then can be rapidly cleaned and dissected under direct vision by retracting the neck of the pancreas anteriorly (Fig 74–9). The dissection is continued until it connects to the portal vein dissection from above. This technique is much simpler, quicker, and associated with less blood loss than the traditional technique of finding the superior mesenteric vein by opening the greater omentum, and entering the lesser sac and dissecting the inferior surface of the body of the pancreas.[23]

Most experienced pancreaticobiliary surgeons, at this point, will proceed with a pancreaticoduodenectomy without obtaining a tissue diagnosis. The clinical presentation, the results of preoperative CT scan and cholangiography, and the operative findings of a palpa-

ble mass in the head of the pancreas surpass the ability of an intraoperative biopsy in defining the diagnosis of malignancy. Although transduodenal needle biopsies can provide a tissue diagnosis in a high percentage of patients, it remains possible that small, potentially curable cancers may be missed by this technique. Therefore, in light of the improved operative morbidity and mortality following pancreaticoduodenectomy, surgical resection without a prior tissue diagnosis is appropriate.

Having excluded regional and distant metastases and demonstrated no tumor involvement of major vascular structures, the surgeon can proceed with pancreaticoduodenectomy with a high degree of certainty that the tumor is resectable. Currently, in most series, a pylorus-preserving pancreaticoduodenectomy is the procedure of choice. The duodenum is at first mobilized and divided approximately 2 cm distal to the pylorus. If a classic Whipple procedure is to be performed, the stomach is divided to include approximately 40% to 50% of the stomach with the resected specimen. The gastroduodenal artery is exposed, ligated, and divided near its origin at the common hepatic artery. It is always important to confirm prior to ligation that the structure to be ligated is indeed the gastroduodenal and not either a replaced right hepatic or even, in some cases, the hepatic artery. The neck of the pancreas then is divided, taking care to avoid injury to the underlying SMV and portal vein. The next step is to dissect the portal vein and SMV from the uncinate process and the head of the pancreas. There are several small venous branches between these sites that must be ligated and divided carefully (Fig 74–10). It is at this point that the surgeon may discover that the tumor may extend from the uncinate process to involve the vein. If the tumor involvement is localized, a segment of the vein wall may be excised en bloc with the tumor and the vein repaired primarily or with a vein patch. Alternatively, an en bloc resection of the SMV-portal vein with reconstruction and with a vein graft may be performed. Although advocates of this technique have reported acceptable results, morbidity and mortality are clearly increased. Furthermore, the chance of long-term survival is small.[24]

At this point, the fourth portion of the duodenum and the proximal jejunum are mobilized, with the proximal jejunum divided approximately 10 cm distal to the ligament of Treitz. The proximal jejunum and the fourth portion of the duodenum are passed under the superior mesenteric vessels to the right, and the uncinate process then is dissected from the superior mesenteric artery. The tissue between the uncinate process and the superior mesenteric artery contains several small arterial vessels. Therefore, this tissue is best divided between clamps and individually ligated. The course of the superior mesenteric artery should be identified clearly in order to avoid injury to this structure. At

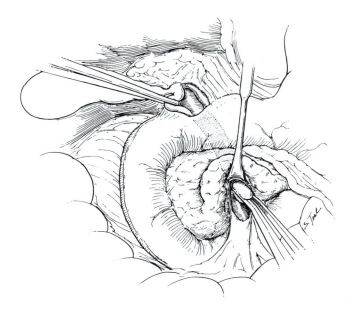

Figure 74–9. The SMV and portal veins are separated from the neck of the pancreas by dissection above and below the pancreas. The dissection should be limited to the anterior surface of these vessels, since there are usually no venous branches in this plane. (From Crist DW, Cameron JL. The current status of the Whipple operation for periampullary carcinoma. *Adv Surg* 1992;25:21)

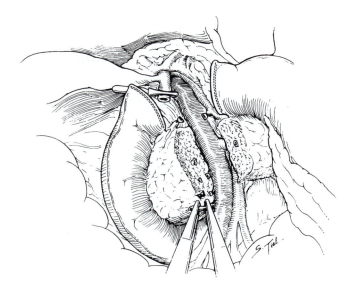

Figure 74–10. The portal and superior mesenteric veins are dissected from the uncinate process of the pancreas and the small venous branches between the veins and the uncinate process are ligated and divided carefully. (From Crist DW, Cameron JL. The current status of the Whipple operation for periampullary carcinoma. *Adv Surg* 1992;25:21)

this point, the specimen, consisting of the gallbladder and common bile duct, the head and neck and uncinate process of the pancreas, the entire duodenum and proximal jejunum (and the distal stomach for a traditional Whipple procedure) is now freed completely and removed from the operative field.

There are a number of techniques for restoring gastrointestinal continuity following a pancreaticoduodenal resection. In the most common technique, the end of the divided jejunum is placed in a retrocolic position, with creation of a pancreaticojejunostomy, followed by hepaticojejunostomy and a duodenojejunostomy or gastrojejunostomy. The pancreaticojejunostomy is the most problematic anastomosis in the reconstruction, with traditionally much of the morbidity and mortality associated with this operation related to problems with this anastomosis. A number of techniques to manage the pancreatic remnant can be used, including end-to-end and end-to-side pancreaticojejunostomy, either stented or unstented. More recently, attention has focused on the use of an end-to-side pancreaticogastrostomy as an alternative for management (Fig 74–11). A recent prospective comparison from The Johns Hopkins Hospital would suggest that the perioperative results are similar with pancreaticogastrostomy and pancreaticojejunostomy.[25]

Our preferred technique for either a pancreaticojejunostomy or pancreaticogastrostomy involves invagina-

tion of the end of the pancreas into the bowel. This requires an adequate mobilization of about 2 to 3 cm of the pancreatic remnant to ensure a length for invagination. A two-layer anastomosis is performed, usually with the outer layer completed with interrupted silk sutures and the inner layer with either interrupted or continuous absorbable suture that incorporates the pancreatic duct. If an end-to-side pancreaticojejunostomy is performed, the outer layer is performed between the pancreatic capsule and parenchyma and the jejunum while the inner layer of absorbable sutures is placed between the pancreatic duct and a small opening in the antimesenteric border of the jejunum. This anastomosis may be stented with a small pediatric feeding catheter that can either be brought out through the jejunum and abdominal wall as an external stent or be left within the bowel lumen to be passed later through the alimentary tract.

The biliary-enteric anastomosis is performed in one layer with absorbable suture approximately 10 cm distal to the pancreaticojejunostomy. Stenting the anastomosis with either the preoperatively placed transhepatic biliary catheter or with an operatively placed T tube usually is used to decompress the jejunal limb during the postoperative period. Approximately 15 cm distal to the biliary-enteric anastomosis, an end-to-side duodenojejunostomy or gastrojejunostomy is performed. It is very important that closed-suction Silastic drains be placed adjacent to the pancreaticojejunostomy and hepaticojejunostomy.

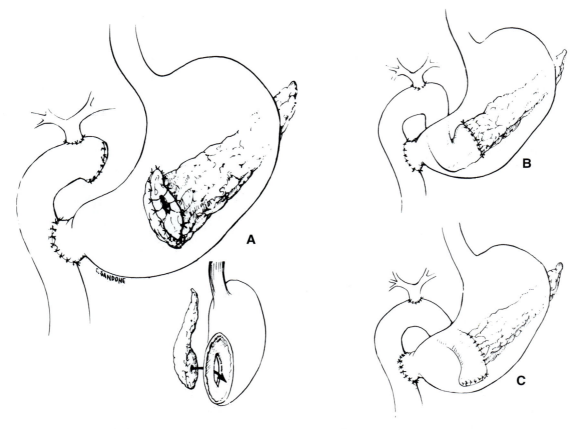

Figure 74–11. Schematic illustration of A: pancreaticogastrostomy; B: end-to-end pancreaticojejunostomy; and C: end-to-side pancreaticojejunostomy. Insert: detailed pancreaticogastrostomy, indicating the location of the posterior gastrostomy. (From Yeo CJ, Cameron JL, Maher MM, et al. A prospective randomized trial of pancreaticogastrostomy versus pancreaticojejunostomy after pancreaticoduodenectomy. *Ann Surg* 1995;222:580

The postoperative management following pancreaticoduodenectomy consists of nothing by mouth, short-term nasogastric and biliary decompression, parenteral analgesia, and a short course of perioperative prophylactic antibiotics. On the fourth or fifth postoperative day, a cholangiogram via the transhepatic biliary catheter or T tube and an upper gastrointestinal series with water soluble contrast material is performed. If no anastomotic leak is demonstrated and gastric emptying is satisfactory, the biliary stent can be internalized and a liquid diet can be instituted. The diet should be advanced slowly, watching for evidence of delayed gastric emptying or increased output from the perianastomotic drains. These drains are removed when the patient is tolerating a regular diet with no evidence of an anastomotic leak.

EXTENT OF RESECTION

The classic pancreaticoduodenectomy performed for decades included a distal gastrectomy. In 1978, Traverso and Longmire described the pylorus-preserving modification of the Whipple procedure.[26] Preserving antral and pyloric function, the pylorus-preserving Whipple procedure reduces the incidence of troublesome postgastrectomy symptoms; a number of studies have documented that gastrointestinal function is better preserved in the pylorus-sparing modification than in the traditional operation.[27,28] Another advantage of the pylorus preservation is the marked decrease in the incidence of marginal ulceration which is only about 5% with the pylorus-preserving procedure versus up to 20% following the classic Whipple resection. In addition, compared to the classic Whipple operation, the pylorus-preserving procedure is less time-consuming and technically easier to perform. Concerns exist in the use of the pylorous-preserving Whipple procedure for the management of periampullary tumors because of the possibility of compromising the already small surgical margins of resection. This question has been addressed by a number of authors, and there appears to be no difference in survival among those treated with the pylorus-sparing Whipple procedure and those managed by the traditional Whipple resection.[29,30]

The extension of the Whipple procedure for pancreatic carcinoma to include a total pancreatectomy with removal of the spleen and more extensive regional lymph nodes has been advocated by some. The overall poor long-term survival for pancreatic cancer following the standard Whipple operation was the impetus for the concept of extending resection to a total pancreatectomy. Advocates cite eliminating multicentric disease as well as eradicating the spread of the disease to the distal pancreas by either direct extension, intraductal seeding, or lymphatic permeation. In addition, it is felt that the operation is a better cancer operation, including a wider en bloc resection of the pancreas as well as regional lymph nodes. Another advantage is the elimination of the pancreaticojejunal anastomosis, which is a major cause of morbidity and mortality following the Whipple operation. Despite these rational arguments, there has been no evidence that a total pancreatectomy offers any survival advantage for those patients with carcinoma of the head of the pancreas undergoing the procedure. Furthermore, there is no reduction in morbidity and mortality for those patients managed by a total pancreatectomy.[31-33] The major disadvantage of the total pancreatectomy is the inevitable total loss of pancreatic endocrine function, often with resultant brittle diabetes. Therefore, total pancreatectomy should be reserved for those patients with histologic evidence of tumor at the margin resection or those with gross multicentric disease.

The concept of an even wider radical resection, or superradical pancreatectomy also has been advocated. These procedures include an extensive regional lymph node and soft tissue resection and may include resection of the portal vein with reanastomosis or graft placement. Reports from Japanese centers have suggested a potential improvement in long-term survival[34-38] (Table 74-1). However, these results have been uncontrolled

TABLE 74-1. LONG-TERM SURVIVAL AFTER PANCREATICODUODENECTOMY FOR ADENOCARCINOMA OF THE PANCREAS

Author	Year	Number of Patients	5 Year Survival (%)
STANDARD RESECTION			
Grace[42]	1986	13	25
Braasch[40]	1986	14	17
Trede[43]	1990	133	24
Cameron[41]	1991	81	21
Yeo[44]	1995	201	21
EXTENDED RESECTION			
Ishikawa[34]	1988	59	9
Tashiro[38]	1991	17	6
Nagakawa[36]	1991	61	26
Satake[37]	1992	57	28

TABLE 74-2. RECENT OPERATIVE EXPERIENCES WITH PANCREATICODUODENECTOMY

Author	Year	Number of Patients	Operative Mortality (%)
STANDARD RESECTION			
Grace[42]	1986	45	2.2
Braasch[40]	1986	87	2.2
Trede[43]	1990	118	0
Cameron[41]	1991	80	1.3
Cameron[45]	1993	145	0
Fernadez-del Castillo[46]	1995	142	0
EXTENDED RESECTION			
Ishikawa[34]	1988	59	10
Tashiro[a 38]	1991	19	5
Nagakawa[36]	1991	61	6
Ishikawa[35]	1992	35	6
Satake[37]	1992	57	7

[a]Includes portal vein resection

and do not appear significantly better than recent Western reports.[39-44] Finally, the more extensive procedure and particularly major vascular resection is associated with increased perioperative morbidity and mortality (Table 74-2).

POSTOPERATIVE RESULTS FOLLOWING PANCREATICODUODENECTOMY

During the 1960s and 1970s many centers reported operative mortality following pancreaticoduodenectomy in the 20% to 40% range, with postoperative morbidity rates as high as 40% to 60%. During the last decade, a dramatic decline in operative morbidity and mortality following pancreaticoduodenectomy has been reported at a number of centers, with operative mortality rates in the range of 2% to 3%. Some centers have even reported large series in excess of 100 patients without a perioperative death.[41,43,45] The reasons behind this decline appear to be (1) fewer, more experienced surgeons performing the operation on a more frequent basis, using less time and with less blood loss; (2) improved preoperative and postoperative care; (3) better anesthetic management; and (4) aggressive nutritional support. Although selection bias may have contributed to these improvements, recent data also extend the improved operative mortality rates to patients in excess of 70 years of age (Table 74-3). A poor functional status, however, as measured by the Karnofsky index, can be an independent risk factor for increased perioperative morbidity and mortality. Finally, there does appear to be an increase in operative mortality and morbidity in the extended procedures including extended resection of lymph nodes and soft tissue on the portal vein (Table 74-2).

TABLE 74–3. EFFECT OF AGE ON MORBIDITY AND MORTALITY FOLLOWING PANCREATICODUODENECTOMY

	Age ≤ 69 Years (%) n=108	Age ≥70 Years (%) n=37	P Value
30 day Mortality	0	0	NS
Complications:			
None	52	38	NS
Delayed gastric emptying	32	46	NS
Pancreatic fistula	19	22	NS
Intra-abdominal abscess	10	5	NS
Bile leak	6	3	NS
Blood transfusion (Units)	1.36	1.27	NS
Postoperative length of stay (days)	19.3	18.8	NS

(Modified from Cameron JL, Pitt HA, Yeo CJ, et al. One hundred and forty-five consecutive pancreaticoduodenectomies without mortality. Ann Surg 1993;217:430)

Complication rates following pancreaticoduodenectomy remain high, however, usually in excess of 25% to 35%. Pancreatic fistula remains the most common serious complication following pancreaticoduodenectomy, with its incidence ranging from 5% to 20%. In the past, the development of pancreatic fistula following pancreaticoduodenectomy was associated with mortality rates of 10% to 40%. Although the incidence of pancreatic fistula following pancreaticoduodenectomy remains stable, the overall mortality associated with it has been diminished owing to improved management. Control of the anastomotic leak with careful placement of closed-suction drains in the area of the pancreatic anastomosis is a major step in minimizing the morbidity of a pancreatic leak. Important supportive measures include careful maintenance of fluid and electrolyte balance, parenteral nutrition, and meticulous care of the drainage site to avoid skin excoriation and autodigestion by activated pancreatic enzymes. The use of the somatostatin analog, octreotide, which does not decrease pancreatic secretion, also may be useful in the management of a postoperative pancreatic fistula, although there are no well-controlled studies. Perioperative use of octreotide does not decrease the incidence of fistula formation following pancreaticoduodenectomy.[46,47]

A prospective randomized trial of pancreaticogastrostomy versus pancreaticojejunostomy after pancreaticoduodenectomy has been recently reported from The Johns Hopkins Hospital.[42] In this study, the incidence of postoperative anastomotic leak as well as other complications and overall length of hospital stay were similar for the two procedures. This study did define factors significantly increasing the risk of pancreatic fistulas. Univariate logistic regression analysis identified ampullary or duodenal disease, soft pancreatic texture, longer operative time, greater red blood cell transfusions, and lower volume of patients treated by the surgeon as factors increasing the risk of pancreatic leak. By multivariate analysis, only lower surgical volume and ampullary and duodenal disease in the resected specimen were associated with pancreatic fistulas.

The most frequent complication following pylorus-preserving pancreatic resection is delayed gastric emptying, with an incidence in the 20%–50% range.[48] The cause of this complication is unknown, and in most patients mechanical obstruction should be ruled out by either contrast studies or endoscopic evaluation. Management of delayed gastric emptying includes gastric decompression and maintenance of parenteral or enteral nutrition. In most cases, delayed gastric emptying is temporary and resolves spontaneously after a variable period of time, resulting simply in a delay in hospital discharge. The use of prokinetic agents such as metoclopramide or erythromycin may be useful in the treatment of postoperative delayed gastric emptying. Furthermore, erythromycin, a motilin antagonist and prokinetic agent, has been shown by a recent prospective randomized study to improve gastric emptying, as measured by both liquid and solid radionucleotide studies.[49] These results did not translate into shortened hospital stay, but it is hoped that with improvement in the prokinetic agents, the incidence of this complication may be reduced.

Although a number of factors appear to contribute to the overall improvement in results following pancreaticoduodenectomy, a high volume of procedures concentrated in the hands of experienced surgeons seems to be of primary importance. Almost all recent large series with improved perioperative results following pancreaticoduodenectomy have come from referral centers concentrating on pancreatic and biliary diseases. A recent analysis compared a single high-volume medical center with the remainder of hospitals in the same state.[50] Hospital mortality (13.5% vs 2.2%), mean length of total hospital and intensive care unit stay, and total hospital costs were all significantly lower in the high-volume provider. Another recent report from the Memorial Sloan-Kettering Cancer Center would further support this observation.[51] In this review, perioperative mortality and length of hospital stay following pancreaticoduodenectomy was significantly lower at institutions with high patient volumes. The operative mortality rate in low-volume hospitals approached 19%, not too dissimilar to operative mortalities reported from earlier eras. These observations would support the regionalization of management of pancreatic cancer in such high-volume institutions for both overall results and cost containment.

MANAGEMENT OF ADENOCARCINOMA OF THE BODY AND TAIL OF THE PANCREAS

Approximately 25% to 30% of pancreatic cancers arise in the body and tail of the pancreas. Unfortunately, the role of surgical resection for these patients is much more limited than for that of cancers of the head of the pancreas due largely to the extent of the disease present at the time of symptomatic presentation. Most patients are unable to undergo resection because of major vascular involvement of the superior mesenteric/splenic vein junction with the portal vein or the celiac axis. If the preoperative arteriogram and venous phase studies are normal, and there is no evidence of liver metastases, exploration and attempted resection is appropriate. Since in most cases, there is no indication for surgical palliation, diagnostic laparoscopy may be performed prior to laparotomy. If at laparoscopy or laparotomy, there is no evidence of metastatic disease to the liver or peritoneal implants, the local extent of disease should be determined. The lesser sac is opened and the SMV is identified as it passes under the neck of the pancreas, in a similar fashion as described previously for pancreaticoduodenectomy. If this vessel is normal, the celiac axis should be explored for evidence of tumor involvement. If no evidence of extensive local disease is found, the spleen and distal pancreas are mobilized and an en bloc resection is performed. The resection should be extended as proximally as possible, with the transected pancreas simply oversewn. The tumor bed should be marked with the placement of clips for postoperative radiation therapy. If, as in most cases, the tumor cannot be resected, a biopsy should be obtained, and chemical splanchnicectomy with alcohol should be performed for pain management. In some cases, a gastrojejunostomy may be indicated because of the potential for obstruction of the proximal jejunum or fourth portion of the duodenum by tumor at the ligament of Treitz.

A review of the management of 113 patients with adenocarcinoma at the Johns Hopkins Hospital between 1972 and 1989 was reported in 1992.[52] In that series only 41% underwent surgical exploration with 8% of patients undergoing resection. In the last 6 years of the study, the percentage of patients not undergoing operation increased significantly from 32% to 53%, reflecting better preoperative staging. The percentage of patients resected increased from 5% to 10% over the same time period (not significant). The median survival for all patients was less than 4 months, and 7 months in those patients undergoing pancreatic resection. One 3-year and one 6-year survivor were observed. A series from The Mayo Clinic during the same time period reported similar findings with a 10 month median survival: a 2 year survival rate of 15% and a 5 year survival rate of 8%.[53] It would appear that aggressive preoperative staging should be performed for patients with pancreatic carcinoma of the body and tail of the gland, but that distal pancreatectomy, when indicated, does offer some hope for long-term care.

■ LONG-TERM SURVIVAL FOR PANCREATIC AND PERIAMPULLARY CARCINOMA

Survival following resection for periampullary carcinoma is highly dependent on the site of origin of the tumor (Fig 74–12). Survival following resection of distal bile duct, ampullary, and duodenal carcinoma has always been significantly longer than that for pancreatic carcinoma, with some series reporting a 5 year survival in the range of 30% to 60%.[54–56] Size of the tumor, regional nodal metastasis, neural invasion, and degree of

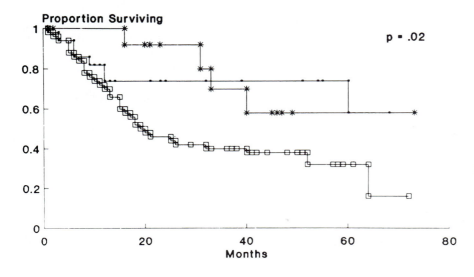

Figure 74–12. Kaplan-Meier survival curves after pancreaticoduodenectomy at the Memorial Sloan-Kettering Cancer Center. All patients had negative nodes. •: ampulla (n=32); □: pancreatic adenocarcinoma (n=88); *: duodenum (n=14). (From Ashley SW, Brennan MF, Reber HA. Surgery for tumors of the pancreas. In: Bluvd KJ, Karakousis CP, Copeland EM (eds), *Atlas of Surgical Oncology.* Philadelphia, PA: WB Saunders; 1995:485)

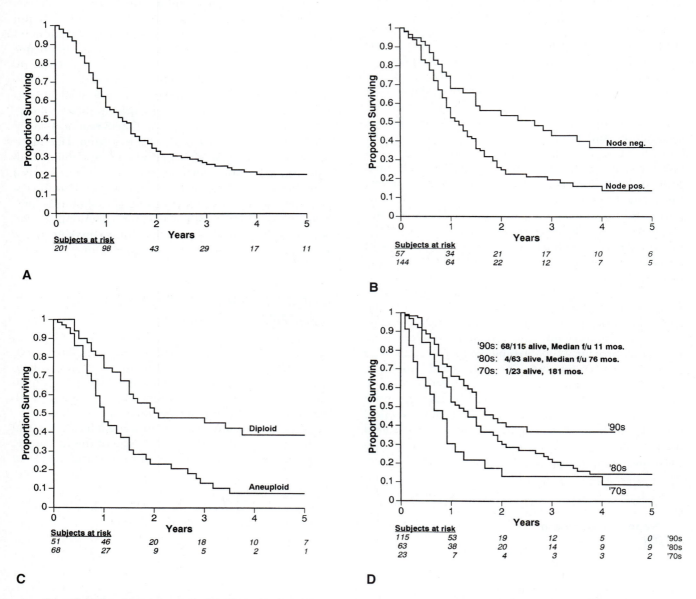

Figure 74–13. Actuarial survival curves for 201 patients with adenocarcinoma of the head of the pancreas undergoing pancreaticoduodenectomy at the Johns Hopkins Hospital from 1970 to 1994. **A.** Actuarial survival for all 201 patients. **B.** Actuarial survival rates for node-negative and node-positive patients. **C.** Actuarial survival rates; as influenced by DNA status, among 119 patients. **D.** Actuarial survival rates by decade.(From Gudjousson B. Cancer of the pancreas: 50 years of surgery. *Cancer* 1987;60:2284)

differentiation appear to influence survival in most series. Although long-term survival following local resection for invasive carcinoma of the ampulla has been observed, in general, pancreaticoduodenectomy remains the procedure of choice for most patients.

Historically, 5 year survival rates for patients with adenocarcinoma in the head of the pancreas managed by pancreaticoduodenectomy have been reported in the range of 5%. However, a number of recent studies have suggested an improved survival for patients following pancreaticoduodenectomy (Table 74–1). In 1987, Crist and colleagues reported a 5 year survival rate of 18% among 50 patients with adenocarcinoma at the head of the pancreas.[57] Moreover, the 5 year survival for 13 patients with negative lymph nodes was 48%. Similar results have been reported by Braasch and associates in 1986,[39] Trede and colleagues in 1990,[42] and Geer and Brennan in 1993.[58] In 1995, Yeo and associates updated the Hopkins' series to 201 patients with adenocarcinoma of the head of the pancreas managed by pancreaticoduodenectomy.[25] The actuarial 1, 3, and 5 year survivals for these patients was 57%, 26%, and 21%, respectively, with a median survival of 15.5 months (Fig 74–13). A number of variables were evaluated by both univariate and multivariate analysis in an attempt to identify factors predictive of long-term survival. Factors significantly favoring long-term survival by univariate analysis included tumor diameter less than 3 cm, negative nodal status, diploid tumor DNA content, tumor S phase fraction less than 18.9%, pylorus-preserving resection, less than 800 mL intraoperative blood loss, less than two units blood transfused, negative resection margins, and the use of postoperative adjuvant chemotherapy and radiation therapy. Multivariate analysis indicated the strongest predictors of long-term survival were diploid tumor content, tumor diameter less than 3 cm, negative nodal status, and negative resection margins. Finally, the decade of resection was a strong predictor of survival with patients undergoing resection in the decade of the 90s faring better than previous decades.

The data from this study further support the importance of image cytometric DNA measurements as a prognostic factor in pancreatic carcinoma. In this series, patients undergoing pancreatic resection with diploid tumors had a median survival of 24 months and an actuarial 5 year survival of 39%, significantly better ($P = .002$) than the 11.5 month survival seen with aneuploid tumors. DNA tumor content was the most powerful prognostic factor favoring long-term survival in that multivariate analysis.

■ ADJUVANT THERAPY

At present, the general consensus of most surgeons treating pancreatic and periampullary carcinoma is that any future improvement in the management of this disease will involve improved adjuvant therapy. The role of adjuvant radiation therapy is emphasized by the pattern of relapse after surgical resection, since over half of the patients resected develop local regional recurrence without evidence of distant metastases.

In 1985, the Gastrointestinal Tumor Study Group reported encouraging results from a prospective randomized trial to evaluate the efficacy of adjuvant radiation and chemotherapy following curative resection for adenocarcinoma at the head of the pancreas.[59] Forty-three patients were allocated randomly to either adjuvant therapy with radiation and 5-fluorouracil or no adjuvant therapy. Median survival for the 21 patients who received adjuvant therapy was 20 months and three (14%) survived 5 years or longer. Among the 22 patients who received no adjuvant therapy, median survival was 11 months, and only one patient (4.5%) survived 5 years. These results have been subsequently confirmed and provide strong support for the concept of postoperative combined adjuvant therapy.[60] Although no prospective trials had yet been completed for other periampullary carcinomas, most groups favor a similar adjuvant regiment for all but the most favorable of these tumors as well.

Presently, a number of clinical trials are underway, including preoperative chemoradiation protocols. Preliminary results suggest that neo-adjuvant therapy can be completed without increasing subsequent morbidity and mortality of surgical resection.[61] However, limited available follow-up suggests that although improvement in local control of the disease is obtained, long-term survival rates owing to distant failure is not improved from historical controls.[62,63] Studies of intraoperative radiation therapy added to external beam irradiation have been reported and although suggesting the possibility of enhanced local control, long-term survival has not been improved.

■ PALLIATION OF PANCREATIC AND PERIAMPULLARY CARCINOMA

Unfortunately, only a minority of patients with carcinoma of the pancreas are suitable for resection and the possibility of cure by the time diagnosis is made. Thus, the optimal palliation of symptoms to maximize the quality of life is of primary importance in many patients. Obstructive jaundice is the most common symptom of periampullary cancer. In recent years, nonoperative palliation has become available as an option for managing these patients. Four prospective randomized studies have been completed in which surgical biliary bypass has been compared with nonoperative biliary stenting for malignant obstructive jaundice (Table 74–4). The conclusions of these studies are similar, demonstrating that both techniques are equally effective in relief of

TABLE 74–4. RESULTS OF PROSPECTIVE RANDOMIZED TRIALS OF NONOPERATIVE VERSUS SURGICAL PALLIATION FOR MALIGNANT BILIARY OBSTRUCTION

	Bornman[78] 1986		Shepard[79] 1988		Anderson[80] 1989		Smith[81] 1994	
	Stent	Surgery	Stent	Surgery	Stent	Surgery	Stent	Surgery
N	25	25	23	25	25	25[a]	100	101
% Success	84	76	82	92	96	88	95	94
Major complications (%)	28	32	30	56	36	20	11	29[b]
30 day mortality (%)	8	20	9	20	20	24	8	15
Hospital stay (days)	18	24[c]	5	13[d]	26	27	19	26
Late complications								
Jaundice/cholangitis (%)	38	16	30[e]	0	0	0	36	2
Gastric outlet obstruction (%)	14	0	9	4	0	0	10	5
Survival (weeks)	19	15	22	18	12	14	21	26

[a]Six patients randomized to surgical arm did not undergo surgical palliation. In one patient extensive tumor precluded palliative bypass. Five other patients underwent endoscopic stent placement. Data presented based on randomization.
[b]$P < .05$
[c]Median post-procedural hospital stay was significantly shorter in stented patients; however, when readmissions for late complications were considered, there was no longer a significant difference.
[d]Both initial and total hospital days were less in the stented group.
[e]13% required two admissions for late biliary complications.

TABLE 74–5. POSTOPERATIVE COMPLICATIONS IN 118 PATIENTS UNDERGOING SURGICAL PALLIATION

Complication	Number	%
Wound infection	12	10
Cholangitis	10	8
Delayed gastric emptying	9	8
Biliary anastomotic leak	4	4[a]
Cardiovascular	4	3
Respiratory	4	3
Genitourinary	4	3
Miscellaneous	5	4

[a]Represents percentage of patients undergoing biliary anastomosis
(*Modified from Lillemoe KD, Sauter P, Pitt HA, et al. Current status of surgical palliation of periampullary carcinoma. Surg Gynecol Obstet 1993;176:1*)

TABLE 74–6. COMPARATIVE RESULTS BETWEEN PERCUTANEOUS AND ENDOSCOPIC STENT PLACEMENT AND SURGICAL BYPASS IN PATIENTS WITH MALIGNANT OBSTRUCTION OF THE COMMON BILE DUCT

	Percutaneous stent (n=490)		Endoscopic stent (n=689)		Surgical bypass (n=1807)	
	Range	Mean	Range	Mean	Range	Mean
30 day mortality (%)	6–33	9	0–20	14	0–31	12
Hospital stay (days)	13–18	14	3–26	7	9–30	17
Success rate (%)	76–100	92	82–100	90	75–100	93
Early complications (%)	4–67	16	8–34	21	6–56	31
Late complications (%)	7–38	28	13–45	28	5–47	16

(*Modified from Watanapa P, Williamson RCN. Surgical palliation for pancreatic cancer: developments during the past two decades. Br J Surg 1991;79:8*)

jaundice. Nonoperative palliation, however, appears to be associated with lower complication rates, lower procedure-related mortality rates, and shorter initial periods of hospitalization. There appears to be no advantage with respect to long-term survival.

Advocates of surgical palliation, however, criticize these studies on two counts. First, the 30 day mortality rates in the surgical arms of these studies range from 15% to 24%, which is much higher than many recent surgical series. A recent series of patients undergoing surgical palliation of periampullary carcinoma at Johns Hopkins reported a hospital mortality of 2.5% and overall postoperative complication rate of 37%, with nearly all complications being non-life-threatening (Table 74–5).[64] Similar results also have been reported by other institutions with hospital mortality rates between 2% and 4%.[65–67] The second reason to favor surgical palliation is that nonoperative palliation is frequently associated with late complications of gastric outlet obstruction and recurrent jaundice, resulting in the need for rehospitalization (Table 74–6).

Recently, larger diameter expandable metallic stents have been developed with encouraging results (Fig 74–14). Prospective studies show that these stents can be placed in patients with distal bile duct obstruction owing to periampullary carcinoma, with an incidence of acute complication similar to that for plastic endoprosthesis.[68–70] Long-term results favor the metallic stents with a decreased late occlusion rate, prolonged stent pa-

tency, and a decrease in endoscopic interventions. Finally, preliminary results from case reports and small series describe the use of larger diameter biliary-type metallic stents for the treatment of duodenal obstruction. Further experience with these techniques will be necessary before their role can be completely defined.

Surgical palliation offers the only chance for long-term palliation of all three major symptoms of pancreatic carcinoma: obstructive jaundice, duodenal obstruction and pain. Biliary bypass can be performed as either a cholecystojejunostomy or choledochohepaticojejunostomy. Both a randomized prospective study and a collective review favor the use of the bile duct for better long-term results without associated increased perioperative morbidity or mortality.[71,72] In the experience at Hopkins, recurrent jaundice developed in only 2% of patients prior to death.

The ability to perform a gastrojejunostomy to treat or prevent gastric outlet obstruction is currently the only palliative procedure that cannot be performed nonoperatively. In a review of more than 8000 patients reported in the English literature from 1965 to 1980, it was reported that the creation of a gastrojejunostomy did not increase the operative mortality rate.[73] Moreover, if a gastrojejunostomy was not performed, 13% of patients had subsequent duodenal obstruction requiring a gastrojejunostomy before death, and nearly one in five of the remaining patients died with symptoms of duodenal obstruction. In a review of more than 950 patients in the

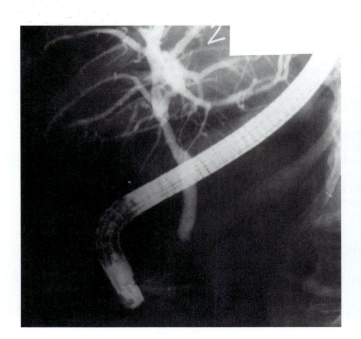

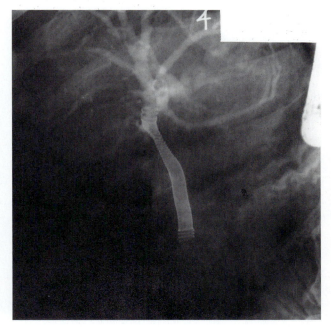

A   **B**

Figure 74–14. A. ERCP showing distal bile duct obstruction owing to pancreatic cancer. **B.** ERCP showing a metallic expandable stent in place.

more recent literature, the percentage requiring a gastrojejunostomy at a later date was 21%.[67] Finally, in an analysis of more than 1600 reported cases, 17% of patients who underwent biliary bypass alone developed duodenal obstruction at a mean of 8.6 months after operation and required subsequent gastric bypass.[70] In none of these reviews did performance of a gastrojejunostomy at the original operation increase the operative mortality. However, in patients requiring a second operation, mortality rates are higher, approaching 25%.

The ability of a gastrojejunostomy to adequately palliate duodenal obstruction has been questioned. In one study, 25 of 36 patients with radiographic evidence of duodenal obstruction died in the hospital after gastrojejunostomy.[74] Furthermore, nine of the eleven survivors experienced a mean interval of 56 days between gastrojejunostomy and resumption of eating. These results are not typical, however, of most other series. In the Hopkins experience, using a retrocolic gastrojejunostomy in 79% of patients, a strong trend toward both a decreased incidence of delayed postoperative gastric emptying and late gastric outlet obstruction was observed when compared to the standard antecolic technique. The incidence of late gastric outlet obstruction prior to death in patients undergoing a gastrojejunostomy was only 4%, with two of those patients manifesting symptoms only in the terminal state.

The final major advantage of operative palliation is in the management of pain. A recent prospective randomized study has demonstrated that intraoperative celiac axis injection with 50% alcohol can both successfully relieve pain in patients, and prevent the development of pain in patients without pain at the time of exploration.[8] (Fig 74–15) The performance of a celiac axis injection was not associated with significant morbidity, mortality, or a prolongation of hospital stay. Standard pain assessment completed until death showed a significant reduction in both pain scores and narcotic use. In addition, a surprising benefit revealed by the study was a prolonged survival in those patients undergoing chemical splanchnicectomy who had significant preoperative pain (Fig 74–16).

The management of pain in patients dying of carcinoma of the pancreas is one of the most important aspects of their care. The appropriate use of oral agents can be successful in most patients. Patients with significant pain should receive their medication on a regular schedule and not on an as-needed basis. The use of long-acting morphine derivative compounds appears to be best suited for such treatment. The use of percutaneous neurolytic block of the celiac axis, either using fluoroscopic or CT guidance, is also successful, in the vast majority of patients, at eliminating pain.[75] In those rare patients in whom percutaneous techniques are not possible, thoracoscopic splanchnicectomy has been shown to effectively relieve pain.[76] Finally, although not well demonstrated by objective measures, it appears that external beam radiation therapy has a beneficial effect on pancreatic cancer pain.

The decision to perform nonoperative versus surgi-

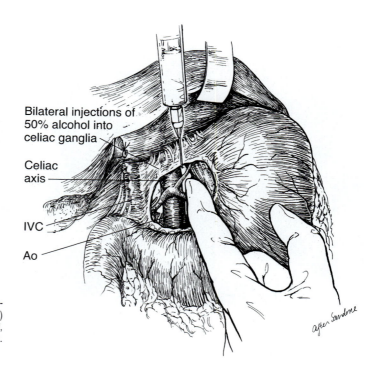

Figure 74–15. Chemical splanchnicectomy is performed using a syringe and a 22-gauge spinal needle. Twenty cc of 50% alcohol is injected on each side of the aorta (Ao) at the level of the celiac axis (IVC: inferior vena cava). (Redrawn from Lillimoe KD, Sauter P, Pitt HA, et al. Current status of surgical palliation of periampullary carcinoma. *Surg Gynecol Obstet* 1993;176:1)

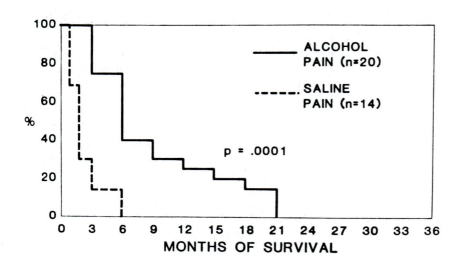

Figure 74–16. Kaplan-Meier survival curves determined from the time of hospital discharge in patients with significant preoperative pain. Alcohol represents patient receiving alcohol chemical splanchnicectomy compared to saline controls. (From Lillimoe KD, Sauter P, Pitt HA, et al. Current status of surgical palliation of periampullary carcinoma. *Surg Gynecol Obstet* 1993;176:1)

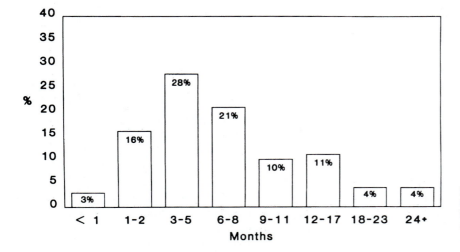

Figure 74–17. Distribution of survival for 118 patients with unresectable periampullary carcinoma undergoing surgical palliation. (From Lillimoe KD, Sauter P, Pitt HA, et al. Current status of surgical palliation of periampullarycarcinoma. *Surg Gynecol Obstet* 1993;176:1)

cal palliation for periampullary cancer is influenced by a number of factors, including the patient's symptoms, overall health status, predicted procedure-related morbidity and mortality, and projected survival. Finally, an aggressive surgical approach will allow occasional resection for potential cure in patients who might otherwise be considered to have a low probability of resection. It would appear that, currently, surgical palliation can be completed with acceptable perioperative morbidity and mortality. Those complications that do occur are seldom life-threatening and, importantly, the mean hospital stay is usually in the range of 7 to 10 days. The avoidance of late complications of recurrent jaundice, duodenal obstruction, and disabling pain would support the argument in favor of surgical palliation in those patients expected to survive 6 months or more. In the series from Johns Hopkins, the mean survival of 118 patients undergoing surgical palliation was 7.7 months (Fig 74–17) with less than one in five patients requiring readmission to the hospital.[8] A recent analysis would suggest that criteria such as advanced age, male sex, liver metastases and large tumor diameters are unfavorable prognostic factors which would favor a nonsurgical approach.[77]

■ RADIATION AND CHEMOTHERAPY FOR UNRESECTABLE PANCREATIC AND PERIAMPULLARY CARCINOMA

The goals of treatment of unresectable pancreatic and periampullary carcinoma include palliation of symptoms and prolongation of life (albeit usually only by months). Although much clinical investigation has been undertaken, the standard treatment for locally advanced, unresectable pancreatic cancer remains external beam radiation therapy in combination with 5-fluorouracil as a radiosensitizer. Although refinements in drug delivery and radiation techniques and higher doses have evolved, no other technique has yet proven superior.

A major area of investigation currently centers on intraoperative irradiation and interstitial implantation of radioactive seeds, followed by high-dose photon beam irradiation. The use of interstitial implants primarily with ^{125}I has been advocated, but results have been disappointing and morbidity and mortality have been considerable.[78] Intraoperative radiation therapy has several advantages, including treatment of larger tumors, more uniform dose delivery of radiation to a broader field, and less trauma to the pancreas and surrounding tissues. The experience with this technique at the Massachusetts General Hospital has demonstrated a median survival of 13 months with excellent local control and excellent pain management.[79] Irradiation to the duo-

denum can result in late gastrointestinal ulceration with bleeding, obstruction, and perforation in over 30% of patients; therefore, a protective gastrojejunostomy should be added.

The status of chemotherapy for unresectable pancreatic cancer has been difficult to assess due to the problem of assessing objective response rates. A number of clinical investigations have been undertaken with modest increments in response rates observed with the combination of multiple agents. However, at this time no regimen has been demonstrated to be beneficial based on a large, randomized trial. Therefore, at present, most patients wishing to receive chemotherapy for unresectable pancreatic carcinoma should do so within the framework of a controlled trial. Finally, based on epidemiologic and experimental data, several investigators have employed endocrine therapy with both antiestrogens and anti-androgens, although, currently, clinical trials have not demonstrated significantly improved survival.

■ CONCLUSION

Periampullary and pancreatic carcinoma represent a significant clinical problem. Although traditionally pancreatic cancer has been associated with a dismal prognosis, recent advances in diagnosis and management, both surgical and nonsurgical, have led to overall improvement in the management of these conditions. Aggressive evaluation with appropriate staging should be performed on all patients. Surgical management with either resection for cure by a pancreaticoduodenectomy or operative palliation should be performed by surgeons experienced in the management of this disease to minimize morbidity and mortality. Following resection, postoperative adjuvant radiation and chemotherapy should be offered to most patients for improved long-term survival.

REFERENCES

1. Whipple AO, Parsons WB, Mullins CR. Treatment of carcinoma of the ampulla of Vater. *Ann Surg* 1935;102:763
2. Boring CC, Squires TS, Tong J, et al. Cancer statistics in 1994. *CA Cancer J Clin* 1994;44:7
3. Webb TH, Lillemoe KD, Pitt HA, Jones RJ, Cameron JC. Pancreatic lymphoma: is surgery mandatory for diagnosis or treatment? *Ann Surg* 1989;209:25
4. Gold EB. Epidemiology of and risk factors for pancreatic cancer. *Surg Clin North Am* 1995;75:819
5. Gordis L. Consumption of methylxanthine-containing beverages and risk of pancreatic cancer. *Cancer Lett* 1990; 52:1

6. Gold EB, Cameron JL. Chronic pancreatitis and pancreatic cancer. *N Engl J Med* 1993;328:1485

7. Hahn SA, Kern SE. Molecular genetics of exocrine pancreatic neoplasms. *Surg Clin North Am* 1995;75:857

8. Lillemoe KD, Sauter P, Pitt HA, et al. Current status of surgical palliation of periampullary carcinoma. *Surg Gynecol Obstet* 1993;176:1

9. Rosa JA, Van Linda BM, Abourizk NN. New-onset diabetes mellitus as harbinger of pancreatic carcinoma. *J Clin Gastroenterol* 1989;11:211

10. Steinberg W. The clinical utiliity of the CA 19-9 tumor-associated antigen. *Am J Gastroenterol* 1990;85:350

11. Friess H, Buchler M, Averbach B, et al. CA 494—a new tumor marker for the diagnosis of pancreatic cancer. *Int J Cancer* 1993;53:759

12. Lillemoe KD. Current management of pancreatic carcinoma. *Ann Surg* 1995;221:133

13. Pitt HA, Gomes AS, Lois JF, et al. Does preoperative percutaneous biliary drainage reduce operative risk or increase hospital cost? *Ann Surg* 1985;201:545

14. Lygidakis NJ, Van Der Heyde MN, Lubler MJ. An evaluation of preoperative biliary drainage in the surgical management of pancreatic head carcinoma. *Acta Chirurgica Scandinavia* 1987;153:665

15. Dooley WC, Cameron JL, Pitt HA, et al. Is preoperative angiography useful in patients with periampullary tumors? *Ann Surg* 1990;211:649

16. Rosch T, Braig C, Gain T, et al. Staging of pancreatic and ampullary carcinoma by endoscopic ultrasonography: comparison with conventional sonography, computed tomography, and angiography. *Gastroenterology* 1992;102:188

17. Warshaw AL, Tepper JE, Shipley WU. Laparoscopy in the staging and planning for pancreatic cancer. *Am J Surg* 1986;151:76

18. Warshaw AL, Gu ZY, Wittenberg J, Waltman AC. Preoperative staging and assessment of resectability of pancreatic cancer. *Arch Surg* 1990;125:230

19. Crile G Jr. The advantages of bypass operations over radical pancreaticoduodenectomy in the treatment of pancreatic carcinoma. *Surg Gynecol Obstet* 1970;130:1049

20. Shapiro TM. Adenocarcinoma of the pancreas: a statistical analysis of bypass vs Whipple resection in good risk patients. *Ann Surg* 1975;182:715

21. Gudjousson B. Cancer of the pancreas: 50 years of surgery. *Cancer* 1987;60:2284

22. Crist DW, Cameron JL. The current status of the Whipple operation for periampullary carcinoma. *Adv Surg* 1992;25:21

23. Cameron JL. Rapid exposure of the portal and superior mesenteric veins. *Surg Gynecol Obstet* 1993;176:395

24. Roder JD, Stein JH, Siewert JR. Carcinoma of the periampullary region: who benefits from portal vein resection? *Am J Surg* 1996;171

25. Yeo CJ, Cameron JL, Lillemoe KD, et al. Pancreaticoduodenectomy for cancer of the head of the pancreas: 201 patients. *Ann Surg* 1995;221:721

26. Traverso LW, Longmire WP Jr. Preservation of the pylorus in pancreaticoduodenectomy. *Surg Gynecol Obstet* 1978;146:959

27. Hunt DR, McLean R. Pylorus-preserving pancreatectomy: functional results. *Br J Surg* 1989;76:173

28. Kozuschek W, Reeth HB, Waleczek H, et al. A comparison of long-term results of the standard Whipple procedure and the pylorus-preserving pancreaticoduodenectomy. *J Am Cancer Soc* 1994;178:443

29. Grace PA, Pitt HA, Longmire WP. Pancreatoduodenectomy with pylorus preservation for adenocarcinoma of the head of the pancreas. *Br J Surg* 1986;73:647

30. Tsao JI, Rossi RL, Lowell JA. Pylorus-preserving pancreatoduodenectomy: is it an adequate cancer operation? *Arch Surg* 1994;129:405

31. Kummerle F, Ruckert K. Surgical treatment of pancreatic cancer. *World J Surg* 1984;8:889

32. Andren-Sandberg A, Ihse I. Factors influencing survival after total pancreatectomy in patients with pancreatic cancer. *Ann Surg* 1983;198:605

33. Sarr MG, Behrns KE, van Heerden JA. Total pancreatectomy: an objective analysis of its use in pancreatic cancer. *Hepatogastroenterology* 1993;40:418

34. Ishikawa O, Ohigashi H, Sasaki Y, et al. Practical usefulness of lymphatic and connective tissue clearance for the carcinoma of the pancreas head. *Ann Surg* 1988;208:215

35. Ishikawa O, Ohigashi H, Imaoka S, et al. Preoperative indications for extended pancreatectomy for locally advanced pancreas cancer involving the portal vein. *Ann Surg* 1992;215:231

36. Nagakawa T, Konishi I, Ueno K, et al. Surgical treatment of pancreatic cancer: the Japanese experience. *Int J Pancreatol* 1991;9:135

37. Satake K, Nishiwak AL, Yokomatsu H, et al. Surgical curability and prognosis for standard versus extended resection for T carcinoma of the pancreas. *Surg Gynecol Obstet* 1992;175:259

38. Tashiro S, Uchmo R, Hiraoka T, et al. Surgical indication and significance of portal vein resection in biliary and pancreatic cancer. *Surgery* 1991;109:481

39. Braasch JW, Deziel DJ, Rossi RL, et al. Pyloric and gastric preserving pancreatic resection: experience with 87 patients. *Ann Surg* 1986;204:411

40. Cameron JL, Crist DW, Sitzmann JV, et al. Factors influencing survival following pancreaticoduodenectomy for pancreatic cancer. *Am J Surg* 1991;161:120

41. Grace PA, Pitt HA, Tompkins RK, et al. Decreased morbidity and mortality after pancreaticoduodenectomy. *Am J Surg* 1986;151:141–149

42. Trede M, Schwall G, Saeger H. Survival after pancreaticoduodenectomy: 118 consecutive resections without an operative mortality. *Ann Surg* 1990;211:447

43. Yeo CJ, Cameron JL, Maher MM, et al. A prospective randomized trial of pancreaticogastrostomy versus pancreaticojejunostomy after pancreaticoduodenectomy. *Ann Surg* 1995;222:580

44. Cameron JL, Pitt HA, Yeo CJ, et al. One hundred and forty-five consecutive pancreaticoduodenectomies without mortality. *Ann Surg* 1993;217:430

45. Fernandez-del Castillo C, Rattner DW, Warshaw AL. Standards for pancreatic resection in the 1990s. *Arch Surg* 1995;130:295

46. Buchler M, Friess IL, Klempa I, et al. Role of octreotide in

the prevention of postoperative complications following pancreatic resection. *Am J Surg* 1992;163:125

47. Montorsi M, Zayo M, Mosea F, et al. Efficacy of octreotide in the prevention of pancreatic fistula after elective pancreatic resections: a prospective, controlled, randomized trial. *Surgery* 1995;117:26

48. Warshaw AL, Torchiana DL. Delayed gastric emptying after pylorus-preserving pancreaticoduodenectomy. *Surg Gynecol Obstet* 1985;160:1

49. Yeo CJ, Barry K, Sauter PK, et al. Erythromycin accelerates gastric emptying after pancreaticoduodenectomy: a prospective, randomized placebo-controlled trial. *Ann Surg* 1993;218:229–38

50. Gordon TA, Burkyson GP, Tielsch JM, Cameron JL. The effects of regionalization on cost and outcome for one general high-risk surgical procedure. *Ann Surg* 1995;221:43

51. Lieberman MD, Kilburn H, Lindsey M, Brennan MF. Relation of perioperative deaths to hospital volume among patients undergoing pancreatic resection for malignancy. *Ann Surg* 1995;222:638

52. Nordback IH, Hruban RH, Boitnott JK, et al. Carcinoma of the body and tail of the pancreas. *Am J Surg* 1992;164:26

53. Dalton RR, Sarr MG, van Heerden JA, Colby TV. Carcinoma of the body and tail of the pancreas: is curative resection justified? *Surgery* 1992;111:489

54. Sperti C, Pasquali C, Piccoli A, et al. Radical resection for ampullary carcinoma: long-term results. *Br J Surg* 1994;81:668

55. Allema JH, Reinders ME, vaGulik TM, et al. Results of pancreaticoduodenectomy for ampullary carcinoma and analysis of prognostic factors for survival. *Surgery* 1995;117:247

56. Monson JRT, Donohur JH, McEntee GP, et al. Radical resection for carcinoma of the ampulla of Vater. *Arch Surg* 1991;126:353

57. Crist DW, Sitzmann JV, Cameron JL. Improved hospital morbidity, mortality and survival after the Whipple procedure. *Ann Surg* 1987;206:358

58. Geer RJ, Brennan MF. Prognostic indicators for survival after resection of pancreatic adenocarcinoma. *Am J Surg* 1993;165:68

59. Kalser MH, Ellenberg SS. Pancreatic cancer: adjuvant combined radiation and chemotherapy following curative resection. *Arch Surg* 1985;97:28

60. Gastrointestinal Tumor Study Group. Further evidence of effective adjuvant combined radiation and chemotherapy following curative resection of pancreatic cancer. *Cancer* 1987;59:2006

61. Evans DB, Rich TA, Byrd DR, et al. Preoperative chemoradiation and pancreaticoduodenectomy for adenocarcinoma of the pancreas. *Arch Surg* 1992;127:1335

62. Yeung RS, Weese JL, Hoffman JP, et al. Neoadjuvant chemoradiation in pancreatic and duodenal carcinoma: a phase II study. *Cancer* 1993;72:2124

63. Evans D, Abbruzzese J, Lee J, Cleary K, Rich T. Preoperative chemoradiation and pancreaticoduodenectomy for adenocarcinoma of the pancreas. *Proc Am Soc Clin Onc* 1994;13:226

64. Lillemoe KD, Cameron JL, Kaufman HS, et al. Chemical splanchnicectomy in patients with unresectable pancreatic cancer. *Ann Surg* 1993;217:447

65. Potts JR III, Broughan TA, Hermann RE. Palliative operations for pancreatic carcinoma. *Am J Surg* 1990;159:73

66. deRooij PD, Rogatko A, Brennan MF. Evaluation of palliative surgical procedures in unresectable pancreatic cancer. *Br J Surg* 1991;78:1053

67. Singh SM, Longmire WP Jr, Reber HA. Surgical palliation for pancreatic cancer: the UCLA experience. *Ann Surg* 1990;212:132

68. Davids PHP, Groen AK, Rauws EAJ, et al. Randomized trial of self-expanding metal stents versus polyethylene stents for distal malignant biliary obstruction. *Cancer* 1992;340:1488

69. Knyrim K, Wagner HJ, Starck E, et al. Metall oder Kunstoffendoproshesen bei malignem Verschulssiktersus. Ein randomisierter und prospektiver Vergleich. *Dtsch Med Wochenschr* 1992;11:847

70. Carr-Locke DL, Ball TJ, Connors PJ, et al. Multicenter randomized trial of Wallstent biliary endoprosthesis versus plastic stents. *Gastrointest Endosc* 1993;39:310

71. Sarfeh IJ, Rypins EB, Jakowatz JG, et al. A prospective, randomized clinical investigation of cholecystoenterostomy and choledochoenterostomy. *Am J Surg* 1988;155:41

72. Watanapa P, Williamson RCN. Surgical palliation for pancreatic cancer: developments during the past two decades. *Br J Surg* 1991;79:8

73. Sarr MG, Cameron JL. Surgical management of unresectable carcinoma of the pancreas. *Surgery* 1982;91:123

74. Weaver DW, Wiencek RG, Bouwmann DL, et al. Gastrojejunostomy: is it helpful for patients with pancreatic cancer? *Surgery* 1987;102:608

75. Brown DL, Bulley CK, Quiel EL. Neurolytic celiac plexus block for pancreatic cancer pain. *Anesth Anal* 1987;66:869

76. Worsey J, Ferson PF, Keenan RJ, et al. Thoracoscopic pancreatic enervation for pain control in irresectable pancreatic cancer. *Br J Surg* 1993;80:1051

77. van der Bosch RP, van der Schelling GP, Klinkengill JHG. Guidelines for the application of surgery and endoprostheses in the palliation of obstructive jaundice in advanced cancer of the pancreas. *Ann Surg* 1994;219:18

78. Merrick HW III, Dobelbower RR Jr. Aggressive therapy for cancer of the pancreas: does it help? *Gastroenterol Clin North Am* 1990;19:935

79. Shipley WU, Wood WC, Tepper JE, et al. Intraoperative electron beam irradiation for patients with unresectable pancreatic carcinoma. *Ann Surg* 1984;200:289

75

Operations on the Pancreas

Howard A. Reber

■ PANCREATIC RESECTIONS

PANCREATICODUODENECTOMY (THE WHIPPLE PROCEDURE; THE PYLORUS-PRESERVING WHIPPLE PROCEDURE)

Either a bilateral subcostal or a long midline incision provides adequate exposure. The operation is carried out in the following sequence: (1) mobilization of the duodenum and the head of the pancreas, with identification of the superior mesenteric vein, (2) mobilization of the common bile duct and the portal vein above the pancreas, (3) elevation of the neck of the pancreas from the superior mesenteric and portal veins, (4) division of the stomach or, if the pylorus and stomach are to be preserved, the duodenum, (5) division of the common bile duct and neck of the pancreas, (6) dissection of the divided pancreas from the mesenteric vessels, (7) mobilization/division of the proximal jejunum, (8) division of the mesoduodenum and attachments of the uncinate process to the superior mesenteric artery, and removal of the specimen, and (9) reconstruction of gastrointestinal continuity.

The lateral peritoneal attachments of the duodenum are incised, and the duodenum, head of the pancreas, common bile duct, and portal vein are mobilized by blunt dissection posteriorly (Fig 75–1). Next the gastrocolic omentum is divided to expose the anterior surface of the pancreas; the hepatic flexure of the colon is mobilized and retracted inferiorly (Fig 75–2). The superior mesenteric vein is identified as it courses under the pancreas. A plane is developed between the anterior surface

of the vein and the undersurface of the neck of the pancreas, but the separation of the two is not pursued further at this time (Fig 75–3). Attention is turned to the hepatoduodenal ligament where the distal common bile duct is freed circumferentially and isolated with a small penrose drain (Fig 75–4). The hepatic artery is palpated in the hepatoduodenal ligament, and the vessel is isolated. It is dissected free for a sufficient distance so that the gastroduodenal and right gastric arteries may be identified and divided (Fig 75–5). These vessels are doubly ligated, since postoperative bleeding from this source can be fatal. The anterior aspect of the portal vein is identified at the upper border of the pancreas. A plane is developed for the subsequent separation of the posterior aspect of the neck of the pancreas from the portal vein, a critical step in determining resectability. The points for resection of the gastric antrum are selected on both greater and lesser curves, and the necessary dissection in both the gastrohepatic and gastrocolic omenta is done. The stomach is divided with a stapler, the proximal portion is packed away superiorly, and the distal portion is retracted inferiorly and to the right of the patient (Fig 75–6). Then the common bile duct is divided, and a bulldog clip is placed temporarily to occlude the proximal portion.

Now the neck of the pancreas is separated completely from the superior mesenteric and portal veins behind it. The dissection is performed bluntly using the index finger, a small piece of gauze held in the tip of a clamp, or a Kelly clamp itself (Figs 75–6 and 75–7). It usually should be carried out from the inferior border of the

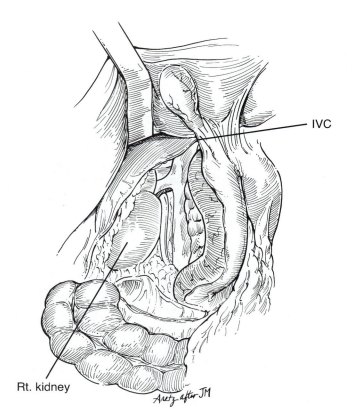

Figure 75–1. Division of the duodenocolic ligament and gastrocolic omentum and continuation of the retroperitoneal dissection. The third part of the duodenum and head of the pancreas are mobilized. (Redrawn from Braasch S, Tompkins N (eds). *Surgical Diseases of the Biliary Tract and Pancreas.* St Louis, MO: Mosby; 1994)

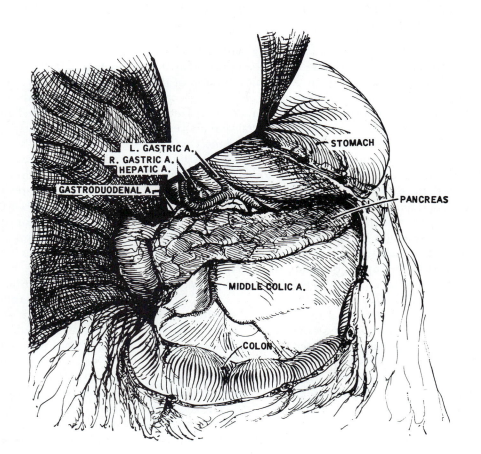

Figure 75–2. Division of the gastrocolic omentum provides exposure of the entire anterior surface of the pancreas. (From Jordan GL Jr. In: Howard JM, Jordan GL Jr, Reber HA (eds), *Surgical Diseases of the Pancreas.* Philadelphia, PA: Lea & Febiger; 1987)

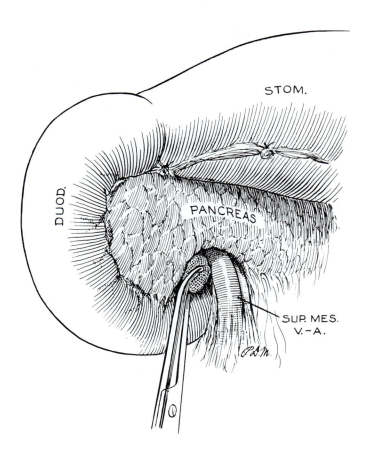

Figure 75–3. The neck of the pancreas is being elevated from the superior mesenteric vein following incision of the overlying peritoneum. A small pledget of gauze held in a right-angle clamp is used for this delicate dissection, which will eventually be carried out completely under the neck of the pancreas.

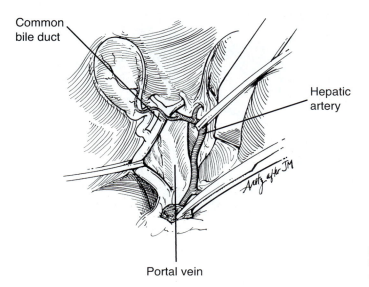

Figure 75–4. Dissection of the hepatic artery, bile duct, and exposure of the anterior surface of the portal vein. (Redrawn from Braasch S, Tompkins N (eds). *Surgical Diseases of the Biliary Tract and Pancreas.* St Louis, MO: Mosby; 1994)

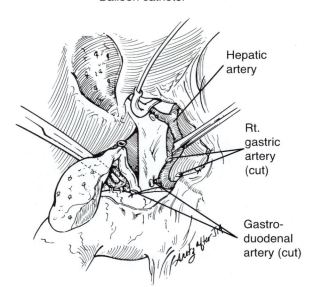

Balloon catheter

Hepatic artery

Rt. gastric artery (cut)

Gastro-duodenal artery (cut)

Figure 75–5. Cholecystectomy and transection of the bile duct. All soft and lymphatic tissues in the hepatoduodenal ligament are swept away from the porta hepatis to the specimen, skeletonizing the portal vein. (Redrawn from Braasch S, Tompkins N (eds). *Surgical Diseases of the Biliary Tract and Pancreas.* St Louis, MO: Mosby; 1994)

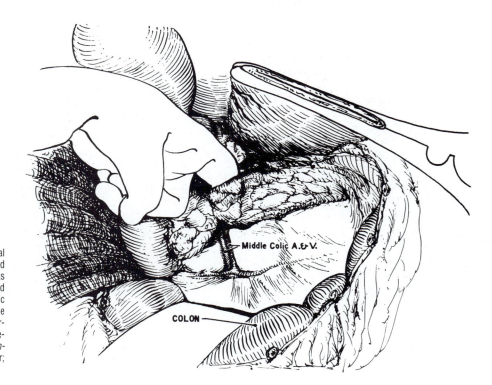

Middle Colic A. & V.

COLON

Figure 75–6. The plane between the portal vein and the pancreas is now fully developed by blunt dissection, freeing the pancreas from the anterior surface of the portal and superior mesenteric veins. The middle colic vein serves as an anatomic landmark at the inferior margin of the pancreas. (From Jordan GL Jr. In: Howard JM, Jordan GL Jr, Reber HA (eds), *Surgical Diseases of the Pancreas.* Philadelphia, PA: Lea & Febiger; 1987)

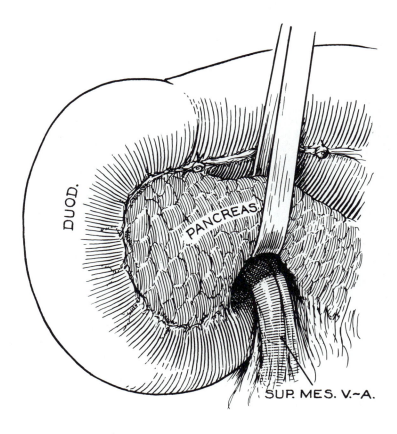

Figure 75–7. The neck of the pancreas has been completely mobilized, and a small Penrose drain has been passed beneath it. The drain is useful for subsequent manipulation of this structure.

pancreas, but when resistance is encountered, it may be useful to alternate the dissection from both the superior and inferior borders. It is unusual to encounter any vessels during this dissection, since most of the tributaries enter the vein from its lateral and posterior aspects. However, some resistance to the dissection is not uncommon when the operation is done for chronic pancreatitis. This is owing to inflammatory adherence of the pancreas to the vein. When the dissection is complete, a penrose drain is passed through the opening that has been created (Fig 75–7). Next, hemostatic transfixion sutures are placed through the pancreatic tissue to occlude the transverse arteries before the pancreas is divided (Fig 75–8). Two are placed in the superior and two in the inferior border of the gland on either side of the proposed line of transection. During this maneuver, the neck of the gland is elevated by slight traction on the penrose drain so that the underlying vessels are protected. The pancreas then is divided either sharply or with electrocautery. Bleeders are controlled with suture ligatures of 4-0 or 5-0 prolene. The pancreatic duct is identified.

Now the separation of the pancreas from the lateral

aspect of the superior mesenteric and portal veins is begun (Fig 75–9). The small vessels that are encountered are friable and tear easily. They should be ligated in continuity (4-0 silk) and then divided. This is safer than the application of clamps, which should be avoided.

When the separation is complete, a moist laparotomy pad is laid over this field. The transverse colon is elevated superiorly and the small bowel is retracted to the right to expose the third and fourth portions of the duodenum and the ligament of Treitz. The peritoneal attachments of these segments of the duodenum as well as the ligament are incised (Figs 75–10 and 75–11). The proximal jejunum is divided with a stapler at a point where the vascular arcades will allow the creation of an adequate length of bowel for the subsequent anastomoses. The fourth portion of the duodenum is dissected from the posterior abdominal wall, and the transected proximal jejunum then is passed under the superior mesenteric vessels and delivered to the area of previous dissection (Fig 75–18). An alternative approach is to transect the proximal jejunum above the transverse mesocolon *after* delivering it under the mesenteric vessels, while still in continuity with the duode-

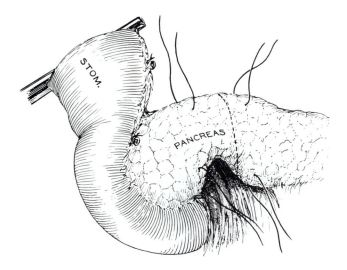

Figure 75–8. The superior and inferior pancreatic longitudinal arteries have been encircled with transfixion sutures of 3-0 silk proximal and distal to the point where the pancreas will be divided.

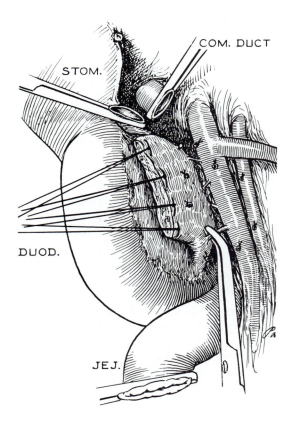

Figure 75–9. Small vessels entering the superior mesenteric and portal veins from the head of the pancreas have been ligated and divided. (It is safer to ligate these vessels in continuity and then to divide them, rather than apply clamps as shown above.) With traction on the divided common duct above and the divided jejunum below, the uncinate process is elevated and separated from the superior mesenteric and portal veins. The uncinate process will be divided between paired right-angle clamps.

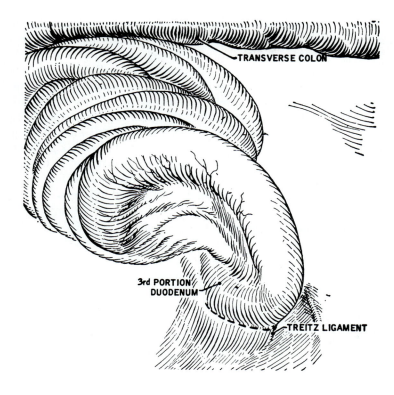

Figure 75–10. The small bowel is retracted superiorly and to the right to expose the third and fourth portions of the duodenum. The ligament of Treitz and the peritoneal reflection of the third portion of the duodenum are divided. (From Jordan GL Jr. In: Howard JM, Jordan GL Jr, Reber HA (eds), *Surgical Diseases of the Pancreas.* Philadelphia, PA: Lea & Febiger; 1987)

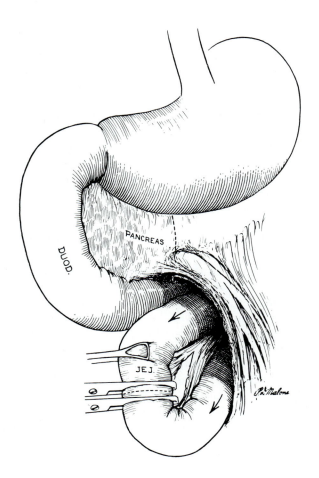

Figure 75–11. The ligament of Treitz has been incised beneath and to the right of the superior mesenteric artery and vein. The ventral and dorsal leaflets of Treitz have been incised superiorly to the uncinate process. The proximal jejunum has been drawn underneath the mesenteric vessels. Two branches of mesenteric vessels supplying the proximal jejunum have been divided and ligated. The jejunum is then also divided.

num. This is usually possible after an extensive Kocher maneuver and the freeing of the ligament of Treitz earlier in the operation. It may be preferable since it can be done during the dissection of the pancreas from the great vessels, and does not require changing retractors and losing exposure.

Now the only remaining attachments are the mesoduodenum and the mesentery of the uncinate process which are usually short, thickened and quite vascular (Fig 75–12). This part of the procedure may be associated with some blood loss until the specimen has been removed. If the tissue is thick, the best approach is to successively divide it between clamps, applying suture ligatures to the tissue that will remain. If the tissue is less thick, and the operation is being done for benign disease, a stapler (eg, TA 55) may be placed across it and the specimen transected leaving the stapled mesentery behind. If this technique is used, the stapler must be applied very carefully to avoid injury to the superior mesenteric artery and vein. Then a continuous hemostatic locking suture of 2-0 or 3-0 Prolene is placed along the entire margin of this area. (When the operation is done for cancer, the entire uncinate process should be removed. When it is done for chronic pancreatitis, it is acceptable to leave some of the uncinate process behind. This may be done if the tissue is particularly adherent to the superior mesenteric vein and the dissection is difficult.) The operative field is copiously irrigated with saline, and a cholecystectomy is performed if it has not been done earlier. Gastrointestinal reconstruction then is begun.

The pancreaticojejunal anastomosis is performed first, in a retrocolic fashion. The jejunum can either be brought through a hole in the transverse mesocolon, or behind the superior mesenteric artery and vein. The author prefers the technique of an end-to-side pancreaticojejunostomy, although an end-to-end anastomosis also works well (Fig 75–13). An end-to-side reconstruction is required if the pancreas remnant is large. The anastomosis is performed in two layers, interrupted 3-0 silk for the outer and continuous 3-0 Maxon for the inner. A pancreatic duct anastomosis is not required, and the incidence of pancreatic fistula formation is <5% with the technique described. Fistula is even less likely when the operation is done for chronic pancreatitis. An alternative technique preferred by some surgeons is an end-to-side pancreaticojejunostomy with a duct anastomosis (Fig 75–14).

The choledochojejunal anastomosis is performed next at a sufficient distance from the pancreas to avoid tension on the suture lines, but not so long to allow kinking of the bowel. I prefer a single layer anastomosis using interrupted sutures of 4-0 Maxon. For the posterior row, the knots are placed within the lumen of the duct. Tension is taken off the suture line by suturing the

small bowel on either side of the anastomosis to the capsule of the liver. If the duct is smaller than 1 cm in diameter, the author usually stents the anastomosis with a small T tube inserted through the wall of the bile duct proximal to the anastomosis. The distal limb is situated in the small bowel. The tube is removed 4 weeks later.

Finally, a retrocolic gastrojejunostomy is constructed approximately 18 inches distal to the choledochojejunostomy, in a standard two-layer fashion (Fig 75–15). Two closed suction drains are placed close to the pancreatic and hepatic duct anastomoses, and after the abdomen is irrigated again, it is closed in layers.

Pylorus-Preserving Whipple Resection

A modification of this operation is the *pancreaticoduodenectomy with preservation of the stomach and pylorus*. If this is done, the gastroduodenal and right gastric arteries are preserved, if possible (Fig 75–16). The duodenum is transected, usually 3 to 4 cm distal to the pylorus, and reanastomosed to the jejunum at the point where a gastrojejunostomy would have been done in the standard operation. The remaining aspects of the procedure are no different. The postoperative recovery may be complicated by delayed gastric emptying in some patients, but this resolves eventually.

PANCREATIC HEAD RESECTION

Beger and his colleagues from Ulm, Germany have described an operation in which the head of the pancreas is resected, and the entire stomach and duodenum are preserved. The body and tail of the pancreas as well as a thin rim of pancreatic tissue in the C loop of the duodenum also remain.

The procedure is begun with mobilization of the duodenum, head of the pancreas, common bile duct, superior mesenteric and portal veins as for a standard pancreaticoduodenectomy. Important steps before the resection is begun include the separation of the neck of the pancreas from the underlying mesenteric and portal vein and the dissection of the common hepatic artery along the superior edge of the pancreas (Fig 75–17). Hemostasis of the cut surfaces of the remaining pancreas must be meticulous, and is accomplished with numerous transfixion sutures of 4-0 or 5-0 Prolene. The subtotal resection of the head is carried out after transection of the neck, as for the standard Whipple procedure. The dissection is carried from the superior mesenteric vein toward the intrapancreatic common bile duct (Fig 75–18). As the uncinate process is resected, the mesoduodenal vessels should be preserved (Fig 75–19). Although the gastroduodenal artery usually is preserved, this is not necessary for adequate duodenal blood flow. The intrapancreatic common bile duct may be protected as the dissection proceeds by inserting a

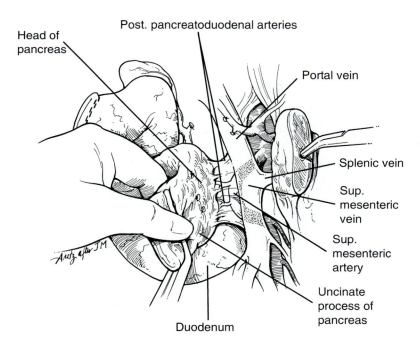

Head of pancreas

Post. pancreatoduodenal arteries

Portal vein

Splenic vein

Sup. mesenteric vein

Sup. mesenteric artery

Uncinate process of pancreas

Duodenum

Figure 75–12. Dissection of the retropancreatic vessels. Surgeon's left hand grasps and retracts pancreatic head to the right. (Redrawn from Braasch S, Tompkins N (eds). *Surgical Diseases of the Biliary Tract and Pancreas.* St Louis, MO: Mosby; 1994)

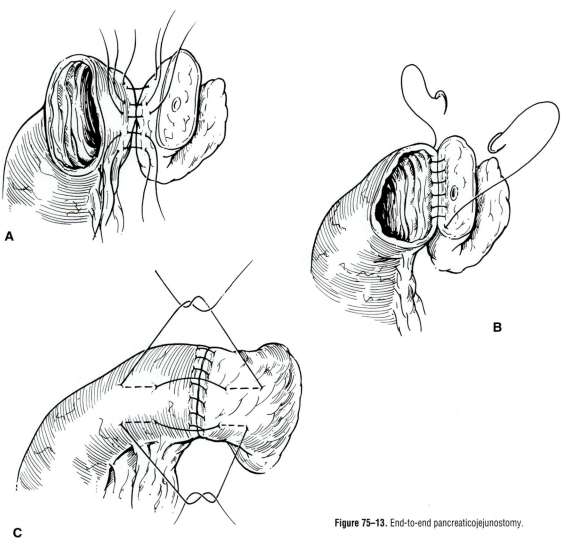

A

B

C

Figure 75–13. End-to-end pancreaticojejunostomy.

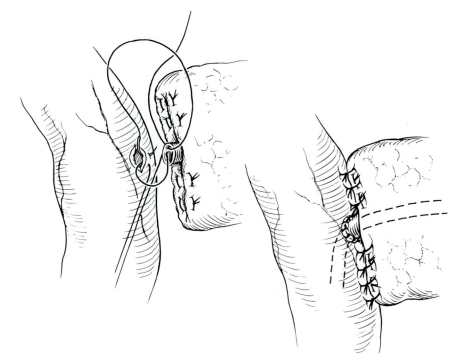

Figure 75–14. Technique of end-to-side pancreaticojejunostomy with mucosa-to-mucosa ductal anastomosis. The transected end of the pancreas is closed except
for the pancreatic duct. A meticulous mucosa-to-mucosa anastomosis is made between the duct and a small
opening in the jejunum. The pancreas is approximated
to the jejunum by an anterior and a posterior row of interrupted sutures of silk. (From Jordan GL Jr. In:
Howard JM, Jordan GL Jr, Reber HA (eds), *Surgical Diseases of the Pancreas.* Philadelphia, PA: Lea & Febiger;
1987)

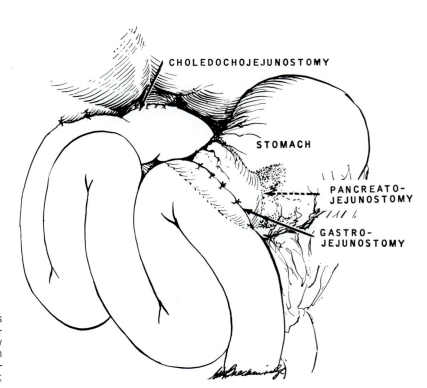

Figure 75–15. An illustration of the complete anastomoses shows
the relative positions of the pancreaticojejunostomy, the choledochojejunostomy, and the gastrojejunostomy. The T-tube that may
be inserted in the bile duct is not shown in this drawing. (From
Jordan GL Jr. In: Howard JM, Jordan GL Jr, Reber HA (eds), *Surgical Diseases of the Pancreas.* Philadelphia, PA: Lea & Febiger;
1987)

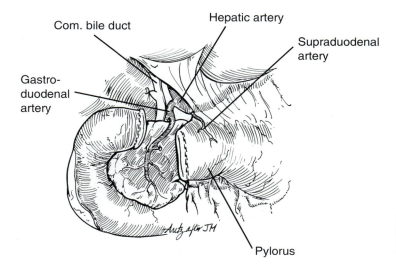

Figure 75–16. Site of section and arterial supply of duodenum in pylorus-preserving pancreatoduodenectomy. (Redrawn from Braasch S, Tompkins N (eds). *Surgical Diseases of the Biliary Tract and Pancreas.* St Louis, MO: Mosby; 1994)

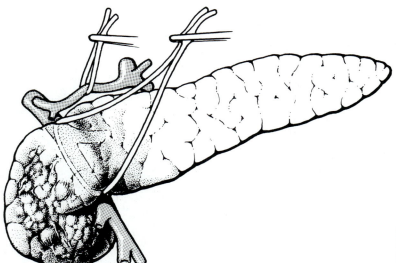

Figure 75–17. The first steps in resection of the head of the pancreas. The hepatic artery has been isolated, and the neck of the pancreas has been elevated from the underlying superior portomesenteric vein. (Courtesy of HG Beger)

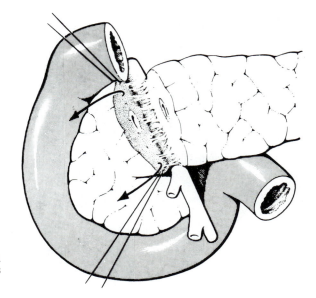

Figure 75–18. The dissection proceeds as the pancreatic neck, now transected, is reflected to the right. The venous tributaries from the pancreas to the vein are carefully ligated and divided, and the vein is freed completely on its anterior and right lateral aspect. (Courtesy of HG Beger)

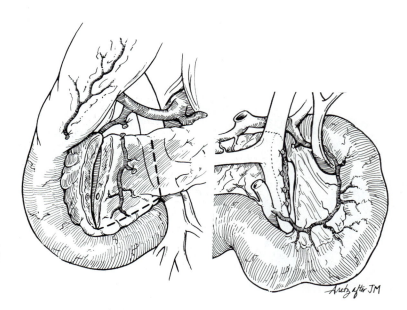

Figure 75–19. Beger duodenal-preserving resection of the head of the pancreas (for chronic pancreatitis). Inset shows posterior pancreatic capsule still intact after resection (dorsal view). (Redrawn from Braasch S, Tompkins N (eds). *Surgical Diseases of the Biliary Tract and Pancreas.* St Louis, MO: Mosby; 1994)

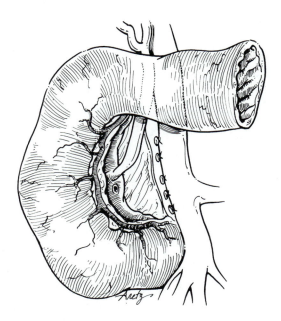

Figure 75–20. The head of the pancreas has been removed. Both the duodenopancreatic vascular arcade and the dorsal pancreatic capsule have been preserved. Anterior view. (Courtesy of HG Beger)

Bakes dilator through a proximal choledochotomy. The metal tip can be felt through the duct wall. When the bile duct has been compressed by the fibrotic pancreas, it often is decompressed by the resection. If not, a choledochojejunostomy(duodenostomy) should be done in addition to the pancreaticojejunostomy. A rim of pancreatic tissue between 5 and 10 mm thick should remain along the duodenal margin, and between the wall of the duodenum and the common bile duct (Fig 75–20). A 3 to 4 mm thick capsule of the pancreas also is preserved posteriorly, anterior to the inferior vena cava. The pancreatic juice is drained by a Roux-en-Y limb of jejunum both to the body of the gland on the left side of the patient and to the cut edge of the pancreas that remains attached to the duodenum. If the pancreatic duct is dilated, a lateral pancreaticojejunostomy is fashioned instead (Fig 75–21).

NINETY-FIVE PERCENT DISTAL PANCREATECTOMY

Ninety-five percent distal pancreatectomy entails the removal of all of the pancreas except for a thin rim of tissue which lies within the C loop of the duodenum and, usually, the spleen.

The operation is begun by dividing the gastrocolic and colosplenic ligaments, retracting the splenic flexure of the colon inferiorly. The duodenum and the head of the pancreas are mobilized, and the peritoneum along the inferior border of the body and tail

of the pancreas is incised. The body and tail then are freed by blunt dissection from the posterior abdominal wall in this avascular retroperitoneal plane (Fig 75–22). The dissection should extend from the superior mesenteric vein to the hilum of the spleen. The splenic artery then should be identified along the superior border of the pancreas near its origin from the celiac axis (Fig 75–23). It should be divided and doubly ligated with vascular suture at that point. The spleen should then be freed from its attachments to the diaphragm, and the gastroepiploic and short gastric vessels should be divided and ligated. The spleen and the attached pancreas then are retracted to the patient's right. On the undersurface of the pancreas, the inferior mesenteric vein can be seen where it enters the splenic vein. This confluence should be preserved if possible, and the splenic vein ligated and divided distal to that point. If the inferior mesenteric vein enters the superior mesenteric vein directly, the

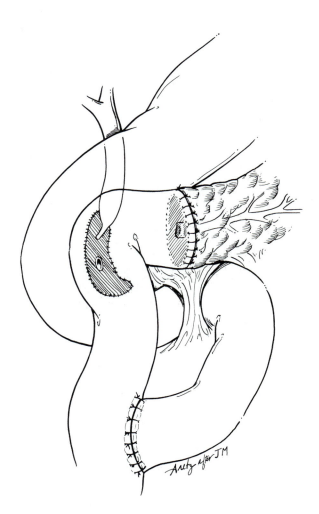

Figure 75–21. Beger duodenal-preserving resection of the head of the pancreas (for chronic pancreatitis). (Redrawn from Braasch S, Tompkins N (eds). *Surgical Diseases of the Biliary Tract and Pancreas.* St Louis, MO: Mosby; 1994)

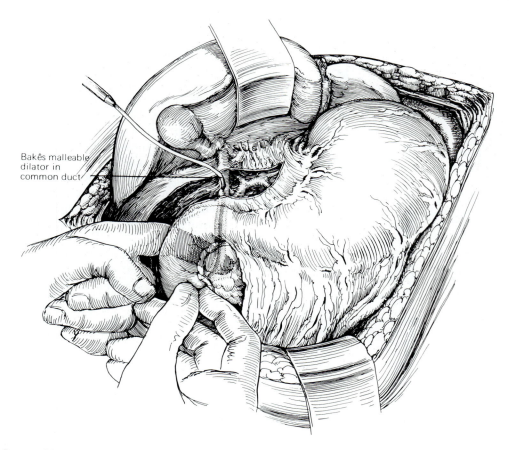

Bakês malleable
dilator in
common duct

Figure 75–22. Exposure of the pancreas. (From Frey CF. In: Malt R (ed), *Surgical Techniques Illustrated, A Comparative Atlas: Surgery for Chronic Pancreatitis.* Philadelphia, PA: WB Saunders; 1985)

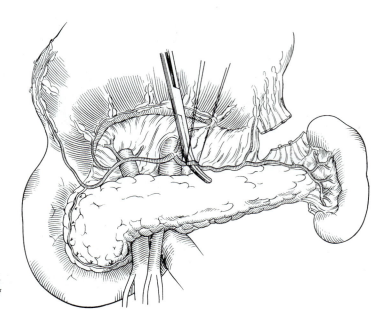

Figure 75–23. Pancreatectomy (I). (From Reber H. Partial subtotal pancreatectomy for chronic pancreatitis. In: Nyhus LM, Baker RJ, Fischer J (eds), *Mastery of Surgery,* Boston, MA: Little Brown; 1996)

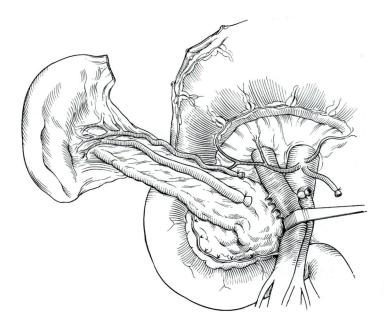

Figure 75–24. Pancreatectomy (II). (From Reber H. Partial subtotal pancreatectomy for chronic pancreatitis. In: Nyhus LM, Baker RJ, Fischer J (eds), *Mastery of Surgery.* Boston, MA: Little Brown; 1996)

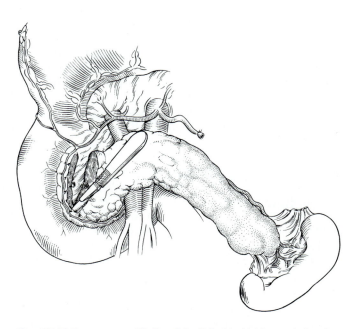

Figure 75–25. Pancreatectomy (III). (From Reber H. Partial subtotal pancreatectomy for chronic pancreatitis. In: Nyhus LM, Baker RJ, Fischer J (eds), *Mastery of Surgery.* Boston, MA: Little Brown; 1996)

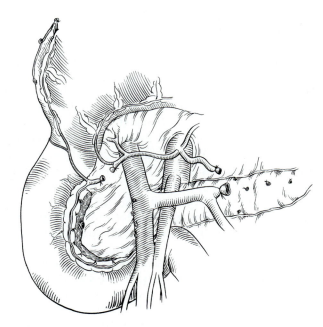

Figure 75–26. Pancreatectomy (IV). (From Reber H. Partial subtotal pancreatectomy for chronic pancreatitis. In: Nyhus LM, Baker RJ, Fischer J (eds), *Mastery of Surgery.* Boston, MA: Little Brown; 1996)

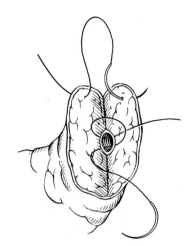
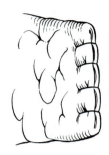

Figure 75–27. Technique for closure of transected pancreas. (From Reber H. Partial subtotal pancreatectomy for chronic pancreatitis. In: Nyhus LM, Baker RJ, Fischer J (eds), *Mastery of Surgery*. Boston, MA: Little Brown; 1996)

splenic vein is ligated and divided at the point where it joins the superior mesenteric vein. In any case, the pancreas is dissected from the superior mesenteric vein, first on its anterior aspect and then on the right lateral aspect. This part of the dissection requires meticulous isolation, ligation, and division of a number of small friable veins. Here the mesentery of the uncinate process, or the uncinate itself, in patients with benign disease, should be ligated in continuity and divided (Fig 75–24).

The dissection of the pancreas then proceeds from left to right in a fashion similar to that described previously for an isolated resection of the pancreatic head. The freed pancreas and spleen are returned temporarily to their normal position. A superficial incision is made into the pancreatic tissue following the curve of the duodenum and about 5 to 10 mm away from it (Fig 75–25). Gradually this incision is deepened, stopping at intervals to suture ligate bleeding vessels with 4-0 or 5-0 Prolene. One hand behind the duodenum and pancreatic head helps to orient the surgeon as the dissection proceeds. The common bile duct should be protected during this part of the operation, and it may be advantageous for identification to insert a metal dilator into it through a proximal choledochotomy.

The specimen then can be removed. The cuff of remaining pancreatic tissue contains the superior and inferior pancreaticoduodenal vascular archade which assures an adequate blood supply to the duodenum. At least one of these vessels should be preserved during the resection. The pancreatic duct stump should be identified, its patency to the duodenum assured, and it should be ligated securely. The splenic bed and remaining pancreas are drained with soft closed-suction drains, and the abdomen is closed in layers (Fig 75–26).

DISTAL PANCREATECTOMY

Distal pancreatectomy is an imprecise term that describes resection of variable amounts of the tail, or body and tail, of the pancreas, in which the head of the gland is preserved.

The operation is carried out in a similar fashion as described for a 95% pancreatectomy, but the dissection from left to right is stopped at or before the juncture of the splenic and superior mesenteric veins. The pancreas is transected at an appropriate level, and an end-to-end pancreaticojejunostomy may be fashioned. In the event that the remaining pancreas is normal and the main duct drains without obstruction into the duodenum, a pancreaticojejunostomy is unnecessary. Then the duct should be ligated and the cut end of the pancreas closed with interrupted mattress sutures of nonabsorbable material (Fig 75–27). A closed-suction drain should be placed close to this point, and the abdomen closed in layers.

■ PANCREATICOJEJUNOSTOMY

THE PUESTOW PROCEDURE

The operation can be performed easily through a bilateral subcostal incision, although many surgeons prefer a midline approach. If a midline incision is used, exposure of the tail of the pancreas may be more difficult in patients where the gland tends to be more vertical in its orientation. The pancreas should be exposed widely from the head to the tail, by taking down the gastrocolic ligament and some of the short gastric vessels to the spleen. A Kocher maneuver should be performed. Often the posterior wall of the stomach is adherent to the anterior surface of the pancreas, probably as a result of repeated episodes of inflammation in the lesser sac.

These avascular attachments must be divided so that the entire anterior aspect of the pancreas is exposed. Thus freed from the pancreas, the stomach is retracted cranially. It is not necessary to free the pancreas posteriorly or to incise its inferior or superior margins in the body or tail. It is generally not necessary to expose the superior mesenteric vein where it runs under the neck of the pancreas.

In most cases, a preoperative pancreatogram will have been obtained; if not, it can be done at this time. The dilated duct is often palpable as a longitudinal depression on the anterior surface of the gland. The duct in the body may be punctured with a 20-gauge needle attached through extension tubing to a syringe containing undiluted radiopaque contrast material. The pancreatic juice is usually under considerable pressure, and it is advisable to allow some of it to drain out before the contrast is injected. Between 2 and 5 mL usually fill the ductal system, and a radiograph then is taken. Points of obstruction, communication with pseudocysts, and general ductal anatomy are noted.

With the tip of the needle still in the duct lumen, but now disconnected from the syringe and tubing, the duct is incised using the needle as a guide. The author prefers electrocautery because of the ease with which hemostasis can be achieved by electrocoagulation, but incision with a scalpel is preferred by some. In either case, suture ligation of bleeding vessels (4-0 Prolene) is occasionally needed, but this part of the operation is never associated with significant blood loss. Once the duct lumen is visible, the needle is removed and replaced with a right-angled clamp (Fig 75–28). The incision into the duct is

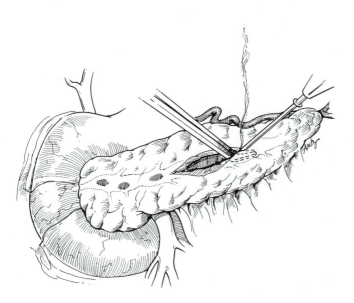

Figure 75–28. The duct is opened with electrocautery using a right angle clamp within the lumen as a guide.

extended toward the head and caudally into the tail of the gland by cutting through the tissue overlying the instrument. If calcifications are present, they are removed. Often they are attached firmly to the wall of the duct in which they are found. It is important that all of the larger ducts in the head of the pancreas be opened and emptied of debris. If there is an accessory duct present, it too should be opened. This dissection is continued until it is possible to pass a probe through the pancreatic duct into the duodenal lumen. This assures that no significant ductal obstructions remain. The incision into the pancreas itself should be extended to within about 1 cm from the duodenum, avoiding possible damage to the duodenum or the pancreaticoduodenal vessels, and allowing for a technically comfortable jejunal anastomosis. Because the ducts in the head of the gland run posteriorly, if the head is thickened, an incision deep into the pancreatic parenchyma is required. In this case, or whenever the duct is situated deeply so that there is much overlying pancreas, it is useful to excise some of that tissue. This makes it easier to achieve hemostasis, the anastomosis is easier to construct, and it probably also increases the chances that the pancreaticojejunal anastomosis will remain open.

"CORING" OF THE HEAD OF THE PANCREAS

When the head of the pancreas is particularly enlarged (A-P diameter >4 cm as seen on CT scan), the tissue in the head should be "cored out." This is done after opening the pancreatic duct from the tail into the head of the gland, as is done for the conventional Puestow operation. Interrupted 4-0 Prolene sutures are placed into the pancreatic tissue about 1 cm from the duodenal edge. These sutures are hemostatic and also mark the line of incision into the pancreas. The tissue is resected piecemeal, with the surgeon's left hand behind the head of the pancreas in order to judge the depth of the dissection and protect deeper structures. Stones are removed and cystic spaces are entered; parts of the ductal structures are actually removed with the tissue. The location of the retropancreatic superior mesenteric–portal vein is always apparent during this dissection, because the pancreatic duct invariably dives deeply posteriorly just to the patient's right of those vessels (Fig 75–29). The pancreatic tissue adjacent to the mesenteric vein marks the medial limit of the resection, although some of the deeper uncinate process can be removed. If the intrapancreatic portion of the bile duct was compressed by the pancreas, the obstruction is often relieved by the resection of this tissue. This must be confirmed, either by cholangiography or by the passage of a metal dilator through the duct from above. Indeed, even if the duct is of normal caliber, it may be helpful to pass a dilator through a proximal choledochotomy so that the posi-

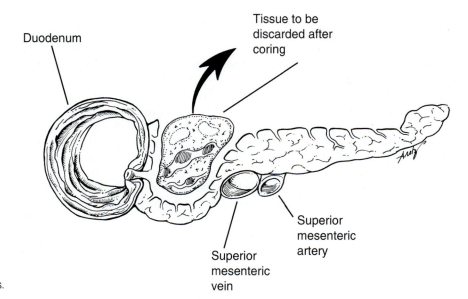

Figure 75–29. Coring of the head of the pancreas.

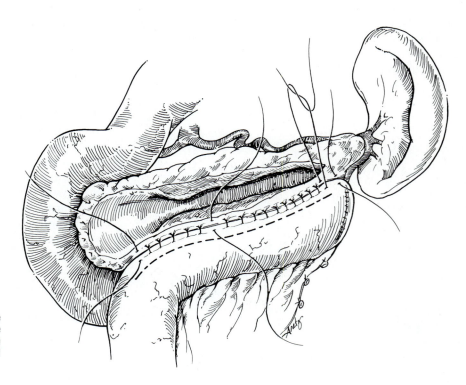

Figure 75–30. The pancreatic duct has been opened for the length of the pancreas. Tissue has been cored out from the head of the gland. The anastomosis to the pancreas is begun with interrupted 3-0 silk sutures. The jejunum will be opened along the *dashed line* after the silk sutures are tied.

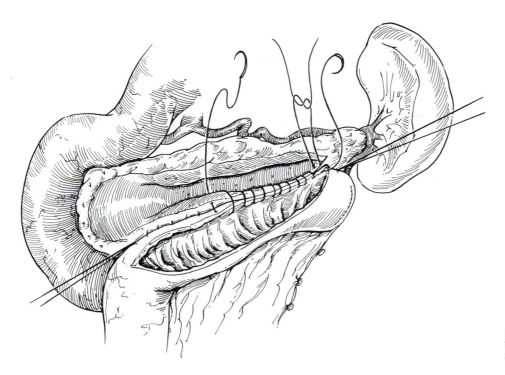

Figure 75–31. The posterior row of interrupted sutures have been placed. The two inner continuous sutures are begun (see text for details).

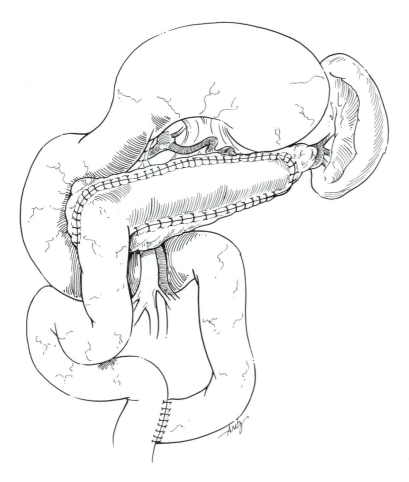

Figure 75–32. This is the appearance of a completed pancreaticojejunostomy.

tion of the intrapancreatic pancreatic bile duct can be determined, and injury to it can be avoided. With experience, this may not be necessary. Resection of the head of the pancreas ends when the posterior wall of remaining pancreas is pliable (3 to 4 mm thick) and the sensation of a hard mass in the head is no longer present anywhere.

When this portion of the operation is completed, we pack several gauze pads inside the length of the opened duct (if any oozing of blood is still present, this promotes coagulation), and then construct the Roux-en-Y jejunal segment. This is done in the usual fashion, the end is stapled closed, reinforced with a row of interrupted 3-0 silk mattress sutures, and the bowel is brought through a hole in the transverse mesocolon. It makes no difference whether the stapled end of this bowel is positioned toward the head or the tail of the pancreas; whichever position can be achieved with less tension is chosen. The two-layer anastomosis is begun with a posterior row of interrupted 3-0 silk sutures spaced about 8 to 10 mm apart (Fig 75–30). Seromuscular bites are taken in the bowel; in the pancreas the sutures enter the peritoneum overlying the gland and extend perhaps 5 mm or so into the pancreas itself. They do **not** enter the pancreatic duct. This first row of sutures is begun in the tail of the gland and proceeds toward the head along the inferior edge of the pancreas. When this row is complete, an incision is made with electrocautery into the jejunum for an appropriate distance according to the length of the opened duct. The inner row of sutures then is placed. We use a continuous row of 3-0 absorbable material such as Maxon. Here the suture is placed through the full thickness of the bowel, and into the pancreas so that it emerges within a millimeter or so of the cut edge of the duct, but still not inside it. Two such continuous sutures are required to complete the inner layer of the anastomosis. Then the outer row of silk sutures is placed along the cranial edge of the pancreas, again starting at the tail and working toward the head (Fig 75–31). Sometimes, if the incision into the pancreas was carried very close to the duodenum, some of the seromuscular silk sutures may actually be placed into the medial wall of the duodenum rather than the pancreas. This is acceptable. Gastrointestinal continuity then is restored by anastomosing the proximal jejunum to the defunctionalized segment about 40 cm distal to the point where the bowel comes through the opening in the mesocolon (Fig 75–32). The defects in the transverse mesocolon and the small bowel mesentery are closed. A closed-suction drain made of Silastic is placed along the length of the pancreaticojejunal anastomosis, and the end is brought out through a stab wound in the right flank. The drain is pulled after the patient resumes oral intake, usually on postoperative day 4 or 5.

■ INTERNAL DRAINAGE OF PANCREATIC PSEUDOCYSTS

Internal drainage of pseudocysts is done by creating an opening between the wall of the cyst and either the duodenum, the posterior wall of the stomach that is adherent to it, or a Roux-en-Y limb of jejunum. The latter technique is adaptable to cysts in various locations, multiple cysts, and also can be used to drain a cyst along with the pancreatic duct, as in a Puestow procedure.

CYSTGASTROSTOMY

A cystgastrostomy may be appropriate when the cyst develops in the lesser sac behind the stomach. Through a bilateral subcostal or midline incision, the anterior wall of the stomach is opened between stay sutures, directly on top of the palpable cyst (Fig 75–33). The liquid nature of the cyst may be confirmed by aspiration with an 18-gauge needle on a syringe, and some of the fluid should be sent for bacterial culture. The thickness of the combined cyst/posterior gastric wall also can be estimated by the depth of the needle, and an incision then is made through this tissue with electrocautery until the cyst lumen is entered. A full thickness biopsy of the cyst wall should be sent for frozen section examination, and after the cyst is evacuated of fluid and debris, the opening is enlarged to a diameter of 3 to 4 cm. The biopsy will avoid misdiagnosis of a malignant cystic neoplasm, which should be excised instead. When the diagnosis is confirmed, the adherent posterior gastric and anterior cyst wall should be sewn together with nonabsorbable suture (eg, 3-0 Prolene) as a continuous locking stitch, which ensures hemostasis (Fig 75–34). On occasion, the wall of the cyst contains large vessels, usually veins, which may bleed briskly. These should be suture ligated with vascular suture. When the anastomosis is complete, the anterior wall of the stomach is closed in the usual way with staples or sutures.

CYSTDUODENOSTOMY

Rarely, the cyst presents in the head of the pancreas, presses upon the duodenum, and is so deep within the duodenal parenchyma, that drainage into the duodenum seems appropriate. Then, following a generous Kocher maneuver to mobilize the head of the pancreas with the contained cyst, a longitudinal incision is made in the lateral wall of the duodenum. With a needle, fluid is aspirated from the cyst in order to localize it, the medial duodenal and adjacent cyst walls are incised, and a continuous suture which sews the two together is placed (Fig 75–35). With this approach, one must take care to avoid injury to the pancreatic and bile ducts. The duodenotomy then is closed in two layers in the same direction as the original incision. The closure must be meticulous, taking small bites of tissue, and with avoid-

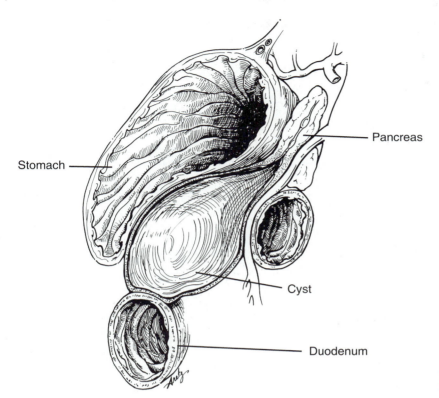

Stomach

Pancreas

Cyst

Duodenum

Figure 75–33. The anterior wall of the stomach opened directly on top of the palpable cyst.

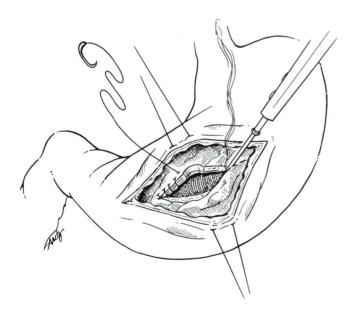

Figure 75–34. After cyst evacuation, the opening is enlarged to 3- to 4-cm diameter. Adherent posterior gastric and anterior cyst wall is sewn with nonabsorbable suture.

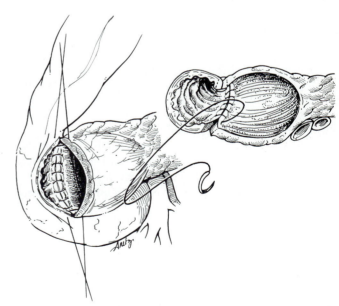

Figure 75–35. The medial duodenal and adjacent cyst walls are incised and sewn together with continuous suture.

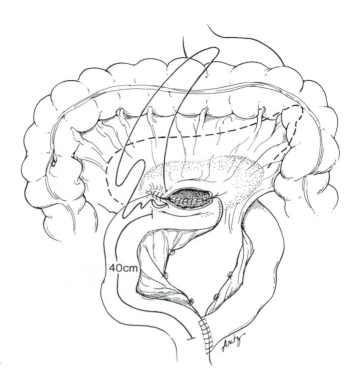

Figure 75–36. Cystjejunostomy.

ance of significant narrowing of the lumen. A closed suction drain, which is removed after the patient is eating, is placed near the duodenal suture line.

CYSTJEJUNOSTOMY

If the cyst presents in an area away from the stomach and duodenum (eg, transverse mesocolon), a Roux-en-Y limb of jejunum should be constructed and brought up to the cyst wall, which must be cleaned of overlying tissue. A dependent site on the cyst is chosen for the anastomosis, and the same maneuvers as described for cystgastrostomy are performed (Fig 75–36). However, because the jejunum is not adherent to the cyst wall, the anastomosis is done in two layers with interrupted 3-0 silk sutures on the outside and continuous locking 3-0 Prolene on the inside. The proximal jejunum is anastomosed to the side of the Roux limb at least 40 cm distal to the cystjejunostomy. After copious irrigation of the operative area, a closed-suction Silastic drain is placed near the anastomosis.

■ DEBRIDEMENT OF INFECTED PANCREATIC NECROSIS

Patients with infected pancreatic necrosis need debridement of the necrotic material and external drainage. Preoperative CT scans indicate the areas of involvement and provide a roadmap that guides the exploration.

The abdomen is opened through a bilateral subcostal incision, and free peritoneal fluid is evacuated. Any loculated areas of fluid also should be broken up and aspirated. The transverse colon is elevated to expose the transverse mesocolon, where the inflammatory process in the lesser sac may have extended. If the process has eroded through the mesocolon, the lesser sac should be entered at that point, and necrotic material evacuated. The middle colic vessels must be preserved. Occasionally, this maneuver opens the lesser sac widely enough so that the entire pancreas can be effectively debrided. More often, the lesser sac must be opened through the gastrocolic ligament as well. If the transverse mesocolon is not involved, the gastrocolic ligament approach to the lesser sac is preferred. This provides better exposure, and avoids the risk of injury to the middle colic vessels. Sometimes the gastrocolic ligament is fused with the inflammatory process in the lesser sac, which makes it difficult to select a safe area to begin the dissection. Then it is useful to make a small hole in the transverse mesocolon through which an index finger can be inserted into the lesser sac. This serves as a guide to prevent injury to the transverse colon when the gastrocolic ligament is entered.

All necrotic material should be removed back to the point where some bleeding is provoked. This usually is done effectively with a ring forceps and piecemeal removal of dead tissue (Fig 75–37). Each area is irrigated copiously and packed with laparotomy pads to promote

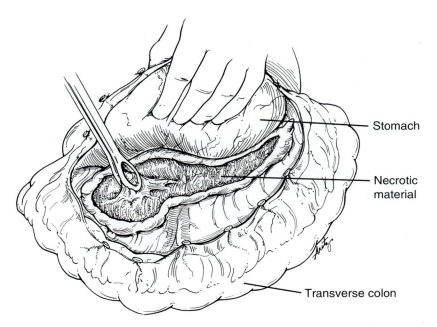

Stomach

Necrotic
material

Transverse colon

Figure 75–37. The necrotic material is debrided.

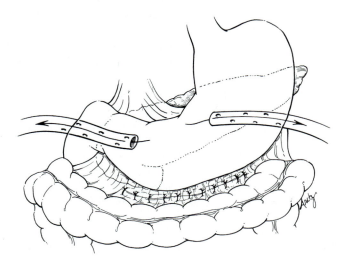

Figure 75–38. When debridement is complete the opening in the gastrocolic ligament is closed and two Silastic suction catheters are placed over the pancreas in the lesser sac.

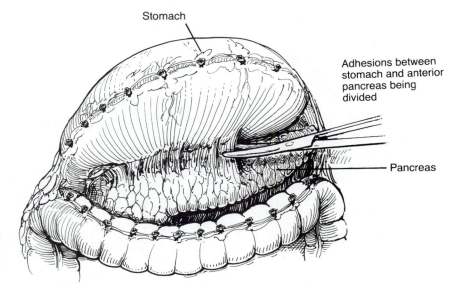

Stomach

Adhesions between
stomach and anterior
pancreas being
divided

Pancreas

Figure 75–39. Exposure of the anterior surface of the pancreas. The gastrocolic ligament has been divided, and the stomach has been elevated. (From Ashley SW, Reber HA. Surgery for endocrine tumors of the pancreas. In: Bland KI, Karakousis CP, Copeland EM III (eds), *Atlas of Surgical Oncology*. Philadelphia, PA: WB Saunders; 1995)

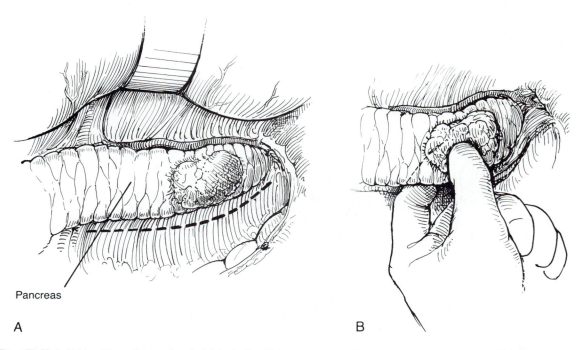

Pancreas

A

B

Figure 75–40. A. Division of the peritoneum along the inferior border of the pancreas so that the body and tail of the gland can be elevated off the retroperitoneum.
B. This permits palpation of the distal pancreas between the thumb and forefinger. (From Ashley SW, Reber HA. Surgery for endocrine tumors of the pancreas. In: Bland KI, Karakousis CP, Copeland EM III (eds), *Atlas of Surgical Oncology*. Philadelphia, PA: WB Saunders; 1995)

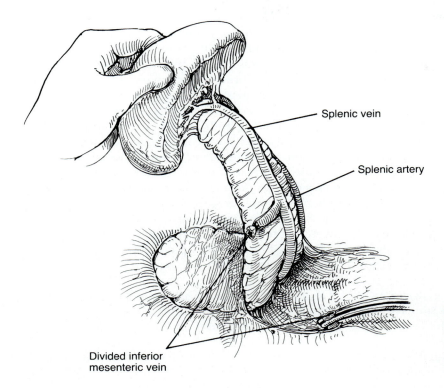

Splenic vein

Splenic artery

Divided inferior
mesenteric vein

Figure 75–41. Division of the splenic ligaments and vasa brevis permits elevation of the spleen and tail of the pancreas so that the posterior surface of the gland can be completely visualized and palpated. (From Ashley SW, Reber HA. Surgery for endocrine tumors of the pancreas. In: Bland KI, Karakousis CP, Copeland EM III (eds), *Atlas of Surgical Oncology*. Philadelphia, PA: WB Saunders; 1995)

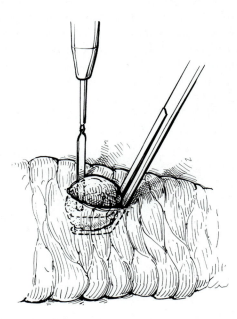

Figure 75–42. Using a combination of blunt dissection and cauterization, a small lesion is "shelled-out" of the parenchyma. (From Ashley SW, Reber HA. Surgery for endocrine tumors of the pancreas. In: Bland KI, Karakousis CP, Copeland EM III (eds), *Atlas of Surgical Oncology*. Philadelphia, PA: WB Saunders; 1995)

coagulation, while other involved areas are sequentially debrided. If significant hemorrhage follows overaggressive debridement, the bleeding points should be suture-ligated with vascular suture. When all of the affected areas have been exposed and debrided, large soft Silastic sump drains are placed to each. To drain only the lesser sac, two drains are required (Fig 75–38). These should be arranged so that they do not lay directly on bowel, which could result in the development of a fistula later. A feeding jejunostomy usually is placed, since these patients often cannot eat for long periods, and enteral nutrition is important to maintain gut mucosal integrity and function.

■ ISLET CELL TUMORS

Because of the multifocal nature of these neoplasms, the entire pancreas should be mobilized and carefully examined. The gastrocolic omentum is first divided and the lesser sac is entered. The splenic and hepatic flexures are mobilized. Adhesions between the posterior stomach and pancreas are divided and the stomach is elevated exposing the anterior surface of the pancreas (Fig 75–39).

Islet cell lesions may have a flesh-colored appearance or bluish tinge and often can be identified by inspection alone. Deeper lesions may not be visible, however, and it is always necessary to completely mobilize the gland so that it can be carefully palpated between the thumb and forefinger. An extensive Kocher maneuver is performed to permit palpation of the posterior head and uncinate process. Endocrine tumors are typically somewhat firmer than the normal pancreatic parenchyma. Next, the peritoneal reflection along the inferior border of the pancreas is incised and the body and tail are elevated

from the retroperitoneum from below so that they too can be palpated (Fig 75–40). In some patients, because of its proximity to the spleen, the tail of the gland cannot be adequately examined by this maneuver alone. Then the spleen and tail of the pancreas can be mobilized and elevated together out of the retroperitoneum (Fig 75–41). This requires division of the splenic ligaments and vasa brevia, which allows entrance into the plane between the splenic vessels and Gerota's fascia.

In most patients, the tumor can be identified by these maneuvers, along with intraoperative ultrasound. Ultrasound also can provide information regarding the relationship of the tumor to the major vessels and to the pancreatic and bile ducts. If the ducts are intimately associated with the tumor, resection may be required. Otherwise, simple enucleation of the tumor may suffice. The choice of operation also depends on the location of the tumor in the pancreas. A distal pancreatectomy may be indicated for lesions of the body or tail; a pancreaticoduodenectomy might be required for a tumor in the head.

Enucleation of these tumors is performed with a combination of blunt and sharp dissection. Larger vessels and ductal structures must be sutured with nonabsorbable material (Fig 75–42). The edges of the cavity that remains can be reapproximated with interrupted 3-0 silk sutures. The defect should be drained with a closed-suction drain.

In an effort to avoid a Whipple resection, even some lesions deep in the head of the pancreas may be enucleated. If there is concern about injury to the pancreatic duct, the resultant cavity can be managed by drainage into a Roux-en-Y loop of jejunum. However, if the lesion is large, if the main pancreatic duct must be transected, and especially if there is concern that it might be malignant, pancreaticoduodenectomy is indicated.

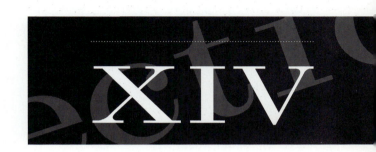

XIV

SPLEEN

76

The Spleen

Seymour I. Schwartz

■ HISTORICAL BACKGROUND

The spleen was regarded by Galen as "an organ of mystery," by Aristotle as unnecessary, by Pliny as an organ that might hinder the speed of runners and also as an organ that produced laughter and mirth, a concept reasserted in the Babylonian Talmud. The first recorded splenectomy was performed for splenomegaly on a 24 year–old Neapolitan woman in 1549 by Adrian Zacarelli. The first successful partial splenectomy for trauma was reported by Franciscus Rosetti in 1590. Thus, partial splenectomy for trauma antedated total splenectomy for trauma, first performed by Nicolaus Matthias in 1678 in Capetown, South Africa, on a patient whose spleen protruded through a flank wound. The first splenectomy for trauma in the United States was reported by O'Brien, a Royal Navy surgeon, in 1816. In 1866, Sir Thomas Spencer Wells gave an account of the first successful splenectomy in England.

Although Billroth, reporting on an autopsy in 1881, felt that a splenic injury might have healed spontaneously, as recently as 1927 Hamilton Bailey asserted that "surgical aid is always needed." During the first two decades of the 20th century, however, proponents began to appear championing the use of judicious tamponade of the organ and suture repair was reported to be successful. Zikoff, in Russia, is credited with the first successful repair of a lacerated spleen in 1895. The first successful partial splenectomy for trauma in modern times was reported by Campos Christo in 1962.

The role of the spleen in relation to infection has been considered for many years. Countering early experiments that showed no adverse effects of splenectomy on infection, Morris and Bullock, conducting controlled experiments with rat plague bacillus in 1919, concluded that removal of the spleen "robs the body of its resistance." Until relatively recently, however, most physicians and surgeons have felt that splenectomy did not compromise the host defense against infection. The first of the recent reports was that of King and Shumacker in 1952, chronicling an increased susceptibility to infection in children following splenectomy for hemologic disorders. In 1973, Singer's review of the literature emphasized the increase in postsplenectomy sepsis in infants and children.

■ ANATOMY

The spleen arises by mesenchymal differentiation along the left side of the dorsal mesogastrium in juxtaposition to the anlage of the left gonad in the 8-mm embryo. In the healthy adult, the weight of the spleen ranges between 75 and 100 gm. It resides in the posterior portion of the left upper quadrant lying deep to the ninth, tenth, and eleventh ribs, with its long axis corresponding to that of the tenth rib. Its convex, superior, and lateral surfaces are immediately adjacent to the undersurface of the left leaf of the diaphragm. The configuration of the concave, medial surface of the spleen is a consequence of impressions made by the stomach, pancreas, kidney, and splenic flexure of the colon (Fig 76–1).

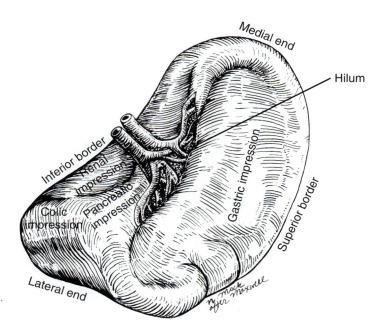

Figure 76–1. Gross anatomy of the spleen.

The position of the spleen is, in part, maintained by several suspensory ligaments, including the gastrosplenic, splenophrenic, splenocolic, and splenorenal ligaments (Figs 76–2 and 76–3). The gastrosplenic ligament contains the short gastric vessels that course to the splenic hilum from the greater curvature while the remaining ligaments are generally avascular, except in patients with portal hypertension or myeloproliferative disorders.

The splenic artery, a branch of the celiac artery, provides the spleen with arterial blood. A varying degree of branching occurs proximal to the hilus. Frequently, a branch to the inferior pole originates centrally. The major venous drainage flows through the splenic vein, which usually receives the inferior mesenteric vein centrally, and then joins the superior mesenteric vein to form the portal vein.

Accessory spleens, made of blood, sinuses, and malpighian bodies, have been classified into two types: (1) the more uncommon is a constricted part of the main organ to which it is bound by fibrous tissue, and (2) the more common distinct, separate mass. The latter has been reported in 14% to 30% of patients; a higher incidence of this has been reported in patients with hematologic disorders. These accessory organs that receive their blood supply from the splenic artery are present in decreasing order of frequency in the hilus of the spleen, the gastrosplenic and the splenocolic ligaments, the gastrosplenic ligament, and splenorenal ligament, and the greater omentum (Fig 76–4). Accessory spleens may also occur in the pelvis of the female, either in the presacral region or adjacent to the left ovary, and in the scrotum in juxtaposition to the left testicle.

The spleen is made up of a capsule that is normally 1 to 2 mm thick, and trabeculae that surround and invaginate the pulp. The parenchyma (Fig 76–5) is made up of "white pulp" that functions as an immunologic organ, "red pulp" that phagocytizes particulate matter from the blood, and a marginal zone. The white pulp, which is central and surrounds a central artery, is made of lymphatic nodules with germinal centers and periarterial lymphatic sheaths that constitute a reticular network filled with lymphocytes and macrophages. Peripheral to the white pulp is the marginal zone that contains end arteries arising from the central artery and from peripheral peniciliary arteries. The marginal zone contains lymphocytes and macrophages and some red blood cells that have exited from terminal arteries. The marginal zone also contains the marginal sinus that filters material from the centrally located white pulp. Locally produced immunoglobulins enter the marginal zone, eventually coursing to the bloodstream.

Peripheral to the marginal zone is the red pulp. This pulp consists of cords and sinuses that contain cellular elements of blood in transit. Most of the blood flow passing through the spleen courses though an "open" circulation in which the blood passes from arterioles to reticular cell-lined networks of the splenic cords and then to the sinuses. In addition, there is a "closed" circulation with direct arterial venous connections.

The vascular supply of the spleen enters along the trabeculae. The intrasplenic arteries first pass through the white pulp where branches come off almost perpendicularly, contributing to the skimming effect by which the plasma exits, whereas most red cells pass to

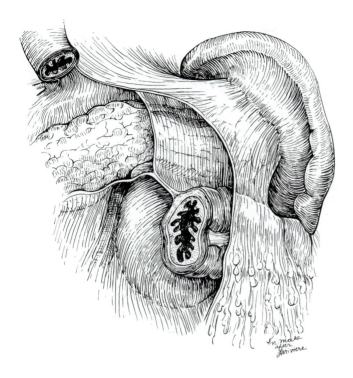

Figure 76–2. Anatomy of the spleen showing complicated peritoneal reflections in the region of the hilus.

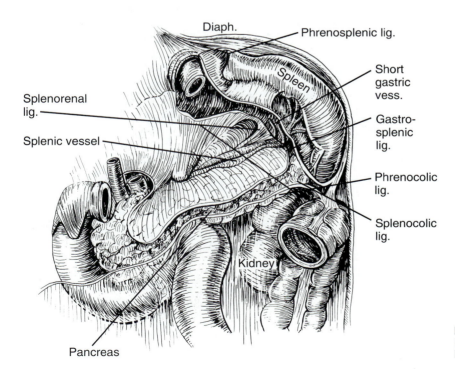

Figure 76–3. Ligaments of the spleen. (From Schwartz SI. Spleen. In: Schwartz SI, Shires GT, et al (eds), *Principles of Surgery,* 5 ed. New York, NY: McGraw-Hill, 1989)

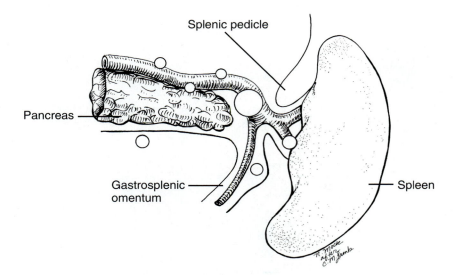

A

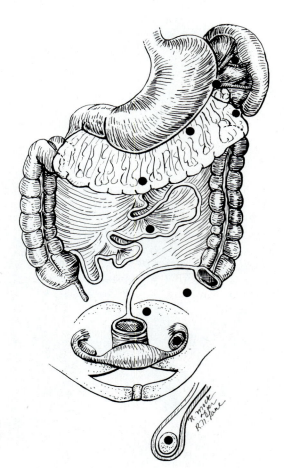

Figure 76–4. A. The more common locations of accessory spleens. Accessory spleens are also found in the left ovary, in the left testicle along the course of the left ureter, and in the lesser sac and greater omentum. **B.** Locations of accessory spleens. Note position of presacral and paraureteric spleniculi.

B

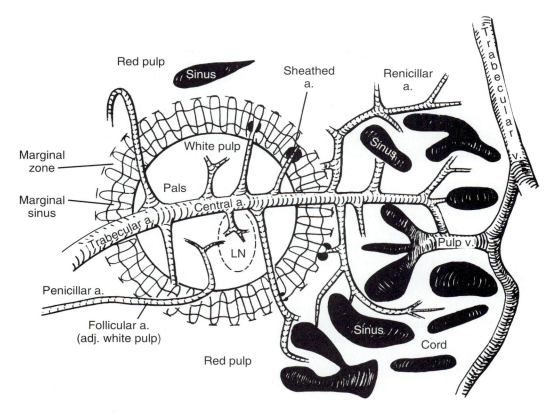

Figure 76–5. Diagram illustrating splenic compartments and potential vascular supply routes. A: artery or arteriole; V: vein; LN: lymphatic nodule which may include germinal center; PALS: periarterial lymphatic. (From Barnhart MI, Lusher JM The human spleen as revealed by scanning electron microscopy. *Am J Pediatr Hematol Oncol* 1976;1:131

the red pulp cords. It is in the red pulp at the point of passage from cords to sinuses that deformability and flexibility are demanded of the red cells so that they can squeeze through. The normally biconcave discs elongate and become thinner. Almost 90% of cells slowly make their way through open circulation, whereas 10% pass more rapidly through direct arteriovenous conduits. The resultant cumulative flow through the spleen averages 300 mL/min.

■ PHYSIOLOGY

Although the spleen is not necessary for life, it performs important functions that are generally divided into two major categories: (1) those related to cellular elements in the circulating blood and (2) those that are immunologic in nature.

The cellular functions include hematopoiesis, storage, "pitting," and "culling." Hematopoiesis, which supplies erythroid, myeloid, lymphoid cells, and platelets in fetal life, essentially ceases by the seventh intrauterine month. In human beings, the spleen does not serve as an important reservoir for blood cells, except platelets.

At any given time, about one-third of the total platelet mass is in the spleen.

Pitting refers to the removal of rigid structures such as Heinz bodies, Howell-Jolly bodies, and hemosiderin granules from red cells. The process involves the removal of nondeformable intracellular substances from deformable cells. The rigid body is phagocytized while the deformable cytoplasmic mass passes into the sinus and returns to the general circulation. The postsplenectomy blood smear is characterized by the presence of circulating erythrocytes with Howell-Jolly and Pappenheimer bodies (siderotic granules). Nucleated cells also have their nuclei removed in the same fashion.

Culling is the term applied to the spleen's ability to remove red cells that are aged or abnormal. Normally, as the red cell ages after a life span of approximately 120 days, it loses osmotic balance and membrane integrity, and therefore deformability. When these cells lose their deformability they are phagocytized by native macrophages. The spleen does not represent the only site for red cell destruction, and there is no difference in red cell survival following splenectomy. Naturally deformed cells and red cells that are affected by disease states also are removed by phagocytosis. In those circumstances in which there is a superabundance of reticulocyte formation, these cells are remodeled in the spleen and exit as mature cells. In the normal adult, the spleen is the most important site of selective erythrocyte sequestration. During its 120 day life cycle, the red cell spends an estimated minimum of 2 days within the spleen which, when normal, contains about 25 mL red blood cells.

The neutrophil has a half-life of about 6 hours; hence 85% of neutrophils either emigrate at random into tissues or are destroyed within 24 hours. Although the role of the spleen in the destruction of neutrophils under normal conditions is not well quantified, in some hypersplenic states the role of the spleen is augmented, with resulting neutropenia. This augmented removal can occur because of splenic enlargement and accelerated sequestration of granulocytes or because of enhanced splenic removal of altered granulocytes, as seen in immune neutropenias.

There is significant interaction between the platelets and splenic cells. Normally, about one-third of the platelet mass is pooled in the spleen, and this pool exchanges freely with the circulating platelets that have a life span of about 10 days. With splenomegaly, a large proportion of platelets is sequestered in the spleen (up to 80%) and this, coupled with accelerated platelet destruction in the spleen, accounts for thrombocytopenia. Splenic phagocytosis of platelets occurs in normal states, but in pathologic states, such as immune thrombocytopenia (ITP), it is greatly accelerated.

In addition to the phagocytosis of antibody-coated cells, the immunologic functions of the spleen include antibody synthesis (especially IgM), generation of lymphocytes, and production of tuftsin, opsonins, properdin, and interferon.

THE ASPLENIC STATE

The spleen plays a role in the phagocytic clearance of bacteria, especially encapsulated bacteria such as pneumococci and *Haemophilus influenzae,* particularly if the host has deficient concentrations of opsonizing antibodies. The spleen also produces specific IgM antibody to blood-borne bacteria. It is generally believed that if sufficient opsonins are present and the reticuloendothelial (RE) system is normal, the spleen probably plays a relatively small role in the clearance of blood-borne organisms. Any dysfunction of the RE system, such as caused by hematologic disease or immunosuppressive therapy, increases the likelihood of sepsis.

In a series reported by Albrechtsen and Ly of 221 patients with hematologic disease, late postsplenectomy pulmonary infection was seen in 8 patients. All but one was either on immunosuppressive therapy or had advanced malignancy. No neutrophil defect or impairment of serum opsonin or chemotactic activity could be demonstrated after incidental or traumatic splenectomy in the study by Deitch and O'Neal of 24 healthy adult patients. Also, screening for complement activation by classic and alternative pathways did not reveal any defects resulting from splenectomy in 12 patients who underwent incidental splenectomy. A study by Schwartz and associates of 93 adult patients subjected to splenectomy revealed only 2 cases of fulminant sepsis documented during 1090 person-years of follow-up. The incidence of any type of serious infection was 7 per 100 person-years. Patients undergoing splenectomy in association with a malignant lesion had higher subsequent infection rates, and patients receiving immunosuppressive or radiation therapy were also at higher risk.

Children who have undergone splenectomy should be protected with *pneumococcus* and *H influenzae* vaccine and they should receive penicillin until age 18. *Pneumococcus* vaccine should also be administered to splenectomized adult patients. Equivalent response to pneumococcal antigens has been demonstrated for patients vaccinated after splenectomy compared with those vaccinated with the spleen in place. Patients with diseases associated with high infection rates, such as thalassemia, sickle cell anemia, autoimmune hemolytic anemia, and thrombocytopenia, should not be denied splenectomy, but should be under close postsplenectomy surveillance. Malangoni and associates reviewed reports dealing with sepsis after splenectomy for trauma and defined a rate of serious infection of one per 331.5 years.

■ RUPTURE OF THE SPLEEN

See also Chapter 22.

ETIOLOGY

The causes of splenic rupture, in which the organ's parenchyma or capsule is disrupted, include penetrating trauma, nonpenetrating or blunt trauma, operative trauma, and, rarely, a spontaneous event. Rupture of the spleen may be caused by puncture wounds due to stabbings or missiles. The trajectory of the penetrating wound may pass through the anterior abdominal wall, the posterior abdominal wall, the flank, or transthoracically, piercing the pleural space and diaphragm. Isolated splenic injury may be present, or organs in juxtaposition may be involved; this would include the stomach, left kidney, pancreas, and root of the mesentery. Nonpenetrating or blunt trauma represents an increasing etiologic factor in splenic rupture. The spleen, alone or in combination with over viscera, is the most frequently injured organ, following blunt trauma to the abdomen or lower thoracic cage. In this circumstance, splenic trauma is an isolated event in only 30% of patients. Other organs that may be injured, in decreasing order of frequency, include chest (rib fracture), kidney, spinal cord, liver, lung, craniocerebral structures, small intestine, large intestine, pancreas, and stomach.

Operative trauma to the spleen most commonly occurs during operation on adjacent viscera. The spleen has been injured in approximately 2% of patients whose operations involved viscera in the left upper quadrant. Subtotal gastrectomy and abdominal repair of a diaphragmatic hernia are high on the list of operations associated with splenic trauma. In these situations, injury usually results from retractors placed against the organ in order to obtain exposure.

Although spontaneous rupture of the normal spleen has been reported in approximately two dozen cases, it is a much more common event when the spleen is involved with a hematologic disorder. Spontaneous rupture, or rupture associated with minor trauma, is the most common cause of death for patients with infectious mononucleosis; this is second only to malaria as a cause of spontaneous splenic rupture. The complication of splenic rupture occurs most frequently in weeks 2 to 4 in the patient with infectious mononucleosis. Splenic rupture has also been reported in patients with sarcoidosis, acute and chronic leukemia, hemolytic anemia, congestive splenomegaly, polycythemia vera, candidiasis, and splenic abscess.

PATHOLOGY

The spectrum of lesions associated with trauma to the spleen include linear and stellate lacerations, capsular tears, puncture wounds, subcapsular intrasplenic hematomas, avulsion of the organ from its vascular pedicle, and laceration of the short gastric vessels within the gastrosplenic omentum. The spleen is an extremely friable vascular organ, and even minor trauma may result in significant bleeding, particularly if the spleen is enlarged or diseased. Most injuries result in transverse ruptures as a consequence of the internal architecture of the spleen, which is arranged on a transverse plane. Injuries through this plane usually do not cross any major segmental arteries. Experimentally, it has been shown that injuries coursing along the blood supply heal by primary intention, whereas those traversing segmental vessels are attended by infarction of the involved segment but persistent viability of the remainder of the organ.

The vascular anatomy of the spleen favors spontaneous cessation of bleeding following trauma. Large and small arteriovenous anastomoses permit segments of the organ to be bypassed, particularly in states of shock. The complex arterial–capillary venous circulation and arterial–capillary sinus circulations result in a meshwork that facilitates platelet aggregation and clot formation. When lacerations occur along the horizon-

TABLE 76–1. SPLENIC ORGAN INJURY SCALE

Class I	Nonexpanding subcapsular hematoma <10% surface area. Nonbleeding capsular laceration with <1 cm deep parenchymal involvement.
Class II	Nonexpanding subcapsular hematoma 10–50% surface area. Nonexpanding intraparenchyml hematoma <2 cm in diameter. Bleeding capsular tear or parenchymal laceration 1–3 cm deep without trabecular vessel involvement.
Class III	Expanding subcapsular or intraparenchymal hematoma. Bleeding subcapsular hematoma or subcapsular hematoma >50% surface area. Intraparenchymal hematoma >2 cm in diameter. Parenchymal laceration >3 cm deep or involving trabecular vessels.
Class IV	Ruptured intraparenchymal hematoma with active bleeding. Laceration involving segmental or hilar vessels producing major (>25% splenic volume) devascularization.
Class V	Completely shattered or avulsed spleen. Hilar laceration which devascularizes entire spleen.

(From Cogbill TH, Moore EE, et al. Nonoperative management of blunt splenic trauma: a multicenter experience. *J Trauma* 1989;29:1312)

tal axis, control of the arterial supply to individual segments is technically feasible. An injury scale has been proposed (Table 76–1).

Splenic rupture may be acute, delayed, or occult. Acute rupture, which is attended by immediate intraperitoneal bleeding, occurs in >90% of cases of blunt trauma to the spleen. Delayed rupture, with an interval of days or weeks between the injury and intraperitoneal bleeding, has been reported in approximately 10% of cases of blunt trauma. The quiescent period referred to as the "latent period of Baudet" persists for <7 days in half of these patients, and <2 weeks in three-quarters of them. Occult rupture is a term applied to traumatic pseudocysts of the spleen when injury to the organ previously had not been diagnosed. This is an extremely rare event.

Another pathologic lesion related to splenic trauma is splenosis; this is the result of autotransplantation of fragments of the traumatized spleen onto the peritoneal surface. Patients with splenosis are generally asymptomatic, but the lesion may stimulate the formation of adhesions, which, in turn, may lead to intestinal obstruction. It is not known whether splenosis protects against the infection that has been associated with the asplenic state. At least two deaths, caused by overwhelming infection following traumatic rupture of the spleen, have been reported in patients who were proven to have splenosis.

CLINICAL MANIFESTATIONS

The signs and symptoms produced by splenic rupture vary according to the severity and rapidity of intra-abdominal hemorrhage, the presence of other organ injuries, and the interval between the injury and the examination. Most patients present with some degree of hypovolemia and, therefore, have tachycardia and hypotension. This can be accentuated by raising the head of the bed. Usually, there is generalized abdominal pain, which, in one-third of cases, is localized in the left upper quadrant. Pain at the tip of the shoulder (Kehr sign) is evidence of diaphragmatic irritation, but it occurs in less than one-half the patients. This may be produced by placing the patient in a Trendelenberg position. Tenderness in the left upper quadrant is a frequent physical sign, and a mass or a percussible area of fixed dullness in this region (Ballance sign) has been described but is rarely detected.

DIAGNOSTIC STUDIES

Serial determinations of the hematocrit may suggest continued intraperitoneal bleeding. Increases in the white blood count to levels frequently greater than $15,000/mm^3$ are to be anticipated. Routine abdominal radiographs may demonstrate fractured ribs, which should arouse suspicion of injury to the spleen. More specific findings, which may be noted on abdominal films, include: (1) elevated, immobile left diaphragm, (2) enlarged splenic shadow, (3) medial displacement of the gastric shadow with serration of the greater curvature owing to dissection of blood into the gastrosplenic omentum, and (4) widening of the space between the splenic flexure and the preperitoneal fat pad. Ultrasonography may define blood in the peritoneum and has been shown to be sensitive to as little as 300 mL accumulation. Computed tomography (CT) scanning may demonstrate a splenic rupture; the same may be effected by splenic radionuclide scan, but in both instances false-positives may be caused by congenital clefts (Fig 76–6). The diagnosis may be established

angiographically by visualization of: (1) disruption of the parenchyma, (2) radiopacity in the peritoneal cavity, and (3) early filling of the splenic vein (Fig 76–7).

Treatment

Spontaneous rupture of a diseased organ usually requires splenectomy. By contrast, iatrogenic lacerations that are detected intraoperatively generally can be repaired. Concern with the risk of asplenic sepsis has led to an altered approach to penetrating and blunt splenic trauma. In many recent series it has been reported that observation, without operative intervention, is possible in 85% of the cases of splenic rupture in children. These cases are observed for 7 to 14 days and delayed rupture rarely occurs. Operation is mandated if there is suggestion of injury of other intra-abdominal organs. In adult series, approximately one-third of the spleens have been salvaged. Although splenectomy as a life-saving procedure is the standard in many cases, splenic repair can be successfully effected for the majority of parenchymal injuries. Nonoperative management is appropriate if the patient is hemodynamically stable, requires fewer than 2 units of blood (for an adult), and has minimal peritoneal signs. If an operation is mandated, splenic repair and salvage is preferred only if hemostasis is achieved, if greater than a third of the splenic mass can be preserved, and if there is no other significant intraperitoneal injury.

A midline incision is recommended for the management of splenic trauma, and the chest should be prepared at the same time to permit extension of the incision. A clot is usually detected in the left upper quadrant, and if this is not apparent, the spleen should be exposed gently to avoid inadvertent trauma. If there is no apparent active bleeding from the traumatized spleen, no further therapy is indicated. If minor bleed-

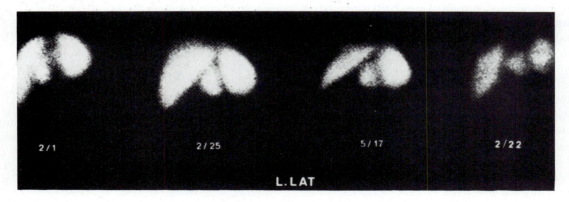

Figure 76–6. Initial left lateral scan (2/1) in patient who fell on stairs shows a wide band of decreased activity through spleen. Subsequent scans show that the band persists, with only minor narrowing. (From Fischer KC, Eraklis A, et al: Scintigraphy in follow-up of pediatric splenic trauma treated without surgery. *J Nucl Med* 1978;19:3)

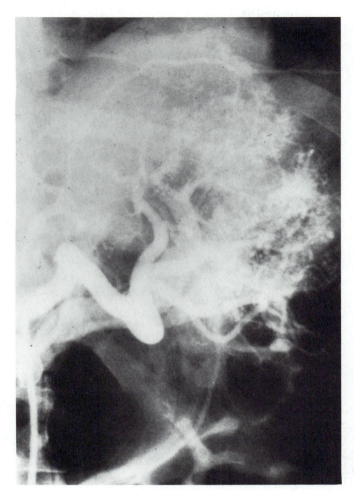

Figure 76–7. Splenic angiogram showing early filling of splenic vein diagnostic of parenchymal rupture.

ing is noted, it may be managed by the application of micronized collagen or oxidized cellulose, absorbable sutures passed through the capsule, or suturing the omentum to the area of laceration to effect tamponade. The techniques of splenorrhaphy and splenic preservation are discussed later.

■ LOCAL SPLENIC DISORDERS

ANEURYSMS OF THE SPLENIC ARTERY

The lesion was first mentioned by Baussier in 1770. St. Leger Brockman described one of the first surgical cases in 1930. The first radiologic diagnosis was made by Lindboe 2 years later.

The splenic artery is the most common site of an intra-abdominal aneurysm when the abdominal aorta is excluded. The incidence in autopsy series ranges be-

tween 0.02% and 0.16%. The lesion occurs most frequently in women, usually as a consequent of atherosclerosis. In a series of 125 cases collected by Sherlock and Learmonth, the average diameter of the aneurysmal sac was 3.4 cm and the largest was 15 cm. The main splenic artery was involved in 81% of the cases, while 26% were multiple. Eighty-seven percent of splenic artery aneurysms occurred in women, and 92% of the women had been pregnant an average of 4.5 times.

A splenic artery aneurysm usually is discovered in the sixth decade as an incidental finding. Eighty-three percent of patients are asymptomatic at the time of diagnosis. The remainder present with epigastric, left upper quadrant, or flank pain. The pain usually cannot be attributed conclusively to the lesion. The physical examination is usually normal, and a bruit is detectable in <10% of cases. A calcified lesion is noted on plain film of the abdomen in 70 percent of the patients (Fig 76–8).

Rupture usually is manifested by sudden abdominal pain. In 12.5% a warning hemorrhage occurs, with temporary cessation of bleeding. Rupture into the colon, stomach, and intestine may take place, but intraperitoneal rupture is by far the most common presentation. The risk of rupture in a calcified aneurysm is small, occurring in only 1 of 34 patients; the patient was followed for 1 to 19 years, and that aneurysm was 7 cm in diameter. When rupture occurs in the nonpregnant female, it is usually contained in the lesser sac, resulting in a patient mortality rate of <5%. Rupture in the pregnant female, however, has been associated with a 70% maternal and a 95% fetal mortality. Sixty-nine % of the ruptures during pregnancy occur during the third trimester.

Criteria for operation are not firm, but it is generally believed that removal is not required for the asymptomatic lesion that is <2 cm detected on a radiograph. Symptomatic aneurysms, and those that are >2 cm in diameter, should be removed if the patient is a reasonable risk. An aneurysm detected in a female who anticipates pregnancy should be removed; one detected early in pregnancy should be resected before the third trimester. Lesions proximal to the hilus of the spleen can be managed by proximal and distal ligation, with resection of the involved segment, if possible. Proximal ligation is reasonable, since the spleen will not become ischemic following central ligation of the main splenic artery. Distal lesions and multiple lesions generally necessitate splenectomy.

CYSTS

In 1929, Andral first described a splenic cyst; this was a dermoid cyst found at autopsy. Pean performed the first recorded splenectomy for cyst in 1867. Cysts are generally subdivided into those of nonparasitic etiology and those that are caused by echinococcus.

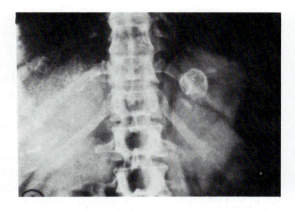 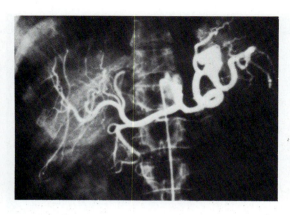

A   **B**

Figure 76–8. A. Plain abdominal roentgenogram demonstrating "signet-ring" pattern of calcification in left upper quadrant. Diameter is 3.0 cm. **B.** Selective celiac artery arteriogram of same patient demonstrating saccular splenic artery aneurysm. (From Trastek VF, Pairolero PC, et al, Splenic artery aneurysms *Surgery* 91:694)

Nonparasitic Cysts

This category is made up of cysts devoid of cellular lining (pseudocysts), simple cysts, epidermoid cysts, and dermoid cysts.

Pseudocysts comprise 70% to 80% of nonparasitic cysts of the spleen; most result from trauma and represent the resolution of a subcapsular or intraparenchymal hematoma. Malaria, infectious mononucleosis, tuberculosis, and syphilis are all predisposing factors. The pseudocysts vary in size, can reach large proportions, and contain as much as 3 L of a dark, turbid fluid. In over 80% of the cases the lesion is unilocular (Fig 76–9); the cyst wall is dense and smooth. Microscopically the wall consists of fibrous tissue without an internal epithelial lining.

Pseudocysts occur more frequently in women, children, and young adults. Many patients recall a history of trauma. One-third of the patients are asymptomatic. The most frequent complaint is left upper quadrant pain radiating to the left shoulder or chest. Symptoms related to pressure on the stomach occur less frequently. Physical examination usually reveals a smooth mass in the left upper quadrant that can be seen on routine abdominal films (Fig 76–10). A focal calcification may be noted. Ultrasonography, CT, and arteriography will define the cystic nature of the lesion. Splenectomy is curative, and cases also have been managed by unroofing and draining the area, preserving the bulk of splenic parenchyma.

Simple congenital cysts, lined by flattened or cuboidal cells, may originate from infolding of peritoneal mesothelium during splenic development. These lesions are usually small and asymptomatic. Large simple cysts present with the same manifestations as pseudocysts and have the same radiographic appearance. Smaller lesions found incidentally do not require excision; larger lesions are removed by total or partial splenectomy.

About 10% of cystic lesions are lined by squamous epithelium; 100 cases of this lesion have been reported. These cysts are usually round and unilocular and may be very large. They are filled with yellow or brown turbid fluid. The cyst is dense and the diagnosis is established by microscopic definition of the stratified squamous lining. Examination of multiple cuts may be required to demonstrate the pathology.

Epidermoid cysts of the spleen occur in children and in young adults in 75% of the cases. About two-thirds of the patients have been female. The clinical manifestations are dependent upon the size and are similar to those of the pseudocysts, as are the radiologic findings. Splenectomy, or partial splenectomy, effects a cure, as it does for simple cysts.

True dermoid cysts of the spleen are exceedingly rare; fewer than ten cases have met the pathologic criteria of a squamous epithelium with dermal appendages such as hair follicles and sweat glands. Splenectomy is indicated.

Echinococcal Cysts

Hydatid disease occurs epidemically in south central Europe, South America, Australia, and Alaska. Two-thirds or more of the splenic cysts are caused by *echinococci*. The parasitology of echinococcal disease is presented in the section on liver disease. *Echinococcus granulosus*, the most commonly implicated species, usually results in a unilocular cyst composed of an inner germinal layer (endocyst) and an outer laminated layer (ectocyst) surrounded by a fibrous capsule. Unlike the nonparasitic cysts, these are filled with fluid under positive pressure, and also contain daughter cysts and infective scolices.

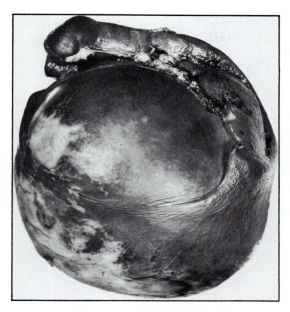

Figure 76–9. Pseudocyst of the spleen. The patient was a girl 11 years of age. Splenectomy was successfully performed. (Courtesy of Dr R Dick, Royal Free Hospital, London, England)

Echinococcal cysts are usually asymptomatic unless they reach a size causing pressure symptoms or become secondarily infected or rupture.

As a diagnostic tool, the Casoni skin test is sensitive but not specific. The passive hemagglutination test provides the best diagnostic specificity and sensitivity and is preferable to flocculation and complement fixation tests. The abdominal film may show a partially calcified mass in the left upper quadrant. Ultrasound and CT scan may demonstrate a cystic mass that is septated and contains daughter cysts.

Splenectomy is the treatment of choice because there is no effective medical therapy. Care should be taken to avoid spilling the contents of the cyst. The lesions can be sterilized by instilling a 3% sodium chloride solution. If intraperitoneal spillage occurs during the course of dissection, an anaphylactic hypotension may occur and require intravenous epinephrine to treat the shock.

SPLENIC ABSCESSES

Splenic abscesses occur more frequently in the tropics, where there is a higher incidence of sickle cell anemia, with associated thrombosis of parenchymal vessels and consequent infarction. In North America and the European countries, intrasplenic abscess is usually a consequence of bacteria associated with endocarditis or postoperative infection, frequently in a patient with a hematologic disorder. Seventy-five percent of splenic abscesses are caused by bacteremia; 15% are the result

of trauma, and 10% represent direct extension from a neighboring process. Pyogenic abscesses occur in addicts taking intravenous drugs. The organisms most frequently implicated are *Staphylococcus aureus, streptococci,* and gram-negative bacilli. Splenic fungal microabscesses have been reported in immunocompromised patients. Concurrent neutropenia is a contributing factor. Ketoconazole may afford prophylaxis. Amphotericin, usually accompanied by splenectomy, has been therapeutic.

Patients present with asthenia, weight loss, high fever, and rigors. Pain is most pronounced in the left upper quadrant, and there may be restriction of respiratory excursions. Spread or transdiaphragmatic rupture may result in empyema. The diagnosis may be established by sonogram (Fig 76–11) or by CT scan.

Splenectomy should be performed if feasible. Frequently, however, the extent of the perisplenic inflammatory process compromises removal of the organ, in which case splenotomy and drainage is indicated. Percutaneous ultrasonographically directed insertion of a pigtail catheter for drainage represents an alternative approach. With drainage and appropriate antibiotics, recent mortality rates of <10% have been reported.

BENIGN NEOPLASMS

Hemangioma is the most common benign neoplasm of the spleen, but fewer than 100 cases have been reported. The lesion may be focal, multiple, or involve the

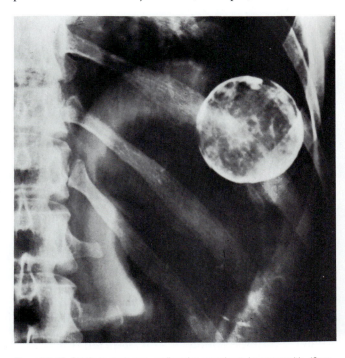

Figure 76–10. Calcified splenic cyst, confirmed at operation to be nonparasitic. (Courtesy of Dr R Dick, Royal Free Hospital, London, England)

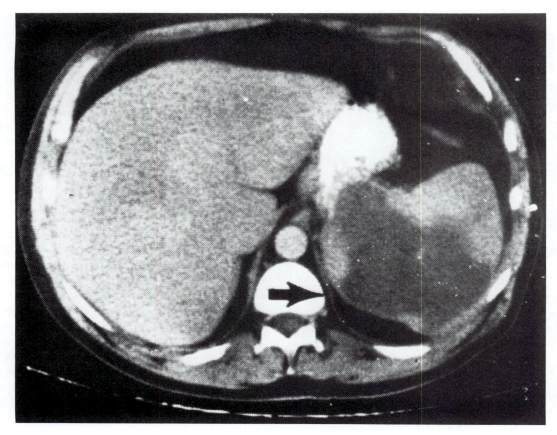

Figure 76–11. CT scan of abdomen with oral medium, demonstrating splenic abscess. (From Linos DA, Nagorney DM, et al. 1983 Splenic abscess–The importance of early diagnosis. *Mayo Clin Proc* 1983;58:261)

entire organ. Marked enlargement resulting in a splenic weight of 13 000 gm has been reported. The vast majority of lesions are the cavernous type. Most splenic hemangiomas remain asymptomatic; they cause symptoms when they reach sufficient size to encroach on adjacent organs. Spontaneous rupture may occur and has been reported in 25% of Husni's review of 56 cases.

There may be pancytopenia or isolated thrombocytopenia caused by platelet trapping in the cavernous spaces of the lesion. X-ray examination may reveal a soft tumor mass with anterior displacement of the stomach and downward displacement of the kidney and splenic flexure of the colon. CT scan demonstrates an enlarged spleen. The diagnosis can be established by ultrasonography or magnetic resonance imaging (MRI), or by angiography, which demonstrates the "laking" effect in the capillary phase. This is identical to that noted for hepatic hemangiomas. The "laking" effect is often accompanied by early filling of the splenic vein, characteristic of an arteriovenous shunt.

Surgical intervention is not indicted for small, asymptomatic, incidentally detected hemangiomas. The treatment is splenectomy for the larger and symp-

tomatic hemangiomas, including those that have ruptured intraperitoneally. In one series of cases complicated by rupture, 79% survived splenectomy and were cured, 14% died preoperatively, and 7% died postoperatively.

Lymphangioma of the spleen is made up of a malformation of lymphatics and occurs much less frequently than hemangioma. The lesion may be part of a generalized lymphangiomatosis. Cystic spaces of varying sizes containing clear gelatinous fluid may account for a splenic weight of 2000 to 3000 gm. Microscopically, endothelium-lined spaces constitute the major portion of the lesion.

Symptoms, when present, are related to the size of the tumor. CT scan reveals a lesion with a density approximating that of water. Angiography demonstrates splaying of the blood vessels and the absence of lakes, characteristic of hemangiomas. Splenectomy is indicated for symptomatic lesions.

Other benign tumors that have rarely required splenectomy include hamartoma, with fewer than 50 reported cases, and an occasional case of lipoma and fibroma.

PRIMARY MALIGNANT TUMORS

Lymphoma with primary involvement of the spleen is rare. Primary *hemangiosarcoma*, although rare, is now regarded as the most frequent primary malignant tumor of the spleen. Less than 100 cases have been reported. The tumor arises from endothelial or primitive mesenchymal cells. The average weight of the spleen in one series was 1700 gm. The lesions grow rapidly and metastasize to regional lymph nodes, marrow, liver, and lungs. Most patients are middle-aged, and symptoms are related to the mass effect of the lesion, in addition to general weight loss and cachexia, ascites, and pleural effusions. Angiographic findings are similar to those noted for hemangiomas. Splenectomy is indicated but is rarely curative. Four cases of fibrosarcoma of the spleen have also been reported.

METASTATIC TUMORS

Recent autopsy series have refuted the concept that metastases to the spleen are rare. Metastatic involvement of the spleen was present in 9% of autopsy patients with epithelial malignancies. Celiotomy for undiagnosed splenomegaly, however, rarely reveals metastatic deposits in the absence of known, generalized metastases. Rarely, spontaneous rupture of the spleen with consequent intraperitoneal hemorrhage may be owing to metastatic deposits. It is only in this situation that splenectomy may be indicated.

■ HEMATOLOGIC DISORDERS

The role of splenectomy in the management of hematologic disorders has greatly increased in recent years. In general, removal of the spleen in these disorders affects its role in cellular sequestration and destruction and also its role as an immunologic organ. In 1887, Sir Thomas Spencer Wells, the renowned gynecologist, performed a therapeutic splenectomy in a patient with what subsequently proved to be hereditary spherocytosis. The first splenectomy for autoimmune hemolytic anemia was performed in 1911 by Micheli; 6 years later Schloffer, responding to the suggestion of a fourth year medical student, Kaznelson, removed a spleen for idiopathic thrombocytopenic purpura.

ANEMIAS

The two major categories of anemia that benefit from splenectomy are (1) intracellular defects, including membrane abnormalities, enzyme defects, and hemoglobinopathy, and (2) extracellular defects, particularly autoimmune hemolytic anemia.

Hereditary Spherocytosis

Hereditary spherocytosis is a hemolytic anemia caused by an inherited disorder of the red cell membrane; this category also includes hereditary elliptocytosis (ovalocytosis) and stomatocytosis. The disorder is a prime example of a loss of cellular deformity, based on an inherited defect of the red cell membrane resulting in an excessive splenic trapping and consequent hemolysis. In addition to the fundamental abnormality found in the erythrocyte membrane, the cells also demonstrate an increased osmotic fragility; in other words, lysis occurs at a higher than normal concentration of sodium chloride.

The role of the spleen in this disorder is related to the inability of the spherocytes to pass through the splenic pulp. The cells that escape from the spleen are more susceptible to trapping and disintegration during each successive passage. The red cells entering the circulation from the bone marrow in patients with hereditary spherocytosis are normal; they become spherical within the circulation, and the spleen further conditions them by means of its unique environment, making them more spheroidal and susceptible to destruction in subsequent passages through the organ.

Hereditary spherocytosis is transmitted as an autosomal dominant trait and is the most common of the symptomatic familial hemolytic anemias. In rare instances, the disease occurs in patients whose parents appear to be unaffected. Hereditary spherocytosis primarily affects people of European origin and is rare in the black population.

The salient clinical features are anemia, jaundice, and an enlarged spleen. The symptoms and findings may vary greatly in severity, but it is unusual for the anemia to be extremely severe. The jaundice usually parallels the severity of anemia and generally is not intense; it is related to an increased red cell destruction, with the production of amounts of bile pigment that cannot be cleared totally by the liver and, regardless of intensity, is unaccompanied by pruritus or bradycardia. Bile pigment is not present in the urine unless there is associated biliary obstruction by pigmented gallstones or hepatic damage following severe hemolytic crises.

Periodic and sudden increases in the intensity of anemia and jaundice may occur, and this circumstance may be accompanied by abdominal pain, pyrexia, vomiting, and tachycardia. These so-called minor crises often follow intercurrent infections, emotional stress, fatigue, or exposure to cold and may last for a few hours to several days. Occasionally there may be a sudden, sometimes fatal, acute illness representing a major crisis. This usually follows an acute viral infection. The crises are characterized by a marked increase in the severity of the anemia, thrombocytopenia, leukopenia, and increased jaundice. Cholelithiasis has been reported in 60% of patients with hereditary spherocytosis but is unusual in children under 10 years of age. Gallstones usually are of the pigment variety, presumably developing as a result of an increased bilirubin concentration within the bile. Splenomegaly is almost invariable, and it may be the cause of pressure symptoms within the abdomen. Chronic leg ulcers represent an unusual complication; although their pathogenesis has not been defined, they tend to heal quickly after splenectomy.

The diagnosis can be established by an evaluation of a peripheral bloodstream that demonstrates small, spherocytic-shaped erythrocytes that appear thick. The degree of spherocytosis varies from case to case, but usually more than 80% of the red cells demonstrate this characteristic. In most patients, the hematocrit is in the range of 30%, and the reticulocyte count is usually increased to levels between 5% and 20%. The serum bilirubin is rarely greater than 5 mg/dL, and most if it is unconjugated. The red blood cell survival in these patients, as in all patients with hemolytic anemia, is reduced. The normal half-life of the red cell is 25 to 30 days, whereas a half-life of <20 days is indicative of increased hemolysis.

In 1992 Gansslen reported clinical cure following splenectomy in nine patients; his results led to the establishment of this procedure as the principal method of treatment. The results of removal of the spleen in almost all series have been uniformly good and associated with a low operative mortality and morbidity. Within a few days following removal of the spleen, the erythrocytes achieve a normal life span and the intensity of jaundice, if present, is reduced. The morphology of the red cell is not altered as the inherent membrane abnormality persists. An established diagnosis of hereditary spherocytosis is now generally accepted as an indication for splenectomy. Even if the hemolytic process is compensated, the longer it is allowed to continue, the greater the potential for complications such as crises or gallstone formation. There have been differences of opinion regarding the timing of operation, and it is now generally recommended that the procedure be delayed until the fourth year of life. It is appropriate to perform an ultrasound before splenectomy, and the gallbladder should always be examined at the time of operation. If gallstones are present, the gallbladder should be removed at the time of splenectomy. It is also important to search for accessory spleens because this may be the cause of failure to respond to splenectomy in this disease.

Hereditary Elliptocytosis and Other Membrane Defects

Hereditary elliptocytosis (ovalocytosis) is transmitted as a simple Mendelian trait on a gene linked to the Rh blood type. It occurs in approximately 0.04% of the population. Oval erythrocytes constitute up to 25% of the total red cell population in many patients with macro-cytic and hypochromic microcytic anemia. This is also true in patients with sickle cell anemia, thalassemia, and hemoglobin C disease. In patients with hereditary elliptocytosis, however, the oval- and rod-shaped forms constitute about 80% to 90% of the red cell population.

This disorder usually exists as a harmless trait, but in about 12% of the cases there is an active, variably compensated hemolytic anemia. The presence of hemolysis often is a familial characteristic, and it has been suggested that excessive hemolysis occurs only when the gene for elliptocytosis is present in the homozygous form, or is modified in some other way.

The majority of patients with hereditary elliptocytosis are Caucasians and the signs and symptoms are directly related to the severity of the hemolysis. Occasionally an acute hemolytic episode may be precipitated by infection. The clinical syndrome is indistinguishable from that described for hereditary spherocytosis. Gallstones are frequent, and chronic leg ulcers have been reported. The spleen is usually palpably enlarged in symptomatic cases. Diagnosis is established by the smear; Cr-51 studies in symptomatic cases demonstrate decreased red cell survival coupled with splenic sequestration. A reticulocytosis of 20% or higher occurs in patients with overt hemolysis.

Splenectomy is indicated in all symptomatic patients because removal of the organ is almost always followed by lasting effects of decreased hemolysis and corrected anemia, although the morphologic abnormality of the red blood cell remains unchanged. Associated cholelithiasis should be managed as in hereditary spherocytosis.

Hereditary stomatocytosis does not respond as well to splenectomy.

Hereditary Hemolytic Anemia with Red Cell Enzyme Deficiency

This disorder also has been referred to as hereditary nonspherocytic hemolytic anemia. On the basis of auto-hemolysis studies, two forms termed type I and type II have been defined. Type I has been shown to be due to a red cell deficiency of glucose-6-phosphate dehydrogenase (G-6-PD), whereas type II is due to a deficiency of pyruvate-kinase (PK). As a consequence of these enzyme deficiencies, the red cells are unable to utilize glucose at a normal rate, resulting in a disturbed metabolism that renders the cells susceptible to increased hemolysis. Cr 51–tagged red cell studies have demonstrated that the spleen serves as a major site for hemolysis, particularly in patients with PK deficiency.

G-6-PD–deficient hereditary nonspherocytic hemolytic anemia is transmitted as a sex-linked, incompletely dominant factor. PK deficiency is transmitted as a recessive factor affecting both sexes equally, and without racial predominance. Clinically, the two types cannot be differentiated and are usually detected in children who are investigated because of jaundice and anemia. The spleen is rarely enlarged in patients with G-6-PD deficiency, whereas enlargement occurs more frequently with PK deficiency. The survival time of erythrocytes in PK deficiency is reduced to a mean life span averaging approximately half normal, and sometimes the reticulocyte count may be as high as 70%. The reticulocyte count is not increased to the same extent in patients with G-6-PD deficiency. Pigmented gallstones may be associated with both disorders.

Differentiation of the two disorders is important to define therapy. In the G-6-PD deficiency, the rate of hemolysis occurring on incubation of red cells is similar to that of normal cells and, like normal cells, is diminished when glucose is added. With PK deficiency, autohemolysis is greater than normal and is unaffected by the addition of glucose. There are specific screening tests available in most laboratories.

The majority of patients who maintain a hemoglobin greater than 8 g/dL are asymptomatic and do not require therapy. With significant anemia and increasing transfusion requirements, splenectomy should be considered in patients with PK deficiency. The role of splenectomy is not predictable in a given case, and radiolabeled red cell sequestration studies are not accurately predictive of results. Postoperative thrombocytosis may occur if the hemolytic rate is unabated after splenectomy. In some cases this represents a serious sequela that may lead to hepatic, portal, and even caval thrombosis. Thus, the risk–benefit ratio of splenectomy is considerably higher in these disorders than in hereditary membrane disorders.

Heinz Body Hemolytic Anemias (Thalassemia)

The development of intracellular hemoglobin precipitates (Heinz bodies) that damage red cells and contribute to their premature destruction can occur because of thalassemia, unstable hemoglobins, or enzyme deficiencies in the pentose phosphate pathway.

Thalassemia (Mediterranean anemia) is a congenital disorder transmitted as a dominant trait in which the anemia is primarily the result of a defect in hemoglobin synthesis. It has been referred to as Cooley's anemia, erythroblastic anemia, and target-cell anemia. As a consequence of the defect, there are intracellular precipitates (Heinz bodies) that contribute to premature red cell destruction. The hemoglobin-deficient red cells are small, thin, misshapen, and have a characteristic resistance to osmotic lysis.

The disease is classified as alpha, beta, and gamma types, determined by the specific defect in the synthesis rate of the peptide chain. In the United States most patients suffer from beta thalassemia, and there is a quantitative reduction in the rate of beta chain synthesis, resulting in a decrease in the hemoglobin A. The characteristic feature is the persistence of Hb-F and a re-

duction of Hb-A. Gradations of the disease range from heterozygous thalassemia minor to severe homozygous thalassemia major. The latter is manifested by chronic anemia, jaundice, and splenomegaly.

Patients with homozygous thalassemia major usually present with clinical manifestations in the first year of life. In addition to the anemia and consequent pallor, there is usually retarded body growth and enlargement of the head. Intractable leg ulcers may be noted, and intercurrent infections are particularly common. Some patients present with repeated episodes of left upper quadrant pain related to splenic infarction. Cardiac dilatation occurs and, in advance stages, there is subcutaneous edema and effusion into the serous cavities. Intercurrent infections occur frequently, often leading to death in the more severe cases. These infections may be associated with aplastic crises. Gallstones have been reported in up to 24% of cases.

Therapy is directed only at symptomatic patients, those having thalassemia major or intermedia. In these patients, transfusions are usually required at regular intervals. Since most children with thalassemia major accommodate to low hemoglobin levels, transfusions are given when the hemoglobin level is less than 10 g/dL. Although splenectomy does not influence the basic hematologic disorder, it may eliminate or reduce the hemolytic process responsible for accelerated destruction of normal donor red cells within the patient's circulation and thus reduce transfusion requirements. In general the best results associated with splenectomy have been obtained in older children and in young adults with large spleens in whom excessive splenic sequestration of red cells has been demonstrated. Occasionally, splenectomy may be indicated because of mechanical symptoms associated with marked splenomegaly or repeated episodes of abdominal pain owing to splenic infarction.

Patients with homozygous beta thalassemia have an overall increased susceptibility to bacterial infection, but the immunoglobulin levels cannot be demonstrated as consistently abnormal. It is difficult to evaluate the effect of splenectomy per se on the risk of infection in these patients. A review of 130 splenectomized thalassemic patients, in whom the incidence of infection was assessed, revealed that 21 patients developed severe infection following splenectomy, seven of these within 2 years of the operation, and most in a 5 to 10 year period. The majority of studies indicate that there is no difference in the risk of infection before or after operation, and the overall benefit–risk ratio seems to favor the performance of splenectomy when appropriate indications are present.

Sickle Cell Disease

Sickle cell anemia is a hereditary hemolytic anemia, seen predominantly in blacks, and characterized by the presence of crescent-shaped erythrocytes that, because of a lack of deformability, are trapped in the splenic cords. In this disorder, the normal hemoglobin A is replaced by hemoglobin S. Under conditions of reduced oxygen tension, hemoglobin S molecules undergo crystallization within the cell; this, in turn, elongates and distorts the cell. The sickle cells themselves increase the blood viscosity and circulatory stasis, thus establishing a vicious cycle. Sickling occurs so rapidly that blood flow through both the fast and slow compartments of the spleen is obstructed, and, as a consequence, a series of microinfarcts develop. In most adult patients only a fibrous area of the spleen remains, but autosplenectomy is preceded by splenomegaly in about 75% of patients.

In addition to serving as the site of destruction for damage of nondeformable erythrocytes, there are other splenic functional abnormalities in sickle cell anemia. These include (1) an abnormal role that the spleen plays as a red cell reservoir in these patients, (2) a reduced antibody production by the spleen, and (3) reduction in the spleen's ability to filter bacteria, especially streptococccal pneumonia.

There are two situations in sickle cell anemia where the spleen is a pathologic red cell reservoir. The first is a form of chronic hypersplenism that usually occurs in childhood or adolescence and is manifested by reduced red cell survival, leukopenia, and thrombocytopenia. In these patients, for some unknown reason, there is a failure to undergo autosplenectomy, and in this rare circumstance splenectomy will correct the leukopenia and thrombocytopenia and also will decrease the rate of red cell survival. The second abnormality has been termed *acute splenic sequestration* and is marked by sudden splenic enlargement associated with worsening anemia and profound hypotension. It usually occurs in the first five years of life in an SS child; streptococcal pneumonia infection may act as a precipitating event in these patients. The acute splenic sequestration is usually effectively treated with packed red cell transfusion. If there is a propensity for recurrence, splenectomy may be indicated.

Although the sickle cell trait occurs in approximately 9% of the black population, the majority of patients are asymptomatic. Sickle cell anemia is observed in 0.3% to 1.3% of blacks. Depending upon the vessels affected by vascular occlusion, the patients may have bone or joint pain, priapism, neurologic manifestations, or skin ulcers. Abdominal pain and cramps owing to visceral stasis are frequent. Rarely, thrombosis of the splenic vessels may result in the complication of splenic abscess manifested by splenomegaly, splenic pain, and spiking fever.

For most patients with sickle cell anemia, only palliative therapy is available. Recent studies have shown that sodium cyanate will prevent sickling of hemoglobin S. Adequate hydration and partial exchange transfusion may help the crisis. In the circumstance of splenic abscess, incision and drainage of the abscess cavity may be required. Splenectomy is of benefit in only a few patients in whom excessive splenic sequestration of red cells, leukocytes, or platelets can be demonstrated.

Anemias Due to Extracellular Defects

These include fragmentation hemolytic diseases and immune hemolytic anemia. The most frequent cause of fragmentation hemolysis is associated with a regurgitant stream through and around a heart valve prosthesis. Aortic valves are more common sites than mitral valves. Fragmentation also can be the result of microangiopathic disease. In this circumstance, hemolytic anemia results from red cell fragmentation in small blood vessels. Heterogeneous disorders, such as disseminated carcinoma, collagen vascular disease, disseminated intravascular coagulation as associated with abruptio placentae and purpura fulminans, giant hemangiomas, and thrombotic thrombocytopenic purpura, all have sufficient vascular damage to lead to red cell fragmentation within these vessels.

Immune Hemolytic Anemia

This is a disorder in which the life span of presumably normal erythrocytes shortens when exposed to an endogenous hemolytic mechanism. The first description of the disease is credited to Chauffard and Troisier who, in 1908, demonstrated autohemolysins in the serum of several patients with acute hemolytic anemia. Three years later Micheli performed the first planned, successful splenectomy, thus stimulating the application of splenectomy for hematologic disease in general.

The etiology of the disorder has not been defined, but an immune mechanism seems to be fundamental. There is an antibody coating of blood cells that predisposes them to increased phagocytosis by reticuloendolethial cells in the spleen and other organs. IgG antibodies bind to the red cell, and complement becomes fixed. Phagocytosis occurs primarily in the spleen and is initiated by the binding of the Fc portion of the IgG molecule to the corresponding macrophage surface Fc receptor. In this process, phagocytosis may be partial and remove only a portion of the red cell membrane, but it results in spherocytes that have increased rigidity and are more sensitive to destruction in the splenic microcirculation.

The diagnosis of immune hemolytic anemia is made in a patient with anemia and reticulocytosis who has a positive antiglobulin test. The direct antiglobulin reaction (Coombs' test) is characteristically positive, but recently Coombs-negative reactions in these patients have been reported. Both warm and cold antibodies have been described. Warm antibodies, which react best at 37° C, occur more frequently. They are "incomplete" antibodies because they produce agglutination of normal erythrocytes when exposed to antiglobulin serum but do not cause agglutination in a saline medium. Cold antibodies are potentiated by temperatures below 37° C and act as "complete" agglutinating antibodies.

Although immune hemolytic anemia may occur or be encountered at any age, it is more frequent after 50 years of age and occurs twice as often in females. The onset may be insidious, and the course of the disease may be chronic. The disease, however, may develop abruptly and be fulminant; chills, fever, backache, and other symptoms of rapid blood destruction may occur. The acute cases occasionally develop as a complication of viral illnesses.

Symptoms and signs vary with the severity of the hemolytic process, and mild jaundice is often present. The spleen is palpably enlarged in half the cases, and gallstones are demonstrated in one-quarter of the cases. In the most severe cases, patients may have hemoglobinuria followed by renal tubular necrosis. The diagnosis of hemolysis is made by demonstrating anemia and reticulocytosis, accompanied by increased products of red cell destruction in the blood, urine, and stool. The distinguishing feature of the disease is the demonstration by direct and indirect Coombs' test of an autoantibody on the patient's own red cells, in the patient's serum, or in both. Platelets are usually normal, but occasionally autoimmune hemolytic anemia and idiopathic thrombocytopenic purpura occur together (Evans' syndrome).

In some patients the disorder tends to run an acute, self-limited course. Steroids constitute the first approach to patients requiring therapy. In the "warm" antibody–immune hemolytic anemias, splenectomy should be considered (1) if the steroids have been ineffective, (2) if excessive doses of steroids are required to maintain remission, (3) if toxic manifestations of steroids become apparent, and (4) if steroids are contraindicated for other reasons. A favorable response to splenectomy is anticipated in about 80% of selected splenectomized patients. The demonstration of excessive splenic sequestration of Cr 51–tagged red cells offers a guide to the selection of patients who may respond to splenectomy. More important than splenic sequestration alone is the ratio of spleen–liver sequestration; ratios greater than 2:1 and preferably 3:1 usually indicate a favorable response to splenectomy. Using these criteria, improvement following splenectomy has risen to approximately 80%. Splenectomy is rarely beneficial in diseases associated with cold antibodies.

PURPURAS

Idiopathic Thrombocytopenic Purpura

Idiopathic thrombocytopenic purpura (immune thrombocytopenic purpura) (ITP), the most common hematologic indication for splenectomy, is an acquired disorder characterized by destruction of platelets exposed to circulating IgG antiplatelet factors. It is known that the spleen is the source of IgG specific for platelets; following splectomy in these patients there is a normalization of platelet-associated IgG levels. In ITP, the spleen is also an important organ for platelet destruction by macrophagic phagocytosis. The fact that 30% of circulating platelets are in the spleen at all times provides a high concentration upon which a high antiplatelet antibody concentration of the spleen can act.

Female patients outnumber males 3:1. The most common presenting sign is petechiae or ecchymosis or both; bleeding gums, vaginal bleeding, mild gastrointestinal (GI) bleeding, and hematuria also may occur. In some patients, the purpuric manifestations take an almost cyclic course, with exacerbations occurring at the time of the onset of menses. The incidence of central nervous system bleeding ranges between 2% and 4% and usually occurs early in the course of disease. The spleen is rarely palpable.

The platelet count is generally less than 50 000/mm^3 and at times approaches 0. With markedly reduced platelet counts the bleeding time may be prolonged, but the clotting time remains normal. There is usually no significant anemia or leukopenia, with the exception of the uncommon circumstance in which there is combined autoimmune hemolytic anemia. Bone marrow reveals a normal or increased number of megakaryocytes.

Idiopathic thrombocytopenic purpura in children has an excellent prognosis and rarely requires surgical intervention. In adults, the disease is usually more persistent and a sustained response to steroid therapy occurs in only about 15% of cases. Between 75% and 80% of patients subjected to splenectomy, however, respond permanently and require no further steroid therapy. In most patients the platelet count rises to over 100 000/mm^3 in 7 days. Rarely, return to normal can take months. A positive effect of splenectomy is noted even in those patients in whom the platelet count does not return to normal because recurrent bleeding rarely takes place.

Steroids constitute the initial form of therapy. Some patients respond to plasmapheresis and/or infusions of high doses of gammaglobulin. Splenectomy should be performed in patients who have not responded to glucocorticoid treatment within 6 weeks or who have responded to glucocorticoids and then have become thrombocytopenic when the dosage is reduced. Rarely, either intracranial bleeding or profound gastrointestinal (GI) hemorrhage may require intensive intravenous corticoid treatment and emergency splenectomy.

Failure to respond to glucocorticoids does not indicate that splenectomy will be unsuccessful and should not disuade one from performing splenectomy. Radioactive chromium–labeled platelet sequestration studies are of little practical value in selecting patients. Platelet transfusions are never given preoperatively and are reserved for an occasional patient who continues to bleed diffusely following removal of the spleen. In patients undergoing splenectomy for ITP, a careful search should be made for accessory spleens, present in 18% to 30% of these patients. Rudowski reported 15 patients with ITP who underwent reoperation for persistent or recurrent thrombocytopenia coupled with an accessory spleen that had been defined by technetium scan. In 13 of these cases, the accessory spleen was found and removed. The platelet count became normal in 12 of the 13, and recurrent bleeding did not develop in the remaining patient.

Either ITP or immune hemolytic disease may proceed to or be concomitant with the manifestations of systemic lupus erythematosus. The indications for splenectomy in these patients are the same as in the idiopathic diseases. The majority of patients with systemic lupus erythematosus who are operated on specifically for thrombocytopenia respond with elevation of platelet counts. Patients with the acquired immune deficiency syndrome (AIDS) have an increased incidence of ITP that responds equally well to splenectomy.

Thrombotic Thrombocytopenic Purpura

Thrombotic thrombocytopenic purpura (TTP) is a disease of the arterioles or capillaries that undergo widespread, subintimal hyalinization and consequent occlusion. It is associated with marked trapping of platelets, particularly in the spleen (Fig 76–12). The etiology has not been defined precisely, but immune mechanisms have been suggested. Approximately 5% of reported cases occur during pregnancy.

A pentad of clinical features is present in virtually all cases and consists of fever, purpura, hemolytic anemia, varied neurologic manifestations, and signs of renal disease. Splenomegaly has been reported in approximately 20% of cases. Pertinent laboratory findings include anemia, reticulocytosis, thrombocytopenia, leukocytosis, elevated serum bilirubin, proteinuria, hematuria, and azotemia. The peripheral blood smear reveals pleomorphic normochromic red cells that are fragmented and distorted and may include triangular cells, helmet cells, schistocytes, and polychromatic macrocytes. The degree of thrombocytopenia varies during the course of the illness, with a profound decrease in platelets often developing within hours of onset.

The majority of patients with this disease experience a rapid onset and fulminant course. Recovery has been

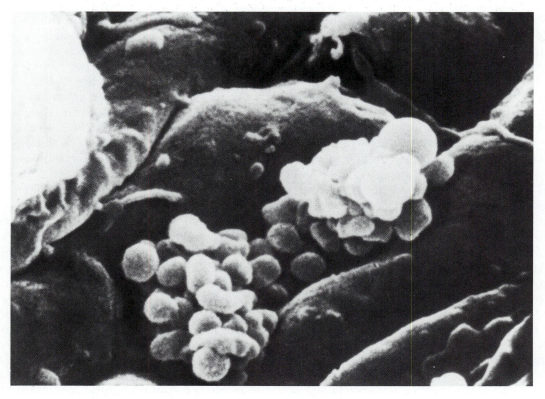

Figure 76–12. Electron microscopic scan of spleen removed from patient with ITP. Note clumping of platelets.

reported for patients treated with heparin, exchange transfusions, fresh blood, dextran, antimetabolites, and massive doses of steroids. Most patients are now managed by plasmapheresis. The combination of plasmapheresis and splenectomy has achieved a high degree of success.

OTHER HYPERSPLENIC DISORDERS

Secondary Hypersplenism

Pancytopenia may be a consequence of portal hypertension. Thrombocytopenia is present in approximately one-third of patients with portal hypertension resulting from schistosomiasis and in one-fourth of patients with portal hypertension resulting from nutritional cirrhosis. The portal hypertension results in delayed passage and engorgement of the vascular spaces within the spleen, which, in turn, leads to accelerated destruction of the circulating cells as they course through the organ.

Hypersplenism per se is rarely an indication for operative intervention in patients with portal hypertension. Splenectomy alone generally will not permanently reduce portal hypertension in patients in whom the primary disorder is cirrhosis. Splenectomy, however, may be curative of portal hypertension in patients with isolated splenic vein thrombosis or myeloid metaplasia. In patients who undergo a decompressive procedure for bleeding esophagogastric varices, regardless of the procedure performed, the hypersplenism usually is corrected.

In patients with lymphomas and chronic lymphocytic leukemia, splenectomy is carried out when the organ is sufficiently enlarged to cause symptoms, or when cytopenia is severe while the marrow is apparently adequate. In patients with very large spleens and chronic lymphocytic leukemia, improvement may be substantive even with reduced numbers of hematopoietic cells in the marrow. In these patients, the hematologic response is favorable in the majority of patients subjected to splenectomy. In most patients the neutropenia and thrombocytopenia are improved, and the hemolytic response is controlled. There is little evidence that splenectomy alters the course of chronic myelogenous leukemia, but is may be applicable in an occasional patient whose platelet count is markedly reduced. Splenectomy improves cytopenia and survival in patients with hairy cell leukemia, particularly if there is splenomegaly. Splenectomy is now regarded as secondary therapy for this disease because patients without splenomegaly and few hairy cells in the peripheral blood smear do well without any treatment.

Splenectomy offers significant increase in the neutrophil count in neutropenic patients with Felty's syndrome (splenomegaly, neutropenia, arthralgia) but is generally reserved for neutropenic patients with serious or recurrent infections, increasing transfusion requirements, or marked thrombocytopenia. The arthralgia is not affected, but leg ulcers, when present, usually heal. Similarly, although splenectomy does not alter the course of the disease in sarcoidosis or Gaucher's disease, it may play a palliative role for patients with symptomatic splenomegaly and may be indicated for control of secondary hypersplenism. In children with Gaucher's disease, partial splenectomy has been performed to reverse the hypersplenism and to reduce the incidence of postsplenectomy sepsis.

Porphyria erythropoietica, a congential disorder of pyrrole metabolism, is characterized by excessive deposition of porphyrins in tissue, photosensitivity, and bullous dermatitis. Red cell destruction in the spleen results in anemia that is improved by splenectomy. Systemic mast cell disease (SMCD) is manifested by urticaria pigmentosa and mast cell infiltration of tissues. Splenectomy may be indicated for severe thrombocytopenia to permit chemotherapy.

MYELOPROLIFERATIVE DISORDERS

The myeloproliferative disorders, including myeloid metaplasia and myelofibrosis, represent panproliferative processes manifested by increased connective tissue proliferation of the bone marrow, liver, spleen, and lymph nodes and a simultaneous proliferation of hematopoietic elements in the liver, spleen, and long bones. The disease is closely related to polycythemia vera, idiopathic thrombocytosis, and myelogenous leukemia. The presenting symptoms are symptomatic splenomegaly and anemia.

The laboratory hallmark is a peripheral smear that demonstrates red cell fragmentation and shows many immature forms of numerous teardrop and elongated shapes. The white blood count is in the range of 50 000/mm^3 and may reach extremely high levels. Immature myeloid cells are found in the peripheral smear. Thrombocytopenia is present in about one-third of the patients and thrombocytosis, with white blood counts of >1 million, is observed in about one-fourth of the patients.

Although splenectomy does not alter the course of the disease, the procedure is indicated for the control of anemia and for increasing transfusional requirements, leukopenia, or thombocytopenia, in addition to the symptoms attributable to splenomegaly. The spleen may reach very large proportions in patients with myeloproliferative disorders. The mortality and morbidity rates for patients with myleoid metaplasia who undergo splenectomy are higher than those reported for splenectomy for other hematologic disorders. Postoperative thrombocytosis or thrombosis of the splenic vein extending to the portal and mesenteric veins occurs more commonly in these patients. The incidence of this complication can be reduced by using alkylating agents preoperatively and employing drugs to prevent platelet aggregation and thrombosis during the perioperative period.

Portal hypertension has been described as being due either to hepatic involvement of sufficient degree to be obstructive to the portal circulation or to an increased forward blood flow through the splenoportal system. In the latter circumstance splenectomy alone effects a significant reduction in portal hypertension and has resulted in disappearance of varices. In this group of patients, it is appropriate to measure pressure in an omental vein before splenectomy; if portal hypertension is defined, the pressure should be measured once again subsequent to removal of the organ, in order to define the etiology of portal hypertension, ie, hepatic sinuosidal obstruction or increased afferent flow.

HODGKIN'S DISEASE

In addition to the role that splenectomy plays in the palliation of patients with Hodgkin's disease who have symptomatic splenomegaly or hypersplenism, removal of the spleen as part of a diagnostic laparotomy functions significantly in the definition of the extent of Hodgkin's disease.

The diagnosis of Hodgkin's disease is generally established by histologic evaluation of a clinically suspect area of lymphadenopathy or splenomegaly. The possible sites of involvement include the cervical supraclavicular nodes, mediastinal nodes, axillary nodes, iliac and ileofemoral nodes, periaortic nodes, and the spleen itself. In the overwhelming majority of patients suspected of Hodgkin's disease, the diagnosis is substantiated by a peripheral node biopsy.

Although the predominant neoplastic cell appears to be a histocytic type, the typical large multinucleated cell, traditionally called the Sternberg-Reed cell, is regarded as essential for the diagnosis. Currently, four major histologic types have been categorized: (1) lymphocyte predominant, (2) nodular sclerosing, (3) mixed cellularity, and (4) lymphocyte depletion. Lymphocyte-predominant lesions have the lowest incidence of mediastinal and abdominal involvement; nodular sclerosing lesions demonstrate a distinct predilection for cervical, mediastinal, and abdominal nodes. The 5 year survival rate for patients with lymphocyte predominance approaches 90%; those with lymphocyte depletion and a mixed cellularity have a 5 year survival of 40%. Nodular sclerosing lesions are associated with an intermediate survival time.

The application of celiotomy, splenectomy, liver biopsy, retroperitoneal and hepatoduodenal node biopsy, in addition to marrow biopsy, as diagnostic tools for Hodgkin's disease, is based on several considerations.

The first is that the lesion usually begins as a single focus and spreads in a predictable manner along adjacent lymphoid channels. The second is that therapy may be dictated by the stage. The third, and most important, is that previous methods of evaluating the stage, including physical examination, laboratory studies, and radiologic studies, have significant indices of inaccuracy.

Stage I Hodgkin's disease is limited to one anatomic area, either one lymph node region or a localized extralymphatic organ or site. In stage II there is involvement of two or more lymph node regions on the same side of the diaphragm, or solitary involvement of an extralymphatic organ or site and one or more lymph node regions on the same side of the diaphragm. In stage III there is involvement of lymph node regions on both sides of the diaphragm, which may also be accompanied by involvement of the spleen (IIIs). In stage IV there is diffuse or disseminated involvement of one or more extralymphatic organs or tissues, with or without associated lymph node involvement. Each stage is divided into two groups: A, based on the absence of specific symptoms, and B, based on the presence of fever, night sweats, or weight loss >10% of normal body weight.

The definition of intra-abdominal areas involved by Hodgkin's disease is difficult, as clinical appraisal of this region is, at best, imprecise. Neither periaortic nor iliac nodes are generally palpable, and the palpability of both the liver and spleen is related, to a large extent, to the habitus of the patient as well as to the organ size. More important, it is now well established that both splenic and hepatic involvement may occur in the absence of specific organomegaly. Liver function tests and scintillation scanning procedures only infrequently provide unequivocal evidence of hepatic involvement. Inferior venacavography, CT, and lymphangiography have been applied to define infradiaphragmatic nodal involvement.

Surgical staging was introduced in 1968 at the Stanford University Medical Center. Since that time there have been several studies demonstrating a lack of correlation between clinical assessment and subsequent operative and histopathologic findings. The spleen was involved by Hodgkin's disease in 39% of patients explored; in half of these it was the only site of intra-abdominal involvement. Preoperative determinations of splenic involvement based on palpability or radiographic and isotopic splenomegaly have proved to be imprecise. There has been approximately 30% error relying on these indices; spleens that had been adjudged clinically normal proved to have involvement with Hodgkin's disease. Conversely, spleens that were thought to be abnormal failed to demonstrate involvement with Hodgkin's histologically, in approximately 38% of cases. Forty percent of patients thought to have hepatic involvement, based on hepatomegaly or abnor-

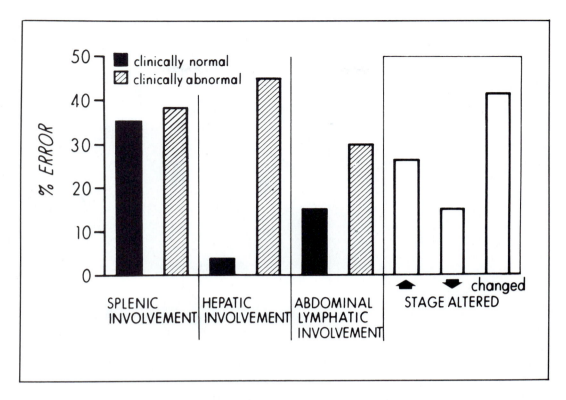

Figure 76–13. Correlation between operative "staging" and clinical assessment. (From Schwartz SI, Cooper RA Jr. Surgery in diagnostic and treatment of Hodgkin's disease. In: *Advances in Surgery,* vol 6, Chicago IL: Medical Year Book; 1972)

mal liver function tests, proved to have no evidence of Hodgkin's disease in the organ, while approximately 4% of patients whose livers were normal clinically, based on function studies, had Hodgkin's disease involvement. The preoperative assessment of lymphatic involvement by CT or lymphangiography has an index of error of approximately 15% with normal preoperative studies, and 30% of those lymph nodes thought to be involved proved to have no involvement. Overall, operative staging of Hodgkin's disease has altered the stage in 43% of cases, increasing it in approximately 28% of cases and decreasing it in 14% (Fig 76–13).

There is disagreement regarding the applicability of operative staging for Hodgkin's disease. The consensus is presently that with lymphocyte-predominant lesions and no evidence of mediastinal involvement, staging is not applicable. With nodular sclerosing lesions that clinically are staged IA and IIA, surgical staging is considered appropriate.

In reference to the routine staging for non-Hodgkin's lymphoma, a difference of opinion also pertains. Veronesi and associates conclude that diagnostic laparotomy and staging should be carried out in centers in which the information can be translated into aggressive treatment but believe that it should not have the wide adoption that Hodgkin's staging has had. Chabner

and associates reported that percutaneous and peritoneoscopically directed biopsies were reasonable alternatives to staging for non-Hodgkin's lymphoma and that the presence or absence of subdiaphragmatic disease could be established in >80% of the patients by nonsurgical procedures, including lymphangiography, marrow biopsy, and percutaneous liver biopsy. The yield of staging procedures was highest in patients with nodular lymphomas and lowest in patients with histiocytic lymphomas.

Surgical Staging

A variety of incisions may be used. Generally, a long subcostal incision, approximately two fingerbreadths below the left costal margin, extending from a point just to the right of the midline to a point above the anterior iliac crest, will facilitate dissection of the lower periaortic and iliac nodes. A midline incision is preferable when ovariopexy to preserve ovarian function is performed. The iliac crest marrow biopsy is taken through a separate incision, using an osteotome.

After the peritoneal cavity is entered, the liver is first assessed for grossly apparent lesions, and a wedge biopsy is performed in both the left and right lobes. We no longer do needle biopsies in addition to the wedge biopsy because we have never experienced a case in

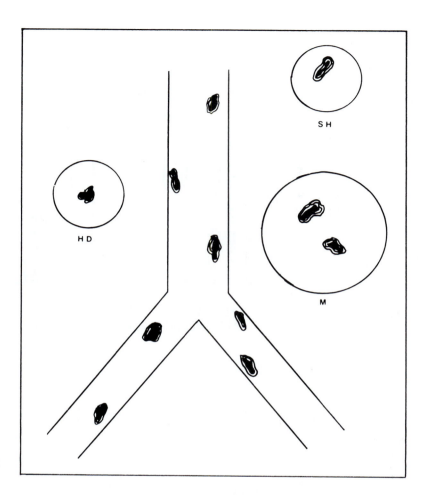

Figure 76–14. Mapping of nodes excised during Hodgkin's staging. HD: hepatoduodenal ligament; SH: splenic hilus; M: mesentery.

which needle biopsy results were positive in the face of negative wedge biopsy results. Both wedge biopsies should be carried out before general abdominal exploration and before retractors are placed on the liver, in order to avoid confusion of histologic evaluation because prolonged application of the retractor rapidly results in cellular infiltration.

Attention is next directed to removing the spleen. The splenectomy is carried out in the fashion described later. In most instances, lesions can be defined on gross examination. If marked adenopathy limits the dissection of hilar vessels, it may be expeditious to enter the lesser sac through the gastrocolic omentum and to ligate the vessels more centrally as they course along the superior surface of the pancreas.

The biopsy sites for periaortic nodes may be selected by palpation at laparotomy or based on the finding of CT or lymphangiography. Representative nodes from areas that either look or feel suspicious should be removed, and these areas should be marked with clips. The nodes should be sent for pathologic study sepa-

rately, with their locations indicated. This can be facilitated by drawing a map on a piece of paper and submitting the nodes positioned on the map to the pathologist (Fig 76–14). Because the greatest yield is from the region of the twelfth thoracic and first lumbar vertebrae, the colon is retracted craniad in all instances, and the ligament of Treitz is transected to provide ready access to the upper retroperitoneum (Fig 76–15). The retroperitoneal incision is carried down to the bifurcation of the iliac vessels and may be extended into the pelvis, if nodes are palpable in that region. Biopsy of representative mesenteric nodes is also done. It is imperative that a representative node be removed from the hepatoduodenal ligament because cases have been recorded in which nodes in this region were involved in the absence of other nodal involvement.

In young females, ovariopexy by suturing the ovaries to one another in the midline, posterior to the uterus, preserves ovarian function by obviating subsequent radiation damage to these organs.

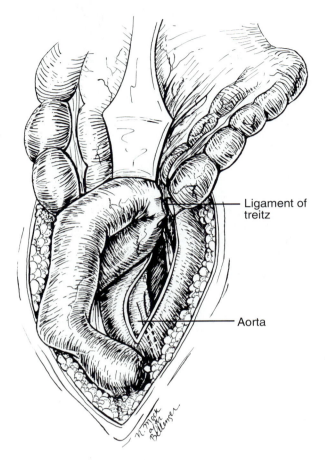

Figure 76–15. Retroperitoneal node dissection. The ligament of Treitz has been transected to permit exposure of T12 and L1 area, which provides the highest yield of suspicious nodes. (From Schwartz SI, Cooper RA Jr, Surgery in the diagnostic and treatment of Hodgkin's disease. In: *Advances in Surgery*, vol 6, Chicago IL. Medical Year Book 1972)

Ligament of treitz

Aorta

■ SPLENECTOMY

PREOPERATIVE PREPARATION

In most instances, there is no specific treatment required for the preoperative management of patients undergoing splenectomy. Patients with a past history of multiple transfusions and those with autoimmune hemolytic anemia may require a longer preoperative stay because of difficulties in blood typing and cross-matching. Platelets should not be administered preoperatively to patients with idiopathic thrombocytopenic purpura because these cells will not survive. In those patients with myeloproliferative disorders who have a tendency to develop thrombosis, it is beneficial to medicate the patient with low-dose heparin, 5000 units twice daily, and aspirin on the day before surgery, and to continue this regimen for 5 days postoperatively. In elective cases, Pneumovax and *Haemophilus Influenzae* vaccine are administered approximately 10 days to 2 weeks before op-

eration and, in emergency cases, it is given immediately preoperatively. A nasogastric tube is used during the operation to decompress the stomach and to facilitate ligation of the short gastric veins. The tube can be inserted intraoperatively and removed immediately at the end of the procedure.

OPERATIVE TECHNIQUE

A variety of incisions may be used, depending upon the nature of the disease and the personal preference of the surgeon. They include upper midline incision, left paramedian incision, and left oblique subcostal incision, which may be extended to the right upper quadrant as a "hockey-stick" and a combined abdominothoracic approach.

The midline incision is the one most applicable in cases of suspected rupture of the spleen, because it is made rapidly and affords satisfactory access to the spleen and other viscera that may have been traumatized. This incision generally is preferred when splenectomy is performed as part of a staging procedure in order to facilitate dissection of the lower para-aortic and iliac nodes and ovariopexy.

The left paramedian incision is preferred by many surgeons. The left rectus muscle is retracted laterally. The incision should reach to, or extend beyond, the costal margin craniad and about 5 cm below the umbilicus caudad. A variant of this incision is the left vertical muscle-splitting incision, which divides the inner portion of the left rectus muscle in a vertical plane, starting at the costal margin itself and extending down below the level of the umbilicus.

This author's preference is the left oblique subcostal incision, which should begin to the right of the midline and proceed obliquely outward and downward about two fingerbreadths below the costal margin. In the case of patients with ITP and small spleens, the oblique muscles do not have to be divided. With larger spleens, the oblique muscles are divided in the course of their fibers laterally, and if additional exposure is required, a "hockey-stick" extension is used transecting the right rectus muscle.

In the case of marked splenomegaly with significant diaphragmatic adhesions, some surgeons have advised a thoracoabdominal incision with the patient's left side elevated between 45° and 60°. The incision represents an extension from a transverse left upper quadrant incision into the eighth intercostal space, transecting the eighth costal cartilage and dividing the diaphragm. It is this author's opinion that this incision should be avoided because it is associated with a higher incidence of morbidity. We have been able to remove spleens as large as 7.5 kg (17 lb) through a left subcostal incision extended into the right upper quadrant.

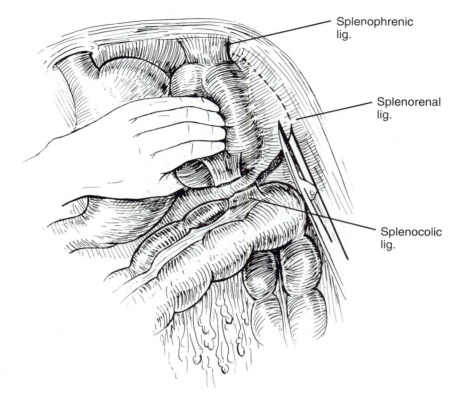

Splenophrenic lig.

Splenorenal lig.

Splenocolic lig.

Figure 76–16. Transection of ligamentous attachments. (From Schwartz SI, Splenectomy and splenorrhaphy. In: *Modern Techics in Surgery.* Mount Kisco, NY: Futura; 1980)

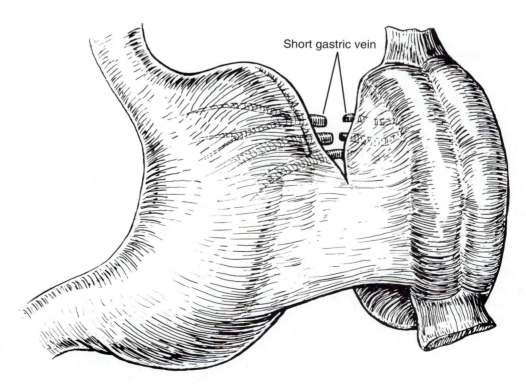

Short gastric vein

Figure 76–17. Ligation of short gastric veins. (From Schwartz SI, Splenectomy and splenorrhaphy. In: *Modern Techics in Surgery.* Mount Kisco, NY: Futura; 1980)

Usually splenectomy is performed by a technique of mobilization and dissection down to an ultimate pedicle of splenic artery and vein. Exploration with the right hand, following the convex surface of the organ, will define the extent of ligamentous attachments. In the case of splenic trauma, a hematoma frequently has dissected these attachments and rapid delivery of the organ into the wound is facilitated. In the case of elective splenectomy, the first step is transection of the ligamentous attachments (Fig 76–16). This includes the splenophrenic ligament at the superior pole and the splenocolic and splenorenal ligaments at the inferior pole posteriorly. Once the splenophrenic ligament has been completely transected, the spleen can be sufficiently mobilized to identify, and to permit interruption of, two or three short gastric veins that run from the spleen to the greater curvature of the stomach (Fig 76–17). It is important not to incorporate the gastric wall in these ligations. If there is any question of this circumstance, a Lembert suture should be placed in the gastric wall to cover the area with serosa and to avoid the complication of gastric fistulization.

After the ligamentous attachments and short gastric vessels have been transected, dissection is directed toward the hilus of the spleen. The inferior pole of the spleen may be attached to the stomach by a gastrosplenic ligament that requires transection. Once this is divided, all that remains are the main splenic artery and vein. With small spleens, such as those encountered in patients with ITP, the three-clamp method of Federoff has been advocated by Maingot (Fig 76–18). It is generally preferable, however, in all instances, and certainly in the case of an enlarged spleen, to individually ligate the splenic artery or arterial branches and splenic vein or venous branches. The splenic artery is managed by the technique of double ligation and suture ligature (Fig 76–19). In the case of myeloid metaplasia, with markedly enlarged spleens, it is frequently necessary to use a vascular clamp on the splenic vein and to close the lumen with a continuous vascular suture.

It is during the hilar dissection that care must be taken to avoid damage to the tail of the pancreas. If the tail of the pancreas has been transected inadvertently, the anterior and posterior capsule should be approximated with nonabsorbable suture material. In rare circumstances in which adhesions apparently preclude safe delivery of the spleen into the wound by means of transecting the ligamentous attachments, the lesser sac is entered through the greater omental fold, and the splenic vessels are individually isolated, ligated, and divided before attempting to deliver the spleen into the wound (Fig 76–20).

Following removal of the spleen, hemostasis is checked in three major areas: the inferior surface of the diaphragm, the greater curvature of the stomach in the region of the short gastric vessels, and the region of the hilus. This is readily accomplished, inserting two Mikulicz pads into the left upper quadrant and first exerting downward and medial traction on the stomach and hilar region. This permits visualization of the undersurface of the diaphragm. The pads are then moved caudad to permit visualization of the greater curvature of the stomach and the short gastric vessels that have been divided. The final step is uncovering the hilar dissection to determine any evidence of bleeding.

If the tail of the pancreas has not been injured, drainage is not performed on a routine basis. It has been our policy to drain the subphrenic region in patients with myeloproliferative disorders and markedly enlarged spleens accompanied by evidence of portal hypertension and collateralization of the ligamentous attachment. In this circumstance, we have used soft, rubber drains exiting through a stab wound into a closed-system Hollister bag. If the tail of the pancreas has been inadvertently injured, a sump drain is brought out through a stab wound.

An integral part of the procedure of splenectomy for hematologic disease consists of a thorough laparotomy to identify accessory spleens that must be removed. These are present in 18% to 30% of patients with hematologic disease. The more common locations of the accessory spleens are in the region of the hilus and the gastrosplenic ligament, gastrocolic ligament, and the greater omentum, mesentery, and presacral space. Accessory spleens have been found in juxtaposition to the left ovary and left testicle. The overwhelming majority of accessory spleens are located in the region of the splenic hilus (Fig 76–4).

Partial Splenectomy

After complete mobilization of the spleen, the hilar vessels to the segment to be removed are ligated and divided. Demarcation of the devascularized segment defines the line of parenchymal dissection. After this segment has been removed, hemostasis of the remaining raw surface is achieved with argon coagulation, microfibrillar collagen, or oxydized cellulose. At least 30% of the spleen should be preserved.

SPLENORRHAPHY AND AUTOTRANSPLANTATION

The techniques to preserve splenic tissue and function are dictated by the extent of damage. Small lacerations can be managed by compression and the application of a hemostatic agent, such as oxidized cellulose, or micronized collagen (Fig 76–21). Hemostasis associated with significant disruptions of the splenic capsule and parenchyma can generally be managed with absorbable sutures that traverse the capsule and incorporate the parenchyma. In this circumstance, the horizontal mat-

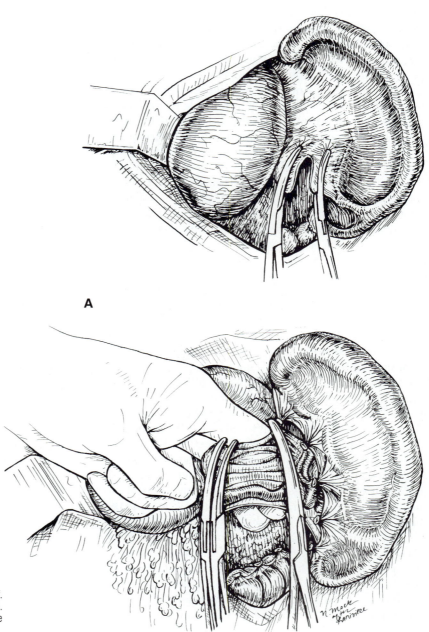

A

B

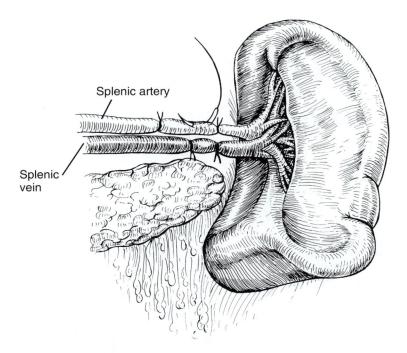

Splenic artery

Splenic
vein

Figure 76–19. Management of hilus. (From Schwartz SI, Splenectomy and splenorrhaphy. In: *Modern Technics in Surgery*. Mount Kisco, NY: Futura;1980)

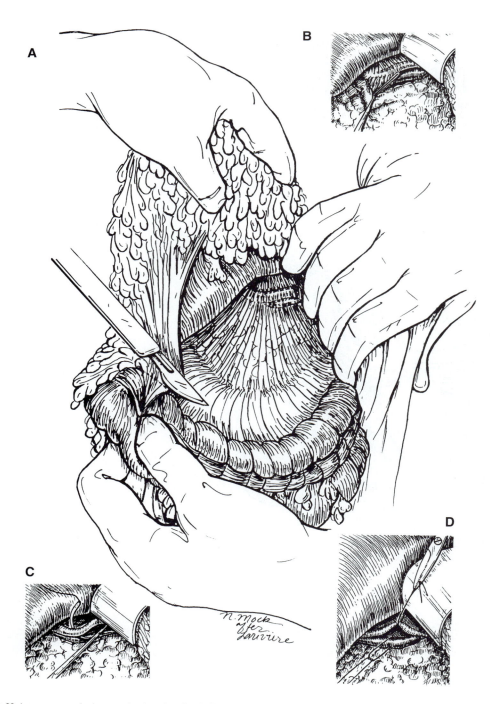

Figure 76–20. In some cases of splenomegaly where the spleen is firmly attached to the diaphragm by numerous adhesions, this approach through the omental bursa to the splenic artery and vein (above the superior border of the pancreas) is sometimes selected. The splenic artery and vein should be cautiously dissected free from their bed before applying silk ligatures proximally and distally to them (firmly but not too tightly) and then dividing each vessel between the ligatures. Following this procedure, the bulky tethered spleen is carefully mobilized from the diaphragm, tail of the pancreas, stomach, and colon before ligating its pedicle once again and removing the organ.

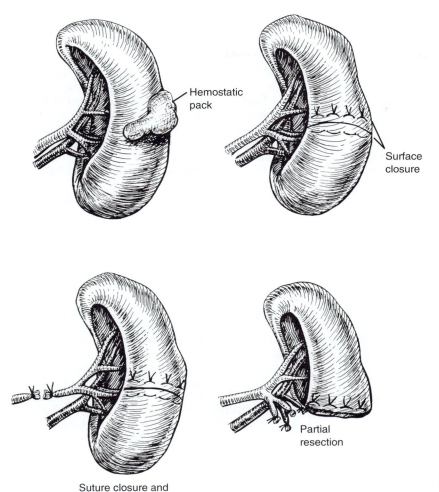

Figure **76–21.** Preservation of traumatized spleen. (From Schwartz SI, Splenectomy and splenorrhaphy. In: *Modern Technics in Surgery*. Mount Kisco, NY: Futura;1980)

tress suture is advantageous because it minimizes cutting through tissue. In the case of more profound bleeding, the splenic artery can be ligated in the hilus, following which the transcapsular suture is inserted and tied. If trauma is localized to one pole of the spleen, this area should be resected and the edges approximated with a series of mattress sutures. The omentum may be used to fill large defects, or to suture over the injury site to provide tamponade.

In order to determine which of these techniques is applicable, and to effect the splenic repair and preservation, it is essential that the ligamentous attachments are transected to permit mobilization of the organ and thorough inspection of all surfaces.

In the event of trauma sufficient to require splenectomy, some investigators have reported salutory effect with implantation. The spleen is cut into slices that are approximately 0.5 cm in diameter, and these slices then are placed in an omental pocket so that there is drainage into the portal venous system. Viability of these implants has been demonstrated, and the tuftsin, opsonin complement, and IgM levels have all returned to normal. Most authors have shown that the combination of lack of sufficient tissue mass and the development of a vascularization distinctly different from the normal splenic circulation preclude adequate phagocytosis of encapsulated bacteria.

COMPLICATIONS

Early postoperative bleeding must be closely monitored, particularly in patients with thrombocytopenia or myeloproliferative disorders. In these patients it is an error to indict hematologic abnormalities as the cause of bleeding, and it is generally safer to reexplore the patients early and to evacuate a hematoma to reduce the incidence of subphrenic abscess. The most common site of bleeding is a short gastric vessel. Left lower lobe atelectasis is another complication; it occurs more frequently following splenectomy than other abdominal procedures. Much has been written about the incidence of deep venous thrombosis following splenectomy, but most large series have not substantiated this finding. In unusual cases, the platelet count may rise to very high levels, at times greater than 2 million/mm^3, but no specific therapy other than hydration is generally indicated. If medical therapy is thought to be appropriate, a drug that inhibits platelet aggregation, such as acetylsalicylic acid or dipyridamole, can be used. Thrombosis of the splenic vein, with extension into the portal vein and superior mesenteric vein, is an extremely rare complication, occurring mostly in patients with myeloproliferative disorders or in those with sepsis as a consequence of intra-abdominal abscess.

The increased incidence of fulminant sepsis related to *pneumococcus* or to *H influenzae* following splenectomy is an established fact, but it occurs more commonly in patients who are immunosuppressed or have diseases with a propensity for infection. All patients subjected to splenectomy should be treated with Pneumovax, and younger patients should receive long-term antibiotic prophylaxis against *H influenzae* sepsis until they reach adulthood.

SELECTED READINGS

Akwari OE, Itani KMF, et al. Splenectomy for primary and recurrent immune thrombocytopenic purpura (ITP): current criteria for patient selection and results. *Ann Surg* 1987; 206:529

Albrechtsen D, Ly B. Complications after therapeutic splenectomy for hematologic disease in adults. *Acta Chir Scand* 1980;146:577

Babb RR. Aneurysm of the splenic artery. *Arch Surg* 1976; 111:924

Barnhart MI, Lusher JM. Structural physiology of the human spleen. *Am J Pediatr Hematol Oncol* 1979;1:311

Barnhart MI, Lusher JM. The human spleen as revealed by scanning electron microscopy. *Am J Hematol* 1976;1:243

Benbassat J, Gilon D, Penchas S. The choice between splenectomy and medical treatment in patients with advanced agnogenic myeloid metaplasia. *Am J Hematol* 1990;33:128

Bernard RP, Bauman AW, et al. Splenectomy for thrombotic thrombocytopenic purpura. *Ann Surg* 1969;169:616

Boxer MA, Braun J, et al. Thromboembolic risk of postsplenectomy thrombocytosis. *Arch Surg* 1978;113:808

Broe PJ, Conley CL, et al. Thrombosis of the portal vein following splenectomy for myeloid metaplasia. *Surg Gynecol Obstet* 1981;152:488

Buntain WL, Lynn HB. Splenorrhaphy: changing concepts for the traumatized spleen. *Surgery* 1979;86:748

Cannon WB, Nelson TS. Staging of Hodgkin's disease: a surgical perspective. *Am J Surg* 1976;132:224

Chabner BA, Johsnon RE, et al. Sequential nonsurgical and surgical staging of non-Hodgkin's lymphoma. *Ann Intern Med* 1976;85:149

Chen LT. Microcirculation of the spleen: an open or closed circulation? *Science* 1978;201:157

Christo MC: Segmental resections of the spleen: report on the first eight cases operated on. *Hospital (Rio)* 1962;62:575

Chulay JD, Lankerani MR. Splenic abscess: report of 10 cases and review of literature. *Am J Med* 1976;61:513

Cogbill TH, Moore EE, et al. Nonoperative management of blunt splenic trauma: a multicenter experience. *J Trauma* 1989;29:1312

Coon WW. Felty's syndrome: when is splenectomy indicated? *Am J Surg* 1985;149:272

Coon WW. Splenectomy for idiopathic thrombocytopenic purpura. *Surg Gynecol Obstet* 1987;164:225

Coon WW, Liepman MK. Splenectomy for agnogenic myeloid metaplasia. *Surg Gynecol Obstet* 1982;154:561

Deitch EA, O'Neal B. Neutrophil function in adults after traumatic splenectomy. *J Surg Res* 1982;33:98

Delpero JR, Houvenaeghel G, et al. Splenectomy for hypersplenism in chronic lymphocytic leukaemia and malignant non-Hodgkin's lymphoma. *Br J Surg* 1990;77:443

Ein SH, Shandling B, et al. The morbidity and mortality of splenectomy in children. *Ann Surg* 1977;185:307

El-Khishen MA, Henderson JM, et al. Splenectomy is contraindicated for thrombocytopenia secondary to portal hypertension. *Surg Gynecol Obstet* 1985;160:233

Emond AM, Morais P, et al. Role of splenectomy in homozygous sickle cell disease in childhood. *Lancet* 1984;1:88

Engelhard D, Ciridalli G, et al. Splenectomy in homozygous beta thalassemia: a retrospective study of 30 patients. *Br J Hematol* 1975;31:391

Feliciano DV, Bitondo CG, et al. A four-year experience with splenectomy versus splenorrhaphy. *Ann Surg* 1985;201:568

Ferguson CM. Splenectomy for immune thrombocytopenia related to human immunodeficiency virus. *Surg Gynecol Obstet* 1988;167:300

Fowler RH. Nonparasitic benign cystic tumors of the spleen. *Int Abst Surg* 1953;96:209

Friedman B, Darling G, et al. Splenectomy in the management of systemic mast cell disease. *Surgery* 1990;107:94

Gadacz T, Way LW, et al. Changing clinical spectrum of splenic abscess. *Am J Surg* 1974;128:182

Gill PG, Souter RG, et al. Splenectomy for hypersplenism in malignant lymphomas. *Br J Surg* 1981;68:29

Glatstein E, Vosti KL, et al. Serious bacterial infections in pediatric Hodgkin's disease: relative risks of radiotherapy, chemotherapy and splenectomy. *Proc Am Soc Clin Oncol* 1976;17:252

Golumb HM, Catovsky D, et al. Hairy cell leukemia: clinical review based on 71 cases. *Ann Intern Med* 1978;89 (pt 1):677

Gordon DH, Schaffner D, et al. Postsplenectomy thrombocytosis: its association with mesenteric, portal, and/or renal thrombosis in patients with myeloproliferative disorders. *Arch Surg* 1978;113:713

Grimfors G, Bjorkholm M, et al. Type-specific anti-pneumococcal antibody subclass response to vaccination after splenectomy with special reference to lymphoma patients. *Eur J Haematol* 1989;43:404

Guzzetta PC, Ruley EJ, et al. Elective subtotal splenectomy:

indications and results in 33 patients. *Ann Surg* 1990; 211:34

Helton WS, Carrico CJ, et al. Diagnosis and treatment of splenic fungal abscesses in the immune-suppressed patient. *Arch Surg* 1986;121:580

King H, Shumacker HB Jr. Splenic studies. I, susceptibility to infection after splenectomy performed in infancy. *Ann Surg* 1952;136:239

Lawthorne TW Jr, Zuidema GD. Splenic abscess. *Surgery* 1976; 79:686

Linos DA, Nagorney DM. Splenic abscess—the importance of early diagnosis. *Mayo Clin Proc* 1983;58:261

Longo WE, Baker CC, et al. Nonoperative management of adult blunt splenic trauma. Criteria for successful outcome. *Ann Surg* 1989;210:626

Lucas CE. Splenic trauma: choice of management. *Ann Surg* 1991;213:98

Malangoni MA, Dillon LD, et al. Factors influencing the risk of early and late serious infection in adults after splenectomy for trauma. *Surgery* 1984;96:775

Martin JK, Clark SC, et al. Staging laparotomy in Hodgkin's disease. *Arch Surg* 1982;117:586

Molin MR, Shackford SR. The management of splenic trauma in a trauma system. *Arch Surg* 1990;125:840

Moore FA, Moore EE, et al. Risk of splenic salvage after trauma: analysis of 200 adults. *Am J Surg* 1984;148:800

Moore RA, Brunner CM, et al. Felty's syndrome: long term follow-up after splenectomy. *Ann Intern Med* 1971;75: 381

Nallathambi MN, Ivatury RR, et al. Pyogenic splenic abscess in intravenous drug addiction. *Am Surg* 1987;53:342

Necheles TF, Allen DM, et al. The many forms of thalassemia: definition and classification of thalassemia syndromes. *Ann NY Acad Sci* 1969;165(art 1):5

Necheles TF, Finkel HE, et al. Red cell pyruvate kinase deficiency: the effect of splenectomy. *Arch Intern Med* 1966; 118:75

O'Grady JP, Day EJ, et al. Splenic artery aneurysm rupture in pregnancy. *Obstet Gynecol* 1977;50:627

Owens JC, Coffey RJ. Collective review: aneurysm of the splenic artery, including a report of 6 additional cases. *Surg Gynecol Obstet: Int Abstr Surg* 1953;97:313

Pinna AD, Argiolu F, et al. Indications and results for splenectomy for beta thalassemia in two hundred and twenty-one pediatric patients. *Surg Gynecol Obstet* 1988;167:109

Ross ME, Ellwood R, et al. Epidermoid splenic cysts. *Arch Surg* 1977;112:596

Rubin M, Yampolski I, et al. Partial splenectomy in Gaucher's disease. *J Pediatr Surg* 1986;21:125

Rudowski WJ. Accessory spleens: clinical significance with particular reference to the recurrence of idiopathic thrombocytopenic purpura. *World J Surg* 1985;9:422

Salky BA, Krell I, et al. Splenectomy for thrombotic thrombocytopenic purpura. *Mt Sinai J Med* 1983;50:56

Schneider PA, Rayner AA, et al. The role of splenectomy in multimodality treatment of thrombotic thrombocytopenic purpura. *Ann Surg* 1985;202:318

Schwartz PE, Sterioff S, et al. Postsplenectomy sepsis and mortality in adults. *JAMA* 1982;248:2279

Schwartz SI. Myeloproliferative disorders. *Ann Surg* 1975;182: 464

Schwartz SI. Physiology of the spleen and the role of splenectomy in hematologic disorders. In: Condon RE, DeCosse J (eds), *Surgical Care II.* Philadelphia, PA: Lea & Febiger; 1985:118–125

Schwartz SI. Splenectomy and splenorrhaphy. In: *Modern Technics in Surgery.* Mt. Kisco, NY: Futura; 1980

Schwartz SI. Splenectomy for thrombocytopenia. *World J Surg* 1985;9:416

Schwartz SI, Adams JT, et al. Splenectomy for hematologic disorders. In: *Current Problems in Surgery.* Chicago IL: Year Book Medical Publishers, Inc; 1971

Schwartz SI, Cooper RA Jr. Surgery in the diagnosis and treatment of Hodgkin's disease. In: *Advances in Surgery,* vol 6. Chicago IL: Year Book Medical Publishers, Inc; 1972

Schwartz SI, Lichtman MA. Surgical considerations in hematologic patients. In: Lichtman MA (ed), *Hematology for Practitioners.* Boston MA: Little, Brown; 1978:421

Sherman R. Perspectives in management of trauma to the spleen: 1979 Presidential Address, American Association for the Surgery of Trauma. *J Trauma* 1980;20:1

Singer DB. Postsplenectomy sepsis. *Perspect Pediatr Pathol* 1973; 1:285

Sirinek KR, Evans WE. Nonparasitic splenic cysts. *Am J Surg* 1973;126:8

Taylor, MA, Kaplan HS, Nelsen TS. Staging laparotomy with splenectomy for Hodgkin's disease: The Stanford Experience. *World J Surg* 1985;9:449

Trastek VF, Pairolero PC, et al. Splenic artery aneurysms. *Surgery* 1982;91:694

Tyler DS, Shaunak S, et al. HIV 1–associated thrombocytopenia: the role of splenectomy. *Ann Surg* 1990;211:211

Van Norman AS, Nagorney DM, et al. Splenectomy for hairy cell leukemia: a clinical review of 63 patients. *Cancer* 1986; 57:644

VerHeyden CN, Beart RW, et al. Accessory splenectomy in management of recurrent idiopathic thrombocytopenic purpura. *Mayo Clin Proc* 1978;53:442

Veronesi U, Musumeci R, et al. Value of staging laparotomy in non-Hodgkin's lymphomas (with emphasis on the histiocytic type). *Cancer* 1974;33:446

Wanachiwanawin W, Piankijagum A, et al. Emergency splenectomy in adult idiopathis thrombocytopenic purpura: a report of seven cases. *Arch Intern Med* 1989;149:217

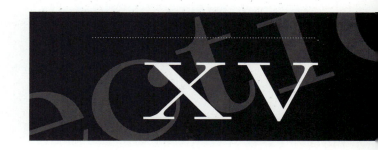

XV

PEDIATRICS

77

Infantile Pyloric Stenosis and Pyloric Mucosal Diaphragm

Lewis Spitz ▪ *Robin Abel*

▪ INFANTILE PYLORIC STENOSIS

HISTORICAL BACKGROUND

Fabricius Hildanus is credited with the first description, in 1646, of pyloric stenosis in an infant. This infant survived after having been given thickened feeds. Further descriptions of the condition appeared in 1717 by Blair, in 1758 by Weber, and in 1777 by Armstrong. Renewed interest in the condition, which at the time carried an 80% mortality rate, arose after the detailed clinical and pathologic report by Harold Hirschsprung, in 1888. The preferred method of treatment during this period was medical, using a combination of gastric lavage, antispasmodic drugs, dietary manipulations, and application of local heat, in an attempt to overcome the "pyloric spasm."

The first successful surgical procedure is attributed to Lobker, who, in 1898, carried out an anterior gastroenterostomy on an infant 10 weeks of age. Pylorectomy carried a 100% mortality rate and the Heineke-Mikulicz procedure, a 95% mortality rate; gastrojejunostomy was successful in less than half the patients on whom it was attempted. The Loreta procedure of instrumental pyloric divulsion, first attempted on an infant by Nicoll in 1899, appeared to be successful only in the hands of Burghard. Fredet, in 1908, advocated longitudinal submucous division of the thickened pyloric muscle, but complicated the procedure by at-

tempting to suture the divided thickened musculature transversely. Four years later, Ramstedt was attempting this procedure in a severely emaciated infant when the infant suddenly collapsed. Because Ramstedt was unable to complete the transverse suture, the stomach was rapidly returned to the peritoneal cavity and the abdomen closed. To Ramstedt's surprise, the infant made an uninterrupted recovery. Ramstedt then repeated the procedure, without transverse suturing, in subsequent cases with unqualified success. The development and success of the Ramstedt pyloromyotomy was a major breakthrough for surgery in infancy and undoubtedly contributed to the establishment of modern pediatric surgery as an independent surgical discipline. The procedure for pyloric stenosis has remained virtually unchanged since 1912. (The reader is referred to the articles by Ravitch[1] and Benson[2] for detailed descriptions of the history of pyloric stenosis.)

INCIDENCE

The incidence of pyloric stenosis among white infants is two or three cases per 1000 live births, whereas black infants are less frequently affected. The male-to-female ratio is 4:1, and there is an increased incidence among firstborn infants. A strong familial pattern of inheritance has been established.[3] Sons of male index patients have a 5.5% chance of developing pyloric stenosis, whereas daughters have a 2.4% chance. The figures are more striking for female index patients: 18.9% of sons and 7% of daughters develop pyloric stenosis. The condition has been described in more than one member of a family, including twins and triplets, and in three, four, five and even seven siblings in the same family. In the United Kingdom, a real increase in the incidence of pyloric stenosis was noted in the 1970s.[4,5] In all these studies there was an increase in the male to female ratio of the affected children.

ETIOLOGY

Despite numerous theories, the cause of pyloric stenosis remains obscure. Many theories have been postulated, and the possible causes can be conveniently divided into five groups: (1) genetic and environmental factors, (2) work hypertrophy, (3) neuronal abnormalities, (4) elevated gastrin levels, and (5) neuropeptide activity.

Genetic and Environmental Factors

The increased incidence in male infants and in white infants and the strong familial pattern of inheritance were noted above. There is a relatively low incidence in infants in the A blood group, and breast-fed infants are apparently more prone to the condition than formula-fed infants. A seasonal variation has been noted, with a preponderance of cases in autumn and spring.

Work Hypertrophy

Heinische was the first investigator to produce hypertrophic pyloric stenosis experimentally in rabbits by attaching glass beads on rubber bags filled with lead shot to the gastric fundus.[6] Gastric peristalsis was decreased, except in the antrum where it was enhanced. Lynn proposed that milk curds propelled by the gastric musculature against a pyloric canal in spasm produced edema of the pyloric mucosa and submucosa and narrowed the pyloric canal.[7]

Neuronal Abnormalities

Belding and Kernohan described a decrease in the number of ganglion cells and nerve fibers in the pylorus, which they ascribed to degenerative changes.[8] Friesen and associates postulated an immaturity of myenteric ganglion cells.[9] Other workers have failed to find any significant changes in the morphologic features of the ganglion cell.

Gastrin

The role of gastrin in the genesis of hypertrophic pyloric stenosis has received much attention. Dodge and Karim successfully induced hypertrophic pyloric stenosis in puppies by prolonged perinatal administration of pentagastrin.[10] They further implicated maternal stress as the primary factor mediated by an increase in the release of the hormone gastrin.[10] The role of gastrin as an etiologic factor in pyloric stenosis remains unresolved despite numerous recent reports on the subject. Immunoreactive gastrin levels have been found to be either normal or raised.[11–15] Spitz and Zail concluded that the raised serum gastrin levels were largely owing to antral distension caused by the pyloric obstruction and could not be directly implicated as an etiologic factor in this condition.[15] Werlin and associates measured serum gastrin levels in cord blood of infants who subsequently developed pyloric stenosis and found no difference in comparison with control specimens.[16] The current consensus is that gastrin has only a small role or none in infantile pyloric stenosis.

Neuropeptides

Tam demonstrated intense neurone-specific enolase activity in the ganglion cells of the pylorus in infants with pyloric stenosis and concluded that his findings suggested that the neurones were either immature or severely degenerated.[17] A decrease in substance P immunoreactivity suggested possible involvement of the peptidergic innervation in the pathogenesis of pyloric stenosis.

Reduced enkephelin and vasoactive intestinal peptide (VIP)-containing nerve fibers have been demonstrated within the pyloric smooth muscle of infantile hypertrophic pyloric stenosis (IHPS), whereas there is an increase in the number of VIP-containing nerve fibers within the myenteric plexus.[18] Reduced numbers of nerve fibers containing enkephelin gastrin-releasing peptide, neuropeptide Y, somatostatin, substance P and vasoactive intestinal peptide have been demonstrated within the circular muscle layer.[19] Changes in the VIP function have been implicated in the etiology of pyloric stenosis.[20] Abnormally dilated tortuous nerve fibers, that had reduced nitric oxide synthase activity, within the circular muscles layer, have been demonstrated by Vanderwinden[21,22] and proposed to be the cause of "pylorospasm."

PATHOLOGY

Macroscopically

The pyloric musculature is thickened and elongated, giving the external surface a shiny grey appearance. The muscle layers of the body of the stomach become hypertrophied in response to pyloric outlet obstruction. It generally is accepted that the increase in volume of the pyloric musculature is owing to a true hypertrophy, that is, an increase in the size of the muscle fibers rather than an increase in their numbers. The hypertrophy causes a cervix-like projection into the duodenum with a fornix where the duodenal mucosa is reflected over the distal surface of the tumor. It is in this area, where the mucosa is adherent to the muscle, that a perforation is prone to occur at operation.

Microscopically

Ultrastructural changes recorded in the smooth muscle include swelling, necrosis, nuclear abnormalities, glycogen accumulation, and the presence of dense gramiles. Neurological, ultrastructural changes included an increased variability of axon diameter and degenerative changes. An increase in the number of small diameter axons was taken as evidence of regeneration. Changes within the perikarya and glial cells were seen less often.[23,24]

CLINICAL MANIFESTATIONS

Symptomatology

It is classic for an infant with pyloric stenosis to be seen first between 2 and 4 weeks of age, with projectile vomiting occurring 10 to 20 minutes after a feeding. Several cases have been reported in which the onset of symptoms occurred on the first day or two of life; however, at the other end of the spectrum, presentation may be delayed until 6 to 9 months of age. The vomitus contains milk, and, although it may be yellow as a result of carotene concentrated from colostrum or milk formula, is virtually never stained with bile. The infant does not appear to be in any discomfort and will readily refeed immediately after vomiting. As the stomach becomes dilated and the muscle flaccid in the decompensatory stage of the infant whose condition is undiagnosed, vomiting becomes regurgitant in type and may occur only once or twice every 24 hours. Approximately 10–15% of infants develop hematemesis in the form of "coffee grounds" in the vomitus. The source of the blood loss, originally attributed to stasis gastritis, has been revealed to be the result of ulcerative esophagitis secondary to gastroesophageal reflux. Takeuchi found that every child with pyloric stenosis had gastroesophageal reflux on 24 hour pH monitoring.[25]

Constipation or the passage of small, green "starvation" stools is usual.

Failure to thrive or frank weight loss occurs as a result of inadequate caloric intake.

Associated anomalies occur in 6–20% of patients. They include esophageal atresia, Hirschsprung's disease, anorectal anomalies, and intestinal malrotation.

Physical Examination

The clinical features of dehydration, depressed anterior fontanelle, sunken eyes, loss of turgor in the skin, and dry mucous membranes, appear when fluid loss is in excess of 5% of total body water. This is found in only 10–15% of patients, the remainder being relatively well hydrated on admission. A biochemical disturbance is present to a greater or lesser extent in most infants. This consists of a metabolic alkalosis in combination with hypochloremia and hypokalemia. In the early stages, the kidneys are able to compensate by reabsorbing hydrogen and chloride ions in exchange for sodium, potassium, and bicarbonate. However, as the body stores of sodium and especially potassium become depleted, these ions are selectively retained while hydrogen is excreted in the urine, thereby aggravating the alkalotic state.

Visible gastric peristalsis is best observed shortly after a feed and appears as a wave of peristalsis passing across the upper abdomen from left to right. This sign is not pathognomonic of pyloric stenosis and may be observed in any wasted infant, irrespective of the cause of obstruction.

Palpation of a pyloric tumor is the crucial diagnostic feature of pyloric stenosis. Careful examination will reveal its presence in 90% of cases. The tumor characteristically is described as "olive shaped" and firm, and lies deep within the right upper quadrant of the abdomen, beneath the liver edge. It is best palpated during the early stages of a small feeding or immediately after a vomiting episode, when the pylorus is in spasm and the abdominal muscles of the infant are relaxed. A full stomach tends to overlie and obscure the tumor. Unfortunately, the ability to palpate a pyloric tumor clinically is diminishing with the increasing use of ultrasound as a diagnostic tool.[26–28]

Once the pyloric tumor has been palpated, further diagnostic investigations are unnecessary. Jaundice has been noted in 2–3% of infants with pyloric stenosis. The hyperbilirubinemia is largely of the unconjugated type and resolves rapidly after relief of the pyloric obstruction. An absolute decrease in hepatic glucuronyl transferase activity has been shown to exist in association with pyloric stenosis and may be considered an early manifestation of Gilbert's syndrome,[29,30] since jaundice resolves rapidly following pyloromyotomy, before full feeds are established.

Radiographic Examination

Radiographic examination is required only when a pyloric tumor cannot be palpated. The plain abdominal x-ray film shows a distended stomach with an air-fluid level and an absence of gas beyond the pylorus (Fig 77–1). The following features should be sought on barium meal examination:

1. String sign, which indicates the convex, narrow, elongated pyloric canal (Fig 77–2)
2. Double-track appearance, which is the result of the enfolding of mucosa into the pyloric canal
3. Gastric hyperperistalsis and delayed gastric emptying
4. Mushroom effect of the pyloric mass indenting the duodenal cap

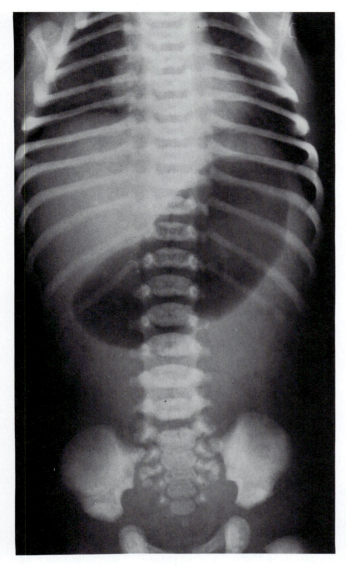

Figure 77–1. Plain abdominal radiograph showing a dilated gas-filled stomach with little air passing through into the distal portion of the intestine.

Ultrasonography has replaced barium meal examination as the diagnostic method of choice in pyloric stenosis. The pyloric tumor appears as a well-defined muscular echogenic mass with a central lucent zone, comprising the pyloric mucosal folds and aperture (Fig 77–3).

The diagnostic size of the tumor varies with the age of the child. Pyloric muscle thickness of 3 mm or more is diagnostic in children up to 30 days of age. A statistically significant length of the pylorus has not yet been identified.[31,32] If the thickness of the pyloric muscle measures 4 mm or more, a diagnosis of pyloric stenosis can be made confidently. There is no consensus of opinion regarding the length of the pyloric

tumor in establishing the diagnosis. A pyloric wall <4 mm thick does not exclude the diagnosis of pyloric stenosis and, if the clinical features are strongly suggestive, a contrast meal radiographic examination should be carried out.

Differential Diagnosis

In the absence of a palpable pyloric tumor, the following conditions should be considered:

1. *Feeding problems.* Faulty feeding technique or attempts at overfeeding can produce vomiting, but the pattern of the vomiting is unlikely to mimic the classic picture of pyloric stenosis.
2. *Gastroesophageal reflux.* Incompetence of the lower esophageal sphincter is common in early infancy and produces vomiting, which may occasionally be truly projectile in nature.
3. *Infections.* Urinary tract infection, pneumonia, and meningitis cause vomiting, but the infant is listless and lethargic and generally shows other signs of infection, such as hypothermia or hyperthermia, peripheral vasoconstriction, grunting respiration, and jaundice.
4. *Adrenal hyperplasia.* The presence of plasma hyperkalemia should alert the clinician to this diagnosis.

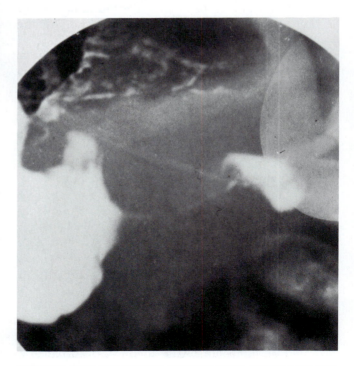

Figure 77–2. Barium meal examination showing the narrow, elongated pyloric canal (string sign) passing convexly upward, toward the duodenal cap.

MANAGEMENT

Preoperative Preparation

The operation for pyloric stenosis is *never* an emergency. However, rehydration and correction of acid-base and electrolyte imbalance are urgently required. The mildly dehydrated infant may be rehydrated orally by substituting a glucose-saline solution for breast or formula feeding. The moderately or severely dehydrated alkalotic infant is managed best by intravenous infusions, which achieve accurate and rapid correction of the fluid and electrolyte disturbance. Plasma chloride concentration of 106 mmol/L is a reliable guide for the assessment and correction of hypochloremic alkalosis.[33] Initial infusion consists of either isotonic saline solution or plasma at a rate of up to 20 mL/kg of body weight during a period of 1 hour. Once urinary output has been established, potassium chloride (20 to 30 mmol/L) is added to the infusate of 5% glucose in 0.9% saline solution. Fluids are administered at a rate of 150 to 180 mL/kg of body weight per 24 hours until rehydration is complete. This may take as long as 48 to 72 hours to achieve. It is important to correct potassium depletion, prior to general anesthesia, because of the hazard of cardiac arrhythmia and to correct alkalosis because of the risk of respiratory center depression. One metabolic derangement exacerbates the risks of the other.[34] During the period of intravenous fluid ad-

ministration, all oral intake is suspended and the stomach contents are evacuated by gentle saline lavages.

Anesthesia

Although local anesthesia has been used successfully, it is generally recommended that where there is an acceptable standard of pediatric anesthetic expertise, general endotracheal anesthesia is preferred. Immediately before the induction of anesthesia, the stomach should be emptied of its contents by the passage of a nasogastric tube, which remains in situ until the end of the procedure. After the intubation, and with the infant closely monitored, an adequate oxygen supply can be guaranteed and the danger from inhalation of vomitus eliminated. It is essential to preserve body heat before, and particularly during, the operation to prevent the development of hypothermia. This is best achieved by using swaddling, thermostatically controlled warm air mattresses and a regulated, ambient operating room temperature.

Operative Technique

Many different incisions have been used for pyloromyotomy. A paramedian incision is not only cosmetically unacceptable but is also more prone to dehiscence. The transverse incision (Fig 77–4A) consists of either a muscle-

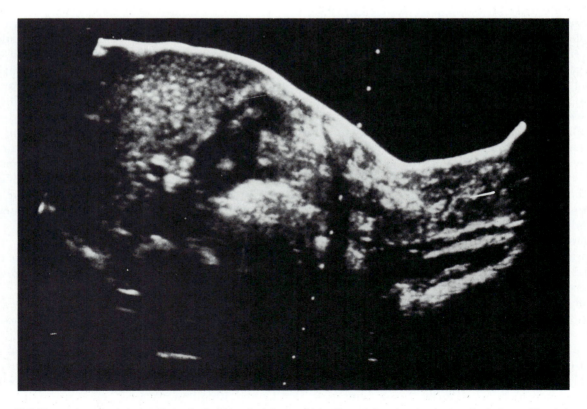

Figure 77–3. Ultrasound scan in pyloric stenosis, showing the thickened pyloric musculature with a central sonolucent area representing the lumen of the pyloric canal.

cutting or muscle-splitting (gridiron) procedure in the line of the fibers. The latter is the more secure from the point of view of dehiscence but involves more extensive dissection and exposes wider tissue planes to potential wound sepsis. We prefer a transverse incision, with the rectus muscle divided in the line of the incision. The incision is placed high in the right upper quadrant of the abdomen, over the anterior surface of the liver. The subcutaneous tissues and muscle fibers are divided with electrocautery to restrict blood loss.

The peritoneum is opened in the line of the incision, and the body of the stomach is identified and delivered into the wound. No attempt should be made to grasp the pyloric tumor, because the result will be serosal tears and hemorrhage. If the stomach is tensely distended, it may be difficult to hold, and the anesthetist should be asked to aspirate the air via a nasogastric tube. When the stomach is not readily identifiable, the introduction of 20 to 30 mL of air into the stomach via the nasogastric tube will achieve just sufficient distension of the body of the stomach to facilitate its identification. Alternatively, the transverse colon may appear first when the peritoneal cavity is opened. Gentle traction on the transverse mesocolon will draw the greater curvature of the stomach into the operative field.

The greater curvature of the stomach is held in a moist gauze swab, and by drawing it over to the left and applying traction on the antrum, the surgeon delivers the pyloric tumor out of the incision (Fig 77–4B). The distal extent of the tumor is marked by the pyloric vein of Mayo. Proximally, the tumor is less obviously defined as it merges into the hypertrophied musculature of the antrum of the stomach. The relatively avascular middle zone on the anterior surface of the tumor is selected for the incision, which extends longitudinally from the pyloroduodenal junction to the antrum (Fig 77–4C). The muscle fibers are split down to the mucosa, with the use of the handle of a scalpel or a MacDonald dissector (Fig 77–4D). The hypertrophied muscle should be split through the entire extent of the pylorus. This is best achieved by means of a pyloric spreader (Denis Browne or Benson and Lloyd) or a blunt hemostat (Figs 77–4E–F, and 77–5). Particular care must be exercised at the pyloroduodenal junction, where the deeper muscle fibers invaginate into the duodenal bulb. The overlying duodenal mucosa is firmly adherent to the muscle layer and is torn easily if the splitting procedure is carried too far distally. A duodenal perforation is not a catastrophe unless it remains unrecognized. Injecting air into the stomach and squeezing it through into the duodenum will make a perforation of the duodenum obvious. Any such perforation should be closed by direct suture with 5.0 polyglycolic acid suture (Dacron). The defect may be closed with a patch of omentum, but because this structure is relatively underdeveloped in the young infant, insufficient omentum may be available for this procedure. Slight hemorrhage from the pyloromyotomy is invariable owing to venous congestion, which will resolve with gentle pressure for a few minutes or by returning the pylorus into the peritoneal cavity, thereby relieving the pressure on the veins by the abdominal incision. The incision may be closed either in layers or en masse with 3-0 polyglycolic acid sutures. The skin is closed with a subcuticular suture, which results in a cosmetically acceptable scar and avoids the distress of having to remove skin sutures from a wriggling, crying infant.

In recent years, intra-abdominal pyloromyotomy has gained favor, either as an open procedure following transfixion of the pylorus, or as a laparoscopic procedure.[35–37] The possible advantages associated with these techniques need to be assessed carefully. The risks associated with an increased anesthetic time and the number of assistants required for the latter technique also need to be evaluated. Similarly, the efficacy of endoscopic balloon dilation requires evaluation before it can be recommended.[38,39]

Postoperative Care

The nasogastric tube may be removed soon after the infant has recovered from the anesthetic. However, if perforation had occurred, nasogastric decompression is required for 24 hours. Many feeding regimens, varying from commencing feedings within 4 hours of operation to delaying feeding for 24 hours, have been advocated. It has been clearly shown that gastric peristalsis is abolished for up to 24 hours postoperatively. The incidence of vomiting after pyloromyotomy ranges from 50% to 86%.[40] Following pyloromyotomy, using applied potential tomography, gastric motility gradually returns to normal by the seventh day.[41] Acid reflux owing to gastroesophageal reflux is commonly associated with pyloric stenosis. Pyloromyotomy cures acid reflux in 95% of cases.[25] A policy that involves delaying feeding for at least 12 hours and propping the infant in an upright position within 6 hours of surgery has significantly reduced the incidence of postoperative vomiting. The feeding regimen shown in Table 77–1 has been found to be highly successful.

The feeding program progresses rapidly through each stage as the feedings are tolerated. In the majority of cases, the infant is ready for discharge from the hospital within 48 hours following operation.

The mortality rate for pyloric stenosis is extremely low, <1%. Most deaths are due to anesthetic complications, particularly in the electrolytically depleted, poorly prepared infant. Wound dehiscence and sepsis are, unfortunately, not so rare, and incidence of between 0–5% and 9–15%, respectively, are seen in the United Kingdom. Wound sepsis primarily owing to *Staphylococcus aureus* has been found to be related to the

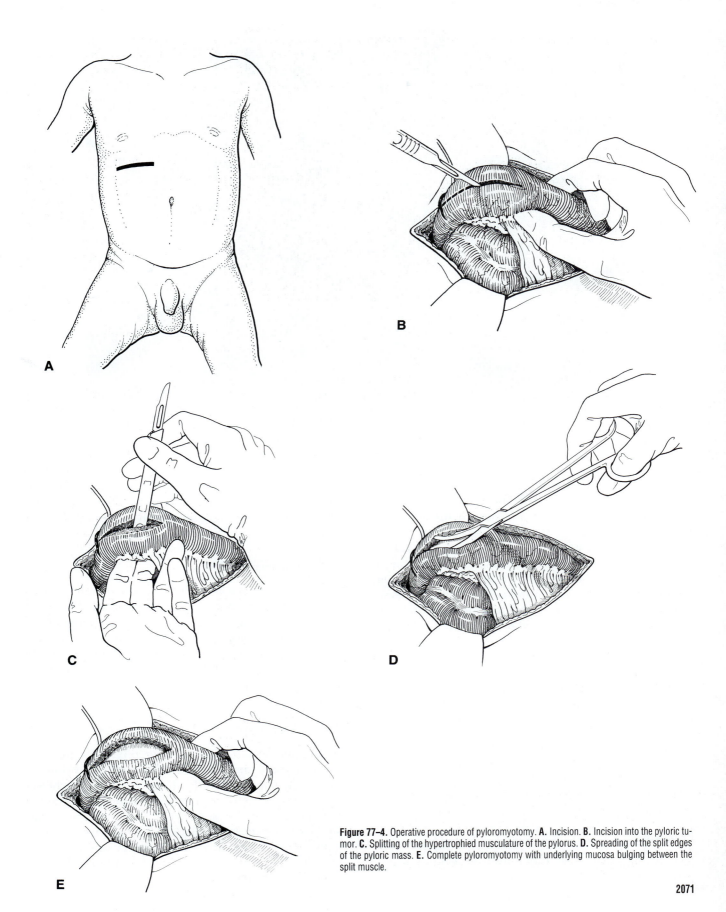

Figure 77–4. Operative procedure of pyloromyotomy. **A.** Incision. **B.** Incision into the pyloric tumor. **C.** Splitting of the hypertrophied musculature of the pylorus. **D.** Spreading of the split edges of the pyloric mass. **E.** Complete pyloromyotomy with underlying mucosa bulging between the split muscle.

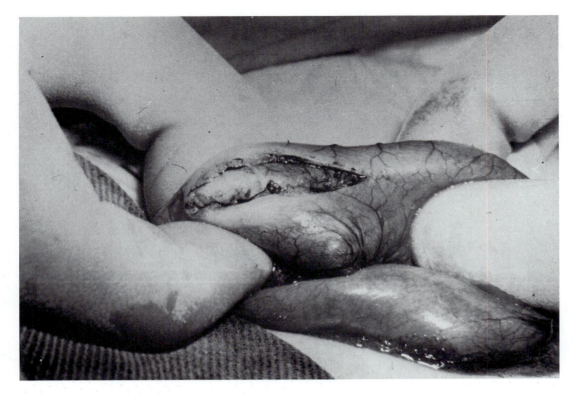

Figure 77–5. Appearance of the pylorus after pyloromyotomy. Note the thickened musculature of the pylorus and the exposed mucosa bulging into the incised pylorus.

age of the child, the duration of the period of vomiting, and surgical technique, particularly in the malnourished infant.[42]

Medical treatment for pyloric stenosis has been abandoned in favor of the more definite, simpler, and more effective surgical treatment. The gradual feeding, administration of antispasmodics (atropine, scopolamine), and gastric lavage that form the basis of medical therapy require dedicated nursing and involve prolonged periods of hospitalization.

■ PYLORIC MUCOSAL DIAPHRAGM

HISTORICAL BACKGROUND

Pyloric mucosal diaphragm was first described by Parsons and Barling in 1933.[43] The first successful surgical correction was reported by Touroff and Sussman in 1940. Since then, sporadic reports and various reviews have appeared in the literature.

PATHOLOGY

The diaphragm is more commonly prepyloric or antral, rather than pyloric, in location. It generally is perfo-

rated and may cause an incomplete obstruction at the gastric outlet. The condition may be associated with IHPS.[44,45]

CLINICAL MANIFESTATIONS

With partial obstruction, clinical presentation begins at birth, with persistent nonbilious vomiting. Upper abdominal distension and visible gastric hyperperistalsis soon develop. Although the diagnosis is usually made in the neonatal period, it may be delayed until adult life. These patients then have a lifelong history of early satiety and fullness, associated with episodes of nausea and vomiting.

DIAGNOSTIC STUDIES

In complete obstruction in the neonate, the plain abdominal x-ray film reveals a dilated gas-filled stomach with no air passing into the distal portion of the bowel. The plain film is of no diagnostic value in incomplete obstructions. In these cases, barium contrast studies show a thin, sharp, transverse filling defect approximately 1 to 2 cm proximal to the pyloric canal. Recently, ultrasound has been used in the diagnosis of antral webs.[46]

TABLE 77–1. OPTIMUM FEEDING REGIMEN

Stage	Volume of Feed (mL)	Type of Feed	Interval
I	15	Glucose saline solution	3 hours
II	30	Half-strength formula or breast	3 hours
III	60	Half-strength formula or breast	3 hours
IV	90	Full strength formula or breast	4 hours

The presence of an antral web should be confirmed on gastroscopy before proceeding to surgery.

TREATMENT

The membrane should be excised at its attachment to the gastric wall via a generous gastrotomy incision. The raw mucosal surface should be closed with interrupted sutures. The gastrotomy may be closed in a transverse direction if an adequate gastric outlet cannot otherwise be guaranteed.

REFERENCES

1. Ravitch MM. The story of pyloric stenosis. *Surgery* 1960; 48:1117

2. Benson CD. Infantile pyloric stenosis. *Prog Pediatr Surg* 1970;1:63

3. Carter CO, Evans KA. Inheritance of congenital pyloric stenosis. *J Med Genet* 1969;6:233

4. Knox EG, Armstrong E, Haynes R. Changing incidence of hypertrophic pyloric stenosis. *Arch Dis Child* 1983;58:582

5. Webb AR, Lari J, Dodge JA. Infantile hypertrophic pyloric stenosis in South Glamorgan. *Arch Dis Child* 1983;58:586

6. Heinische HM. Die sog: Pylorishypertrophic in Tierversuch. *Klin Wochenschr* 1967;45:1251

7. Lynn HB. The mechanism of pyloric stenosis and its relationship to preoperative preparation. *Arch Surg* 1960;81:453

8. Belding HH, Kernohan JW. A morphology study of the myenteric plexus and musculature of the pylorus with special reference to changes in hypertrophic pyloric stenosis. *Surg Gynecol Obstet* 1953;97:323

9. Friesen SR, Boley JA, et al. Myenteric plexus of the pylorus: its early normal development and its changes in hypertrophic pyloric stenosis. *Surgery* 1956;39:21

10. Dodge JA, Karim AA. Induction of pyloric hypertrophy by pentagastrin. *Gut* 1976;17:280

11. Rogers IM, Drainer IK, et al. Plasma gastrin in congenital hypertrophic pyloric stenosis: a hypothesis disproved? *Arch Dis Child* 1975;50:467

12. Moazam F, Kolts BE, et al. In pursuit of the etiology of congenital hypertrophic pyloric stenosis. *J Pediatr Gastroenterol Nutr* 1982;1:97

13. Hambourg MA, Mignon M, et al. Serum gastrin levels in hypertrophic pyloric stenosis in infancy. *Arch Dis Child* 1979;54:208

14. Bleicher MA, Shandling B, et al. Increased serum immunoreactive gastrin levels in idiopathic hypertrophic pyloric stenosis. *Gut* 1978;19:794

15. Spitz L, Zail SS. Serum gastrin levels in congenital hypertrophic pyloric stenosis. *J Pediatr Surg* 1976;11:33

16. Werlin SL, Grand RJ, Drum DE. Congenital hypertrophic pyloric stenosis: the role of gastrin reevaluated. *Pediatrics* 1978;61:883

17. Tam PK. An immunochemical study with neuron-specific enolase and substance P of human enteric innervation: the normal developmental pattern and abnormal deviations in Hirschsprung's disease and pyloric stenosis. *J Pediatr Surg* 1986;21:227

18. Malmfors G, Sundler F. Peptidergic innervation in infantile hypertrophic stenosis. *J Pediatr Surg* 1986;21:303

19. Wattchow DA, Cass DT, Furness JB, et al. Abnormalities of peptide containing nerve fibers in infantile hypertrophic pyloric stenosis. *Gastroenterology* 1987;92:443

20. Grisoni E, De Augustin JC, Kalhan SC. Vasoactive intestinal polypeptide causes relaxation of the pyloric sphincter in rabbits. *J Pediatr Surg* 1993;28:1117

21. Vanderwinden JM, Mailleux P, Schiffmann SN, et al. Nitric oxide synthase activity in infantile hypertrophic pyloric stenosis. *N Eng J Med* 1992;327:511 (published erratum appears in *N Engl J Med* 1992;327(17):1252) (see comments)

22. Vanderwinden JM, De Laet MH, Schiffman SN, et al. Nitric oxide synthase distribution in the enteric nervous system of Hirschsprung's. *Gastroenterology* 1993;105:969

23. Dieler R, Schroder JM. Myenteric plexus neuropathy in infantile hypertrophic pyloric stenosis. *Acta Neuropathol* 1989;78:649

24. Dieler R, Schroder JM, Skipnik H, et al. Infantile hypertrophic pyloric stenosis: myopathic type. *Acta Neuropathol* 1990;80:295

25. Takeuchi S, Tamate S, Nakahira M, et al. Esophagitis in infants with hypertrophic pyloric stenosis: a source of hematemesis. *J Pediatr Surg* 1993;28:59

26. Macdessi J, Oates RK. Clinical diagnosis of pyloric stenosis: a declining art. *BMJ* 1993;306:553

27. Rollins MD, Shields MD. Clinical diagnosis of pyloric stenosis (letter). *BMJ* 1993;306:1065

28. Tam PK, Chan J. Increasing incidence of hypertrophic pyloric stenosis. *Arch Dis Child* 1991;66:530

29. Lippert MM. Jaundice with hypertrophic pyloric stenosis (letter; comment) *J Pediatr* 1990;117:168

30. Roth B, Staz A, Heinisch HM. Jaundice with hypertrophic pyloric stenosis: a possible manifestation of Gilbert syndrome (letter; comment). *J Pediatr* 1990;116:1003

31. Lamki N, Athey PA, Round ME, et al. Hypertrophic pyloric stenosis in the neonate—diagnostic criteria revisited. *Can Assoc Radiologists J* 1993;44:21

32. Deluca SA. Hypertrophic pyloric stenosis. *Amer Family Physician* 1993;47:1771

33. Goh DW, Hall SK, Gornall P, et al. Plasma chloride and alkalaemia in pyloric stenosis. *Br J Surg* 1990;77:922

34. Bissonette B, Sullivan PJ. Pyloric stenosis. *Can J Anesth* 1991;38:668

35. Donnellan WL, Cobb LM. Intraabdominal pyloromyotomy. *J Pediatr Surg* 1991;26:174

36. Alain JL, Grousseau D, Terrier G. Extramucosal pyloromyotomy by laparoscopy. *J Pediatr Surg* 1991;26:1191

37. Tan HL, Najmaldin A. Laparoscopic pyloromyotomy for infantile hypertrophic pyloric stenosis. *Pediatr Surg Int* 1993;8;376

38. Tam PK, Carty H. Nonsurgical treatment for pyloric stenosis (letter). *Lancet* 1989;2:393

39. Hayashi AH, Giacomantonio JM, Lau HY, et al. Balloon catheter dilatation for hypertrophic pyloric stenosis. *J Pediatr Surg* 1990;25:1119

40. Spitz L. Vomiting after pyloromyotomy for infantile hypertrophic pyloric stenosis. *Arch Dis Child* 1979;54:886

41. Nour S, Mangnall Y, Dickson JA, et al. Measurement of gastric emptying in infants with pyloric stenosis using applied potential tomography. *Arch Dis Child* 1993;68:484

42. Rao N, Youngson GG. Wound sepsis following Ramstedt pyloromyotomy. *Br J Surg* 1989;76:1144

43. Parsons LG, Barling S, *Diseases of Infancy and Childhood,* Oxford, England: Oxford Medical; 1933;739

44. Leach JL, Johnson III JF. Antral web: association with hypertrophic pyloric stenosis. *Pediatr Radiol* 1993;23:206

45. Bell MJ, Ternberg JL, et al. Prepyloric gastric antral web: a puzzling epidemic. *J Pediatr Surg* 1978;13:307

46. Chew AL, Friedwald JP, Donovan C. Diagnosis of congenital antral web by ultrasound. *Pediatr Radiol* 1992;22:342

78

Neonatal Intestinal Obstruction and Intussusception in Childhood

Jay L. Grosfeld ■ *Karen W. West*

Instances of intestinal obstruction in the newborn infant account for a large proportion of surgical admissions to a neonatal intensive care unit. The spectrum of bowel obstruction is varied (Table 78–1) and, because of the complexity of care, these patients are best treated in tertiary neonatal referral centers where pediatric specialties (surgery, neonatology, radiology, anesthesiology, pathology, cardiology, nephrology, and nursing staff) are available.

■ INTESTINAL OBSTRUCTION IN THE NEWBORN INFANT

GENERAL PRINCIPLES

Signs of Intestinal Obstruction

Signs of intestinal obstruction in the newborn infant include bilious vomiting (blockage below the ampulla of Vater), abdominal distention, failure to pass meconium in the first 24 hours of life, and maternal polyhydramnios. Bilious vomiting is considered a pathologic finding and the cause should be investigated. The degree of distention will depend on the level of the obstruction (eg, infants with ileal atresia will have more distention than those with duodenal atresia). The fetus swallows 25% to 40% of the amniotic fluid pool and urinates in utero to return some fluid to the amniotic cavity. Any high alimentary tract obstruction (more commonly duodenum, high jejunum) may prevent the swallowing of amniotic fluid resulting in polyhydramnious (>2000 cc). The fetus does not normally defecate in utero, but does pass 200 to 250 gm of viscid, greenish-black meconium in the first 24 hours of life. Failure to pass meconium may be associated with a low bowel obstruction.

Care of the Surgical Neonate

In all newborn infant surgical cases, prevention of heat loss is important. Not only are the children transported in temperature controlled isolettes, but in the operating rooms the extremities are wrapped in cotton or plastic, the ambient room temperature is increased to 80°F to 85°F, the head (proportionately larger surface area in the newborn) is placed in a plastic cap, a warming blanket is placed under the infant, and accessory warming lights are utilized to prevent hypothermia resulting from conductive and evaporative losses and possible acidosis. Warmed, humidified anesthetic agents also are employed. The gastrointestinal tract is decompressed with an oral-gastric tube (neonates are obligate nose breathers) in order to reduce abdominal distention and possible respiratory compromise, to prevent emesis and potential life-threatening aspiration during transportation and upon intubation in the operating room setting.

The intravenous fluids required will depend on the patient's state of hydration and underlying diagnosis. Infants with gastroschisis with an associated bowel atresia and/or meconium peritonitis will often require 175

TABLE 78–1. NEWBORN ALIMENTARY OBSTRUCTIONS

GASTRIC
  Pyloric atresia
  Antral web
DUODENAL
  Atresia—stenosis
  Malrotation
  Annular pancreas
  Anterior portal vein
SMALL BOWEL
  Structural
    Atresia
    Duplication cysts
    Vitelline duct remnants
    Internal hernias
  Mechanical
    Meconium ileus
    Milk curd syndrome
  Acquired
    Sepsis
    Necrotizing enterocolitis
COLONIC
  Colonic atresia
  Hirschsprung's disease
  Anorectal atresia
  Small left colon syndrome
  Meconium plug
  Neuronal colonic dysplasia

to 200 cc/kg/24 hrs owing to the chemical peritonitis affecting the fetal bowel exposed to the amnionic fluid in utero. In contrast, the fluid requirement for an infant with a patent ductus arteriosus is 60 to 80 cc/kg/24 hrs. Table 78–2 offers suggested fluid requirements for the pediatric patient based on body mass. Intravenous fluids include a 10% dextrose infusion to prevent hypoglycemia. Sodium and chloride are the major extracellular ions and potassium is the main intracellular ion. Sodium requirements are 2 to 4 mEq/kg/day in the newborn and levels are managed by following serum values (130 to 145 mEg/dL), monitoring urine output and specific gravity. Urine output should be at least 0.5 to 1.0 cc/kg/hr. Additional intravenous potassium of 2 mEq/kg/day is not given until good urinary output has been established. Ten percent calcium gluconate is also added to the intravenous (IV) fluids at a rate of 0.5 to 0.9 mm/kg/day to prevent hypoglycemia and the possibility of apnea in the newborn. Rapid volume expansion can be achieved with plasmanate infusions at 10 to 20 cc/kg (being careful to avoid hypoglycemia).

If overhead warming lights or bililights are required, the transdermal evaporative losses will increase and the intravenous fluid rate will need upward adjustment by as much as 10%. Gastric losses should also be replaced on a cc for cc basis, with the regular intravenous fluids or 0.45% Normal Saline (N/S), if clear, and a dextrose containing lactated Ringer's solution, if bilious.

Careful records of the amount of blood removed for necessary laboratory studies are maintained so that blood losses can be assessed more accurately and replaced (newborn blood volume is 80 cc/kg). Important baseline data include the serum electrolytes, complete blood profile including platelet counts, blood urea nitrogen, serum creatinine, and calcium levels obtained by using standard microtechniques.

Intramuscular vitamin K (1 mg intramuscularly) is administered and broad-spectrum antibiotics instituted intravenously (often ampicillin, 100–200 mg/kg/day and gentamicin, 5 mg/kg/day). Appropriate drug levels are monitored and dosages adjusted accordingly.

Subsequent nutrition is important, especially in infants with complicated intestinal anatomy and prolonged ileus patterns in whom total parenteral nutrition (TPN) is required. Full-term infants require 100 to 120 calories/kg/day for consistent weight gains of 10 to 30 gm/day. This need will vary according to the overall metabolic rate and should be reassessed on a daily basis. TPN solutions are designed to contain 1 to 3 gm/kg of protein and dextrose concentrations which should not exceed 20 mg/kg/min (usually 17% to 20% glucose concentration is adequate). To prevent fatty acid deficiency, intralipid solutions (1 to 3 gm/kg/day) should be used on a daily basis. Careful monitoring of serum bilirubin (fatty acids may displace the bilirubin bound to albumin and thereby increase the risk of kernicterus) and triglycerides is mandatory in the early postnatal period.

GASTRIC OUTLET OBSTRUCTION

In instances of a gastric outlet obstruction, the prenatal ultrasound may document the presence of polyhydramnios and fetal gastric dilatation.

Coupled with the presence of a scaphoid abdomen, a palpable mass in the left upper quadrant (dilated stomach), and emesis of clear nonbilious tenacious secretions, the diagnosis of pyloric atresia or a prepyloric diaphragm should be considered. These defects are more commonly owing to a failure of recanalization, but also may result from an intrauterine vascular insult (as in the case of small bowel atresias). Some instances of pyloric atresia are familial and may be associated with epidermolysis bullosa (a blistering skin lesion that is caused by a defect in the lamina lucida between the basal cell and lamina densa layers) that also may affect the mucosal surfaces (mouth, bladder, bowel, etc).

In patients with gastric enteric obstruction, abdominal radiographs will show a dilated air-filled stomach (single bubble) with no distal bowel gas. A water soluble or dilute barium contrast study will confirm the diagno-

TABLE 78–2. FLUID REQUIREMENTS BASED ON BODY MASS IN THE PEDIATRIC PATIENT

Weight (kg)	cc/kg/hr	cc/kg/day
0–2	3	75
2–10	4	100
10–20	2	50
>20	1	20

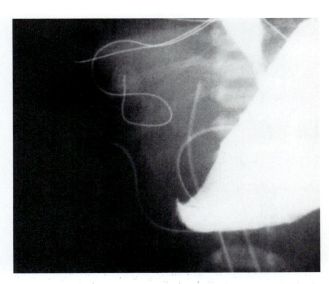

A   **B**

Figure 78–1. In this newborn with nonbilious emesis, the dilute barium contrast identified the pyloric atresia anomaly. Note the lack of distal gas in the intestinal tract.

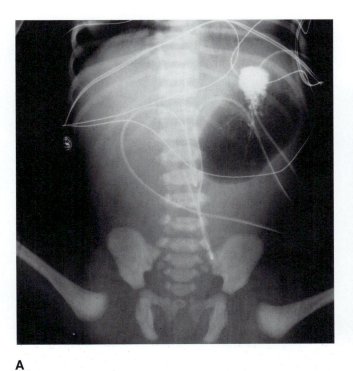

Type I   Type II

Type III

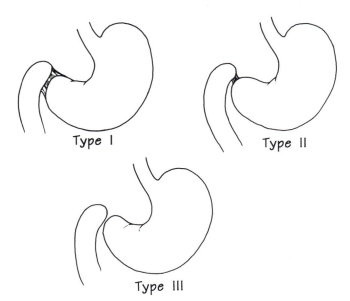

Figure 78–2. In cases of type 1 prepyloric atresia, the seromuscular continuity is present and the mucosal atretic area must be excised.

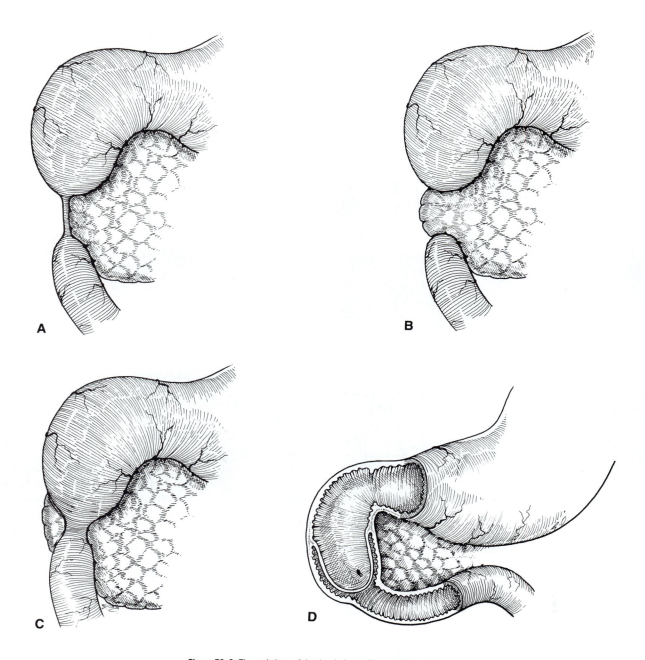

A

B

C

D

Figure 78–3. The variations of duodenal obstruction are pictured above.

sis (Fig 78–1). A transverse incision is made in a supra-umbilical location and the dilated stomach identified. In type 1 atresia, seromuscular continuity is usually present (Fig 78–2) and a mucosal atresia is noted. In type 2 atresia, a fibrous band exists between the stomach and the duodenum. This is excised and an end-to-end anas-tomosis (one or two layer) is performed with inter-rupted 5-0 sutures. Prolonged gastric atony owing to the relatively longstanding fetal congenital obstruction may make the placement of a temporary gastrostomy tube useful. Postoperatively, nutritional support is required until gastric function returns.

DUODENAL OBSTRUCTION

The duodenum begins to develop during the fourth week from the caudal portion of the foregut, the cranial part of the midgut, and the splanchnic mesenchyme associated with the primitive gut. The common bile duct enters the duodenum at the junction of the distal foregut with the midgut. The proliferation of the epithelial cells during the fifth and sixth weeks narrows the lumen of the duodenum and is the solid cord phase of development. Failure of complete recanalization (described by Tandler in 1902) during the eighth to tenth week will result in the various forms of duodenal obstructions encountered. (External compression, in the form of an anterior portal vein (persistent primitive vitelline vein) or annular pancreas (persistent ventral primordium), is associated with duodenal stenosis. True atresias usually occur between the second and third portions of the duodenum and have been classified into three types by Gray and Skandalakis. A type 1 atresia has an intact diaphragm comprised of mucosa and submucosa layers with a continuous seromuscular layer. This so-called windsock deformity may extend into the distal duodenum for several centimeters beyond the point of origin and there will be a size discrepancy between the first and second portions of the duodenum. A fibrous cord connects the two segments in the type 2 defects and there is a complete separation of the two ends in the type 3 variation (Fig 78–3). Associated findings include Down syndrome (20% to 30%), prematurity (20% to 47%), maternal polyhydramnios (30% to 50%), and congenital heart disease (33%). Duodenal atresia is present in approximately 1/10 000 births. A midline work-up should include a cranial ul-trasound, echocardiogram (ECHO), renal ultrasound, and vertebral films to determine the presence of other early developing associated anomalies in these infants. The presence of the "double-bubble sign" on abdominal radiograph results from the fluid levels in the dilated stomach and the first portion of the duodenum and the lack of distal bowel gas (Fig 78–4).

Intravenous fluids and broad-spectrum antibiotics are administered. The surgical approach is through a right upper quadrant transverse incision. When a duodenal web is encountered, the membrane can be located more easily by advancing the indwelling oral-gastric tube through the pylorus until the obstructing membrane is encountered. As the catheter is advanced, there will be an indentation on the side wall of the duodenum where the web originates. A longitudinal duodenotomy is made slightly proximal to the origin of the web to allow for the identification of the web and to determine the location of the ampulla. It is important to locate the ductal opening (facilitated by milking the gallbladder and noting the entrance of bile into the duodenal lumen) prior to either excision of the web or bypass of the membrane with a duodenoduodenostomy (Fig 78–5). The duodenal incision is closed transversely to prevent narrowing of the lumen.

In cases of duodenal stenosis associated with an anterior portal vein or an annular pancreas, the area of obstruction is bypassed with a side-to-side duodenoduodenostomy. The annular pancreas should not be divided, in order to prevent the formation of a pancreatic fistula and the division of any intraluminal pancreatic tissue. A catheter should be passed distally through the duodenum and into the proximal small intestine to be certain that a concomitant second distal web is not

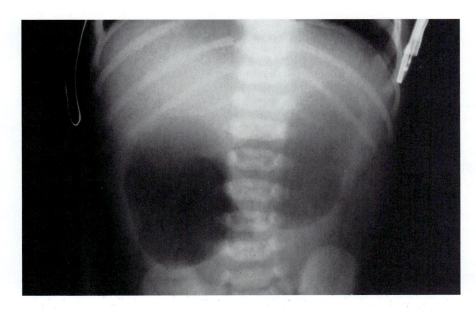

Figure 78–4. This double-bubble sign noted on plain radiograph is a typical finding in cases of duodenal atresia.

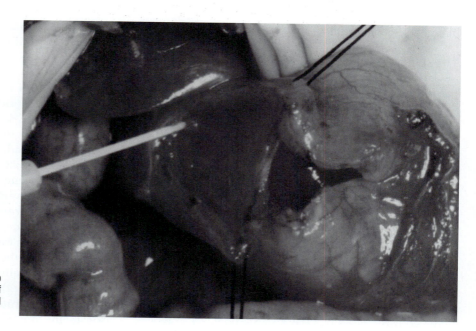

Figure 78–5. In cases of duodenal webs, it is important to locate the ampulla prior to excision of the web or bypass of the web with a duodenoduodenostomy. In this case a small angiocath is used to cannulate the duct to prevent injury.

present. In cases associated with malrotation, a Ladd's procedure also should be performed at this time.

The procedure of choice for duodenal atresia is duodenoduodenostomy (interrupted single- or two-layer anastomosis) that is constructed using the most dependent portion of the proximal atretic segment to minimize stasis (Fig 78–6). Kimura proposed the construction of a diamond-shaped anastomosis in order to create a larger intraluminal orifice. With this technique, an extensive Kocher maneuver is performed to mobilize the proximal megaduodenum. A transverse incision then is made in the dependent portion of the proximal duodenum and a longitudinal incision of the same length is made in the narrow distal duodenum. By matching the midportion of the longitudinal distal duodenotomy to the corner of the proximal transverse incision, a two-layer anastomosis can be performed with interrupted 5-0 suture. This modification is reported to have fewer problems with duodenal stasis and, like the side-to-side technique, eliminates the potential problem of blind-loop syndrome associated with a duodenojejunal anastomosis. In cases of associated malrotation, a Ladd's procedure should be performed. This includes division of the abnormal fixation bands across the duodenum, mobilization of the cecum and right colon, appendectomy, and arranging the bowel so that the small intestine is on the right side of the abdomen, the cecum is in the left lower quadrant next to the sigmoid, and the entire colon is on the left side of the celomic cavity. The abdomen then is closed in layers with absorbable or nonabsorbable 4-0 suture.

In some cases, a prolonged gastric ileus may require the use of TPN and gastric drainage (using either oral-gastric tube or gastrostomy). Some pediatric surgeons use transpyloric and transanastomotic feeding tubes to institute enteral feedings more quickly, thereby avoiding some of the potential complications of TPN (sepsis, biliary dysfunction, etc).

Long-term complications following repaired duodenal atresia include stasis in the proximal megaduodenum. To eliminate this problem, Ein and associates have suggested that an imbrication of the duodenum be performed at the time of the original operation. Other authors, including Adzick and associates, have advocated the performance of a tapering duodenoplasty at the time of the initial anastomosis, in cases where the proximal duodenum measures more than 5 cm. With this technique, a red rubber catheter is placed into the dilated duodenum and a GIA stapling device (US Surgical Corporation, Norwalk, CT) is positioned so the anterolateral aspect of the bowel wall can be excised without injury to the blood supply or the ductal system. Interrupted Lembert silk sutures are used to oversew the staple line (Fig 78–7).

Although mortality in this patient population has been reduced to 5% to 8% (usually owing to complicated congenital cardiac disease), late complications may be observed, including foregut motility disorders (gastroesophageal reflux, duodenal stasis, duodenal-gastric reflux), gastritis, and biliary tract disorders (including cholecystitis and cholelithiasis), suggesting that long-term follow-up is extremely important.

MALROTATION

In 1898, Mall described the embryology of intestinal rotation and Dott reported the clinical complications associated with anomalies of rotation and gut fixation in

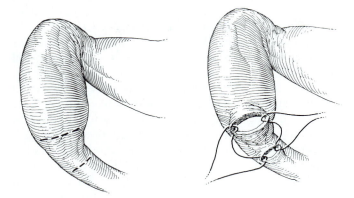

Figure 78–6. Forms of repair for a duodenal atresia defect; includes a side-to-side duo-denoduodectomy.

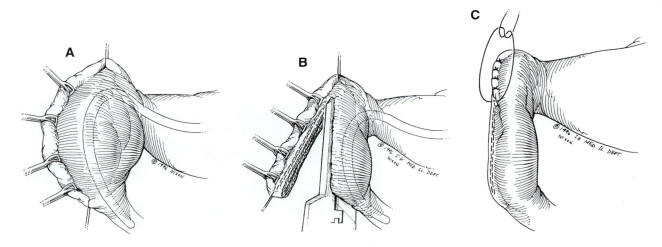

Figure 78–7. A tapering duodenoplasty may be indicated at the time of original repair if the proximal duodenum measures >5 cm.

1923. In 1936, Ladd described the surgical treatment of malrotation in 21 cases, based on an understanding of the embryology. The foregut is supplied by the celiac artery, the midgut by the superior mesenteric artery, and the hindgut by the inferior mesenteric artery. The cephalic end of the midgut is the duodenojejunal or prearterial loop and the caudal end is the ileocecal or postarterial loop. During the sixth week of gestational development, the gut herniates through the umbilical ring and continues to elongate. During this process, it also rotates 270° in a counterclockwise fashion around the superior mesenteric artery (SMA). This creates the normal location of the second portion of the duodenum to the right of the SMA, the third portion posterior to the SMA, and the junction of the duodenum and the jejunum to the left of the artery. By 12 weeks, the gut begins to return to the celomic cavity and during the following eight weeks, the mesentery will attach to the posterior abdominal wall along a diagonal plane between the duodenojejunal junction in the left upper quadrant and the cecum in the right lower quadrant. Anomalies of rotation and fixation can occur during any or all three embryologic stages. When present, a Meckel's diverticulum (persistent vitelline duct remnant) denotes the junction of the cranial and caudal portions of the gut.

Problems of fixation occur in 1/500 live births and are associated with abdominal wall defects (omphalocele and gastroschisis), duodenal atresia, and congenital diaphragmatic (Bochdalek) hernias. They also can occur de novo. More than two-thirds of cases become symptomatic in the newborn period with bilious emesis often associated with a midgut volvulus. There is a male predominance. The older child is likely to present with intermittent abdominal pain and bilious emesis. At the completion of the rotation process, the bowel becomes fixed to the posterior abdominal wall. This includes the attachment of the second and third portions of the duodenum and the ascending and descending colon at the line of Toldt. The root of the mesentery also becomes fixed beginning at the ligament of Treitz toward the ileocecal valve. This broad-based fixation stabilizes the base of the mesentery and prevents a volvulus around the SMA.

Newborns with malrotation may present in several ways. If there is a partial duodenal obstruction owing to Ladd's bands, the abdomen may be soft to palpation and bilious emesis might be the only presenting sign. Erect, recumbent, and decubitus abdominal radiographs will show a dilated stomach (owing to the partial obstruction at the duodenal level) and a decreased amount of distal bowel gas. In a stable child, an upper gastrointestinal series will confirm the diagnosis and reveal a partial or complete duodenal blockage ("spiral-beak" or "corkscrew" appearance) (Fig 78–8). Additionally, a barium enema contrast study would reveal an abnormal location of the cecum in the right upper quadrant or midabdomen, or an obstruction of the transverse colon, in instances of a partial volvulus.

In cases where an intrauterine midgut torsion has occurred, the child is born with abdominal distention and bilious gastric aspirates in the delivery room. Abdomi-

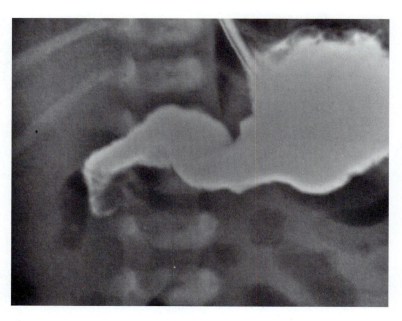

Figure 78–8. A. This barium contrast study has the spiral beak or corkscrew appearance which is diagnostic of a malrotation with volvulous. Additional contrast findings include a dilated stomach with a decrease in the amount of distal gas. *Continued*

A

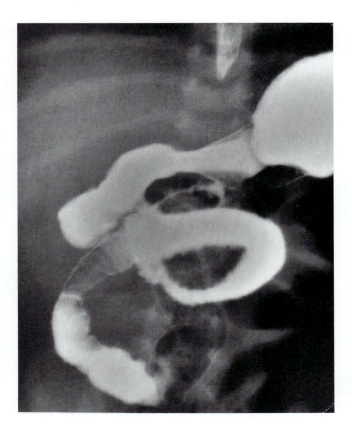

B

Figure 78–8, cont'd. B. Malrotation is present without evidence of obstruction.

nal radiography may reveal a dilated stomach and a gasless abdomen in cases of a persistent twist, or there may be dilated proximal small bowel loops indicative of an acquired small bowel atresia resulting from mesenteric ischemia.

Acute torsion of the small bowel postnatally around the narrowed vascular pedicle may result in abdominal distention, bilious emesis, and passage of blood per rectum (owing to ischemic bowel mucosa). There may be evidence of peritonitis, in this case, and an emergency operation is performed after adequate fluid resuscitation has been instituted. Contrast studies in children with peritoneal signs are not warranted.

The surgical approach in infants with anomalies of rotation with fixation is a transverse supraumbilical incision. If a volvulus is present, the bowel is eviscerated and the mesentery derotated in a counterclockwise fashion (Fig 78–9). Warmed, moist laparotomy sponges are placed over the bowel and the viability is assessed. In cases where the entire small bowel remains ischemic, the abdomen is closed and a second-look procedure performed in 24 to 48 hours to ascertain any improvement in bowel viability. Infusion of low molecular weight dextran during this time, prior to reoperation, may be useful. When demarcation of ischemic or necrotic segments is clear, the involved bowel will be resected and it then becomes the decision of the surgeon to place a temporary enterostomy (in cases where peritonitis or fecal soilage is present) or to attempt a primary anastomosis.

The Ladd's bands (duodenal cecal peritoneal attachments) are divided and the duodenum straightened so the bowel descends into the right lower quadrant. In some infants, duodenojejunal bands also may be encountered and are similarly lysed. An appendectomy (either standard or inversion technique) is performed and the cecum placed into the left lower quadrant. This will broaden the base of the mesentery to prevent recurrent torsion and the small bowel will now occupy the midabdomen and right abdomen.

JEJUNOILEAL ATRESIA AND STENOSIS

Although Goeller first described ileal atresia in 1684 and Voisin performed an enterostomy for an intestinal atresia in 1804, it was not until 1911 that Fockens performed the first successful anastomosis for this condition. Most cases of intestinal atresia and stenosis are related to the occurrence of late intrauterine mesenteric vascular accidents causing sterile necrosis and resorption of the involved bowel. Support for a vascular etiology of these defects is based on animal experiments by Barnard and Louw, Curtois, Abrams, Koga and others and upon clinical observations of atresias associated with midgut volvulus, tight abdominal wall defects causing ischemia of the extracelomic intestines, and internal hernias. The incidence of intestinal atresia has been reported from 1/350 to 1/5000 live births and is equally distributed between the sexes. Unlike duodenal atresia, the association of Down syndrome in cases of jejunoileal atresia is uncommon. With advances in prenatal ultrasound diagnosis, TPN, improved anesthetic management, innovative surgical techniques, and neonatal intensive care, the survival for these infants has gradually improved from 10% in 1950 to >90% presently.

Classification

In 95% of cases, there is a true atresia (Greek word for "blind-end") in which there is a congenital intralumenal obstruction. In the remaining cases, there is an intraluminal narrowing or partial obstruction (stenosis) (particularly associated with gastroschisis defects and following medically treated necrotizing enterocolitis). The types of atresias have been characterized by Louw and Barnard, and later modified by Grosfeld, to include the variations encountered (Fig 78–10). In Type 1 defects, there is a mucosal or membranous atresia with an intact bowel wall and mesentery. There are two blind ends

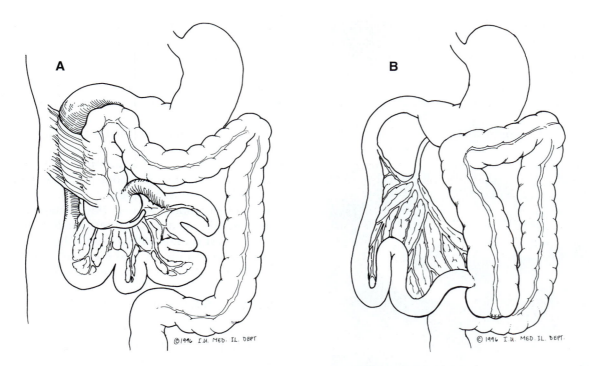

Figure 78–9. A. Initially the bowel is detorsed in a counterclockwise fashion as shown. **B.** The Ladd's bands are carefully divided and the mesentery broadened to prevent subsequent episodes of torsion. The cecum is placed in the left lower quadrant and an appendectomy is performed.

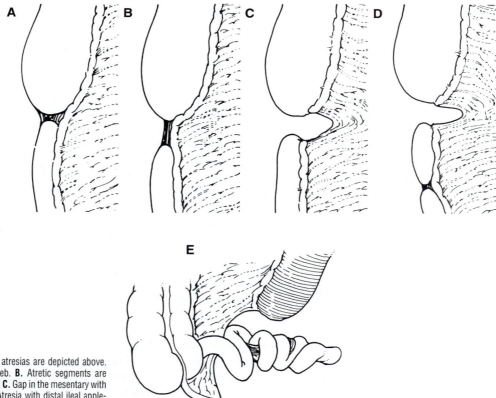

Figure 78–10. The various types of intestinal atresias are depicted above. **A.** Serosal continuity with an intralumenal web. **B.** Atretic segments are joined by a fibrous cord with no mesenteric gap. **C.** Gap in the mesentary with atresia. **D.** Multiple or "sausage" atresias. **E.** Atresia with distal ileal apple-peel deformity.

with a fibrous cord and an intact mesentery in the Type 2 variation. Type 3a defects have a complete separation of the blind ends with a V-shaped mesenteric defect; type 3b is the "apple-peel" deformity with an extensive mesenteric defect and the blood supply of the entire distal small bowel is supplied in a retrograde fashion by the ileocolic or right colic artery. There is a reported familial tendency in this group as well as a recognized association with prematurity, malrotation, associated anomalies, and short-bowel syndrome. Type 4 is characterized by multiple sausage-shaped atresias and also may be familial. These anomalies are distributed evenly between the jejunum and ileum with the proximal jejunum involved in 31%, the distal jejunum in 20%, proximal ileum in 13%, and distal ileum in 36% of cases. Although a single atresia is most common, multiple defects are reported in 6% to 20% of cases.

Diagnosis and Treatment

Clinical findings in cases of jejunoileal atresia include bilious emesis, maternal polyhydramnios, abdominal distention, failure to pass meconium in the first 24 hours of life, and jaundice (increased enterohepatic circulation owing to the small bowel atresia). The lower the level of obstruction, the more distended the abdomen becomes; palpable bowel loops and visible peristaltic waves through the thin abdominal wall may be observed. If the bowel loops noted on abdominal radiograph are larger than thumb-sized, this may be indicative of a bowel obstruction, especially if air-fluid levels are noted. If abdominal distention is noted at birth in conjunction with respiratory compromise from an elevated diaphragm, the diagnosis of antenatal perforation and the presence of giant cystic meconium peritonitis (GCMP) should be considered. In cases of GCMP, calcifications may be noted on the plain abdominal radiographs. Intraluminal calcifications (mummification) may be observed when an antenatal volvulus has occurred. Since it is difficult to discern between small and large bowel on the abdominal radiograph of a newborn infant, a contrast barium enema should be performed. The barium enema often shows a small unused microcolon, if the atresia has occurred early in gestation, and will document an associated malrotation in up to 10% of cases. This contrast study also helps to differentiate between instances of small bowel atresia, colonic atresia, Hirschsprung's disease, and meconium ileus syndromes as the cause for the abdominal distention and obstruction.

Operative Management

The infant is taken to the operating room after appropriate fluid repletion and the administration of broad-spectrum antibiotics (ampicillin 100 mg/kg/day, gentamicin 5 mg/kg/day). Owing to the presence of abdominal distention and intestinal obstruction, an "awake" intubation is performed to minimize the possibility of aspiration. The operative approach is through a transverse abdominal incision and the pathology encountered will determine the type of repair attempted. The bowel is eviscerated and the distal bowel evaluated for the presence of a second atresia. This can be accomplished by placing a purse-string suture in the distal segment, inserting an angiocatheter through the suture, and injecting sterile saline into the lumen. Once the integrity of the distal bowel has been ascertained, attention then is turned to the primary problem, resection of the atresia and construction of the anastomosis. If the overall bowel length is assessed as being normal (200 to 250 cm in the full-term infant) (as in most cases of ileal atresia), then several centimeters of the bulbous proximal atretic segment can be excised at a 90° angle, the distal atretic segment divided at a 45° angle, between infant Bainbridge bowel clamps, and an end-oblique anastomosis constructed using one or two layers of interrupted 5-0 suture (Fig 78–11). In cases where resection of the bulbous proximal jejunum is not advisable because of short bowel length, a tapering antimesenteric jejunoplasty using a GIA stapling device (US Surgical Corp, Norwalk, CN) can be performed up to the level of the ligament of Treitz. Alternatively, an imbricating jejunoplasty (as advocated by deLorimer) can be accomplished at this time (Fig 78–11). Both techniques seem to improve the motility of the proximal atretic segment by reducing the circumference of the lumen and improving peristalsis, shortening postoperative ileus, and avoiding dependence upon TPN. The imbrication technique preserves absorptive surfaces, which may be of importance in short bowel cases but may become unraveled with time (Fig 78–12). Associated abnormalities of fixation and rotation also are addressed at this time.

In cases where bowel viability is in question or there is significant soiling present owing to peritonitis, a primary anastomosis is not attempted, and temporary enterostomies are created. The type of enterostomy performed depends upon the preference of the surgeon and the underlying condition, but a double-barreled modified Mikulicz stoma brought out through the abdominal wound, using interrupted silk sutures, is performed easily and obviates the need for an intra-abdominal anastomosis. This technique also allows for the assessment of bowel viability and for eventual distal bowel feedings prior to enterostomy closure. With the side-by-side stomas, placing an enterostomal pouch is not a problem and a limited laparotomy will be required for the eventual enterostomy take-down.

Postoperative complications may be related to prolonged ileus, associated short bowel syndrome, dependence on TPN, motility disorders affecting the proximal

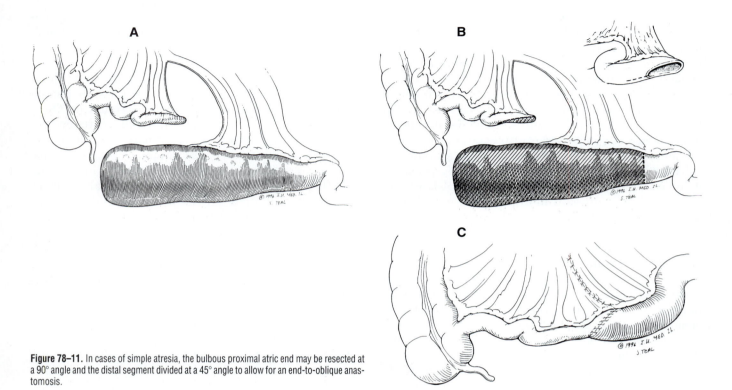

Figure 78–11. In cases of simple atresia, the bulbous proximal atric end may be resected at a 90° angle and the distal segment divided at a 45° angle to allow for an end-to-oblique anastomosis.

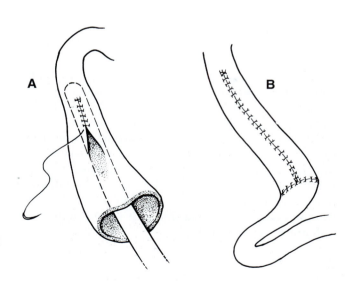

Figure 78–12. When there is a concomitant shortgut situation, the dilated proximal bowel should be lavaged and a tapering enteroplasty, using a resection or an imbricating technique, is required to preserve length.

atretic segment, and adhesion formation. Although a gastrostomy may be placed at the time of the original laparotomy, adequate gastric decompression can be accomplished safely using an oral gastric tube. In cases associated with short bowel syndrome in which continuous drip feedings to facilitate adaptation of intestinal microvilli may be required long-term, placement of a Stamm gastrostomy should be considered.

Postoperatively, careful attention to nutrition is imperative and should follow the guidelines discussed at the beginning of this chapter. When there has been a prolonged ileus, a contrast study should be performed to delineate the difference between a motility disorder and an anastomotic complication (stricture). Since cystic fibrosis may be associated with jejunoileal atresia in 10% to 12% of cases, a sweat chloride determination should be performed in all these patients prior to discharge from the hospital.

DUPLICATION CYSTS

There are two types of duplication cysts (tubular or spherical) that can occur anywhere along the gastrointestinal tract and usually are located along the mesenteric border of the bowel. The spherical or cystic duplications may be separate from the bowel lumen, while the tubular defects will often communicate with the lumen. Duplication cysts are lined by gastrointestinal mucosa and the presence of ectopic gastric mucosa can lead to peptic ulceration and bleeding; one or more muscle layers can be shared with the associated bowel wall. Embryologically these can arise from persistent intestinal diverticuli seen in the sixth to eighth week of gestational life. If these outpocketings are trapped between the leaves of the mesentery, a duplication cyst may develop. Additional theories relate to the failure of complete separation of the neural endoderm and gut ectoderm during the fourth week of intrauterine life. If a connection persists and both ends obliterate, a cystic lesion can form; if a communication persists with the ectoderm, a tubular defect would result.

Diagnosis and Treatment

Most duplication cysts (60% to 70%) are located in the small bowel. With the increased availability of prenatal ultrasound, these lesions are being diagnosed in utero and referred for treatment early, before the findings of a palpable mass or symptoms of obstruction owing to volvulus occur. When ectopic gastric mucosa is present, gastrointestinal bleeding may occur in the older child. The palpable mass will move with the mesentery (in the absence of torsion) and therefore change locations as the infant is moved from side to side. Ultrasound findings include a well-defined cystic mass with a discrete mucosal lining (Fig 78–13). In instances of bleeding, a technetium pertechnitate (^{99m}Tc) nuclear medicine study often will locate the areas of ulcerated ectopic gastric mucosa.

Operative Management

At operation, the cystic lesions simply are excised, often with the normal segment of intestine sharing a common muscular wall and intestinal continuity established with an end-to-end interrupted anastomosis. While short-segment tubular defects may be similarly excised; the long-segment duplication defects may present problems if total resection will result in a short bowel length. In these cases, a GIA stapling device (US Surgical Corp, Norwalk, CT) may be used to restore a single lumen by dividing the common wall. Care must be made to exclude the presence of gastric mucosa if this method is

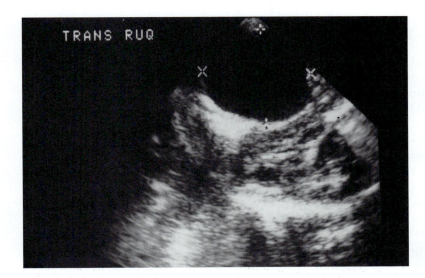

Figure 78–13. This ultrasound of an antenatally diagnosed duplication cyst shows a discrete mucosal lining within the cystic mass.

employed. Alternatively, submucosal mucosectomy can be completed in the duplication, which will then allow for the collapse and adherence of the muscular wall upon itself, avoiding the need to resect the normal bowel. Mucosal mucosectomy is also a very useful technique in the management of cystic duplications attached to the duodenum where resection would require pancreaticoduodenectomy.

MECONIUM ILEUS

Cystic fibrosis (CF) or mucoviscoidosis occurs in 1/2000 live births and is an autosomal recessive defect. In 1905, Landsteiner noted the association of obstructing insipissated meconium in the distal small bowel and concominant pancreatic abnormalities. Although initially believed to be the result of pancreatic achylia in these infants, the insipissated meconium has a 5 to 10 times higher concentration of albumen than normal children. There is also a significant increase in the amount of intraluminal glutamyltranspeptidase (GGTP) and 5'-nucleotidase, which are both produced in the liver. The albumen is derived from the swallowed amniotic fluid and becomes more concentrated as it passes distally. It is now known that the gene for CF occurs on the long arm of chromosome 7 and, in 70% of cases will be associated with a delta F508 mutation (based on work at the University of Michigan and University of Toronto). Screening for CF now includes a sweat chloride test (measures an elevated chloride level in the sweat), and a search for the F508 mutation.

Diagnosis and Treatment

A family history of cystic fibrosis associated with abdominal distention and radiographic evidence of a small bowel obstruction at birth is highly suggestive of meconium ileus. There are two types of meconium ileus (complicated and uncomplicated). In the uncomplicated form, there is a simple mechanical (obturator) obstruction of the small bowel owing to the presence of insipissated meconium. Distal to this point of obstruction, the bowel is small, unused, and filled with small pellets (concretions) of viscid meconium. Proximal to the obstruction, the lumen is dilated and filled with thickened putty-like meconium. The abdominal radiographs will show dilated proximal loops of bowel of similar size without air-fluid levels. There may be a "soap-bubble" or "ground-glass" appearance in the right lower quadrant as bubbles of air get trapped in the thick intralumenal contents. The diagnosis can be confirmed with a barium enema which will show the obstructing pellets in the small, unused proximal portion of a microcolon and the distal small bowel. The initial treatment of choice for simple uncomplicated meconium ileus is nonoperative manage-

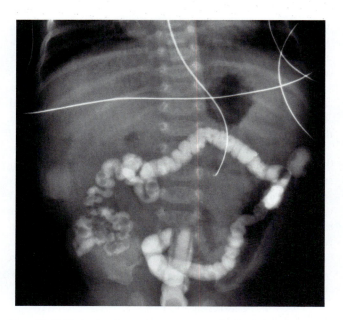

Figure 78–14. The inspisated meconium appears as small pellets in the colon and distal small bowel in this child with cystic fibrosis and meconium ileus. After the diagnostic barium study, a gastrograffin enema is used in an attempt to clear the obstructing meconium.

ment, as developed by Noblett. The installation of hypertonic hydrophilic contrast (diatrizoate meglumine) into the colon and distal small bowel draws fluid into the lumen and assists in the evacuation of the meconium (Fig 78–14). Prior to the gastrograffin enema (usually diluted to 20% to 30%), a bolus of 10 to 20 cc/kg of intravenous fluids is administered and the maintenance fluid rate increased to 1.5X the baseline to prevent potential problems related to hypovolemia induced by the fluid shift from the intravascular to the intralumenal compartments. Usually within 24 to 48 hours, there is a clearing of the obstructing meconium pellets and the abdominal distention resolves. Occasionally, a second gastrograffin enema is required to complete the evacuation. Additionally, a 5% solution of N-acetyl-cysteine (Mucomyst, 5 to 10 cc every 6 to 8 hours) may be administered via an oral gastric tube to assist in the clearing of the thicker proximal putty-like material. Enteral feedings are initiated when stools are passed on a consistent basis.

Meconium ileus may be complicated by associated giant cystic meconium peritonitis (owing to an antenatal perforation), a volvulus (owing to twisting of bowel at the site of the obstructing pellets and the dilated proximal segment), atresia of the distal small bowel (CF children account for 12% of ileal atresias), and perforation. In infants with a meconium pseudocyst, abdominal distention usually is observed at birth. If the processus vaginalis is patent, there may be dark greenish-black staining of the scrotal skin or labia majora. Occasionally, meconium is seen in the vagina owing to spillover through the fallopian tubes. Gastrograffin enema is contraindicated in complicated cases of meconium ileus; surgical intervention is required in all cases of complicated meconium ileus, as well as those simple cases in which more than two Gastrograffin enemas fail to relieve the obstruction.

Operative Management

In 1948, Hiatt and Wilson described a number of infants with meconium ileus who survived this previously fatal condition when an enterotomy was created and the obstructing thick meconium was irrigated from the bowel lumen. In 1953, Gross reported the use of resection and

Mickulicz enterostomy formation to relieve the blockage. Since then, several other techniques have been described to manage cases of complicated meconium ileus (Fig 78–15). The Bishop-Koop method involves resection and anastomosis of the proximal dilated segment to the distal bowel in an end-to-side fashion, with the distal bowel brought out as an end ileostomy to provide a portal for continued postoperative irrigation. Others have suggested the placement of tube enterostomy for postoperative irrigations. In most cases where atresias are not present, a simple purse-string enterotomy can be performed and the meconium irrigated, initially with saline and subsequently with Gastrograffin or N-acetylcysteine solutions. These agents may be left within the lumen to be excreted rectally as bowel function returns.

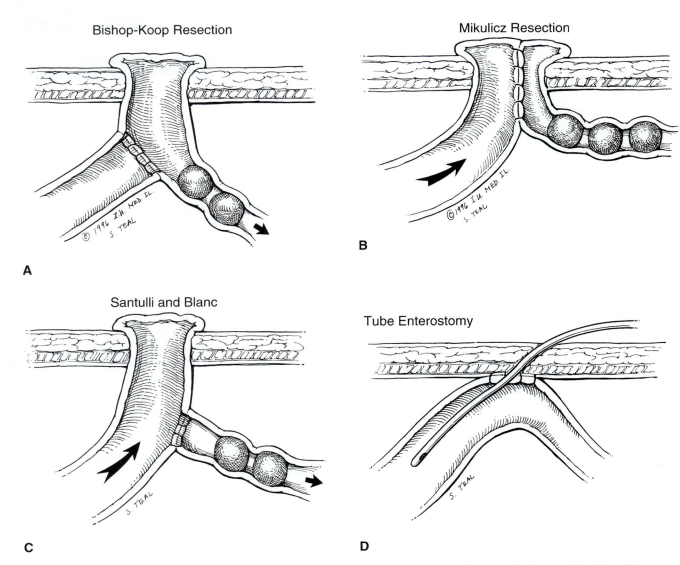

Figure 78–15. Various types of intestinal resections with anastomosis which are possible in the treatment of complicated meconium ileus are depicted above. When possible intestinal continuity is restored at the time of initial operation.

Other reports describe irrigation through the appendiceal stump, thereby eliminating the need for separate enterotomies in the small bowel. Swenson advocated a primary anastomosis after resection of the dilated segment and intraluminal irrigation.

In instances of giant cystic meconium peritonitis, the abdomen is evacuated of the pseudomembrane and the antenatal perforation identified. In the face of extensive abdominal soiling, a double-barrel ostomy is formed using silk sutures at the facial level; the abdominal wall is closed with nonabsorbable monofilament suture. The timing for reanastomosis is dependent upon the response of the individual infant in question. Supportive treatment includes TPN in conjunction with enteral feedings (often using elemental formulas because of associated short-bowel syndrome) and appropriate pancreatic enzyme replacement.

The overall 1 year survival for these infants has increased from 10% in the early 1950s to 90% presently. The long-term survival in children with CF is dependent upon the degree of associated pulmonary compromise.

NECROTIZING ENTEROCOLITIS

Although the exact etiology of necrotizing enterocolitis (NEC) remains unknown, this condition is associated with prematurity, low birth weight, episodes of hypoxia and hypotension, and the presence of intraluminal gut flora. Ninety percent of cases occur in premature infants; NEC may develop in 1% to 2% of all neonatal intensive care admissions. It has long been accepted that hypoxia or hypotension may result in splanchnic vasoconstriction (diving reflex), decreased mesenteric blood flow, and subsequent intestinal mucosal ischemia. However, in 20% of infants with NEC, no hypoxic event can be documented. NEC has also been observed following intestinal rotovirus infections (resulting in mucosal injury), respiratory distress syndrome, hyperviscosity syndrome, congenital heart disease, and after initiation of early intestinal feedings. Iatrogenic factors that have been implicated in the occurrence of NEC include the use of umbilical artery catheters, the need for exchange transfusions, and the administration of medications including indomethacin (for nonsurgical closure of a patent ductus), aminophyllim, and vitamin E. Premature infants have impaired humoral immunity owing to decreased levels of IgA (in the lamina propria) and circulating IgM. Cytotoxic, free radical anions (superoxide), cytokines [tumor necrosis factor (TNFa) and platelet activating factor (PAF)], bacterial endotoxins, interleukins, bowel immaturity, and an increased permeability to macromolecules may also play a role in the pathogenesis of this complex disease process.

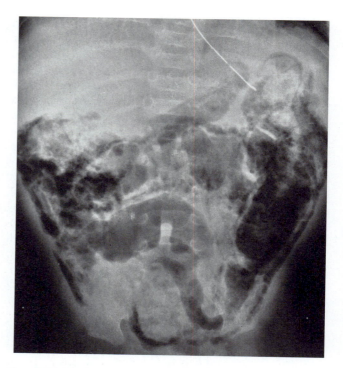

Figure 78–16. In this radiograph, pneumotosis intestinalis is noted in a neonate with necrotizing enterocolitis.

Diagnosis and Treatment

The initial clinical symptoms of NEC usually include increased gastric residuals (often bilious), abdominal distention, and the passage of a bloody stool. Radiographic findings include pneumatosis intestinalis, portal vein air loops, or free intraperitoneal air (Fig 78–16). The only absolute indication for surgical intervention is the presence of free air. Initially, oral feedings are stopped and the infant is managed with gastric decompression, vigorous intravenous rehydration, broad-spectrum antibiotics, and close observation of the clinical course (monitoring of the WBC, platelet counts, blood gas tension and pH, and evaluation of serial abdominal radiographs). Evidence of abdominal wall erythema or a palpable abdominal mass (usually indicative of perforation and peritonitis) and failure to respond to medical management (underlying ischemic gut), associated with clinical deterioration, are other indications for laparotomy. The presence of portal vein air often is associated with advanced disease and, in conjunction with clinical instability, is a relative indication for operative intervention. In the unstable micropremature infant (400 to 700 gm) with suspected perforation, simple abdominal drain placement at the bedside (isolette), under local anesthesia, may be a useful initial surgical procedure to decrease distention, drain fecal content, improve respiration, and allow time for coagulation factors to be corrected and perfusion to improve.

Laparotomy is performed through either a transverse supraumbilical or an infraumbilical incision, if free intraperitoneal air develops or clinical deterioration and progressive acidosis develops. Special emphasis is placed on avoiding injury to the thin liver capsule, which can bleed excessively in the face of sepsis and coagulopathy. In cases where nearly the entire bowel appears nonviable (NEC totalis), the abdomen simply is closed and the infant is supported and re-explored in 24 to 48 hours, if still alive. Occasionally, there is improvement in viability and appropriate resection can be accomplished with the formation of enterostomies. The most common area of bowel involvement is the distal ileum and the right colon. At operation, all frankly necrotic bowel is resected and exteriorization performed, although there are some advocates of primary end-to-end anastomosis, if there is no fecal contamination of the peritoneal cavity and if there is no question of intestinal viability in the remaining bowel. In most infants, there is considerable contamination and patchy involvement of residual bowel and we would recommend resection and exteriorization. Timing of the eventual enterostomy closure depends upon the clinical course of the infant, the length of remaining bowel and his or her ability to tolerate enteral feedings. It is important to obtain a distal intestinal contrast study prior to attempting closure of an enterostomy to be sure that no colonic strictures are present (noted in 10% to 12% of cases). Following the initial procedure, these patients may continue to consume platelets for up to 10 to 14 days, are predisposed to intracranial hemorrhage (assessed by cranial ultrasound examination), and require close monitoring of their fluid status to prevent cardiac compromise owing to increased shunting through an associated patent ductus arteriosus. Nutritional support is imperative because enteral feedings cannot be instituted for 7 to 10 days. Antibiotics are continued postoperatively and may be adjusted according to the results of intraoperative cultures. When the extent of resection will leave the infant with an ultrashort gut syndrome (<20 cm of small bowel with no ileocecal valve), the patient will be dependent on drip feedings of elemental formulas and TPN until bowel adaptation occurs or small bowel transplantation is required. Long-term morbidity is related to hepatic dysfunction from dependence upon TPN, recurring TPN-related episodes of catheter sepsis, and nutritional deficiencies, including the development of rickets.

The overall survival for infants with NEC has improved significantly for those treated both medically (80%) and surgically (70%). Candidates for surgical intervention already have failed medical therapy and are significantly higher risk patients. The highest mortality in NEC is observed in very low birth weight infants (<100 gm) who are <27 weeks gestation at diagnosis, and those with NEC totalis.

■ INTUSSUSCEPTION OF CHILDHOOD

Idiopathic intussusception is a frequent cause of bowel obstruction in children under the age of two years and may be associated with pathological lead points in older children (>5 yrs). In the late 1600s, Paul Barbette described the invagination of one segment of bowel into another, and Sir Jonathan Hutchison reported the first successful surgical reduction in 1871. He detailed the description of intermittent crampy abdominal pain in a toddler associated with bloody stools and prolapse of the ileum out the rectum. When attempts to reduce the prolapsed bowel by dangling the child by the feet and multiple enemas was unsuccessful, a laparotomy was performed and a satisfactory reduction accomplished.

In most cases, intussusception is a process without a true lead point and occurs when a proximal segment of bowel (intussusceptum) becomes telescoped into a distal segment (intussuscipiens) pulling the associated mesentery along with it. As bowel wall edema develops subsequent lymphatic and venous congestion result in passage of "currant jelly stools." Ischemia of the intussusceptum is possible when the diagnosis is delayed. Most cases are of the ileocolic type and occur in otherwise healthy children, with a male predominance. There is often (10% to 15%) an association with a preceding viral illness (upper respiratory illness or gastroenteritis). The resultant viremia may increase the size of the lymphoid tissue of the terminal ileum and induce hypertrophy of the Peyer's patches. These hypertrophied lymphoid patches then may act as a potential lead point for the intussusception.

In the older child, a true pathological lead point may be encountered and include instances of lymphomas, Meckel's diverticulum, hamartomatous polyps, hemangiomas, and even an inverted appendiceal stump. Small bowel intussusceptions are encountered in children with Henoch-Schonlein purpura and are probably owing to a submucosal hematoma. In the postoperative patient with signs of an early small bowel obstruction (<7 days after surgery), a postoperative small bowel intussusception should be considered.

DIAGNOSIS AND TREATMENT

Intussusception is characterized by the sudden onset of intermittent crampy abdominal pain during which the child draws up his or her legs and may be inconsolable. Between these episodes the child may appear comfortable. As the symptoms persist and the time interval between these painful episodes shorten, the toddler may

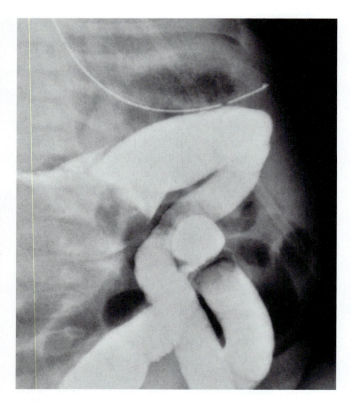

Figure 78–17. Although the hydrostatic barium enema or air enema can be utilized in the safe reduction of an ileocolic intussusception, this study illustrates a transverse colonic perforation.

hours, in infants <6 months of age, with evidence of complete bowel obstruction on plain abdominal radiographs. Attempting hydrostatic reduction under ultrasound guidance has recently gained popularity, as has air reduction techniques initially developed in China. During air reduction, the column of insufflated air is monitored so as not to exceed 80 mm Hg in infants <6 months of age and 120 mm Hg in older infants, for periods of <3 minutes. A satisfactory reduction is noted when the cecal mass disappears and the distal small bowel becomes distended with air. In controlled studies, similar results now are obtained with both hydrostatic barium and air reduction. Successful nonoperative reduction is recorded in 55% to 80% of cases.

Surgical intervention is required when hydrostatic or air reduction techniques have failed. Laparotomy is performed through a transverse muscle-cutting incision in the right lower quadrant to allow for mobilization of the right colon. The intraluminal mass is identified and manual reduction is attempted by retrograde milking of the intussuscipiens proximally (Fig 78–18). Although there is edema at the ileocecal valve, careful handling of the colonic tissue will prevent serosal splitting. In cases where the reduction is successful, an appendectomy also is performed and the peritoneal band between the distal ileum and cecum (Jackson's veil) carefully divided. If there is underlying ischemia and reduction is not possible, a limited resection should be performed

become increasingly lethargic. The classically described triad of abdominal pain, a palpable abdominal mass, and currant jelly stools is only encountered in 15% of reported series. Emesis (often bilious) is seen in over 80% of cases and as many as 40% will be referred for evaluation of sepsis, lethargy, or even suspected of having meningitis.

A high index of suspicion is required in these patients to obviate the need for intraoperative intervention. The abdominal radiographs may show air-fluid levels with a paucity of gas in the right lower quadrant. If a palpable mass is present, it is often sausage-shaped and located in the right upper quadrant and the right lower region is relatively empty. A barium enema is employed to diagnose the entity and to attempt hydrostatic radiographic reduction. Prior to sending the child to the radiology suite for the attempted reduction, intravenous hydration is instituted, a nasogastric tube inserted, broad-spectrum antibiotics are administered and the infant is sedated. The contrast material is elevated 36 inches above the table and the reduction is monitored carefully by flouroscopy. The risk of perforation (Fig 78–17) during this procedure ranges from 1% to 3% and is more likely to occur with symptom duration >72

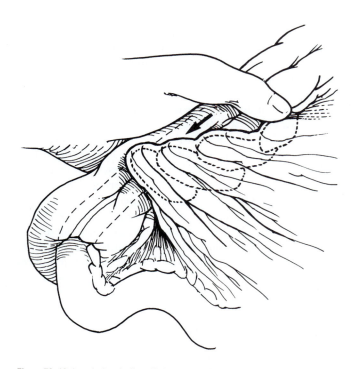

Figure 78–18. In reducing the ileocolic intussusception is milked proximally to avoid a serosal tear in the surrounding intussuscipiens.

with a primary end-to-end anastomosis. This usually is accomplished with an interrupted two-layer technique. In most cases, intussusception is not protected within a normal segment of bowel so that, as the irreducible necrotic lead point is accompanied by peritonitis, a primary anastomosis is reasonable. If there is a perforation and significant fecal soiling of the peritoneal cavity caused by attempts at nonoperative reduction, then the decision to place enterostomies may depend on the hemodynamic status of the patient at the time of the procedure. The stomas can be brought out safely through the incision and early closure (10 days) is suggested.

The incidence of recurrent intussusception following hydrostatic reduction ranges from 8% to 10%. Following intraoperative reduction, the recurrence rate is very low (0% to 3%). The associated morbidity and occasional mortality noted in infants and children with intussusception is directly related to delays in diagnosis. We have had no deaths following either nonoperative or operative reduction of intussusception in 9 of 120 patients. However, two children with unrecognized intussusception arrived in the emergency room in extremis and succumbed. The diagnosis was observed at a postmortem study.

SELECTED READINGS

Pyloric Obstruction

Bennett RJ Jr. Atresia of pylorus. *Am J Dig Dis* 1937;4:44

Bull MJ, Norins AL, et al. Epidermolysis bullosa-pyloric atresia: an autosomal ressive syndrome. *Am J Dis Child* 1983; 137:449

Ducharme JC, Bonsousan AL. Pyloric atresia. *J Pediatr Surg* 1975;10:149

Hayashi AH, Galliani CA, et al. Congenital pyloric atresia and junctional epidermolysis bullosa: a report of long-term survival and a review of the literature. *J Pediatr Surg* 1991;26: 1341

Olsen L, Grotte G. Congenital pyloric atresia: report of a familial occurrence. *J Pediatr Surg* 1976;11:187

Thompson NW, Parker W, et al. Congenital pyloric atresia. *Arch Surg* 1968;97;792

Duodenal Obstruction

Adzick NW, Harrison MR, et al. Tapering duodenoplasty for megaduodenum associated with duodenal atresia. *J Pediatr Surg* 1986;21:311

Boyden EA, Cope JG, et al. Anatomy and embryology of congenital intrinsic obstruction of the duodenum. *Am J Surg* 1967;114:190

Browne AF, Clatworthy HW. Congenital duodenal obstruction. In: Scott HW, Sawyer JL (eds), *Surgery of the Stomach, Duodenum and Small Intestine.* Boston, MA: Blackwell; 1987

Dewan PA, Guiney EJ. Duodenoplasty in the management of duodenal atresia. *Pediatr Surg Int* 1990;5:253

Ein SH, Shandling B. The late nonfunctioning duodenal atresia repair. *J Pediatr Surg* 1986;21:798

Ernst NP. A case of congenital atresia of the duodenum treated successfully by operation. *BMJ* 1916;1:1644

Fonkalsrud EW, DeLorimier AA, et al. Congenital atresia and stenosis of the duodenum: a review compiled from the members of the Surgical Section of the American Academy of Pediatrics. *Pediatrics* 1969;43:79

Gray SW, Skandalakis JE. *Embryology for Surgeons.* Philadelphia, PA: WB Saunders; 1972

Grosfeld JL, Rescorla FJ. Duodenal atresia and stenosis: reassessment of treatment and outcome based on antenatal diagnosis, pathologic variance, and long-term follow-up. *World J Surg* 1993;17:301

Hancock BJ, Wiseman NE. Congenital duodenal obstruction: the impact of an antenatal diagnosis. *J Pediatr Surg* 1989;24:1027

Jona JZ, Belin RP. Duodenal anomalies and the ampulla of Vater. *Surg Gynecol Obstet* 1976;143:565

Kimura K, Mukahara N, et al. Diamond shaped anastomosis for duodenal atresia: an experience with 44 patients over 15 years. *J Pediatr Surg* 1990;25:977

Kokkonnen ML, Kalina T. Duodenal atresia—late followup. *J Pediatr Surg* 1988;23:216

Knechtle SJ, Filston HC. Anomalous biliary ducts associated with duodenal atresia. *J Pediatr Surg* 1990;25:1266

Miro J, Bard H. Congenital atresia and stenosis of the duodenum: the impact of a prenatal diagnosis. *Am J Obstet Gynecol* 1988;158:555

Moore KL, Persaud TVN. *The Developing Human.* Philadelphia, PA: WB Saunders; 1993;237–251

Nixon HH, Tawes R. Etiology and treatment of small intestinal atresias: analysis of a comparison with 62 duodenal atresias. *Surgery* 1971;69:41

Spigland N, Yazbeck S. Complications associated with surgical treatment of congenital intrinsic duodenal obstruction. *J Pediatr Surg* 1990;25:1127

Tandler J. Entwicklungsgeschichte des menschlichen duodenum. *Marhol Jahrb* 1902;29:187

Tchirkaw G, Highmnan LM, et al. Cholelithiasis and cholecystitis in children after repair of congenital duodenal anomalies. *Arch Surg* 1980;115:85

Touloukian RJ, Hobbins JC. Maternal ultrasonography in the antenatal diagnosis of surgically correctable fetal anomalies. *J Pediatr Surg* 1980;15:373

Reid IS. Biliary tract abnormalities associated with duodenal atresia. *Arch Dis Child* 1973;48:952

Rescorla FJ, Grosfeld JL. Intestinal atresia and stenosis: analysis of survival in 120 cases. *Surgery* 1985;98:668

Rowe MI, Buckner D, et al. Windsock web of the duodenum. *Am J Surg* 1968;116:444

Webb CH, Wangensteen OH. Congenital intestinal atresia. *Am J Dis Child* 1931;41:262

Weber TR, Lewis JE, et al. Duodenal atresia: a comparison of techniques of repair. *J Pediatr Surg* 1986;21:1133

Duplications

Akers DR, Fuvara BE, et al. Duplications of the alimentary tract: report of three unusual cases associated with bile and pancreatic ducts. *Surgery* 1972;71:817

Bishop HC, Koop CE. Surgical management of duplications of the alimentary tract. *Am J Surg* 1964;107:434

Bower RJ, Sieber WK, et al. Alimentary tract duplications in children. *Ann Surg* 1978;188:669

Grosfeld JL, O'Neill JA Jr, et al. Enteric duplications in infancy and childhood: an 18 year review. *Ann Surg* 1970; 172:83

Gross RE, Holcomb GW Jr, et al. Duplications of the alimentary tract. *Pediatrics* 1952;9:449

Hoffman M, Sugerman HJ, et al. Gastric duplication cyst communicating with aberrant pancreatic duct: a rare cause of recurrent acute pancreatitis. *Surgery* 1987;101:369

Holcomb GW, Bheissari A, et al. Surgical management of alimentary tract duplications. *Ann Surg* 1989;209:167

Ilstad ST, Tollerud DJ, et al. Duplications of the alimentary tract clinical characteristics, preferred treatment and associated malformations. *Ann Surg* 1988;208:184

Ladd WE, Gross RE. Abdominal surgery in infancy and childhood. Philadelphia, PA: WB Saunders; 1941

Middledorf K. Zur Kenntniss der angeborenen Sacraugeschwuiste. *Arch Pathol Anat* 1885;101:37

Malrotation

Andrassy RJ, Mahour GH. Malrotation of the midgut in infants and children: a 25 year review. *Arch Surg* 1981;116:158

Brandt ML, Pokorny WJ, et al. Late presentations of midgut malrotation in children. *Am J Surg* 1985;150:767

Brennon WS, Bill AH. Prophylactic fixation of the intestine for midgut malrotation. *Surg Gynecol Obstet* 1974;138:181

Dott NN. Anomalies of intestinal rotation: their embryology and surgical aspects. *Br J Surg* 1923;11:251

Filston, HC, Kirks DR. Malrotation: the ubiquitous anomaly. *J Pediatr Surg* 1981;16:614

Gaines PA, Saunders AJ, et al. Midgut malrotation diagnosed by ultrasound. *Clin Radiol* 1987;38:51

Gibson MF. Familial multiple jejunal atresia with malrotation. *J Pediatr Surg* 1987;22:1013

Krasna KH, Becker JM, et al. Low molecular weight dextran and reexploration in the management of ischemic midgut volvulus. *J Pediatr Surg* 1978;13:480

Ladd WE. Surgical diseases of the alimentary tract in infants. *N Engl J Med* 1936;215:705

Mall FG. Development of the human intestine and its position in the adult. *Bull Johns Hopkins Hosp* 1898;9:197

Ornstein MY, Lund RJ. Simultaneous occurrence of malrotation volvulus and intussusception in an infant. *Br J Surg* 1981;68:440

Potts SR, Thomas PS, et al. The duodenal triangle: a plain film sign of midgut malrotation and volvulus in the neonate. *Clin Radiol* 1985;36:47

Powell DM, Othersen HB, et al. Malrotation of the intestines in children: the effect of age on presentation and therapy. *J Pediatr Surg* 1989;24:777

Rescorla FJ, Shedd FJ, et al. Anomalies of intestinal rotation in childhood: analysis of 442 cases. *Surgery* 1990;108:710

Snyder WH, Chaffin L. Embryology and pathology of the intestinal tract: presentation of 40 cases of malrotation. *Ann Surg* 1954;140:368

Stauffer UG, Herrmann P. Comparison of late results in patients with corrected intestinal malrotation with and without fixation of the mesentry. *J Pediatr Surg* 1980;15:9

Stewart DR, Colodny AL, et al. Malrotation of the bowel in infants and children: a 15 year review. *Surgery* 1976;79:716

Torres AM, Ziegler MM. Malrotation of the intestine. *World J Surg* 1993;17:326

Jejunoileal Atresia

Abrams JS. Experimental intestinal atresia. *Surgery* 1968;64:185

Benson CD, Lloyd JR, et al. The surgical and metabolic aspects of massive small bowel resection in the newborn. *J Pediatr Surg* 1967;2:227

Benson CD, Lloyd JR, et al. Resection and primary anastomosis in the management of stenosis and atresia of the jejunum and ileum. *Pediatrics* 1960;26:265

Boggs TR, Bishop H. Neonatal hyperbilirubinemia associated with high obstruction of the small bowel. *J Pediatr* 1965;66:349

Cloutier R. Intestinal smooth muscle response to chronic obstruction: possible application in jejunoileal atresia. *J Pediatr Surg* 1975;10:3

deLorimier AA, Fonkalsrud EW, et al. Congenital atresia and stenosis of the jejunum and ileum. *Surgery* 1969;65:819

deLorimier AA, Harrison MR. Intestinal imbrication for atresia and pseudo-obstruction. *J Pediatr Surg* 1983;18:734

Dickson JAS. Apple peel small bowel: an uncommon variant of duodenal and jejunal atresia. *J Pediatr Surg* 1970;5:595

Grosfeld JL, Ballantine TVN, et al. Operative management of intestinal atresia and stenosis based on pathologic findings. *J Pediatr Surg* 1979;13:368

Lloyd JR, Clatworthy HW. Hydramnios as an aid to the early diagnosis of congenital obstruction of the alimentary tract: a study of the maternal and fetal factors. *Pediatrics* 1958;21:903

Louw JH, Barnard CN. Congenital intestinal atresia: Observations on its origin. *Lancet* 1955;2:1065

Louw JH. Resection and end-to-end anastomosis in the management of atresia and stenosis of the small bowel. *Surgery* 1967;62:940

Martin LW, Zerella JT. Jejunoileal atresia: proposed classification. *J Pediatr Surg* 1976;11:399

Nixon HH. Intestinal obstruction in the newborn. *Arch Dis Child* 1955;30:13

Pokorny WJ, Harberg FJ, et al. Gastroschisis complicated by intestinal atresia. *J Pediatr Surg* 1981;16:261

Pari P, Fujimoto T. New observations on the pathogenesis of multiple intestinal atresias. *J Pediatr Surg* 1988;23:221

Randolph JG, Zollinger RM, et al. Mikulicz resection in infants and children: a 20-year survey of 196 patients. *Ann Surg* 1963;158:481

Rowe MI, Buckner D, et al. Windsock web of the duodenum. *Am J Surg* 1968;116:444

Santulli TV, Blanc WA. Congenital atresia of the intestine: pathogenesis and treatment. *Ann Surg* 1961;154:939

Seashore JH, Collins FS, et al. Familial apple peel jejunal atresia: surgical, genetic, and radiographic aspects. *Pediatrics* 1987;80:540

Touloukian RJ. Intestinal atresia and stenosis. In: Holder TM,

Ashcraft KW (eds), *Pediatric Surgery*. Philadelphia, PA: WB Saunders; 1980

Touloukian RJ, Hobbins JC. Maternal ultrasonography in the antenatal diagnosis of surgically correctable fetal abnormalities. *J Pediatr Surg* 1980;15:373

Touloukian RJ, Walker GJ. Normal intestinal length in preterm infants: an autopsy study. *J Pediatr Surg* 1983;18:720

Turneck RR, Brereton RJ, et al. Primary anastomosis in apple-peel bowel syndrome. *J Pediatr Surg* 1991;26:718

Weber TR, Vane DW, et al. Tapering enteroplasty in infants with bowel atresia and short gut. *Arch Surg* 1982;117:684

Weitzman JJ, Vanderhoof RS. Jejunal atresia with agenesis of the dorsal mesentery with "Christmas tree" deformity of the small intestine. *Am J Surg* 1966;111:443

Meconium Ileus

Bishop HC, Koop CE. Management of meconium ileus: resection, Roux-en-Y anastomosis and ileostomy irrigation with pancreatic enzymes. *Ann Surg* 1957;145:410

Buchanan DJ, Rapoport S. Chemical comparison of normal meconium and meconium from a patient with meconium ileus. *Pediatrics* 1952;9:304

Caniano DA, Beaver BL. Meconium ileus: a fifteen year experience with forty-two neonates. *Surgery* 1987;102:699

Collins FS, Riordan J, et al. The cystic fibrosis gene: isolation and significance. *Hosp Pract* 1990;25:47

Ein SH, Shandling B, et al. Bowel perforation with nonoperative treatment of meconium ileus. *J Pediatr Surg* 1987;22:146

Farber SJ. The relation of pancreatic achylia to meconium ileus. *J Pediatr* 1944;24:387

Fitzgerald R, Colon K. Use of the appendix stump in the treatment of meconium ileus. *J Pediatr Surg* 1989;24:899

Harberg FJ, Senekjian EK, et al. Treatment of uncomplicated meconium ileus via T-tube ileostomy. *J Pediatr Surg* 1981;16:61

Holsclaw DS, Eckstein HB, et al. Meconium ileus. *Am J Dis Child* 1965;109:101

Kalayoglu M, Sieber WK, et al. Meconium ileus: a critical review of treatment and eventual prognosis. *J Pediatr Surg* 1971;6:290

Landsteiner K. Darmverschluss durch eingedictes Meconium Pankreatitis. *Zentralbl Allg Pathol* 1905;16:903

Noblett H. Meconium ileus. In: Ravitch MM, Welch KJ, Benson CD, Aberdeen E, Randolph JG (eds), *Pediatric Surgery*. Chicago, IL: Year Book; 1979

Nguyen LT, Youssef S, et al. Meconium ileus: is a stoma necessary? *J Pediatr Surg* 1986;21:766

Olim CB, Ciuti A. Meconium ileus: a new method of relieving obstruction. *Ann Surg* 1954;140:736

O'Neill JA, Grosfeld JL, et al. Surgical treatment of meconium ileus. *Am J Surg* 1970;119:99

Park RW, Grand RJ. Gastrointestinal manifestations of cystic fibrosis: a review. *Gastroenterology* 1981;81:1143

Rescorla FJ, Grosfeld JL, et al. Changing patterns of treatment and survival in neonates with meconium ileus. *Arch Surg* 1989;124:837

Rescorla FJ, Grosfeld JL. Contemporary management of meconium ileus. *World J Surg* 1993;17:318

Riordan J, Rommens JM, et al. Identification of the cystic fibrosis gene: cloning and characterization of complimentary DNA. *Science* 1989;245:1066

Rommens, JM, Iannuzzi MC, et al. Identification of the cystic fibrosis gene: chromosome walking and jumping. *Science* 1989;245:1059

Rowe MI, Furst J, et al. The neonatal response to Gastrografin enema. *Pediatrics* 1971;48:29

Shaw A. Safety of N-acetylcysteine in the treatment of meconium obstruction in the newborn. *J Pediatr Surg* 1969;4:119

Santulli TV, Blanc WA. Congenital atresia of the intestine: pathogenesis and treatment. *Ann Surg* 1961;154:939

Venugopal S, Shandling B. Meconium ileus: laparotomy without resection, anastomosis, or enterostomy. *J Pediatr Surg* 1979;14:715

Wagget J, Bishop HC, et al. Experience with gastrografin enema in the treatment of meconium ileus. *J Pediatr Surg* 1970;5:649

Necrotizing Enterocolitis

Caplan MS, Sun XM, et al. Role of platelet activating factor and tumor necrosis factor-alpha in neonatal necrotizing enterocolitis. *J Pediatr* 1988;23:557

Cheu H, Sukarochana K, et al. Peritoneal drainage for necrotizing enterocolitis. *J Pediatr Surg* 1988;23:557

Cikrit D, Mastandrea J, et al. Significance of portal vein air in necrotizing enterocolitis, analysis of 53 cases. *J Pediatr Surg* 1985;20:425

Cikrit D, Mastandrea J, et al. Necrotizing enterocolitis: factors affecting mortality in 101 surgical cases. *Surgery* 1984;96:648

Clark DA, Miller MJ. Intraluminal pathogenesis of necrotizing enterocolitis. *J Pediatr* 1990;117:564

Czyrko C, delPin CA, et al. Maternal cocaine abuse and necrotizing enterocolitis: outcome and survival. *J Pediatr Surg* 1991;26:414

Ein SH, Shandling B, et al. A 13-year experience with peritoneal drainage under local anesthesia for necrotizing enterocolitis perforation. *J Pediatr Surg* 1990;25:1034

Griffiths DM, Forbes DA, et al. Primary anastomosis for necrotizing enterocolitis: a 12 year experience. *J Pediatr Surg* 1989;24:515

Grosfeld JL, Rescorla FJ, et al. Short bowel syndrome in infancy and childhood: analysis of survival in 60 cases. *Am J Surg* 1986;151:41

Grosfeld JL, Cheu H, et al. Changing trends in necrotizing enterocolitis. *Ann Surg* 1991;214:300

Halac E, Halac J, et al. Prenatal and postnatal corticosteroid therapy to prevent neonatal necrotizing enterocolitis: a controlled trial. *J Pediatr* 1990;117:132

Harberg FJ, McGill CW, et al. Resection and primary anastomosis for necrotizing enterocolitis. *J Pediatr Surg* 1983;18:743

Kliegman RM. Neonatal necrotizing enterocolitis: bridging the basic science with the clinical disease. *J Pediatr* 1990;117:833

Kosloske AM. Pathogenesis and prevention of necrotizing enterocolitis: a hypothesis based on personal observation and a review of the literature. *Pediatrics* 1984;72:1086

Lawrence G, Bates J, Gaul A. Pathogenesis of neonatal necrotizing enterocolitis. *Lancet* 1982;i:137

Musemeche C, Kosloske A, et al. Comparative effects of ischemia, bacteria, and substrate on the pathogenesis of intestinal necrosis. *J Pediatr Surg* 1986;21:536

Musemeche CA, Reynolds M. Necrotizing enterocolitis following intrauterine blood transfusion. *J Pediatr Surg* 1991; 26:1411

O'Neill JA. Necrotizing enterocolitis in Grosfeld JL (ed), *Common Problems in Pediatric Surgery*. St Louis, MO: Mosby Year-Book; 1991

Powell RW, Dyess DL, et al. Necrotizing enterocolitis in multiple-birth infants. *J Pediatr Surg* 1990;25:319

Robinson MJ, Clayden GS, Smith MS. Xanthines and necrotizing enterocolitis. *Arch Dis Child* 1980;55:494

Rotbart HA, Nelson WL, et al. Neonatal rotavirus-associated necrotizing enterocolitis: case control study and prospective surveillance during an outbreak. *J Pediatr* 1988;111:87

Sun XM, Hsueh W. Bowel necrosis induced by tumor necrosis factor in rats is mediated by platelet activating factor. *J Clin Invest* 1988;81:1328

Telsey A, Merrit T, et al. Cocaine exposure in a term neonate: necrotizing enterocolitis as a complication. *Clin Pediatr* 1988;27:547

Touloukian RJ, Posch JN, et al. The pathogenesis of ischemic gastroenterocolitis of the neonate: selective gut mucosal ischemia in asphyxiated neonatal piglets. *J Pediatr Surg* 1972; 7:194

Walsh MC, Kleigman RM. Necrotizing enterocolitis: treatment based on staging criteria. *Pediatr Clin North Am* 1986; 33:179

Weber TR, Lewis JE. The role of second-look laparotomy in necrotizing enterocolitis. *J Pediatr Surg* 1986;21:323

Intussusception

Barbette P. *Oeuvres chirurgiqes et Anatomiques*. Geneva, Switzerland: Francois Miege; 1674:522

Bolia A. Case report: diagnosis and hydrostatic reduction of an intussusception under ultrasound guidance. *Clin Radiol* 1985;36:655

Bramson RT, Blickman JG. Perforation during hydrostatic reduction of intussusception: proposed mechanism and review of literature. *J Pediatr Surg* 1992;27:589

Ein SH. Leading points in childhood intussusception. *J Pediatr Surg* 1976;11:209

Ein SH, Mercer S, et al. Colon perforation during attempted barium enema reduction of intussusception. *J Pediatr Surg* 1981;16:313

Fiorito ES, Recalde Cuestas LA. Diagnosis and treatment of acute intestinal intussusception with controlled insufflation of air. *Pediatrics* 1959;24:241

Freund H, Hurvitz H, et al. Etiologic and therapeutic aspects of intussusception in childhood. *Am J Surg* 1977;134:272

Franken EA, Smith WL, et al. The use of glucagon in hydrostatic reduction of intussusception. *Radiology* 1983; 146:687

Guo JB, Ma S, et al. Results of air pressure enema reduction of intussusception: 6,396 cases in 13 years. *J Pediatr Surg* 1986; 12:1201

Hedlund GL, Johnson FJ, et al. Ileocolic intussusception: extensive reflux of air preceding pneumatic reduction. *Radiology* 1990;174:187

Holsclaw DS, Racmans C, et al. Intussusception in patients with cystic fibrosis. *Pediatrics* 1971;48:51

Hirschsprung H. Et tilfaelde at subakut tarminvagination. *Hospitals-Tidende* 1976;3:321

Hutchinson J. A successful case of abdominal section for intussusception. *Proc R Med Chirsoc* 1873;7:195

Jinzhe Z, Yenxia W, et al. Rectal inflation reduction of intussusception in infants. *J Pediatr Surg* 1986;21:30

Konno T, Suzuki H, et al. Human rotavirus infection in infants and young children with intussusception. *J Med Virol* 1982; 2:265

Mercer S, Carpenter B. Mechanism of perforation occurring in the intussusception. *Can J Surg* 1982;25:481

Mollitt DL, Ballantine TVN, et al. Postoperative intussusception in infancy and childhood: analysis of 119 cases. *Surgery* 1979;86:402

Nissan S, Levy E. Intussusception in infancy caused by hypertrophic Peyer's patches. *Surgery* 1966;59:1108

Palder SB, Ein SH, et al. Intussusception: barium or air? *J Pediatr Surg* 1991;26:271

Reijnen JAM, Festen C, et al. Intussusception-factors related to treatment. *Arch Dis Child* 1990;65:871

Rosenkrantz JG, Cox JA, et al. Intussusception in the 1970s: indication for operation. *J Pediatr Surg* 1977;12:367

Ravitch MM. Intussusception in infancy and childhood. *N Engl J Med* 1958;259:1058

Ravitch MM: McCune RM. Reduction of intussusception by hydrostatic pressure: an experimental study. *Bull Johns Hopkins Hosp* 1948;82:550

Shiels WE, Bisse GS, et al. Simple device for air reduction of intussusception. *Pediatr Radiol* 1990;20:472

Stringer DA, Ein SH. Pneumatic reduction: advantages, risks, and indications. *Pediatr Radiol* 1990;20:475

Wayer ER, Campbell JB, et al. Management of 344 children with intussusception. *Radiology* 1973;107:597

West KW, Stephens B, et al. Intussusception: current management in infants and children. *Surgery* 1987;102:781

West KW, Stephens B, et al. Postoperative intussusception: experience with 36 cases in children. *Surgery* 1988;104:781

79

Hirschsprung's Disease

Eric W. Fonkalsrud

In 1887, Harald Hirschsprung presented the first classic description of colonic distention and muscular hypertrophy proximal to a smaller normal-sized rectum at postmortem examination in two infants who had experienced severe constipation and abdominal distention since birth.[1] Despite isolated reports of the histologic absence of ganglion cells in affected patients in subsequent years, controversy regarding the etiology of the condition continued until 1948, when the clinicopathologic correlation between aganglionosis and incomplete colonic obstruction was established.[2,3]

Congenital aganglionic megacolon (Hirschsprung's disease) currently is recognized as a malformation in which there is a neurogenic form of intestinal obstruction associated with an absence of ganglion cells in the myenteric (Auerbach's) and submucosal (Meissner's) plexuses. There is an associated absence of both submucosal and intermuscular nerve plexi, and an increase in the size and prominence of nerve fibers. Neuroblasts are recognized intramurally in the esophagus by the sixth week of gestation and may be recognized in the rectum by the twelfth week. Maturation of neuroblasts into ganglion cells occurs through the period of fetal development, but may continue into the second year of life. The ganglion cells and associated nerve plexi are believed to be responsible for the relaxation phase of peristalsis and for the relaxation of the internal anal sphincters.[4] Spasm, lack of relaxation, and/or lack of propulsive peristalsis may account for the functional obstruction caused by the aganglionic intestine. Histopathologic studies have demonstrated an increase in the enzyme acetylcholinesterase in aganglionic colon.[5] An absence of the gut hormones vasointestinal peptide, substance P, and somatostatin has been noted in aganglionic bowel. Elevated class II histocompatibility antigen levels have been demonstrated in aganglionic intestine from patients with Hirschsprung's disease.

Congenital aganglionosis occurs in approximately 1 in every 5000 live births without racial predilection, and is about four times more frequent in males than in females. Hirschsprung's disease is commonly a solitary anomaly in a full-term, otherwise healthy infant. Prematurity is uncommon. Associated anomalies occur in approximately 15% of patients.[6] Congenital heart disease and Down's syndrome each occur in 4% to 5% of patients. Hirschsprung's disease has a definite family history, although a genetic inheritance pattern has not been established clearly. The risk of a second child being born with Hirschsprung's disease in a family in whom the first infant had the anomaly ranges from 6% to 12%, being more frequent if the first child had long segment aganglionosis. Occasional patients with Hirschsprung's disease have other neuropathic disorders, including Klippel-Feil syndrome, cochlear deafness, Ondine's curse (sleep apnea), neurofibromatosis and neuroblastoma.

The aganglionic segment of intestine extends for varying distances proximally from the anal sphincter and may involve as little as the lower rectum, or as much as the entire colon. In some instances, the aganglionic segment may extend to varying lengths of small intestine. It is generally believed that "skip areas," in which segments of intestine may contain ganglion cells between areas of aganglionosis, do not occur. Furthermore, it is generally recognized that aganglionosis is an all-or-none phenomenon and that ganglion cells, as well as nerve plexi, are either present or absent.[7]

The transition from normally innervated intestine to the aganglionic segment is usually abrupt, although occasionally there may be an intervening segment of hypoganglionosis. There is no apparent anatomical explanation for the often observed lack of correlation between the extent of aganglionosis and the severity of symptoms. It has been noted that infants in whom severe symptoms occurred early tended to have larger numbers of nerve fibers in the aganglionic intestine than those patients with milder symptoms. The extent of aganglionosis in most large reports shows that the anomaly extends only to the low sigmoid colon or lower in 76%, may involve varying lengths of the descending colon in 10%, extends to the transverse colon in 3%, and involves the total colon and varying lengths of small intestine in >10% of patients.[6]

■ CLINICAL PRESENTATION

Approximately half the patients with Hirschsprung's disease in the United States are diagnosed in the neonatal period; most of the remainder are recognized before two years of age. The clinical course almost invariably is characterized by delay in initial spontaneous passage of meconium for over 36 hours. Complete obstruction with vomiting and abdominal distention may occur shortly after birth. Other patients may experience repeated episodes of obstruction relieved either spontaneously or by enemas. Others may have mild symptoms of constipation for weeks or months, followed by acute intestinal obstruction. Diarrhea with foul liquid stools may be an early symptom. Cecal perforation with pneumoperitoneum rarely may be the initial finding in infants. Both acute appendicitis and the meconium plug syndrome in the neonate may be associated with Hirschsprung's disease.

In older children, a lifelong history of infrequent stools, marked abdominal distention, poor nutrition, and a large fecal mass are common features. Children with functional constipation are more likely to have fecal soiling, anal pain and bleeding.

The most serious complication of aganglionosis is enterocolitis, which occurs in 10% to 30% of patients and which may produce foul-smelling, watery, and often bloody stools (Fig 79–1). Enterocolitis is believed to be caused by stasis with bacterial proliferation and translocation resulting in mucosal inflammation and eventual transmural necrosis above the aganglionic segment, and usually involving the entire colon. *Clostridium difficile* has been implicated as an important pathogenic or-

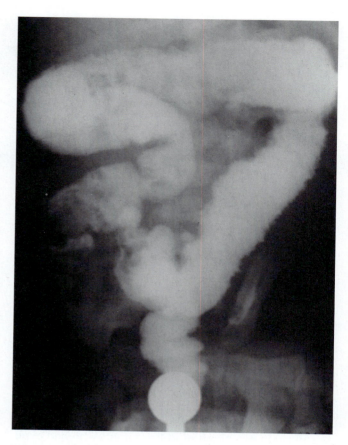

Figure 79–1. Radiographic contrast enema in a 2 week–old male infant with enterocolitis associated with Hirschsprung's disease. Note irregular appearance of mucosal folds.

ganism. This condition may lead to early perforation, septicemia, and death, if untreated. The mortality related to enterocolitis continues to be approximately 25%. Prompt treatment with antibiotics, intravenous fluid resuscitation, and rectal tube decompression, with cautious irrigation followed by colostomy proximal to the transition zone, are imperative.

■ DIAGNOSIS

Although plain abdominal radiographs may indicate colonic distention with absence of air in the rectum and suggest Hirschsprung's disease, a contrast enema, using a thin barium-water mixture, is more helpful. The site of transition between the narrow aganglionic segment and the dilated normally innervated bowel often may be identified, even in infants. Barium retention in the colon for 2 to 3 days or longer, however, may be the only suggestive sign of the disease. In older patients, the colonic distention above the transition zone may be massive (Fig 79–2). Infants with total colonic agan-

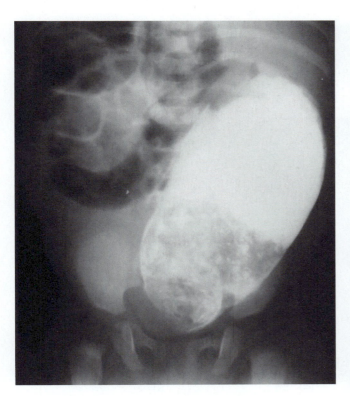

Figure 79–2. Radiographic contrast enema in a 10 week–old male infant with Hirschsprung's disease. Note fecal impaction and marked distention of sigmoid and lower left colon above transition zone.

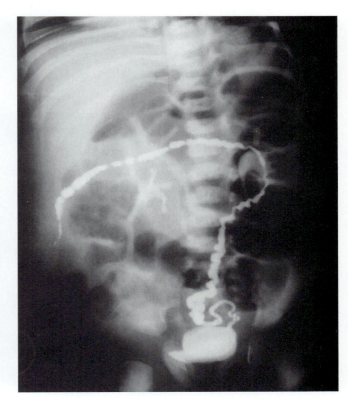

Figure 79–3. Radiographic contrast enema in a 24 hour–old male with total colonic aganglionosis. Note characteristic appearance of microcolon.

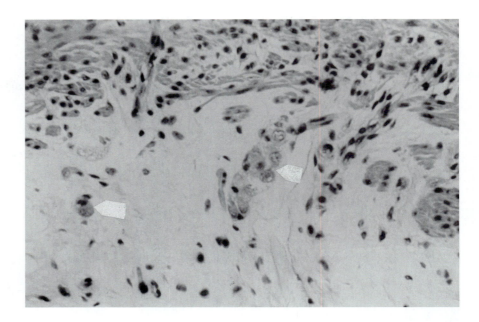

A

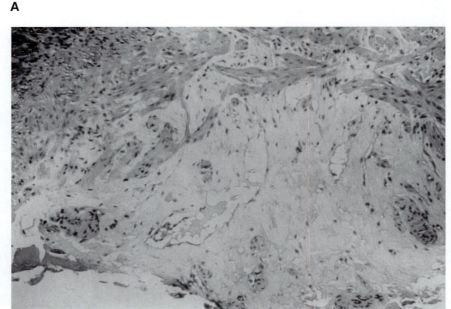

Figure 79–4. A. Suction biopsy specimen of rectal submucosa from a 2 month–old male with constipation but normal appearing ganglion cells, as indicated by *arrows* (hematoxylin and eosin ×100). **B.** Similar biopsy from a 3 week-old male with Hirschsprung's disease, as noted by complete absence of ganglion cells (hematoxylin and eosin ×60).

B

glionosis will show a microcolon pattern with an apparent transition zone in the terminal ileum in most instances (Fig 79–3). For these patients, prompt ileostomy at the site of the transition zone is imperative.

The diagnosis of Hirschsprung's disease may only be established conclusively by examining a rectal submucosal biopsy and noting the absence of ganglion cells and nerve plexi. The biopsies should be taken at least 2 cm proximal to the dentate line. This suction biopsy procedure commonly is performed without anesthesia and has few complications. The examination must be done with permanent stains and is not amenable to frozen section techniques (Fig 79–4, A, B). The more extensive full rectal muscle biopsy is necessary only in rare circumstances. Other studies which are confirmatory, but not considered diagnostic of Hirschsprung's disease, include increased acetylcholinesterase staining of neurofibrils and the demonstration, by anorectal manometry, of an absent rectoanal inhibitory reflex, indicating a lack of relaxation of the internal sphincter.

The differential diagnosis of Hirschsprung's disease in the neonate includes meconium plug syndrome, meconium ileus, ileal or colonic atresia, hypothyroidism, intestinal dysmotility syndromes, and ileus related to maternal narcotic addiction. In older infants and children, functional constipation, intestinal pseudoobstruction, neuronal intestinal dysplasia, and other dysmotility syndromes should be considered. Rectal mucosal biopsy should rule out each of these other conditions.

■ TREATMENT

Although an occasional undiagnosed patient with aganglionosis may reach adolescence, or even adulthood, with only chronic constipation as a major symptom, almost all will require operative treatment during infancy or early childhood. For infants, a proximal diverting colostomy is recommended by the majority of surgeons, although a few have favored the definitive pull-through procedure, in the neonatal period. We almost routinely perform a proximal transverse end colostomy placing the distal oversewn end in the abdomen; a biopsy is taken at the site of the stoma to confirm the presence of ganglion cells. It is unusual for the transition zone to be located in the transverse colon. Although some surgeons favor performing serial biopsies to precisely identify the transition, the colon is almost always too dilated to perform a satisfactory functional stoma within 10 cm of the transition. Furthermore, it may be inadvisable to perform serial biopsies in a sick infant undergoing operation on an emergency basis when the appropriate pathologist may not be available. The definitive pull-through operation generally is performed when the patient weighs approximately 12 to 15 pounds. A longer period of diversion does not appear to enhance the technical ease of the operation and may delay the development of continence. The colostomy may be closed at the same operation, or two months later, if there is any concern about the technical aspects of the pull-through procedure.

For older infants and children, the decision to construct an initial colostomy generally is based on the severity of the fecal impaction and the size of the colon immediately proximal to the transition zone, and the state of the overall health and nutrition of the patient. For these patients, a loop or double-barrel colostomy may be preferred in order to permit frequent irrigation of the diverted colon through the mucous fistula. Colostomy prolapse, however, occasionally occurs with loop or double-barrel stomas and may require urgent surgical correction (Fig 79–5).

Each of the definitive pull-through operations removes a portion of the aganglionic rectosigmoid as well

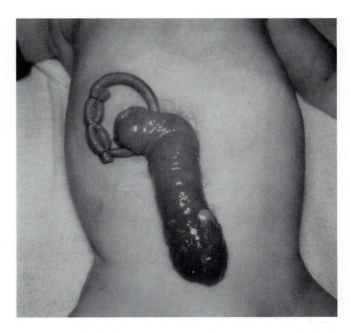

Figure 79–5. Colostomy prolapse in a 3 month-old male following construction of loop transverse colostomy for Hirschsprung's disease. Note that prolapse comes from the distal side of stoma in most cases.

as the most dilated portion of the colon immediately proximal to the transition zone (Fig 79–6). The choice of the Soave (endorectal), Duhamel-Martin (retrorectal), or the Swenson (rectosigmoidectomy) procedure is based on the surgeon's preference and experience, rather than by compelling differences in outcome.

Although the Swenson procedure was the original curative pull-through procedure for Hirschsprung's disease,[8] it has fallen into relative disfavor because it appears to be technically more problematic and to have a higher incidence of postoperative complications, particularly pelvic infection or anastomotic leak. If precisely performed, however, it can be predictably curative. The rectum is mobilized by meticulous dissection close to the rectal wall down to the sphincter mechanism (2 cm above the dentate line anteriorly and 1 cm posteriorly). The aganglionic intestine is resected with temporary closure of both the distal aganglionic rectum and the proximal, normally innervated, colon. The closed rectal stump is everted through the anus and a precise two-layer anastomosis of the pulled through normal colon to the everted rectum is performed transanally. The completed anastomosis then retracts back into the pelvis.

A large number of pediatric surgeons prefer to use the Duhamel pull-through procedure with Martin modification[9,10] (Fig 79–7, A through D). This operation eliminates much of the pelvic dissection used in the Swenson procedure and preserves the aganglionic rec-

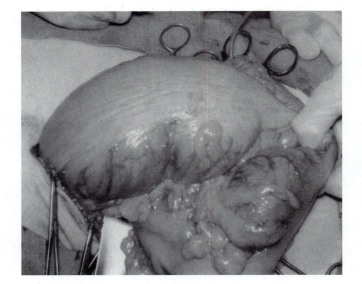

Figure 79–6. Appearance of hypertrophic and markedly dilated sigmoid colon in 5 month-old male with rectal aganglionosis. Colostomy is technically difficult to perform in dilated hypertrophic colon.

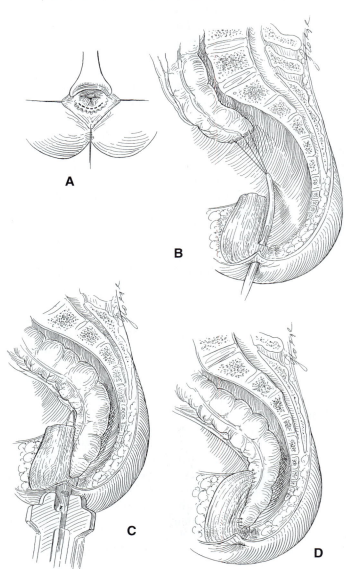

Figure 79–7. For the Duhamel pull-through operation, the dilated sigmoid colon is resected down to the peritoneal reflection. **A.** A curvilinear incision is made through the full thickness of the posterior rectal wall approximately 5 mm above the dentate line. **B.** The left colon is drawn through the space posterior to the rectum and sutured to an opening in the posterior wall of the rectum with interrupted absorbable stitches. **C.** A GIA stapling device is inserted with one blade in the rectum and the other in the colon. **D.** The upper end of the rectum is sutured to the side of the colon to complete the anastomosis.

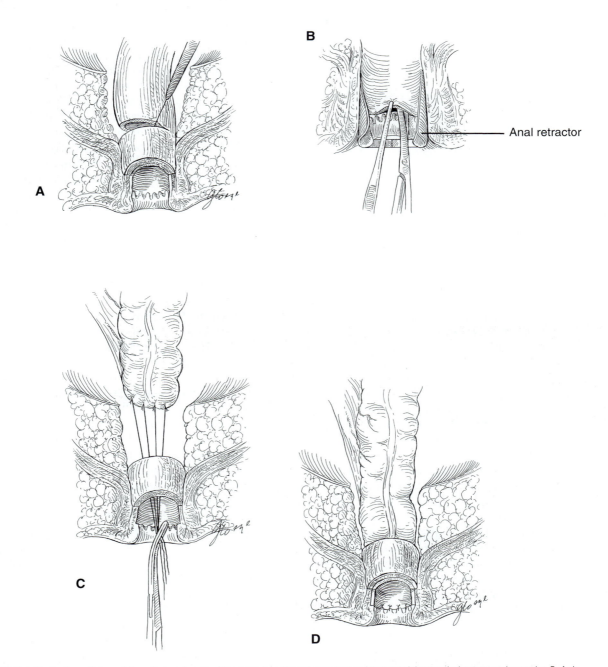

B — Anal retractor

Figure 79–8. A. For the Soave-Boley pull-through procedure, the dilated sigmoid colon and upper rectum are resected down to the levator muscle complex. **B.** A circumferential incision is made through the rectal mucosa at the upper edge of the anal crypts. The mucosa is dissected from the muscularis up to the line of rectal transaction using scissors or electrocautery. **C.** The left colon is drawn through the rectal muscle canal. **D.** The left colon is sutured to the anal mucosa and underlying muscularis with interrupted absorbable stitches.

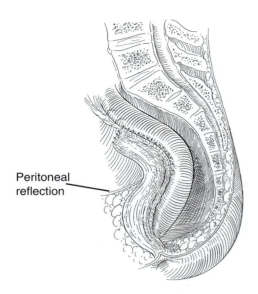

Peritoneal
reflection

Figure 79–9. For total colonic aganglionosis, the aganglionic distal ileum and entire colon down to the upper sigmoid are resected. The most distal ganglionic ileum is drawn through the posterior pelvis and anastomosed to the side of the distal rectum, as described for the Duhamel procedure. A long stapled anastomosis is constructed over a distance of 12 to 15 cm (Martin procedure).

tum and adjacent nerves to the bladder and genitalia. The proximal normal colon is brought through a retrorectal tunnel and then through an incision in the posterior half of the distal rectal wall, slightly above the dentate line. The posterior wall of the rectum above this level and the anterior wall of the pull-through colon then are anastomosed with a stapling device, which produces a wide anastomosis between the colon and the rectum. The upper end of the rectum is sutured to the colon to avoid producing a blind rectal segment.

Many surgeons use the endorectal pull-through procedure with rectal mucosal stripping as initially recommended by Soave[11] and modified by Boley.[12] With this procedure, the mucosa of the lower rectum is removed down to the dentate line (Fig 79–8, A through D). After resection of the aganglionic rectum above the levator muscles and the sigmoid colon, the normally innervated left colon is brought through the remaining rectal muscle cuff and is sutured to the anal mucosa. This procedure is technically less demanding than either the Swenson or Duhamel procedures and has the advantage of only one suture line to the anus with a protecting muscular cuff.

Some surgeons, particularly in Europe, prefer the Rehbein procedure.[13] This procedure is basically a low anterior resection performed from above, leaving 2 to 3 cm of rectum above the dentate line. In contrast, in the Swenson technique, the anastomosis is performed lower and from the perineal approach. Proponents for anorectal myotomy as the primary treatment for low Hirschsprung's disease have found few supporters in recent years.

A water soluble radiographic contrast study of the rectum usually is performed to identify any intestinal leaks or sinus tracts before colostomy closure. Although many surgeons close the colostomy at the time that the pull-through operation is constructed, it is imperative for optimal success of the procedure that anastomotic leaks be avoided and that the pull-through operative procedure be constructed carefully at the initial operation.

If a pelvic anastomotic leak or abscess develops after the pull-through procedure, prompt return to a colostomy or ileostomy is usually imperative in order to avoid extensive scarring in the pelvis, which might preclude a subsequent good result from the pull-through procedure. Closure of the colostomy may be performed 4 to 6 months after the pelvic inflammation and leak or sinus tracts have resolved. The most successful reconstruction after extensive pelvic leak or persistent sinus, in our experience, has been to resect the pull-through segment of colon and rectum in the pelvis to within 2.5 cm of the dentate line and then remove the rectal mucosa, as with a modified Soave-Boley procedure. The proximal normal colon then is brought through the short rectal muscle cuff to the anus, where it is anastomosed with interrupted absorbable sutures. A silastic drain is placed into the lower pelvis and brought through the lower abdominal wall for a few days.

In 1979, a survey of American surgeons with experience in Hirschsprung's disease indicated a preference for the Swenson procedure by 23%, the Duhamel procedure by 30%, and the endorectal pull-through by 47%.[6] This study concluded that all the operative procedures were used successfully for the treatment of congenital aganglionosis, but that the Swenson procedure was associated with a slightly higher incidence of complications. Most authors indicate the importance of close postoperative follow-up to avoid anastomotic strictures and to encourage the development of a regular bowel pattern with defecatory movements at least once daily. For patients who experienced persistent constipation and who have a tight anal sphincter, daily dilation for a few months may be helpful. For those who have persistent rectal stenosis, it is likely that the anastomosis was performed a bit higher in the rectal wall than might be desired. In such cases, anorectal myotomy may be helpful.

For infants with total colonic aganglionosis, we prefer to operate when the patient weighs approximately 15 pounds, at which time the aganglionic ileum and entire colon down to the midsigmoid are resected. The ganglionic ileum is anastomosed to the low rectum in the same manner as performed with the Duhamel procedure, followed by continuation of the ileal anastomosis with a stapling device to the upper rectum and sigmoid (Fig 79–9). This operative technique has permitted maximal storage capacity to minimize stool frequency and still permits optimal colonic emptying.[14]

The most common complications following the pull-through operations include anastomotic leak, anastomotic stricture, intestinal obstruction, pelvic abscess, and wound infection. Mortality from Hirschsprung's disease is rare in modern practice, unless enterocolitis is a presenting clinical feature or there is some associated disorder such as cardiac disease. Unique to Hirschsprung's disease is the problem of postoperative enterocolitis, which may manifest similar features to those mentioned previously. Enterocolitis tends to be less virulent in the postoperative patient than in the unoperated infant. The incidence of postoperative enterocolitis is approximately 15% in most series. However, the frequency has decreased in recent years.

The vast majority of children who have undergone the pull-through operation in infancy or early childhood and who do not experience major operative complications will develop normal bowel control by 2 to 3 years of age and have 1 to 2 defecatory movements daily. Prompt dilation of rectal anastomotic strictures and avoidance of proximal colonic distention with suppositories, or low enemas, if necessary, are helpful if the patient is to develop near-normal bowel habits during the first year following operation. Long-term results appear good for all the pull-through procedures. Eighty to ninety percent of patients have excellent or normal bowel function when evaluated 5 years after surgery, regardless of the procedure used.

REFERENCES

1. Hirschsprung H. Stuhltragheit neurgeborner in folge von dilatation und hypertrophic des colons. *Sahrb Sinkerh* 1887;27:1–8

2. Whitehouse FW, Kernahan JW. Myenteric plexus in congenital megacolon. *Arch Intern Med* 1948;82:75–81

3. Zuelzer WW, Wilson JL. Functional intestinal obstruction on a congenital neurogenic basis in infancy. *Am J Dis Child* 1948;75:40–46

4. Frigo GM, Del Tacco J, Lecchini S, et al. Some observations on the intrinsic nervous mechanism in Hirschsprung's disease. *Gut* 1973;14:35–41

5. Elema JJ, de Vries JA, Vos LJJ. Intensity and proximal extension of acetylcholinesterase activity in the mucosa of the rectosigmoid in Hirschsprung's disease. *J Pediatr Surg* 1973;8:361–366

6. Kleinhaus S, Boley SJ, Sheraw M, et al. Hirschsprung's disease: a survey of the members of the surgical section of the American Academy of Pediatrics. *J Pediatr Surg* 1979;14:588–594

7. Ehrenpreis T. *Hirschsprung's Disease*. Chicago, IL: Year Book Medical; 1970

8. Swenson O, Bill AH. Resection of rectum and rectosigmoid with preservation of the sphincter for benign spastic lesions producing megacolon: an experimental study. *Surgery* 1948;24:313–316

9. Duhamel B. Retrorectal and transanal pull-through procedure for the treatment of Hirschsprung's disease. *Dis Colon Rectum* 1964;7:455–460

10. Martin LW, Altemeier WA. Clinical experience with a new operation (modified Duhamel procedure) for Hirschsprung's disease. *Ann Surg* 1962;156:678–682

11. Soave F. A new surgical technique for treatment of Hirschsprung's disease. *Surgery* 1964;56:1007–1011

12. Boley SJ. New modification of the surgical treatment of Hirschsprung's disease. *Surgery* 1964;56:1015–1019

13. Rehbein F, Marger R, Kundert JG, et al. Surgical problems in congenital megacolon (Hirschsprung's disease). *J Pediatr Surg* 1966;1:526–530

14. Martin LW. Surgical management of total colonic aganglionosis. *Ann Surg* 1972;176:343–349

80

Imperforate Anus

Eric W. Fonkalsrud

Although imperforate anus has been recognized since antiquity, it was not until the 20th century that a distinction was made between high and low malformations. The radiologic invertogram described in 1930 was the first diagnostic study to delineate the difference between high and low anomalies with fair accuracy.[1] In 1953, Stephens performed the first objective anatomic studies of human specimens and described several variations of the basic malformations, as well as associated genitourinary anomalies.[2] He also recognized the importance of the puborectalis muscle sling as a key factor in achieving fecal continence and suggested that a sacral surgical approach be used to define this muscle before performing corrective surgery for high anomalies.

Anorectal malformations occur in approximately one in every 3,000 live births, with a slight preponderance in males. By the fifth gestational week, the fetal cloaca is identifiable with the adjacent hindgut, allantois, and vestigial tailgut. With the formation of the urorectal septum, the cloaca is divided into a dorsal rectum and a ventral urogenital sinus. Developmental arrest at any one of several stages during normal embryogenesis appears to account for the anatomic variations seen with anorectal anomalies.

In 1984, an international classification of anorectal malformations was established based on the sex of the patient and the level at which arrest of the rectal descent had occurred[3] (Table 80–1). From an anatomic as well as functional standpoint, the anomalies can be grouped according to whether the lower end of the rectum is supralevator (high), partially translevator (intermediate), or fully translevator (low). The location of the lowermost point of the rectum may be classified in relation to the pubococcygeal line and the "I" (ischium) point,[4] represented by the lowest fourth of the ossified ischium when viewed on an inverted lateral roentgenogram (Fig 80–1). When the rectum ends above the pubococcygeal line, it is considered high (Fig 80–2); when it ends below the pubococcygeal line, but not below the "I" point, it is intermediate and has entered the upper funnel portion of the levator mechanism but has not passed completely through the puborectalis muscle. When the rectum extends below the "I" point, it has penetrated the entire levator mechanism and is considered to be a low defect (Fig 80–3). Some degree of intrinsic hypoplasia of the striated muscle complex occurs with virtually all anorectal malformations, although the physiologic effects may be variable. Fecal continence is determined largely by the degree of competence of the muscular funnel surrounding the rectum.

With experience, identification of the level of the distal end of the rectum as high or low often may be made on the basis of external appearance and verified by radiographic or imaging studies. Approximately 55% of anomalies are of the low type which, in the male, often may be identified by the presence of a perineal membrane, deep anal dimple, or hypertrophied midline raphe extending to the scrotum (Figs 80–4; 80–5, A, B). Patients with complete absence of any anal dimple and the presence of a flat natal fold who have no external sphincter contraction on stimulation of the perineum

TABLE 80–1. INTERNATIONAL CLASSIFICATION OF ANORECTAL MALFORMATIONS

MALE
  High
    Anorectal agenesis
      Rectoprostatic urethral fistula[a]
      Without fistula
    Rectal atresia
  Intermediate
    Rectobulbar urethral fistula
    Anal agenesis without fistula
  Low
    Anocutaneous fistula[a]
    Anal stenosis
  Rare malformations

FEMALE
  High
    Anorectal agenesis
      Rectovaginal fistula
      Without fistula
    Rectal atresia
  Intermediate
    Rectovestibular fistula
    Rectovaginal fistula
    Anal agenesis without fistula
  Low
    Anovestibular fistula[a]
    Anocutaneous fistula[a,b]
    Anal stenosis
  Cloacal malformations
  Rare malformations

[a]Common anomaly.
[b]Includes fourchette fistulae or vulvar fistulae.

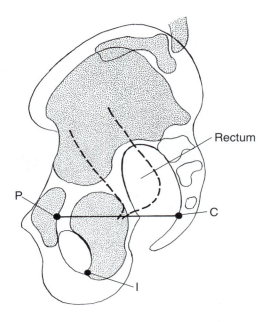

Figure 80–1. Cross-section of neonatal pelvis showing line from midpubis (P) to coccyx (C), which defines the upper limit of the anorectal muscle complex and puborectalis muscle sling. When the rectum extends below the lower ischium (I), it has penetrated the entire levator mechanism. *Dashed line* shows common location of high imperforate anus in a male with rectourethral fistula.

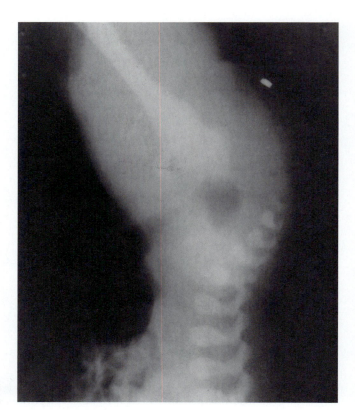

Figure 80–2. Inverted lateral radiograph in newborn male showing long distance between lower end of rectal air column and optimal location of anus, identified by radiopaque marker.

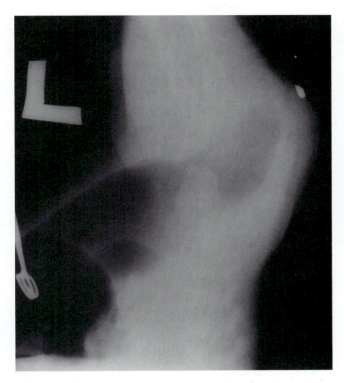

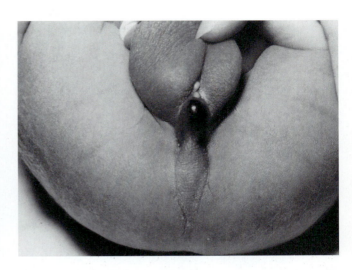

Figure 80–4. Low imperforate anus with hypertrophied midline raphe and anteriorly placed anal membrane.

Figure 80–3. Lateral inverted radiograph in a male infant showing rectal air column to extend below the pubococcygeal line and through the rectal muscle complex almost to the anal dimple.

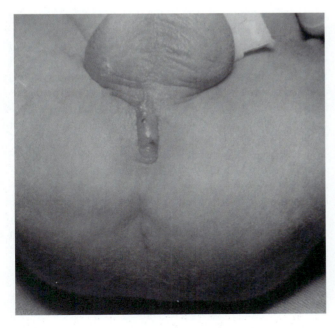

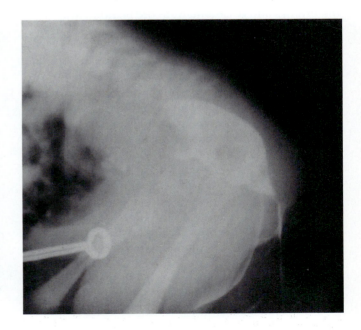

A   **B**

Figure 80–5. A. Low imperforate anus in a male, with dilated midline raphe extending to scrotum. Note small anal dimple and flat natal fold. **B.** Radiographic contrast sinogram through midline raphe showing low-lying rectum.

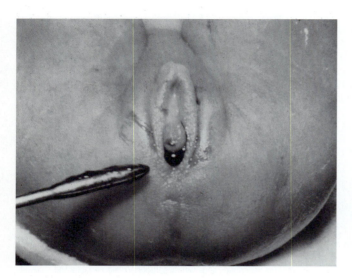

Figure 80–6. A female infant with low imperforate anus and rectovulvar fistula located in posterior fourchette, showing meconium draining.

are likely to have high anomalies. The presence of a fistula extending from the lowermost portion of the rectum to the region of the perineal body usually indicates a low imperforate anus. Regardless of gender, external fistulas may not become apparent until 12 to 24 hours of age, when meconium moves distally into the rectum. Fistulous tracts from the lower rectum in males with high anomalies usually extend to the bulbous portion of the urethra and occasionally, to the bladder. More than 90% of male and female patients with high lesions have a fistula extending from the rectum.

In the female, the anal orifice may be stenotic, anteriorly placed (anocutaneous fistula), or in the very posterior vulvar fourchette, all of which are considered low lesions (Fig 80–6). When the rectum extends more anteriorly and lies adjacent to the vagina as a narrow rectovestibular fistula extending distally from a dilated rectum above, the anomaly is considered intermediate in location (Fig 80–7, A through D). When the perineum shows only two orifices (vagina and urethra), the rectal fistula enters the posterior wall of the vagina and is usually considered a high lesion. Occasional females will have only one perineal orifice; the rectum enters the side of the vagina posteriorly and the urethra enters anteriorly to form a "cloacal anomaly," which is invariably a high defect. The intermediate category of anomalies is primarily for descriptive purposes, since clinical management is often the same as for high lesions.

Approximately 60% of infants with imperforate anus, particularly those with high defects, will have associated anomalies, the VACTERL (vertebral, anal, cardias, tracheal, esophageal, renal, and limb) associations being most important. The most common associated anomalies are in the spine, urinary tract, trachea, esophagus, heart, gastrointestinal tract, and skeletal system. A thorough search should be made for associated malformations in order to manage all major defects in a logical and orderly sequence. Sacral dysplasia and agenesis are associated with sacral autonomic dysfunction with a poor prognosis for fecal continence and a high incidence of neurologic urologic dysfunction. A variety of other spinal cord malformations have been associated with high anorectal anomalies, including tethered cord, and certain myelodysplastic syndromes. Tracheoesophageal fistula occurs in about 10% of infants with anorectal anomalies. Renal or lower genitourinary tract malformations are the most common associated defects and may take virtually any form. Screening for both upper and lower tract anomalies is essential. A broad range of cardiac anomalies also are reported in 9% of infants with high anorectal defects. Thus, screening echocardiography is considered routine.

The primary goal of the diagnostic evaluation is to place the anomaly into a high or low category. Evaluation of the location of the lowest point in the rectum may be accurately obtained within 6 to 8 hours after birth. At this stage, a radiologic invertogram is performed after placing a thin smear of barium paste on the perineal skin at the optimal location for the anal orifice (Figs 80–2 and 80–3). Crying or straining may cause caudal prolapse of the rectal pouch and diminish the accuracy of the study. More detailed and dynamic visualization of the distal rectal pouch may be provided by real-time ultrasound. Computed tomography (CT) or magnetic resonance imaging (MRI) scans of the pelvis can define more clearly the location and degree of hypoplasia of the muscle structures and configuration of the sacrum, and may assist in identifying urinary tract anomalies. When a patient is suspected of having a low imperforate anus that cannot be identified clearly by noninvasive studies, insertion of a #18 needle into the perineum at the site of the anal dimple to aspirate meconium may be helpful. If meconium is aspirated, water soluble contrast may be inserted and a radiograph taken to demonstrate the anatomy clearly (Fig 80–5B). Such manipulation should be very limited and not extend inward from the skin more than 1 cm in order to minimize the risk of injury to the delicate neuromuscular structures. Any child not clearly found to have a low anomaly should be considered to have an intermediate or high lesion. Renal ultrasound examination and voiding cystourethrography together provide a fairly comprehensive evaluation of both the upper and lower urinary tracts for malformations.

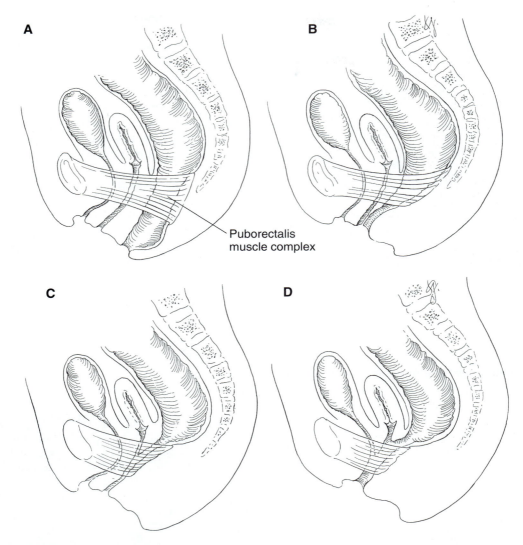

Figure 80–7. Four of the most common types of imperforate anus malformations in females. **A.** Lateral view of female infant with imperforate anus and rectovulvar fistula with anal orifice in posterior fourchette. **B.** Rectovestibular fistula adjacent to vaginal wall extending distally from dilated rectum. **C.** Rectovaginal fistula into posterior vagina at upper edge of puborectalis muscle complex. **D.** Cloacal anomaly with one external pelvic orifice; rectal fistula enters vagina posteriorly and urethra enters anterior wall of vagina.

■ SURGICAL MANAGEMENT

Treatment of anorectal malformations is always surgical, but is not life threatening, with a delay of 12 to 24 hours occasionally simplifying the diagnostic evaluation. Infants with anal stenosis (covered anus) can be managed by progressive dilation of the anus with Hegar dilators in the nursery using appropriate analgesia. Most other low malformations will require a relatively simple surgical procedure in the perineum without the need for a proximal diverting colostomy.

In females with an anteriorly placed anus external to the vulva, a "cut-back" anoplasty will commonly relieve the obstruction without disturbing the continence mechanism (Fig 80–8). When the fistulous orifice is more anteriorly placed in the posterior vulvar fourchette, circumferential mobilization of the fistula with transposition to the site of the anal dimple and external sphincter with reconstruction of the perineal body is often the operation of choice. By probing the rectal orifice in a distal direction, one can frequently demonstrate that the rectal bulb has descended posteriorly and lies close to the true external sphincter mechanism. The anatomy can often be verified by a radiologic contract study before undertaking surgical reconstruction. Occasional fistulas that open to the rectovestibular location may

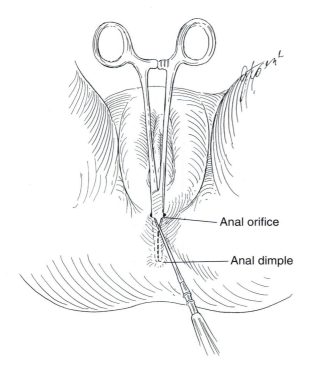

Figure 80–8. Cutback procedure for anteriorly placed anus located posterior to vulvar fourchette.

the fecal stream from the urinary fistula and also to allow decompression and cleaning of the dilated distal rectum. Radiographic contrast placed into the mucous fistula will clearly outline the lowermost rectum and the location of its communication with the genitourinary tract (Fig 80–9).

The pull-through procedure commonly is performed between 6 and 12 months of age, when the body weight is over 12 to 15 pounds. The first reconstructive operation is very important, with minimal margin for error. The posterior sagittal anorectoplasty described by de Vries and Peña is currently used by many surgeons in the United States.[5] The skin is incised from coccyx to anal dimple and all muscles are divided down to the rectum, with care taken to identify each muscle layer (Fig 80–10 A, B, and C). A nerve stimulator is used to map the striated muscle complex precisely for purposes of symmetric division as well as reconstruction. The distal rectum is mobilized and the fistula to the urethra or vagina is divided and repaired under direct vision. The rectum then is brought down to the level of the anal skin in the desired location. Because the lower rectum frequently is dilated, which might obviate subsequent re-

have a low rectum and lend themselves to the transposition procedure. However, most fistulas are classified as intermediate anomalies.

Daily anal dilation with a size 24- to 32-French (Fr) catheter for a few weeks following repair of a low imperforate anus will help to prevent stricture formation and rectal distention, which occasionally lead to fecal impaction and long-term constipation. Glycerine suppositories and oral lubricants or stool softeners may assist in producing adequate daily fecal output.

Although occasional female infants with rectovestibular or rectovaginal fistulas may pass some meconium spontaneously, these patients require a formal repair, which is usually deferred 4 to 6 months. Attempts to dilate such fistulas may injure the thin, closely adherent vaginal wall or surrounding structures. The presence of a high anomaly often may be verified, in the female, by performing a vaginogram and, in the male, by performing a retrograde urethrogram.

Infants with intermediate or high malformations require a diverting colostomy. For patients in whom we are quite sure that a perineal approach will be sufficient to correct the anomaly, a sigmoid colostomy is preferred. For those patients in whom a laparotomy with mobilization of the rectum from above is anticipated, a right transverse colostomy is preferred. An end colostomy with a mucous fistula is recommended to divert

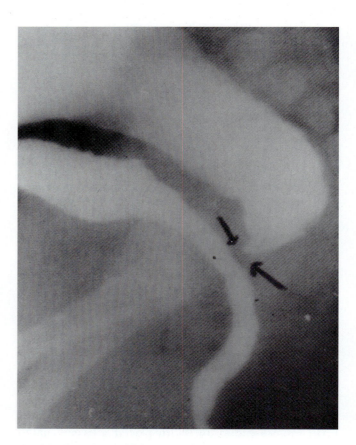

Figure 80–9. Contrast radiograph following injection into sigmoid colonic mucous fistula of a male infant. Note the location of rectourethral fistula.

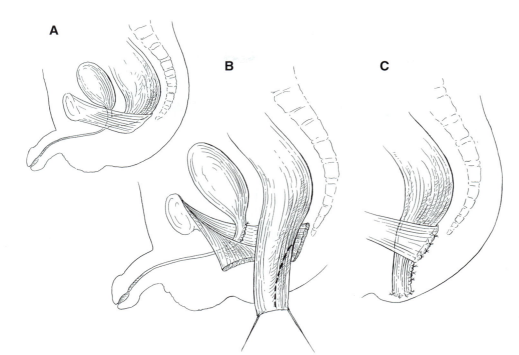

Figure 80–10. Posterior sagittal anorectoplasty technique commonly used for definitive repair of high imperforate anus malformations. **A.** High imperforate anus malformation in male infant showing puborectalis muscle sling around lower end of rectum. **B.** Puborectalis and anorectal muscle complex are divided in the midline posteriorly. The rectum is mobilized and the rectourethral fistula is closed. The lower end of the rectum is drawn to the perineal skin. A wedge of the distal rectum is excised to reduce the diameter sufficient to fit beneath the reconstructed puborectalis muscle complex. **C.** Completed repair with closure of the puborectalis and anorectal muscle complex.

closure of the perineal muscles, a "tapering rectoplasty" is performed posteriorly by resecting a wedge of rectal wall. A rectal lumen of at least 1.5 cm diameter should remain at the level of the anal anastomosis. The end of the rectum is sutured to the skin circumferentially; the perineal muscles are then carefully reapproximated in layers with interrupted sutures.

The sacroabdominoperineal approach for the pull-through procedure also has been used successfully by many surgeons during the past 25 years.[6,7] The anal dimple is identified with a nerve-muscle stimulator and an opening is made in this location. The skin from the anal dimple to the coccyx then is incised and the underlying muscles exposed, but not divided (Fig 80–11A, B, and C). The puborectalis-levator muscle sling is identified and a space is developed from the anal dimple up through the perineal muscle complex and puborectalis sling. This muscle tunnel is dilated gently with a blunt-tipped clamp and is marked by placing a small drain through the entire muscle complex. The colon and rectum then are mobilized from the abdomen through a lower midline incision. The dissection in the pelvis is carried 1 to 2 cm below the peritoneal reflection, staying close to the muscularis in order to avoid injury to adjacent nerves. The rectal muscularis is incised circumferentially and the mucosa is removed from the lower remaining segment of rectum. The fistula extending to the urethra or bladder is oversewn from within the short rectal segment. A clamp then is extended up from the perineal wound through the per-

ineal muscle complex and puborectalis muscle sling such that the tip elevates the lower end of the remaining muscular rectal segment. An opening is made in the midportion in order to avoid injury to the urinary tract. A urethral catheter is used for careful identification of the urethra and for postoperative urinary drainage, for all such operations. The space through the lower rectal segment and puborectalis muscles is dilated gently with a blunt clamp, with care taken to avoid overdistending or tearing the perineal muscles. The rectosigmoid colon then is directed through the rectal segment and the muscular sling and sphincter mechanism to the anus. The end of the pull-through segment is attached to the skin circumferentially with interrupted absorbable sutures. The mesentery of the colon is attached to the posterior abdominal wall to prevent internal herniation.

Approximately 6 weeks after the pull-through operation, the colostomy is closed through a transverse elliptical abdominal incision around the stoma. Any protruding mucosa from the previous coloanal anastomosis may be resected as a small perineal anoplasty at that time, and anal skin can be tucked upward to form an anal canal. Subsequent dilation of the rectum is often necessary for several weeks to avoid stenosis.

The majority of patients with low anorectal anomalies will develop good fecal continence postoperatively, providing that the perineal muscles and rectum are not injured and that major infection does not occur. Most patients will benefit from periodic anal dilation and

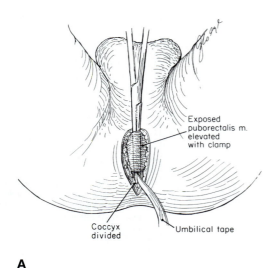

A

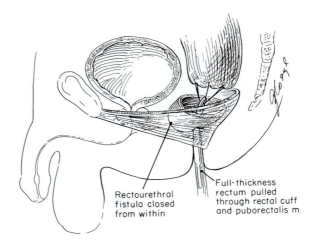

B

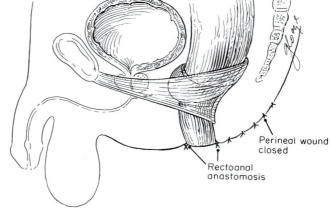

C

Figure 80–11. Sacroabdominoperineal technique for repair of high imperforate anus anomalies. **A.** Perineal incision from anal dimple to coccyx exposing puborectalis muscle complex which is gently elevated with a blunt clamp. **B.** Lower end of rectum is divided and mucosa is removed. The rectourethral fistula is closed from within the small rectal segment. **C.** A space is developed through the lower rectal segment and beneath the puborectalis muscle to the new anus. After gentle dilation of this space, the rectosigmoid is drawn through to the anal skin.

close follow-up to ensure that constipation with fecal impaction does not occur.

The long-term results from the different techniques for formal repair of high or intermediate imperforate anus anomalies are still under evaluation. Our preference is to use the posterior sagittal anorectoplasty for reconstruction of the female perineum and for intermediate anomalies in male patients. The combined sacroabdominoperineal approach is preferred for both males and females with high defects.

The cause of death in most children with imperforate anus is related to associated congenital anomalies and varies from 11% to 34%.[4] The numerical grading system is based on the presence or absence of fecal leakage, rectal sensation, and normal levator indentation on contrast studies.[8] Other authors have stressed the importance of meticulous physiologic assessment with manometric studies, electromyography, and perineal electrostimulation.[9] Thirty-three percent to eighty percent of patients are classified as having good results, 7% to 43% as having fair results, and 8% to 46% as having poor results.[9] In general, female patients have much better fecal continence than do males postoperatively. Those patients with an intact sacrum have much better continence than those with two or more segments missing.

For children who have fair or poor continence following operation, motivation of the patient has been determined to be a major factor and generally will cause improvement with time. Encouragement to defecate after major meals to make maximum utilization of the gastrocolic reflex has assisted greatly in achieving continence in some children. Others may benefit from glycerine suppositories or occasional cleansing enemas following meals. Biofeedback training has been beneficial for some patients. It is important to avoid development of a fecal impaction during the postoperative period. Children should be evaluated on a frequent basis during the first several years of life in order to obtain optimal results.

REFERENCES

1. Wangensteen OH, Rice CO. Imperforate anus: a method of determining the surgical approach. *Ann Surg* 1930;92: 77–81

2. Stephens FD. Imperforate rectum: a new surgical technique. *Med J Aust* 1953;1:202–206

3. Stephens FD. Wingspread Conference on Anorectal Malformations, Racine, WI, May 1984.

4. Stephens FD, Smith ED. *Anorectal Malformations in Children.* Chicago, IL: Year Book Medical; 1971.

5. de Vries P, Peña A. Posterior sagittal anorectoplasty. *J Pediatr Surg* 1982;17:638–643

6. Kieswetter WB. Imperforate anus II. The rationale and technique of the sacro-abdomino-perineal operation. *J Pediatr Surg* 1967;2:106–111

7. Stephens FD, Smith ED. *Anorectal Malformations in Children.* Chicago, Year Book Medical; 1981.

8. Kelly JH. The clinical and radiologic assessment of anal continence in childhood. *Austr NZ J Surg* 1972;42:62–67

9. Templeton JM Jr, Dietshelm JA. High imperforate anus: quantitative results of long-term fecal continence. *J Pediatr Surg* 1985;20:645–652

81

Extrahepatic Biliary Atresia

Edward R. Howard

Atresia means *without a lumen* and in patients with biliary atresia, bile flow is obstructed by occlusion or even complete destruction of part or all of the extrahepatic bile ducts. The incidence throughout the world is approximately 1 in 14,000 live births. The occlusion of the bile ducts is accompanied by a variable degree of intrahepatic damage that can progress to cirrhosis and liver failure, in untreated cases. Historically, cases were classified as *correctable* or *noncorrectable,* depending on the presence or absence of residual proximal segments of bile ducts. The term *correctable* implied that a patent segment of proximal duct could be treated by a conventional biliary-enteric anastomosis (hepaticojejunostomy). *Noncorrectable* suggested that the atretic process was so extensive that all attempts at surgical correction would fail.

The introduction of a new surgical technique, portoenterostomy, in the 1960s, invalidated the traditional classification. Effective biliary drainage has now been achieved in a large number of cases that would have previously been described as noncorrectable.

■ HISTORICAL NOTE

The first major review of 49 cases was published by Thomson in 1891 and 1892 and concluded that, whatever the etiology of biliary atresia, it was characterized by a progressive, destructive inflammatory lesion of the bile ducts.[1] Thomson noted that "the children themselves are either jaundiced at birth, or they become so within the first week or so of life; otherwise they are healthy and well nourished." He reported that most children died from spontaneous hemorrhage within the first few months of life.[1]

Holmes analyzed more than 100 case reports and first suggested that surgical treatment might be effective in biliary atresia.[2] He estimated that 16% of cases might be correctable by surgery. Ladd described 20 more cases; 11 patients underwent operation, and eight were considered to be correctable (40%).[3] However, although six recovered from the operation, a review of these case reports suggests that two were examples of choledochal cysts, two were cases of hepatitis with hypoplastic ducts, and two were rare examples in which the atretic segments were confined to the distal portion of the common bile duct. Surgical success was rare. Hays and Snyder reported, in 1963, that in most American series, <5% of patients survived beyond early childhood.[4] These poor results led to trials of partial hepatic resection, insertion of tubes into the hepatic parenchyma, thoracic duct lymph drainage to the esophagus and hepatic lymph drainage to the jejunum. However, these techniques failed to prolong survival. In 1959, Kasai and Suzuki described a new radical operation for noncorrectable atresia based on the histologic observation that remnants of the extrahepatic ducts at the porta hepatis frequently contained ductules measuring up to 300 μm in diameter.[5] It was suggested that anastomosis of this tissue to bowel could result in effective bile drainage. Approximately 85% of extrahepatic biliary atresia cases classified as noncorrectable now are treated routinely with the Kasai portoenterostomy procedure.[6]

The 4 year survival rate in untreated cases of biliary atresia is approximately 2%, but portoenterostomy performed before the age of 7 weeks has resulted in early jaundice-free survival in more than 90% of cases. Past 7 weeks of life, the long-term results of surgery are poor. A large number of patients with effective bile drainage have now been recorded in the literature, with the oldest post-portoenterostomy survivor older than 33 years of age. Survival figures have been further enhanced by hepatic transplantation in patients who do not respond to portoenterostomy, or who develop liver failure later in life.

■ ETIOLOGY

An early theory suggested that biliary atresia might be the result of a failure of recanalization of the biliary tract in the early embryo. This theory was challenged by Landing, who introduced the concept of *infantile cholangiopathy*.[7] He suggested that the biliary tract was affected by, for example, a viral infection in the late prenatal or perinatal period. This hypothesis links neonatal hepatitis, biliary atresia, and choledochal cyst because of similarities in the histological changes observed in the liver. However, although a viral etiology has been suggested on several occasions, viral studies remain inconclusive. For example, Morecki and associates showed antibodies to type III reovirus in 68% of a group of infants with biliary atresia, compared with 8% of age-matched controls.[8] In a similar study, Dussaix and associates showed no difference between subjects and controls.[9] Additional investigations have focused on abnormalities in the metabolism of L-proline, which affects growth of the biliary tract, and monohydroxy bile acids, which cause bile duct inflammation.

CONGENITAL FACTORS

The association of biliary atresia with other congenital anomalies suggests a genetic factor in at least a number of cases. The associated anomalies, which occur in approximately 20% of cases, include polysplenia, asplenia, situs inversus, and anomalies of the portal vein. Some of the more frequent anomalies are listed in Table 81–1. A recent report showed poorer survival in children with associated defects.[10] The presence of these defects has suggested that a disturbance of organogenesis in the embryo at approximately 30 to 40 days postfertilization is involved because of the timing in the stage of development of the affected organs.

Biliary atresia has been described in association with trisomy 17, 18, and 21. However, twin studies do not suggest a simple genetic factor, since atresia has been reported to affect a single sibling of both monozygotic and dizygotic pairs. Another review of 11 instances of familial biliary atresia concludes that the evidence suggested a combined etiology of genetic susceptibility and environmental insult.

Anatomical anomalies of the common bile duct have been observed with retrograde cholangiographic examinations. Chiba and associates showed abnormally long common pancreatico-biliary channels in 28 cases of atresia, although the abnormality was not detected in a group of seven infants with neonatal hepatitis.[12] Similar observations have been made by others and are reminiscent of the changes found in approximately 70% of patients with choledochal cysts.[13]

■ PATHOLOGY

Histology of the extrahepatic ducts shows a destructive inflammatory process with inflammatory cells of all types and a variable degree of fibrosis (Fig 81–1). The inflammatory process is not confined to the bile ducts and gallbladder but also affects the periductal tissues. Increased vascularity is a prominent feature often seen at surgery. Hyperplastic lymph nodes and enlarged extrahepatic lymphatics also are found in the region of the porta hepatis.

Typical intrahepatic changes observed during the first few weeks of life include a mixture of cholestasis and portal tract expansion. There is bile duct and canalicular plugging with bile, and intracellular features of hepatocyte and macrophage staining with bile pigment. Proliferation of bile ducts is seen in the portal tracts and is accompanied by an inflammatory response.

Percutaneous liver biopsies are performed for diagnosis, but occasionally, the presence of significant numbers of giant cells and areas of hepatocellular necrosis can lead to a misdiagnosis of neonatal hepatitis. Progression of the disease in the untreated case leads rapidly to increasing periportal fibrosis and to biliary cirrhosis.

TABLE 81–1. CONGENITAL ANOMALIES ASSOCIATED WITH BILIARY ATRESIA

Cleft palate, esophageal atresia
Annular pancreas, duodenal atresia
Jejunal atresia
Situs inversus, malrotation
Polycystic kidney
Splenic anomalies
    Polysplenia
    Asplenia
Portal vein anomalies
    Preduodenal
    Cavernomatous transformation
    Absent
Cardiac anomalies
    Immotile cilia (Kartagener's syndrome)

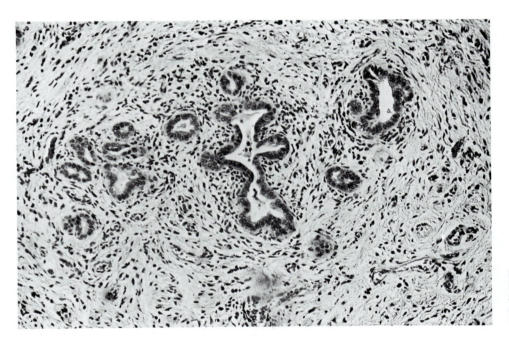

Figure 81–1. Microscopic appearance of residual bile duct tissue excised from the porta hepatis of a 3 month–old infant with noncorrectable biliary atresia. Small ductules lined by cuboidal epithelium are visible within the fibrous tissue. (H&E)

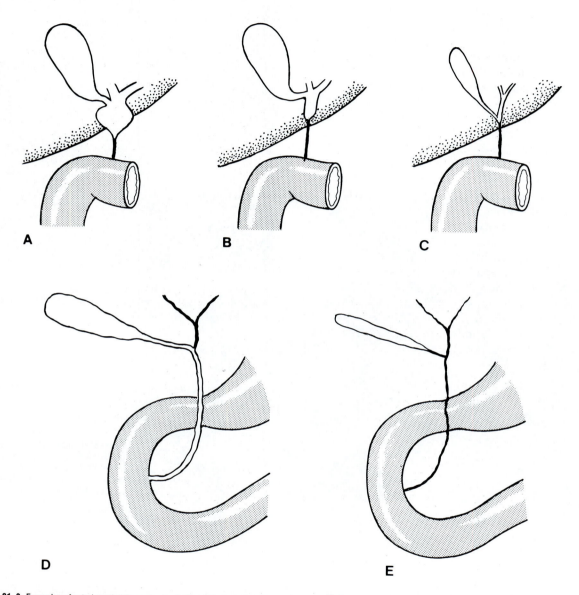

Figure 81–2. Examples of extrahepatic biliary atresia. **A, B,** and **C** are types of correctable atresia in which there is occlusion of the distal common bile duct. **D** and **E** represent the more common varieties of noncorrectable atresia with occlusion of the proximal bile ducts.

Intrahepatic bile ducts remain patent during the first 2 to 3 months after birth. Studies of the bile ducts at the porta hepatis have revealed that the major intrahepatic ducts divide into many small branches, which terminate in the residual extrahepatic inflammatory ductal tissue. Gautier and associates classified this residual tissue into three types: type 1 tissue showed no residual ductal tissue and few inflammatory cells; type 2 tissue contained small residual lumina lined with cuboidal epithelium but with a diameter of <50 μm; and type 3 tissue retained obvious central structures resembling residual bile ducts with at least some areas of columnar epithelium.[14] Bile staining was reported in 68% of type 3 tissue, mostly within macrophages.

Surgery is most effective before 7 weeks of age, since the intrahepatic ducts undergo progressive destruction in the newborn period. *Early and rapid investigation, diagnosis, and treatment are therefore mandatory.* It should be noted that intrahepatic bile ducts do not develop normal morphology after surgery, even in the presence of good bile flow, although some reduction in hepatic fibrosis and inflammatory cell infiltrates has been shown.[15] In failed cases, the intrahepatic ducts tend to become cystic, particularly in the region of the porta hepatis.

Although morphology of the extrahepatic bile ducts varies widely in biliary atresia, the Japanese Society of Pediatric Surgeons identified three principal types, which form the basis of the classification now in general use (Fig 81–2):

- Type 1: Atresia of the common bile duct
- Type 2: Atresia of the common hepatic duct
- Type 3: Atresia of the right and left ducts

In a Japanese survey of 643 cases, 566 (88%) were type 3, 64 (10%) were type 1, and only 13 (2%) were type 2 lesions.

Subdivisions of this classification depend on the details of the morphology of the gallbladder and distal common bile duct, as well as the histologic features of the tissue at the porta hepatis. Noncommunicating segments may occur in any area of the biliary tract and may suggest, to the inexperienced surgeon, a false diagnosis of choledochal cyst or of type 1 atresia.

■ DIAGNOSIS AND EVALUATION

CLINICAL MANIFESTATIONS

Affected infants are usually born at term with normal birth weight and may feed and gain weight appropriately during the first few weeks of life. A small female preponderance has been reported in most series. Jaundice and acholic stools are observed within the first two weeks of life in 80% of patients, with liver and spleen

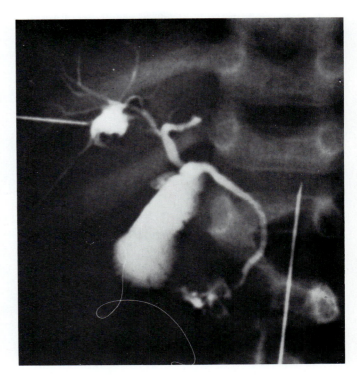

Figure 81–3. Percutaneous cholangiogram of a 5 month–old infant with hepatitis syndrome. Contrast material flows freely into the duodenum. Bile duct size is compared with the 19-gauge needle lying over the spine.

enlargement also common findings. Coagulopathy and abnormal bleeding caused by vitamin K deficiency are occasional presenting features. Failure to thrive is seen in the later stages of the disease and may be accompanied by ascites secondary to hepatic fibrosis or cirrhosis.

Conjugated hyperbilirubinemia in infancy also can be a presenting sign of the infective, metabolic, and other medical causes of neonatal hepatitis syndrome (Fig 81–3), as well as surgical causes of jaundice such as inspissated bile syndrome, intrahepatic hypoplasia, choledochal cyst, and spontaneous perforation of the bile duct.

Although surgery performed before 7 or 8 weeks of age is an important factor in achieving good bile flow, in 50 consecutive cases referred to one hospital, the median age at operation was 10 weeks.[16] An identical finding was reported from a review of 816 cases collected from more than 100 institutions in North America.[17]

■ DIAGNOSTIC STUDIES

Examination of the stools in a jaundiced infant is important, since white or acholic stools are suggestive of biliary atresia.

Techniques used to investigate conjugated hyper-bilirubinemia in infants include the following:

- Screening test for infection, metabolic disorders, and genetic disorders, especially α_1-antitrypsin deficiency
- Liver biopsy
- Ultrasonography
- Radionucleide hepatobiliary imaging
- Percutaneous or endoscopic cholangiography
- Duodenal intubation for bile
- Laparoscopy and liver biopsy
- Operative cholangiography

There is no single definitive test for atresia and even liver biopsy may be equivocal in up to 10% of cases. Standard liver function tests do not differentiate clearly between medical and surgical causes of conjugated hyper-bilirubinemia in early infancy. Screening tests do identify infective, metabolic, or genetic causes in approximately 30% of cases of hepatitis syndrome; the remainder, identified on biopsy, are termed *idiopathic*. A choledochal cyst may present as persistent jaundice in this age group, but the diagnosis is usually made without difficulty on ultrasound examination.

Hepatobiliary excretion scans, using technetium labeled imino diacetic acid compounds (eg, isopropyl-imino-diacetic acid [DISIDA]), are now commonly used for diagnosis. A 3 day course of phenobarbitone helps to increase the sensitivity of the test, and visualization of the bowel with isotope would exclude the diagnosis of biliary atresia.

Intrahepatic hypoplasia, which is found in association with patent extrahepatic ducts, must be considered in the differential diagnosis. Liver biopsy typically shows less fibrous tissue than in cases of extrahepatic atresia, although intrahepatic bile ducts are either reduced in number or are absent from the portal triads. This syndrome is often associated with characteristic facial features and vertebral and cardiac anomalies.[18,19] It is compatible with survival into adult life.

■ SURGICAL TREATMENT

Surgical treatment of biliary atresia used to be divided into two stages. The first stage was a minilaparotomy performed through a small transverse incision in the right hypochondrium, followed by inspection of the liver and biliary tract and operative cholangiography. A liver biopsy completed the procedure. Definitive surgery was reserved for the second procedure, performed a few days later. In most cases, this two-stage management is unnecessary. Atresia often can be diagnosed from the characteristic appearance of the gallbladder, and the extent of the atretic process rules out cholan-

giography in more than 75% of cases. Open liver biopsy has now been superseded by preoperative percutaneous biopsy, followed by radical resection of the occluded biliary tract and reconstruction with a Roux-en-Y loop of jejunum.

Current procedures are based on the original Kasai procedure,[6,20] based on the observation of residual microscopic bile channels in the fibrous tissue of the porta hepatis. The technique now is applied to the majority of cases, including the 15% to 20% who are found at laparotomy to have cystic bile-containing structures in the porta hepatis and in whom conventional bile duct–to-bowel anastomoses have been applied in the past (correctable atresia). However, surgical results for this latter group have been disappointing, and the more radical Kasai approach now is recommended for all cases except those with a long residual segment of proximal bile duct.

PREOPERATIVE PREPARATION

Vitamin K (phytomenadione) (1 mg/day) is administered for 4 days and oral neomycin (50 mg/kg/day in six divided doses) for 24 hours before surgery. One unit of blood is cross-matched, and oral fluids are withheld, beginning three hours before inducing anesthesia. An adequate intravenous line is inserted and a nasogastric tube is passed. The infant is placed supine on a thermostatically controlled warming pad. X-ray facilities must be available for operative cholangiography. Intravenous antibiotics (cephalosporins) are started with the induction of anesthesia and are continued for 5 days. An oral cephalosporin then is substituted for a further 3 weeks as prophylaxis against possible attacks of ascending cholangitis.

THE KASAI PORTOENTEROSTOMY

A transverse abdominal incision across the right rectus muscle is made over the palpable liver edge, and the inferior surface of the right lobe of the liver is exposed (Fig 81–4). The appearance of the liver is recorded as well as the presence or absence of ascites and portal hypertension. A search is made for other anomalies such as polysplenia or asplenia. The gallbladder in biliary atresia is often thick walled, contracted, and hidden within a cleft in the liver parenchyma. In these circumstances, operative cholangiography is usually impossible and aspiration of the gallbladder should produce clear mucus. *However, operative cholangiography is mandatory whenever bile is found in the gallbladder.*

To perform cholangiography, the fundus of the gallbladder is incised within a purse-string suture and a small polythene catheter is inserted. Two or three milliliters of contrast material (25% Hypaque) are injected into the gallbladder, and x-rays are taken. The demonstration of patent hepatic and common bile ducts terminates the procedure (Fig 81–5). In some cases, the cystic and distal common bile ducts remain patent and contrast flows into the duodenum but not into the proximal bile ducts (Fig 81–6). Once atresia is confirmed, the abdominal incision is extended across the left rectus muscle.

The liver is now mobilized fully by dividing the falciform ligament, the left and right triangular ligaments, and the two diverging peritoneal reflections on the right lobe of the liver. The liver is delivered out of the peritoneal cavity and is supported by the anterior abdominal wall. This maneuver is useful in allowing accurate dissection of the porta hepatis and the subsequent anastomosis (Fig 81–7).

Large lymph nodes frequently obscure the extrahepatic ducts, which are identified most easily by an initial mobilization of the gallbladder from its liver bed. The vascularity of the gallbladder bed usually is increased, and bleeding is controlled by diathermy and ligatures.

The cystic artery is ligated and divided and the cystic duct traced to its junction with the fibrotic common bile duct. The distal portion of the common duct is divided between ligatures at the level of the upper border of the duodenum (Fig 81–4D).

Dissection of the extrahepatic bile duct remnants then is performed toward the porta hepatis. Meticulous tying with fine ligatures close to the ducts will prevent the development of postoperative ascites from leakage of lymph. The hepatic artery and portal vein are identified during the dissection, and the ductal system is traced above the bifurcation of the latter. Magnifying glasses will facilitate the dissection.

Rarely, a long patent segment of proximal duct (correctable atresia) that can be used for a hepaticojejunostomy is discovered. In the majority of cases, however, the dissection proceeds above and behind the bifurcation of the portal vein and hepatic artery, and the tissue is transected at its junction with, and parallel to, the capsule of the liver (Figs 81–4E and 81–8). Angled scissors have been designed for the accurate performance of this part of the operation, (Fig 81–9).

The aim of the operation is to expose remnants of the hepatic bile ducts or to transect bile ductules that may be identified on histologic examination of the excised tissue. Any bleeding from the porta hepatis should be controlled by direct pressure, since cautery may damage the microscopic ducts.

A Roux-en-Y loop of jejunum is prepared. The jejunum is transected between staples just distal to the duodenojejunal flexure. The distal end is passed in a retrocolic manner to the hilum of the liver and an end-to-side anastomosis is fashioned accurately between the cut edges of the tissue in the porta hepatis and the jejunal loop with interrupted sutures of 5-0 or 6-0 polydioxanone (PDS). The accessibility of the anastomosis is im-

proved by positioning all of the posterior sutures before they are tied (Fig 81–4F). The jejunum can then be "railroaded" into position and the sutures tied seriatim.

Intestinal continuity is reestablished by anastomosing the proximal jejunum to the distal loop approximately 40 cm from the porta hepatis. A small drain is placed in the supraduodenal area before closure of the abdomen.

The frequent occurrence of ascending cholangitis after operation is, in part, owing to ascending infection from the bowel. Surgical attempts to minimize the problem have included rearrangements of the biliary-enteric anastomoses and the inclusion of stomas for the drainage of bile which may be re-fed to the patient to prevent excessive fluid and electrolyte loss. The stomas are closed after 1 year. These techniques have been illustrated diagrammatically (Fig 81–10). However, complications associated with stoma formation include a significant incidence of bleeding from varices, which develops at the mucocutaneous junctions, and an increase in the difficulty of any transplant procedure should this become necessary at a later stage. Therefore, the routine use of these procedures is no longer advised. Saeki and associates devised an alternative technique in which a valve is fashioned within the Roux loop by removing a segment of the seromuscular layer of the bowel wall and intussuscepting the denuded mucosa as a nipple.[21]

Anastomosis of the gallbladder to the transected tissue in the porta hepatis (portocholecystostomy, Fig 81–10F) has been used in the 15% to 20% of patients who have a patent distal common bile duct. However, a possible reduction in the incidence of cholangitis must be compared with an increased number of technical complications which have included obstruction of the mobilized gallbladder and prolonged biliary leakage.

POSTOPERATIVE MANAGEMENT

Intravenous fluids, antibiotics and nasogastric aspiration are continued until satisfactory bowel function returns. Oral antibiotics (cephalosporin) are continued for three weeks and phenobarbitone and cholestyramine are prescribed to encourage bile flow. The administration of vitamins D and K is continued for many months. Histologic analysis of the tissue excised from the porta hepatis may help to predict prognosis. If ductules with diameters >150 μm are observed, then there is a good chance of satisfactory bile drainage. The drainage, however, may not be effective for several weeks (Fig 81–11). Any sign of cholangitis in the immediate postoperative period must be treated rapidly with a broad-spectrum antibiotic. Bacteremia should be identified by blood cultures and culture of liver biopsy material. Common infecting organisms include *Proteus, Klebsiella,* and *Escheria coli.*

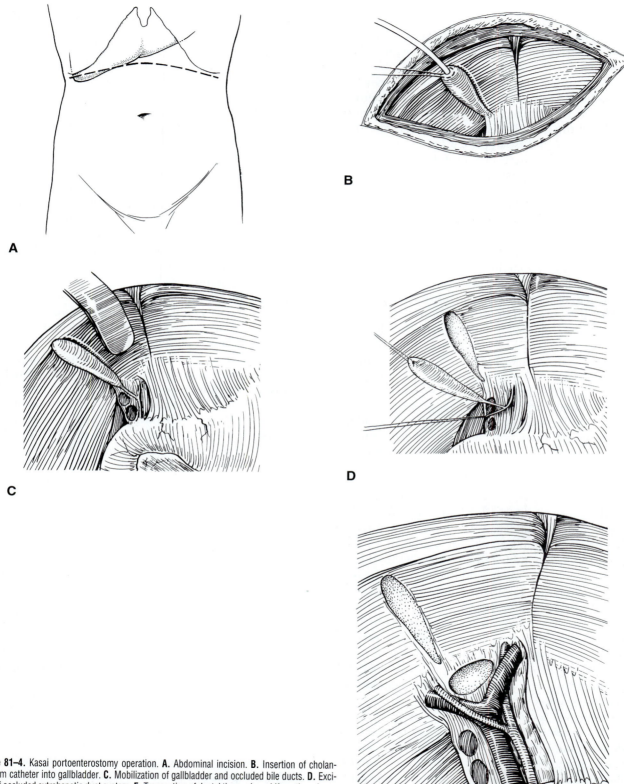

Figure 81–4. Kasai portoenterostomy operation. **A.** Abdominal incision. **B.** Insertion of cholangiogram catheter into gallbladder. **C.** Mobilization of gallbladder and occluded bile ducts. **D.** Excision of occluded extrahepatic duct system. **E.** Transection of ductal tissue above bifurcation of portal vein flush with liver capsule. *Continued*

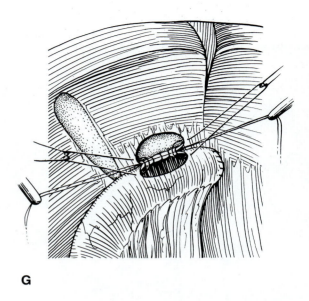

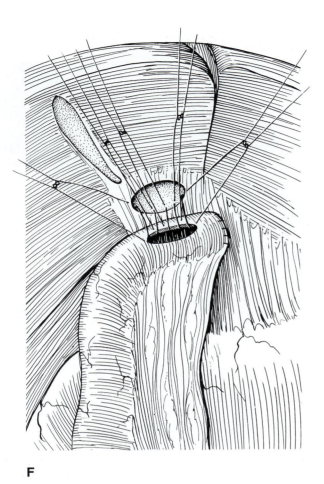

G

F

Figure 81–4, cont'd. F. Anastomosis of Roux-Y loop (30 cm) of jejunum to porta hepatis-posterior layer. **G.** Anterior sutures begun to complete the anastomosis.

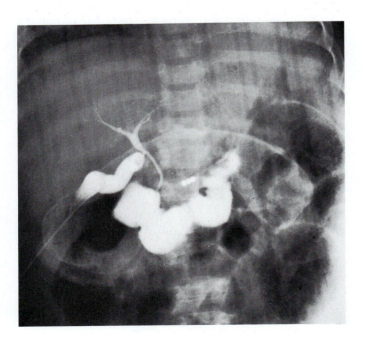

Figure 81–5. Operative cholangiogram of a 3 month–old infant with hypoplastic but patent extrahepatic bile ducts.

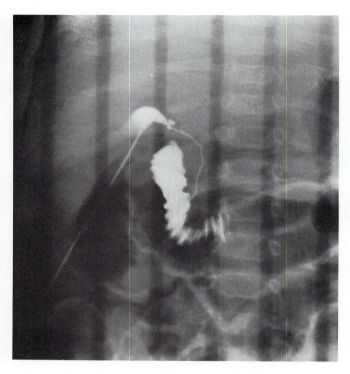

Figure 81–6. Operative cholangiogram of a 3 month–old infant with atresia of the common hepatic duct. The cystic and common bile ducts are patent.

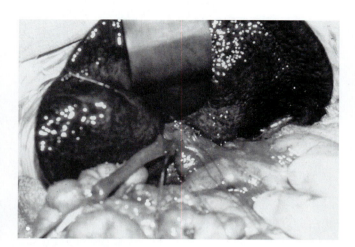

Figure 81–7. Operative view of the liver in a case of biliary atresia. The liver has been mobilized and rotated into the abdominal wound to expose the structures of the porta hepatis.

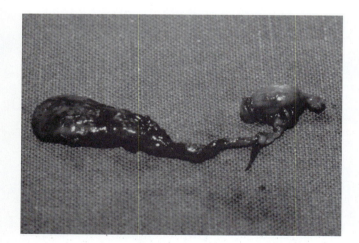

Figure 81–8. Complete specimen of gallbladder and atretic hepatic ducts excised during a portoenterostomy operation. Note the prominent swelling of fibrous tissue that has replaced the hepatic ducts in the porta hepatis.

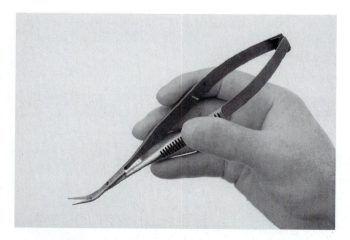

Figure 81–9. Portoenterostomy scissors, with flat angled blades, designed for accurate transection of tissue in the porta hepatis. (From Davenport M, Howard ER. Portoenterostomy scissors: a new instrument for surgery in the porta hepatis. *Ann R Coll Surg Engl* 1992;74:68)

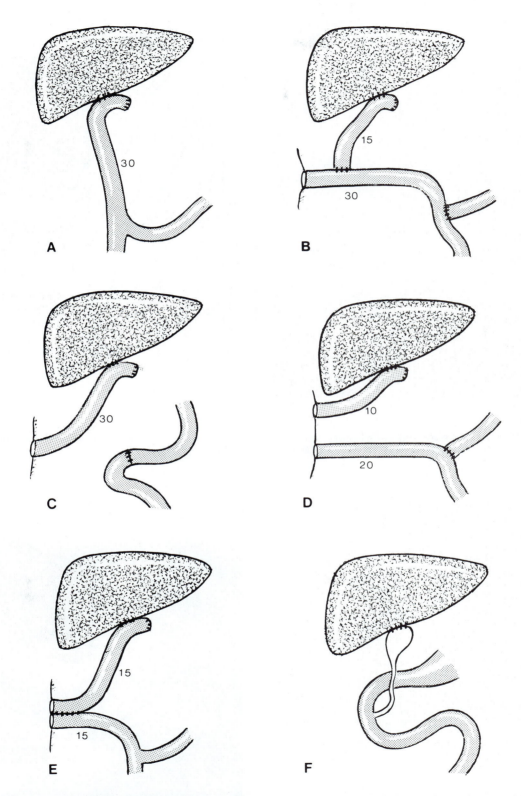

Figure 81–10. Diagrams of some of the suggested modifications to the original portoenterostomy operation. The recommended lengths of bowel segments (cm) are indicated. **A.** Original Kasai portoenterostomy. **B.** Kasai[6] modification to prevent ascending cholangitis. **C, D,** and **E.** Operations suggested by Sawaguchi,[33] Suruga, and Lilly and Altman[29], respectively. **F.** Portocholecystostomy utilizing a patent gallbladder and distal common bile duct.

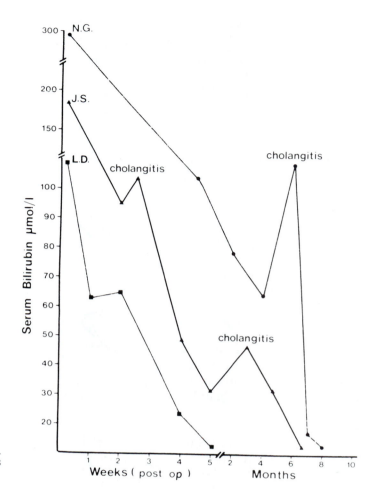

Figure 81-11. Fall in serum bilirubin after three portoenterostomy operations. Episodes of ascending bacterial cholangitis in two cases were accompanied by rises in bilirubin.

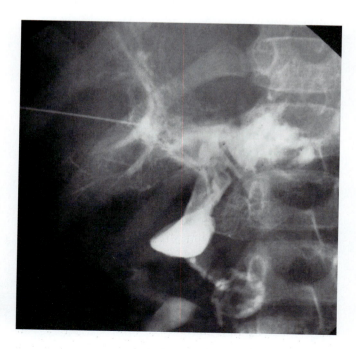

Figure 81-12. Percutaneous cholangiogram in a 7 year-old girl with recurrent jaundice who had been treated with portoenterostomy at 6 weeks of age. The cholangiogram shows good flow of contrast into the Roux loop which is narrowed distally by adhesions. Note the very abnormal intrahepatic bile ducts.

TABLE 81–2. BILIARY ATRESIA: ENDOSCOPIC ASSESSMENT OF VARICES IN LONG-TERM SURVIVORS FROM FIVE SERIES

	No. of Cases	Varices (%)	Bleeding (%)
Akiyama[24]	37	65	20
Okamoto[30]	28	50	32
Valayer[31]	45	31	0
Ohi[32]	27	48	?
Stringer[22]	58	67	28
Totals	195	52	

TABLE 81–3. IMPROVEMENT IN RESULTS OF THE PORTOENTEROSTOMY OPERATION FROM ONE CENTER: 1953 TO 1988

	No. of Cases	Alive—No Jaundice
1953–1961	26	2 (7.6%)
1962–1971	78	13 (16.6%)
1972–1981	91	42 (46.0%)
1982–1988	56	34 (60.7%)

(Modified from Ohi R, Hanamatsu M, et al. Progress in the treatment of biliary atresia. World J Surg 1985;9:285)[32]

LONG-TERM COMPLICATIONS OF SURGERY

Episodes of cholangitis, beyond the immediate perioperative period, occur in 25% to 50% of patients. The attacks are recognized from the triad of pyrexia, rising serum bilirubin, and recurrence of acholic stools. Prompt treatment with intravenous fluids and intravenous antibiotics is essential because of the deterioration in liver function that may follow each attack. Fig 81–11 shows the postoperative progress in three cases and the rises in serum bilirubin that accompanied each episode of infection. These infections are most frequent 6 to 9 months after surgery, and an episode more than 2 years after treatment should suggest a possible obstruction in the Roux drainage loop and perhaps the necessity for reoperation. Assessment of the Roux loop is achieved with a combination of radionucleide scanning and percutaneous cholangiography (Fig 81–12). Prophylactic antibiotics have not been shown to have any significant effect on the long-term prevention of ascending cholangitis.

Many survivors after portoenterostomy eventually show evidence of portal hypertension (Table 81–2) and Stringer and associates observed significant varices in 67% of their long term cases.[22] Bleeding from varices occurred in 28% of children. The problem was greatest in those who never lost their jaundice after portoenterostomy. Postoperative cholangitis also increases portal hypertension through progressive hepatic fibrosis. Injection sclerotherapy is the best primary management for bleeding varices in these children. Esophageal transection and other devascularization procedures have had significant complications and are not recommended as a substitute to injection sclerotherapy.

Occasionally, bleeding will occur from ectopic sites such as anastomoses in the bowel and cutaneous stomas. In these cases, portosystemic shunts are required. These shunts are probably best performed with a mesocaval interposition of the segment of internal jugular vein.[13]

Reexploration of the porta hepatis in cases of failed portoenterostomy is not recommended. The results are poor and complications include severe ascites and liver failure. Since liver transplantation is made more hazardous by repeated exploration of the abdominal cavity, it should be avoided except for the occasional case involving obstruction of the Roux loop of jejunum.

RESULTS OF SURGERY

Prior to portoenterostomy, long-term survival was very rare, except for cases of type 1 atresia. In 1981, Hays and Kimura analyzed 84 patients who had undergone portoenterostomy between 5 and 20 years previously.[23] Only three of the patients were jaundiced and the majority were capable of normal school and social activities. Hepatomegaly was noted in 37% and splenomegaly in 17%. Akiyama and associates reported a long-term survival in 16% of 2013 patients treated in Japan.[24]

A more recent review by Karrer and associates, from more than 100 institutions in North America, included 5 and 10 year follow-up data on 670 children. The survival after portoenterostomy for these two groups was 48% and 30%, respectively, and the authors compared these results with a 3 year survival of <10% in a group of children who were not offered corrective surgery. This survey confirmed that age at operation is the most influential factor in prognosis and showed a survival rate of 62.5% for infants treated before 30 days, 43.6% for those treated between 31 and 60 days, and only 28.6% for those treated after 90 days of life.[17]

It is clear that the results of portoenterostomy have gradually improved and this was illustrated in a report that showed that the number of jaundice-free children rose from 7.6% in the period 1953–1961 to 85% in 1987–88 (Table 81–3).[25] The current probability of 5 year survival after portoenterostomy in our own unit is 60%.

HEPATIC TRANSPLANTATION

Hepatic transplantation is now an accepted treatment modality for patients who either fail to completely respond to portoenterostomy, or for those whose condition deteriorates at a later stage. The results have improved with advances in immunosuppression and with improvements in surgical technique. Biliary atresia represents the most common single indication for pediatric transplantation, Starzl and associates reported 217 cases out of a total series of 400 pediatric patients.[26] Previous surgery does not seem to affect the results and Millis and associates found no significant differences in intraoperative blood loss, postoperative biliary tract complications, or retransplantation between a group of children with a previous portoenterostomy and a group of eight who were treated primarily with transplantation.[27] The 6 month survival rate was 82% in children with a previous portoenterostomy and 62% for those without. The 3 year actuarial survival for all children was 75%.

At the moment, portoenterostomy is accepted as the initial treatment for biliary atresia. It is performed best before 7 weeks of age. Rapid diagnosis should be a first priority. There are many reports of long-term survivors, and the original operation without stoma formation is now recommended. Revision operations should be avoided and transplantation offered to those patients who fail to achieve a favorable outcome with portoenterostomy, or those who develop severe complications at a later age.

REFERENCES

1. Thomson J. On congenital obliteration of the bile ducts. *Edinb Med J* 1892;37:604
2. Holmes JB. Congenital obliteration of the bile duct: diagnosis and suggestions for treatment. *Am J Dis Child* 1916;11:405
3. Ladd WE. Congenital atresia and stenosis of the bile duct. *JAMA* 1928;91:1082
4. Hays DM, Snyder WH. Life-span in untreated biliary atresia. *Surgery* 1963;54:373
5. Kasai M, Suzuki S. A new operation for "noncorrectable" biliary atresia; hepatic portoenterostomy. *Shujitsu* 1959;13:733
6. Kasai M. Treatment of biliary atresia with special reference to hepatic portoenterostomy and its modifications. *Prog Pediatr Surg* 1974;6:5
7. Landing BH. Considerations of the pathogenesis of neonatal hepatitis, biliary atresia and choledochal cyst: the concept of infantile obstructive cholangiopathy. *Progr Pediatr Surg* 1974;6:113
8. Morecki R, Glaser JH, Horwitz MS. Etiology of biliary atresia: the role of reo 3 virus. In: Daum F (ed), *Extrahepatic Biliary Atresia*. New York, NY: Marcel Dekker;1983:1
9. Dussaix E, Hadchouel M, et al. Biliary atresia and reovirus type 3 infection. *N Engl J Med* 1984;311:658
10. Davenport M, Savage M, et al. Biliary atresia splenic malformation syndrome. *Surgery* 1993;113:662
11. Cunningham ML, Sybert VP. Idiopathic extrahepatic biliary atresia: recurrence in sibs in two families. *Am J Med Genet* 1988;31:421
12. Chiba T, Ohi R, Mochizuki I. Cholangiographic study of the pancreaticobiliary ductal junction in biliary atresia. *J Pediatr Surg* 1990;25:609
13. Howard ER. *Surgery of Liver Disease in Childhood*. Oxford, England: Butterworth-Heinemann;1991
14. Gautier M, Eliot N. Extrahepatic biliary atresia: morphological study of 98 biliary remnants. *Arch Pathol Lab Med* 1981;105:397
15. Dessanti A, Ohi R, et al. Short term histological liver changes in extrahepatic biliary atresia with good postoperative bile drainage. *Arch Dis Child* 1985;60:73
16. Mieli-Vergani G, Howard ER, et al. Late referral for biliary atresia—missed opportunities for effective surgery. *Lancet* 1989;i:421
17. Karrer FM, Lilly JR, et al. Biliary atresia registry, 1976 to 1989. *J Pediatr Surg* 1990;25:1076
18. Porter SD, Soper RT, et al. Biliary hypoplasia. *Ann Surg* 1968;167:602
19. Alagille D, Odiévre H, et al. Hepatic ductular hypoplasia associated with characteristic facies, vertebral malformation, retarded physical, mental and sexual development and cardiac murmur. *J Pediatr* 1975;86:63
20. Kasai M, Mochizuki I, et al. Surgical limitations for biliary atresia: indications for liver transplantation. *J Pediatr Surg* 1989;24:851
21. Saeki M, Nakano M, et al. Effectiveness of an intussusceptive antireflux valve to prevent ascending cholangitis after hepatic portoenterostomy in biliary atresia. *J Pediatr Surg* 1987;26:800
22. Stringer MD, Howard ER, Mowat AP. Endoscopic sclerotherapy in the management of esophageal varices in 61 children with biliary atresia. *J Pediatr Surg* 1989;24:438
23. Hays DM, Kimura K. Biliary atresia: new concepts of management. *Curr Probl Surg* 1981;18:546
24. Akiyama H, Saeki M, Okata T. Portal hypertension after successful surgery for biliary atresia. In: Kasai M (ed), *Biliary Atresia and its Related Disorders*. Amsterdam, Netherlands: Excerpta Medica; 1983:276
25. Ohi R, Nio M, et al. Long-term follow-up after surgery for patients with biliary atresia. *J Pediatr Surg* 1990;25:442
26. Starzl TE, Demetris AJ, Van Thiel D. Liver transplantation. Part 1. *N Engl J Med* 1989;321:1014
27. Millis JM, Brems JJ, et al. Orthotopic liver transplantation for biliary atresia. *Arch Surg* 1988;123:1237
28. Davenport M, Howard ER. Portoenterostomy scissors: a new instrument for surgery in the porta hepatis. *Ann R Coll Surg Engl* 1992;74:68
29. Lilly JR, Altman RP. Hepatic portoenterostomy (the Kasai operation) for biliary atresia. *Surgery* 1975;78:76
30. Okamoto E, Toyosaka A, Okasora T. Surgical treatment of portal hypertension in biliary atresia. In: Kasai M (ed), *Biliary Atresia and its Related Disorders*. Amsterdam, Netherlands: Excerpta Medica;1983:283
31. Valayer J. Biliary atresia and portal hypertension. In: Daum F and Fisher SE (eds), *Extrahepatic Biliary Atresia*. New York, Marcel Dekker;1983:105
32. Ohi R, Hanamatsu M, et al. Progress in the treatment of biliary atresia. *World J Surg* 1985;9:285
33. Sawaguchi S, Akiyama H, Nakajo K. Long-term follow-up after radical operation for biliary atresia. In: Kasai M and Shiraki K (eds), *Cholestasis in Infancy*. Tokyo, University of Tokyo Press;198;371

XVI

GYNECOLOGICAL PROCEDURES

82

Gynecologic Pelvic Procedures

F.J. Montz ■ *Jonathan S. Berek*

Earlier in the 20th century, the majority of gynecologic surgery was performed by general surgeons who had a special interest in the disease processes of the female reproductive organs. However, the compartmentalization of surgical subspecialties has become much more elaborate. In 1930, the American Board of Obstetrics and Gynecology was established and, since then, numerous international certifying organizations also have formed. Many of the pioneers of gynecologic surgery, such as Bonney, opposed the separation of gynecologic surgery from general surgery and the subsequent creation of a distinct specialty joined with obstetrics.[1]

The division of abdominal and pelvic surgery into two unique disciplines is arbitrary because pathologic processes that affect the pelvic reproductive organs often involve nonreproductive pelvic organs or upper abdominal organs.[2] Similarly, it is common for diseases affecting nonreproductive pelvic organs to involve the adjoining uterus, fallopian tubes, and ovaries.[3] Therefore, it is imperative that the general surgeon have a clear understanding of selected "gynecologic" operations and be knowledgeable about the management of common intraperitoneal gynecologic neoplasms found incidentally at laparotomy.

In this chapter, we present the three most relevant situations the general surgeon needs to be familiar with: the en bloc removal of the female reproductive organs when they are secondarily involved with a gastrointestinal malignancy; the unanticipated gynecologic adnexal mass; and vesicovaginal, enterovaginal, or rectovaginal fistulas.

■ EN BLOC RESECTION OF PELVIC ORGANS WHEN INVOLVED WITH GASTROINTESTINAL MALIGNANCY

Colorectal cancer, with its propensity for both local and lymphatic spread, invades adjacent organs in 3.1% to 11.8% of cases.[3–5] When an abdominoperineal resection is undertaken to control an apparently localized colorectal malignancy, it is recommended that if there is any suggestion of involvement of the rectovaginal septum, but no evidence of intraperitoneal metastasis or distal disease, a hysterectomy and a partial, posterior vaginectomy be performed to facilitate adequate tumor removal.[6] Thus, the surgeon responsible for the operative management of colorectal cancer must understand the principles guiding the extirpation of the reproductive organs in these patients.

The essential skills required to effectively perform any surgical procedure in the pelvis mandate a thorough understanding of applied female pelvic anatomy and a mastering of a few, selected surgical techniques.

ESSENTIALS OF FEMALE PELVIC ANATOMY (FIG 82–1)

The main blood supply to the female reproductive organs is via the ovarian and uterine arteries. The ovarian arteries arise directly from the abdominal aorta distal to the level of the renal arteries. With the associated veins and lymphatics, the ovarian arteries run in the retroperitoneal space, lateral to the aorta and vena cava. Approximately at the level of the pelvic brim, the vessels are enveloped by peritoneum and develop the suspensory

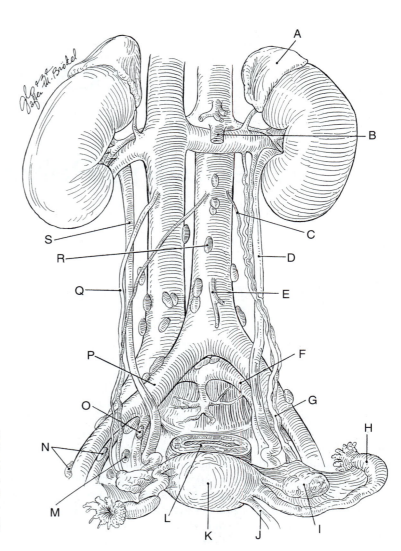

Figure 82–1. Essential female retroperitoneal and pelvic anatomy A: Adrenal glands. B: Superior mesenteric artery. C: Left ovarian artery. D: Left ureter. E: Inferior mesenteric artery. F: Left common iliac vein. G: Left ovarian vessels. H: Left fallopian tube. I: Left ovary. J: Left round ligament. K: Uterine corpus. L: Transected sigmoid colon. M: Right obturator lymph nodes. N: Right external iliac lymph nodes. O: Right hypogastric lymph nodes. P: Right common iliac artery. Q: Right ovarian vein. R: Para-aortic lymph node. S: Right ureter. (Redrawn from Hacker NF, Moore JG. Introduction. In: Hacker NF, Moore JG, (eds), *Essentials of Obstetrics and Gynecology.* 2nd ed. Philadelphia, PA: WB Saunders; 1992)

ligament of the ovary, also known as the infundibulopelvic ligament. It is at this site, where the vessels cross over the common iliac artery and the ureter and enter the pelvis, that the ovarian vessels are most easily identified and safely ligated. The uterine arteries arise from the anterior division of the internal iliac (hypogastric) artery approximately 2 cm from the bifurcation of the iliac artery distal to the separation of the internal iliac into anterior and posterior divisions and immediately proximal to the origin of the superior vesical artery. These arteries then course superior to the ureter as the latter runs lateral to the cervix and enters the trigone of the bladder. The uterine artery can be ligated safely in several specific sites, depending on the indication.

These two (ovarian and uterine) arterial sources anastomose near the uterine cornua. The ovarian vessels anastomose with vessels of the uterovarian ligament that attaches the ovary to the dorsal aspect of the uterus,

run caudad to the fallopian tube, and there anastomose with blood vessels ascending from the uterine artery.

Because of the proximity of the pelvic ureter to the ovarian and uterine vessels and because it courses through the parametrium as it descends toward the trigone, the ureter is vulnerable to injury. The pelvic surgeon must accurately appreciate the course of the ureter and be proficient at identifying its location. As the ureter courses through the retroperitoneal space it enters the pelvis at the brim, crossing ventral to the common iliac artery just caudad to the iliac artery bifurcation. At this site, the ureter is dorsal to the ovarian vessels at the origin of the infundibulopelvic ligament. It is at this location that the ureter is most likely to be injured during pelvic surgery.[7–9] If the ureter is not identified here, it can be inadvertently incorporated into a pedicle when the ovarian vessels are being ligated cephalad to the ovary.

After entering the pelvis, the ureter continues in the medial leaf of the broad ligament and courses under the uterine artery, approximately 0.7 to 1.5 cm lateral to the isthmus of the uterus (the site where the uterine corpus and the cervix meet). This is also a common site of ureteral injury because it may be clamped inadvertently when ligating the uterine artery medial to the ureter.

The ureter completes its pelvic course by transversing the parametrium lateral to the cervix. It then enters the bladder trigone approximately at the level of the anterior vaginal fornix. It is here that the third common site of ureteral injury exists. If the bladder and the ureter have not been adequately mobilized from the cervix and anterior vagina, they both can be injured at time of separation of the cervix from the attached vagina.

THE RETROPERITONEAL APPROACH TO PELVIC ORGAN RESECTION

The use of the retroperitoneal approach permits the mobilization of the pelvic organs without interference from intraperitoneal disease processes. Often, the retroperitoneal space functions as a "surgical sanctuary," in other words, the pelvic vessels and the ureters are in a region to which intraperitoneal disease often does not extend. The retroperitoneal approach was championed by Hudson[2] for use in the completion of one of the most difficult of pelvic resections: extensive ovarian cancer that has obliterated the cul-de-sac and has agglutinated the adjacent peritoneal surfaces. Using such a technique, tumors that had been previously deemed unresectable can be safely removed.

In order to accomplish this technique, critical steps must be appreciated:

1. The peritoneal incision must be made lateral to the external iliac vessels over the psoas muscles. This facilitates the use of the pelvic peritoneum as a "retractor," mobilizing the pelvic contents and tumor mass off the sidewall and avoiding injury to the pelvic vessels.

2. The ureter, ovarian vessels, and internal iliac vessels must be identified and their courses traced.

3. The ureter should be freed from the medial leaf of the broad ligament using an atraumatic technique. The specific location where it should be freed depends upon the extent of peritoneal involvement. Usually this dissection occurs two or more centimeters cephalad to the site where the ureter runs under the uterine artery. (Fig 82–2a)

4. The uterine artery should be sacrificed at the point where it crosses the ureter. This allows lateral displacement of the ureter so that the sur-

geon can follow its course in the bladder. Dissection of the ureter under the uterine artery should be accomplished with a right-angle clamp placed medially to the ureter to avoid injury to the bladder which is located laterally and ventrally.

5. After mobilization of the ureter and bladder from the cervix and vagina, the vagina should be sharply entered anteriorly in the midline, perpendicular to its longitudinal axis. The vaginal incision should be continued posteriorly until the posterior vaginal wall is reached. We prefer to clamp the vagina and ligate the individual pedicles because, at this site, they are attached to the suspensory ligaments (uterosacral and cardinal). (Fig 82–2b)

6. The posterior vaginal wall should be incised carefully to avoid injury to the rectum. The rectovaginal septum should be identified so that the vagina can be dissected to the introitus, if necessary, when removal of the rectum or anal canal is to be performed. The retroperitoneal operation is completed with transection of the sigmoid colon or rectum, distal to the involved cul-de-sac.

7. In those instances when the posterior vagina must be resected to assure an adequate margin, the rectovaginal septum need not be entered. The vagina can be incised at 4 and 8 o'clock, ventral to the insertion of the uterosacral ligaments. Using a "clamp, cut, and tie" technique, the incision can be extended to the introitus, and if necessary, the perineal body and the anus can be resected en bloc. Because the vagina is well vascularized with the majority of the blood supply arising from the descending vaginal branch of the uterine artery and the ascending collateral branches from the pudendal vessels and surrounding structures, blood loss can be extensive if the vagina is not clamped prior to its incision.

8. The pelvis is dependent and a common site for fluid to collect. When drainage is used, we prefer to place closed-suction drains (ie, Jackson-Pratt) in the sacral hollow or pararectal gutters in an attempt to evacuate any blood, ascites, or lymph that may pool at these sites. Routine drainage of the pelvis, however, is not warranted.

9. After transection of the uterosacrocardinal ligament complex, it is not uncommon for a patient to have a transient dystonic bladder. To facilitate management of this problem, we prefer to perform a suprapubic cystotomy. We create a 0.5 cm cystotomy in the dome of the bladder

and place a 16F silastic Foley catheter that allows adequate bladder drainage with less discomfort and lower risk of bacterial contamination than with a transurethral catheter. The suprapubic catheter is particularly useful in instances when return of normal bladder function is delayed until after the patient has been discharged. The suprapubic catheter is removed when postvoid residuals are consistently less than 75 cc.

10. We encourage the maintenance of a functional vagina in all but rare cases. In those instances when the vagina is not being excised, the cuff can be closed using interrupted sutures. By closing the vagina in this manner, maximal length can be maintained. It is important to incorporate the uterosacralcardinal ligament complex into the lateral aspect of the vagina when it is being closed so as to maintain satisfactory apical support and to prevent vaginal prolapse.

If the posterior vaginal wall has been resected, we encourage that an omental J flap be developed and placed into the cul-de-sac. A split thickness skin graft (STSG) can be harvested, placed into the vaginal defect distal to the J flap and maintained in place using a vaginal stent (ie, Heyer-Schulte).[11] (Fig 82–3) When a graft is placed, the vagina should be made as large as possible because there is a natural contraction of all STSGs that can lead to a small, fibrotic, nonfunctional vagina. Alternatively, the transverse rectus abdominous muscle can be used for the creation of a neovagina (Fig 82–4). Muscle pedicles offer the advantages of a graft with an independent blood supply, one that eliminates the need for an STSG donor site, one with minimal shrinkage, and a graft that helps to fill the pelvic defect.[12]

CONTROVERSIES IN THE MANAGEMENT OF WOMEN WITH GASTROINTESTINAL MALIGNANCIES METASTATIC TO THE PELVIC ORGANS

Sterilization of Women Who May Desire Fertility

There has been a growing number of women who are deciding to delay childbearing until their fifth decade. Such a delay finds these women developing serious and life-threatening diseases that are uncommon in younger women. It is imperative that the patient be informed (prior to surgery) that there is a potential, however small, risk that she may be rendered sterile by her cancer operation. Appropriate psychosocial support should be provided when the decision is made to proceed with a hysterectomy.

Because of the theoretical increase in risk of development of endometrial cancer in women who have colorectal cancer (there is a common hereditary link: the Lynch 2 syndrome[13]), the uterus should be removed in those premenopausal women with colon cancer who have been sterilized or have completed their families. If

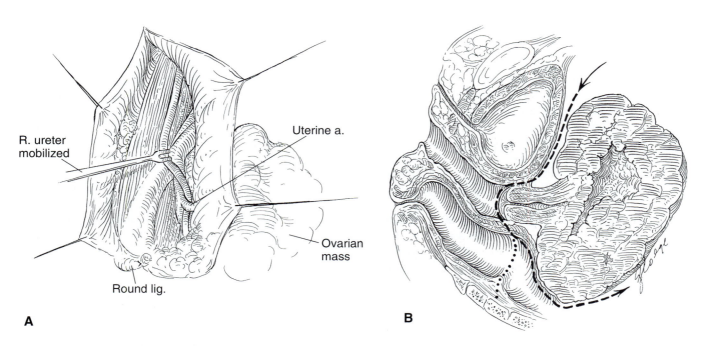

Figure 82–2. A. Retroperitoneal approach to resection of a cul-de-sac/pelvic mass. The peritoneum has been incised over the right psoas muscle and the retroperitoneum entered. The ureter has been mobilized off the medial leaf of the broad ligament in preparation for ligation of the uterine artery as it crosses the ureter. **B.** The vagina is entered anteriorly and the uterus and pelvic mass, with or without attached sigmoid colon, are resected in a retrograde fashion.

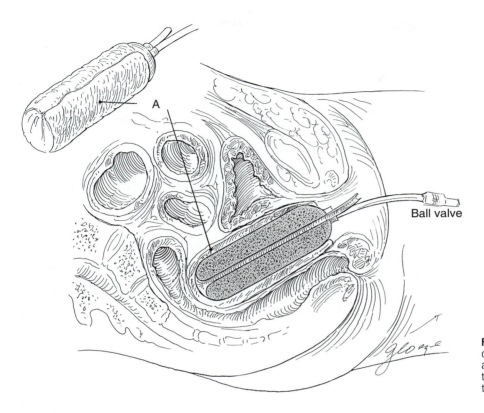

Figure 82–3. Split thickness skin graft used for formation of neovagina. The cutaneous epithelium (A) is shaped into a cylinder, over a stent, with the epithelial surface against the stent. The skin covered stent is placed into the defect that remains after resection of the vagina.

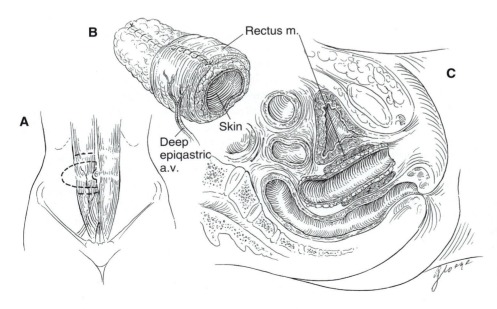

Figure 82–4. Transverse rectus abdominus muscle island flap used for formation of neovagina. **A.** The rectus abdominus muscle with overlying skin segment and inferior epigastric blood supply intact is utilized. **B.** The island is "tubularized" with the cutaneous epithelium on the inner surface. **C.** The neovagina is placed into the pelvic defect with minimal tension on the vascular pedicule.

the patient is uncertain about her future fertility, the surgeon must attempt to conserve the intact reproductive organs.

Oophorectomy in Premenopausal Women and Postoperative Hormone Replacement

There are many premenopausal women for whom maintenance of fertility is not an issue, but preservation of adequate estrogenization is essential. In the premenopausal woman in whom gonadal resection is required as a part of therapy for a gastrointestinal malignancy, immediate hormone replacement is recommended. Estrogen alone is appropriate when the uterus has been removed. If a hysterectomy is not performed, a progestin should also be given to minimize the risk of endometrial hyperplasia or malignancy. Hormone replacement therapy should be continued indefinitely unless a specific contraindication develops.

In the postmenopausal patient, we recommend continuation of the hormone replacement regimen used prior to surgery. We delete progestins if a hysterectomy has been performed. In women who have not received postmenopausal hormone replacement, the potential benefits of hormonal treatment should be discussed. These women should also have a diet rich in calcium and Vitamin D, as well as appropriate supplementation. They should perform weight-bearing exercise and, if there is a significant decrease in libido, androgen therapy may be considered.

■ MANAGEMENT OF THE ADNEXAL MASS

Of all the gynecologic disease processes that the general surgeon might confront intraoperatively, adnexal masses are the most common, especially those arising in the ovaries. Thus, surgeons must have a basic understanding of the physiologic and pathologic changes of the ovary so that appropriate action can be taken based on incidental findings at laparotomy performed for other indications.

The changes that can occur in the female reproductive adnexa can be classified by the status of the patient: premenarchal, menarchal, or postmenopausal. In those women in the reproductive age group, the adnexal changes can be either self-limiting physiologic or neoplastic processes. The symptoms of the patient and the physical signs of the mass can help to specifically characterize the process.

ADNEXAL MASSES IN THE PREMENARCHAL FEMALE

The premenarcheal ovary is quiescent. Therefore, most pelvic masses discovered in children are neoplastic. The most common neoplasms (85%) in these patients arise

from the pluripotent germ cells, and are benign cystic teratomas (dermoids). Malignant germ cell tumors (dysgerminomas, immature teratomas, endodermal sinus tumors, and mixed germ cell tumors) occur in this age group but are uncommon.[14] Other ovarian neoplasms are relatively uncommon, and lesions of gonadal stroma origin (eg, granulosa theca tumors, Sertoli-Leydig cell tumors) are rare. Paratubal cysts, the majority of which are mesonephric in origin, may be found attached to, or near, the fallopian tube. These tumors are frequent incidental findings and are very rarely malignant.

As a child approaches the age of menarche (mean 12.9 years in the United States[15]), she is more likely to have physiologic changes as ovulation begins. The surgeon must recognize these physiologic changes so that ovaries are not unnecessarily biopsied (or removed!).

ADNEXAL MASSES IN THE REPRODUCTIVE AGE PATIENT

In these women, 85% of adnexal masses that are found by pelvic examination (usually 3 cm or greater in diameter) represent normal physiologic changes of the female gonad. Cystic changes in the gonad can be found in most women of reproductive age that are neither pregnant or taking oral contraceptives.[16] The most common findings are follicular cysts, corpus lutea, or luteal cysts, all of which have typical gross appearances. Follicular cysts are usually multiple, between 1 to 5 cm in diameter, thin-walled and contain a clear straw-colored fluid. Corpus lutea are usually 3 cm in diameter, consist of the yellow-orange convoluted stromal tissue (from which their name originated), have relatively thin walls, and often contain a small amount of hemorrhagic fluid. Generally, lesions that are >3 cm in diameter are called a "corpus luteum cyst." These masses contain a central cavity with blood of varying ages.

True neoplasms in this age group are responsible for <15% of adnexal masses. The most common neoplasms arise from ovarian germ cells as found in the premenarcheal patient. Benign cystic teratomas predominate. Malignancies of either the germ cell, stromal, or epithelial origin are uncommon in this age group, with about 5% of lesions in those under 30 years of age being malignant, while 10% in patients 30 to 50 years of age are malignant.[17,18] Adnexal masses that are not ovarian also are formed in the reproductive-age patient. Paratubal cysts can occur, as can pedunculated uterine leiomyomata. When a fallopian tube mass is found, an ectopic pregnancy or a hydrosalpinx must be excluded, as both are more common in women who have antecedent histories of sexually transmitted diseases or salpingitis.

ADNEXAL MASSES IN THE POSTMENOPAUSAL FEMALE

The further past menopause, the less likely that an incidental mass found in the adnexa, especially the ovary, will represent a physiologic process. Menopause does not occur instantaneously and sporadic ovulation can occur for a period of months around the time of menopause. The majority of adnexal masses in the postmenopausal woman are, however, neoplastic processes, predominately of epithelial origin. The older the patient, the more likely that an adnexal mass will be malignant, with women in their eighth decade having a 70% chance that a mass will represent a cancer.[19] Most small masses that are appreciated at time of surgical exploration for a nongynecologic process are not malignant. However, the ovaries are a common site for metastasis from other malignancies and metastatic cancer accounts for 15% of all malignant lesions of the ovary. In a woman with a known breast or gastrointestinal malignancy, these cancers are the most likely extragenital primary to metastasize to the ovary.

MANAGEMENT DECISIONS

When an adnexal mass is discovered at the time of laparotomy, there are two questions that must be answered: (1) does this represent a malignant process, and (2) can the adnexa be salvaged? The most prudent course is to obtain intraoperative consultation with a respected and skilled gynecologic surgeon. This is often not possible and the surgeon will have to independently make the management decision. In the premenopausal patient, as most masses are benign and it is uncertain that the mass needs to be removed, we recommend that, if the mass is isolated to one ovary, it should be removed by cystectomy (see description) and sent for frozen section. If the mass is benign, postoperative referral to a gynecologist is encouraged. If the mass is malignant, surgical staging must be performed to document any spread of disease and to determine the need for further therapy. Small, pedunculated peritubal cysts should be removed completely, and frozen section pathology analysis is unnecessary as malignancy is rare. Masses of the fallopian tube must also be carefully evaluated, and if there is an ectopic pregnancy, a salpingostomy should be carried out conserving the tube to minimize the disruption of fertility.

In the postmenopausal patient in whom ovarian conservation is not a major issue, most masses are neoplastic, and many are malignant. The performance of a cystectomy is not appropriate and an adnexectomy should be performed. Frozen section should be obtained and, if a malignancy is present, a thorough operative staging (pelvic and paraaortic lymph node sampling, omentectomy, selected pelvic and abdominal washings and peritoneal biopsies) is essential. If no malignancy is found, the management of the contralateral adnexa and the uterus must be carefully considered. In those patients from whom appropriate surgical consent has not been

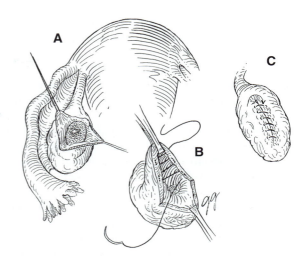

Figure 82–5. Ovarian cystectomy. **A.** The ovarian capsule is incised at the antimesenteric portion with care being taken to avoid the underlying mass. **B.** After the mass is enucleated and meticulous hemostasis obtained, the deep aspect of the defect is closed using 4-0 PGA suture, avoiding the ovarian capsule. **C.** The unclosed edge is approximated using similar suture in a "baseball" stitch manner, burying the raw edges.

obtained, the remaining reproductive organs should be preserved. If the patient has agreed in writing to have a hysterectomy and salpingo-oophorectomy, however, the operation should be performed, provided that the operation can be accomplished without undue morbidity. The reason for this recommendation is to eliminate recurrent neoplasms in the contralateral ovary and in the uterus, the most common site of a gynecologic cancer. Also, postmenopausal hormone replacement is simplified because only estrogen therapy needs to be given and progestins can be omitted as there is no longer a concern for the problem of "unopposed estrogen" therapy. If the performance of a contralateral salpingo-oophorectomy and hysterectomy is deemed unsafe or morbid, it is preferable not to undertake this procedure.

OPERATIVE TECHNIQUES

Ovarian Cystectomy (Fig 82–5)

In the majority of premenopausal patients, ovarian cystectomies can be performed without compromising gonadal function even when the ovaries are large and no normal ovarian tissue is apparent. The operation is carried out in the following manner:

1. Start the dissection at the antimesenteric portion of the gonad.
2. Make a sharp, straight incision through the ovarian capsule, but not into the underlying mass, allowing the development of a plane superficial to the neoplasm.

3. Use gentle traction and blunt dissection, following the tissue plane that has been developed.
4. Extend the incision on the ovarian capsule as needed to remove the cyst en bloc.
5. When the base of the mass has been reached and it is otherwise free from the surrounding ovary, the pedicle is cross-clamped, the mass sharply excised, and the pedicle suture ligated using a 3-0 polyglycolic acid (PGA) suture.
6. The ovarian defect is lavaged and meticulous hemostasis obtained to avoid a hematoma.
7. Reconstruction of the ovary is undertaken, resisting the temptation to resect the thin "shell" of ovary encasing the neoplasm. We prefer to repair the deep part of the defect with interrupted "u" stitches, using 4-0 PGA suture. The remaining unclosed edge is closed using the same suture in a baseball-stitch manner, burying the traumatized edge and therefore minimizing adhesion formation.

Oophorectomy

There are instances when preservation of an ovary is not advisable. In the premenarchal and women of reproductive age in whom the ovary has undergone prolonged torsion with associated devascularization and necrosis, the ovary must be removed. If the fallopian tube has not been significantly compromised, it can be conserved. In the postmenopausal patient, the affected ovary and fallopian tube should be removed.

Oophorectomy can be performed safely using the following steps:

1. The disruption of the blood supply to the fallopian tube must be minimized. The ovarian vessels of the infundibulopelvic ligament must be conserved. Using a narrow-ended clamp (ie, tonsil clamp), the hilus of the ovary should be closely "hugged" (Fig 82–6).
2. The adjacent pedicles should be ligated using a Hainey technique with 2-0 PGA suture. Clamps should be removed slowly while the suture is being tightened to avoid slippage and retroperitoneal bleeding. If bleeding occurs, it may be extensive, requiring a retroperitoneal exploration and potential loss of the entire adnexa.

Adnexectomy

For perimenopausal or postmenopausal women with disease in the ovary or tube, adnexectomy is the recommended operation. Sometimes an adnexectomy must be performed in women who desire preservation of their fertility, such as in those who have a unilateral tubo-ovarian abscess refractory to medical management, and those with adnexal torsion when the tube

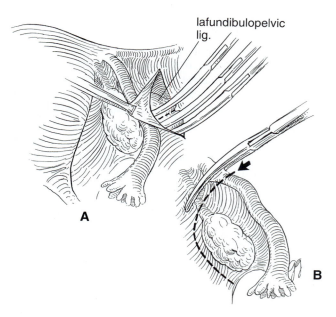

Figure 82–6. Oophorectomy using a hugging technique. Care is taken to avoid injury to the tube or disruption of its blood supply.

and ovary have both been compromised to a degree that precludes salvage. A thorough knowledge of retroperitoneal anatomy and careful adherence to surgical principles permits the safe performance of an adnexectomy even when the anatomy has been distorted by extensive disease.

The following steps should be carried out: (Fig 82–7)

1. The peritoneum is incised lateral to the adnexa, parallel to the infundibulopelvic ligament and the fallopian tube. We prefer to begin just lateral to the external iliac artery over the psoas muscle. The incision in the peritoneum is extended cephalad over the pelvic brim and caudad to the level of the round ligament. On the left side, care must be taken to avoid the sigmoid colon as it enters the pelvis. The peritoneal incision is extended lateral to the most proximal aspect of the sigmoid so that is has been adequately mobilized and will not be injured during ligature of the ovarian vessels.
2. After the peritoneum has been incised, the ureter should be traced from its site of entry into the pelvis to its entry into the paracervical tissues.
3. Under direct visualization, a fenestration should be made in the medial leaf of the broad ligament between the ovary and the ureter. This window should be extended cephalad to the pelvic brim and caudad to the para-uterine blood vessels.

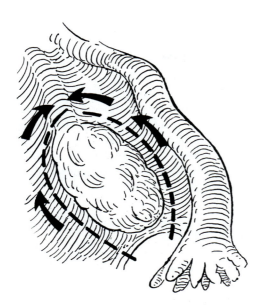

Figure 82–7. Adnexectomy. A. The peritoneum over the psoas muscle, lateral to the infundibulopelvic ligament is incised, exposing the retroperitoneal anatomy. The infundibulopelvic ligament is clamped with the ureter under direct visualization. **B.** The fallopian tube and uretero-ovarian ligament are clamped near the uterus, the pedicle transected in an antegrade fashion and the specimen delivered.

4. The infundibulopelvic ligament is clamped with the ureter under direct visualization. The ligament, with the ovarian vessel included, is transected between the distal clamps, assuring that all ovarian tissue is removed.

5. A free 2-0 PGA tie is passed cephalad to the most proximal clamp and tied while the clamp is released. A second suture ligature of the same material is passed through the ligament between the prior suture and the distal clamp. The suture is passed in front of and in back of the pedicle and tied tight while the clamp is being removed.

6. The peritoneum surrounding the proximal fallopian tube and the utero-ovarian ligament is incised to make the remaining pedicle as small as possible. Care must be taken to avoid the often engorged uterine veins that are found in the region of the uterine cornua.

7. The fallopian tube is double clamped, transected between the clamps and the proximal clamp suture ligated with 2-0 PGA. The utero-ovarian ligament is ligated similarly. We prefer to transect these two structures separately to avoid unintentional incorporation of periuterine vessels that may cause "back bleeding" and hematoma.

INTRAOPERATIVE STAGING

Thorough surgical staging must be performed in patients in whom the frozen section demonstrates the presence of a primary ovarian malignancy. This operation will "upstage" 70% of presumed stage I ovarian malignancies, and the information obtained is critical to make informed management decisions.[20,21]

1. *Any free fluid, especially in the pelvic cul-de-sac, should be submitted for cytologic evaluation.*

2. *If no free fluid is present, peritoneal "washings" should be performed* by instilling and recovering 50 to 100 mL of saline from the pelvic cul-de-sac, each paracolic gutter, and from beneath each hemidiaphragm. Obtaining the specimens from under the diaphragms can be facilitated with the use of a red rubber catheter attached to the end of a bulb syringe.

3. *A systematic exploration of all the intra-abdominal surfaces and viscera is performed,* proceeding in a clockwise fashion from the cecum cephalad along the paracolic gutter and the ascending colon to the right kidney, the liver and gallbladder, the right hemidiaphragm, the entrance to the lesser sac at the paraaortic area, across the transverse colon to the left hemidiaphragm, down the left gutter and the descending colon to the rectosigmoid colon. The small intestine and its mesentery from the ligament of Trietz to the cecum should be inspected.

4. *Any suspicious areas or adhesions on the peritoneal surfaces should be biopsied. If there is no evidence of disease, multiple intraperitoneal biopsies should be performed.* The peritoneum of the pelvic cul-de-sac, both paracolic gutters, the peritoneum over the bladder, and the intestinal mesenteries should be biopsied.

5. *The diaphragm should be sampled either by biopsy or by scraping with a tongue depressor and making a cytologic smear.* Biopsies of any irregularities on the surface of the diaphragm can be facilitated by use of the laparoscope and the associated biopsy instrument.

6. *The omentum should be resected from the transverse colon, a procedure called an infracolic omentectomy.* The procedure is initiated on the underside of the greater omentum, where the peritoneum is incised just a few millimeters away from the transverse colon. The branches of the gastroepiploic vessels are clamped, ligated, and divided, along with all the small branching vessels that feed the infracolic omentum. If the gastrocolic ligament is palpably normal, it does not need to be resected.

7. *The retroperitoneal spaces should be evaluated to evaluate the pelvic and paraaortic lymph nodes.* The retroperitoneal dissection is performed by incision of the peritoneum over the psoas muscles. This may be done on the ipsilateral side only for unilateral tumors. Any enlarged lymph nodes should be resected and submitted for frozen section. If no metastases are present, a formal pelvic lymphadenectomy should be performed.

TABLE 82–1. FIGO STAGING FOR PRIMARY CARCINOMA OF THE OVARY (1988)

Stage I		Growth limited to the ovaries.
	Stage Ia	Growth limited to one ovary; no ascites containing malignant cells. No tumor on the external surface; capsule intact.
	Stage Ib	Growth limited to both ovaries; no ascites containing malignant cells. No tumor on the external surfaces; capsules intact.
	Stage Ic	Tumor either Stage Ia or Ib but with tumor on the surface of one or both ovaries; or with capsule(s) ruptured; or with ascites present containing malignant cells or with positive peritoneal washings.
Stage II		Growth involving one or both ovaries with pelvic extension.
	Stage IIa	Extension and/or metastases to the uterus and/or tubes.
	Stage IIb	Extension to other pelvic tissues.
	Stage IIc[a]	Tumor either Stage IIa or IIb but with tumor on the surface of one or both ovaries; or with capsule(s) ruptured; or with ascites present containing malignant cells or with positive perineal washings.
Stage III		Tumor involving one or both ovaries with peritoneal implants outside the pelvis and/or positive retroperitoneal or inguinal nodes. Superficial liver metastases equals stage III. Tumor is limited to the true pelvis, but with histologically proven malignant extension to small bowel or omentum.
	Stage IIIa	Tumor grossly limited to the true pelvic with negative nodes but with histologically confirmed microscopic seeding of abdominal peritoneal surfaces.
	Stage IIIb	Tumor of one or both ovaries with histologically confirmed implants of abdominal peritoneal surfaces, none exceeding 2 cm in diameter. Nodes negative.
	Stage IIIc	Abdominal implants >2 cm in diameter and/or positive retroperitoneal or inguinal nodes.
Stage IV		Growth involving one or both ovaries with distant metastases. If pleural effusion is present, there must be positive cytologic test results to allot a case to Stage IV. Parenchymal liver metastasis equals stage IV.

[a]These categories are based on findings at clinical examination and/or surgical exploration. The histologic characteristics are to be considered in the staging, as are results of cytologic testing as far as effusions are concerned. It is desirable that a biopsy be performed on suspicious areas outside the pelvis. *In order to evaluate the impact on prognosis of the different criteria for allotting cases to stage Ic or IIc, it would be of value to know if rupture of the capsule was (1) spontaneous or (2) caused by the surgeon and if the source of malignant cells detected was (1) peritoneal washings or (2) ascites. (From Berek JS, Hacker NF. *Practical Gynecologic Oncology*, 2nd ed. Williams and Wilkins. Baltimore 1994,336.)

LONG-TERM FERTILITY ISSUES

Unquestionably, one of the most pressing concerns in the mind of the patient of reproductive age or the parents of the premenarchal patient is what effect adnexal surgery will have on the future ability to have children. The answer is not straightforward, as there are many variables that impact the type of procedure necessary. The patient and her family can be informed that though removal of a single ovary and tube with preservation of the contralateral adnexa does impact on fertility, future successful pregnancy is likely.[22]

■ VAGINAL FISTULAS

CAUSES AND INCIDENCE

Historically, the most common cause of vesicovaginal and rectovaginal fistula is obstetric, usually following a protracted second stage of labor or a traumatic delivery. Although obstetric causes persist as the most common predisposing event for genitourinary fistulas in countries where access to obstetric care is limited, they have been surpassed by other causes in industrialized societies. Presently, approximately 80% of vesicovaginal fistula occur after a gynecologic surgery, following an abdominal hysterectomy, in 75% of patients, and a vaginal hysterectomy in the majority of the remaining instances.[23] Interestingly, fistulas are uncommon after radical pelvic dissections. Those individuals who have had infections after a difficult surgery for benign disease are at the highest risk. Vesicovaginal fistulas may occur in women who have had a malignant disease process that has extended to the bladder, most commonly occurring in cervical cancer patients.[24] The fistula may result de novo from malignancy or from radiation-induced necrosis of the bladder base.[25]

Rectovaginal fistulas are still most frequently a sequelae of obstetric trauma, usually after an unsuccessful or inadequate repair of an episioproctotomy or a third- or fourth-degree perineal laceration. Less commonly, rectovaginal fistulas result from radiation-induced injury, iatrogenic injury at hysterectomy, or inflammatory bowel disorders.

PREOPERATIVE EVALUATION

Prior to any attempt at surgical management, it is essential that the exact locale of the fistula be identified and that the total number of fistula be confirmed as it is not uncommon that multiple defects have developed.

It is essential when evaluating the patient with a presumed vesicovaginal fistula to assure that the ureters are intact. We therefore prefer to perform an excretory urogram followed by a cystogram, which are usually adequate for localization of the defect and confirmation of the integrity of the upper urinary tract.

Sometimes it is beneficial to perform a "triple swab" test. This simple, inexpensive office investigation often can locate fistula that have been difficult to identify. Three tampons are placed in a row in the vagina so that the first is at the vaginal apex, the second is in the mid-vagina and the third is near the introitus. The bladder is filled with 150 cc of normal saline into which one ampule of methylene blue has been diluted. After the dye has been instilled, the patient is asked to ambulate, valsalva, and micturate. The tampons are then removed one at a time. The concentrated blue fluid will stain the tampon that is positioned in proximity to the fistula as well as the fistula tract, making it relatively easy to identify. The fistula location should be confirmed by cystoscopy at the time of surgery.

Rectovaginal fistulas, particularly those that occur after obstetric trauma and when attempts at repair have not been undertaken, are relatively easy to localize by clinical examination and do not require preoperative radiographic evaluation. In those patients in whom the location is unclear or there is concern that the fistula involves proximal small or large bowel, radiographic contrast studies are indicated and may be helpful in identifying the fistula site. Some patients develop successive enterovaginal fistula after pelvic radiation, multiple prior surgeries or inflammatory bowel disease, in which case the origin of the fistula cannot be identified. These patients present major management challenges.

SURGICAL MANAGEMENT

Vesicovaginal Fistula

How a vesicovaginal fistula is repaired is related to the site of the fistula, the etiology (eg, postoperative, radiation-induced, etc), and whether prior repair attempts have been made. It is critical to remember that the first repair is the one that is most likely to be successful. Cavalier suboptimal attempts must never be undertaken and attention to operative detail is imperative.

Although, traditionally, it has been felt that repair of a vesicovaginal fistula should not be undertaken for at least 6 months after diagnosis, this attitude is changing, based on reports from the 1970s.[26–28] We prefer to attempt surgical correction as soon as any associated soft-tissue infection has cleared. Some patients have fistulas (<5 mm occurring after a hysterectomy without prior pelvic irradiation) that will close spontaneously when treated only with transurethral bladder drainage. If the patient has become "dry" after catheter placement, the bladder should be allowed to remain "at rest" for 1 month. Prior to removing the catheter, the bladder subsequently can be instilled with indigo-carmen in saline to confirm fistula closure.

There are four criteria that are essential to maximize the chance that a fistula will be repaired successfully:

1. The fistula tract must be excised.
2. The vaginal mucosa must be mobilized widely around the fistula.
3. The closure must be completed without tension.
4. The bladder must be drained adequately after the fistula repair.

These guidelines are to be followed regardless of the approach taken (abdominal or vaginal) or the surgical technique used.

Primary Fistula

In the majority of cases in which there has been no prior repair, we prefer to correct the fistula using a transvaginal approach. In those instances when the fistula is located at the vaginal apex and exposure is suboptimal or when the vagina is very fibrotic, an abdominal route should be used.

The surgeon must be comfortable that the ureters are protected and their integrity is not compromised during the repair. When the fistula is small and midline, fistula repair can be performed without placement of ureteral stents. When the fistula is large or lateral, we prefer to place retrograde ureteral stents prior to the repair. These stents, usually a 5F double pigtail, can be placed retrograde by direct visualization through the fistula, when there is a large defect, or with a cystoscope, occluding the fistula with an Alyce clamp, when there is a small fistula.

Vaginal Repair (Fig 82–8)

The following steps should be used for the vaginal repair:

1. The fistula tract is sharply excised en toto.
2. The vaginal mucosa is mobilized from the site of the fistula to assure closure with minimal tension. This distance is usually at least 1.5 cm, and may be more.
3. The bladder wall is closed in two layers. The first is a running, inverting 3-0 chromic or plain suture; the second is an imbricating 3-0 PGA suture.
4. The vaginal epithelium is tailored to allow closure without overlap and approximated with 3-0 PGA suture.
5. In selected patients in whom the fistula occurs at the apex of the vagina after hysterectomy, a modified Latzko procedure can be performed.[29,30] This operation is performed as outlined above, but the mobilization of the vagina epithelium is done so that the anterior and posterior vaginal walls are approximated for a small (2 to 3 cm) distance and a partial colpocleisis is carried out.

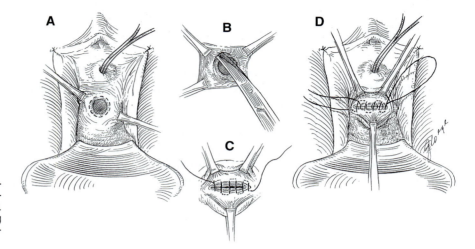

Figure 82–8. Primary vaginal repair of a vesicovaginal fistula. **A.** Fistula tract is sharply encised entoto. **B.** The vaginal mucosa is mobilized off of the underlying bladder. **C.** The bladder wall is closed in two layers; the first being a running inverting suture. **D.** The second being an imbricating suture.

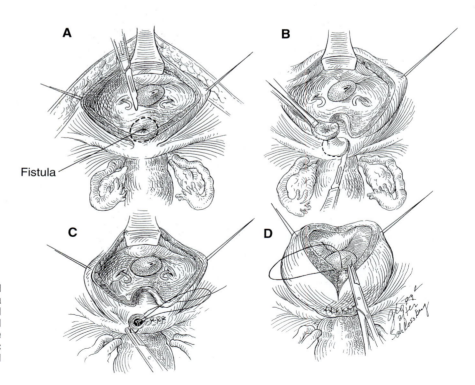

Fistula

Figure 82–9. Primary abdominal repair of a vesicovaginal fistula. **A.** The dome of the bladder is incised. **B.** The fistula tract removed en toto. A transurethral catheter and bilateral ureteral stints have been placed. **C.** The vagina is closed with 3-0 absorbable continuous running suture. **D.** The bladder is closed in two layers, the first being 3-0 chromic running suture inverting the mucosa (shown). The second layer is interrupted 3-0 PGA suture.

6. Suture line integrity is assured by filling the bladder with 200 mL of distilled methylene blue.
7. A transabdominal suprapubic catheter is placed. A Bannano-style or Silastic catheter can be inserted to assure adequate bladder drainage.

Success rates for primary vaginal repairs of vesicovaginal range from 93% to 100%.

Abdominal Repair (Fig 82–9)

We recommend performance of an abdominal repair as initial surgery for a vesicovaginal fistula in those patients in whom other abdominal surgery is indicated (ie, surgical staging of a malignancy, management of an associated bowel obstruction), or if the fistula involves the distal ureter and ureteroneocystomy must be performed. If the fistula is near the trigone, even if other abdominal surgery is to be completed, it may be more efficient to perform a transvaginal fistula repair.

The following steps should be used:

1. Once intraperitoneal access has been established, the dome of the bladder is incised in a vertical manner to the site of the fistula.
2. The full thickness of the fistula is excised sharply, and the vagina dissected from the posterior bladder wall.
3. The vagina is closed with 3-0 absorbable continuous running suture.
4. The bladder is closed in two layers: the mucosa closed with a 3-0 chromic or plain running suture inverting the mucosa into the bladder; the second layer is an interrupted 3-0 PGA suture.
5. A suprapubic catheter (16 Silastic Foley) is placed through a separate bladder incision via the space of Retzius.
6. Incision integrity is assured by instilling the closed bladder with 200 mL of diluted methylene blue.
7. An omental J flap from the transverse colon is developed and interposed between the vagina and the repaired bladder.[31]

Success rates using this technique, even when the patients are at high risk for failure, is approximately 90%.[32,33]

Recurrent or Postirradiation Vesicovaginal Fistulas

Recurrent fistulas or those that occur after pelvic radiation offer unique surgical challenges. Often, extensive scarring and distorted anatomy have occurred. The tissues may have extensive fibrosis and microvascular occlusion, both of which hinder postrepair healing. In these patients, a layer or cushion of well-vascularized tissue must be interposed between the vaginal and vesicular walls that have been repaired so that neovascularization can be promoted. When the procedure is performed abdominally, a substantial omental flap can be used. If omentum is unavailable because it has been previously removed, a transverse rectus abdominis muscle flap (TRAM), without the attached skin, can be used.[34] TRAM flaps, with their generous blood supply (via the inferior epigastric vessels) and extensive mobility, are uniquely suited for interposition between the vagina and other organs serving as a well-vascularized "cushion."

If a vaginal approach is used, we prefer to perform a Martius bulbocavernosus fat pad graft[35] (Fig 82–10). The vaginal repair is performed using the technique described above. After closure of the vesicle wall, the fat pad graft is developed in the following manner:

1. The lateral margin of the labia major is incised.
2. The fat pad overlying the bulbocavernosus muscle is mobilized, attempting to gain as broad a pad as possible.
3. The dorsal aspect of the pad is transected. The length of the pad should be no more than twice the breadth of the base to avoid necrosis of the end of the pedicle.
4. A tunnel is developed from the space between the repaired bladder base and the mobilized vaginal wall.
5. The fat pad is drawn through this tunnel, under minimal tension, and fixed to the contralateral aspect of the bladder past the line of fistula repair. It is stabilized in place with interrupted 3-0 PGA sutures.
6. The vaginal epithelium is widely mobilized and closed without tension using interrupted 3-0 PGA sutures. We use the delayed absorbable sutures to maintain strength over an extended period, although the suture material may be associated with vaginal discharge.

Postoperative Care

In all vesicovaginal fistula repairs, the bladder is "rested" for at least 14 days after primary repair and 1 month in women who have recurrent fistulas or fistulas after radiotherapy. Prior to catheter removal, we instill 200 mL of dilute methylene blue to confirm adequate healing. If a leak occurs, a catheter is re-inserted for 2 more weeks and the procedure repeated. Should leakage persist, we conclude that the repair has failed and prepare for a subsequent attempt. Prior to removal of the catheter, we perform serial clamping for 3 hours to check postvoid residuals to assure that functional micturition has been restored. The patient should be able to empty the bladder with a postvoid residual consistently <75 mL. If ureteral catheters have been placed, they can be removed in the office, using a cystoscope.

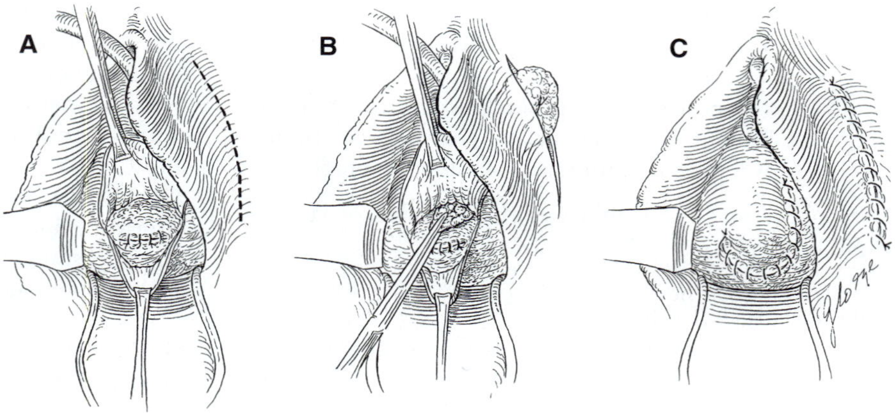

Figure 82–10. Martius Bulbocavernous fat pad graft for recurrent vesicovaginal fistula. **A.** After repair of the bladder wall, but prior to closure of the vagina, an incision is made on the lateral aspect of the labia majus. **B.** The fat pad overlying the bulbocavernous muscle is mobilized and the dorsal aspect transected. This pad is brought through a deep subcutaneous tunnel and fixed to the contralateral aspect of the bladder, past the fistula repair. **C.** The labial and vaginal incisions are closed without tension using 3-0 PGA sutures.

Patients are admonished to not insert anything in the vagina for 6 weeks. If the vagina has healed adequately by then, coitus is permitted and tampons may be inserted.

Enterovaginal Fistula

Enterovaginal fistulas are rare. Most result from inflammatory bowel disease, prior pelvic surgery (ie, hysterectomy), or pelvic irradiation. Regardless of the etiology, management is challenging, often frustrating, and complicated.

Localization of the fistula site is imperative prior to attempted surgical correction. Radiographic techniques (ie, upper gastrointestinal series follow-through and a barium enema) combined with endoscopic investigations of the lower gastrointestinal tract are the preferable methods. However, the exact site often cannot be localized because multiple adherent loops of affected small bowel are present at the site. The phlegmon interferes with identification of the fistula site and complicates surgical repair.

When an enterovaginal fistula occurs in a woman who has inflammatory bowel disease, medical management must be undertaken aggressively prior to surgical intervention. Intensive nutritional support, such as total parenteral nutrition, and drugs such as sulfasalazine and corticosteroids, are used. After months of medical therapy, surgical repair must be performed transabdominally because morbidity and failure rates are high. Careful dissection of intestinal loops is necessary to minimize enterotomies, since any small bowel injury is a potential site of subsequent bowel perforation or enterocutaneous fistula. The resected segment of bowel should be as short as possible, including only the injured portion. In some patients, we prefer to conserve the injured bowel and perform a bypass to drain the mucous produced in the fistula tract. The rationale for this approach is that the conserved bowel can act as a barrier between the vagina and other adherent small bowel loops that can also develop a fistula. If the segment of small bowel is severely injured or suffers from significant vascular compromise, it must be resected.[36]

Patients who develop postirradiation enterovaginal fistulas should be approached in a manner similar to patients with fistulas resulting from inflammatory bowel disease. Those who have radiation-induced enterovaginal fistulas often are compromised nutritionally and benefit from bowel rest and parenteral nutrition. Surgical management is the same as described for patients with inflammatory bowel disease because simple resections and closures have a high failure rate. If a recurrence of the primary malignancy is discovered intraoperatively, than a palliative diversion should be performed. Because the majority of patients who develop postradiation enterovaginal fistulas have undergone therapy for invasive cervical cancer, only a small central pelvic recurrence can be managed with an exenteration, whereas all other patients are likely to recur and succumb to their disease. Therefore, the most limited palliative operation should be performed to maximize patient comfort and function while minimizing morbidity. In some cases, the creation of an enterostomy with a mucus fistula avoids extensive surgery and bowel resection while palliating the distal fistula.

Simple enterovaginal fistulas in the patient not compromised by inflammatory bowel disease or prior pelvic irradiation are uncommon. Management is straightforward and must include an attempt at nonsurgical management (ie, 6 weeks to 2 months of bowel rest with either total enteral or total parenteral nutrition). If the fistula does not heal spontaneously, surgical repair is indicated. A transabdominal approach with resection of the involved loop of bowel and a layered closure of the vagina is the preferred technique.

Rectovaginal Fistulas

The majority of rectovaginal fistulas are sequelae of birth trauma with unsuccessful episiotomy repair or perineal laceration. Diagnosis is straightforward when the patient complains of incontinence of flatus or stool. The extent of the anatomic defect correlates with the complaints of the patient. Women who are continent of stool (whether formed or liquid) but incontinent of flatus will have the smallest defects, while those that are incontinent of formed stool have the largest. Women who are incontinent of flatus and liquid stool have defects that are of intermediate severity. On physical examination, a low fistula can be visualized simply by spreading the labia, while a higher fistula will be noted on vaginal speculum examination.

In some patients the fistula will not be readily identified. These patients are more likely to complain only of incontinence of flatus or liquid stool. Typically, they have undergone prior attempts at fistula repair or have developed fistulas in association with a chronic inflammatory disease process (eg, lupus, Crohn's disease). There also is a subset of patients who do not have fistulas per se, but have an inadequate anal sphincter and may present with similar symptoms.

Identification of both the vaginal and rectal defects is essential for successful repair. Proctoscopy, radiographic contrast studies, and methylene-blue rectal expansion studies should be performed to confirm the location of the tract. If no fistula is identified, the degree of rectal sphincter function should be assessed. Clinical impression of sphincter tone by rectal examination is not an adequate evaluation, and thus a defecogram and electromyogram of the perineal and rectal sphincter muscles must be done.

The potential for successful repair can be maximized by appropriate preparation. If patients who have nutritional compromise, preoperative nutritional support should be given prior to surgery. We prefer total enteral nutrition using an elemental diet. In those unable to tolerate enteral diets, parenteral feeding may be necessary. Prior to surgery, a complete 3 day mechanical and antibiotic bowel preparation should be performed in the usual fashion. The colon must be completely emptied, cleansed, and sterilized prior to surgery.

Primary Rectovaginal Fistula

The timing of fistula repair has changed considerably in recent years. The experience of Hankins and others[37] demonstrated that early repairs could be performed, with success rates equivalent to those after late repairs (6 weeks or longer). Preoperatively, the patient should be given antibiotics and local care (eg, frequent sitz baths). When all signs of infection have resolved, evidence of fistulitis has abated, and fresh granulation tissue is present, the repair can be performed. The time from development of a symptomatic fistula to repair, in most patients, will be 10 days to 3 weeks when treated in this manner.

The specific surgical technique used depends on the location of the fistula. As with vesicovaginal fistula, care must be taken to assure adequate mobilization of all layers of the perineum, vagina, and rectum so that the closure is performed without tension on the suture line.

Complete Perineal Breakdown (Fig 82–11)

We prefer to perform a Warren flap in patients who have complete re-epithelized granulation tissue.[38] The following steps are taken:

1. An inverted U incision is made in the vagina, outlining the flap of vaginal epithelium.
2. Using sharp dissection, the flap is mobilized caudad from the underlying rectum.
3. The ends of the external anal sphincter muscle are identified. Typically, the ends of the anal sphincter will be retracted laterally. They must be freely mobilized, brought into the midline, and sutured together using interrupted suture. We prefer to place at least three separate 0 Maxon sutures on the sphincter capsule.
4. The puborectalis muscles then are approximated in the midline using interrupted 0 PGA suture.
5. To maximize vaginal length, the perineal body is reinforced by reapproximating the transverse perineal muscle fascia using 0 PGA on a large needle.
6. The vaginal incision is repaired from the apex with a continuous running 3-0 chromic suture. At the introitus, the suture is passed into the subcutaneous tissue deep to the perineal skin, which is closed using a subcutaneous stitch. The perineal skin is repaired with a subcuticular stitch.

Any redundant skin tag that remains is excised and the defect closed using interrupted 3-0 chromic sutures. In those patients in whom an early repair is performed, the same basic technique is used. A thorough resection of any granulation tissue and a layered rectal repair must be performed without tension. We recommend closure of the rectum in two layers: a running 3-0 absorbable suture in the mucosa layer and an interrupted 3-0 PGA in the seromuscular layer.

Small (≤0.5 cm) Rectovaginal Fistula

The following steps should be taken:

1. A circular incision is made through the vaginal epithelium but not into the rectum.
2. The vaginal epithelium layer is mobilized approximately 1.5 cm around the fistula sight.

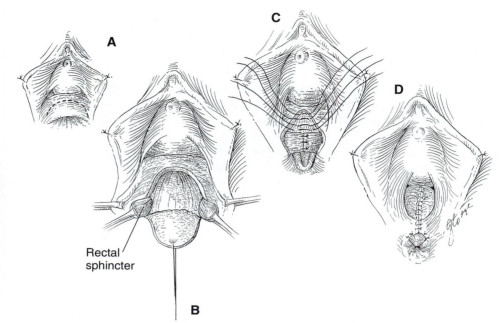

Figure 82–11. Warren flap repair of complete perineal breakdown. **A.** An inverted U incision is made in the vagina, outlining the flap of vaginal epithelium to be mobilized. **B.** The flap is mobilized off the rectum using sharp dissection and the ends of the rectal sphincter identified. **C.** The sphincter is reapproximated with minimal tension using O Maxon sutures through the sphincter capsule. The puborectalis muscles are approximated using 0 interrupted PGA suture. **D.** The vaginal incision is closed using a continuous 3-0 chromic suture. Any redundant skin tag remaining is excised and the defect closed using interrupted 3-0 chromic sutures.

Rectal sphincter

3. An imbricating pursestring suture of 3-0 PGA is placed around the fistula, closing and burying the tract.
4. A second purse-string suture is placed.
5. The vagina is closed without tension using interrupted 3-0 absorbable sutures.

Large Fistula

To properly repair a large defect, the following steps should be used:

1. Using sharp dissection, the entire fistula tract is resected.
2. The rectum is mobilized laterally, proximally, and distally from the vaginal epithelium at least 1.5 cm in all directions. The epithelium should be freed as much as necessary to minimize tension on the closure.
3. The rectum is closed in two layers. An inverting running 3-0 absorbable suture is used in the mucosa and the muscularis is closed with inverting interrupted 3-0 PGA.
4. The pararectal fascia is approximated in the midline using 2-0 PGA interrupted sutures.
5. If the fistula is distal in the vagina, the puborectalis muscles are approximated with interrupted 0 PGA sutures.
6. The vaginal epithelium is trimmed and closed with interrupted 3-0 absorbable sutures.

If there is a large rectovaginal fistula at the vaginal apex and the uterus is absent, it can be repaired using a

modified Latzko technique in the following manner (Fig 82–12):

1. The vagina around the fistula tract is incised and the tract left in vivo.
2. The surrounding vaginal epithelium, approximately 1.5 cm in radius, is undermined and excised.
3. The fistula is inverted into the rectal lumen using two layers of interrupted suture, the first a 3-0 absorbable suture in the rectal mucosa, and the second a 3-0 PGA suture in the muscularis and pararectal fascia. These sutures are placed horizontally.
4. The vagina is closed over the inverted rectal lumen (as a partial colpocleisis) with interrupted horizontal 3-0 absorbable sutures.

Women undergoing their first attempted repair of a rectovaginal fistula, when appropriately selected, adequately prepared, and who receive meticulous surgical technique, should expect cure rates of $\geq 90\%$.[39–42]

Recurrent or Postirradiation Fistula

In women whose fistulas are recurrent or occur after pelvic irradiation, we recommend a Martius graft technique (as described above, in the vesicovaginal fistula repair section). The technique is modified to transect the ventral portion of the bulbocavernosus muscle and labial fat pad, "swinging" the pedicle graft dorsally (instead of ventrally as repairing a vesicovaginal fistula).[42] An important decision is whether or not to perform a di-

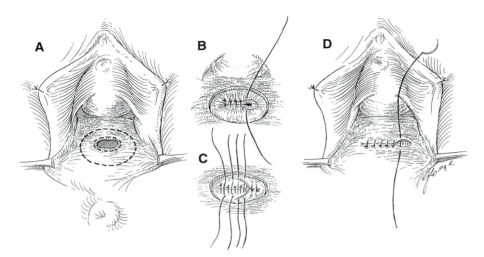

Figure 82–12. Repair of large rectovaginal fistula in upper vagina using a modified Latzko technique. **A.** The vagina around fistula tract is incised and the tract left in vivo. **B.** The fistula is inverted into the rectal mucosa, using 3-0 chromic suture. **C.** A second layer of 3-0 interrupted PGA suture is placed, inverting the muscularis and pararectal fascia. **D.** The vagina is closed over the inverted rectal lumen as a partial colpocleisis using interrupted 3-0 chromic suture.

verting colostomy. Our preference is to not perform a colostomy in individuals undergoing their first repair with a Martius graft. However, in those patients who have significant medical problems (eg, HIV seropositivity, transplant recipients, poor diabetes control), a diverting colostomy should be performed prior to the repair with the Martius graft.

Perioperative Care

Rigid guidelines must be followed to maximize the chance of a successful repair. All patients should receive prophylactic perioperative antibiotics, including at the time of surgery and for 2 to 3 days after operation. The bowel should be rested for 10 days using a no-residue diet and oral Lomotil. After 10 days, the perineum is inspected and if there are no signs of infection or incision breakdown, the Lomotil is discontinued, and oral Colace, Milk of Magnesia (MOM), and a regular oral diet reinstituted. Metamucil (two tablespoons every morning in a large glass of orange juice) is also given. At time of discharge from the hospital, the patient is continued on the above regimen (without the MOM) and advised to insert nothing into the vagina. At 6 weeks postoperative the patient is re-examined. If healing is adequate, vaginal activity may be resumed and the medications discontinued.

Vaginal Stenosis After Fistula Repairs

Other than recurrence of the fistula, the most common postoperative problem is vaginal foreshortening and narrowing. In the premenopausal woman who has not received pelvic irradiation, the vaginal caliber can be maintained readily because it is very distensible and stretches with use. In postmenopausal patients, those who have received pelvic irradiation, or in patients who have had several prior repairs, vaginal stenosis and/or foreshortening occurs frequently.

In order to minimize the occurrence of this problem, we recommend the prophylactic use of vaginal dilators, preferably the rigid plexiglass type. These dilators have the advantages of being available in several sizes of variable width and length and of being sufficiently rigid. Estrogen cream can be used as a lubricant with the dilator. We also prescribe the nightly insertion of 2 gm of estrogen cream into the vagina.

Vaginal intercourse is often the best way to maintain or increase vaginal caliber. The patient and her partner must proceed carefully because the vagina is often very tender. Initial unpleasant experiences might induce pain and the couple will be hesitant to attempt further coitus. With encouragement from a supportive health care professional and the assistance of a sensitive partner, satisfactory vaginal intercourse often can occur. In those patients in whom the vagina has become exceptionally stenotic, making vaginal intercourse impossible and dilation unsuccessful, vaginal reconstruction should be considered. However, in these women the potential for bladder or rectal morbidity associated with the reconstruction is considerable.

REFERENCES

1. Stallworthy JA. Surgery of Endometrial Cancer in the Bonney Tradition. Annals of the Royal College of Surgeons of England. 1971;48:29–305
2. Hudson CN. Surgical treatment of ovarian cancer. *Gynecol Oncol* 1973;1:370–375
3. Heslov SF, Frost DB. Extended resection for primary colorectal carcinoma involving adjacent organs or structures. *Cancer* 1988;62:1637–1640
4. McGlone TP, Bernie WA, Elliorr DW. Survival following extended resection for extracolonic invasion by colon cancer. *Arch Surg* 1982;117:595–599
5. Bonfanti G, Bozzetti F, Doci R et al. Results of extended

surgery for cancer of the rectum and sigmoid. *Br J Surg* 1982;69:305–307

6. Cohen AM, Shank B, Friedman MA. Colorectal cancer. In: DeVita, VT Jr, Hellman S, Rosenberg SA (eds), *Cancer; Principles and Practice of Oncology*, 3rd ed. Philadelphia, PA: JB Lippincott; 1989:942

7. Daly JW, Higgins KA. Injury to the ureter during gynecologic surgical procedures. *Surg Gynecol Obstet* 1988;167:19–22

8. Mann WJ, Arato M, Patsner B, Stone ML. Ureteral injuries in an obstetrics and gynecology training program: etiology and management. *Obstet Gynecol* 1988;72:82–85

9. Mann WJ. Intentional and unintentional ureteral surgical treatment in gynecologic procedures. *Surg Gynecol Obstet* 1991;172:453–456

10. Berek JS, Hacker NF, Lagasse LD. Vaginal reconstruction performed simultaneously with pelvic exenteration. *Obstet Gynecol* 1983;63:318–323

11. Benson C, Soisson AP, Carlson J, et al. Neovaginal reconstruction with a rectus abdominis myocutaneous flap. *Obstet Gynecol* 1993;81:871–875

12. Lynch HT, Krush AJ. Differential diagnosis of the cancer family syndrome. *Surg Gynecol Obstet* 1973;136:221–224

13. Norris HJ, Jensen RD. Relative frequency of ovarian neoplasms in children and adolescents. *Cancer* 1972;30:713

14. Frisch RE, Revelle R. Height and weight at menarche and a hypothesis of menarche. *Arch Dis Child* 1971;46:695–697

15. Holt VL, Daling JR, McKnight B, et al. Functional ovarian cysts in relation to the use of monophasic and triphasic oral contraceptive. *Obstet Gynecol* 1992;79:529–531

16. Killackey MA, Neuwirth RS. Evaluation and management of the pelvic mass: a review of 540 cases. *Obstet Gynecol* 1988;71:319–322

17. Hernandez E, Miyazawa K. The pelvic mass: patient's age and pathologic findings. *J Reprod Med* 1988;33:361–365

18. Koonings PP, Campbell K, Mishell DR, Grimes DA. Relative frequency of primary ovarian neoplasms: a 10 year review. *Obstet Gynecol* 1989;74:921–924

19. Young RC, Decker DG, Wharton JT, et al. Staging laparotomy in early ovarian cancer. *JAMA* 1983;250:3072–3075

20. McGowan L, Lesher LP, Norris HJ, Barnett M. Misstaging of ovarian cancer. *Obstet Gynecol* 1985;65:568–570

21. Lee RA, Symmonds RE, Williams TJ. Current status of genitourinary fistula. *Obstet Gynecol* 1988;72:313–319

22. Bradshaw KD, Guzick DS, Grun B, et al. Cumulative pregnancy rates for donor insemination according to ovulatory function and tubal status. *Fertil Steril* 1951;48:1051–1054

23. Hopkins MP, Morley GW. Squamous Cell Cancer of the cervix: prognostic factors related to survival. *Int J Gynecol Cancer* 1991;1:173–177

24. Borronow RC, Rutledge F. Vesicovaginal fistula, radiation, and gynecological cancer. *Am J Obstet Gynecol* 1971;111:85–90

25. Collins CG, Collins JH, Harrison BR, et al. Early repair of vesicovaginal fistula. *Am J Obstet Gynecol* 1971;111:524–28

26. Persky L, Herman G, Geurrier K. Nondelay in vesicovaginal fistula repair. *Urology* 1979;13:273–275

27. Hankins GD, Hauth JC, Gilstrap LC, et al. Early repair of episiotomy dehiscence. *Obstet Gynecol* 1990;75:48–51

28. Latzko W. Postoperative vesicovaginal fistula. *Am J Surg* 1942;58:211–227

29. Tancer ML. Observations on prevention and management of vesicovaginal fistula after total hysterectomy. *Surg Gynecol Obstet* 1992;175:501–506

30. Turner-Warwick RT, Wynne EJC, Handley-Ashken M. The use of the omental pedicle graft in the repair and reconstruction of the urinary tract. *Br J Surg* 1967;54:849–53

31. O'Conor VJ Jr. Review of experience with vesicovaginal fistula repair. *J Urol* 1980;123:367–373

32. Wen AJ, Malloy TR, Carpiniello VL, et al. Repair of vesicovaginal fistula by a suprapubic transvesical approach. *Surg Gynecol Obstet* 1980;150:57–62

33. Robertson CN, Fiefkohl R, Webster GD. Use of the rectus abdominis flap in urological reconstructive procedures. *J Urol* 1986;135:963–965

34. Martius J. Operations for urinary incontinence. In: McCall M, Bolten KA (eds), *Operative Gynecology*. Boston, MA: Little, Brown; 1956

35. Levenback C, Gershenson DM, McGehee R, et al. Enterovesical fistula following radiotherapy for gynecologic cancer. *Gynecol Oncol* 1994;52:269–300

36. Hankins GDV, Hauth JC, Gilstrap LC, et al. Early repair of episiotomy dehiscence. *Obstet Gynecol* 1990;75:48–51

37. Warren JC. A new method of operation for the relief of rupture of the perineum through the sphincter and rectum. *Trans Am Gynecol Soc* 1982;7:322–328

38. Russell TR, Gallagher DM. Low rectovaginal fistulas: approach and treatment. *Am J Surg* 1977;134:13–18

39. Hibbard LT. Surgical management of rectovaginal fistulas and complete perineal tears. *Am J Obstet Gynecol* 1978;130:139–142

40. Rothenberger DA, Goldberg SM. The management of rectovaginal fistula. *Surg Clin North Am* 1983;63:61–79

41. Tancer ML, Lasser D, Rosenblum N. Rectovaginal fistula or perineal and anal sphincter disruption, or both after vaginal delivery. *Surg Obstet Gynecol* 1990;171:43–46

42. White AJ, Buchsbaum HJ, Blythe JG, Lifshitz S. Use of the bulbocavernosus muscle (Martius procedure) for repair of radiation induced rectovaginal fistulas. *Obstet Gynecol* 1982;60:114–118

INDEX